The Clinical Practice of
Neurological and Neurosurgical Nursing

The Clinical Practice of
Neurological and Neurosurgical Nursing

FIFTH EDITION

Joanne V. Hickey
PhD, RN, ACNP, APRN, BC, CNRN, FAAN, FCCM

Professor of Clinical Nursing
The University of Texas—Houston
Houston, Texas

◆ LIPPINCOTT WILLIAMS & WILKINS
A **Wolters Kluwer** Company
Philadelphia • Baltimore • New York • London
Buenos Aires • Hong Kong • Sydney • Tokyo

Acquisitions Editor: Alan Sorkowitz
Editorial Assistant: Daniel Pepper
Senior Project Editor: Tom Gibbons
Senior Production Manager: Helen Ewan
Design Coordinator: Brett MacNaughton
Manufacturing Manager: William Alberti
Indexer: Maria Coughlin
Compositor: Cadmus
Printer: Courier-Westford

5th Edition

9 8 7 6 5 4 3 2 1

Library of Congress Cataloging-in-Publication Data
The clinical practice of neurological and neurosurgical nursing/[edited by] Joanne V. Hickey.— 5th ed.
     p. cm.
   Includes bibliographical references and index.
   ISBN 0-7817-2660-3 (cloth: alk. paper)
   1. Neurological nursing. I. Title: Neurological and neurosurgical nursing. II. Hickey,
Joanne V.
   [DNLM: 1. Nervous System Diseases—nursing. 2. Neurosurgery—nursing.]
RC350.5.C55 2003
610.73′68—dc21
                                                                                    2002016019

Care has been taken to confirm the accuracy of the information presented and to describe generally accepted practices. However, the authors, editors, and publisher are not responsible for errors or omissions or for any consequences from application of the information in this book and make no warranty, express or implied, with respect to the content of the publication.

The authors, editors, and publisher have exerted every effort to ensure that drug selection and dosage set forth in this text are in accordance with the current recommendations and practice at the time of publication. However, in view of ongoing research, changes in government regulations, and the constant flow of information relating to drug therapy and drug reactions, the reader is urged to check the package insert for each drug for any change in indications and dosage and for added warnings and precautions. This is particularly important when the recommended agent is a new or infrequently employed drug.

Some drugs and medical devices presented in this publication have Food and Drug Administration (FDA) clearance for limited use in restricted research settings. It is the responsibility of the health care provider to ascertain the FDA status of each drug or device planned for use in his or her clinical practice.

To neuroscience patients and their families who have the lived experience of neurological illness.

To the many nurses who compassionately and competently care for neuroscience patients, making a difference in so many meaningful ways.

And as always ... it is you, my family—my husband Jim, daughter Kathan, son Christopher and their families—who have given and continue to give my life meaning, direction, and purpose through your continued love and support. It is family that is the most precious of gifts and the substantive denominator of life. And my grandchildren, Jenna, Matthew, Max, and Joanna, who are wonderful and special gifts that are the linkage from the past to the future.

About the Author

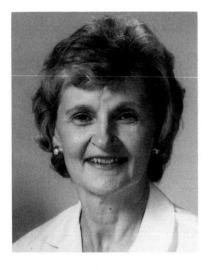

Dr. Hickey received her diploma in nursing from Roger Williams General Hospital School of Nursing in Providence, Rhode Island; her BSN from Boston College in Boston, Massachusetts; her MSN from the University of Rhode Island in Kingston, Rhode Island; her MA in counseling from Rhode Island College; her PhD from the University of Texas at Austin, Texas; and her postmaster's certificate as an acute care nurse practitioner from Duke University, Durham, North Carolina. She is certified in neuroscience nursing (CNRN) by the American Board of Neuroscience Nursing, and is board certified as an acute care nurse practitioner (APRN,BC) by the American Nurses Credentialing Center. She is a fellow in the American Academy of Nursing (FAAN) and a fellow in the American Academy of Critical Care Medicine (FCCM).

Dr. Hickey has focused her career on education, practice, research, and publications in the neurosciences and neuroscience patient populations. She has been a faculty member in a number of schools of nursing. At Duke University, she developed and directed their first acute care nurse practitioner program. She has had clinical appointments at Massachusetts General Hospital in Boston and Duke University Medical Center in Durham, where she was Attending Nurse, Neuroscience Nursing. Her neuroscience research interests include cerebrovascular problems and increased intracranial pressure, and she was an American Foundation of Nursing Research Scholar in 1992 for research on preparing family caregivers for recovery from stroke.

The Clinical Practice of Neurological and Neurosurgical Nursing, now in its fifth edition, has received the AJN Book of the Year Award and has been repeatedly cited by the Brandon and Hill listing of recommended books in nursing. The text has been translated into Japanese. Dr. Hickey is also senior editor of *Advanced Practice Nursing: Changing Roles and Clinical Applications,* Second Edition, published in 2000 by Lippincott Williams & Wilkins and edited by Dr. Hickey, Ruth Ouimette, and Sandra Venegoni. She serves on a number of editorial and advisory boards.

Dr. Hickey has been a member of the American Nurses Association, the American Association of Critical Care Nurses, the American Association of Neuroscience Nurses, and the Society of Critical Care Medicine. She serves on a number of national boards and commissions, including the American Nurses Credentialing Center, Board on Certification for Acute Care Nurse Practitioners, Commission on Certification, and Board of Directors. Dr. Hickey is a frequent national and international speaker and consultant on topics in neuroscience patient management, neuroscience nursing practice, and advanced practice nursing.

Contributors

The following individuals contributed to chapters in the fifth edition:

ROSEMARY BROWN, MSN, RN, CNRN
Clinical Nurse Specialist
Duke University Healthcare System
Rex Medical Center
Raleigh, North Carolina
Chapter 27 • Management of Chronic Pain:
A Neuroscience Perspective

DEIDRE BUCKLEY, MS, RN, ANP-C
Nurse Clinician, MGH Brain Aneurysm/AVM
 Center
Massachusetts General Hospital
Boston, Massachusetts
Chapter 24 • Cerebral Aneurysms
Chapter 25 • Arteriovenous Malformations and Other
 Cerebrovascular Anomalies

NANETTE H. HOCK, MSN, RN, CNRN
Senior Clinical Research Coordinator
Guidant Corporation
Santa Clara, California
Chapter 26 • Stroke and Other Cerebrovascular
 Diseases

STEPHEN W. JANNING, PharmD
Senior Regional Medical Scientist
North America Medical Affairs
GlaxoSmithKline
Raleigh, North Carolina
Chapter 11 • Pharmacological Management
 of Neuroscience Patients

TIMOTHY F. LASSITER, PharmD, MBA
Clinical Pharmacist
Neuroscience Intensive Care Unit
Duke University Hospital
Durham, North Carolina
Chapter 11 • Pharmacological Management
 of Neuroscience Patients

MELANIE S. MINTON, BSN, RN, MBA, CNRN
Coordinator—Continuing Education University
 of Texas Health Science Center at Houston
 School of Nursing
Critical Care Educator, Bayshore Medical
 Center
Pasadena, Texas
Chapter 17 • Neurological Critical Care

Reviewers

The following individuals reviewed chapters from the fourth edition and made recommendations for revisions for the fifth edition.

DEIDRE BUCKLEY, MS, RN, ANP-C
Nurse Clinician, MGH Brain Aneurysm/AVM
   Center
Massachusetts General Hospital
Boston, Massachusetts
   Chapter 28 • Cerebral Aneurysms
   Chapter 29 • Arteriovenous Malformations and Other
      Cerebrovascular Anomalies

CAROLINE GHANBARI, RD, CSM, LD
Clinical Dietitian Specialist III
Memorial Hermann Hospital
Houston, Texas
   Chapter 9 • Nutritional Support for Neuroscience
      Patients

NANETTE H. HOCK, MSN, RN, CNRN
Senior Clinical Research Coordinator
Guidant Corporation
Santa Clara, California
   Chapter 27 • Stroke and Other Cerebrovascular
      Diseases

JANE MAHONEY, DNS, RN, CS
Assistant Professor
University of Texas Health Science Center—
   Houston
Houston, Texas
   Chapter 13 • Behavioral and Psychological Responses
      to Neurological Illness

NORMA D. MCNAIR, MSN, RN, CCRN, CNRN, CS
Clinical Nurse Specialist
   Neuroscience/Orthopedics
UCLA Medical Center
Los Angeles, California
   Chapter 21 • Craniocerebral Injuries
   Chapter 22 • Vertebral and Spinal Cord Injuries

PATRICIA MURPHY, PhD, APN, FAAN
APN Ethics/Bereavement
UMDNJ—University Hospital
Newark, New Jersey
   Chapter 4 • Ethical and Legal Issues
      in Neuroscience Nursing

LEEANN SIMS, MS, RN, CRRN-A
Clinical Nurse Specialist
Legacy Rehabilitation Institute of Orgeon
Portland, Oregon
   Chapter 14 • Rehabilitation of Neuroscience Patients

MARIE WOODWARD, MSN, RN, CNAA
MD Anderson Cancer Center
Department of Neuro-Oncology/Neurosurgery
Houston, Texas
   Chapter 25 • Brain Tumors

JAMIE L. ZOELLNER, MSN, RN, ACNP-C
Neurosurgical Nurse Practitioner
Myrtle Beach, South Carolina
   Chapter 18 • Management of Patients Undergoing
      Neurosurgical Procedures

Preface

As with prior editions, this revision has been influenced by the significant changes that have occurred in science and practice since the last edition, and the nurse's continuing need for the best-quality, up-to-date, patient-centered information. I remain committed to the goals, purposes, scope, and intended audience of the text as discussed in the prefaces of all the other editions. This edition continues to focus on the care of the adult neuroscience patient. It is intended to be a ready reference and reliable resource for practicing nurses in beginning and advanced practice roles, nursing students, nursing faculty, and other health professionals.

With the publication of the fifth edition of *The Clinical Practice of Neurological and Neurosurgical Nursing*, a new norm of clinical reasoning and decision making is emerging for all health care professionals. Known as evidence-based practice (EBP), this new approach integrates the best research evidence with clinical expertise and patient values. EBP challenges health care providers to rethink how they critically evaluate the enormous body of scientific knowledge and its application to patient care. Although the value of clinical expertise and judgment is not abandoned, patient preference enjoys a higher status. In addition to EBP and technological innovation, various other trends identified in earlier editions continue to have a strong influence on practice. These trends include:

- The knowledge explosion
- Information technology that continues to reshape how we practice
- Interdisciplinary practice
- Cost-benefit decision making
- The increasing level of critical illness in hospitals
- The level of care being provided in alternative settings
- The aging of the population resulting in increased prevalence of chronic illness

On one end of the spectrum, the rate of emergence of fundamental new knowledge about the nervous system, injury, recovery, and overall management of patients has had obvious beneficial implications for practice in the acute care setting. On the other end of the spectrum, community-based care and home care for many neuroscience problems is growing. Technology in the home can provide the means for home discharge for persons previously destined for life-long institutional care. Amidst all this emphasis on technology, it must not be forgotten that information is also needed to address chronic health problems that require equally powerful but "low-tech" strategies, such as assessment and modification of risk factors, health promotion, disease prevention, and symptom-management strategies for optimal health and quality of life. The cornerstone of management is patient education for lifestyle changes and self-management. Empowerment of patients and families with knowledge and active decision-making roles regarding their own health care is a most effective cost-saving and quality-promoting approach that needs to be developed and expanded.

Efficacy in today's health care environment is evaluated in terms of cost containment and measurable outcomes. In those areas where they have been developed, this edition relies on widely accepted clinical guidelines, protocols, algorithms, and clinical care maps as the standards for efficacious care.

The extensive revision of content in this edition reflects practice changes in the management of neuroscience patients that have resulted from the growth of knowledge since the last edition. All chapters were carefully reviewed and extensively revised to reflect evidence-based practice and best practice. New chapters have been added and, in some cases, existing chapters merged. Many more tables, charts, and figures aid in clarifying information, and more information is presented in a quick-to-use tabular format. Various colleagues recommended a format highlighting collaborative problems rather than nursing diagnoses, citing the increased number of nurses practicing in interdisciplinary collaborative-practice models. I have used both formats in the presentation of nursing management to meet the multiple needs of nurses. The recommended bibliographies have been curtailed. With the enormous amount of new information published monthly, citations quickly become outdated. The references cited support the treatment and management protocols presented in the chapter and are recommended for review. Websites are listed as resources for current information. Use caution when consulting websites as they are as vulnerable as the published literature to becoming outdated.

The following section-by-section discussion highlights the revisions incorporated in this new edition:

- **Section 1, Neuroscience Nursing: A Perspective on Practice,** provides an updated perspective of changes in neuroscience nursing practice and forecasts trends. Chapter 2 examines the health care continuum for neuroscience patients and the care options for transition in levels of care that have greatly expanded, especially in the area of subacute care. Placement issues related to neuroscience patients are addressed with an emphasis on continuity of care. The multiple models of practice for neuroscience nurses within current practice settings are explored. The clinical reasoning chapter is expanded to provide a focus on outcomes of care. The ethics chapter is revised to focus on palliative and end-of-life care. The goal is to assist nurses in recognizing the need for palliative care and for supporting a peaceful and pain-free death for patients who are no longer candidates for aggressive treatment.
- **Section 2, Assessment and Evaluation of Neuroscience Patients,** includes expansion of the content on neuroanatomy and neurophysiology. The chapter on diagnostics is expanded with detail provided on the clinical applications of tests such as transcranial Doppler and continuous electroencephalographic monitoring. The chapters on neurological physical examination and neurological assessment are revised and expanded to reflect the needs of advanced practice nurses for greater depth of knowledge on data collection and analysis of findings.
- **Section 3, General Considerations in Neuroscience Nursing,** updates several chapters related to basic therapeutics and supportive care such as nutritional support, fluid and electrolyte management, behavioral and psychological responses, and rehabilitation. A comprehensive overview of the pharmacological management of neuroscience patients is addressed in Chapter 11, which has been revised to provide the reader with an overview of practical information related to drug therapy.
- **Section 4, Common Management Problems and Approaches to Neuroscience Patients,** addresses management of the unconscious patient, intracranial hypertension, and preoperative neurosurgical care. The nutrition chapter reflects the current standards of nutritional support for various categories of neuroscience patients, such as the neurotrauma patient, and expands on the assessment of nutritional status in collaboration with the clinical dietician. The intracranial hypertension chapter is based on new standards and guidelines for practice. A chapter has been added on management of patients requiring neurological intensive care; the chapter focuses on prevention of secondary injury. Neurological physiological monitoring as a basis for targeted therapy is discussed. This chapter is coauthored by a nurse with extensive experience and knowledge in neurological critical care.
- **Section 5, Nursing Management of Patients With Injury to the Neurological System,** focuses on patients with injury to the brain, spinal cord, and peripheral nerves. The chapter on brain injury includes the recently published evidence-based guidelines for management of severe injury. The spinal cord injury chapter includes the American Spinal Injury Association (ASIA) Motor and Sensory Assessment Form and ASIA Impairment Scale. The classification of vertebral fractures is expanded, and the "three-column approach" is used to determine need for surgical intervention. The chapter on back and disc injury uses national guidelines as a basis for discussion and addresses patient education as an important means of assisting the patient to achieve optimal outcomes.
- In **Section 6, Nursing Management of Patients With Neoplasms of the Neurological System,** nursing management of patients with nervous system tumors is addressed. The expanded options and treatment protocols for treating brain tumors and spinal cord tumors are presented. Currently used chemotherapeutic agents effective in the management of central nerovus system neoplasms are discussed.
- Cerebrovascular problems are addressed in **Section 7, Nursing Management of Patients With Cerebrovascular Problems.** The paradigm for management of stroke has shifted to include a strong emphasis on prevention. Recent research-based information on pathophysiological alterations and changes in management practices are reflected in the chapter on stroke. American Heart Association (AHA) guidelines provide the foundation for discussion. The chapters on cerebral aneurysms and arteriovenous malformations (AVMs) are also updated to incorporate AHA's most recent guidelines. Excellent pictures of surgical aneurysm clipping and of AVMs are added to assist the reader in appreciating the pathology associated with these conditions.
- Finally, **Section 8, Nursing Management of Patients With Pain, Seizures, Infections, Degenerative Diseases, and Peripheral Nerve Diseases of the Neurological System,** addresses these special neurological problems. Chapters in this section have undergone major revision to include more community-based care and the newest treatment approaches, such as is evident in the chapter on seizures. The headache chapter discusses a multidimensional approach to management and new knowledge about migraine management. The chapter on seizures incorporates the newest drug therapy, clinical guidelines, and patient education. The central nervous system infections chapter has been revised to include content on meningitis and encephalitis and to add content on AIDS. The chapter on neurodegenerative diseases uses a chronic illness management approach, specifically the trajectory of illness model, to discuss the multiple conditions involved. Discussion of each disease is expanded to include symptom management and new pharmacotherapeutics designed to enhance the quality of life for the patient and family. A new chapter on peripheral nerve disease has been added because nurses frequently care for patients with these problems. Entrapment neuropathies, such as carpal tunnel syndrome, and neuropathies related to chronic illness, such as diabetic neuropathies, are included in this chapter.

Nurses engaged in practice at different levels of acuity, including intensive care units, emergency departments, neuroscience specialty units, and other general units that provide care to neuroscience patients, should find this text a helpful and reliable reference. Throughout *The Clinical Practice of Neurological and Neurosurgical Nursing*, pathophysiology is correlated with nursing management to provide a rationale for care and to identify patient outcomes. Caring for patients with neurological problems and disabilities requires special knowledge and skills to support optimal functional level, quality of life, and patient outcomes. This book is written in an effort to respond to the diverse needs of the many committed nurses who provide compassionate, competent, quality care to patients and their families.

Joanne V. Hickey

Acknowledgments

Writing is a demanding and all-consuming process that competes for time and creative energy with family, work, and professional commitments. Yet, somehow, major writing projects like *The Clinical Practice of Neurological and Neurosurgical Nursing*, Fifth Edition, are completed. Many wonderfully supportive and helpful colleagues have sustained me during the writing of this book and have challenged me to think new things and find new ways to capture the essence of clinical practice. Patients and their families are the center of this text, for they are the real teachers of what is most helpful to support a functional and acceptable quality of life. My thinking over the years about neuroscience patient management and neuroscience nursing practice has evolved from these interactions and the privilege of caring for neuroscience patients in a variety of settings with talented and committed health professionals. I am indebted to all of these numerous people who have touched my life.

This project would not have been completed without the support of my family, and especially my husband and best friend, Jim Hickey. It is he who sustained me through the many challenges faced in this enormous writing project and good-naturedly shared the major limitations placed on our life with the long evening and weekend writing schedule. He has been my in-house editor, painstakingly reading chapter after chapter, making excellent recommendations on grammatical and sentence structure. Words cannot acknowledge how he enabled me to complete this work. And my four grandchildren were my pleasant distraction from writing. Jenna, the oldest and an enthusiastic kindergartner, has waited patiently while Grandma finished the book so we could proceed with some planned fun projects.

Finally, I would like to gratefully acknowledge and thank the contributors and the many reviewers who shared their expertise and ideas with me that strengthened the quality of the manuscript. They are listed elsewhere in this book.

Contents

CHAPTER 6

Diagnostic Procedures and Laboratory Tests
for Neuroscience Patients 93

Joanne V. Hickey

CHAPTER 7

The Neurological Physical Examination 117

Joanne V. Hickey

CHAPTER 8

Neurological Assessment 159

Joanne V. Hickey

■ SECTION 3

General Considerations in Neuroscience
Nursing 185

CHAPTER 9

Nutritional Support for Neuroscience Patients 187

Joanne V. Hickey

C H A P T E R   3 2

Peripheral Neuropathies   693
Joanne V. Hickey

C H A P T E R   3 3

Cranial Nerve Diseases   703
Joanne V. Hickey

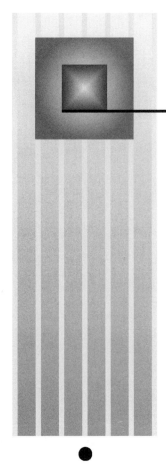

S E C T I O N **1**

Neuroscience Nursing: A Perspective on Practice

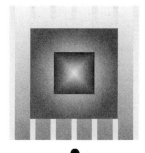

C H A P T E R **1**

Neuroscience Nursing: The Dawn of the 21st Century

Joanne V. Hickey

▥ NEUROSCIENCE NURSING PRACTICE: COMING OF AGE

The explosion of new knowledge coming from basic and clinical research has expanded the scientific foundation for significant developments in neuroscience nursing. As a result, neuroscience nursing has emerged as one of the fastest growing areas of specialty practice. The impact of new knowledge on practice is evident in the strides made in neurology, neurosurgery, neuropharmacology, and neuropsychology and the increased complexity of the knowledge base required for clinical reasoning and decision making. New treatment options raise questions about access, quality, cost, and ethical implications. Meanwhile, health care trends are encouraging many neuroscience nurses to become subspecialists in the care of specific neuroscience populations and to assume new roles as advanced practice nurses. With the assumption of new roles come new levels of responsibility and accountability.

Evidence-Based Practice

Practice, theory, and research, the familiar interrelated cornerstones of professional nursing, imply that practice be based on sound theoretical principles forged from solid research evidence. This necessity is ever more important as current fiscal pressures on the health care delivery system increase demands for accountability from health professionals to be cost-effective while delivering quality care. In the early 1990s, the term **evidence-based medicine** (EBM) was defined as an approach to medical practice and teaching that is based on knowledge of the evidence upon which practice is founded and the strength of that evidence.[1] Although EBM focuses on the results of clinical reports of human experiments, it acknowledges that trials are built on the pivotal work of laboratory research and upon preliminary observational studies in animals and humans.[2] Evidence-based practice is a model for practice and teaching. The term **best practice** combines evidence-based practice, clinician's judgment, and the patient's preference.

EBM and Best Practice Have Their Counterparts in Nursing Practice

Evidence-based nursing (EBN) is an approach to practice and teaching that emphasizes knowledge of the evidence upon which practice is based and the strength of that evidence. Like EBM, EBN is a model of practice and teaching. For many years, nursing has supported research-based practice and encouraged nurses to critically evaluate research for utilization into practice. Like medicine, nursing is striving to identify and deliver best practice. The evidence-based and best practice approach to practice by both medicine and nursing is a way of providing cost-effective, competent, quality care. In addition to incorporating the existing scientifically based knowledge from research, it reaffirms the importance of clinical expertise in decision-making.[4]

Population-Based Care and Disease Management

Population-based care and disease management are other important trends in practice. **Population-based care** is the use of an epidemiological approach to a population to identify health care needs. A population may be defined by characteristics such as age, socioeconomic status, culture/ethnicity, gender, risk factors, or disease. When the unique characteristics of a targeted population are examined, the health care needs of the population can be matched to a cost-effective, quality program of care.[5,6] **Disease management** is a comprehensive, integrated approach to care based on a disease's natural course with the goal of preventing exacerbations through prevention strategies and proactive case management.[5] Population-based care utilizes knowledge of the natural course of the disease and disease management strategies. For example, in Parkinson's disease understanding of the relationship between the characteristic rigidity of the disease and the high risk of falls suggests the need to integrate a fall prevention component into the program of care for all persons with Parkinson's disease.

Neuroscience Nursing Practice

Neuroscience nurses provide EBN and best practice in meeting patient needs. The application of scientific knowledge to population-based practice and disease management is being integrated into care. Neuroscience nurses not only utilize scientific knowledge but also generate new knowledge through the conduct of research. Nursing research is the foundation for building a scientific knowledge base for practice. The National Institute for Nursing Research (NINR) within the National Institutes of Health has been important in setting research priorities and supporting nursing research efforts on a national level. A number of NINR research priorities focused on neuroscience problems are providing opportunities for neuroscience nurses to conduct research. Many other organizations also fund neuroscience research, making neuroscience practice a fertile area for both independent and collaborative research.

The neurosciences constitute the fastest-growing life science field in the United States, a growth reflected in neuroscience nursing practice. Research opportunities beckon to those willing to seize the opportunity. The decade of the brain culminated with significant breakthroughs in understanding neurological diseases, but there is much more to do. This new knowledge is being slowly integrated into practice through EBM and EBN. Being a neuroscience nurse has always been challenging and stimulating. It will continue to be so in the 21st century.

TOWARD A GLOBAL COMMUNITY

The world around us continues to change rapidly into a smaller, more accessible global community. For thousands of years mankind was engaged in the slow transformation from nomadic hunter-gatherers and warriors to communities of farmers dependent for survival on the soil, a strong extended family, and community networks. This was the agricultural revolution. During this time health care was home care provided by the family, sometimes with the assistance of a midwife or doctor. This was followed by a rise of the industrial civilization, which began with the 19th century and was well under way in the middle 1800s. Jobs shifted from the farms to the city factories, where a variety of industries manufactured products that the general population craved. The massive rural to urban shift brought with it the major societal change in family structure from an extended family to a nuclear family, creating radical social, political, economic, and health care delivery changes. Rampant communicable diseases and deplorable workplace conditions posed major health problems. Extended families were not available to care for sick family members, and health care shifted to hospitals. As the causes of common communicable diseases were understood, effective treatment options became available. People began to live longer and, as a result, chronic illness replaced communicable disease as the prevalent health problem in the population.

Today we live in an information society, and our economy has shifted. White-collar workers outnumber blue-collar workers. A manufacturing economy is rapidly being replaced by an economy based on services, using information and knowledge. The workplace is becoming smaller as information businesses grow in importance and computer technology allows easy access to the information superhighway. The emphasis in the Information Age is on knowledge work, knowledge-intense organizations, interdisciplinary collaboration, and accountability.[7] This is an era that offers great opportunities for nursing, for patients, and for health care in general. With the promise comes the upheaval of rapid transition and ongoing change. As knowledge workers in this recast health system where knowledge becomes outdated rapidly, nurses are subject to a high-intensity intellectual environment. The breadth of change experienced today is a sign that we are moving into a new era.[8] That era is still undefined.

The fiber of American culture is undergoing radical changes as the current political, economic, and societal structures that were erected to support an industrial-wave economy are collapsing or being reformed to meet the needs of an information society. Concurrently, the health care industry is undergoing major changes as it struggles to align itself with the needs and demands of contemporary society and a new evolving world paradigm. The only thing certain for the future of health care is change, like it or not.

TRENDS SHAPING HEALTH CARE DELIVERY

Powerful political, economic, demographic, sociological, technological, and health trends are shaping the health care delivery system as the nation endeavors to meet the growing health needs and expectations of its diverse people. These trends are summarized in Chart 1-1 and are discussed briefly below to provide a framework for understanding their influence on the health care system. Due to the overlapping nature of the trend categories, some of the discussion relates to more than one category. For efficiency, trends have been placed in the most logical category.

Political Trends

To some extent, national political trends reflect deeply held attitudes of the country's middle-class electorate. However, these attitudes are filtered through the prisms of multitudes of special interest groups that lobby politicians. The policies, laws, and regulations that result from this process have tremendous impact on economic, demographic, sociological, and technological trends. For this reason, we should be aware of the importance of the political process in promoting or retarding general trends in society.

POWER, SPECIAL INTEREST GROUPS, AND THE BALANCE OF POWER

Politics is the art and science concerned with guiding or influencing policy. It is also the art and science concerned with winning and maintaining control over a government or

---

Chart 1-1 • Trends Influencing the Reshaping of the Health Care Delivery System

POLITICAL

Health policy
Power and lobbying (governmental and nongovernmental impact)
Impact of government regulations
  Demand for quality
  Measurement of outcomes
  Nongovernmental impact
  International perspective

ECONOMICS

Cost containment
Financing and reimbursement practice

DEMOGRAPHICS

"Graying" of America
Immigration and consequent cultural diversity

SOCIOLOGICAL

Consumer activism
Lifestyle changes
Women's movement (also gender, ethnicity differences)
Quality of life
Caregiver stress

TECHNOLOGICAL

Proliferation of scientific knowledge
Computer technology
Information superhighway

HEALTH CARE

Chronicity
Aging of population and health providers
Influence of trauma centers and specialized units
Increased specialization in medical and nursing practice
Increased emphasis on rehabilitation and health promotion

---

an organization. Politics has to do with *power*, and who has the power or assumes the most central position to influence, control, and shape the outcome of decisions. Regardless of how small or large the group or organization, a struggle for power is a dynamic force underlying the relationship and how it develops. Power struggle, power balance, and the exchange of power are ongoing processes that make the world go round.

Being elected or appointed to public or private office provides the holder with power that, if seized, can be used as the bearer sees fit. Health care, as a major industry in the United States involving billions of dollars annually, is a potent reservoir of power. There are those within the industry who wield tremendous power and represent the special interests of insurers, hospital corporations, health providers such as nurses and physicians, and manufacturers of equipment and supplies. There are also consumer groups that express the views and the special interests of consumers. Elected and appointed persons make laws and rules governing health care; their decisions are influenced by the lobbying of diverse special interest groups that try to exert their influence on decisions regarding health care. In this ongoing process, the essential players and pivotal issues can change rapidly under the influence of local and national events and media coverage.

IMPACT OF REGULATIONS

There continues to be a broad political health care mandate for the nation: comprehensive, affordable, quality health care for all Americans. The struggle for political power revolves around how "comprehensive," "affordable," and "quality" are ultimately defined and interpreted. For example, the Joint Commission on Accreditation of Healthcare Organizations (JCAHO) defines quality as measurable, prescribed patient care outcomes that require documentation. For the consumer, quality is often defined by the friendliness of the staff or a positive outcome from care.

Cost of care continues to rise, partially because of requirements mandated by regulatory organizations such as the Health Care Financing Administration (HCFA), which administers Medicare and Medicaid.[9,10] There is an increasing public sentiment to decrease the burdensome requirements of the entitlement programs, to allow states to pilot different approaches to cost containment, and to require able people to work rather than depend on government-funded health care. These and other controversial issues will be decided in a variety of political arenas and will continue to shape the American health care system. In addition, regulatory agencies have a significant impact on how practitioners practice, who can be reimbursed for professional services, and at what level of reimbursement. These are important considerations for advanced practice nurses.

ECONOMIC TRENDS

Cost Containment

Cost containment and affordability continue to be driving forces affecting all aspects of health care delivery. The cost containment strategies of the 1980s, including diagnosis related groups (DRGs) and utilization review, have had mixed results. Increases in hospital acuity levels and paperwork requirements tended to offset any real cost savings accomplished. The cost-control strategies for the 1990s are being spearheaded by managed care and large health networks. In managed care environments there are, theoretically, savings because primary care physicians act as gatekeepers to more expensive specialists such as neurologists and neurosurgeons. What is not clear are the long-term implications for costs if optimal patient outcomes have not been achieved and patients eventually require even more expensive care. Of principal importance are the criteria by which patients are triaged to specialists and the competence of those performing the triage functions.

Maturing managed care markets, focused on cost containment, are developing more community-based care. Subacute care options, home health care, hospice care, and various outpatient services are being expanded and justified based on cost savings. Another essential trend with cost-saving implications is reimbursement for preventive, health promotion, and rehabilitative services. Preventive and health promotion measures keep people healthy or identify problems in the early, less costly intervention stage. Rehabilitation assists people to be as functional and as independent as possible, thus limiting disuse syndromes, disabilities, and other problems requiring more expensive care.

Financing and Reimbursement

Fees for health care services in the United States are largely set by formulas promulgated by the federal and state governments for Medicare (elderly) and Medicaid (poor) and by third-party insurers for group and individual insurance. Current estimates indicate that approximately 40 million people in the United States have no medical insurance and little or no ability to pay for services. The cost for their care must be absorbed by the system, mostly through nonprofit hospital emergency rooms. The younger cohorts of the population, together with their employers, are balking at the dramatic increases in Medicare and health insurance costs that they must bear.

People are being asked to choose intelligently among a large assortment of health care plans and health care packages. They are also being required by their employers to assume a greater portion of health care premiums. A more ominous trend is that many employers are no longer offering health care benefits as a condition of employment. Rather than hiring permanent employees, they now fill positions with temporary or part-time employees who are not given health care benefits. These economic trends are central to the health care delivery debate and place pressure for reform squarely in the political arena.

▥ DEMOGRAPHICS

There are two major demographic trends impacting on health care in the US: the graying of America associated with the baby boom phenomenon and increasing life span for many, and increasing cultural diversity associated with increased immigration.

The Graying of America

Many believe that the changing age profile of America will be the greatest force shaping health care for the next 40 years. The nation's baby boomers, those 76 million people born between 1946 and 1964, will drive the nation's health care consumption curve up steeply as they enter the age spectrum where the manifestations of chronic illness predominate. As of the year 2000, people aged 45 to 54 years number 36 million. By the year 2030, those who are 65 years of age and older will account for 20% of the population, a greater percentage than children.[4] Those 85 years of age and older are the fastest-growing segments of the population.

The graying of America is occurring not only because the absolute numbers entering these age groups are growing, but also because a larger percentage are surviving to older ages. Life expectancy has increased steadily for several decades, largely as a result of (1) improved economic conditions for older Americans, coupled with improved access to affordable, quality health care; (2) strides made in the treatment of many diseases of old age, especially cancer and heart disease, which have extended life significantly; and (3) a new appreciation of the benefits of a healthy lifestyle, including diet, personal habits, exercise, and stress reduction. Nevertheless, with aging eventually comes an overall increase in chronic illnesses such as coronary artery disease, osteoarthritis, and Alzheimer's disease. The greatly increased prevalence of these diseases and others will impose an increased burden on the system and require a redirection of scarce societal resources toward these needs. Although management of chronic illness is causing a major shift in health care to meet the needs of people who are living longer, at some point the common good may require that some of the resources devoted to elder care be allocated to other segments of society. Equity in distribution of health care resources will need to be addressed.

Related ethical decision making is likely to focus on the care provided for the growing number of chronically ill elderly who have a substantially decreased quality of life. It is well documented that the use of health care resources is highest during the last year of life and that these resources are often expended with little or no gain in quality or quantity of life. The underdevelopment of less costly community-based care and support services to assist the elderly and their families in managing their needs in their homes has led to utilization of the high-cost alternative, hospital care. Independent healthy elderly, on the other hand, need help with continued health promotion and preventive measures to keep them healthy and independent. There is a growing realization that the impending stress posed by the graying of America on the health care system has serious consequences for the future health of all sectors of the U. S. economy.

Immigration and Cultural Diversity

The second major demographic trend to shape health care into the 21st century is the greatly increased infusion of multiple ethnic and culturally diverse groups into the United States. This reality is changing the economics, process, and structure of health care delivery. The primary migration from Western Europe in the first half of the century has been replaced by an influx of people from Asia, Africa, and Central and South America. Smaller but growing numbers are coming from the Moslem countries of the Middle East and the newly configured countries of the former Soviet Union. A relatively small number come through the traditional and legal immigration channels. Many now come through special immigration programs for political refugees. Immigrant populations are often of a lower socioeconomic group. By almost every measure, the health of minorities is worse than that of the non-Hispanic white population.[11,12,13] These disparities are addressed in *Healthy People 2010*.

Immigrant groups bring with them ethnic and cultural values that include belief-value systems about health and illness throughout the life cycle. The values and rituals of Western medicine are often held suspect by members of these groups and may be rejected in favor of their own ethnic and folk medicine. Health care professionals must nevertheless understand and respect their cultural values and strive to develop cultural competence and implement programs that are culturally sensitive as well as effective. Education of both health care providers and health care recipients with the goal of easing the transition and blending of native culture and American culture is necessary if mutual needs are to be addressed.

SOCIOLOGICAL TRENDS

Unlike temporary fads and fashions, deep-rooted trends in attitudes and values develop over generations in reaction to shared experiences on community, national, and global levels. They therefore have a tremendous impact on the ways in which people interact with societal institutions. Of the numerous sociological trends influencing society in general and the course of health care in particular, the following few are discussed briefly because of their relevance to practice: consumer activism, lifestyle changes, the women's movement, quality of life, and caregiver stress.

Consumer Activism

Individual values and attitudes toward health are formed, in part, by the information to which one is exposed. As more and more information has become widely available, consumers have become more active in choosing, evaluating, and criticizing the products and services available to them, including health care.

Television, the print media, and now the Internet are the principal sources of consumer health information. Computer technology and the Internet are growing in importance, especially among the better-educated segments of society. For example, Medline and on-line computer health bulletin boards are now easily accessible by the public, and many people are using them to become informed about their health and medical problems. The quality of the information varies, and consumers are not always able to discern the accuracy and completeness of the information. As a result, more consumers are actively participating in making decisions about their health and health care options. They no longer do what they are told to do by the health provider without question or discussion of options. Consumers are also interested in alternative, nontraditional health care such as herbal therapy, homeopathic treatment, and relaxation therapies. Advance directives are becoming more common. The demand for information and involvement in decision making has created a new industry of educational material for the consumer.

Lifestyle Changes

Broad dissemination of information about the health implications of smoking, alcohol and drug abuse, diet, exercise, stress, and sexual practices has had an enormous impact on behavior. These lifestyle changes are decreasing disease frequency and severity. Failure to heed health promotion and disease prevention initiatives, however, continues to be a serious public health problem. For example, obesity, including childhood obesity, continues to increase. Smoking by adolescents continues to rise while smoking in general declines.[14] With so many serious chronic diseases associated with smoking and obesity, these are ominous trends. As women have become more engaged in high-stress occupations, negative lifestyle factors such as poor diet, infrequent exercise, and increased stress are afflicting them as grievously as they have been afflicting men. Positive lifestyle changes are also apparent. Exercise, weight control, low-fat and low-cholesterol diets, and stress reduction are all health promotion and disease prevention basics embraced by a growing number of Americans. The outcome of these conflicting trends on mortality and morbidity is uncertain. Either way, they will be felt in practice settings.

The Women's Movement

An important social and political trend labeled "feminism" or "equal rights for women" has been steadily growing in the United States for the last three decades and has gradually changed the role of women in society. In line with this trend, women's health is being recognized as a legitimate specialty practice, more programs designed to meet the special health needs of women across the life cycle are being established, and more health providers are practicing in this specialty area. In addition, research funds are being allocated to support women's health issues such as breast cancer screening and treatment. Coronary artery disease in women, previously neglected because of a gender bias in medical thinking, is now receiving the attention it deserves.

Quality of Life

In many cases, technology now allows for extension of life indefinitely even though the quality of that life may be minimal or nonexistent. Patients and family members have become more attuned to factoring quality of life into their decisions about health care and extraordinary means of maintaining life. New interest in end-of-life care is shedding new light on palliative care and decisions to control the intensity of care. Resolution of these issues, which are addressed in Chapters 4, has far-reaching implications for the future cost of health care, personal and clinical decision making, and the way health professionals practice.

Caregiver Stress

The caregiver role is being assumed by an increasing number of family members who provide care in the home. Caring for someone with multiple deficits and needs on a 24-hour-a-day basis is an overwhelming responsibility. Successful resuscitation of trauma victims and patients experiencing other acute neurological events often results in a patient's survival with multiple deficits. Improved management is leading to longer survival for patients with chronic neurological diseases, such as stroke, multiple sclerosis, and Parkinson's disease. Such patients have needs that can place a tremendous burden on the family caregiver. Recognition of family caregiver stress and their needs has increased support services in the community for both patients and family caregivers. Effective strategies of support groups such as the Brain Injury Association and Alzheimer's disease groups have helped to focus attention on and secure funds for the care of persons with neurological deficits. Many groups with worthwhile goals are competing for limited resources to fund programs for special patient populations. Great opportunities exist for neuroscience nurses to work with these groups to develop programs that address the special needs of patients and their family caregivers.

TECHNOLOGICAL TRENDS

The information society in which we live is characterized by a proliferation of information about world, national, and local issues, all of which are rapidly disseminated to anyone able to read a newspaper, watch television, or access the Internet. Information technology is changing how we live, work, and learn. The Internet opens portals for the general population to detailed specialized information on almost any subject, which previously would have required time-consuming dedicated research to obtain. Moreover, information is disseminated so rapidly that today's sensational product or treatment is already widely known by the time it is reported in conventional media. Even a casual observer cannot help but be amazed by the discoveries and new technologies that are emerging in almost every area of scientific study.

The areas impacted by the great technology explosion have already been mentioned in previous sections. Diseases are being diagnosed at an earlier stage, new interventions are being developed for previously untreatable diseases (notably, genetically based diseases), less invasive interventions are emerging, and more precise and effective interventions with fewer complications and residual effects are becoming available for common medical problems To cope with these events, medicine and nursing continue to become more specialized as the time and practice requirements to become expert in certain procedures and equipment become more

time consuming. Interventional neuroradiology and interventional cardiology are recent examples. At the same time, health care settings are becoming more specialized. The new, experimental, and highly advanced interventions of the future will only be available at a relatively few, highly specialized centers.

Technology is also having a dramatic effect on rehabilitation. Development of new, high-tech prosthetic devices, as well as the opportunity that new interventions offer for saving and restoring function, will have a profound effect on the quality of life of many patients who have sustained trauma or who have chronic diseases.

NATIONAL AGENDA FOR HEALTH

Governmental, private, and professional organizations are forging many new initiatives in an attempt to influence the future direction of health care in the nation. Two of the more ambitious and promising are *Healthy People 2010* and Prevention Guidelines.

Healthy People 2010

The quintessential document outlining a comprehensive plan for the health care of the nation was *Healthy People 2000*,[15] an unprecedented cooperative effort bringing together a wide spectrum of interests including government and business, voluntary and professional organizations, and private individuals. We now have *Healthy People 2010*, which builds on *Healthy People 2000* and reflects the scientific advances that have taken place over the past 20 years in preventive medicine, surveillance, vaccine and therapeutic development, and information technology.[14] It also mirrors the changing demographics of the country, the changes that have taken place in health care, and the growing impact of global forces on our national health. *Healthy People 2010* incorporated input from a broad cross-section of people. Its two central goals are to:

1. Increase quality and years of healthy life
2. Eliminate health disparities

The first goal acknowledges that we are growing older as a nation, and the second goal addresses the diversity of our population. Like *Healthy People 2000*, *Healthy People 2010* is committed to the single overarching purpose of promoting health and preventing illness, disability, and premature death. Organized around 467 objectives in 28 focus areas, health improvement opportunities are outlined for the first decade of the 21st century. For the first time, a set of Leading Health Indicators will assist individuals and communities target desirable outcomes. An underlying premise of *Healthy People 2010* is that the health of the individual is almost inseparable from the health of the larger community and that the health of every community in every state and territory of the United States determines the overall health status of the Nation.[14] This vision is summarized as *Healthy People in Healthy Communities*.

All health care professionals should review the entire publication to appreciate the magnitude of the national health agenda. Health promotion and disease prevention are important aspects of every nurse's practice, neuroscience nurses included. From the ICU to community-based care, health promotion, risk assessment, and disease prevention strategies must be incorporated into practice regardless of setting. Primary prevention is the ultimate goal, but secondary and tertiary prevention are also necessary to provide optimal outcomes and quality of life for persons with health problems.

PREVENTION GUIDELINES

The Guide to Clinical Preventive Services, 2nd edition, provided by the United States Preventive Services Task Force, is an established reference for clinicians needing evidence-based recommendations on preventive care.[16] Included for more than 80 targeted conditions are health screening schedules for early detection of disease, immunizations and prophylactics to prevent disease, and counseling to modify risk factors that lead to disease. Recommendations in each chapter reflect a standardized review of current scientific evidence and include a summary of published clinical research regarding the clinical effectiveness of each preventive service.[16] Neuroscience practitioners will find this book helpful as they assume more responsibility for prevention. For example, specific information is included on modification of risk factors for stroke including management of hypertension and high cholesterol levels.

Primary care has become a central component of federal, state, local, and private initiatives to reorganize health care, highlighting preventive care as a component within the context of primary care. The term *primary care,* introduced in the 1960s from Europe, traditionally specified four main components: the provision of first-contact care, person-focused care over time, comprehensive care, and coordinated care. In the 1990s, the traditional definition seemed inadequate for the contemporary complexities in health care delivery and the more multidisciplinary, collaborative models of practice. As a result, the Institute of Medicine (IOM) refined the definition of primary care as follows:[17]

"the provision of integrated, accessible health care services by clinicians who are accountable for addressing a large majority of personal health care needs, developing a sustained partnership with patients, and practicing in the context of family and community."

What will happen to specialty practice?[18] While specialty practice will continue, how the generalist and specialist interface will change. In neuroscience specialty practice we will need to be more attuned to the holistic needs of our patients while working collaboratively with primary care providers to achieve optimal outcomes for our patients across a seamless continuum of care.[19]

HEALTH CARE REFORM AND IMPLICATIONS FOR NEUROSCIENCE PATIENTS AND PRACTICE

Reformation of the Health Care System

The health care system and how health care professionals practice continues to change significantly. These changes will have a major impact on both neuroscience patients and neuroscience nursing practice.

Three terms commonly used to provide a framework for understanding health care reform are restructuring, reengineering, and redesigning.[20] *Restructuring* refers to rebuilding, reorganizing, reconfiguring, reconstructing or changing the *structure* of an organization or system. In the context of health care, restructuring refers to the reconfiguring of the organization or institution and is usually diagrammatically illustrated on the organizational chart. *Reengineering* is the fundamental rethinking and radical redesign of *processes* to achieve dramatic improvements in critical, contemporary measures of performance such as cost, quality, service, and speed. In health care, it is "starting over" and rethinking all of the processes involved in providing care. The term *redesigning* focuses on the revision in appearance, function, or content of *what people in an organization do.* In health care it is redesigning that answers the question, who does what in providing care and services to patients. Reengineering and redesigning of practice have the utmost impact on nurses and nursing practice.

RESTRUCTURING OF HEALTH CARE

Dramatic and innovative changes are underway in the structuring of health care facilities as they attempt to respond to the forces and trends of the marketplace. Many smaller hospitals have closed, victims of economic perils. Through mergers and purchase arrangements, other hospitals have become part of larger networks. The surviving tertiary hospitals have become giant intensive care units (ICUs) and part of integrated delivery systems. Hospital stays are shorter, and patients are going home "quicker and sicker" with needs that extend beyond the walls of the hospital into the community.

Most hospitals are either downsizing, often called "rightsizing," or merging with other health care organizations. Mergers encourage collaboration among previously competing independent facilities with the goal to capture a mutually profitable market share from a limited pool of patients. In many mergers, services that were previously duplicated in the independent facilities are consolidated or reapportioned to eliminate duplication. This is true not only for medical services but also for administrative, purchasing, janitorial, and other nonmedical services. Some mergers and buyouts are designed to create major comprehensive regional health care networks to provide a continuum of care from primary preventive care through centralized tertiary care called *integrated delivery systems (IDS).* These large regional networks, which often serve both rural and urban areas, use advanced systems of communication and transportation to facilitate consultations and referrals and to enable health providers to schedule periodic clinics in facilities located where patients live. Comprehensive care networks also offer community-based care (home care, hospice care), ambulatory clinics, subacute care, and tertiary care.

Restructuring changes the components of an organizational chart, and how the components relate to one another. Decentralization, begun in the 1980s, continues in vogue, with the business concepts of matrix structure and product lines added to better delineate responsibility and accountability for managers. Newer product line categories, such as "hotel services," are now included in the organizational structure, reflecting the new emphasis on creature comforts for patients and their families. Health care facilities are striving to meet the needs of patients by becoming user-friendly, comfortable environments, unlike the old inflexible structures that required patients and families to conform.

Restructuring: Implications for Neuroscience Patients and Practice

The health care paradigm for the 21st century is shifting from an acute care model to a two-pronged acute care and chronic care model. In this context, it is significant that so many neurological problems are either chronic in nature—for example, Parkinson's disease and multiple sclerosis—or result in chronic, long-term functional disabilities—for example, head injury, spinal injury, and stroke. The needs of patients with chronic illness differ significantly from those of patients with acute problems. Home care, for instance, is more desirable for most neurological patients and their families and is less expensive than institutional care. To meet these realities, the structures for chronic illness management within the health care system and health networks must be expanded, more fully developed, and better defined.

For neuroscience patients, acute/critical care management is available in Neuroscience ICUs and other specialty units. The Neuro ICU is a high-tech environment utilizing sophisticated computerized equipment for patient support and monitoring, staffed by highly skilled physicians and nurses with very specialized training. Other specialty units, such as Acute Stroke Units, focus on supporting acute care and early rehabilitation through a multidisciplinary team of specialists. The intermediate units of hospitals are shrinking in size. In all units, length of stay is growing shorter and patients are often being discharged with unmet rehabilitative and other needs. Access to specialists' care and specialty units is a major concern emerging from health care reform.

▎▎▎▎ REENGINEERING OF HEALTH CARE

Health care reengineering focuses on the processes involved in providing care and services to patients and their families. According to Hammer and Champy, reengineering begins with the question, why do we do what we do, and why do we do it in the way we do?[20] Particularly in health care, the answer is often "that's the way we have always done it

here," or "that's our policy." How we develop standards of care or care maps; how we develop and regulate visiting hours, admission, discharges, and transfers; and how we teach patients and families are examples of processes that can be conducted in many ways, some more reasonable, sensible, humanistic, and successful than others.

Many confusing and imprecise terms are used to describe health care reform. Often, they refer to new processes in the delivery of care intended to increase efficiency through coordination, collaboration, cost control, and refinement of whatever measurable outcomes seem appropriate at the time. Managed care, an essential concept in health care reform, is an example (see Chapter 2). Other process-focused reengineering initiatives intended to control cost are managed competition, health alliances, and capitation. One could argue that health alliances are also new structures within health care and, therefore, are examples of restructuring. Although it is true that alliances may be viewed as conceptual structures, the primary purpose is a reengineering of business processes. For that reason, alliances should be considered a reengineering rather than a restructuring initiative.

Reengineering: Implications for Neuroscience Patients and Practice

Almost all patients, including neuroscience patients, will receive care under managed care contracts. Many patients will receive all of their care, including prevention, health promotion, acute and chronic illness management, and rehabilitative services, through giant health care networks. Nurses caring for neuroscience patients will work collaboratively with case managers to expeditiously provide the care patients and families need using clinical pathways or care maps. Nurses will be responsible and accountable for achieving predetermined measurable outcomes for patients. More and more health services will be shifted from the relatively high-cost institutional arena to community settings. Community-based care will continue to grow and expand, and this will include further development of home care for neurological patients.

Multidisciplinary clinical pathways, with accompanying guidelines and protocols, are being used to guide neuroscience practice with the goal of achieving predetermined measurable outcomes along a trajectory of illness. Additional practice guidelines are being introduced as a result of the work of national consensus conferences and specialty organizations. With the increased use of limited drug formularies, practitioners have fewer options and must choose from cost-effective drugs with proven quality-outcome measures.

Traditional policies and procedures are being reexamined. Services emphasizing the comfort of patients and families are becoming prominent as health care organizations compete for patients. Settings of care are being reexamined. More patients are receiving high-tech care in the home and in community-based facilities rather than in hospitals. Patients and families are assuming more responsibility for care. In addition, health care is focusing on disease prevention and health maintenance in all health care services rendered. Neuroscience nurses, as an integral part of teams making these critical decisions about care, should be in the vanguard of those reaching out to provide community and home-based care for neurological patients.

REDESIGNING OF HEALTH CARE

Who does what in the health care arena? This is the essence of what is meant by redesign. For nursing, the issue concerns staffing. Optimum staff mix has been a matter of debate for many years, regardless of whether the unit is within a hospital, a clinic, or a community-based program. The optimistic trend in the 1980s was toward an all-RN staff with each holding, at minimum, a BSN degree. With a substantial portion of operating budgets devoted to nursing personnel salaries, the new focus of redesign envisions a staff mix model that includes both licensed and unlicensed nursing care providers.

Embedded within the above redesign process is the unresolved issue of what is the appropriate differential practice for nurses educationally prepared at the associate, baccalaureate, and graduate levels. Integrative tri-level models of professional differentiated practice have been proposed by many with little success.[21] Moreover, both master's-prepared and doctoral-prepared nurses have traditionally been lumped together for purposes of describing nurses with graduate education. The roles of advanced practice nurses (APN)s, particularly clinical nurse specialists and nurse practitioners, continue to evolve in the redesign climate.

Redesigning: Implications for Neuroscience Patients and Practice

Since the question of who should do what for patients is central to redesign, roles, responsibilities, and accountability for neuroscience practice will continue to evolve. This is true for physicians as well as for nurses and other health professionals. Redistribution of roles and responsibilities will occur depending on education, experience, and the environment. In the early 1900s the blood pressure cuff, heralded as a cutting-edge innovation, was introduced in the United States. Taking a blood pressure was the sole responsibility of the physician. Now, most nonlicensed personnel take and record blood pressure, usually with the use of automatic electronic equipment. While giving up responsibility for some activities, physicians assume new responsibilities. This is also true of nurses.

As staff mix changes and nurses become responsible for supervising nonlicensed personnel, nurses must become involved in decisions regarding these personnel. These decisions include identification of activities that can be safely delegated, educational requirements to safely and competently execute assumed duties, and requirements for supervision and monitoring of personnel to assure quality and accuracy. For example, nonlicensed personnel can safely assist a neurological patient with eating *if* the patient has been assessed for swallowing and found to have no difficulty. However, *if* the patient is at high risk for aspiration,

then the nurse should attend to the patient. Neurological patients can change rapidly, and the nurse must assume responsibility for making ongoing decisions about delivery of safe care.

Many APNs are assuming new roles in neuroscience practice as nurse practitioners and clinical nurse specialists. They are practicing in tertiary settings on Neuro ICUs, on intermediate units, in neuro clinics, in rehabilitation programs, and in community-based programs such as home care. These nurses are assuming responsibility for diagnosing some neurological problems and for prescribing treatment plans. Many chronic neurological problems can be well managed by APNs who combine a holistic nursing framework with a medical framework. As medical residents in specialty practice decrease due to a shift to primary care in the United States, this trend is expected to grow. As this trend takes hold there will come the realization that differentiation of roles for nurses is the key to providing cost-effective, quality care.

Neuroscience nurses working at the bedside are being cross-trained in other clinical areas so that they can move between areas as staffing needs increase and decrease. With a trend toward more community-based care, fewer RNs will be practicing in hospitals; however, this trend will be balanced by a growing need for nurses with neuroscience skills in community-based care, especially home care. A discussion of changing models of practice is found in Chapter 2.

LIVING IN THE PRESENT WHILE PREPARING FOR THE FUTURE

Professional life at the beginning of the 21st century involves dealing with a rapidly changing present while preparing for a future wherein change may come quickly and frequently. No longer can a nurse depend on her or his basic education to prepare for years of practice. A characteristic of a profession is the responsibility for and commitment to lifelong learning. To provide the most current evidence-based practice, nurses must update and maintain their knowledge, skills, and abilities to provide competent care. Computer literacy is essential to practice if one wishes to access information efficiently. Computer technology and the Internet provide easy access to libraries, databases, bulletin boards, and countless other resources in the world. Without computer skills a nurse will be without the basic tools to sustain a viable professional life. Critical thinking skills and computer literacy are the keys to survival in the 21st century. The challenge for nurses will be stimulating and provide opportunities for further professional development of the specialty of neuroscience nursing practice.

REFERENCES

1. Evidence-Based Medicine Working Group. (1992). Evidence-based medicine: A new approach to teaching the practice of medicine. *JAMA, 268*, 2420–2425.
2. Cook, D. J., Sibbald, W. J., Vincent, J. L., & Cerra, F. K. (1996). Evidence based critical care medicine: What is it and what can it do for us? *Critical Care Medicine, 24*, 334–337.

3. Hayes, Sacket, D. L., Gray, J. M., Gook, D. J., & Guyaato, G. H. (1996). Transferring evidence from research into practice. I. The role of clinical care research evidence in clinical decisions. *ACP Journal Club*, A14–A15.

4. Sibbald, W. J. (1998). Some opinions on the future of evidence-based medicine. *Critical Care Clinics, 14*(3), 538–558.

5. Zitter, M. (1997). A new paradigm in health care delivery: Disease management. In W. E. Todd & D. Nash (Eds.), *Disease management: A systems approach to improving patient outcomes* (p. 4). Chicago: American Hospital Publishing Inc.

6. Hickey, J. V. Advanced practice nursing at the dawn of the 21st century. (2000). In J. V. Hickey, R. M. Ouimette, & S. L. Venegoni, (Eds.), *Advanced practice nursing: Changing roles and clinical applications* (2nd ed., p. 26). Philadelphia: Lippincott Williams & Wilkins.

7. Sorrells-Jones, J., & Weaver, D. (1999). Knowledge workers and knowledge-intense organizations, Part 1. *Journal of Nursing Administration, 29*(7/8), 12–18.

8. Wilson, C. K., & Porter-O'Grady, T. (1999). *Leading the revolution in health care: Advancing systems, igniting performance* (2nd ed., pp. 1–39). Gaithersburg, MD: Aspen.

9. Iglehart, J. K. (2001). The American health care system: Medicare. In P. R. Lee & C. L. Estes, *The nation's health* (6th ed., pp. 349–361). Boston: Jones and Bartlett Publishers.

10. Iglehart, J. K. (2001). The American health care system: Medicaid. In P. R. Lee & C. L. Estes, *The nation's health* (6th ed., pp. 389–401). Boston: Jones and Bartlett Publishers.

11. Lee, P. I., & Estes, C. L. (2001). The health of the nation. In P. R. Lee & C. L. Estes, *The nation's health* (6th ed., pp. 1–7). Boston: Jones and Bartlett Publishers.

12. Moss, N. (1999). Socioeconomic disparities in health in US: An agenda for action. In P. R. Lee & C. L. Estes, *The nation's health* (6th ed., pp. 65–78). Boston: Jones and Bartlett Publishers.

13. Collins, K. S., Hall, A., & Neuhaus, C. (1999). *U.S. minority health: A chartbook*. New York: The Commonwealth Fund.

14. U. S. Department of Health and Human Services. (2000). *Healthy people 2010* (pp. 7–8). Washington, D. C.: U. S. Government Printing Office.

15. U. S. Department of Health and Human Services. (1990). *Healthy people 2000* (p. 6.) (DHHS Publication No. PHS 91-50213). Washington, D. C.: U. S. Government Printing Office.

16. U. S. Preventive Services Task Force. (1996). *Guide to clinical preventive services* (2nd ed.). Baltimore, MD: Williams & Wilkins.

17. Donaldson, M. S. , Yordy, K. D., Lohr, K. N. , & Vanselow, N. A. (Eds.) for the Institute of Medicine. (1996). *Primary care: American's health in a new era*. Washington, D. C.: National Academy Press.

18. Kassirer, J. P. (1994). Access to specialty care. *New England Journal of Medicine, 331*(17), 1151–1152.

19. Baer E, D. (1999). Philosophical and historical bases of advanced practice nursing roles. In M. D. Mezey & D. O. McGivern (Eds.), *Nurses, nurse practitioners* (3rd ed., pp. 72–91). New York: Springer.

20. Hammer, M., & Champy, J. (1993). *Reengineering the corporation*. New York: Harper Business.

21. Baker, C. M., Lamm, G. M., Winter, A. R., Robbeloth, V. B., Ransom, C. A., Conly, F., Carpenter, K. C., & McCoy, L. E. (1997). Differentiated nursing practice: Assessing the state-of-the-science. *Nursing Economics, 15*(5), 253–262.

RESOURCES
Professional

Published Material (Classics)

Recreating Health Professional Practice for a New Century: The Fourth Report of the Pew Health Professions Commission (1998). http://futurehealth.ucsf.edu/pubs.htlm

Websites

The Best Practice Network. http://www.best4health.org

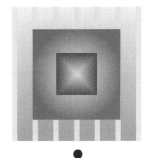

C H A P T E R **2**

The Health Care Continuum and Transitions in Levels of Care

Joanne V. Hickey

This chapter briefly discusses the continuum of care, transitions in levels of care, and models of practice in the dynamic health care system in the context of neuroscience nursing practice. The configuration of a health care system is driven by the needs of society and by economic and other resources allocated to support the system. All these factors have some impact on neuroscience nursing practice.

HEALTH CARE FINANCING

Over the last 50 to 60 years, a complex system of financing and delivering health care has evolved in the United States. About 40 million Americans have no health insurance. Insured Americans have health insurance that varies from minimal benefits to comprehensive coverage. The United States government is the major purchaser of health care through its Medicare program. Health insurance organizations, the "third party payers," have become the universal vehicles through which health care providers are paid. Health insurers have also become powerful controllers and interpreters of services and reimbursement provided under the provisions of a contract. Control of services is intended to restrain cost and maintain quality of care. However, differences in opinion about application of cost-effective policies have created a discontinuity among the receivers, providers, and payers of health services.

Over the years, health insurance benefit packages have become increasingly comprehensive for some and limited for others. Copayments are rising, and services previously covered in full now require a deductible. Despite these changes, it is questionable whether the system can be sustained, particularly as a greater proportion of the population ages. Those without health care insurance and with no financial assets receive some health care free of charge through Medicaid, the government program for the poor. Others without health insurance who do not qualify for Medicaid receive limited and sporadic care, often through hospital emergency departments with the cost transferred to the health insurance system. Managed care was introduced in an attempt to address escalating costs and quality issues.

Managed Care

The managed care revolution in the health care delivery system has seen changes in corporate structures, health care policy, and demographics. All have contributed to the evolution of managed care.[1] In the last century, society has transformed from rural to urban, from an individual to institutional focus, and from an agrarian to an industrial-information and service economy. During the same period, changes among physicians have included transition from general practitioner to specialist, from solo to group practice, and from direct payment for care to group insurance.

The term *managed care* represents a host of different, sometimes conflicting, ideas about health care delivery and financing. It is a system of health care delivery that monitors usage and cost of services and measures performance (p. 1).[1] The goal is a system that delivers value by providing access to cost-effective, high-quality care. Managed care systems are oriented toward outcomes, focusing on cost, health indicators, quality of life, and patient satisfaction. Insurers typically emphasize cost while acknowledging that achieving optimal health, quality of life, and patient satisfaction have a significant impact on cost. As managed health care systems have developed, the methods employed for achieving goals have come to include:

- Analyzing processes and results of medical treatment to achieve specific outcomes
- Developing and communicating practice guidelines for effective and cost-effective care
- Building networks of providers to improve the cost effectiveness of health care delivery
- Seeking continuous quality improvement
- Facilitating access to preventive services and early diagnosis and treatment
- Supporting patients and their families in finding the most appropriate treatments available
- Assuming a coordinator role among the complex networks of payers, providers, and patients to enhance communication and continuity of care

Managed care integrates the financing and delivery of health care through contracts with selected health care providers and hospitals that provide comprehensive health care services to enrolled members of a health care plan.[2] The provider network is the single most important feature distinguishing a managed care from an indemnity (fee-for-service) plan.[3] Other characteristics of managed care plans are lower hospital use (both admission rates and length of stay), greater use of less costly procedures and tests, greater emphasis on disease prevention and screening, and comparable quality and enrollee satisfaction. Central components of a managed care environment include projected length of stay designation, use of case managers and care maps, and the requirement for approval before care is provided. Projected length of stay is guided by diagnostic related groups (DRGs) and the experience of the insurer. Hospital use is minimized by providing services on an outpatient basis as often as possible. Managed care relies heavily on case managers assigned to each patient to provide continuity of care through timely, coordinated care. Case managers work with the health care team and patient and must approve care and specific use of resources before implementation.

Continuity of care is a concept that describes the ideal result of well-coordinated care throughout a person's illness and across health care settings. It is the expeditious process of providing uninterrupted, cohesive, continuous, seamless care that is maintained throughout the transition points of illness, including the transition from institutional care to community-based care.[4] *Coordination of care* implies that there is an active and effective coordinator (often the case manager) working with the health team. The coordinator sees the "big picture" and identifies specific patient needs, initiates action to meet those needs, and integrates these actions to promote *appropriate and timely* use of resources and services. The coordinator must be able to communicate information to the appropriate people (e.g., patient, family, service providers) regarding what is specifically needed, why it is needed, and the expected measurable outcomes to be achieved. The person responsible and accountable for coordination must also be effective in follow-up to monitor the progression of activities and be able to identify when course modification or implementation of an alternative plan is necessary to achieve optimal outcomes.

Health care markets vary greatly from one another, and many factors influence market penetration by managed care plans and the manner of their maturity. As managed care markets continue to develop and move toward consolidation of services into large integrated systems, we can expect to see more care provided within the framework of managed care.

ORGANIZATION OF HEALTH CARE

In this section, health care is discussed from the perspectives of acuity, location of health care delivery, focus of care, and health promotion-disease prevention.

Acuity of Care

One can view health care as two systems, acute-critical care and chronic illness care. The purposes and underpinnings of the two systems are in sharp contrast to each other. *Acute*

illness is characterized by an abrupt onset of a disease process with the potential for single-system or multisystem complications. Treatment often takes days or weeks, and significant changes in condition can occur within hours or days. Patients require critical-acute care because they are physiologically unstable, technologically dependent, at high risk for complications, and/or require close monitoring. The vulnerability for complications is compounded by comorbidity, particularly in the elderly who are often living with many chronic health problems that increase the complexity of illness and need for care. Care is usually provided within hospital settings where a wide variety of acute care services and cutting-edge treatment options are offered by multidisciplinary specialists working together in sophisticated high-tech environments to achieve a *cure* or the best outcomes for critically ill patients. In this physician-dominated model, the attending physician assumes the primary role of decision-maker and directs the overall plan of care. Patients and families are included in decision making to the degree it is possible, but the physician primarily maintains control over care. Acute care, and particularly critical care, is the most expensive care provided, and access is uneven depending on location and health insurance of the recipient.

Chronic illness is an irreversible condition characterized by an accumulation or latency of disease states or impairments that have an impact on a person's functional abilities and quality of life. Persons with chronic illness need supportive care and self-care management strategies to maintain function and prevent further disability.[5] Chronic illness tends to involve multiple, long-term diseases that span many years or a lifetime and follow an uncertain course. A major focus of management is stabilization of the disease, and often includes palliation. Because *cure is usually not possible*, the goal of care is adaptation, that is, to learn to live with the illness in the least intrusive way and to maintain the highest functional level and quality of life for as long as possible. Care is provided mainly in a low-tech, community-based, primary care model with consultation from specialists as needed. The patient is the primary decision maker and coordinator of care, thus maintaining a high level of control. Emphasis in chronic illness management is on empowering the patient with knowledge through education and counseling to optimize self-management, adaptation, and symptom management.

How illness is viewed shapes care. A key transition point in illness comes when a patient moves from an acute care model to a chronic illness model, thus redefining the illness and needed care. The *chronic illness trajectory model*, proposed by Corbin and Strauss,[6] provides a comprehensive framework for understanding chronic illness and the roles of health care providers, the patient, and family in management. This model is particularly helpful for understanding the nurse's role in symptom management, rehabilitation, education, and support, and as an advocate for the patient and the family. The trajectory model is based on the fundamental idea that chronic illnesses have a course or trajectory that changes over time. The course can be shaped and managed by the collaborative effort of the patient, family, and health care providers to support optimal outcomes. Although shaping may not change the direction of the illness, the course of the illness can be extended and stabilized, and symptoms may be controlled and managed. The shaping process is complicated by the use of technology, which has a potential impact on the patient's personal identity, well-being, and activities of daily living.

The success of the United States' health care system in developing effective acute and critical care models has resulted in many people surviving acute episodes they might otherwise not have survived. These people survive with chronic health problems that must be managed for the remainder of their lives. The quality of their management directly influences their quality of life and that of their families. Both the acute/critical care and the chronic illness models are essential to meet the needs of modern society. The challenge remains the development of good models to provide seamless care as the patient moves from one level of care to another, and to do this in a cost-effective way while providing quality care. The role of the *case manager* has emerged as the person responsible for coordinating timely, cost-effective care that often includes transitions in care. Neurological patients require both acute/critical care and chronic illness care because those who survive major neurological trauma often do so with complex, long-term chronic health problems that must be addressed.

Environments of Health Care Services

Health care is provided as either institutional-based care or community-based care. *Institutional-based care* is available at hospitals, nursing homes, and other full-time facilities where patients stay until discharged to another type of institution, to community-based care, to their homes, or until they die. Within hospitals, more specialty units have developed, such as chronically/critically ill units, ventilatory-dependent units, stroke step-down units, and collaborative care units. These units are designed to meet the needs of special patient populations efficiently and cost effectively.

Community-based care, available usually in the community where the patient resides, is provided in the home or at a site where the patient goes for care in his or her community as an outpatient and then returns home. Community-based care is generally less expensive than institutional care and is often preferred by and more convenient for the patient and family. The cost savings are particularly attractive to third-party payers. More and more high-tech care, traditionally provided only in institutions, is becoming available in the community. Home health care services, in particular, are expanding to include more infusion therapy, ventilatory support, rehabilitation, and other services traditionally associated with institutional care. The phenomenal growth of services in the community has led to corresponding complex organizational structures to support community-based care.

Although patients with neurological conditions have always been managed in the community, their number is greatly increasing and the interventions involved in their care are much more complex. Successful community-based management of a neuroscience patient with complex needs requires appropriate support and careful monitoring. An example is day-care programs that offer cognitive retraining programs for cognitively impaired adults, thus improving the client's quality of life and functional level. Another example is a weekly exercise program for persons with Parkinson's disease to improve muscle strength, balance, and

education. High-tech care for neurological problems, such as ventilatory support, is becoming increasingly available in the home but requires high-level support by appropriately skilled health professionals for it to be successful.

Sick Care to Health Care

The shift in focus from sick care to health care is apparent as the emphasis in processes of care shift to primary care. The provisional definition of primary care adopted by the Institute of Medicine (IOM) is as follows:

Primary care is the provision of integrated, accessible health care services by clinicians who are accountable for addressing a large majority of personal health care needs, developing a sustained partnership with patients, and practicing in the context of family and community.[7]

According to the IOM report, primary care is *comprehensive care*, that is, care of any and all health problems at a given stage of a person's life. It includes ongoing care of patients in various care settings, such as hospitals, nursing homes, clinicians' offices, community sites, schools, and homes.[7] The assumption was made by the committee that primary care is the logical foundation of an effective health care system because primary care can address most health problems of the population. The diagnosis and treatment of some neurological problems will be managed exclusively by primary care physicians or collaboratively with neurologists and neurosurgeons. This positions the primary care physician as the gatekeeper for care, including referrals for specialty neurological care. Within the context of primary care, disease prevention, health promotion, and health maintenance are fundamental components.

Disease Prevention, Health Promotion, and Health Maintenance

Three levels of prevention are generally recognized for disease and disability:[8]

1. *Primary prevention:* any intervention that prevents a pathologic process from occurring. Examples include immunization or identification and control of risk factors, such as smoking, with the ultimate goal of preventing vascular disease such as stroke.
2. *Secondary prevention:* intervention after a pathologic process has begun, but before symptoms occur. For example, prescription of aspirin for patients who have had a stroke may prevent a second stroke.
3. *Tertiary prevention:* prevention of progressive disability or other complications in individuals with established disease. For example, community management of patients with Parkinson's disease or multiple sclerosis includes prevention of complications such as injury due to falls and decreased levels of mobility.

Health promotion and *health maintenance* are related terms that refer to the advocacy and provision of programs and strategies that have been demonstrated through research and practice to be beneficial in maintaining optimal health and preventing disease and disability. For instance, low-fat diet, exercise, and sensible personal habits are essential for all people to live healthy and productive lives. Health promotion is everyone's job regardless of practice setting.

Primary care physicians are the gatekeepers for coordinating care and referring patients to other specialists. As primary care physicians become more involved in managing care of neurological patients, there will be an increased emphasis on maintaining and promoting health. This will be beneficial in preventing exacerbation of neurological conditions due to problems in other body systems and in preventing effects on other systems due to poorly managed neurological conditions. Primary care physicians and neuroscience health professionals are forging new partnerships. At the same time, neurological specialists will continue to assume leadership roles in coordinating and managing the care of patients with complex neurological problems, those requiring acute care management or hospitalization, and those needing long-term management of chronic illness. The neurological specialist assuming this role may be a physician or an advanced practice nurse.

The efficient and economical movement of patients along the continuum of care remains focused on outcomes. The criteria for deciding when patients should be moved from one level of care to another will change based on research findings related to key indicators and transition points of diseases and illnesses. Transitions in health status are occurring more rapidly, necessitating quick and efficient responses in health care service to provide transitional care and control costly delays in services.

THE CONTINUUM OF HEALTH CARE

A continuum is a coherent whole characterized by a progression of elements varying by degrees, and one that is anchored on each end by significantly different elements or opposite elements. This is true of the health care continuum anchored at one end by high-tech critical care and at the other end by "no-tech" self-care. Between these two poles is an array of levels of care. Some are recent entrants; others are familiar terms that have been redefined, such as long-term care. New options, particularly in the subacute arena, are emerging, often in response to cost-containment mandates and unmet patient needs.

Levels of Care

Definitions and interpretations relating to skilled nursing care, intermediate care, long-term care, and custodial care are changing. These changes are creating confusion in decision making for reimbursement and availability of services. To make informed decisions about services offered and insurance coverage provided, each particular agency's policies must be investigated closely (Table 2-1).

This section addresses acute care and subacute care. A number of texts provide comprehensive coverage of levels of care. The reader is directed to these resources for further

discussion. For purposes of this chapter, *acute care* includes acute care hospitals, inpatient acute rehabilitation hospitals, transitional hospitals, and all services within these hospitals (e.g., emergency services). *Subacute care* includes skilled nursing facilities (SNFs), hospice care, rehabilitation units that are not considered acute, home health, and specialty pharmacy providers.[9]

Acute Care Facilities

Acute Care Hospitals

Acute care hospitals are discussed elsewhere in this chapter. Acute care facilities provide a wide range of services and specialty care. JCAHO guidelines apply to these facilities.[10]

Inpatient Acute Rehabilitation Hospitals

Included in this category are inpatient acute rehabilitation hospitals and units within hospitals that provide short-term comprehensive intensive rehabilitation programs designed to achieve a high level of independence and functional return. The number of these facilities is limited, and stays are expensive and goal oriented. To optimize use of these scarce resources, patients are carefully screened for admission. Insurance criteria reflect Medicare requirements and addresses three major areas:[9]

1. Selected diagnoses (e.g., stroke, head trauma, spinal cord trauma, neurological disorders).
2. The primary problem must include a recent functional loss (e.g., cognitive, mobility, bowel/bladder, communication dysfunctions) in a person previously independent.
3. A physician must document the expected significant functional improvement to be achieved within a reasonable time frame.

Candidates must also meet these other admission criteria: be medically stable; possess the mental ability to follow one- or two-step commands; and be able to withstand at least 3 hours of therapies, daily, 5 times per week. Therapy can consist of any combination of physical therapy (PT), occupational therapy (OT), and speech therapy (ST). Progress toward achieving stated goals is monitored closely. The patient may be discharged from the rehabilitation program for several reasons, including:[9]

Achievement of stated goals
Lack of progress toward stated goals after a reasonable trial period
Onset of a severe complication necessitating transfer to an acute care setting
Onset of a complication that requires discontinuation of the comprehensive rehabilitation program for more than 1 week

Transitional Hospitals

Transitional hospitals are acute care hospitals for medically stable patients with long-term rehabilitative needs and care that are too complex for SNFs. They differ from traditional acute care hospitals in that they have fewer specialists and

▦ Table 2-1 • COMMON CATEGORIES OF CARE AND EXAMPLES OF SERVICES PROVIDED

TYPE OF CARE	EXAMPLES OF CARE PROVIDED
Skilled nursing care is based on a progression of complexity of a patient's medical and functional needs. • The level of skilled nursing care is the most intensive in a skilled nursing facility (SNF).	See section on SNF.
Intermediate care provides moderate assistance with activities of daily living (ADLs) and often restorative nursing supervision for some activities. • These patients require more care than those receiving custodial care (distinction may be blurred). • Insurers do not usually pay for this level of care unless skilled care is also required.	• Transfer from bed to chair or toilet by a single staff member. • Assistance with ambulation. • Moderate assistance with ADLs. • Routine medication and treatment with little assessment or monitoring. • Intermittent incontinence care. • Interactive although may have episodes of confusion, agitation, or emotional outbursts.

Long-term care (LTC) is a term that was once used as an equivalent to **nursing home care.** It now refers to a level of care in which chronically impaired persons, dependent on others, receive care in various settings.
• Care is provided in homes, foster homes, day care centers, and various other institutional and noninstitutional settings.
• The goal of LTC is to promote or maintain as much independence and quality of life as possible.
• There is no single regulatory defining condition of LTC, but the key elements are chronicity and dependency of the patient.*
• LTC is usually financed through individual patient insurance policies and personal funds, although state aid may finance some patients.
	A broad spectrum of services is provided, depending on the needs of the patient and family. For example, services within a category such as adult day care can vary.
	• Adult day care may provide three levels of care: core (unskilled assisted living); enhanced (skilled nursing care that requires little supervision or support, e.g. dressing change); and intensive (maximum that includes skilled nursing care as well as therapies that require significant supervision and support).†
	• Generally two types of candidates for LTC; those who require care for:
	  • Complex care and a long convalescence
	  • Chronic and multiple medical, mental health, and social problems
	• Some patient with conditions, such as quadriplegia or mental retardation, live in group homes where all their needs are met in a supervised environment.
	• Services may include terminal care.

Custodial care is primarily to help patients with their personal care needs (e.g., ADLs); this care can be safely and reasonably provided by persons without professional skills or training. • May also be referred to as personal care, supervisory care, or assisted living • Requires the lowest skilled personnel for care • Ambulates independently with or without assistive devices • Takes own medication (no sliding scales) • Medicare will not pay for custodial care alone; however, it will pay if skilled care is also needed.	• Transfer from bed to chair or toilet with standby assistance • Minimal assistance for ADLs • Continent, but may need assistance with catheter or colostomy care • Socially interactive; may have episodes of confusion or agitation, but do not require restraints or control of behavior • For example, assisted living provides many levels of care to fill the gap in services between independent living and nursing home care. Services vary but generally may include group meals to some skilled nursing care

* Williams, S. J., & Torrens, P. R. (1993). *Introduction to health services.* New York: Delmar.

† Tellis-Nayak, M. (1998). The postacute continuum of care: Understanding your patient's options. *AJN, 98*(8), 44–48.

provide only basic diagnostic and surgical equipment. Major surgeries are not done (minor procedures such as tracheotomies and tube placements are available). The staffing of nurses is similar to that of other acute care hospitals. These hospitals admit stable patients with complex medication and treatment needs. Examples of patients admitted include ventilator-dependent patients, including those requiring weaning; patients needing extensive wound care; patients recovering from coma; and patients requiring cognitive or neurobehavioral rehabilitation.

Subacute Care

According to JCAHO,[11] subacute care is a separate and distinct inpatient program that provides highly skilled rehabilitation care or medically intensive care for patients following an acute event or significant change in condition.

Candidates for subacute care are those patients who do not require surgery or invasive procedures but do require frequent assessment and longer patient stays. Subacute care facilities provide care to patients who have an acute illness or injury but are not in the acute phase and who need a level of care more intensive than traditional nursing or home care, but less intensive than hospital care.[11] They fill the gap between acute hospital care and long-term care.

The National Subacute Care Association offers the following definition: subacute care is a comprehensive, cost-effective inpatient level of care for patients who:[12]

Have had an acute event from injury, illness or exacerbation of a disease process

Have a determined course of treatment

Though stable, require diagnostics or invasive procedures, but not intensive procedures requiring an acute level of care

The severity of the patient's condition requires:

Active physician direction with frequent on-site visits
Professional nursing care
Significant ancillary services
An outcomes-focused interdisciplinary approach using a professional team
Complex medical and/or rehabilitation care

The International Healthcare Association outlines four categories of subacute care:[13]

1. *Transitional subacute care units* (average length of stay, 5 to 30 days). Patients require 5.5 to 8 hours per day of nursing care. These types of units or facilities serve as a hospital step-down unit and can significantly reduce high-cost acute care hospitalization by substituting less costly care. Patients include those who may need ventilator weaning (Guillain-Barré syndrome), those recovering from stroke or head injury, and those with medically complex conditions. The goal of care is discharge to the home or to less expensive care such as long-term care or an assisted living arrangement.
2. *General subacute care units* (average length of stay, 10 to 40 days). The major difference between the general subacute and transitional unit is patient acuity. Patients need approximately 3.5 hours of nursing care and 1 to 3 hours of rehabilitation therapies daily. Some patients may require intravenous (IV) therapy or dressings. The goal of care is the same as that for transitional subacute care.
3. *Chronic subacute care units* (average length of stay, 60 to 90 days). These units provide care for patients with little hope of recovery or functional independence such as ventilator-dependent patients who have failed attempts at weaning, long-term comatose patients, and those with progressive neurological disease. Patients need approximately 3.5 hours of nursing care and 1 to 3 hours of therapies daily. The goal of care is stabilization so patients can go home or to a long-term care facility or have a peaceful death.
4. *Long-term transitional subacute facilities* (average length of stay, 25 days or more). These facilities are usually licensed as long-term care hospitals rather than as nursing facilities. Typical patients include acute, ventilator-dependent patients, and those with medically complex conditions who require 6.5 to 9 hours of nursing care daily. The goal of care is stabilization of medical conditions with possible discharge to complex home care or continued long-term care.

Skilled Nursing Facilities

Skilled nursing facility units include both free-standing and hospital-based units providing skilled nursing care. Most include rehabilitative services in addition to restorative nursing care. Many have specialty units such as dementia units. Patients may require maximum assistance with activities of daily living (ADLs), bowel and bladder incontinence, and altered level of consciousness from confusion to coma. These needs alone will not qualify a patient for SNF insurance coverage. To be approved for payment, there must be a clear need for skilled licensed professional care on a daily basis for reasons of patient safety and economy. Examples of care provided include:

Daily medication administration of parenteral injections, sliding scale insulin, or IV fluids
Daily wound care requiring aseptic technique
Enteral tube feeding and tube care (e.g., nasogastric [NG] tube, duodenostomy, jejunostomy) with initial teaching and care
Tracheostomy care with initial teaching and care
Frequent monitoring and assessment by licensed personnel to prevent deterioration or complications
Treatment for decubitus ulcer treatment (i.e., grade 3 or lower) and severe skin conditions
Administration of inhalers such as bronchodilator therapy
Early postoperative care and teaching of stomal care, Hickman catheters, and other tubes
PT, OT, or ST
Diabetic teaching for patients who have been newly diagnosed

Hospice Care

Hospice care, which has its roots in Great Britain, began in the United States in the 1970s. The underlying philosophy of hospice care is that terminally ill patients have a right to maintain their final days of life comfortably and with dignity. The setting for hospice care may be the home, where the patient is surrounded by a familiar environment and family and friends, or it may be in a hospice facility maintained in a home-like atmosphere. Hospice care becomes an option when death is imminent and no further medical treatment is available or when further treatment is no longer desired. The patient is kept comfortable with palliative care and does not undergo aggressive or life-prolonging therapy. Hospice care does not hasten or prolong death but allows for a natural death.

Hospice care is available to Medicare recipients if all three of the following criteria are met: (1) a physician certifies that the patient is terminally ill; (2) the patient (or family) chooses to use the hospice benefit; and (3) the hospice agency is Medicare-certified.[14]

A revision to Medicare hospice regulations in 1995 noted that, "A discharge planning evaluation must include an evaluation of a patient's likely need for appropriate post-hospital services, including hospice services and the availability of those services."[15] Medicare payment for hospice services is based on four levels of care. The per diem rate is adjusted depending on the intensity of services. The four levels of intensity include:[15]

Routine home care
Continuous home care (24 hours in a crisis situation)
Inpatient respite care (not to exceed 5 consecutive days at a time)
General inpatient care (e.g., pain control or other symptom management that would otherwise be difficult to control in other settings)

Rehabilitation Units

Rehabilitation units can be either community-based, free-standing units, or hospital-based units that are not considered acute. These include hospital-based PT departments to which patients come from home or other sites to receive a half-hour or 1-hour session of PT, OT, or ST on an outpatient basis.

Home Health Agencies

Home health agencies provide both skilled and unskilled services to patients in their homes. Services may include the use of technology (e.g., ventilator), therapy (PT, OT), and skilled nursing care. A person who has lived independently before an acute episode of illness often prefers to return home, if possible. With the support of family and friends and with a few added services, this is often possible. A comprehensive medical and social assessment is needed to determine the feasibility of home care, stressing the adequacy of patient safety and support in the home. A very important component of this determination is an evaluation of the primary caregiver to be sure that he or she can safely care for the person at home.

Joint Commission for the Accreditation of Healthcare Organizations (JCAHO) guidelines are outlined in the Comprehensive Accreditation Manual for Home Care.[16] Under Medicare, home health visits are available only if all four criteria are met:[14]

1. The patient is homebound.
2. The care required includes intermittent skilled nursing services and possibly PT, OT, or ST.
3. The patient is under the care of a licensed physician who has a formal home health plan that he or she oversees (the plan is reasonable and necessary and is reviewed at least every 60 days).
4. The home health agency is Medicare-certified.

Specialty Pharmacy Providers

Some patients need around-the-clock pharmacologic intervention, particularly through the parenteral route, for an extended period of time. With the availability of specialty pharmacy providers, it is not necessary or cost-effective to keep the patient in a hospital setting for this purpose alone. Twenty-four hour, around-the-clock pharmacy services provide drugs and drug therapy, ongoing monitoring and evaluation of pharmacy needs, and patient education. For example, IV drugs can be premixed and delivered to the patient's home, at which time the patient is assessed for any problems with administration or reaction to therapy. In this model, patients and families are taught to inject their own medications through an IV line as well as to care for the line. Arrangements are made for the next delivery, and the patient may be referred to the physician if there are any medical concerns.

Summary

Acute and subacute care has been briefly reviewed through a discussion of the major categories under these two broad headings. Demographers project large numbers of older people, many with chronic health problems, who will soon be requiring health care. The health care delivery system will continue to be challenged to provide options to meet the needs for cost-effective care while recognizing the concurrent and comparably important requirement for maximal independence and optimal quality of life.

TRANSITIONS IN CARE

A *transition* is a passage from one state, stage, or place to another; that is, it is a change. Passage suggests movement from one place to another, and the movement is along some path or trajectory. In health care, discharge planning and safe transfer to alternative levels of care are necessary to meet patient-centered health care needs. For many neurological patients, recovery from an acute episode does not mean return to preillness or preinjury states of health. Many neurological patients have unstable, complex needs that must be addressed to support optimal health. This may require a transition in level of care and the environment of care.

Whenever transition occurs, the goal is a smooth movement with bridges in place to facilitate the process and continuity of care. Smooth transition is made easier through coordination of care that anticipates potential problems, removes obstacles, addresses unmet needs, and prevents fragmentation. Coordinated care that prevents fragmentation is called continuity of care. Although a transition may represent some recovery, it often involves a move into an unknown environment and culture and can be unsettling to the patient and family. Transitions in care can occur among various facilities and levels of care. All require a coordinated approach to promote continuity.

Depending on the services available in a facility, a neuroscience patient may move from a high-acuity unit, such as an ICU, to a lesser-acuity intermediate unit. The patient and family must be prepared for the transition through education, anticipatory guidance, and counseling. This includes a brief description of the new unit, the patient population, services available, visiting hours, care providers, and the ratio of nurses to patients. The ratio of nurses to patients in intermediate units is much lower than the 1:1 or 1:2 ratio common in ICUs, and patients and families need to be prepared for the decreased nursing intensity. Reassurance is needed that the transfer is a positive sign of recovery and that needed care will continue to be met by health professionals. A visit to the new unit to meet with a staff representative can alleviate anxiety.

If the patient is going to a special unit, such as one dedicated to rehabilitation or transitional care, the nurse should discuss the new unit's philosophy focus of care with the patient and family. In particular, the expected level of patient and family involvement should be addressed. For example, in a comprehensive rehabilitation program, the focus is on functional recovery and self-care to promote independence. Family members should be prepared to assist the patient with care after discharge. These skills must be taught and practiced in a supportive environment. Continuity of care for a transition within a facility or system is usually easier to coordinate because the system is the same, and there are usually procedures for transferring a patient in place. Transitions to other "outside" care environments can be more complex and require more coordination.

PLANNING FOR TRANSITIONS IN HEALTH CARE SETTINGS

The standards of JCAHO require that discharge planning be part of the care provided to patients and that planning must involve the patient and family. Many different areas of the

JCAHO *Manual of Accreditation* address discharge planning as a necessary part of service to the patient and as a responsibility of health care providers.[11] Discharge planning is the vehicle through which the patient's future health care needs are met within the continuum of health care services.

Discharge planning is a logical, coordinated, multilevel process of decision making and other activities involving the patient, the family or significant other, and a team of multidisciplinary health professionals working together to facilitate a smooth, coordinated transition from one environment to another. The transitional environment may be an acute care facility, a chronic care or rehabilitation hospital, a nursing home, or the patient's home. The purpose of discharge planning is to assist the patient to make a smooth transition from one environment or level of care to another without sacrificing the progress that has already been achieved and to provide for other health care needs that are still unmet. Numerous studies have shown that hospitals and patients benefit from a smooth transition out of the hospital. Benefits cited include improved patient outcomes, increased patient and family satisfaction, decreased length of stay, decreased hospital readmission, enhanced cost effectiveness, decreased complications, and decreased mortality. There are many models of discharge planning. In most, the case managers assume major responsibility for facilitating the process.

DISCHARGE PLANNING FOR NEUROSCIENCE PATIENTS

The discharge planning process for neurologically impaired patients increases in complexity if cognitive or behavioral disabilities are present. Patient-centered discharge planning may involve patients with:

- Multitrauma (injury not only to the nervous system, but also to other body systems)

- Head injuries or spinal cord injuries
- Neurological degenerative diseases (e.g., multiple sclerosis, amyotrophic lateral sclerosis)
- Neurological deficits from infectious processes
- Nervous system neoplasms; and others

The specific needs of each patient must be comprehensively assessed and the discharge planning process individualized to provide the appropriate level of care for optimal outcomes. Although discharge planning may be organized differently for neurological patients than for patients with other problems, the steps in discharge planning are the same (Fig. 2-1). The steps, as with any process, are not compartmentalized, that is, simultaneous activities occur in multiple areas. The case manager model assists in coordinating the discharge planning process, especially with shorter hospital stays accelerating all patient-oriented activities.

Assessment

Given that neuroscience patients are often managed by a multidisciplinary team, they undergo various individual specialty-specific assessments. From the admission history and ongoing assessments collected by the nursing staff, a pool of information is available to begin predicting special needs, rehabilitative potential, and expected patient outcomes. When the patient is medically stable, deficits and needs can be validated, and a complete database for discharge planning can be refined.

Certain socioeconomic and health issues render some patients difficult to place in other levels of care and facilities. These patients include the uninsured, the homeless, drug abusers, patients with acquired immune deficiency syndrome (AIDS), and those with dysfunctional families or without families. For example, a patient admitted with a severe traumatic brain injury may also have a concurrent cocaine-abuse problem. Planning should include provisions

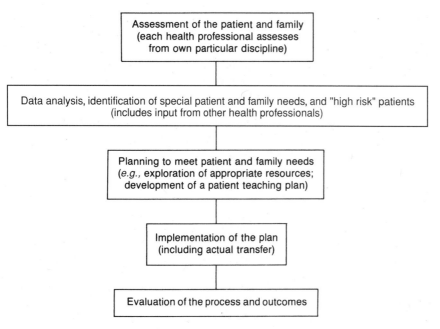

Figure 2–1 • Schematic representation of the steps involved in the discharge planning process.

for special needs, such as drug abuse rehabilitation, as well as for the primary problem and deficits associated with the brain injury. Early identification of high-risk patients and those difficult to place is important so that the multiple issues related to their care can be addressed early and the case manager can be made aware of the complexity of the placement. Before transfer, it may be necessary to submit an application for a Medicare or Medicaid number or undertake some other complicated process. These activities can take time and delay transfer.

Data Analysis and Planning

Health care professionals from each discipline analyze the database to consider the implications for care provided by their discipline. This information is then brought to a multidisciplinary planning conference, and a problem list is generated. A plan of care is then developed based on the problem list.

Based on identification of short-term and long-term outcomes, planning, like the other steps in the discharge process, is ongoing and collaborative. Short-term outcomes are the steps that lead to achievement of long-term outcomes. Flexibility is the key to accommodating those changes likely to occur in the patient's condition. It is impossible to accurately predict the degree of recovery that can occur when the nervous system is injured. At times, the amount of improvement is a pleasant surprise. With other patients, hopes for improvement are not realized. Health care team members need to be prepared to alter the discharge plan based on changes in the patient's condition and a realistic appraisal of potential outcomes.

Collaborative conferences with team members and with the patient and family are absolutely necessary for effective discharge planning. The plan should be documented in writing and updated as necessary. Remember to allow adequate time to complete all pre-transfer activities, including patient and family teaching.

Implementation

Implementation of the discharge plan requires collaboration among many individuals working together to achieve mutual goals. Initially, the case manager, usually a nurse or social worker, contacts a potential transfer facility. Because space in subacute, rehabilitation, and long-term care facilities is limited, often a clinician from the transfer facility will visit the patient to evaluate whether the facility and its programs are suitable for him or her (see previous section on requirements for acute hospital rehabilitation). The clinician assessing the patient must decide whether the patient is:

1. An appropriate candidate for the facility or program and is ready for transfer
2. An appropriate candidate but not ready for transfer so that a re-evaluation is scheduled in a few weeks
3. An inappropriate candidate for transfer to the facility

After acceptance for transfer, it is helpful for the patient, alone or accompanied by the family, to visit the facility to talk with staff members before transfer plans are formalized. After the transfer is formalized, patient information is shared with the receiving nursing staff and other health care providers to promote continuity of care. This may be accomplished through a face-to-face meeting, telephone calls, or written referral forms. A physician from the transferring facility should communicate with the accepting physician to provide the necessary medical management information. For the homebound patient, timely arrangements, well in advance of discharge, should be made for any necessary equipment or community agencies that will be providing services.

The patient and family need emotional and psychological preparation for the transfer. Transfer can be frightening to the patient who has been hospitalized for an extended period. Therefore, much reassurance is needed as the day approaches. Support groups in the community may be helpful to the patient or family. For example, the Brain Injury Association has chapters throughout the country. Information about the purposes of such an organization and contact information should be provided to the patient and family. Printed materials and small group conferences with other patients and families may also be helpful. A discharge handbook or other form of printed material is especially useful because the patient or family member can read it at leisure and then ask questions as necessary.

As caregivers, health care professionals often experience mixed emotions about the discharge of a patient for whom they have cared. Many patients with neurological dysfunction are hospitalized for extended periods of time, with the result that strong bonds are forged between patients and caregivers. Health care professionals should recognize and deal with their feelings.

Evaluation

Evaluation is a critical component in quality assurance. Health care team members should evaluate the discharge planning process to identify any areas that need to be changed or improved. This can be done during team conferences or through periodic reviews. Other foci of evaluation are patient and family satisfaction and benefit from treatment. Information about these topics can be collected at discharge or in a follow-up contact. The quality of the discharge planning system should be monitored through a hospital-wide quality assurance program.

Summary of Discharge Planning

In summary, discharge planning is a complex process of problem solving, ongoing independent and collaborative professional activities, and effective communications directed at helping the patient make a smooth transition from one environment to another without negating any progress toward improved health already made. The new environment may be the home or an acute or subacute level of care that will continue to address unmet care needs. Throughout the discharge planning process, health professionals work with the patient and family to achieve mutually accepted specific goals. Without comprehensive planning, there will be confusion, frustration, discouragement, and fragmentation of effort that will impede achievement of optimal rehabilitation outcomes.

▓ PROVIDING CARE TO PATIENTS AND FAMILIES

Important changes have occurred in how care is provided to patients and their families, and new trends have emerged. Previously mentioned changes in practice connected with managed care include a change from solo practice to group practice, a change from generalist to specialist, and a change to multidisciplinary teams. In *After Reengineering* (1996), Hammer[17] discusses a process-oriented focus for how work is conducted. This approach, which emphasizes teams and collaboration, focuses on outcomes. These changes are apparent in health care settings where multidisciplinary teams provide comprehensive care to patients directed at achieving specific outcomes. The outcomes become the measures of success.

Health care facilities are also being redefined as knowledge-intense organizations staffed by knowledge workers (e.g., nurses, physicians, and other health professionals) who practice primarily in sophisticated interdisciplinary teams. Knowledge work teams differ significantly for other kinds of teams and are composed of multiple specialists.[18–20]

In acute care settings the hospitalist movement has created a team of acute care or critical care specialists who manage patients for a group practice only in the hospital phase of illness.[21,22] Once the patient is ready for hospital discharge, care is provided by other physicians in the group practice. Within hospital settings, intensivists are critical care physicians whose practices are focused in ICUs. With dual certification in critical care and other specialties, these physicians have the expertise to care for critically ill patients with specific systems problems such as neuroscience problems.

The newest frontier for delivery of health care is technology. *Telehealth*, the use of telecommunications equipment and communications networks for transferring health care information between participants at different locations,[23] is beginning to have an impact on how care is provided. *Core Principles on Telehealth* (1998), published by the American Nurses Association, focuses on telehealth as it relates to clinical standards.[24] The publication seeks to identify the appropriate roles and responsibilities for health care professionals in determining standards and guidelines for the practice of telehealth. Along with telemedicine, the use of electronic mail to communicate with patients is emerging.[25] Models have been developed in which patients manage their illness with electronic consultation and support from health professionals. It appears that this methodology will grow rapidly in the next few years, and also that computer-based communications technology in health care will have a phenomenal impact on how care is provided in the next decade. How the technology and standards of practice develop in the next few years remains to be seen.

Collaboration and Collaborative Models of Practice

As traditional practice models in health care delivery give way to more efficient and cost-effective alternatives, the concept of what constitutes effective collaboration among members of a health care team is changing. Collaborative practice is:

> A reciprocal relationship wherein the [providers] assume the greatest responsibilities for patient care within the framework of their respective fields. Although there are areas of overlap, most of the services provided are complementary. A collaborative practice emphasizes joint responsibility in patient care management, with a bilateral process of decision making based on each practitioner's education and ability.[26]

Models of practice can be viewed from the perspective of structure, process, and outcomes. Three models of collaborative practice have been cited:[27]

1. *Hierarchical model:* characterized by unidirectional communications with the physician in the highest position as leader; contact between patient and physician is limited.
2. *Collaborative practice model, type I:* characterized by bidirectional communications among providers; the physician is still the leader; contact between patient and physician is limited.
3. *Collaborative practice model, type II:* patient centered; all providers work both with each other and with the patient; no provider is dominant.

The distinction is also made between multidisciplinary and interdisciplinary teams. A *multidisciplinary team* has *more than one discipline* in its membership. The core multidisciplinary team members may include the nurse, physician, case manager, respiratory therapist, pharmacist, nutritionist, physical therapist, speech therapist, occupational therapist, social worker, and chaplain. Other health care professionals may be included, as needed. In an *interdisciplinary team* there is *collaborative interaction* between members of the different disciplines working together for mutual goals and outcomes. What goes on in the group (process) is the key to differentiating group type. Therefore, not all multidisciplinary teams are interdisciplinary. The collaborative practice model of the 21st century is characterized by interdisciplinary teamwork, the hallmarks of which are effective ongoing communications, cost consciousness, mutual goals, and measurable outcomes.

Collaborative Practice in Neuroscience Patient Care

Many factors influence the manner in which patient-centered care is provided. These include type of patient population, availability of human and material resources, availability of support services, and the focus of care. With a neuroscience population, consciousness and cognition of the patient add special dimensions to the model of practice.

Because of a diminished level of consciousness or altered cognition, it may not be possible to exchange information directly with the patient. A family member may then assume the role of surrogate decision maker for the compromised patient. In this situation, the interdisciplinary team assumes an advocacy role for the patient to ensure that decisions made on the patient's behalf by the family and health team are, to the best of everyone's knowledge, the decisions that the patient would make if he or she were able. Although the communications may be directed toward the family, care is still patient centered.

Many neurological problems affect the personhood, functional level, and independence of the patient. To assist in achieving optimal outcomes, the most successful approach is through patient-centered interdisciplinary collaboration applied across settings and across transitions in illness and care.[28] At one major medical center, an interdisciplinary collaborative model of practice begins in the neuroscience ICU. The cornerstone of this collaboration is interdisciplinary collaborative rounds conducted every morning during which time each patient is reviewed in terms of body systems (e.g., neurological, cardiovascular, respiratory) and patient problems. Goals and clinical targets are set for therapy for the day. The interdisciplinary team includes physicians, nurses, a pharmacist, a nutritionist, and a respiratory therapist.

The attending intensivist, as team leader, guides the review of the patient. The nurse caring for the patient provides a complete assessment based on current data and compares these data with previous data to highlight changes. The acute care nurse practitioner works collaboratively with the physician and care nurse to assess the patient, plan care, and select interventions. The pharmacist makes recommendations on the appropriateness of drug therapy, monitors drug levels, advises on possible drug interactions and side effects, and outlines any special drug administration protocols. The respiratory therapist reports respiratory and ventilatory data, assesses respiratory mechanics, recommends ventilator settings adjustment, and advises on extubation or intubation. The nutritionist calculates target nutritional requirements and monitors albumen, magnesium, and other indicators of nutritional status. Communication is open throughout the patient review, during which time questions are raised and discussed and opinions are shared. After a review of the data, the team enters the patient room and the physician examines the patient. When the examination is completed, the goals for the day are summarized and appropriate orders written. Discharge criteria are set that must be met before the patient can be transferred from the ICU to intermediate care.

After the patient is moved to intermediate care, the structure and processes of the interdisciplinary collaborative model are reformatted to meet the changing acuity needs of the patient. Rounds become briefer and a greater emphasis is placed on rehabilitation and discharge planning. Transition to the community or other levels of care is planned to maintain quality of care, as well as to be cost effective. The hallmarks of interdisciplinary collaborative care are that each patient is valued as a unique individual, care is individualized, and care is patient centered.

MODELS OF NURSING PRACTICE

Neuroscience nursing practice is transforming itself to adjust to the new realities of health care in the 21st century. Neuroscience nurses, regardless of their practice settings, are rethinking their roles and responsibilities to patients, to families, and to their employers. All health care professionals are being asked to integrate health promotion and disease prevention activities such as early identification of risk factors, risk factor modification, and promotion of healthy lifestyles. For neuroscience nurses, who care for patients along the continuum of care from ICUs to home care, managed care environments are forcing more global thinking about how health care is provided and how nursing care is differentiated among the levels of nursing education.

Nurses use models to guide their thinking about patient care and practice. Models also help by placing practice in the context of the overall organizational structure. The theoretical models or conceptual frameworks that guide practice can be broad and describe the philosophy, purposes, and values of a profession such as nursing. Practice models can be narrowly focused to guide thinking and actions regarding specific phenomenon such as intracranial pressure, chronic illness, health promotion, or caregiver stress. Models are often presented as diagrammatic representations of relationships among key components of a phenomenon. Nursing models will continue to be developed and refined through practice-based research.

Quality care provided by competent clinicians is a goal of professional practice. To provide quality care, a supportive environment that includes respect for nursing within the institutional structure and administrative support for nursing must be in place. Hospitals and now long-term facilities that meet high standards of nursing practice can be recognized for their excellence by being designated a *magnet hospital* by the American Nurses Credentialing Center. Three characteristics of nursing practice are found in all magnet facilities: nurse autonomy, nurse control of practice, and collaborative nurse-physician relationships.[29,30] These characteristics contribute to lower nurse turnover rates, greater patient satisfaction, improved patient outcomes, and overall high-caliber patient care. More consumers and payers are becoming aware of the value of a magnet rated facility.

Differentiated nursing practice has been discussed in nursing for many years, and it is gaining renewed attention. The phrase *differentiated nursing practice* describes the sorting of roles, functions, and work of registered nurses according to some identified criteria, commonly education, clinical experience, and competence.[31] Issues related to differentiated nursing practice include optimal nursing care, matching patient needs with nursing competencies, effective use of nursing resources, equitable compensation, career satisfaction, loyalty to employers, and enhanced prestige of the nursing profession.[32] Nurse managers are being challenged to make changes in the organization of work to ensure that high-quality, cost-effective nursing care is provided. Outcomes research on the success and value of differentiated practice is limited, but implementation has occurred in some settings with reported success.[33,34] The complexity of decision making involved in providing care to patients necessitates distinguishing commonalties and differences among nurses prepared at the associate-degree, baccalaureate, master's, and doctoral levels. All levels of academic preparation contribute to the care of neuroscience patients. Determining the best match between patient needs and the knowledge, skills, and abilities of a nurse to provide competent care is challenging.

The American Nurses Association has published scope and standards of practice for both generalists and advanced practice nursing.[35,36] The American Association of Neuroscience Nurses has published a generic description of neuroscience nursing, but it has not differentiated between general and advanced practice nursing. Nurses educated at the graduate level as advanced practice nurses are prepared to implement an advanced model of practice with substantial autonomy and independence.[37] Specialization in practice can be based on advanced practice roles (clinical nurse specialist, nurse practitioner, nurse anesthetist) and on subspecialization in a particular patient population (e.g., neuroscience patients). Practice can be further delineated by a particular neuroscience practice focus such as traumatic brain injury, stroke, or Parkinson's disease. Differentiated nursing practice, within nursing and specifically neuroscience nursing practice, is slowly evolving. The mandate for competency and cost-effective quality care will make this a priority in the next several years. The current nursing shortage and the implications of an aging registered-nurse work force will further challenge models of differentiated practice and how nurses work efficiently with unlicensed personnel.[38]

SUMMARY

This chapter has presented a brief discussion of the realities of practice at the beginning of the 21st century. Change has been rapid and substantive. Caring for neuroscience patients has changed and will continue to be reshaped and redefined. The merit of future changes must be measured by the standard criterion of patient-centered care that meets the health care needs of all populations.

REFERENCES

1. May, C. A., Schraeder, C., & Britt, T. (1996). *Managed care and case management: Roles for professional nursing.* Washington, D.C.: American Nurses Publishing.
2. Iglehart, J. K. (1994). Physicians and the growth of managed care. *New England Journal of Medicine, 331*(17), 1167–1171.
3. Miller, R. H., & Luft, H. S. (1994). Managed care plans: Characteristics, growth, and premium performance. *Annual Review of Public Health, 15,* 437–459
4. Koerner, J., & Burgess, C. S. (1997). Nursing's role and functions in a seamless continuum of care. In S. Moorhead & D. G. Huber (Eds.), *Nursing roles: Evolving or recycled?* (pp. 1–14). Thousand Oaks, CA: Sage Publications.
5. Curtin, L, & Lubkin, I. M. (1995). What is chronicity? In I. M. Lubkin (Ed.), *Chronic illness: Impact and interventions* (3rd ed., pp. 3–25). Boston: Jones and Bartlett Publishers.
6. Corbin, J., & Strauss, A. (1988). *Unending word and care: Managing chronic illness at home.* San Francisco: Jossey-Bass.
7. Donaldson, M., Yordy, K., & Vanselow, E. (1994). *Defining primary care: An interim report.* Washington, DC: National Academy Press.
8. U. S. Preventive Services Task Force. (1996). *Guide to clinical preventive services: Report of the U. S. Preventive Services Task Force* (2nd ed.). Baltimore, MD: Williams & Wilkins.
9. Powell, S. K. (1996). *Case management: A practical guide to a success in managed care* (p. 359). Philadelphia: J. B. Lippincott.
10. Joint Commission on Accreditation of Healthcare Organizations. (1999). *Comprehensive accreditation manual for hospitals.* Oakbrook Terrace, IL: Author.
11. Joint Commission on Accreditation of Healthcare Organizations. (1994). *1995 survey protocol for subacute programs.* Oakbrook Terrace, IL: Author.
12. NSCA. Definition of subacute care. (Online). Available email: *http://www.nsca.net/infi/definition.htm,* Accessed June 27, 1996.
13. Griffin, K. M. (1995). What is subacute care? *AACN News,* April, 6.
14. Health Care Finance Administration. (1994). *The Medicare 1994 handbook* (DHHS Publication No. HCFA 10050). Baltimore, MD: Author.
15. Hamilton, M., & Thomsen, T. (1998). Removing the label. *Continuing Care, 17*(9), 167–168.
16. Joint Commission on Accreditation of Healthcare Organizations. (1996). *Comprehensive accreditation manual for home care.* Oakbrook Terrace, IL: Author.
17. Hammer, M. (1996). *Beyond reengineering.* New York: HarperBusiness.
18. Sorrells-Jones, J., & Weaver, D. (1999). Knowledge workers and knowledge-intense organizations, Part 1: A promising framework for nursing and healthcare. *Journal of Nursing Administration, 29*(7/8), 12–18.
19. Weaver, D., & Sorrells-Jones, J. (1999). Knowledge workers and knowledge-intense organizations, Part 2: Designing and managing for productivity. *JONA, 29*(9), 19–25.
20. Sorrells-Jones, J., & Weaver, D. (1999). Knowledge workers and knowledge-intense organizations, Part 3: Implications for preparing healthcare professionals. *JONA, 29*(10), 14–21.
21. Wachter, R., & Goldman, I. (1996). The emerging role of "hospitalists" in the American health care system. *New England Journal of Medicine, 335*(17), 514–517.
22. Kelley, M. A. (1999). The hospitalist: A new medical specialty. *Annuals of Internal Medicine, 130*(4, Part 2), 373–375.
23. Chaffee, M. (1999). A telehealth odyssey. *American Journal of Nursing, 99*(7), 27–32.
24. American Nurses Association. (1998). *Core principles on telehealth.* Washington, DC: Author.
25. Kane, B., & Sands, D. Z. (1998). Guidelines for the clinical use of electronic mail with patients. *JAMIA, 5,* 104–111.
26. Shortridge, L. M., McLain, B. R., & Gilliss, C. L. (1986). Graduate education for family primary care. In M. D. Mezey & D. O. McGivern (Eds.), *Nurses, nurse practitioners: The evolution of primary care* (pp. 120–134). Boston: Little, Brown.
27. Siegler, E. L., & Whitney, F. W. (Eds.). (1994). *Nurse-physician collaboration: Care of adults and the elderly.* New York: Springer.
28. Counsell, C. M., Guin, P. R., & Limbaugh, B. (1994). Coordinated care for the neuroscience patient: Future directions. *Journal of Neuroscience Nursing, 26*(4), 245–250.
29. Aiken, L. H., Havens, D. S., & Sloane, D. M. (2000). The magnet nursing services recognition program. *American Journal of Nursing, 100*(3), 26–35.
30. Havens, D. S., & Aiken, L. H. (1999). Shaping systems to promote desired outcomes. The magnet hospital model. *Journal of Nursing Administration, 29*(2), 14–20.
31. Boston, C. (Ed.). (1990). *Current issues and perspectives on differentiated practice.* Chicago: American Organization of Nurse Executives.
32. Baker, C. M., Lamm, G. M., Winter, A. R., Robbeloth, V. B., Ransom, C. A., Conly, F., Carpenter, K. C., & McCoy, L. E. (1997). Differentiated nursing practice: Assessing the state-of-the-science. *Nursing Economics, 15* (5), 253–262.

33. Koerner, J. G., & Karpiuk, K. L., (Eds.). (1994). *Implementing differentiated nursing practice: Transformation by design*. Gaithersburg, MD: Aspen.
34. Milton, D., Verran, J., Gerber, R., & Gerber, R. (1992). Differentiated group professional practice in nursing: A demonstration model. *Nursing Clinics of North America, 27*(1), 23–30.
35. American Nurses Association. (1991). *Standards of clinical nursing practice*. Washington, D. C.: American Nurses Publishing.
36. American Nurses Association. (1997). *Scope and standards of advanced practice registered nursing*. Washington, D. C.: American Nurses Publishing.
37. Mitchell, P. H. (1997). Advanced practice and neuroscience nursing. *AACN Clinical Issues, 8*(2), 227–234.
38. Buerhaus, P. I., Staiger, D. O., & Auerbach, D. I. (2000). Implications of an aging registered nurse workforce. *Journal of the American Medical Association, 283*, 2048–2054.

RESOURCES

Professional

Published Material

See References.

Websites

These are but a few helpful websites:
HCFA: Medicare and Medicaid (http://www.hcfa.gov/)

JCAHO Survey Reports Archive:
   (http://sss.nnlm.nih.gov/nnlm/jcahorep/)
Joint Commission Slide Show:
   (http://rampages.onramp.net/~meyerco/jacho.htm)
Long Term Care Minimum Data Set 2.0:
   (http://www.hcfa.gov/medicare/hsqb/mds20/)
Medicaid Information:
   (http://www.hcfa.gov/medicaid/medicaid.htm)
Medicare Information:
   (http://www.hcfa.gov/medicare/medicare.htm)
Medicare Professional/Technical Information:
   (http://www.hcfa.gov/medicare/mcarpti.htm)
Medicare/Medicaid Program Manuals:
   (http://www.hcfa.gov/pubforms/program.htm)
National Subacute Care Association: (http://www.nsca.net/)
ASCA Subacute Care Today:
   (http://www.nsca.net/products/caretoday.htm)
Subacute Unit: (http://www.vmpcares.com/subacu.htm)

Patient and Family

Websites

Medicaid Consumer Information:
   (http://www.hcfa.gov/medicare/mcaicnsm.htm)
Medicare Consumer Information:
   (http://www.hcfa.gov/medicare/mcarpubs.htm)

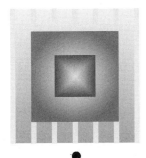

Clinical Reasoning and Outcomes

JOANNE V. HICKEY

The health care system and its practices are rapidly changing. The intellectual demands required to practice nursing in a fast-paced technocratic society are challenging. Nurses are often surrounded by complex technologies that are invariably controlled by computers and connected to exquisite databases. Technologies are constantly being upgraded through software and hardware enhancements. Patient assessment and treatment often involves interfacing with a computer. Sophisticated physiologic monitoring systems provide an integration of waveforms and digital values for various cardiopulmonary and cerebrovascular variables. Decision-making software identifies deviations from set parameters and offers diagnostic and treatment suggestions.

Models of health care delivery are also changing how nurses practice. For example, through telemedicine a patient and health care providers are able to interact although miles physically separate them. More and more technology is found in the home and subacute settings. The nurse receives data from myriad sources to interpret, validate, and process. This complex process requires broad-based scientific knowledge, versatile communication skills in various media, and well-developed critical thinking skills for clinical reasoning. Nurses are among the "information workers" in health care.

Another change in models of practice is that more and more portions of care are being delivered by multidisciplinary teams. Working together as an interdisciplinary team requires collaboration with a focus on patient outcomes that are achievable through collaborative efforts of all disciplines involved. Although each discipline brings discipline-specific expertise and skills to the patient, optimal outcomes are achievable through the work of all health professionals rather than only one. Thus, *multidisciplinary outcomes* encompass the work to be achieved by the entire team working with the patient.

Each of the health professions brings a distinct paradigm to practice. A unique characteristic of the nursing paradigm is a holistic approach to the care to patients and families. This is evident in how nurses think about the care process and how they provide care. This care process is referred to as the nursing process.

NURSING PROCESS

The nursing process, first proposed by Yura and Walsh in the 1970s,[1] provides a unidimensional cognitive model of thinking that includes the five steps of assessment, analysis, planning, implementation, and evaluation. Nursing process is a systematic method of decision making modeled after the scientific method of problem solving. The goal of the nursing process is to identify patient problems using nursing diagnosis and prescribe appropriate nursing interventions.

Development and refinement of the North American Nursing Diagnosis Association taxonomy of nursing diagnoses have been in progress for several years. A nursing diagnosis is defined as "a clinical judgment about an individual, family, or community response to actual or potential health problems/life processes which provide the basis for definitive therapy toward achievement of outcomes for which the nurse is accountable."[2] Most health care professions have specific diagnostic categories that are determined by the given discipline. This is true, to a degree, in nursing. Discipline-specific diagnostic categories influence diagnoses and treatment.[3]

The nursing process concept has been embraced in nursing education and nursing practice as the common denominator and standard for conceptualizing nursing practice and patient care. It has found its way into most nursing textbooks as well as the test construction blueprint for state board licensure examinations. Not all have embraced the nursing process, however. Its adequacy to guide nursing practice, at all levels, has been challenged. Although nursing process has provided a context for nursing practice, it is narrow and restrictive and does not capture the essence or complexity of professional practice in the 21st century. Further, it does not incorporate all the cognitive and intuitive processes that Benner described in *From Novice to Expert*.[4] That classic text describes how nurses think about patients and patient care. Perhaps a broader framework to consider the cognitive processes associated with nursing practice is critical thinking. Jones and Brown[5] state that the nursing process and problem solving are subsumed under critical thinking.

CRITICAL THINKING AND NURSING PRACTICE

The need for nurses with well-developed critical thinking skills has never been more apparent than in the current health care system. Patients are living longer, but with more comorbidity and chronic health problems that have a significant impact on the complexity of care. Cost-containment initiatives and managed care have resulted in shortened hospital stays with patients who are going to subacute care or home care sicker and with more complex needs. More and more care is being provided in the community and home. To move patients through the various levels of care expeditiously and efficiently, nurses are assuming more responsibility and accountability for patient outcomes within compressed time frames. Care is often complex and requires the collaborative effort of a coordinated multidisciplinary team for transitions in illness and care.

Critical thinking skills of nurses drive nursing practice and directly influence the achievement of optimal outcomes for patients. The foundation of professional nursing practice is critical thinking. It involves a philosophical perspective about thinking and cognitive processes characterized by reasoned judgment and reflective thinking. Nurses can be taught the principles of critical thinking beginning in basic nursing programs and on through graduate and continuing education programs. However, these skills are honed in clinical practice in which the nurse must have the intellectual openness and curiosity to question the status quo and accepted explanations and display the courage to explore new possibilities and explanations rigorously. The need for evidence-based practice and "best practice" are important dimensions driving practice of all health providers.

DEFINING CRITICAL THINKING AND RELATED CONCEPTS

Critical thinking is a broad concept that can be applied to all aspects of life. The terms *critical thinking, clinical reasoning,* and *diagnostic reasoning* are sometimes used interchangeably in the literature but need to be distinguished from one another. Much discussion has been directed at defining the elusive concept of critical thinking, and definitions currently exist. However, there are key conceptual elements to critical thinking. Jones and Brown[6] state that critical thinking is not a single way of thinking but a multidimensional cognitive process that demands the skillful application of knowledge and experience in making judgments and evaluations. Critical thinking involves a healthy, reflective skepticism in which complex meanings are analyzed, solutions critiqued, alternatives explored, and contingency-related value judgments made.[5] The critical thinker does not accept conclusions but rather analyzes and evaluates reasons and evidence. Assumptions are made explicit, and unwarranted and irrelevant inferences are rejected. Apparent contradictions are reconciled.[6] The best and most encompassing evidence is cited. Conclusions are the result of reasoned evaluative judgment.[7]

As an example of definitions, the National Council for Excellence in Critical Thinking Instruction defines critical thinking comprehensively as "the intellectually disciplined process of actively and skillfully conceptualizing, applying, analyzing, synthesizing and evaluating information gathered from or generated by observation, experience, reflection, reasoning, or communication as a guide to belief and action" (1992, p. 2).[8] Woods[9] notes that in this definition, the Council suggests two components to critical thinking: (1) a set of information and beliefs *and generating and processing skills and abilities;* and (2) application of those skills and abilities to guide behavior.

Critical thinking is an active process directed toward guiding behavior in every aspect of one's personal and professional life. In nursing, critical thinking is the crux that guides professional practice and patient care. The definition cited also recognizes the importance of the nurse's observation, experience, and reflection to provide context and meaning to information, and reasoning to analyze and synthesize information to make judgments and reach conclusions.

Clinical reasoning encompasses all the thinking and reasoning about patient care, management questions, and treatment decisions one considers in providing care in clinical practice. It is a special type of critical thinking and has been pioneered in medical education. Kassirer and Kopleman[10] define clinical reasoning as the essential function of the physician in which optimal patient care depends on keen diagnostic acumen and thoughtful analysis of the trade-off between the benefits and risks of tests and treatments. They point out that optimal patient outcomes cannot be achieved if reasoning skills are deficient. The outcomes of clinical reasoning are the clinical decisions of diagnosis and treatment that should lead to problem resolution.[11] This is true for nursing and for medicine. For an excellent discussion of clinical reasoning in advanced practice nursing the reader is directed to the chapter entitled "Clinical Reasoning" by Szaflarski.[11] Szaflarski is an advanced practice nurse who has made an important contribution to nursing with her outstanding work in clinical reasoning.

Diagnostic reasoning, a subheading of clinical reasoning, refers to the reasoning that is used to reach a diagnosis. It is a dynamic thinking process that is hypothesis-driven and targeted toward the selection of a hypothesis that best explains clinical evidence.[11] It is the initial stage in the clinical decision-making process and results in the diagnosis of a clinical state, disorder, syndrome, or disease.[11] In medicine, the process of generating and evaluating different diagnostic hypotheses follows five steps: generation of diagnostic hypotheses, refinement of hypotheses, diagnostic testing, causal reasoning, and diagnostic verification.[10,12] Gifford, Mittman, and Vickrey[13] discuss diagnostic reasoning in neurology. Advanced practice nurses such as nurse practitioners follow diagnostic reasoning models in their roles of diagnosing patient problems. In both nursing and medicine, the process of diagnostic reasoning is poorly understood.

After a diagnosis has been established, the next step is **treatment reasoning**. Treatment reasoning begins with the establishment of treatment goals (prevention, curative, supportive), which are based on an assessment of health-related values, perceptions of quality of life, and patient and family preferences early in the initial patient contact. Treatment includes nursing, medical, and surgical interventions (e.g., prevention of falls, drug therapy, skin care, patient education, counseling, physical therapy, exercise prescriptions, speech therapy, procedure, complementary therapies). In considering treatment options a number of factors are considered (e.g., benefit:risk ratio, benefit:cost ratio, potential treatment interactions). In addition, patient preference must be considered. After a treatment has been selected and initiated, treatment monitoring and evaluation regarding modification of current treatment, continuation of current treatment, or inception of additional treatment are needed. Finally, the practitioner must determine whether the problem is resolved and treatment can thereby be discontinued.[11,14–16] Both nurses and physicians engage in these steps as they consider treatment for various patient problems.

From this brief discussion, it is apparent that the clinical reasoning process is the fundamental foundation for diagnosis and treatment decisions related to patient care. Regardless of the discipline, all health care professionals engage in the complex process of clinical reasoning in each patient encounter. Developing and honing these skills are lifelong, challenging processes. In making treatment decisions, knowledge of current evidence-based practice and best practice serve as treatment options to be considered.

EVIDENCE-BASED PRACTICE, BEST PRACTICE, AND OUTCOMES

How patients are treated is becoming increasingly based on the results of peer-reviewed scientific research. Large prospective randomized controlled trials (RTC)s have been the pinnacle in the hierarchy of scientific research. With the advent of powerful computer technology, the means for using complex multivariate statistical analysis techniques for large databases is readily available to most researchers. The easy manipulation of large databases has led to the development of multiple methodologies other than the RTCs for conducting research. Large prospective controlled clinical trials can demonstrate that certain treatments are related to lower morbidity and mortality (e.g., positive outcomes) in a specific population. Metaanalysis, clinical practice improvement,[17] and other comparable methodologies are being increasingly used in clinical studies. The resulting scientific clinical evidence provides the basis for recommending certain treatments for a given population.[15]

The basis of evidence-based practice is found in evidence based medicine. **Evidence-based medicine (EBM)** is "the practice of making medical decision through the judicious identification, evaluation, and application of the most relevant information."[18] **Evidence-based practice (EBP)** is an approach to practice based on knowledge of the evidence on which practice is based, and the strength of that evidence. It is the explicit integration of clinical research evidence with pathophysiologic reasoning, provider experience, and patient preference in providing care.[19] To determine the scientific evidence for practice, a clinician must be able to frame the clinical question, access medical and health care-related information, and assess the validity of that information. Framing the clinical question refers to narrowing the focus of the problem and patient population. Accessing medical and health care-related information is a challenging

proposition in that it requires computer searching of databases and the Internet and keeping up with the literature in your field of practice. After you have identified and collected information, the next step is to determine the validity of clinical research studies, findings from meta-analyses, practice guidelines, algorithms, and cost-effectiveness analyses.[18] This requires knowledge methods for critique of research studies for scientific rigor, evaluation of the credibility of the organizations' publishing guidelines, and appropriateness of the information for the patient problem under consideration.

Although it is encouraging to think that practice is based on science, only about 15% of what we do in practice is. Yet, nurses and other health providers care for patients every day. What is provided on a daily basis is **best practice**, that is, a combination of evidence-based practice, clinician judgment, and patient preference.[20] The goal of EBP and best practice is to improve the underpinnings for clinical reasoning to achieving optimal outcomes for patients.

The effectiveness of the health care delivery system is determined by examining outcomes. From a patient-care perspective, **outcomes** are the consequences or clinical endpoints of care such as a physiological target (e.g., ICP less than 20 mm Hg or serum osmolality of 290), a score on a measurement such as the Barthel scale, or patient satisfaction. An important characteristic of outcomes is that they must be measurable. Otherwise, it would be unclear whether an outcome was achieved. Outcomes are the result of structure and process variables.[21] **Structure** is defined as the system and providers' characteristics within which health care is provided. For example, specific system characteristics in which care is provided may be a health maintenance organization clinic or an intensive care unit. The provider of care may be a multidisciplinary team or by a nurse practitioner. The **processes** of care refer to the technical and interpersonal activities involved in providing care, such as diagnostics, drugs, and communication skills. The demand that health care be cost effective, as well as clinically effective, has had a profound impact on the accountability for use of resources and practice patterns of clinicians. Measuring outcomes of providers and cost of care by the payee is now an integral part of the health care. A focus on outcomes and outcome management will continue to be important determinants of quality of care, effectiveness of care, cost of care, and decisions related to use of health care resources.

In summary, the linkage between clinical reasoning and outcomes is clear. Clinical reasoning must be conducted with clear outcomes in mind. Management of outcomes through use of EBP and best practice contributes to achieving optimal patient outcomes. Outcomes that examine the cost:benefit ratio of care as well as the satisfaction of patients with care completes the picture.

APPLICATION TO NEUROSCIENCE NURSING PRACTICE

What does this all mean for neuroscience nurses? The ramifications of neurological disease and illness have far-reaching implications for the patient, family, and health team.

Neuroscience nurses are integral members of the team and work independently and collaboratively to achieve optimal multidisciplinary outcomes for the patient. Neuroscience nurses cannot be limited by narrow models for processing information and drawing conclusions. Clinical reasoning skills provide the tools to sustain the lifetime practice of nurses in an ever-changing practice environment. Thus, clinical reasoning skills need to be promoted and valued.

REFERENCES

1. Yura, A., & Walsh, M. (1978). *The nursing process: Assessing, planning, implementing, and evaluating* (3rd ed.). New York: Appleton-Century-Crofts.
2. Carpenito, L. (1991). The NANDA definition of nursing diagnosis. In Carroll-Johnson, R. M. (Ed.), *Classification of nursing diagnoses: Proceedings of the ninth conference.* Philadelphia: J. B. Lippincott, pp. 65–71.
3. Carnevali, D. L., & Thomas, M. D. (1993). *Diagnostic reasoning and treatment decision making in nursing.* Philadelphia: J. B. Lippincott.
4. Benner, P. (1985). *From novice to expert: Excellence and power in clinical nursing practice.* Menlo Park, CA: Addison-Wesley.
5. Jones, S. A., & Brown, L. N. (1991). Critical thinking: Impact on nursing education. *Journal of Advanced Nursing, 16,* 529–533.
6. Jones, S. A., & Brown, L. N. (1993). Alternative views on defining critical thinking through the nursing process. *Holistic Nursing Practice, 7*(3), 71–76.
7. Paul, R. (1990). *Critical thinking: What every person needs to survive in a rapidly changing world.* Rohnert Park, CA: Center for Critical Thinking and Moral Critique.
8. National Council for Excellence in Critical Thinking Instruction. (1992)., p. 2. Chicago: Author.
9. Woods, J. H. (1993). Affective learning: One door to critical thinking. *Holistic Nursing Practice, 7*(3), 64–70.
10. Kassirer, J. P., & Kopleman, R. I. (1991). *Learning clinical reasoning.* Baltimore, MD: Williams & Wilkins, pp. 1–46.
11. Szarflarski, N. L. (2000). Clinical reasoning. In J. V. Hickey, R. M. Ouimette, & S. L. Venegoni, (Eds.), *Advanced practice nursing: Changing roles and clinical applications* (p. 111). Philadelphia: Lippincott Williams & Wilkins.
12. Kassirer, J. P. (1989). Diagnostic reasoning. *Annals of Internal Medicine 110,* 893–900.
13. Gifford, D. R., Mittman, B. S., & Vickrey, B. G. (1996). Diagnostic reasoning in neurology. *Neurologic Clinics, 14*(1), 223–238.
14. Barrow, H. S. (1991). Therapeutic decision making. In H. S. Barrows (Ed.), *Developing clinical problem-solving skills* (pp. 162–176). New York: W. W. Norton.
15. Forrow, C., Wartman, S. A., & Brock, D. W. (1988). Science, ethics, and the making of clinical decisions. *Journal of the American Medical Association 259*(21), 3161–3167.
16. Burgus, G. R., & Hamm, R. M. (1995). Clinical practice: How physicians make medical decisions and why medical decision making can help. *Medical Decision Making 22,* 167–180.
17. Horn, S. D. (1999). Provision of outcomes data. *New Horizons: The Science and Practice of Acute Medicine, 7*(5), 198–204.
18. Friedland, D. J. (1998). Introduction. In D. J. Friedland, A. S. Go, M. G. Shlipak, S. W. Bent, S. W. Bent, , L. L. Subak, & T. Mendelson *Evidence-based medicine: A framework for clinical practice,* (pp. 1–8). Stamford, CN: Appleton & Lange.
19. Cook, D. J., & Levy, M. M. (1998). Evidence-based medicine. *Critical Care Clinics 14*(3), 353–358.
20. Byers, J. F., & Brunell, M. L. (1998). Demonstrating the value of the advanced practice nurse: An evaluation model. *AACN Clinical Issues 9*(2), 296–305.
21. Donadedian, A. (1980). The definition of quality and approaches to its assessment, (Vol. 1.). Explorations in quality assessment and monitoring: Ann Arbor, MI: Health Administration Press.

RESOURCES

Professional

Published Material

Sackett, D. L., Straus, S. E., Richardson, W. S., Rosenberg, W., & Haynes, R. B. (2000). *Evidence-based medicine: How to practice and teach EBM.* Edinburgh: Churchill Livingstone.

Websites

Centre for Evidence-Based Medicine: The center was established in Oxford, England as the first of several centers around that country the aim of which is to promote evidence-based health care and provide support and resources. http://cebm.jr2.ox.ac.uk/.

McMaster University EBM Site: McMaster University in Canada sponsors this website that contains a large inventory of evidence-based resources, an online database, user guides, and bibliographies. http://hiru.hirunet.mcmaster.ca/ebm/.

The Cochrane Library: The Cochrane Library is designed to supply high-quality evidence to inform people providing and receiving care, and those responsible for research, teaching, funding and administration at all levels. http://www.cochrane.de/cc/cochrane/cdsr.htm.

Journal of Evidence-Based Medicine: Published bimonthly, it surveys a wide range of international medical journals (at least 70) to identify the key research papers that are scientifically valid and relevant to practice. http://www.bmjpg.com/data/ebm.htm.

Resources for Practicing EBM: A comprehensive and concise bibliography of EBM resources on the web. http://intensivecare.com/EBM.html.

Evidence-Based Nursing: A new high-quality international journal that provides access to the best research related to nursing with the *most* important new evidence within nursing. http://www.bm.jpg.com/data/ebn.htm.

Core Library for Evidence-Based Practice: Assembled by links to full text documents on how to learn about evidence-based practice. http://www.shef.ac.uk/~scharr/ir/core.html.

Centre for Evidence-Based Nursing: As part of the national network of Centres for Evidence-Based Clinical Practice, the University of York in northern England has established a Centre for Evidence-Based Nursing. http://omni.ac.uk/submit-url/archive/0169.html.

The Alberta Clinical Practice Guidelines Program: Supports appropriate, effective, and high-quality medical care in Alberta in western Canada through promotion, development, and implementation of evidence-based clinical practice guidelines. http://www.amda.ab.ca/general/clinical-practice-guidelines/index.html.

Netting the Evidence: A Scharr Introduction to Evidence Based Practice on the Internet: A comprehensive website containing links to other EBM sites, journals, clinical practice guidelines, systematic reviews, and appraisal guides. http://www.shefac.uk/uni/academic/R-Z/scharr/ir/netting.html.

Agency for Healthcare Policy and Research EBM: The AHCPR sponsors many EBM practice centers and has published many clinical practice guidelines on major health problems. The agency has been renamed Agency for Healthcare Research and Quality as of December 6, 1999. http://www.ahcpr.gov.

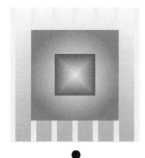

C H A P T E R **4**

Ethical Perspectives and End-of-Life Care

JOANNE V. HICKEY

The ethical dimensions of conduct in professional practice are especially compelling and complex in many situations faced by the neuroscience nurse. The primary focus of this chapter is clinical ethics in neuroscience nursing practice. **Clinical ethics** is primarily concerned with the ethics of clinical practice and the ethical problems that arise in the care of patients. Judicial decisions that have influenced standards of practice are also included. The three main areas discussed in this chapter are (1) the basis for ethical and legal dimensions of practice, (2) a framework for ethical decision making, and (3) selected ethical issues common in neuroscience nursing practice, including end-of-life (EOL) care.

AN ETHICAL PERSPECTIVE OF NEUROSCIENCE PRACTICE

Unique ethical challenges are presented to neuroscience nurses by patients with neurological illnesses and impairments. These patients cross the lifespan, and frequently they experience damage to their personhood that compares with no other illness. Neuroscience nurses must be prepared to care for the young victim of trauma who is left with irreversible paralysis or in a persistent vegetative state, for the middle-aged adult who is newly diagnosed with a progressive neurological disease, and for the elderly person with dementia caused by multi-infarct small strokes. Recovery often does not mean a return to the pretrauma or preillness functional level. These patients may experience complete personality changes or, in other tragic cases, lose the ability to comprehend or communicate information. Although the specific issues involving ethical questions such as determining patient capacity in decision making or decisions about withholding or withdrawing treatments are similar in theory to those identified with many other patients who are seriously ill, the *context* and *circumstances* surrounding neurologically compromised patients are unique.

Use of the term *ethical and legal* is avoided in this chapter to diminish confusion and to avoid the suggestion that ethics and legality are more synonymous than distinctly different. An **ethical perspective** addresses the *moral duties and obligations* to provide optimal care for patients and families. A **legal perspective** speaks to the *minimal standards of care set forth in the judicial system* to which health care providers must adhere. Simply relying on legal precedents does not necessarily imply that ethically grounded care is being provided. However, many issues, including decisions about withholding or withdrawing treatment or surrogate decision making, require addressing both the ethical dimensions and legal precedents for a comprehensive understanding of the complexity of clinical situations. The Quinlan and Cruzan cases are such examples.

A generally recognized phenomenon in health care is the unprecedented development and rapid implementation of new technologies. The appropriate use of technology and its impact on human life are usually secondary, de facto considerations; the lag time between implementation of a new technology and recognition of its broader impact is often the foundation for the associated ethical dilemmas. In addition, sociocultural and economic factors including priorities for allocation of limited health care resources, consensus about self-determination, the cost-effective mandate, and the predominance of managed care environments impact on delivery of care.[1] The dynamics involved in this adjustment process are often addressed in the judicial system—the wrong institution to resolve ethical issues. As a result, there has been an uncomfortable uncertainty about the legalities surrounding many ethical issues, leaving the practitioner to sort them out at the bedside.

The lack of clarity about how to proceed in ethical dilemmas and how to interpret personal wishes and laws has created further problems within the health care system. Before the advent of technology in medical practice, the failure of one or more body system usually limited life well before cognitive capacity was affected. Now, technology is available to keep patients "alive" indefinitely. This includes patients in a persistent vegetative state, in which the "organ of reason" is rendered permanently nonfunctional and unable to make informed consent decisions. This care is very costly and uses a disproportionate amount of limited resources without any potential for positive outcomes for the patient. How does one reconcile the concepts of fair distribution of scarce resources, cost:benefit ratio, and quality of life in these clinical situations?

ETHICS, MORALITY, AND LEGALITY

Ethics

According to the dictionary, *ethics* is defined as the "discipline dealing with moral duty and obligation, a set of moral principles or values, and the principles of conduct governing an individual or a group." Ethics has also been defined as the inquiry into the nature of morality or moral acts and the search for the morally good life.[2] Ethics dates back to the beginning of civilization, when mores and laws were developed to allow different groups of people to live together. Most ethical principles represent cultural and religious values of groups of people and, therefore, differ from culture to culture and from religion to religion. Even within cultures, some subcultures differ significantly in some aspects of their ethics and, therefore, in their standards of behavior.

When the concept of ethics is applied to professional practice, there are basic principles that govern how health care professionals practice within a culture. These principles are usually stated within a code, such as the *Code for Nurses*,[3] which explains to the public the guidelines that will govern how the professional nurse will practice.

Morality

Within the definition of ethics is the word *morality*. **Morality** is defined as "having to do with human activities that are looked upon as good/bad or right/wrong; conforming to the accepted rules of what is considered right (virtuous, just, proper conduct); having the capacity to be directed by an awareness of right and wrong; and pertaining to the manner in which one behaves in relationships with others."[4] Morality comprises also the making of judgments about what is right in given circumstances and the guidance of one's conduct by reason.[5] It suggests doing what seems right while giving equal weight to the interests of each individual who will be affected by one's conduct. Four moral principles that are of particular importance in nursing practice are autonomy, beneficence, justice, and fidelity.

Autonomy is the act of self-governing, self-determining, or self-directing; it involves independence from the will of others, as well as the right to make and follow one's decisions.

The principle of autonomy affirms the nurse's duty to respect the decisions of the patient and the family and to assume the role of a patient/family advocate when necessary.

Beneficence is the charge to do good; it implies the principle of **nonmaleficence,** which is the duty to prevent or avoid doing harm. Many believe that upholding the principle of nonmaleficence is more binding than the duty to do good. For example, although the nurse cannot change the medical diagnosis or injuries incurred, secondary injuries and pain can be controlled.

Justice is defined as fairness, correctness, and impartiality in the application of principles of rightness and of sound judgment. The nurse must treat patients fairly based on their needs and the situation. It suggests an obligation for nurses to distribute their time, expertise, and resources as fairly as possible among patients assigned to their care.[6]

Fidelity is the obligation to be truthful and to keep promises. This principle supports the practice of obtaining informed consent and being honest and genuine in interactions with the patient and family.

Principles are guidelines and, as such, are not absolute in their application to situations. This is also true of moral and ethical principles. It is not uncommon to have more than one principle applicable to a situation simultaneously. Someone must determine which principle takes precedence in the given situation and why. These dilemmas are what make ethical decision making so difficult at times.

Legality

Legality refers to lawfulness or the obligations imposed by law to bind certain behaviors within a society. The professional nurse, licensed to practice in a particular state, is bound by the laws within that state. Each state has its own Nurse Practice Act that defines professional nursing practice within that state. In addition, there are other laws and legal decisions related to health care issues that set a precedent for practice within that state and, often, nationally. An example of a precedent-setting decision is the Karen Quinlan case.[7] In this well-known case, a young woman suffered unexplained apnea and did not receive immediate ventilatory support. She was subsequently placed on a ventilator and remained in a persistent vegetative state. The family petitioned the court to allow the ventilator to be removed so that she could die. Permission was granted. Unexpectedly, she began to breathe spontaneously, and she lived in a persistent vegetative state (PVS) for several years. This case established the precedent that a ventilator could be removed even when the consequence might be death.

Laws and legal precedents related to health care matters may originate at the state or federal levels. The judicial system is divided into municipal, state, and federal courts. The right to appeal to a higher court is provided as a safeguard to protect individual and group rights. Some cases related to health care have reached the U.S. Supreme Court. Laws reflect the values and beliefs of society and thus are subject to review and to change. Although a law is legal, it may not seem moral to some individuals or groups. In a rapidly changing society such as that of the United States, challenges to current laws are common. With respect to health care issues, the changing and competing values and beliefs of a heterogeneous society, along with the unprecedented development of technology, account for the number of health-related issues referred to the courts.

FRAMEWORK FOR ETHICAL DECISION MAKING

Decision Making in General

Decision making includes distinct, logically organized steps that require choosing alternative courses of action. These steps include collecting relevant data, analyzing data, proposing alternative solutions, identifying the pros and cons of each alternative, and selecting the best alternative based on established criteria.

Framework for Ethical Decision Making

Ethical decision making is a dynamic process requiring reflection, discussion, and evaluation of outcomes. Like decision making in general, it should follow the same basic steps. Ethical decisions, as related to health care issues, can be unique in that they involve obligations, responsibilities, duties, rights, and values affecting life-and-death situations. The highly emotional nature of these issues often makes it difficult to separate feelings from facts. It is, therefore, of critical importance for decision makers to separate personal attitudes, beliefs, and feelings from the factual data that are relevant to the particular situation. Without this separation, objectivity is lost.

Many ethical decisions require the input of members of a variety of disciplines and of people to provide a broad, comprehensive perspective of the issues at hand. Members of the interdisciplinary collaborative team must be knowledgeable about the fundamental principles of ethical decision making to guide their analysis of complex decisions. The unique input of each of the team members will reflect their collaborative roles.

Collecting Relevant Data

Data collected should include medical information and patient preferences for treatment. Determination of an accurate diagnosis and prognosis, made by the physician, is critical to the database. In cases of coma, a diagnosis detailing the type of brain damage and the likelihood of recovery is important in planning care. The most important information about treatment preference comes from the patient if he or she is an adult and is mentally capable of making decisions. Consulting the patient in this regard recognizes the patient's right to autonomy and to define quality of life for himself or herself. If the patient is incapable as a result of coma, cognitive deficits, or other causes, then information regarding treatment preferences may be found in a living will or the expression of wishes made to the family or significant other while he or she was well. A surrogate decision maker may be necessary to represent the patient's wishes. The family's preference for treatment is also explored and established. Other data collected include information on state laws, hospital policies, and professional codes related to the particular situation. In some situations, it may be necessary to seek advice from the institutional ethics committee or hospital attorney.

Analyzing Data

After all relevant data have been collected, they are then analyzed. One can apply the question, "What are the duties, rights, and responsibilities of all persons involved?" The moral principles of autonomy, beneficence, justice, and fidelity must be a part of this determination.

Proposing Alternative Solutions

Considering the diagnosis, evidence-based practice, prognosis, treatment preferences of the patient, laws, policies, and other relevant data, alternative actions are then identified.

Identifying the Pros and Cons of Each Alternative

The consequences and benefits of each alternative action are weighed and considered on the bases of treatment preferences, potential outcomes (both desired and consequential), laws, and policies.

Selecting the Best Alternative Based on Established Criteria

Finally, an alternative or action is selected on the basis of treatment preferences, acceptable ethical standards, laws, and policies, and with acceptance of the consequences and benefits of that action. The decision may be not to begin treatment at all but to proceed to palliative care. Physicians are not morally obliged to fulfill patients' requests for actions that they consider ethically objectionable. Physicians have the right to be removed from the care of such patients, although they also have an obligation to arrange for another physician to care for the patient.[8] When clinicians are faced with difficult decisions or disagreements about the best course of action or treatment for a patient, a consultation may be requested from the institutional ethics committee. The purpose of an ethics committee is to review cases impartially and make recommendations. A statement, often written by the chairperson of the group, summarizes the recommendations of the committee as it relates to the *best interest* of the patient within the context of the situation. The criteria of the Joint Commission on Accreditation of Healthcare Organizations (JCAHO) now require a formal mechanism to support ethical decision making.

Process of Ethical Decision Making

Ethical decision making is an integral part of medical and nursing practice, regardless of the setting, and includes both the independent role and the collaborative role of professional practice. However, the responsibilities and participation of physicians and nurses in ethical decision making are dissimilar. Physicians primarily initiate and guide the decisions regarding EOL care, but they are not always the ones to carry out the implementation of decisions. Reckling (1997)[9] commented on the nurses' passive role in decisions to withhold or withdraw life-sustaining treatment. Also noted is physician reluctance to initiate EOL discussions,[10] thus leading to other stresses in ethical decision making. There is need for increased physician and nurse training related to EOL decisions, and nurses need to assume a proactive role in facilitating timely dialogue.[11]

INDEPENDENT ROLE OF THE NURSE

The independent role of the nurse as it relates to ethical decision making generally involves the following:

- Establishing a database, making nursing diagnoses, establishing outcomes, and developing a plan of care
- Orienting the family to the unit and unit policies (e.g., visiting hours, location of telephones and food services)
- Identifying a family spokesperson and scheduling timely updates regarding the patient's condition or progress
- Providing information about the patient's nursing care and response to nursing care
- Seeking information about the patient's or family's care preferences
- Managing pain appropriately to provide and maintain comfort
- Reassuring the family that the patient is receiving sensitive, compassionate care and is comfortable
- Respecting the patient's/family's decisions regarding care
- Supporting the decision of the patient and/or family *not to begin treatment*
- Assuming an advocacy role in behalf of the patient and/or family
- Supporting the patient or family in the grieving process
- Making appropriate referrals to clergy, psychiatric clinical nurse specialists, social workers, or other support resources as necessary
- Documenting the information and support given, other interventions, and patient or family responses
- Follow-up on how family is doing (post-crisis, bereavement)

INDEPENDENT ROLE OF THE PHYSICIAN

Bernat presents both general and specific guidelines for the physician who must make decisions about terminating care for patients with severe, irreversible brain damage.[12] These guidelines are applicable for most neurological and all comatose patients. Accordingly, the role of the physician in the care of a comatose patient includes:

- Making a medical diagnosis of the medical condition and of brain damage (e.g., brain death, persistent vegetative state)
- Making a determination of prognosis based on all available data, evidence-based practice, and experience
- Identifying the patient's preference for treatment, if possible
- Identifying the family's preference for treatment
- Selecting the appropriate level of care
- Making referrals to other physicians, clergy, and other resources as necessary
- Documenting the plan of care and interactions with family to advise them of progress

COLLABORATIVE ROLES

The **collaborative role** of the nurse and physician is based on open, honest, and respectful communications. Ongoing communication with the family is a shared responsibility. The family must be given information and frequent updates regarding the patient's condition and prognosis in a caring, gentle manner. Nurses should know what information has been provided to the family because clarification and reinforcement may be necessary. People in high-stress situations often do not absorb all the information provided to them and therefore may need repetition. Questions raised by the family with the nurse may need to be referred to the physician. The nurse is responsible for notifying the physician of family concerns and the possible need for a family meeting. Depending on the situation, the assistance of other professionals, such as clergy, social workers, or psychiatric or mental health professionals, may be requested to provide support to the patient and family. Discussions with other collaborators can be very helpful in clarifying related issues, not only to the patient and family, but also to the health professionals involved.

The database established by the physician related to the medical diagnosis and prognosis provides information necessary for the nurse's ethical decision-making process. Likewise, information collected by the nurse, as derived from periodic neurological examinations, preferences or responses expressed by the patient or family, and other sources, assists the physician. All information provides a current and updated database for ethical decision making.

Documentation

Written documentation of communications with the family and the decisions made is important to validate that the ethical and legal dimensions of care have been met. The written documentation of both the nurse and the physician helps to keep the professional staff aware of what has transpired in the decision making process and what issues need to be addressed. The physician has the responsibility to provide data about the patient's condition and documentation of decisions for the plan of care. In special situations, such as with "do not resuscitate" (DNR) orders, hospital policy often dictates the frequency of documentation and specific data to be included.

DECISION-MAKING CAPACITY AND ADVANCE DIRECTIVES AND LIVING WILLS

Patient's Capacity to Make Decisions

Discussion about the appropriate use of "competency" has been raised. According to *Guidelines on the Termination of Life-Sustaining Treatment and the Care of the Dying*, the use of competence and incompetence should be restricted to situations in which a formal judicial determination has been made.[13] Under existing law, until such time as a judicial determination of incompetence has been made, individuals are presumed competent to manage their own affairs. The report goes on to promote the use of the notion of decision-making capacity.[13] **Decision-making capacity** refers to a patient's functional ability to make informed health care decisions in accordance with personal values. A person can be legally competent and nonetheless lack the capacity to make a particular treatment decision and vice versa.

Valid consent or refusal assumes adequacy of information provided, absence of coercion, and capacity to make decisions. The accepted standards in designating a patient's decision-making capacity were put forth in the President's Commission report on *Deciding to Forgo Life-Sustaining Treatment*.[14] The criteria include that the patient must be able to understand all information relevant to the decision; communicate with caregivers about the decision; and possess the ability to reason about relevant alternatives against a background of "reasonably stable personal values and life goals."

When cognitive abilities are compromised so that informed consent is no longer possible, the patient is not capable of making decisions. The health care team members then look to a designated family member or significant other as the surrogate to make decisions on behalf of the patient. The decisions made should be guided by the patient's previous expressions of wishes regarding treatment decisions (see discussion later of the substitute judgment standard) and an understanding of the patient's life goals, values, and beliefs and not those of the surrogate. Some states recognize living wills (discussed later in this chapter).

In neuroscience nursing practice, "the organ of reason" is often also the organ of injury and impairment, so that cognitive function is often compromised. The nurse then becomes the patient's advocate to ensure that adequate care is provided within the context of the expressed wishes of the patient as best as they can be determined. There are times when the patient is admitted to a facility in a comatose state, and the nurse has no idea of what the wishes of the patient would be if he or she could convey them. As patient advocates, the health care team is obliged to seek this information as it has been expressed in the past to family members or is found in written documents.

Advance Directives and Living Wills

Advance directives are often misunderstood both by laypeople and health care professionals. Formalized **advance directives** are *written documents* signed by a competent person outlining the extent and form of care in the event of subsequent inability to participate in decision making. A **living will** is an advance directive specifying that, if the person is incapable of participating in decision making, life-sustaining treatments to postpone death should not be used in the event of a terminal illness.[8] The living will is a provision under a state's "Natural Death Act" or "Terminal Care Document." The problem with a living will is that it fails to provide the detailed instructions necessary for care and only applies when the patient is unable to communicate his or her wishes, and then only if death is imminent. It does not imply that the patient wishes to be designated DNR. It lacks the specifics to make decisions from many treatment

options. A more useful directive is the *Durable Power of Attorney for Health Care* (DPAHC), and it is available for use in all states. The DPAHC permits adults to authorize a person to make surrogate medical decisions on his or her behalf if he or she becomes incapable of making decisions.[16]

Studies that have examined patients' advance preferences and the decisions that they or surrogates actually made over time found that treatment preferences are not stable and may change, especially when faced with serious illness.[17] This is important because providers must recognize that previous decisions may be revised because of changes in health status and quality of life. Therefore, advance preferences should be reviewed with the patient with full recognition that decision making is a process and not an endpoint.[18]

The **Patient Self-Determination Act of 1990** supports proxy statutes specifically for health care.[19] It also requires that health care providers elicit and clarify patients' preferences for care and treatment options. This information may be elicited through conversations with the patient or surrogate about the patient's beliefs, values, and life goals. States have different titles for their advance directives, living wills, and durable power of attorney. The formalized designation of a surrogate decision-maker for health care decisions is titled "Designation of a Health Care Power of Attorney" in some states and "Durable Power of Attorney for Health Care" in others. Nurses need to be familiar with the relevant documents and statutes in the state in which they practice. Medicare and Medicaid nursing home certification requires inpatient assessment to determine the status of advance directives and durable power of attorney in those settings. In the absence of any advance directives, the principles of nonmaleficence and best interest become operative.

With readily available technology, the question of appropriate use of technology is often raised. In making decisions about use of technology and other resources, the primary consideration is the expected outcomes of care rather than unqualified entitlement. Laws do not require physicians to provide treatment that is *medically futile* or ineffective. Some state laws include a futility clause about life-sustaining treatment decisions to clarify patients' rights and a mechanism to resolve dispute. The Texas Advance Directive Law of 1999[20] is such an example. Patients have the right to refuse treatment, but they do not have a right to demand and receive interventions that are judged by competent professionals to be of no benefit to them. The role of evidence-based medicine and best practice helps to determine ineffective treatment objectively in relationship to treatment goals and expected outcomes rather than subjective thinking. A second opinion and use of ethical consultation is helpful to resolve differences of opinion, especially when the patient or surrogate opinion is different from that of the physician.

END-OF-LIFE CARE

Nurses have always cared for the dying across the continuum of care. Death has not been a focus of attention for many reasons. For nurses and other health care professionals, death is often viewed as failure; for the general public and policy makers, it is an uncomfortable topic. Death becomes very personal; it is not something that only happens to others, it is something that we will all experience. After years of inattention, American society and American health care are reexamining how we approach dying and death and how we care for people at the end of life.[21] In 1997, the Institute of Medicine published a report on improving care at the end of life with recommendations.[21] This report reinforces the important ongoing work of nurses and how nurses have been addressing this understated problem.

End-of life (EOL) care refers to the comprehensive aspects of care needed by patients and their families as they approach death. These components include palliative care; quality-of-life issues (QOL); pain management; symptoms management; communications; roles/needs of the family; death (e.g., pathophysiology, postmortem care); issues of policy and ethics; and bereavement of family and staff.[22] In a study of patients' perspectives on EOL care, participants identified five domains of quality EOL care: receiving adequate pain and symptom management; avoiding inappropriate prolongation of dying; achieving a sense of control; relieving burden; and strengthening relationships with loved ones.[23]

According to the World Health Organization (WHO), **palliative care** is "the active total care of patients whose disease is not responsive to curative treatment. Control of pain, of other symptoms, and of psychological, social, and spiritual problems is paramount. The goal of palliative care is achievement of the best quality of life for patients and their families"[24] while maximizing comfort and maintaining dignity.[25] Care is provided by an interdisciplinary team of health professionals and trained volunteers. It is apparent that the comprehensiveness of EOL provides a broad framework for considering both care needs for patients and their families and also the societal issues of policies and ethics.

IIII SELECTED ETHICAL ISSUES COMMON IN NEUROSCIENCE NURSING PRACTICE

Although many ethical decisions involve nurses on a daily basis in terms of care, there are several EOL decisions often encountered in practice settings by neuroscience nurses. Those selected for discussion in this section include artificial hydration and nutrition, promotion of comfort and relief of pain, assisted suicide, brain death, and donor organs.

End-of-Life Care Decisions

Several court decisions have clearly addressed the deliberate discontinuation of life-sustaining treatment to allow for a natural death. Life-sustaining treatment can be legally removed from either a patient who is capable or one who is incapable of making decisions. The following cases illustrate this point. In the landmark Quinlan decision of 1976, the court established the right for refusal of life-sustaining treatment by a guardian acting in behalf of a patient who was comatose and, therefore, incapable of making decisions.[26] The request to remove the ventilator was granted based on

the irreversibility of her condition, as well as statements attributed to the patient prior to her illness that indicated an unwillingness to be maintained on life support indefinitely if there was no hope for quality of life. The *Satz v. Perlmutter* case pertains to a fully capable 73-year old patient who depended on a ventilator as a result of amyotrophic lateral sclerosis.[27] He wanted the ventilator to be removed even though he knew death would result. The Florida court ruled that because Mr. Satz was a competent adult, he had a right to refuse life-sustaining treatment. The ventilator was discontinued, and he died within a short period of time.

In 1985, the New Jersey Supreme Court approved the removal of a feeding tube from Ms. Conroy, an elderly nursing home resident with profound dementia. The court ruled that a feeding tube is a medical device and intervention and may be accepted or rejected on behalf of an incompetent patient in the same way as other medical interventions.[28,29] The Brophy decision in 1986 was important in that his care was contested by New England Sinai Hospital. The Massachusetts Supreme Judicial Court allowed Mr. Brophy's family to transfer him to another facility. This act acknowledged the conscientious objection of the staff of New England Sinai Hospital.[30] Finally, in 1990, the U.S. Supreme Court heard the landmark Cruzan case. Nancy Cruzan was a young motor vehicle accident victim who was in a persistent vegetative state. The family wanted to discontinue the feeding tube. The Court affirmed the principle that a feeding tube is a medical device for artificial delivery of hydration and nutrition and is no different from other medical interventions that may be refused by or in behalf of patients.[31]

Professional organizations have published definitive position statements regarding life-sustaining treatment. In 1986, the Council of Ethical and Judicial Affairs of the American Medical Association published the "Statement on Withholding or Withdrawing Life Prolonging Medical Treatment," which stated that such treatment may be withheld from a patient in irreversible coma even when death is not imminent.[32] The Hastings Center, a highly respected source on ethical issues, published "Guidelines on the Termination of Life-Sustaining Treatment and the Care of the Dying."[33] In these guidelines, life-sustaining treatment is defined as "any medical intervention, technology, procedure or medication that is administered to a patient in order to forestall the moment of death whether or not the treatment is intended to affect the underlying disease(s) or biological processes." The position paper of the American Academy of Neurology addressed persistent vegetative state and concluded that nutrition and hydration provided through the enteral route is a medical therapy that can be discontinued.[34,35] Although these publications are not legal documents, they reflect the opinions of those prestigious organizations involved in ethical issues and the delivery of care.

Artificial Hydration and Nutrition

Health care professionals have an easier time of understanding the ethical basis for forgoing ventilators in dying patients than forgoing *artificial hydration and nutrition*.[29] In this context, the term *artificial* refers to providing nutrition by medical devices designed to bypass the mouth through which food and water are normally consumed. Artificially delivered hydration and nutrition refers to water and nutrients provided either directly into the stomach or small intestines or indirectly into the vascular system. First, hydration and nutrition can be administered into the stomach by way of: a nasogastric tube inserted through the nose or mouth, through a surgically inserted gastrostomy tube placed into the stomach or small intestines through the abdominal wall, or by way of a percutaneous endoscopic gastrostomy (PEG) tube inserted into the stomach endoscopically. Second, hydration and nutrition can be administered into the vascular system through a peripheral intravenous (IV) line or into larger vessels or right atria through a central venous catheter.

The American Nurses Association (ANA) published the "Position Statement on Forgoing Artificial Nutrition and Hydration" in 1992.[36] It affirms the principles set forth in the AMA, Hastings Center, and American Academy of Neurology documents. Its central concept is recognition that artificially provided hydration and nutrition, like other interventions, may or may not be justified. As in all other interventions, the anticipated benefits must outweigh the anticipated burdens for the intervention to be justified.

The ANA distinguishes between food and water taken by *mouth* from artificial nutrition and hydration. It also notes that assisting with feeding is a qualitative difference in taking oral nutrition and hydration and not a substantive one. The ANA statement supports the forgoing of tube feedings when there is questionable benefit. The statement also goes on to explain that "competent reflective adults are generally in the best position to evaluate various harms and benefits to themselves in the context of their own values, life projects and tolerance of pain" and that when patients are incapacitated, a surrogate, "preferably designated by the patient," should be relied on to make the decision in behalf of the patient.

Promotion of Comfort and Relief of Pain

Promotion of comfort and relief of pain can be viewed from the perspective of the dying patient and the perspective of acute pain. The ANA published a "Position Statement on Promotion of Comfort and Relief of Pain in Dying Patients" in 1995. It pointed out that when cure or prolongation of life in individuals with serious health problems is no longer possible, the focus of nursing care is on the individual's response to dying and palliative care. Promotion of comfort becomes the primary focus of nursing care. The overriding fear of many patients and families in severe, unrelenting pain during the dying process. Pain is commonly undertreated, and many patients experience inadequate pain control.[37] It is well recognized that severe pain can cause sleeplessness, loss of morale, fatigue, irritability, restlessness, withdrawal, and other serious problems in dying patients.[38,39] Nurses play a key role in both assessment and control of pain either by administering orders for pain or advocating in behalf of the patient for adequate pain control when pharmacologic agents ordered are inadequate to keep the patient comfortable. The assessment and management of pain must be based on an understanding of pathophysiologic, emotional, and spiritual components as well as the knowledge of the particular disease. The ANA says the main goal of nursing intervention for a dying patient should be maximizing comfort through adequate management of pain and discomfort as is in keeping with the expressed desires of the patient. Further, toward that end, the patient should have whatever medication, in whatever dosage, and by whatever route is needed to control the level of pain as perceived by him or her.

Many nurses express concern about the patient's developing tolerance or addiction to analgesics and are fearful of "harming" the patient in that way. The ANA examined authoritative resources and addressed these concerns by saying

Careful titration of pain medication is essential to promote comfort in dying patients. The proper dose is "the dose that is sufficient to reduce pain and suffering."[40] Tolerance to pain medications often develops in patients after repeated and prolonged use. Thus, both adults and children may require very high doses of medication to maintain adequate pain control.[41] These doses may exceed the usual recommended dosages of the particular drug for patients of similar age and weight. Regular dosing of pain medication has been shown to be more effective than PRN use.[42]

The ANA statement goes on to say that pain medications may have sedative or respiratory depressant side effects. This should not be an overriding consideration for dying patients so long as use of pain medication is consistent with the patient's wishes. Pain may continue even when a patient is unresponsive and at the end hours of life when respirations decrease. Pain relief should continue unless there is a reason to believe that the physiologic cause of pain is no longer present. Of particular interest is the following statement: "The increasing titration of medication to achieve adequate symptom control, even at the expense of maintaining life or hastening death secondarily, is ethically justified. Nurses should not hesitate to use full and effective doses of pain mediation for the proper management of pain in the dying patient." Control of pain in the dying patient is an obligation of nurses.

The second focus of acute pain management is in a patient who is not necessarily classified as a "dying patient." Patients with severe headache related to subarachnoid hemorrhage, a brain tumor, stroke, intracranial bleed, or other causes are entitled to adequate pain control. Nurses worry about the reliability of the neurological assessment data if a patient is receiving a narcotic analgesic for pain control. Specifically, concern is expressed about masking the level of consciousness (LOC), mental status, pupillary reflexes, and respiratory function. There is great reluctance to adequately manage pain and discomfort so that many patients are grossly undertreated or not treated at all. A patient may be holding his or her head with severe pain because the nurse is afraid to medicate him or her. Nurses need to consider the physiologic consequences (e.g., increased blood pressure or pulse, increased agitation) of inadequate pain management as well as central nervous system effects with the obligation to keep patients comfortable.

The Clinical Practice Guidelines (p. 29)[37] for acute pain address neurosurgical pain in the following way:

Patients undergoing an operation of the central nervous system frequently show abnormal neurological signs and symptoms that must be closely followed in the postoperative period. These patients may also receive drugs designed to reduce cerebral edema or prevent seizures. A major dilemma in this clinical setting is the need to carefully monitor critical neurological signs, such as pupillary reflexes and the LOC, which may be affected by conventional opioid analgesics used for the relief of postoperative pain. Ideally, postoperative pain control should not interfere with the ability to assess a patient's neurological status, particularly the LOC, or with assessment of motor and sensory function following spinal cord surgery. Therefore, the administration of opioids, benzodiazepines, and anxiolytics, in particular, is relatively contraindicated. However, the clinician must balance the need for analgesia with the requirement for appropriate neurological monitoring. The uncomplicated postcraniotomy patient typically has mild-to-moderate pain and is readily managed by a short period of parenteral medications followed by oral analgesics. Laminectomy and other spinal procedures usually are more painful than craniotomies. Ketorolac, a parenteral NSAID, may be considered in this setting because it has no effect on the LOC or pupillary reflexes. NSAIDs may be contraindicated in some postoperative settings when the risk of coagulopathy or hemorrhage is high, when the need to assess fever is important, or when the degree of pain is higher than the analgesic ceiling of the agent. Furthermore, motor and sensory dysfunction associated with epidural local anesthetics (which are often coadministered with opioids) may obscure important neurological signs. Again remember to balance the need for adequate analgesia while minimizing the confounding central nervous system effects of analgesics and anesthetics.

From this cited information, it is evident that agents used for *acute* pain control must be weighed along with the effects on the central nervous system.

Assisted Suicide

The ongoing publicity of Jack Kevorkian and assisted suicides has caused a moral stir and confusion. People are not ethically obliged to accept life-sustaining treatment.[43] Refusal of such treatment has been ruled legally acceptable in the courts. However, administration of drugs with the intent of causing death, even when requested by a mentally competent person, is considered an act of assisted suicide (voluntary active euthanasia). When the primary intent of an act is to shorten or terminate life, this intent is considered to do harm, based on the ethical principle of nonmaleficence.[18] Based on the interest in physician-assisted suicide in relation to Kevorkian, there are proponents even though it is illegal.

Assisting in a suicide is considered a criminal offense in all U.S. states except Oregon. In 1997, the U.S. Supreme Court, in a 9 to 0 decision, upheld the New York and Washington state laws that said physician-assisted suicide were criminal offenses.[44] The ANA, in a position statement, directs nurses not to support physician-assisted suicide and not to participate in voluntary active euthanasia.[45,46]

Brain Death

Brain death is a *clinical diagnosis* made by a physician. Brain death is defined as irreversible cessation of all functions of the entire brain, including the brain stem.[47–50] The diagnosis of brain death is made based on fulfillment of strict, well-defined clinical criteria of irreversible coma, absence of cortical activity, absence of motor response to pain, loss of brainstem reflexes, and apnea.[51] Ancillary diagnostic tests may be used to support the clinical diagnosis, but they are not strictly required to make the diagnosis. It is critical that the cause of the coma be investigated, and that a cause be identified that is capable of causing irreversible apneic coma when there is no evidence of cerebral or brain-stem function.[52]

Three Key Findings in Brain Death

The three key findings in brain death are coma or unresponsiveness, absence of brain-stem reflexes, and apnea.

Coma or Unresponsiveness. Definite clinical, neuroimaging, or cerebrospinal fluid evidence of an acute central nervous system catastrophic event compatible with death must be found. All reversible causes of coma must be *excluded* before a diagnosis of brain death can be made. Potentially reversible confounding factors of coma include hypothermia (core temperature below 32°C related to blunted brain-stem reflexes); drug intoxication or poisoning; use of neuromuscular blocking agents; severe electrolyte imbalance; severe acid-base abnormalities; and severe metabolic or endocrine imbalance. If barbiturates have been used (e.g., barbiturate-induced coma), the diagnosis of brain death can still be made if the levels of drug are subtherapeutic.[53] In addition, Wijdicks recommends that definite clinical, neuroimaging, or cerebrospinal fluid evidence of an acute central nervous system catastrophic event compatible with brain death must be found.[53]

Absence of Brain-Stem Reflexes. Loss of brain-stem function is incompatible with life. The brain-stem reflexes that are assessed include pupillary reaction to light, corneal reflex, gag reflex, and oculovestibular reflex. All reflexes should be absent in brain death. There should not be a light response to a bright light introduced to the pupil. Most pupils are midposition (4 to 6 mm), although there may be variations from 4 to 9 mm, all of which are compatible with brain death. In addition, pupils may be round, ovoid, or irregularly shaped. The corneal reflex is tested with a wisp of cotton and should be absent. Observe for any grimacing in response to deep pain. The gag reflex is tested with a tongue blade. Along with an absent gag reflex, the cough reflex should also be absent. Ocular movements, as tested by head turning and caloric testing, are absent in brain death. (See Chapter 6 for a description of caloric testing and Chapter 8 for assessment of ocular movement, including precautions to be taken before testing.) Note that sedatives, aminoglycosides, tricyclic antidepressants, anticholinergics, anticonvulsants, and chemotherapeutic agents can diminish or completely abolish caloric response.[53] Loss of brainstem function also results in loss of breathing and vasomotor control, which results in apnea and hypotension.

Apnea. In diagnosing brain death, demonstration of apnea to evaluate respiratory drive (brain-stem function) is critical.[54] Severe hypotension and cardiac arrhythmias (e.g., premature ventricular contractions, ventricular tachycardia) may occur during apnea testing, either spontaneously due to acidosis or related to inadequate precautions. Therefore, there are prerequisites recommended when testing for apnea: (1) core temperature is 36°C (97°F) or higher; (2) systolic blood pressure 90 mm Hg or more; (3) positive fluid balance in the past 6 hours; (4) arterial PCO_2 40 mm Hg or more; and (5) arterial PO_2 200 mm Hg or more.[53,55] Although there may be slight variations in institutional protocol for apnea testing, the following outlines a model apnea testing protocol for the physician to implement:[49] Disconnect the patient from the ventilator (a PCO_2 rise of 3 to 6 mm Hg/min is estimated in the apneic patient).[56]

- Immediately on disconnection, place an oxygen cannula at the level of the carina and administer 100% oxygen at 6 L/min.
- Observe for respiratory movement of the chest/abdomen for 8 minutes (a respiration is defined as abdominal or chest movement that produce adequate tidal volume).
- If there is no respiratory movement and the PCO_2 is 60 mm Hg or higher, the clinical diagnosis of brain death is made.
- If the PCO_2 has not met the target level of 60 mm Hg or higher, apnea testing is repeated after a period of time and confirmatory testing may also be ordered.

Note that the target PCO_2 may be higher in patients with chronic hypercapnia (e.g., severe chronic obstructive pulmonary disease, bronchiectasis, sleep apnea, morbid obesity) because the patient's PCO_2 baseline is higher. If chronic hypercapnia is suspected, additional noninvasive confirmatory tests are strongly recommended.[53]

Reflex Motor Activity

Spontaneous motor responses of spinal origin sometimes called the "Lazarus sign," observed as limb movements, may be seen in brain death.[57] Possible movements seen, especially in younger patients, can include any of the following: rapid flexion of the arms; raising of one or all of the limbs off of the bed; grasping movements; or jerking of one leg. In addition, multifocal vigorous myoclonus may be noted. Although unexpected, these movements are not purposeful and should not be interpreted as such.

Confirmatory Testing

As mentioned earlier, brain death is a *clinical diagnosis* made by a physician. In most instances, the clinical evaluation is conducted two times with an interval of hours (e.g., 6 to 8 hours) elapsing between examinations. Many hospitals have developed guidelines that often include a requirement of two independent clinical evaluations by two different physicians. Figure 4-1 provides a sample guideline. Confirmatory testing is not required to make the diagnosis of brain death in the United States. However, a physician may choose to include confirmatory tests for patients in whom specific components of the clinical evaluation cannot be reliably tested. Confirmatory tests that are accepted based on clinical experience and reliability include conventional angiography, blood-flow studies (e.g. technetium 99m), electroencephalography, and more recently, transcranial Doppler ultrasonography. Absence of blood flow and electrical activity of the brain are confirmatory findings of brain death.

Wijdicks provides an excellent discussion of use, validity, and disadvantages of confirmatory tests and brain death.[53]

After brain death has been confirmed, the patient is pronounced brain dead and all treatment is stopped.[58] The time of death is when the second set of brain death clinical evaluation and possible confirmatory test are met.[59] The organs may be supported for a short period of time if organ harvest is planned.

Organ Procurement

One important result of declaring brain death is the possibility of organ donation. Although kidneys are the most common organs to be donated, other organs, such as the cornea, skin, bone, liver, and heart valves, may be given. When organ donation is considered, donor criteria must be strictly followed. Donor criteria vary depending on the particular organ to be given, but criteria include a specified age range, no history of malignant neoplasms, absence of sepsis or transmittable diseases, and procurement of the organ as quickly as possible, but certainly within a few hours of death. In addition, the medical team involved in the declaration of brain death and the organ harvest team must be kept separate to avoid any special interests. After brain death has been declared and consent has been given for organ donation, the personnel of the organ donor program initiate management. The most common initial physiologic management issues are hypotension, diabetes insipidus, or both.[60] Blood pressure, hydration, and ventilation are supported to provide adequate organ perfusion and oxygenation until surgery. Use of a ventilator, vasopressors and inotropic drugs (e.g., dopamine, dobutamine) to maintain cardiac function and blood pressure, desmopressin to manage diabetes insipidus, and intravenous fluids is necessary to maintain organ perfusion.

The nurse conveys sensitivity and caring for the patient and family by keeping the patient clean and comfortable-looking. Provisions must be made to support the family in their decision for or against organ donation. In addition, the family needs time and privacy to say their goodbyes to their loved one and to begin the bereavement process.

FOSTERING PROFESSIONAL GROWTH IN ETHICAL DECISION MAKING

Professional Development and Ethical Caring

Exploring the ethical dimensions of professional practice is necessary to understand the duties and obligations in providing care. It also may be uncomfortable because it forces us to examine fundamental and personal life-death issues and personal values as moral beings. The JCAHO Standards require a formal mechanism to assist in the resolution of ethical problems in patient care in all facilities. All clinicians are also encouraged to become familiar with the mechanisms that exist within their own institutions.

For those nurses engaged in neuroscience nursing, a number of ethical issues arise in everyday practice that can be

	DATE AND TIME OF EXAM	BODY TEMPERATURE	BLOOD ETHANOL (IF INDICATED)	TOXICOLOGY (IF INDICATED)
1 ST EXAM				
2 ND EXAM				

WRITE A "YES" OR "NO" RESPONSE TO EACH QUESTION	1 ST EXAM	2 ND EXAM
ABSENCE OF CEREBRAL FUNCTIONS IS THE PATIENT IN DEEP COMA, WITHOUT ANY SPONTANEOUS MOVEMENTS OR RESPONSE TO PAINFUL STIMULI ADMINISTERED OVER THE AREAS OF CRANIAL NERVE DISTRIBUTION (e.g. SUPRAORBITAL PRESSURE) AND WITHOUT DECORTICATE OR DECEREBRATE POSTURING? (SPINAL REFLEXES MAY BE PRESENT).		
ABSENCE OF BRAIN STEM FUNCTIONS—CRANIAL NERVE REFLEXES: 1. ARE PUPILS FIXED TO LIGHT?		
2. ARE CORNEAL REFLEXES ABSENT?		
3. ARE OCULOCEPHALIC REFLEXES ABSENT?		
4. ARE COLD WATER OCULOVESTIBULAR REFLEXES ABSENT?		
5. ARE OROPHARYNGEAL RESPONSES ABSENT?		
6. ARE SPONTANEOUS RESPIRATIONS ABSENT?		
APNEA TEST 1. ARE SPONTANEOUS BREATHING MOVEMENTS ABSENT DURING APNEA TESTS?		
2. LIST PaCO2 AT END OF APNEA TEST.		

NAMES AND SIGNATURE OF EXAMINING PHYSICIANS

	PHYSICIAN SIGNATURE	NAME PRINTED
1 ST EXAM	PHYSICIAN SIGNATURE	NAME PRINTED
	PHYSICIAN SIGNATURE	NAME PRINTED
2 ND EXAM	PHYSICIAN SIGNATURE	NAME PRINTED

CONFIRMATORY TEST(S)   DATE, TIME AND RESULTS OF ALL CONFIRMATORY TESTS

_____

_____

_____

CERTIFICATION OF DEATH BY NEUROLOGICAL CRITERIA

HAVING CONSIDERED THE ABOVE FINDINGS, WE HEREBY CERTIFY THE DEATH OF			
PATIENT NAME	DATE	TIME	☐ AM ☐ PM
PHYSICIAN SIGNATURE		NAME PRINTED	
PHYSICIAN SIGNATURE		NAME PRINTED	

Figure 4–1 • A sample checklist for determination of death by neurological criteria. The cause of coma must be established and sufficient to account for the loss of all brain function. Reversible conditions, such as drug sedation, metabolic disturbance, hypothermia (below 32.2° C), neuromuscular blockage, and shock, must be searched for and appropriately treated.

Two separate clinical examinations must be completed, the second no sooner than *six hours after the first*. Each examination must be conducted by two physicians, independent of each other, who shall be licensed to practice medicine in the state. (Note that in this sample form, the institution requires two physicians to examine the patient each time.) The physicians may or may not choose to perform cold calorics.

sources of confusion and discomfort. It is important for the nurse to examine these situations, identify the type of problem that exists, identify the underlying ethical principles that have some impact on the situation, and sort out the components of the clinical situation to arrive at a sense of understanding that will guide clinical practice. Profes-sional development in ethical care must be supported by departments of nursing and health care institutions in several ways; institutional ethics committees, ethics rounds, interdisciplinary ethical educational programs, and discussion groups are helpful in responding to individual patient situations and needs of health professionals.

Institutional Ethics Committee

All health care facilities have some form of an institutional ethics committee. Committee membership is multidisciplinary to represent multiple perspectives and expertise. Often, community representation is sought and may include an ethicist, an attorney, and a lay person. The committee's purposes include education, development of institutional guidelines and standards, concurrent case review, and retroactive case review. Many of the substantive issues center on neurological patients.[58]

Ethics Rounds

Ethics rounds should be conducted on patient care units periodically to support ongoing staff education and to identify patient situations in need of ethical exploration. These rounds have a clinical focus and are usually directed by a group leader with an interest and background in ethics and clinical decision making. Particular patient situations can be reviewed to examine ethical components of care and the bases for decision making. Ethics rounds help to examine and clarify standards of care to address the ethical aspects of care and the rationale for those actions. Other resources can also be identified that may be helpful in resolving ethical matters when there is a need for assistance.

Ethics Educational Programs and Discussion Groups

Interdisciplinary educational programs with a focus in ethics are important to promote professional growth of the staff. They may be focused on the review of new guidelines or patient care situations. Ethics discussion groups are an informal method for discussion of topics of interest related to the ethical dimension of practice. The discussion may or may not address a currently active clinical situation in that facility. Cases reported in the press, recent legal opinions rendered, or the ethical dimensions of a new technology may be among the topics discussed. This forum provides the opportunity to consider a proactive approach to a potential problem. Other issues that may be addressed include clinical situations within the facility that were not adequately resolved in the past and that deserve a fresh review.

Application of the Ethical Dimension to Clinical Practice

Ethical and legal dimensions of nursing practice cut across all clinical areas of practice. Ethics and legality need to be recognized as separate, although often interacting, concerns.[61] For nurses practicing in neuroscience, the complexity of ethical practice is further compounded by the fact that the "organ of reason" is often impaired, thus raising questions about decision-making capability, autonomy, and best interest. Many of the clinical questions confronting the neuroscience nurse are life-and-death situations in which there are no second chances to undo previously made decisions.

This places a tremendous burden of responsibility to do the "right thing." Some situations precipitate an ethical dilemma for the practitioner. It is, therefore, imperative to prepare oneself for this awesome responsibility through ongoing professional education and development.

REFERENCES

1. Riley, J. M., Mahoney, M. J., Fry, S. T., & Field, L. (1999). Factors related to adult patient decision making about withholding or withdrawing nutrition and/or hydration. *The Online Journal of Knowledge Synthesis for Nursing, 6*(3), 1–20.
2. Angeles, P. A. (1981). *Dictionary of philosophy* (p. 82). New York: Barnes & Noble.
3. Pryor-McCann, J. M. (1990). Ethics in critical care nursing. *Critical Care Nursing Clinics of North America, 2*(l), 1–13.
4. Angeles, P. A. (1981). *Dictionary of philosophy* (p. 179). New York: Barnes & Noble.
5. Rachels, J. (1986). *Elements of moral philosophy.* New York: Random House.
6. Angeles, P. A. (1981). *Dictionary of philosophy* (p. 140). New York: Barnes & Noble.
7. *In re Karen Quinlan,* 70 N.J. 10, 335 A. 2d 647 (1976).
8. Nelson, W. A., & Bernat, J. L. (1989). Decisions to withhold or terminate treatment. *Neurologic Clinics, 7*(4), 759–773.
9. Reckling, J. A. B. (1997). Who plays what role in decisions about withholding and withdrawing life-sustaining treatment? *Journal of Clinical Ethics, 8*(1), 30–45.
10. SUPPORT Principal Investigators. (1995). A controlled trial to improve care of seriously ill hospitalized patients: The Study to Understand the Prognoses and Preferences for Outcomes and Risks of Treatment (SUPPORT). *Journal of the American Medical Association, 274*(20), 1591–1598.
11. Terry, P. B., & Korzick, K. A. (1997). Thoughts about the end-of-life decision-making process. *The Journal of Clinical Ethics, 8*(1), 46–49.
12. Bernat, J. L. (1988). Ethical aspects of withdrawing treatment from patients with severe brain damage. In A. H. Ropper & S. F. Kennedy (Eds.). *Neurological and neurosurgical intensive care* (2nd ed., pp. 345–350). Baltimore: Aspen.
13. Hastings Center Report. (1987). *Guidelines on the termination of life-sustaining treatment and the care of the dying* (p. 131). Bloomington, IN: Indiana University Press.
14. President's Commission for the Study of Ethical Problems in Medicine and Biomedical and Behavioral Research. (1983). *Deciding to forego life-sustaining treatment: A report on the ethical, medical, and legal issues in treatment decisions* (p. 121). Washington, D. C.: U. S. Government Printing Office.
15. Hoffinan, N. (1992). Ethical considerations and quality of life. *Cardiovascular Clinics, 22*(2), 243–251.
16. Emanuel, E. J., & Emanuel, L. L. (1992). Proxy decision making for incompetent patients: An ethical and empirical analysis. *Journal of the American Medical Association, 267*(15), 2067–2071.
17. Lee, M. A., Smith, D. M., Fenn, D. S., & Ganzini, L. (1998). Do patients' treatment decisions match advanced statements of their preferences? *The Journal of Clinical Ethics, 9*(3), 258–262.
18. Kyba, F. C. N. (2000). End of life decisions: Legal and ethical quandaries. *Texas Nursing, 74*(3), 6–12.
19. Cranford, R. E. (1984). Termination of treatment in the persistent vegetative state. *Seminars in Neurology, 4,* 36–44.
20. Texas Health and Safety Code, Chapter 166. (1999). Advance directives. (Codification of S.B. 1260, An act pertaining to certain advance directives for medical treatment; providing administrative penalties.)
21. Institute of Medicine. (1997). *Approaching death: Improving care at the end of life.* Washington, D. C.: National Academy of Sciences.

22. Ferrell, B., Virani, R., & Grant, M. (1999). Analysis of end-of-life content in nursing textbooks. *Oncology Nursing Forum, 26*(2), 869–876.

23. Singer, P. A., Martin, D. K., & Kelner, M. (1999). Quality end-of-life care: Patients' perspectives. *Journal of the American Medical Association, 281*(2), 163–168.

24. World Health Organization. (1990). *Cancer pain relief and palliative care*. Technical Report series 804. Geneva: Author.

25. Doyle, D., Hanks, G. W. C., & MacDonald, N. (1998). *Oxford textbook of palliative medicine* (2nd ed.). Oxford: Oxford University Press.

26. *In re Karen Quinlan*, 70 N.J. 10, 335 A. 2d 647 (1976).

27. *Satz v. Perlmutter*, 13 Sept 1978. Florida District Court of Appeal, Fourth District. Southern Reporter, 2nd Series, 362: 160–164.

28. *In re Conroy*, 486 A2d 1209 (N.J. 1985).

29. Price, D. M., & Murphy, P. A. (1994). Tube feeding and the ethics of caring. *Journal of Nursing Law, 1*(4), 53–59.

30. *Brophy v. New England Sinai Hospital, Inc.*, 497 N.E.2d 626 (Mass. 1986).

31. *Cruzan v. Director, Missouri Department of Health*, 497 U.S. 261 (1990).

32. Corbett, T. E. (1986). Council on Ethical and Judicial Affairs, American Medical Association. Statement on withholding or withdrawing life prolonging treatment. *Journal of the American Medical Association, 256*(19), 1263.

33. The Hastings Center. (1987). *Guidelines on the termination of life-sustaining treatment and the care of the dying*. Briarcliff Manor, NY: Author.

34. American Academy of Neurology. (1989). Position of the American Academy of Neurology on certain aspects of the care and management of the persistent vegetative state patient. *Neurology, 39*, 125–126.

35. American Academy of Neurology. (1989). Guidelines on the vegetative state: Commentary on the American Academy of Neurology statement. *Neurology, 39*, 123–124.

36. Committee on Ethics, American Nurses Association. (1992). Guidelines on withholding food and fluids from patients. *Nursing Outlook, 36*, 122–123, 148–150.

37. U. S. Department of Health and Human Services. (1994). *Management of cancer pain: Clinical practice guidelines, #9*. Rockville, MD: Author.

38. Amenta, M., & Bohnet, N. L. (Eds.). (1986). *Palliative care nursing*. Boston: Little, Brown.

39. Melzack, R. (1990). The tragedy of needless pain. *Scientific American, 262*, 27–33.

40. Dalton, J. A., & Fenerstein, M. (1988). Biobehavioral factors in cancer pain. *Pain, 33*, 137.

41. Kachoyenos, M. K., & Zollo, M. B. (1995). Ethics in pain management of infants and children. *Maternal Child Nursing, 20*, 142–147.

42. American Pain Society. (1993). *Principles of analgesic use in the treatment of acute pain and cancer pain* (3rd ed.). Skokie, IL: Author.

43. Beauchamp, T. L. (1996). Refusals of treatment and requests for death. *Kennedy Institute of Ethics Journal, 6*(4), 371–374.

44. Beder, J. (1998). Legalization of assisted suicide: A pilot study of gerontological nurses. *Journal of Gerontological Nursing, 23*(4), 14–20.

45. American Nurses Association. (1994). *Position statement on active euthanasia*. Washington, DC: Author.

46. American Nurses Association. (1996). Position statement on assisted suicide. In *Compendium of ANA position statements*. Washington, DC: Author.

47. Guidelines for the determination of death: Report of the medical consultants on the diagnosis of brain death to the President's Commission for the Study of Ethical Problems in Medicine and Biomedical and Behavioral Research. (1981). *Journal of the American Medical Association, 246*, 2184–2186.

48. Quality Standards Subcommittee of the American Academy of Neurology. (1995). Practice parameters for determining brain death in adults. *Neurology, 45*, 1012–1014.

49. Widjicks, E. F. M. (1995). Determining brain death in adults. *Neurology, 45*, 1003–1011.

50. Cantrill, S. V. (1997). Brain death. *Emergency Medicine Clinics of North America, 15*(3), 713–722.

51. Black, P. M. (1978). Brain death. *New England Journal of Medicine, 299*, 330–344, 393–401.

52. Hughes, R., & McGuire, G. (1997). Neurologic disease and the determination of brain death: The importance of a diagnosis. *Critical Care Medicine, 25*(11), 1923–1924.

53. Wijdicks, E. F. M. (1997). *The clinical practice of critical care neurology* (pp. 320–333). Philadelphia: Lippincott-Raven.

54. Black, P. M. (1988). Guidelines for the diagnosis of brain death. In A. H. Ropper & S. F. Kennedy (Eds.). *Neurological and neurosurgical intensive care* (2nd ed., pp. 323–333). Rockville, MD: Aspen.

55. Ropper, A. H., Kennedy, S. K., & Russell, L. (1981). Apnea testing in the diagnosis of brain death: Clinical and physiological observations. *Journal of Neurosurgery 55*, 942–946.

56. Eger, E. I., & Severinghaus, J. W. (1961). The rate of rise of $PaCO_2$ in the apneic anesthetized patient. *Anesthesiology 22*, 419–425.

57. Ropper, A. H. (1984). Unusual spontaneous movements in brain-dead patients. *Neurology, 34*, 1012–1014.

58. Cranford, R. E. (1989). The neurologist as ethics consultant and as a member of the institutional ethics committee. *Neurologic Clinics, 7*(4), 697–713.

59. Bernat, J. L. (1989). Ethical issues in brain death and multi-organ transplantation. *Neurologic Clinics, 7*(4), 715–728.

60. Power, B. M., Van Heerden, P. V. (1995). The physiological changes associated with brain death—current concepts and implications for treatment of the brain dead organ donor. *Anaesthesia Intensive Care, 23*, 26–36.

61. Wocial, L. D. (1996). Achieving collaboration in ethical decision making: Strategies for nurses in clinical practice. *Dimensions of Critical Care Nursing, 15*(3), 150–159.

RESOURCES

Professional

Published Material

Beresford, H. R. (1999). Medical-legal issues facing neurologists. *Neurologic Clinics, 17*(2), 295–306.

Jecker, N. S., & Schneiderman, L. J. (1995). When families request that "everything possible" be done. *Journal of Medicine and Philosophy, 20*, 145–163.

Kapp, N. O. (1994). Futile medical treatment: A review of the ethical arguments and legal holdings. *Journal of General Internal Medicine, 9*(March), 170–177.

Kopelman, L. M. (1995). Conceptual and moral disputes about futile and useful treatments. *Journal of Medicine and Philosophy, 20*, 109–121.

Latimer, E. J. (1991). Ethical decision-making in the care of the dying and its applications to clinical practice. *Journal of Pain and Symptom Management, 6*(5), 329–336.

Neatherlin, J. S. (2000). Vulnerable populations in neuroscience nursing research. Journal of Neuroscience Nursing, 32(5), 285–289.

Weber, L. J., & Campbell, M. L. (1996). Medical futility and life-sustaining treatment decisions. *Journal of Neuroscience Nursing, 28*(1), 56–60.

Selected Websites

American Nurses Association http://www.nursingworld.org

Hospice and Palliative Nurses Association http://www.HPNA.org

Last acts. A national coalition to improve care and caring at the end of life http://lastacts.org

Joint Commission on Accreditation of Hospitals and Healthcare Organizations http://www.jcaho.org

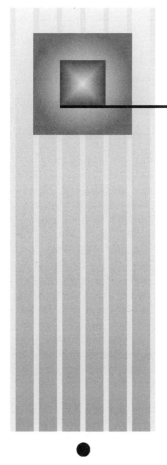

Assessment and Evaluation of Neuroscience Patients

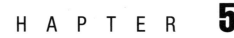

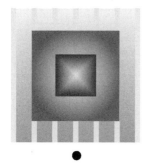

C H A P T E R **5**

Overview of Neuroanatomy and Neurophysiology

JOANNE V. HICKEY

This chapter provides an overview of basic and essential neuroanatomy and neurophysiology as a quick reference to assist the reader in understanding the underlying principles of neurological function and dysfunction as a basis for nursing management. Further discussion of anatomy and physiology is included in many other chapters to enhance understanding. Neuroanatomy and neurophysiology texts should be consulted if more detail is desired.

EMBRYONIC DEVELOPMENT OF THE NERVOUS SYSTEM

The human brain is composed of billions of cells. The nervous system is one of the first recognizable features in embryonic development. From a simple longitudinal invagination on the dorsal portion of the ectodermal layer, a neural groove and neural tube form at about 3 weeks. At the cranial end of the neural tube, rapid and unequal growth occurs, giving rise to the three primary vesicles of the brain. These vesicles, in turn, become five cerebral areas: the telencephalon, the diencephalon, the mesencephalon, the metencephalon, and the myelencephalon (Table 5-1). By 7 weeks, the brain and spinal cord are apparent. At 12 weeks, the brain is the size of a large pea.

Concurrently, cells of the neural tube form two types of cells: spongioblasts, which give rise to the neuroglia (glia) cells, and neuroblasts, which give rise to the nerve cells (neurons). Processes from the neuroblasts form the white matter of the brain. Some of these processes leave the brain and spinal cord to form the fibers of the cranial and ventral roots of the spinal nerves.

Throughout the prenatal period, there is further growth and refinement of the nervous system. All the neurons that a person will ever have are present at birth. These highly specialized cells do not have mitotic capacity and, therefore, are not replaceable. At birth, the brain is about one quarter the size of an adult brain.

CELLS OF THE NERVOUS SYSTEM

From the ectodermal layer, two types of cells develop: neurons and neuroglia cells. **Neurons** are the basic anatomic and functional unit of the nervous system. **Neuroglia cells** provide a variety of supportive functions for the neurons.

Neuroglia Cells

The term *glia* comes from a Greek word meaning "glue" or "holding together." In this regard, the glia cells provide structural support, nourishment, and protection for the neurons of the nervous system. There are 5 to 10 times more neuroglia cells than there are neurons. About 40% of the brain and spinal cord is composed of neuroglia cells.

From a clinical viewpoint, neuroglia cells are important because they can divide by mitosis and are the major source of primary tumors of the nervous system. In the central nervous system (CNS), glia are subdivided into four main types: astrocytes, oligodendrocytes, ependymal cells, and microglia. In the peripheral nervous system (PNS), Schwann cells form myelin sheaths.

Astrocytes have multiple processes extending from the cell body that give it a star-like appearance. Some astrocytic processes may terminate as swellings called *end-feet* on neurons and blood vessels. Functions attributed to astrocytes include providing nutrition for neurons, regulating synaptic connectivity, removing cellular debris, and controlling movement of molecules from blood to brain (part of the blood-brain barrier).

On microscopic examination, **oligodendrocytes** have few branching processes. Oligodendrocytes produce the myelin sheath of the axonal projections of neurons in the CNS. An individual cell can maintain the myelin sheaths of several axons.

Ciliated **ependyma cells** line the ventricular system and the choroid plexuses. They aid in the production of cerebrospinal fluid (CSF) and act as a barrier to foreign substances within the ventricles, preventing them from entering cerebral tissue.

Microglia are minute cells that are scattered throughout the CNS and have a phagocytic function. They remove and disintegrate the waste products of neurons.

Table 5-1 • DEVELOPMENT OF THE PRIMARY VESICLES

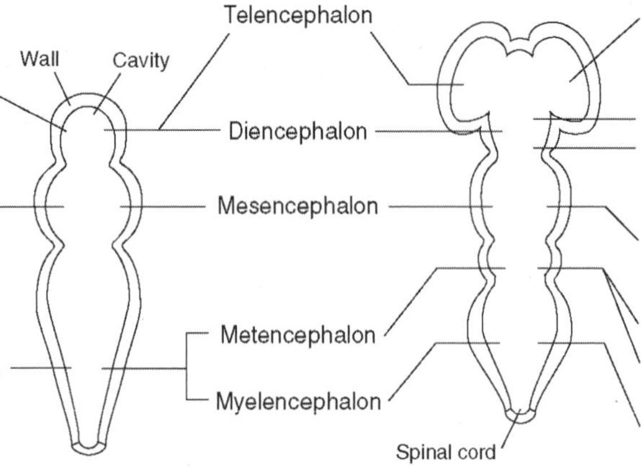

PRIMARY VESICLES	SUBDIVISIONS	STRUCTURES THAT ARISE	VENTRICULAR SYSTEM
Prosencephalon (forebrain)	Telencephalon	Cerebral hemisphere, corpus callosum, basal ganglia, olfactory tracts	Lateral ventricles and part of third ventricle
	Diencephalon	Thalamus Hypothalamus	Most of third ventricle
Mesencephalon (midbrain)	Mesencephalon	Midbrain	Cerebral aqueducts
Rhombencephalon (hindbrain)	Metencephalon	Pons Cerebellum	Fourth ventricle
	Myelencephalon	Medulla oblongata	Fourth ventricle and part of central canal

(Diagram labels: Wall, Cavity, Spinal cord)

Schwann cells function similarly to oligodendrocytes, forming the insulating myelin sheaths around axons to facilitate saltatory conduction of impulses in the PNS.

Neurons

Neurons vary from 5 to 100 μm in diameter. As the basic anatomic and functional unit in the nervous system, the neuron has a number of functions: responding to sensory and chemical stimuli, conducting impulses, and releasing specific chemical regulators.

Neurons are classified as unipolar, bipolar, or multipolar. **Unipolar neurons** possess only one process or pole. This process divides close to the cell body. One branch, called the peripheral process, carries impulses from the periphery toward the cell body. The other branch, called the central process, conducts the impulse toward the spinal cord or the brainstem. **Bipolar neurons** are found only in the spinal and vestibular ganglia, the olfactory mucous membrane, and in one layer of the retina. The anatomic structure is peculiar to the organ in which it is found. Most neurons in the nervous system are **multipolar.** These neurons consist of a cell body, one long projection (the **axon**), and one or more shorter branches (the **dendrites**).

There are three major components of a neuron: a **cell body,** which constitutes the main part of the neuron; a **single axon,** or **axis cylinder,** which consists of a long projection extending from the cell body; and **several dendrites,** which are thin projections extending from the cell body into the immediate surrounding area. The axon carries impulses **away** from the cell body, whereas the dendrites direct impulses **toward** the cell body.

COMPONENTS OF THE CELL BODY

The main organelles of the neuronal cell body include the nucleus, the cell membrane, and the cytoplasm. There are organelles within each of these structures that are important and are mentioned here briefly.

The **nucleus** is a double-membrane structure that contains chromatin and a prominent nucleolus. **Chromatin** is those thread-like structures in the cell nucleus that consist primarily of **deoxyribonucleic acid (DNA)** and protein. DNA contains genes and the genetic code or information about the cell. The **nucleolus** contains **ribonucleic acid (RNA).** RNA is the "messenger" from the genes of the nucleus; it contains the code for synthesis of specific cellular protein.

The **cell membrane** is a triple external membrane primarily consisting of lipoproteins. The cell membrane creates the parameters of the cell body, enclosing the cytoplasm within its border. The main purpose of the cell membrane is to control the interchange of material between the cell and its environment.

The **cytoplasm** contains smooth and rough endoplasmic reticula, Nissl bodies, Golgi apparatus, mitochondria, lysosomes, neurotubules, and neurofibrils. The **endoplasmic reticulum** of the cytoplasm is a network of tubular membranous structures. There are two types of endoplasmic reticulum, smooth and rough. The smooth endoplasmic reticulum serves as the site for enzyme reactions. **Centrioles** are found in the cytoplasm and take part in cell division. **Nissl bodies** are masses of granular (rough) endoplasmic reticulum with ribosomes, which are the protein-synthesizing machinery of the neuron. The endoplasmic reticulum system connects with the nucleus at that portion of the reticulum called the Golgi apparatus. Substances formed in different parts of the cell are transported throughout the cell by means of this system. The **Golgi apparatus** provides for two interrelated functions: further modification of protein by adding carbohydrates and temporary storage and separation of protein types, depending on their function and destination. It is also responsible for the formation of substances important for the digestion of intracellular material.

Mitochondria are structures that serve as the site for production of most cellular energy. Cell nutrients are oxidized to produce carbon dioxide and water. The energy released is used to produce adenosine triphosphate (ATP). **Lysosomes** isolate the digestive enzymes of a cell from the cytoplasm to prevent cell destruction. They are involved in digestion of phagocytosis products and worn-out organelles.

The elongated axons or dendrites can extend 1 meter or more from the cell body. These fibers require protein and other substances produced in the cell body that must be transported from the cytoplasm by a process called *axoplasmic flow*. **Neurotubules** carry out part of axoplasmic transport. **Neurofibrils** are delicate thread-like structures within the cytoplasm and the axon hillock that assist in the transport of cellular material.

CELL PROCESSES: AXONS AND DENDRITES

Axons and **dendrites** constitute the cell processes. Dendrites usually extend only a short distance from the cell body and branch profusely. By contrast, an axon can extend for long distances from the cell body before branching near the end of the projection.

Many axons in the PNS are covered by a myelin sheath composed of a white, lipid substance that acts as an insulator for the conduction of impulses. Nerve fibers enclosed in such a sheath are referred to as **myelinated;** those without the myelin sheath are referred to as **unmyelinated** (Fig. 5-1). As a rule, larger neuron fibers are myelinated, whereas smaller fibers are unmyelinated.

The **myelin sheath** is formed by Schwann cells that encircle the axons. When several **Schwann cells** are wrapped around an axon, their outer layer (sheath of Schwann) encloses the myelin sheath. This outer layer is called the **neurolemma** and is said to be necessary for the regeneration of axons. The myelin sheath itself is a segmented, discontinuous layer that is interrupted at intervals by the **nodes of Ranvier.** The distance from one node to the next is called an **internode.** Each internode is formed by, and surrounded by, one Schwann cell. At the junction between each of the two successive Schwann cells along the axon, a small noninsulated area remains where ions can easily flow between the extracellular fluid and the axon. It is this area that is known as the node of Ranvier. In the CNS, the oligodendroglial cells provide the myelination of the neurons, similar to the role of the Schwann cells in the PNS.

PHYSIOLOGY OF NERVE IMPULSES

Resting Membrane Potential of the Neurons

Although a resting neuron is not conducting an impulse, it is considered to be a charged cell. The difference in electrical charge on either side of the membrane is called the **potential difference** and is related to the unequal distribution of potassium and sodium on either side of the membrane. Normal resting potential of about −80 mV is maintained by the various concentrations of ions in the fluid on either side of the cell membrane.

The cell membrane is both semipermeable and selectively permeable. The area outside the cell is called the interstitial space; the area inside the cell is called the intracellular space. Sodium ions (Na^+) and chloride ions (Cl^-) are found in much greater concentrations in the interstitial space than in the cell. The sodium ion gradient is caused by the powerful sodium pump that continually pumps sodium out of the cell. The potassium ion (K^+) and organic protein material are found in high concentrations within the cell. Potassium is also pumped back into the cell by the potassium pump. The concentration of dissolved ions in a solution is a potential source of energy to drive cellular processes.

Action Potential of the Neuron

The fluid and ions in the intracellular space create a highly conductive solution. The large diameter (10 to 80 μm) allows for unrestricted conduction of impulses from one part of the interior of the cell to the other. Various stimuli can change the permeability of the cell membrane to certain ions, resulting in alterations in the membrane potential (Fig. 5-2). The stimuli must be of sufficient magnitude to conduct an impulse and thus create an **action potential,** which is the fundamental unit of signaling in the nervous system.

Many simultaneous discharges at the synaptic junction must occur to create a sufficient effect on the cell membrane. The membrane potential reverses, and the intracellular surface becomes positive (approximately +20 to +40 mV). When the action potential is realized, there is a sudden reversal of the sodium and potassium relationship across the cell membrane of the axon. This event is called **depolarization.** The neuron receives an influx of sodium and loses potassium to the interstitial space; the time required is only a few milliseconds. With the change in polarity, an impulse is conducted from one neuron to the next at the same amplitude and speed. The cell repolarizes and returns to its resting membrane potential. This sequence of events occurs during the conduction of an impulse in an unmyelinated nerve.

Saltatory Conduction

In myelinated nerves, an action potential hops from one node of Ranvier to the next as a means of rapidly conducting an impulse. This is called **saltatory conduction.** Although ions cannot flow out through the myelin sheath of myelinated nerves, the break in the myelin sheath at the nodes of Ranvier (see Fig. 5-1) provides a perfect route of escape. At this point, the membrane is several times more permeable than many unmyelinated nerves. Impulses are conducted from node to node rather than continuing along the entire span of the axon, as is the case in unmyelinated nerves. Saltatory conduction is advantageous because it increases the velocity of an impulse and conserves energy (because only the nodes depolarize). The velocity of an impulse depends on both the thickness of the myelin and the distance between the internodes. As these two factors increase, the velocity of the impulse also increases.

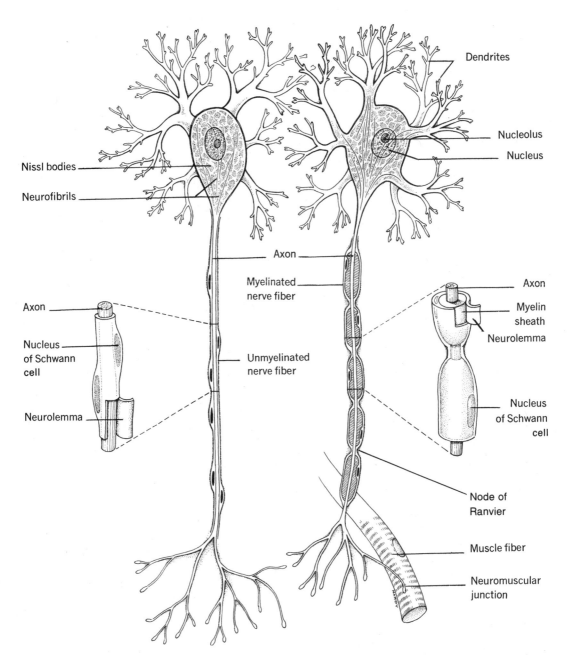

Figure 5–1 • Typical neurons: unmyelinated fiber (*left*); myelinated fiber (*right*). (From Chaffee, E. E., & Lytle, I. M. [1980]. *Basic physiology and anatomy.* Philadelphia: J. B. Lippincott.)

Synapse

The junction between one neuron and the next at which an impulse is transmitted is called the **synapse.** There are three anatomic structures that are necessary for an impulse to be transmitted at a synapse. These include the presynaptic terminals, the synaptic cleft, and the postsynaptic membrane (Fig. 5-3).

Presynaptic terminals are either excitatory or inhibitory. An excitatory presynaptic terminal secretes an excitatory substance into the synaptic cleft, thereby exciting the effector neuron. The inhibitory presynaptic terminal secretes an inhibitory transmitter that, when secreted into the synaptic cleft, inhibits the effector neuron. The excitatory or inhibitory transmitter secretions arise from the synaptic vesicle in the presynaptic terminal of the axon. Mitochondria in the axon supply the adenosine triphosphate (ATP) to synthesize new transmitter secretions. The **synaptic cleft** is the microscopic space (200 to 300 Å) between the presynaptic terminal and the receptor area of the effector cell. The **postsynaptic membrane** is that part of the effector membrane proximal to the presynaptic terminal.

When an action potential spreads over the presynaptic terminal, the membrane depolarizes, emptying some of the contents of the presynaptic vesicles into the synaptic cleft. The released transmitter changes the permeability of the subsynaptic membrane. This results in either excitation or inhibition of the neuron, depending on the type of transmitter substances secreted into the synaptic cleft.

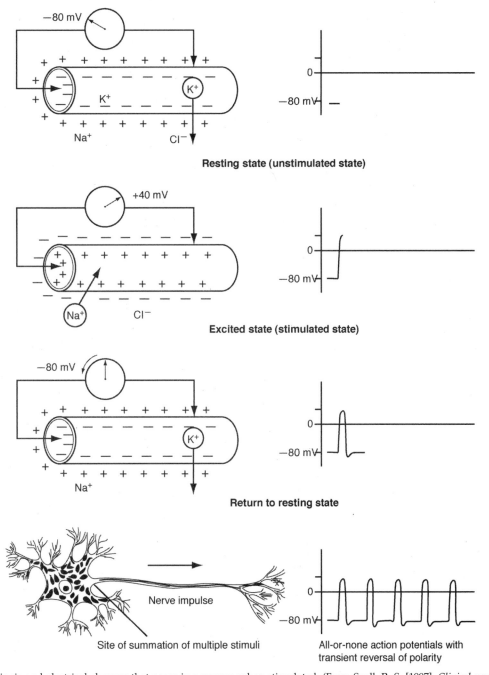

Figure 5–2 • The ionic and electrical changes that occur in a neuron when stimulated. (From Snell, R. S. [1997]. *Clinical neuroanatomy for medical students* [4th ed.]. Philadelphia: Lippincott Williams & Wilkins.)

Neurotransmitters

Chemical substances found in the CNS that excite, inhibit, or modify the response of another cerebral cell or cells are called **neurotransmitters.** The presynaptic terminals of one neuron release the chemical that affects particular postsynaptic cells of another neuron. Generally, each neuron releases the same transmitter at all of its separate terminals. Over 30 neurotransmitters have been identified. They include specific **amines** (acetylcholine, serotonin), **catecholamines** (dopamine, epinephrine, and norepinephrine), **amino acids** (γ-aminobutyric acid [GABA], glutamic acid, glycine, and substance P), and **polypeptides** (endorphins

and enkephalins). Table 5-2 summarizes the major neurotransmitters.

Postsynaptic Membrane—Excitation and Inhibition

The postsynaptic membrane (the dendrite cell body region of the effector neuron) initiates its response to stimuli by decremental conduction through the synapse; that is, the impulse becomes progressively weaker during more prolonged periods of excitation. Stimulation of the effector cell at the dendrite cell body can create an action potential. For

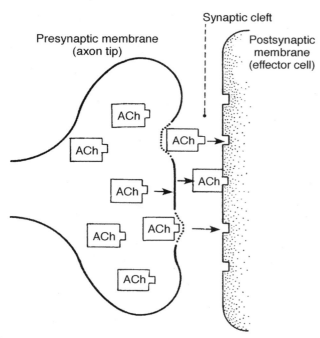

Figure 5–3 • Conduction at synapses. Diagram shows the release of a neurotransmitter (in this case acetylcholine [Ach]) from the presynaptic membrane [axon tip]) into the synaptic cleft, where it bonds to the receptor sites of the postsynaptic membrane (effector cell). (From DeMyer, W. [1998]. *Neuroanatomy* [2nd ed.]. Baltimore: Williams & Wilkins.)

the action potential to be fired, however, the intensity of an impulse must be sufficient to fire the initial segment of axon (just distal to the axon hillock), where the action potential is initiated. It is said that any factor that increases the potential inside the cell body at any given point also increases the potential throughout the cell body.

Because of differences in the cell membrane and shape of the cell, the intracellular voltage necessary to elicit an action potential will vary at different points on the cell membrane. The most sensitive point is the initial segment of the axon, but the impulse must be of sufficient magnitude to depolarize the axon. **Excitation** is the response of the subsynaptic membrane to the neurotransmitter substance that lowers the membrane potential to form an **excitatory postsynaptic potential** (EPSP). The potential is a small depolarization that conducts itself by decrement. The cell membrane is made more permeable to sodium, potassium, and chloride. Sodium ions rush into the neuron, whereas potassium ions leave the cell through the postsynaptic membrane.

Inhibition acts on a cell so that it is more difficult for it to fire. The inhibitory neurotransmitters increase permeability to only potassium and chloride ions at the synaptic membrane. The membrane potential is raised to form the **inhibitory postsynaptic potential** (IPSP).

Presynaptic Inhibition

Another type of inhibition, **presynaptic inhibition,** results from inhibitory knobs being activated on the presynaptic terminal fibrils and synaptic knobs of an axon. When the inhibitory knobs are activated, they secrete a neurotransmit-

ter substance that partially depolarizes the terminal fibrils and excitatory synaptic knobs. As a result, the velocity of the action potential that occurs at the membrane of the excitatory knob is depressed. This action greatly reduces the quantity of excitatory neurotransmitter released by the knob and suppresses the degree of excitation of the neuron.

FUNCTIONS AND DIVISIONS OF THE NERVOUS SYSTEM

The nervous system controls the motor, sensory, autonomic, cognitive, and behavioral functions of the body. It is divided into a hierarchy with three major functional units:

- Spinal cord level—the lowest functional level; controls automatic motor responses, such as reflexes
- Brain stem and subcortical level—the second functional level; controls blood pressure, respirations, equilibrium, and primitive emotions
- Cortical level—the highest level; responsible for cognition (storage of information, thinking, memory, and abstraction)

The nervous system is also divided into the CNS and the PNS. The CNS is composed of the brain and spinal cord. The PNS includes the 12 pairs of cranial nerves (CNs), the 31 pairs of spinal nerves; and the autonomic nervous system, which subdivides into the sympathetic and parasympathetic nervous systems.

CRANIAL AND SPINAL BONES

The purpose of the skull and vertebral column is to protect the most vulnerable parts of the nervous system—the brain and spinal cord.

Skull

The **skull** is the bony framework of the head; it is composed of the eight bones of the cranium and the 14 bones of the face. Knowledge of the anatomy of both the external and internal surfaces of the bones (Figs. 5-4 and 5-5) is helpful in understanding the pathophysiology of craniocerebral trauma.

The **cranium** is defined as that part of the skull that encloses the brain and provides a protective vault for this vital organ. The bones that compose the cranium are the frontal, occipital, sphenoid, and ethmoid, as well as the two parietal and temporal bones.

The **frontal bone** forms the forehead and the front (anterior) part of the top of the skull. The supraorbital arches form the roofs of the two orbits. Frontal sinuses are also located in this bone. The inner table of the frontal bone has a highly irregular bony surface.

The **occipital bone** is the large bone at the back (posterior) of the skull that curves into the base of the skull. The significant markings include the large hole (foramen mag-

▌▌▌ **Table 5-2** • NEUROTRANSMITTERS: SOURCE AND ACTION

NAME	SECRETION SOURCE	ACTION
Amines		
Acetylcholine (ACh) First neurotransmitter identified	Neurons in many areas of brain Large pyramidal cells (motor cortex)	Usually excitatory Inhibitory effect on some of parasympathetic nervous system (e.g., heart by vagus)
Chief transmitter of parasympathetic nervous system (NS)	Some cells of basal ganglia Motor neurons that innervate skeletal muscles Preganglionic neurons of autonomic NS Postganglionic neurons of parasympathetic NS Postganglionic neurons of sympathetic NS	
Serotonin (5-HT) Controls body heat, hunger, behavior, and sleep	Nuclei originating in the median raphe of brain stem and projecting to many areas (especially the dorsal horns of the spinal cord and hypothalamus)	Inhibitor of pain pathway cord; helps to control mood and sleep
Catecholamines		
Dopamine (DA) Affects control of behavior and fine movement	Neurons on the substantia nigra; many neurons of the substantia nigra send fibers to the basal ganglia that are involved in coordination of skeletal muscle activity	Usually inhibitory
Norepinephrine (NE) Chief transmitter of sympathetic nervous system	Many neurons whose cell bodies are located: In brain stem and hypothalamus (controlling overall activity and mood) Most postganglionic neurons of sympathetic NS	Usually excitatory, although sometimes inhibitory Some excitatory and some inhibitory
Amino Acids		
Gamma-aminobutyric acid (GABA)	Nerve terminals of the spinal cord, cerebellum, basal ganglia, and some cortical areas	Excitatory
Glutamic acid	Presynaptic terminals in many sensory pathways; cerebellum mossy fibers	Excitatory
Glycine	Synapses in spinal cord	Inhibitory
Substance P	Pain fiber terminals in the dorsal horns of the spinal cord; also, the basal ganglia and hypothalamus	Excitatory
Polypeptides		
Enkephalin	Nerve terminals in the spinal cord, brain stem, thalamus, and hypothalamus	Excitatory to systems that inhibit pain; binds to the same receptors in the CNS that bind opiate drugs
Endorphin	Pituitary gland and areas of the brain	Binds to opiate receptors in the brain and pituitary gland; excitatory to systems that inhibit pain

NS = nervous system; ANS = autonomic nervous system; CNS = central nervous system.

num) in the base of the skull and also the occipital condyles located on either side of the foramen magnum that fit into depressions on the first cervical vertebra.

The **sphenoid bone** is a wedge-shaped bone thought to resemble a bat's wings. The significant bone markings include a body, lesser wings, greater wings, pterygoid process, the sella turcica (Latin for "Turk's saddle"), and the clivus. The **clivus** is the slanted dorsal surface of the body of the sphenoid bone between the sella turcica and basilar process of the sphenoid bone. The hypophysis (pituitary gland) is located in the region of the sella turcica.

The **ethmoid bone,** largely hidden between the two orbits, contains both perpendicular and horizontal plates as well as two lateral masses. The horizontal plate, also called the cribriform plate, forms part of the base of the skull through which the olfactory nerves (first CNs) travel. The perpendicular plate forms part of the nasal septum, whereas the lateral masses are part of the ethmoid sinuses.

The **temporal bones** are situated at the sides and base of the skull and consist of three anatomic divisions: the squamous, mastoid, and petrous portions. The temporal bone is highly irregular, both on the internal and external surfaces.

The **squamous portion** is very thin just above the auditory meatus. It contains the zygomatic process externally; internally, there are numerous eminences and depressions to accommodate the contour of the cerebrum. Two well-marked internal grooves are evident for the branches of the middle meningeal artery, a common point of trauma with head injury.

The **mastoid portion** is perforated by many foramina, including a larger foramen, the mastoid foramen, which contains a vein that drains the lateral sinus and a small artery to supply the dura mater. The mastoid process is also contained in this portion of the temporal bone.

The **petrous portion** is so named because it is extremely dense and stone-like in its hardness. There is a pyramidal process that is directed inward and is wedged at the base of the skull between the sphenoid and occipital bones. The internal plate of the petrous portion of the temporal bone is proximal to the branches of the middle meningeal artery.

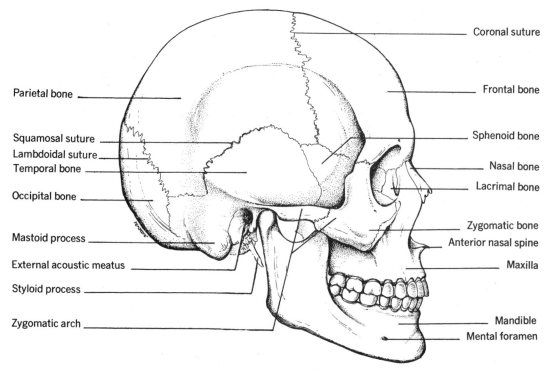

Parietal bone

Squamosal suture
Lambdoidal suture
Temporal bone

Occipital bone

Mastoid process

External acoustic meatus

Styloid process

Zygomatic arch

Coronal suture

Frontal bone

Sphenoid bone

Nasal bone
Lacrimal bone

Zygomatic bone
Anterior nasal spine

Maxilla

Mandible
Mental foramen

Figure 5–4 • Lateral view of the skull.

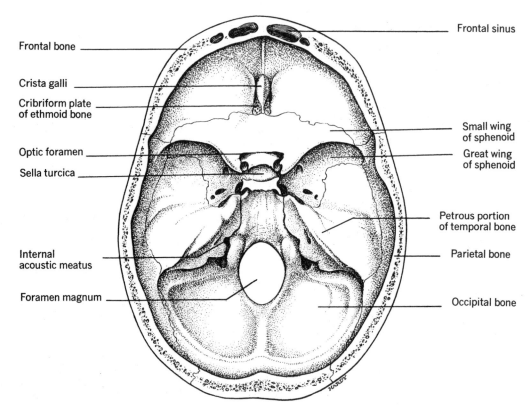

Frontal bone

Crista galli

Cribriform plate
of ethmoid bone

Optic foramen

Sella turcica

Internal
acoustic meatus

Foramen magnum

Frontal sinus

Small wing
of sphenoid

Great wing
of sphenoid

Petrous portion
of temporal bone

Parietal bone

Occipital bone

Figure 5–5 • View of the base of the skull from above, showing the internal surfaces of some of the cranial bones.

The **parietal bones,** which fuse on the top of the skull, form the sides of the skull. Externally, they are smooth and convex; internally, the surface is concave with some depressions to accommodate the convolutions of the cerebrum and the grooves for the middle meningeal artery. With these exceptions, the bone has a regular inner surface.

SUTURES OF THE SKULL

The bones of the skull join at various places, known as suture lines. The four major sutures of the skull include the following (see Fig. 5-4):

Sagittal suture – the midline suture formed by the two parietal bones joining on the top of the skull

Coronal suture (frontoparietal) – connecting the frontal and parietal bones transversely

Lambdoidal suture (occipitoparietal) – connecting the occipital and parietal bones

Basilar suture – created by the junction of the basilar surface of the occipital bone with the posterior surface of the sphenoid bone

SPINE

The spine is a flexible column formed by a series of bones called **vertebrae,** each stacked one on another to support the head and trunk. The vertebral column is made up of 33 vertebrae: 7 cervical vertebrae, 12 thoracic or dorsal vertebrae, 5 lumbar vertebrae, 5 sacral vertebrae (fused into one), and 4 coccygeal vertebrae (fused into one) (Fig. 5-6). Each vertebra consists of two essential parts, an anterior solid segment or **body,** and a posterior segment or **arch.** Two **pedicles** and two **laminae** supporting seven processes (four articular, two transverse, and one spinous) make up the arch (Fig. 5-7).

The cervical vertebrae are smaller than those in any other region of the spine. The first cervical vertebra is called the **atlas,** whereas the second cervical vertebra is known as the **axis.** Each of these two vertebrae has a unique appearance. The axis has a perpendicular projection called the **odontoid process** on which the atlas sits (Fig. 5-8).

The thoracic or dorsal vertebrae are intermediate in size, becoming larger as they descend the vertebral column. The lumbar vertebrae are the largest segments in the spine (see Fig. 5-7).

The vertebral bodies are the largest part of the vertebrae, above and below which flattened surfaces are found for attachment of fibrocartilage. There are apertures for spinal nerves, veins, and arteries. The vertebrae are connected by means of the articular processes and the intervertebral fibrocartilage.

The arch of the vertebrae is composed of two pedicles, two laminae, a spinous process, four articular processes, and two transverse processes. The two **pedicles** are short, thick pieces of bone. The concavity above and below the

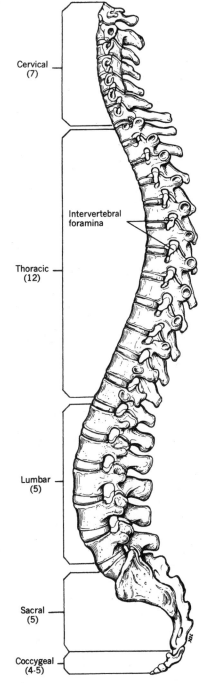

Figure 5–6 • Lateral view of the adult vertebral column.

pedicles creates the intervertebral notches from which the spinal nerves emanate. The two **laminae** are broad plates of bone. They complete the neural arch by fusing in the midline and enclose the spinal foramen, which protects the spinal cord. The upper and lower borders are rough in order to allow for the attachment of the ligamenta subflava. The **spinous process** projects backward from the laminae and serves as the attachment for muscles and ligaments. The four **articular processes** (two on either side) provide stability for the spine. The two **transverse processes** provide stability for the spine and serve as points of attachment for muscles and ligaments.

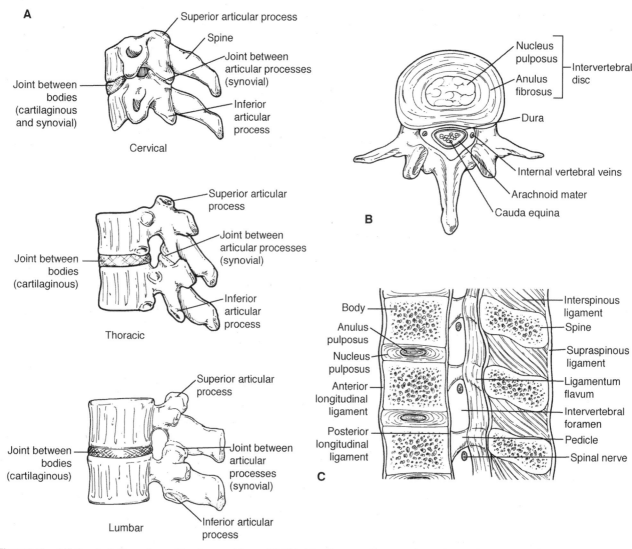

Figure 5–7 • (A) Cervical, thoracic, and lumbar vertebrae. (B) Third lumbar vertebra seen from above, showing the relationship between the intervertebral disc and the cauda equina. (C) Sagittal section through three lumbar vertebrae, showing the ligaments and the intervertebral discs.

LIGAMENTS OF THE SPINE

The most important ligaments of the vertebral column are the anterior and posterior longitudinal ligaments and the ligamenta flava (see Fig. 5-7). The **anterior longitudinal ligament** consists of longitudinal fibers firmly attached to the anterior surface of the vertebral bodies and intervertebral discs. The **posterior longitudinal ligament** is attached to the posterior surface of the vertebral bodies within the spinal canal. The **ligamentum flavum** consists of yellow elastic fibers that connect the laminae of adjacent vertebrae. The attachment pattern is unique in that the attachment is from the lower margin of the anterior surface of the superior lamina to the posterior surface of the upper margin of the inferior lamina.

The **supraspinous ligament** joins the spinous process tips from C7 to the sacrum. The **interspinous ligaments** connect adjacent spinous processes from their tips to their roots. The interspinals fuse with the supraspinals posteriorly and with the ligamentum flavum anteriorly.

Such an arrangement controls vertebral movement to prevent excessive flexion. If violent force in any direction occurs, these ligaments can be ruptured, possibly causing injury to the vertebrae and spinal cord (see Chaps. 19 and 20).

INTERVERTEBRAL DISCS

The **intervertebral discs** are fibrocartilaginous disc-shaped structures located between the vertebral bodies from the second cervical vertebra to the sacrum. They vary in size, thickness, and shape at different levels of the spine. The purpose of the intervertebral disc is to cushion movement. The central core, the **nucleus pulposus,** is surrounded by a fibrous capsule called the **annulus fibrosus.** As a result of aging and trauma, discs lose their water content and the tissue is more prone to injury.

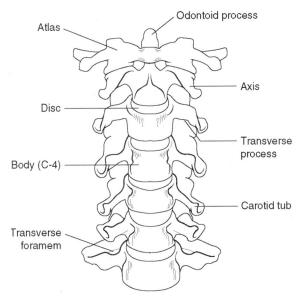

Figure 5–8 • The cervical spine. Note odontoid process of C2 and the atlas, C1, positioned on top of C2.

⦀ MENINGES

Meninges cover both the brain and spinal cord. The layers, from the outermost layer inward, are called the **dura mater,** the **arachnoid,** and the **pia mater** (Fig. 5-9).

The **dura mater** is a double-layer, whitish, inelastic, fibrous membrane that lines the interior of the skull. The outer layer of the dura is actually the periosteum of the bone. The inner layer is the thick membrane that extends throughout the skull and creates compartments. The dura lines various foraminae that exit at the base of the skull. Sheaths for the nerves passing through these foraminae are also formed by the dura.

Four folds of dura (Fig. 5-10) are situated within the skull cavity to support and protect the brain. They include the following:

Falx cerebri, a double fold of dura, descends vertically into the longitudinal fissure between the two hemispheres of the brain and partially divides the frontal lobe into a left and right side.

Tentorium cerebelli is a tent-like double fold of dura that covers the upper surface of the cerebellum, supports the occipital lobes, and prevents them from pressing on the cerebellum. The falx cerebri attaches midline to the tentorium. (The tentorium is an important anatomic point to note. The area above the tentorium is termed **supratentorial,** whereas the area below it is called **infratentorial.** The nursing care given differs based on these two classifications, as discussed in Chap. 18.) In addition, the opening in the tentorium from which the brain stem emerges is called the tentorial notch. Herniation through this opening is called uncal herniation.

Falx cerebelli is found between the two lateral lobes of the cerebellum.

Diaphragma sella is a horizontal process that forms a small circular fold, thus creating a roof for the sella turcica.

The spinal dura is a continuation of the inner layer of the cerebral dura. The outer layer of the dura terminates at the foramen magnum, where it is replaced by the periosteal lining of the vertebral canal. The spinal dura encases the spinal roots, spinal ganglia, and spinal nerves. The spinal dural sac terminates at the second or third sacral level.

The second meningeal layer, the **arachnoid membrane,** is an extremely thin, delicate layer that loosely encloses the brain. The subdural space separates the dura mater from the arachnoid layer. Bleeding within this space (subdural hemorrhage) can occur with head injury. The subarachnoid space is not really a clear space because there is much spongy, delicate connective tissue between the arachnoid and pia mater layers. CSF flows in the subarachnoid space. The cisternum magnum is a space between the hemispheres of the cerebellum and the medulla oblongata. The arachnoid layer of the spinal meninges is a continuation of the cerebral arachnoid (see Fig. 5-9). The arachnoid is a delicate, gossamer network of fine, elastic, fibrous tissue; it also contains blood vessels of varying sizes, which may be damaged by lumbar or cisternal puncture, resulting in hemorrhage.

The innermost layer of the meninges is called the **pia mater.** It is a mesh-like, vascular membrane that derives its blood supply from the internal carotid and vertebral arteries. The pia mater covers the entire surface of the brain, dipping down between the convolutions of the surface. Because the pia covers the gray matter, vascularity increases and minute perpendicular vessels extend for some distance into the cerebrum. The pia mater of the spinal cord is thicker, firmer, and less vascular than that of the brain.

Spaces of the Meninges

Three spaces located within the meninges are important to note. The **epidural** or **extradural space** is a potential space located between the skull and outer layer of the dura layer of the brain. In the vertebral column, the epidural space is between the periosteum and the single dural layer. The **subdural space** is between the inner dura mater and arachnoid layer. This is a narrow space and is the site of subdural hemorrhage with certain injuries. The third space is the **subarachnoid space,** which is between the arachnoid and pia mater layers and contains CSF.

⦀ CEREBROSPINAL FLUID

Cerebrospinal fluid is normally a clear, colorless, odorless solution that fills the ventricles of the brain and the subarachnoid space of the brain and spinal cord. The purpose of CSF is to act as a shock absorber, cushioning the brain and spinal cord against injury caused by movement. The specific gravity of CSF is 1.007 (see Chart 6-2 in Chap. 6 for CSF normal values). CSF differs from other extracellular fluids in the percentage of composition of various factors. It is composed of water, a small amount of protein, oxygen, and carbon dioxide. The electrolytes—so-

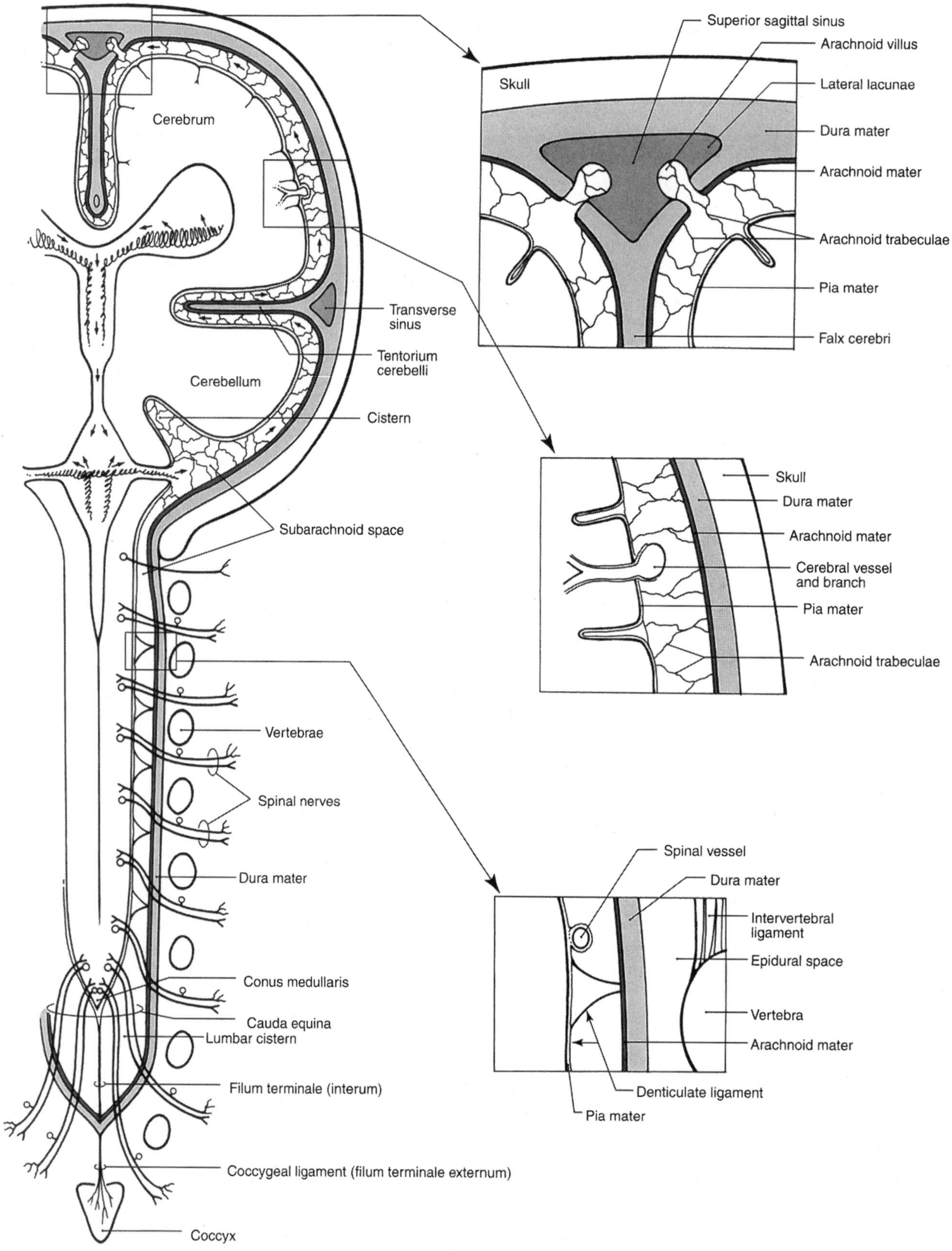

Figure 5–9 • The central nervous system and its associated meninges. The *top right box* shows the superior sagittal sinus and arachnoid villi. Arachnoid villi remove CSF from the ventricles and deposit the CSF into the venous circulation. The *middle right box* shows the layers of tissue from the skull through the three layers of the meninges. The *bottom right box* shows the layers of spinal meninges. (From Haines, D. E. [2000]. *Neuroanatomy: An atlas of structures, sections, and systems* [5th ed.]. Philadelphia: Lippincott Williams & Wilkins.)

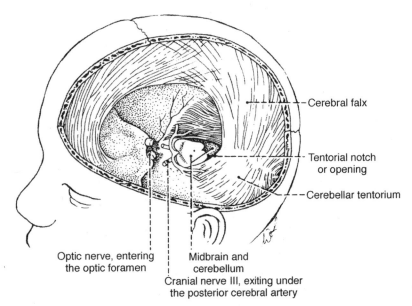

Figure 5-10 • Cranial dura mater folds. With the skull and cerebral hemisphere removed, the falx cerebri and the tentorium cerebelli are shown. Note that cranial nerve III (oculomotor nerve) exits under the posterior cerebral artery. With lateral transtentorial herniation, the oculomotor nerve may be caught between the tentorium and posterior cerebral artery, resulting in dilation of the pupil. (From DeMyer, W. [1998]. *Neuroanatomy* [2nd ed.]. Baltimore: Williams & Wilkins.)

dium, potassium, and chloride and glucose, an important cerebral nutrient—are also present. An occasional lymphocyte may be present. Normally, CSF pressure is in the range of 60 to 180 mm of water pressure in the lateral recumbent position, which is the position assumed for a lumbar puncture. With the patient in the sitting position, a normal lumbar puncture will register 200 to 350 mm of water pressure. Fluctuation in pressure occurs in response to the cardiac cycle and respirations. The amount of CSF in adults is approximately 125 to 150 mL.

FORMATION OF CEREBROSPINAL FLUID

Cerebrospinal fluid, which is produced by active transport and diffusion, is formed from three different sources. The major source of CSF is the secretions from the choroid plexus, a cauliflower-like structure located in portions of the lateral, third, and fourth ventricles (Fig. 5-11). The **choroid plexus** is a collection of blood vessels covered with a thin coating of ependymal cells. CSF is constantly secreted from these surfaces. It is estimated that the amount of CSF produced daily by the choroid plexus is about 500 mL, or 25 mL per hour. A lesser proportion of CSF is secreted from the second source, the ependymal cells, which line the ventricles and blood vessels of the meninges. Finally, CSF is also produced by the blood vessels of the brain and spinal cord. The amount produced from this source is small.

Ventricular System

The two **lateral ventricles,** one on either side of the midline, are located in the lower and inner parts of the cerebral hemisphere. Each lateral ventricle consists of a **central cavity** or **body** and three **horns.** The central cavity is located in the

lower part of the parietal lobe. The **anterior horn** curves forward and outward into the frontal lobe; the **posterior horn** curves backward and inward into the occipital lobe; and the **middle or lateral horn** descends into the temporal lobe. The curved corpus callosum forms the undersurface of the central cavity and the roof of the anterior, middle, and posterior horns.

The singular **third ventricle** is a midline inner brain–cavity structure. The two optic thalami form the side walls. The floor is formed by the tuber cinereum (infundibulum, pituitary), corpora albicantia, and crus cerebri. The ventricle is bounded by the fornix in the front and

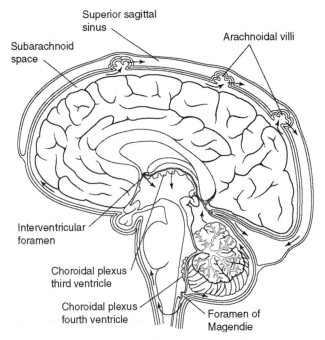

Figure 5–11 • Diagram of the flow of cerebrospinal fluid from the time of its formation from blood in the choroid plexuses until its return to the blood in the superior sagittal sinus.

pineal body in the back. The singular, diamond-shaped **fourth ventricle** is laterally bounded by the pons and the superior cerebellar peduncles. The roof is formed by the superior cerebellar peduncles and medulla. The floor of the fourth ventricle is continuous with the central spinal canal.

Flow of Cerebrospinal Fluid

Cerebrospinal fluid circulation has been termed the "third circulation." It is a closed system. Fluid formed by choroid plexuses in the two lateral ventricles passes into the third ventricle by way of the two foramina of Monro. The single cerebral aqueduct or aqueduct of Sylvius connects the third and fourth ventricles. CSF flows through the two lateral foramina of Luschka and midline through the foramen of Magendie to the cisternal magnum. At this point, the CSF enters the subarachnoid space. The foramen of Magendie allows CSF to circulate around the cord, whereas the foramen of Luschka directs the CSF around the brain (Fig. 5-12).

Expanded areas of the subarachnoid space are called **cisterns.** CSF may be aspirated from some of these areas for analysis. The major cisterns are the **cisterna magnum,** between the medulla and cerebellar region, and the **lumbar cistern,** between vertebrae L-2 and S-2.

Cerebrospinal Fluid Absorption

Most of the CSF produced daily is reabsorbed into the **arachnoid villi,** which are projections from the subarachnoid space into the venous sinuses of the brain (see Fig. 5-11). CSF drains into the superior sagittal sinus. Arachnoid villi are very permeable and allow CSF, including protein molecules, to exit easily from the subarachnoid space into the venous sinuses. CSF flows in one direction through the arachnoid villi (most of which are located in the subarachnoid space of the cerebrum), which have been compared with pressure-sensitive valves. When CSF pressure is greater than venous pressure, CSF leaves the subarachnoid space. As pressures are equalized, the valves close.

CEREBROVASCULAR CIRCULATION

The blood vessels that supply the nervous system form an extensive capillary bed, particularly in the gray matter of the brain. About **20% of the oxygen** consumed by the body is used for the oxidation of glucose to provide energy. The brain is totally dependent on glucose for its metabolism. A lack of oxygen to the brain for 5 minutes can result in irreversible brain damage.

The brain receives **approximately 750 mL/min of blood, or 15% to 20% of the total resting cardiac output.** These figures remain relatively constant because of various control systems affecting the brain. Blood flow rates to specific areas of the brain correlate directly to the metabolism of the cerebral tissue. The brain is supplied by two pairs of arteries: the **two internal carotid arteries** and the **two vertebral arteries.** Cerebral circulation is also divided into the anterior and the posterior circulation. The **anterior circulation** refers to the common carotids and their distal branches including the internal carotid arteries, the middle cerebral arteries, and the anterior cerebral arteries. The **posterior circulation** refers to the vertebral arteries, the basilar artery, and the posterior arteries.

Internal Carotid Arteries

The internal carotid arteries originate from two different vessels: the **left common carotid,** which originates directly from the aorta; and the **right common carotid,** which arises from the **innominate artery** also originating from the aorta. The common carotids branch to form the external and internal carotid arteries. The external carotid artery supplies the face, scalp, and other extracranial structures. The internal carotid artery enters the cranial vault through the foramen lacerum in the floor of the middle cranial fossa. As the internal carotid passes through the bone and dura at the base of the skull and approaches the upper brain, it passes forward through the cavernous sinus just lateral to the pituitary fossa. It curves sharply several times and roughly forms an "S," called the **carotid siphon** (Fig 5-13). Most of the hemispheres, excluding the occipitals, the basal ganglia, and the upper two thirds of the diencephalon, are supplied by the internal carotid arteries (Fig. 5-14).

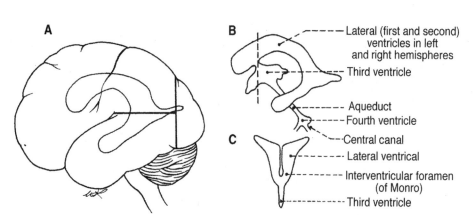

Figure 5–12 • The cerebral ventricles. (*A*) Lateral aspect of the left cerebral hemisphere showing the contour of the lateral ventricles and their relation to the cerebral lobes. (*B*) Lateral outline of the four ventricles. (*C*) Frontal (coronal) section of the lateral and third ventricles at the level of the dotted line (*B*), showing their communicating interventricular foramen. (From DeMyer, W. [1998]. *Neuroanatomy* [2nd ed.]. Baltimore: Williams & Wilkins.)

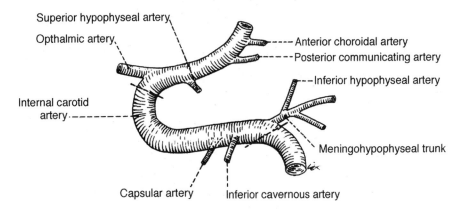

Superior hypophyseal artery

Opthalmic artery

Anterior choroidal artery

Posterior communicating artery

Inferior hypophyseal artery

Internal carotid artery

Meningohypophyseal trunk

Capsular artery

Inferior cavernous artery

Figure 5–13 • Lateral view of the left carotid artery at the siphon or parasellar region. The *lower interrupted line* is where the carotid artery enters the cavernous sinus, and the *upper interrupted line* is where it exits. (From DeMyer, W. [1998]. *Neuroanatomy* [2nd ed.]. Baltimore: Williams & Wilkins.)

The first intracranial branch from the internal carotid artery is the ophthalmic artery. The terminal branches of each carotid include the posterior communicating artery, the anterior cerebral artery, and the middle cerebral artery. Table 5-3 summarizes the major branches of the carotid arteries and the areas supplied (also see Fig. 5-4).

CHARACTERISTICS OF THE CEREBRAL CIRCULATION

The following lists the outstanding characteristics of cerebral circulation:

Cerebral arteries have thinner walls than arteries of comparable size in other parts of the body. Cerebral arteries have an internal elastic tissue and scanty smooth muscle.

The veins (other than sinuses) have even thinner walls in proportion to their size and lack a muscle layer.

The veins and sinuses have **no** valves.

The venous return does not retrace the course of corresponding arteries but follows a pattern of its own.

The dural sinuses are unique to cerebral circulation.

The distribution of the arteries with rich surfaces (arteries anastomosed by localized "end-artery" distribution of branches penetrating the nervous tissue) is distinctive.

Vertebral Arteries

The **vertebral arteries,** originating from the **subclavian arteries,** enter the skull through the foramen magnum, ventrolateral to the spinal cord. The two vertebral arteries unite at the level of the pons to become the singular **basilar artery** (Fig. 5-15). The basilar artery subdivides into the two posterior cerebral arteries that supply part of the cerebrum (Fig. 5-16).

In general, the vertebral arteries and their branches supply the cerebellum, the brainstem, the spinal cord, the occipital lobes, the medial and inferior surfaces of the temporal lobes, and the posterior diencephalon.

Before they begin to supply blood to the brain, the vertebral arteries give off recurrent branches that anastomose with the anterior and posterior spinal arteries and with a posterior meningeal branch. In its intracranial course, the vertebral arteries give rise to direct bulbar arteries to the medulla, the anterior spinal artery, the **posterior inferior cerebellar artery (PICA),** sometimes the posterior spinal artery, and small branches to the basal meninges. The first branch off the basilar artery is the **anterior inferior cerebellar artery (AICA).** The basilar artery is also the origin of the pontine arteries, the internal auditory arteries, the superior cerebellar arteries, and the posterior cerebral arteries. Table 5-4 summarizes the major branches of the vertebral arteries and the areas supplied.

Circle of Willis

The circle of Willis, which is located at the base of the skull, is divided into anterior (carotid portion) and posterior (vertebrobasilar portion) circulation (see Fig. 5-15). The composition of each portion includes these elements:

• Middle cerebral arteries, the anterior cerebral arteries, and the anterior communicating artery, which connects the two anterior cerebral arteries
• Two posterior cerebral arteries; two posterior communicating arteries connect the middle cerebral arteries with the posterior cerebral arteries, thus uniting the internal carotid system with the vertebral-basilar system

The circle of Willis encloses a very small area that is little more than 1 inch square, or about the size of a quarter. Functionally, the carotid circulation and the posterior circulation usually remain separate. At one time, the circle of Willis was thought to be a protective mechanism by which blood was shunted to compensate for alterations in cerebral blood flow or pressure. However, collateral circulation through the circle depends on the patency of its components. The vessels of the circle of Willis, particularly the communicating arteries, may be anomalous. Nevertheless, in *favorable instances,* the circle does permit an adequate blood supply to reach all parts of the brain, even after one or more of the four supplying vessels has been ligated.

Venous Drainage

Unlike venous drainage in other parts of the body, which closely follows an arterial pattern, cerebral venous drainage is chiefly managed by vascular channels created by the two dural

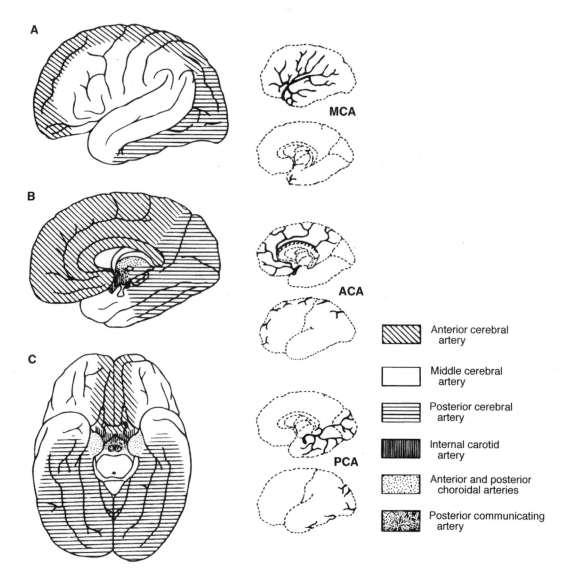

Figure 5–14 • Surface distribution of the anterior, middle, and posterior cerebral arteries. (*A*) Lateral view of the left cerebral hemisphere. (*B*) Medial view of the left cerebral hemisphere. (*C*) Ventral view of the cerebrum. ACA = anterior cerebral artery; MCA = middle cerebral artery; PCA = posterior cerebral artery. (From DeMyer, W. [1998]. *Neuroanatomy* [2nd ed.]. Baltimore: Williams & Wilkins.)

layers called **dural sinuses.** There are no valves in dural sinuses. A few dural sinuses deserve mention; these are included in Table 5-5 along with the areas they supply (Fig. 5-17). **Emissary veins** join extracranial veins with the venous sinuses. **Bridging veins** connect the brain and dural sinuses and are often the cause of subdural hemorrhage. Cerebral veins empty into the dural sinuses which, in turn, empty into the **jugular veins,** which return the blood to the heart.

Meningeal Blood Supply

The meninges are supplied with arterial blood by the anterior, middle, and posterior meningeal arteries. The main route for the arterial supply of the dura mater is through the middle meningeal branches of the external carotid artery. Each vessel ascends through a foramen in the base of the skull and is then situated between the dura mater and the skull. These vessels may be torn as a result of a head injury, thereby causing an epidural hematoma, which requires immediate medical attention.

Blood Supply to the Spinal Cord, Spinal Roots, and Spinal Nerves

The upper cervical cord receives its arterial blood supply from the vertebral arteries through recurrent branches. Below this region, the spinal cord receives its arterial blood supply, in part, from the anterior spinal artery and the two posterior spinal arteries, which arise from the vertebral arteries. The **anterior spinal artery** runs the full length of the cord midventrally, whereas the two **posterior spinal arteries** run full length along each row of the dorsal roots. As these three vessels pass down the cord, they receive feeders from deep cervical, intercostal, lumbar, and sacral arteries. Addi-

Table 5-3 • MAJOR INTERNAL CAROTID ARTERIAL BRANCHES AND THE CEREBRAL AREAS THEY INNERVATE

ARTERY	AREA SUPPLIED
Ophthalmic	Orbits and optic nerves
Posterior communicating (Pcom)	Connects the carotid circulation with the vertebrobasilar circulation
Anterior choroidal	Part of choroid plexuses of lateral ventricles; hippocampal formation; portions of globus pallidus; part of internal capsule; part of amygdaloid nucleus; part of caudate nucleus; part of putamen
Anterior cerebral (ACA)	Medial surfaces of frontal and parietal lobes; part of cingulate gyrus and "leg area" of precentral gyrus
Recurrent artery of Heubner	Special branch of ACA, penetrates the anterior perforated substance to supply part of basal ganglia and genu of internal capsule (also called medial striate artery)
Middle cerebral (MCA) (has several branches)	Entire lateral surfaces of the hemisphere except for the occipital pole and the inferolateral surface of the hemisphere (supplied by posterior cerebral artery)
Lenticulostriate (from MCA)	Part of basal ganglia and internal capsule
Anterior communicating (Acom)	Connects the two ACAs

tional blood supply comes from **radicular arteries** (which supply blood to only one nerve root) and **radiculospinal arteries** (supply blood to about six spinal cord segments). The large **artery of Adamkiewicz** originates from the aorta and enters the cord at about the second lumbar (L2) ventral root level (range, T10 to L2) and supplies most of the caudal third of the cord.

The venous system of the spine includes an intradural and extradural system. The intradural veins follow the pattern of the arteries, whereas the extradural intravertebral veins form a plexus extending from the cranium to the pelvis and having many communications along the way with veins of the neck, thorax, and abdomen.

▌ BLOOD–BRAIN BARRIER

For the CNS to function normally, a very stable environment must be maintained within that body system. The so-called blood–brain barrier (BBB) is a descriptive term for the network of endothelial cells (cells that compose the walls of capillaries) and the projections from the astrocytes located in close proximity to the neuron. Astrocytes are large stellate cells with numerous radiating cytoplasmic processes. Extensions of astrocytes called **perivascular feet** surround the brain capillaries.

Capillaries in the brain, unlike those in other areas, do not have pores between adjacent endothelial cells. Therefore, the brain cannot derive molecules from blood plasma by a non-specific filtering process. Instead, molecules within cerebral capillaries are transported through the endothelial cells by active transport, endocytosis, and exocytosis. This creates a highly selective BBB that guards the entrance into neurons. Before molecules in the blood can enter neurons in the CNS, they pass through both the capillary endothelial cells and the astrocytes. The tight junctions between the endothelial cells and the astrocytes are largely responsible for the BBB. Because of this barrier, most drugs are prevented from affecting the brain and spinal cord.

The movement of substances into the brain depends on particle size, lipid solubility, chemical dissociation, and the protein-binding potential of the drug. In general, drugs that are lipid soluble and undissociated at body pH rapidly enter both the brain and the CSF. When compared with other body organs, the CNS is very slow in its uptake of dyes and both organic and inorganic anions and cations (e.g., sodium, potassium, glutamic acid) from the circulating blood. The barrier is very permeable to water, oxygen, carbon dioxide, other gases, glucose, and lipid-soluble compounds.

▌ BRAIN (ENCEPHALON)

The brain constitutes approximately 2% of body weight. The average weight of the brain of a young male adult is about 1400 g. The brains of older people weigh less, with the average weight being about 1200 g.

The brain is divided into three major areas: the cerebrum, the brain stem, and the cerebellum (Fig. 5-18). The **cerebrum** is composed of the cerebral hemispheres, thalamus, hypothalamus, and the basal ganglia. In addition, the olfactory and optic nerves (CNs I and II) are located in the cerebrum. The **brain stem** includes the midbrain, pons, and medulla. The midbrain, which contains the cerebral peduncles and corpus quadrigemina, is a short segment between the hypothalamus and the pons.

Another means of subdividing the brain is by fossae. The **anterior fossa** contains the frontal lobes; the **middle fossa** contains the temporal, parietal, and occipital lobes; and the **posterior fossa** contains the brainstem and cerebellum.

Cerebrum

The cerebrum comprises **two cerebral hemispheres** that are incompletely separated by the great longitudinal fissure. A **fissure,** also called a **sulcus,** is a large, predictable separation in the cerebral hemisphere. The following are some important fissures that are landmarks in studying the gross anatomy of the brain:

- The **great longitudinal fissure** is a midsagittal fissure that separates the cerebral hemispheres into a left and right side. The hemispheres are joined at the bottom of the fissure by the corpus callosum.
- The **lateral fissure of Sylvius** separates the temporal lobe from the frontal and parietal lobes.
- The **central fissure of Rolando** separates the frontal lobe from the parietal lobe.

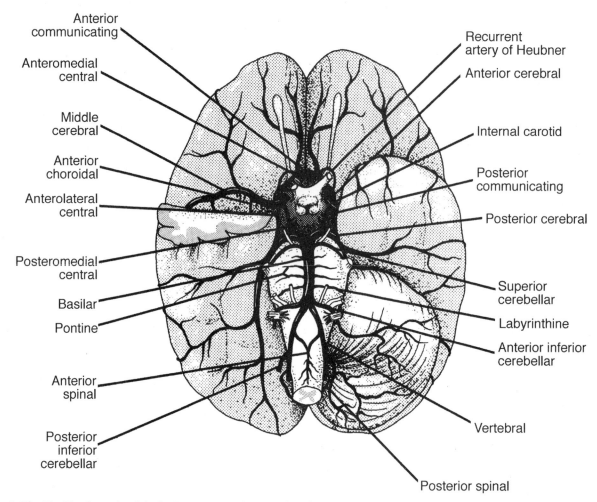

Figure 5–15 • The blood supply of the brain, as seen on the ventral surface. (The right cerebellar hemisphere and the tip of the right temporal lobe have been removed.) (From Barr, M. L., & Kiernan, J. A. [1993]. *The human nervous system* [6th ed.]. Philadelphia: J. B. Lippincott.)

The last major fissure is the **parieto-occipital fissure,** which separates the occipital lobe from the parietal and temporal lobes (Fig. 5-19).

The surface of the hemispheres consists of numerous "wrinkles," or **gyri** (also called **convolutions**). The gyri fold in on one another, thereby substantially increasing the surface area of the brain. Each hemisphere is covered by a cerebral cortex of gray matter that is 2 to 5 mm thick and contains billions of neurons.

Under the cerebral cortex is **white matter,** which serves as an association and projection pathway. The white matter of the cerebral hemispheres contains nerve fibers and neuroglia of various sizes. Three types of myelinated nerve fibers comprise the center of the hemisphere. They are the transverse fibers, the projection fibers, and the association fibers (Fig. 5-20).

- **Transverse (commissural) fibers** are tracts of fibers that interconnect corresponding parts of the *two* hemispheres. The **corpus callosum** is the largest commissure. It is an arch-shaped structure that crosses the great longitudinal fissure.
- **Projection fibers** connect the cerebral cortex with the lower portions of the brain and spinal cord.
- **Association fibers** connect various areas within the *same* hemisphere.

The cerebral hemispheres are composed of pairs of frontal, parietal, temporal, and occipital lobes. **Brodmann** is credited with mapping the cortical areas of the brain based on slight histologic differences of the cells. Almost 100 different areas of the cerebral cortex have been identified. This method of classification provides a basis for the discussion of functional areas of the brain (Figs. 5-21 and 5-22). The following are some Brodmann areas along with their functional classifications:

- **Area 4**—primary motor cortex or primary motor strip
- **Areas 1, 2, and 3**—primary somatic sensory areas
- **Areas 41 and 42**—primary receptive areas for sound
- **Area 17**—primary receptive area for vision

The primary sensory and motor areas perform highly specialized functions.

Other areas of the brain that do not perform primary functions are called **association areas.** Functions of the association areas are more general but nonetheless important. Functional loss of a sensory association area greatly reduces the ability of the brain to analyze characteristics of sensory experience. It should be mentioned that the cerebral cortex is closely associated, both anatomically and functionally, with the thalamus. Many afferent and efferent pathways connect

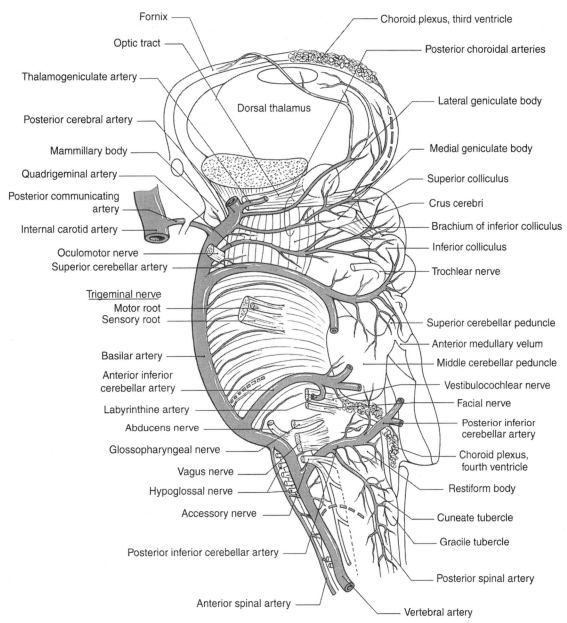

Figure 5–16 • The blood supply to the brainstem and thalamus, showing the relationship of structures and cranial nerves to arteries. (From Haines, D. E. [2000]. *Neuroanatomy: An atlas of structures, sections, and systems* [5th ed.]. Philadelphia: Lippincott Williams & Wilkins.)

with specific parts of the thalamus to perform various complex functions.

GENERAL FUNCTIONS OF THE CEREBRAL CORTEX ACCORDING TO LOBES

Frontal Lobe

The major functions of the frontal lobes are to:

- Perform high-level cognitive functions such as reasoning, abstraction, concentration, and executive control

- Provide for storage of information (memory)
- Control voluntary eye movement
- Influence somatic motor control of activities such as respirations, gastrointestinal activity, and blood pressure
- Motor control of speech in the dominant hemisphere (usually the left hemisphere)

The **motor cortex (area 4),** located anterior to the central fissure, contains giant Betz cells or pyramidal cells that control voluntary motor function. The various muscles are spatially arranged on the strip so that the feet are located in the area of the longitudinal fissure and the muscles of the face are located at the opposite end of the motor strip. Note the large area allocated to the hand (Fig. 5-23).

Areas 6 and **8** of the cortex are called **motor association areas,** or the premotor cortex. There is a connection be-

Table 5–4 • MAJOR VERTEBRAL ARTERIAL BRANCHES AND THE CEREBRAL AREAS THEY INNERVATE

ARTERY	AREA SUPPLIED
Vertebral Branches	
Anterior spinal (only one artery)	Anterior two thirds of spinal cord
Posterior spinals	Posterior one third of spinal cord
Posterior inferior cerebellar (PICA)	Undersurface of the cerebellum; medulla; and choroid plexuses of fourth ventricle
Basilar Artery Branches	
Posterior cerebral (PCA)	Occipital lobes, medial and inferior surfaces of the temporal lobes, midbrain, and choroid plexuses of third and lateral ventricle
Posterior choroidals (from PCA)	
Medial posterior choroidal	Tectum, choroid plexus of third ventricle, and superior and medial surfaces of the thalamus
Lateral posterior choroidal	Penetrating the choroidal fissure and anastomosing with branches of the anterior choroidal arteries
Anterior inferior cerebellar (AICA)	Undersurface of the cerebellum and lateral surface of the pons
Superior cerebellar (SCA)	Upper surface of the cerebellum and midbrain
Pontine	Pons

tween these areas and the oculomotor, trochlear, abducens, glossopharyngeal, vagus, and spinal accessory CNs. Stimulation of the lateral portion of area 6 results in massive generalized movements, such as the turning of the eyes and head, movement of the trunk, and flexion and extension of the extremities, particularly the hands. Area 8 is concerned with the eye field and coordinates eye movement.

Broca's area (areas 44 and 45), located at the inferior frontal gyrus, is classified as an association area because it is critical for motor control of speech. Damage to this area in the dominant hemisphere results in the inability of the patient to express his or her thoughts (non-fluent aphasia).

Parietal Lobe

Posterior to the central fissure is the **primary sensory cortex (areas 1, 2, and 3),** which is arranged in the same topographic scheme as the motor strip, that is, the feet are controlled by an area in the longitudinal fissure, and the muscles of the face are controlled by the temporal region. Area 1 receives fibers responsible for cutaneous and deep sensibility sensations. The fibers in area 2 are concerned with deep sensibility, whereas those in area 3 interpret the cutaneous sensations of touch, position, pressure, and vibration.

Input from the thalamus also reaches the primary sensory cortex. The purpose of the primary sensory cortex is to analyze only gross aspects of sensation and send the results of its interpretation to the thalamus and other cortical areas. It is the function of the **sensory association areas (areas 5 and 7)** to analyze the specific characteristics of sensory input.

In the parietal lobes, sensory input is interpreted to define size, shape, weight, texture, and consistency. Sensation is localized, and modalities of touch, pressure, and position are identified. In addition, a person's awareness of the parts of his or her body are parietal lobe functions. The nondominant parietal lobe processes visuospatial information and controls spatial orientation, whereas the dominant lobe is involved in ideomotor praxis.

Temporal Lobe

The **primary auditory receptive areas (areas 41** and **42)** are located in the temporal lobes. The **auditory association area** occupies a part of the superior temporal gyrus (**area 22**) and is also known as **Wernicke's area.** This area is usually largest in the dominant hemisphere. If Wernicke's area is damaged in the patient's dominant hemisphere, words are heard but they are meaningless to the person (fluent aphasia). Thus, affected persons would be able to verbalize but would unknowingly make many errors in content because of a failure to comprehend what has been said by others or by themselves.

A very important area, called the **interpretive area,** is located in the supramarginal and angular gyri of the temporal lobe. This area is at the junction of the lateral fissure where the temporal, parietal, and occipital lobes meet. It provides an integration of the somatic, auditory, and visual association areas and plays an important role in visual, auditory, and olfactory perception; learning; memory; and emotional affect. Types of thoughts that

Table 5–5 • MAJOR SOURCES OF VENOUS DRAINAGE OF THE CEREBRAL CIRCULATION AND THE AREAS DRAINED

VENOUS STRUCTURE	AREA DRAINED
Superior longitudinal (sagittal) sinus	Superior cortical veins of the convexity of the brain; drains CSF
Inferior longitudinal sinus	Medial surface of the brain
Straight sinus	Joins the superior longitudinal sinus; the vein of Galen drains into the straight sinus
Transverse sinus	Area of the ears; collects blood from superior longitudinal and straight sinuses and drains it into the internal jugular vein
Cavernous sinus (contains several cranial nerves and internal carotid artery)	Inferior surface of the brain, including the orbits

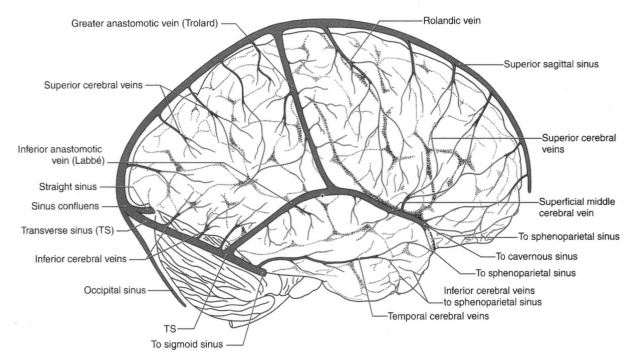

Figure 5–17 • The cranial venous sinuses. Lateral view of the right cerebral hemisphere and part of the venous drainage from the brain. Communications between veins and sinuses or between sinuses are also indicated. (From Haines, D. E. [2000]. *Neuroanatomy: An atlas of structures, sections, and systems* [5th ed.]. Philadelphia: Lippincott Williams & Wilkins.)

might be experienced are greatly detailed memories of past experiences, conversations, artwork, music, and taste. Memory that requires more than one sensory modality is stored, in part, in the angular gyrus of the temporal lobe. Any destruction of the **dominant temporal lobe** and angular gyrus in an adult will result in great impairment of intellectual ability.

Occipital Lobe

The **primary visual cortex** is **area 17** of the occipital lobe. The **visual association areas** are **18** and **19**. Neurons of the **lateral geniculate bodies** give rise to fibers that form the geniculocalcarine tract (optic radiation) to the cortex of the occipital lobes. The major functions of the occipital lobes are visual perception,

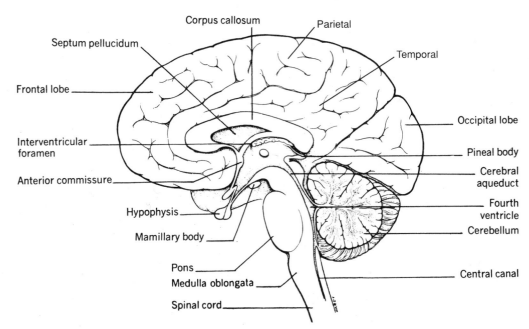

Figure 5–18 • Midsagittal section of the brain. (From Chaffee, E. E., & Lytle, I. M. [1980]. *Basic physiology and anatomy*. Philadelphia: J. B. Lippincott.)

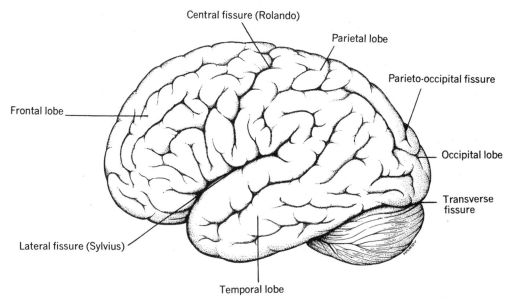

Figure 5–19 • Lateral aspect of the left cerebral and cerebellar hemispheres.

some visual reflexes (i.e., visual fixation) and involuntary smooth eye movements (smooth pursuit system).

DOMINANCE OF A CEREBRAL HEMISPHERE

Cerebral dominance is an important consideration. It is generally accepted that most people have one cerebral hemisphere that has become more highly developedthan the other. At birth, both hemispheres have an equal capacity for development. As a child develops, the attention of the mind is directed to one specific hemisphere, which develops rapidly in relation to the other side. Left hemispheric dominance is found in 90% of the population; these are right-handed people. Surprisingly, most, but not all, left-handed people also have a dominant left cerebral hemisphere. Many "split brain" studies have been conducted on the left and right hemispheres of the brain. The left side of the brain controls language, whereas the right side is the nonverbal or perceptual hemisphere.

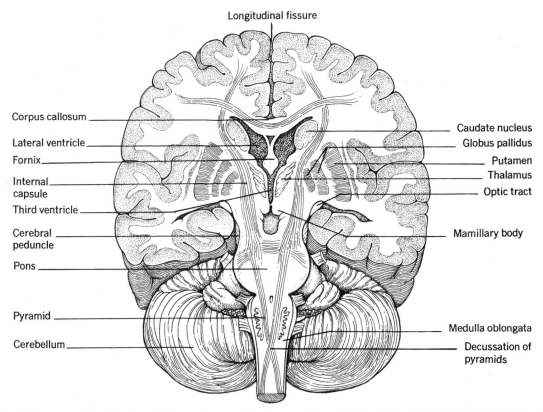

Figure 5–20 • Oblique coronal section through the cerebrum and brain stem. (From Chaffee, E. E., & Lytle, I. M. [1980]. *Basic physiology and anatomy*. Philadelphia: J. B. Lippincott.)

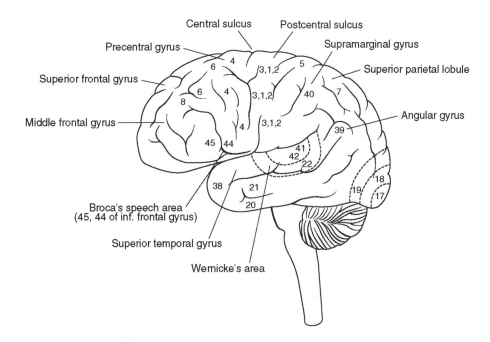

Figure 5–21 • Lateral view of the brain depicting the most significant areas of Brodmann.

CORPUS CALLOSUM

The **corpus callosum,** as mentioned previously, is a thick area of nerve fibers directed transversely, through which every part of one hemisphere is connected with the corresponding part of the other hemisphere. When the fibers of one hemisphere pass into the opposite hemisphere, they permeate the hemisphere in all directions, terminating in the gray matter of the periphery. As a result of this connective process, the two hemispheres are intricately linked.

BASAL GANGLIA

The **basal ganglia** are the several masses of subcortical nuclei located deep in the cerebral hemispheres. Their anatomic parts include the **lenticular nucleus** (composed of the **globus pallidus** and **putamen**), the **caudate nucleus,** the **amygdaloid body,** and the **claustrum.** The lenticular nucleus and the caudate nuclei are collectively called the **corpus striatum.** The lenticular nuclei and the caudate nucleus are functionally

closely related to the thalamus, subthalamus, substantia nigra, and red nucleus. These structures compose the basal ganglia system for motor control of fine body movements, particularly of the hands and lower extremities.

DIENCEPHALON

The **diencephalon,** a major division of the cerebrum, is divided into four regions: the thalamus, hypothalamus, subthalamus, and epithalamus. The thalamus and hypothalamus are the major areas of importance. These four areas are next discussed along with the internal capsule and hypophysis (pituitary gland), which are located in this region.

Thalamus

The **thalamus** consists of a pair of egg-shaped masses of gray matter located in the ventromedial part of the hemispheres that has connections to multiple areas of the

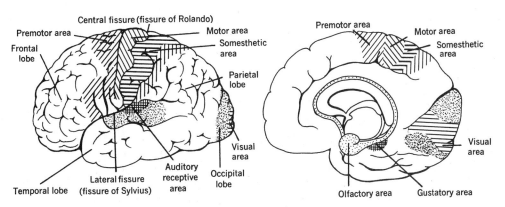

Figure 5–22 • Diagram of the localization of function in the cerebral hemisphere. Various functional areas are shown in relation to the lobes and fissures—lateral view (*left*) and medial view (*right*).

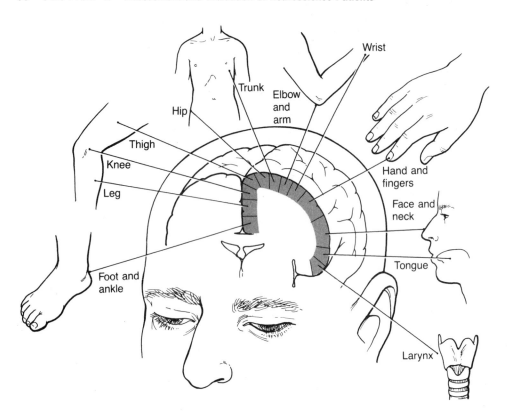

Figure 5–23 • Areas of the brain that control specific areas of the body. Size indicates relative distribution of control. (From Bullock, B. L. [1996]. *Pathophysiology: Adaptations and alterations in function* [4th ed.]. Philadelphia: Lippincott-Raven.)

brain. The thalamus is divided into anterior medial and lateral groups, and each group includes specific nuclei. The lateral border of the thalamus is the posterior limb or the internal capsule, and the third ventricle lies medially to the thalamus. The thalamus is the last station where impulses are processed before they ascend to the cerebral cortex. All sensory pathways (with the exception of olfactory pathways) have direct afferent and efferent connections with the thalamic nuclei. The thalamus plays a role in conscious pain awareness, in focusing of attention, in the reticular activating system, and in the limbic system.

Epithalamus

The **epithalamus** is the most dorsal portion of the diencephalon. It is composed of the pineal body, which is thought to have a role in growth and development. The epithalamus is also involved in the regulation of the primitive "food-getting" reflex.

Hypothalamus

The **hypothalamus** is located in the basal region of the diencephalon, forming part of the walls of the third ventricle. The optic chiasma, the point at which the two optic tracts cross, is located at the rostral area of the hypothalamic floor. The stalk of the pituitary, **infundibulum,** connects the hypophysis with the hypothalamus. The hypothalamus regulates important physiologically based drives such as appetite, sexual arousal, and thirst. It is the center for the

autonomic nervous system, particularly the sympathetic portion. The hypothalamus controls:

Temperature, by monitoring the blood temperature that flows through the hypothalamus and then sending afferent impulses to the sweat glands, peripheral vessels, or muscles (for shivering)

Water metabolism, through the regulation of antidiuretic hormone

Hypophyseal secretions (e.g., growth hormone, follicle-stimulating hormone)

Visceral and somatic activities, by many excitatory-inhibitory functions of the autonomic nervous system (e.g., heart rate, peristalsis, pupillary dilation and constriction)

Visible physical expressions in response to emotions, such as blushing, dry mouth, and clammy hands

Sleep-wakefulness cycle

Circadian rhythms

Subthalamus

The **subthalamus** is located below the thalamus and is closely related to the basal ganglia in function.

▌▌▌ INTERNAL CAPSULE

Many nerve fibers coming from various parts of the cerebral cortex converge at the brain stem, forming the corona radiata. As the fibers enter the thalamus-hypothalamus region, they are collectively termed the **internal capsule.** The internal capsule is a **massive bundle of sensory and motor fibers** connecting the various subdivisions of the brain and spinal cord. Although it includes only a small area of tissue, it is a critical anatomic area that controls major sensory and motor function. It is part of the white matter of the cerebrum and contains both radiation and projection fibers. The internal capsule is formed by fibers of the crus cerebri, with additional fibers from the corpus striatum and optic thalamus laterally.

All afferent sensory fibers going to the cortex pass through the internal capsule in the following succession: the brain stem to the thalamus to the internal capsule to the cerebral cortex. All efferent motor fibers leaving the cortex for the brain stem pass through the internal capsule according to the following schemata: cerebral cortex to the internal capsule to the brain stem.

▥ HYPOPHYSIS (PITUITARY GLAND)

The **hypophysis,** also called the **pituitary gland,** is a small gland that is located above the sella turcica at the base of the brain and is connected to the hypothalamus by the **hypophyseal stalk** (also called the **infundibulum**). The hypothalamus controls pituitary secretions. The hypophysis is divided into two lobes, the anterior and the posterior. The anterior lobe secretes six major hormones related to metabolic function of the body: (1) **growth-stimulating hormone** (GSH), (2) **adrenal-stimulating hormone** (adrenocorticotropin, ACTH), (3) **thyroid-stimulating hormone** (TSH), (4) **prolactin,** (5) **follicle-stimulating hormone** (FSH), and (6) **luteinizing hormone** (LH).

The posterior lobe produces **vasopressin,** also called **antidiuretic hormone** (ADH), and **oxytocin.** ADH controls the rate of water secretion into the urine, thereby controlling the water content of the body. Commonly, abnormal secretion of ADH accompanies intracranial surgery, a pituitary adenoma, or cerebral trauma.

Relationship Between the Hypothalamus and Hypophysis in Neuroendocrine Control

The control center for the autonomic nervous system and the neuroendocrine system is the **hypothalamus.** The following two pathways of hypothalamic connection to the hypophysis enable hypothalamic influence of the endocrine glands: (1) nerve fibers that travel from the supraoptic nuclei and paraventricular nuclei to the posterior lobe of the hypophysis (**hypothalamohypophyseal tract**); and (2) long and short portal blood vessels that connect sinusoids in the median eminence (portion of the hypophysis) and the infundibulum with the capillary plexuses in the anterior lobe of the hypophysis (**hypophyseal portal system**) (Fig. 5-24).

Hypothalamohypophyseal Tract

The precursors of the hormones vasopressin and oxytocin are synthesized in the nerve cells of the **supraoptic** and **paraventricular nuclei.** The precursor material then passes along the axons and is released at the axon terminals, where it is absorbed into the capillaries of the posterior hypophyseal lobe. **Vasopressin** is produced mainly in the nerve cells of the supraoptic nucleus. The functions of vasopressin are to increase water absorption in the

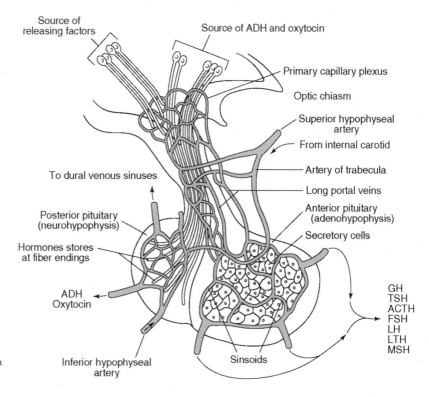

Figure 5–24 • Diagrammatic and schematic representation of hypophysial nerve fiber tracts and the portal system. Releasing factors produced by cell bodies in the hypothalamus trickle down axons to the proximal part of the stalk where they enter the primary capillary plexus and are transported via portal vessels to sinusoids in adenohypophysis for control of secretions. Antidiuretic hormone (ADH) and oxytocin, produced by other cell bodies in the hypothalamus, trickle down axons for storage in the neurohypophysis until needed.

kidney's distal convoluted tubules and to initiate vasoconstriction. The other hormone, **oxytocin,** is produced mainly in the paraventricular nucleus and is responsible for uterine contraction and for stimulating the growth of those cells of the mammary glands responsible for milk production.

Hypophyseal Portal System

The hypophyseal portal system is derived from the superior hypophyseal artery. On entering the median eminence and dividing into capillaries, the capillaries drain into long and short descending vessels that terminate in the anterior lobe of the hypophysis. The release-stimulating hormones and release-inhibiting hormones are delivered to cells of the anterior hypophysis so that the appropriate releasing or inhibiting hormone is synthesized and secreted (e.g., TSH, FSH). Feedback systems from afferent fibers in the hypothalamus, as well as from the target organ, help to regulate the level of the various hormones.

▥ BRAIN STEM (MIDBRAIN, PONS, AND MEDULLA)

The second major subdivision of the brain is the brain stem (Fig. 5-25). Many significant anatomic parts are found in the brain stem and are discussed in relationship to the three major divisions, the midbrain, pons, and medulla.

Midbrain

The **midbrain** is a small, 1.5-cm segment of the upper brain stem lying between the diencephalon and the pons. The midbrain can be divided into the tectum (the roof), the

tegmentum (the posterior portion), and the crus cerebri (the peduncle). The anterior surface extends from the mamillary bodies of the diencephalon to the pons. The **crus cerebri** consists of two rope-like bundles of fibers separated by a deep **interpeduncular fossa.** The rope-like bundles include the corticospinal and corticobulbar tracts centrally and are flanked by corticopontine fibers. Many small penetrating blood vessels emanate in the floor of the interpeduncular fossa. The optic tracts are noted just above the crus cerebri.

The base of the midbrain, also called the **basis pedunculi,** consists of the **cerebral peduncles** (comprising the corticospinal, corticobulbar, and corticopontine tracts) and the substantia nigra. The crus cerebri and tegmentum are collectively called the **cerebral peduncles.** The **substantia nigra** lies between the crus cerebri and peduncles. Because of melanin pigment in the substantia nigra cell bodies, the neurons appear brownish.

On the posterior part of the tectum are four rounded masses: two superior colliculi (optic system) and two inferior colliculi (auditory system). The superior and inferior colliculi are collectively termed the **corpus quadrigemina.** The **superior colliculi** process visual stimuli and also integrate visual and auditory motor reflexes. The **inferior colliculi** are nuclei to relay auditory information.

The **superior cerebellar peduncles** are efferent fibers coming from the dentate nucleus of the cerebellum passing rostrally and near the posterior surface of the midbrain. The crossing of the tracts to the opposite side is called the point of **cerebellar decussation.** The fibers then proceed to the red nuclei and the thalamus.

The **red nuclei** are globular gray masses located at the anterior-central tegmentum. Crossed fibers from the cerebral cortex and superior cerebellar peduncles enter the red nuclei or pass around its edges. The **rubrospinal** and **tectospinal tracts** emanate from this area. They form a relay station for many of the efferent cerebellar tracts. On the lateral surface of the midbrain are the **medial geniculate bodies,** which are the auditory-sensory relay centers. Functionally, the mid-

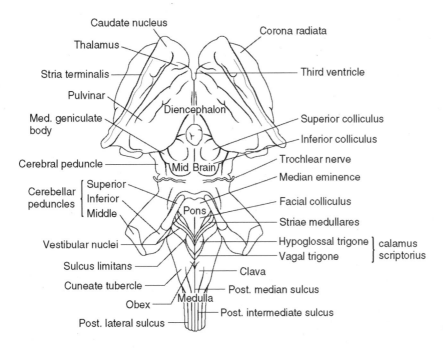

Figure 5–25 • Dorsal view of the brain stem.

brain serves as the pathway for the cerebral hemispheres and the lower brain and as the center for auditory and visual reflexes. CNs III and IV nuclei are located in the midbrain. The midbrain contains the aqueduct of Sylvius.

Pons

The **pons,** about 2.5 cm long, is the bridge between the midbrain and the medulla. The anterior surface of the pons is composed of a band of thick, transverse fibers. The **basal sulcus,** a midline furrow, matches the course of the basilar artery. The anterior area is called the **basis pontis** and is composed of crossing fibers of the middle cerebellar peduncles. The **tegmentum** contains spinothalamic tracts, the lateral lemnisci, the medial longitudinal fasciculi, and part of the reticular formation (regulates consciousness). Several tracts cross through the pons. The inferior, middle, and superior cerebellar peduncles are pathways for the corticospinal tract, and they also connect to the cerebellum. Many other pathways pass through this region connecting higher cerebral regions with the lower levels of the nervous system. The pons contains the fourth ventricle and some control of respiratory function.

Four CNs, V through VIII, have nuclei in the pons. CN V exits laterally from the midpons. At the pontomedullary junction, CN VI exits medially and CNs VII and VIII exit laterally. About 70% of the neurons of CN VI are motor neurons located in the floor of the fourth ventricle; they innervate the lateral rectus muscle. The remaining 30% of neurons are internuclear neurons, whose axons cross midline, ascend in the **medial longitudinal fasciculus (MLF),** and connect with the medial rectus motor neurons on the opposite side. The abducens is the center for conjugate horizontal gaze. CN VI has the longest intracranial course and is, therefore, more vulnerable to injury and dysfunction.

Medulla

The **medulla oblongata,** also approximately 2.5 cm long, is continuous with the spinal cord and level with the foramen magnum and rootlet of the first cervical nerve; it connects with the pons rostrally. On the posterior surface, the point of division between the pons and medulla is an imaginary transverse line that passes between the caudal margins of the middle cerebellar peduncles. Part of the fourth ventricle is located in the medulla. Anteriorly, the pyramidal (corticospinal) tracts decussate or cross; the pyramidal tracts from the left cross to the right side (and vice versa). The point of decussation forms a ridge on either side of the **median fissure.** In the caudal medulla rostral to the pyramidal decussation, axons from the nucleus gracilis and cuneatus loop anterior-medially around the central gray matter as the **internal arcuate fibers.** These fibers cross the midline to the opposite side and continue as the **medial lemniscus.** Laterally, the **olive** is a prominent oval swelling of convoluted bands that includes the inferior olivary nuclei; they receive fibers from the dentate nucleus of the cerebellum, red nucleus, basal ganglia, and cerebral cortex. Axons from the inferior olivary nuclei form the **olivocerebellar tract** (goes from the inferior cerebellar peduncle to the opposite cerebellar hemisphere). The dorsal the spinocerebellar tract is found in a ridge called the **tuberculum cinereum.**

The **MLF** is located in the paramedian area dorsal to the medial lemniscus. The MLF extends rostrally from the cervical cord to the upper midbrain level. It transmits information for the coordination of head and eye movement. In addition to motor and sensory tracts, there are also cardiac, vasomotor, and respiratory centers in the medulla.

CNs IX through XII emanate from the medulla. CNs IX, X, and XI exit the brain stem in the postolivary fissure, whereas CN XII exits from the preolivary fissure.

CEREBELLUM

The **cerebellum,** located in the posterior fossa, is attached to the pons, medulla, and midbrain by the three paired cerebellar peduncles. The organization of the cerebellum allows it to be conceptualized in many ways. The cerebellum consists of three major layers: (1) the cortex, which is the outer gray covering; (2) the white matter, which forms the connecting pathways for efferent and afferent impulses joining the cerebellum with other parts of the CNS; and (3) the four pairs of deep cerebellar nuclei.

The cerebellum can also be divided from side to side and anteriorly to posteriorly. From the anterior to posterior direction, the cerebellum is composed of an **anterior lobe, a posterior lobe,** and a **flocculonodular lobe.** Approaching it from side to side, it is divided into midline structures and lateral structures. The midline of the anterior and posterior lobes is called the **vermis,** and the lateral portions are the **cerebellar hemispheres.** The midline of the flocculonodular lobe is the **nodulus;** the lateral portion is the **flocculus.**

The **anterior lobe** uses impulses from the spinocerebellar proprioception to regulate postural reflexes. The **posterior lobe** controls coordination of voluntary muscle activity and muscle tone. The **flocculonodular lobe** is the primary connection with the vestibular apparatus for coordination of location in space and movements. Afferent and efferent nerve fibers are found in the **inferior, middle,** and **superior cerebellar peduncles.** The **cerebellar peduncles** receive direct input from the spinal cord and brainstem and convey it to the deep cerebellar nuclei (**dentate, globose, emboliform,** and **fastigial nuclei**) and cerebellar cortex. The result is both an excitatory and inhibitory influence on the cerebellar nuclei; the excitatory influences predominate. An excitatory effect on the brainstem and thalamic nuclei maintains a tonic discharge to the motor system.

The cerebellum is integrated into many connective efferent and afferent pathways throughout the brain, thus providing muscle synergy throughout the body. All sensory modalities are circuited through the cerebellum, which provides information about muscle activity. Impulses to provide "corrections" are sent after sensory data are evaluated. In other words, there are many feedback loops in which cerebellar function is the center of the circuit receiving and sending impulses to maintain muscle activity. In summary, the cerebellum controls fine movement, coordinates muscle groups (agonist and antagonist muscles), and maintains balance through feedback loops.

SPECIAL SYSTEMS WITHIN THE BRAIN

Three special systems require further discussion: the reticular formation (RF), the reticular activating system (RAS), and the limbic system.

The **reticular formation (RF)** is a net (reticulum) of a continuous network of nerve cells and fibers from the axis of the CNS that extends from the spinal cord, through the medulla, pons, midbrain, subthalamus, hypothalamus, thalamus, to the cerebrum. The RF is subdivided into lateral, medial, and median columns (Fig. 5-26). The RF receives input from most of the sensory systems and has efferent fibers that descend and influence nerve cells at all levels of the CNS. The exceptionally long dendrites of the neurons of the RF permit input from widely placed ascending and descending pathways. Through its many connections, the RF can: control skeletal muscle activity, control somatic and visceral sensation; control the autonomic and endocrine systems; influence biologic clocks; and the reticular activating system (control the level of consciousness).

The **reticular activating system (RAS)** is a diffuse system that extends from the lower brain stem to the cerebral cortex, from which it disperses (Fig. 5-27). The RAS controls the sleep-wakefulness cycle; consciousness; focused attention; and sensory perception that might alter behavior. The brain stem and thalamic portions of the RAS have different functions. Stimulation of the brain-stem portion results in activation of the entire brain. Wakefulness is controlled by the brain stem. Stimulation of the thalamic portion relays facilitory impulses, causing a generalized activation of the cerebrum and cognition. Stimulation of selective thalamic areas activates specific areas of the cerebral cortex. This selective stimulation plays a role in directing one's attention during certain mental activities.

The **limbic system** is a group of subcortical nuclei and fiber tracts that form a border around the brain stem. The system

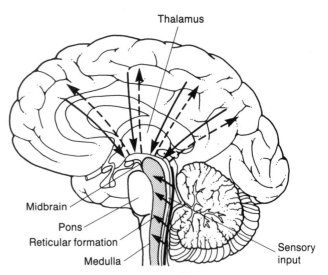

Figure 5–27 • The anatomical components of the reticular activating system related to consciousness.

includes the **hypothalamus,** the **cingulate gyrus,** the **fornix,** the **hippocampus,** the **anterior nucleus** of the **thalamus,** the **uncus,** and the **amygdaloid nucleus** (a part of the basal ganglia). Connections exist with the mamillary bodies, olfactory tract, and the upper RF of the midbrain (Fig. 5-28). The major connections of the limbic system are called the **circuit of Papez.** The complex function of the system involves basic instinctual and emotional drives, such as fear, sexual drive, hunger, sleep, and short-term memory. These emotional reactions are expressed through endocrine, visceral, somatic, and behavioral reactions through neural pathways that connect with the hypothalamus, brain stem, spinal cord, and hypophysis.

SPINAL CORD

The spinal cord is an elongated mass of nerve tissue that occupies the upper two thirds of the vertebral canal and usually measures 42 to 45 cm long in the adult. The spinal cord extends from the upper borders of the atlas (first cervical vertebra) to the lower border of the first lumbar vertebra (Fig. 5-29). As the cord reaches the lower two levels of the thoracic region, the cord becomes tapered and is called the **conus medullaris.** A nonneural filament called the **filum terminale** continues caudally until it attaches to the second segment of the coccyx. The three meninges surround the spinal cord for protection.

The Spinal Cord in Cross Section

When viewed in cross section (Fig. 5-30), the spinal cord appears to be a gray *H* surrounded by white matter. The **gray matter** consists of cell bodies and neuronal projections (axons and dendrites). The **white matter** includes longitudinally running fiber tracts, some of which are myelinated. Each **funiculus** (column) contains ascending and descending tracts. There are two midline sulci, the **anterior median sulcus** and the **posterior median sulcus.** The lateral surface contains both **postero-**

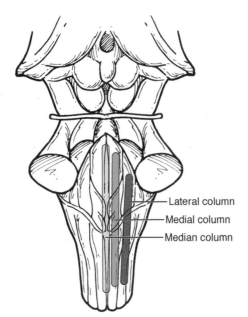

Figure 5–26 • The median, medial, and lateral columns of the reticular formation. (From Snell, R. S. [1997]. *Clinical neuroanatomy for medical students* [4th ed.]. Philadelphia: Lippincott Williams & Wilkins.)

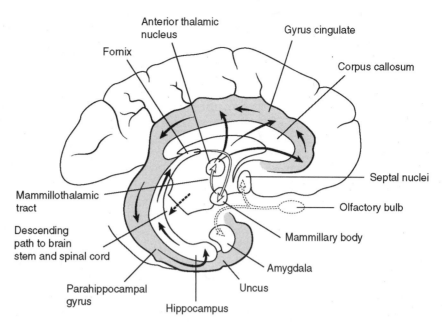

Figure 5–28 • Papez circuit (*arrows*) is depicted in this schematic view of the limbic system. The solid arrows represent the hypothetical circulation of impulses during the experiencing of emotions. The thick dotted arrow indicates the descending path to the brain stem and spinal cord for the expression of emotions. The olfactory afferent fibers (*lightly dotted arrows*) are also shown.

lateral and **anterolateral sulci** that serve to divide the white matter into the anterior, lateral, and posterior funiculi.

Cross-sections of the cord at various levels show striking differences in the shape and extent of gray and white matter. The gray matter of the cord contains the **posterior (dorsal)** and **anterior (ventral) horns. Lateral horns** are smaller in the thoracic and upper lumbar segments because the muscle mass of the trunk is less than that of the extremities, and these horns are made up largely of cell bodies of neurons that innervate skeletal muscles. In the lumbosacral region, the anterior horns are larger than those of the cervical area because of the greater muscle mass in the lower extremities. There is more white matter, compared with gray matter, in the cervical region than in the lumbosacral region. This difference exists because the white matter in the cervical region is made up of connecting fibers that span the entire spinal cord and the brain, whereas the white matter of the lumbosacral cord contains only fibers serving the caudal end of the cord.

On cross-section, the gray matter of the spinal cord is divided into sections I through X, called the **laminae of Rexed (Fig. 5-31)**. Each lamina extends the length of the cord. Numbering of the laminae begins at the most dorsal point of the posterior horn; lamina IX is located at the most ventral point of the anterior horn. Therefore, the posterior horn contains laminae I through VI. Cells receive and send information about sensory input from the spinal nerve. Lamina VII is located in the intermediate gray zone and extends into the anterior horn. Within this area are the nucleus dorsalis and the intermediolateral gray columns. The anterior horn contains laminae VIII and IX. Lamina VIII contains neurons that send commissural axons to the opposite side of the cord. Lamina IX contains alpha and gamma motor neurons that innervate skeletal muscles. The area surrounding the central canal is the site of lamina X.

Spinal Nerves

Spinal nerves are part of the PNS. There are 31 pairs of spinal nerves exiting from the spinal cord, including 8 cervical, 12 thoracic, 5 lumbar, 5 sacral, and 1 coccygeal. Each

spinal nerve has a dorsal root by which afferent impulses enter the cord and a ventral root by which efferent impulses leave. The first pair of cervical spinal nerves leaves the cord above the C-1 vertebra, and spinal nerves of C-2 through C-7 leave by way of the intervertebral foramina, above their corresponding vertebrae. Given that there are seven vertebrae and eight pairs of spinal nerves, the C-8 spinal nerve leaves the cord by way of the intervertebral foramina below the C-7 vertebra. All spinal nerves from T-1 to the caudal end of the cord leave by way of the foramina immediately below the corresponding vertebrae.

In the cervical region, the spinal nerves are almost on a horizontal plane with the corresponding vertebra; however, because the spinal cord is shorter than the vertebral column, the spinal nerves become increasingly oblique as they descend the spinal cord. The lumbar and sacral spinal nerves develop long roots, collectively referred to as the **cauda equina.**

There are two enlargements in the spinal cord to accommodate innervation to the extremities. The cervical (**brachial**) enlargement innervates the upper extremities and extends from the C-5 to the T-1 spinal levels. The lower extremities are innervated by the **lumbosacral** enlargement, which extends from the L-3 to the S-2 levels.

DORSAL (SENSORY) ROOTS

The **dorsal roots (posterior roots)** (see Fig. 5-30) convey sensory input (afferent impulses) from specific areas of the body known as **dermatomes** (Fig. 5-32). There is considerable peripheral overlap between one dermatome and another so that no demonstrable sensory deficit will be found unless the sensory component of two or more spinal nerves is interrupted. Interruption of one sensory nerve root may result in paresthesia or pain in that dermatomal area.

Afferent impulses are directed from the dermatomal area through the dorsal root to the dorsal root ganglia, in which the cell bodies of the sensory component are located. The sensory fibers are of two types:

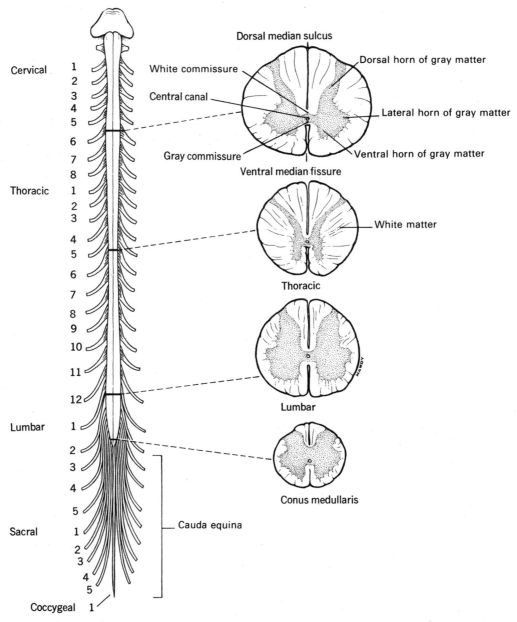

Figure 5–29 • Cross-sectional views of the spinal cord showing the regional variations in the gray matter. (From Chaffee, E. E., & Lytle, I. M. [1980]. *Basic physiology and anatomy.* Philadelphia: J. B. Lippincott.)

General somatic afferent (GSA) fibers, which carry sensory impulses for pain, temperature, touch, and proprioception from the body wall, tendons, and joints

General visceral afferent (GVA) fibers, which carry sensory impulses from the organs within the body (Fig. 5-33 and Table 5-6)

General somatic efferent (GSE) fibers, which innervate voluntary striated muscles and have axons originating from the alpha and gamma motor neurons of lamina IX

General visceral efferent (GVE) fibers, which include the preganglionic and postganglionic autonomic fibers that innervate smooth and cardiac muscle and also regulate glandular secretion (see Fig. 5-33)

▌▌▌ VENTRAL (MOTOR) ROOTS

The **ventral roots** convey efferent impulses from the spinal cord to the body. The motor fibers are of two types:

Impulses to the motor end-plate of voluntary muscle fibers are conveyed by **alpha motor neurons**; impulses to the motor end-plates of intrafusal muscle cells of the neuromuscular spindles are conveyed by **gamma motor neurons.** Both these motor neurons (alpha, gamma) are also called lower motor neurons. Table 5-7 provides a list

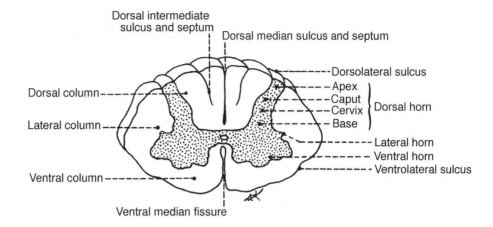

Figure 5–30 • Cross section of the spinal cord. (From DeMyer, W. [1998]. *Neuroanatomy* [2nd ed.]. Baltimore: Williams & Wilkins.)

of myotomes, which are areas of motor innervation to specific muscle groups.

CLASSIFICATION OF NERVE FIBERS

Nerve fibers can be classified by various criteria, including the diameter of the fiber, thickness of the myelin sheath, and speed of conduction of the impulse. Large fibers conduct impulses quickly, and the thicker the myelin sheath, the faster the speed of the impulse conductivity.

Sensory fibers are classified into groups I through IV, depending on their conduction velocities. Group I fibers are the quickest to conduct impulses, whereas group IV fibers have the slowest velocity. Group I is further divided to include I_a fibers (spindle primary afferent) and I_b fibers (from Golgi tendon organs). Group II conveys sensation from the myelinated skin and joint receptors (spindle secondary afferent). Groups III and IV convey impulses from unmyelinated fibers. Another system uses the capital letters A, B, and C to classify both sensory and motor fibers. Type A is either a small, lightly myelinated sensory fiber for touch, pressure, pain, and temperature or alpha

or gamma motor neurons of lamina IX. The greatest diameter and velocity are characteristic of type A fibers. Type B fibers have a smaller diameter and are lightly myelinated preganglionic motor fibers. Type C fibers have a small diameter and are unmyelinated. They include

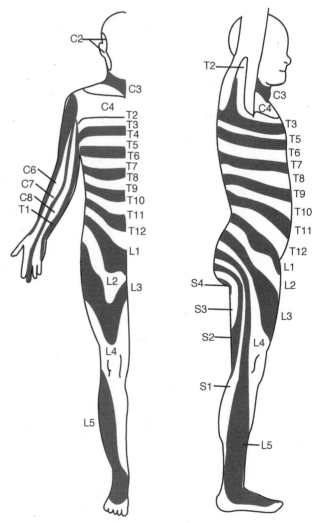

Figure 5–32 • Cutaneous distribution of the spinal nerves (dermatomes). (From Conn, P. M. [1995]. *Neuroscience in medicine.* Philadelphia: J. B. Lippincott.)

Figure 5–31 • The three funiculi of the spinal cord.

Theoretical   **Actual**

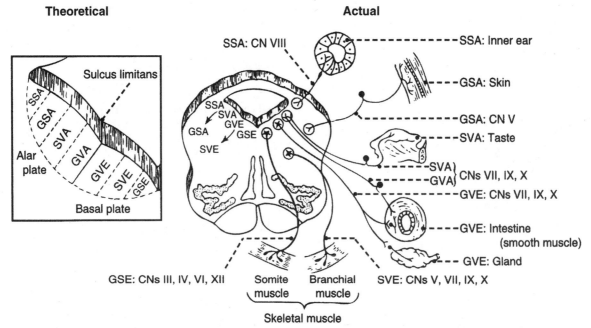

Figure 5–33 • Components of autonomic nervous system in the medulla. (From DeMyer, W. [1998]. *Neuroanatomy* [2nd ed.]. Baltimore: Williams & Wilkins.)

motor postganglionic fibers and sensory fibers for pain and temperature.

Plexuses

A **plexus** is a network of interlacing nerves. Sometimes a plexus is formed by the primary branches of the nerves, such as the cervical, brachial, lumbar, and sacral plexuses. Other

plexuses are formed by the terminal funiculi at the periphery. The following are the major plexuses:

The **cervical plexus** is formed from the ventral branches of the first four cervical nerves of the spine. The resulting branches innervate the muscles of the neck and shoulders. This plexus also gives rise to the **phrenic nerve,** which supplies the diaphragm.

The **brachial plexus** is composed of the ventral branches of the lower four cervical and first thoracic spinal nerves. Important nerves that emerge from this plexus are the radial and ulnar nerves.

The **lumbar plexus** originates from the ventral branches of

Table 5–6 • SENSORY NERVE ROOTS AND THE AREAS THEY INNERVATE (DERMATOME)

SPINAL NERVES	DERMATOME
C-2	Back of head (occiput)
C-3	Neck
C-4	Neck and upper shoulder
C-5	Lateral aspect of shoulder
C-6	Thumb; radial aspect of arm; index finger
C-7	Middle finger; middle palm; back of hand
C-8	Ring and little finger; ulnar forearm
T-1–T-2	Inner aspect of arm and across shoulder blade
T-4	Nipple line
T-7	Lower costal margin
T-10	Umbilical region
T-12–L-1	Inguinal (groin) region
L-2	Anterior thigh and upper buttocks
L-3–L-4	Anterior knee and lower leg
L-5	Outer aspect of lower leg; dorsum of foot; great toe
S-1	Sole of foot and small toes
S-2	Posterior medial thigh and lower leg
S-3	Medial thigh
S-4–S-5	Genitals and saddle area

Table 5–7 • MOTOR NERVE ROOTS (MYOTOMES) AND AREAS THEY INNERVATE

SPINAL NERVES	MUSCLES
C-1 to C-4	Neck (flexion, lateral flexion, extension, rotation)
C-3–C-5	Diaphragm (respirations)
C-5–C-6	Shoulder movement and flexion of elbow
C-5–C-7	Forward thrust of shoulder
C-5–C-8	Adduction of arm from front to back
C-6–C-8	Extension of forearm and wrist
C-7, C-8, T-1	Flexion of wrist
T-1–T-12	Control of thoracic, abdominal, and back muscles
L-1–L-3	Flexion of hip
L-2–L-4	Extension of leg; adduction of thigh
L-4, L-5, S-1, S-2	Abduction of thigh; flexion of lower leg
L-4–L-5	Dorsal flexion of foot
L-5, S-1, S-2	Plantar flexion of foot
S-2, S-3, S-4	Perineal area and sphincters

the 12th thoracic and the first four lumbar nerves. The femoral nerve arises from this plexus.

The **sacral plexus** arises from the ventral branches of the last two lumbar and first four sacral nerves. The sciatic nerve arises from this plexus.

MOTOR SYSTEM

Movement is the result of complex higher-level structures, descending spinal cord tracts, segmental spinal cord circuits, and muscles. The major higher-level structures involved in movement are the cerebral cortex, basal ganglia, cerebellum, brain stem, spinal cord, and final common pathway (Fig. 5-34). Figure 5-35 doe motor pathways.

Nearly all voluntary muscle activity originates from the corticospinal tract (motor cortex, area 4). Other fibers originating in areas 4 and 6 do not initiate voluntary muscle activity, but act as inhibitors or suppressors of the lower motor neurons. Without these controls, lower motor neurons would fire excessively in response to reflex stimuli or discharge spontaneously, resulting in hyperreflexia or spasticity. Other tracts originate in the brain stem and also modify muscle function. The basal ganglia exert an inhibitory effect on lower motor neurons by synapses with the reticular formation. Damage to the basal ganglia results in increased motor tone. The cerebellum's role in movement is indirect through its effect on the vestibular nuclei, red nucleus, and basal ganglia. The tracts affected by these structures include the vestibulospinal, rubrospinal, and reticulospinal tracts. These tracts, in turn, affect the lower motor neurons.

Descending Motor Pathways: Upper Motor Neurons and Lower Motor Neurons

Descending motor pathways are divided into **upper motor neurons (UMNs)** and **lower motor neurons (LMNs). UMNs** are the facilitory and inhibitory descending supraspinal pathways that modify LMNs and are located entirely in the CNS.

UMNs include the neurons themselves and their fibers within the corticospinal tract and corticobulbar tracts originating in the cerebral cortex; the rubrospinal and tectospinal tracts originating in the midbrain; and the reticulospinal and vestibulospinal tracts emanating from the pons and medulla. **LMNs** are located in both the CNS and PNS. Voluntary striated muscles are innervated by alpha and gamma neurons and are the **final common pathway** or final linkage between the CNS and voluntary muscles. LMNs are the GSE components of the spinal nerves and of CNs III, IV, VI, and XII and the special visceral efferent components of CNs V, VII, IX, X, and XI.

Voluntary muscle activity is the sum of neural control of the alpha and gamma motor neurons of muscle and motor components of the CN nuclei. Final neural pathways influence the muscle by way of the myoneural junction. A summary of the major descending motor tracts is found in Table 5-8.

SENSORY SYSTEM

Sensory receptors, which are located throughout the body, convey afferent impulses for interpretation of stimuli. Sensory input may be integrated into spinal reflexes or it may be relayed to the higher centers of the brain by way of ascending pathways. The impulses are analyzed and can influence unconscious and conscious activities by way of efferent responses. There are various types of receptors that convey specific types of stimuli: **exteroceptors** are stimulated by touch, light pressure, pain, temperature, odor, sound, and light; **proprioceptors** convey a sense of position, movement, and muscle coordination; **interoceptors** provide visceral information concerning pain, cramping, and fullness; and **chemoreceptors** are stimulated by chemicals (e.g., lactic acid).

Pain and Temperature

The pain and temperature pathways are so closely related throughout the body that they are treated collectively as one system. The **anterolateral system** is made up of the **anterior spinothalamic, lateral spinothalamic** (Fig. 5-36), and **spinore-**

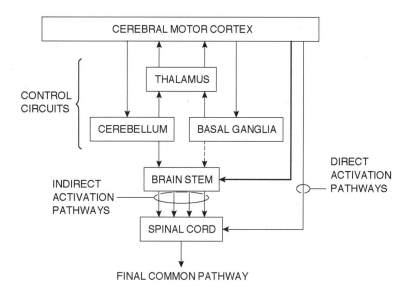

Figure 5–34 • Schematic representation of the motor system. (From Westmoreland, B. F. et al. [1994]. *Medical neurosciences.* Boston: Little, Brown and Company.)

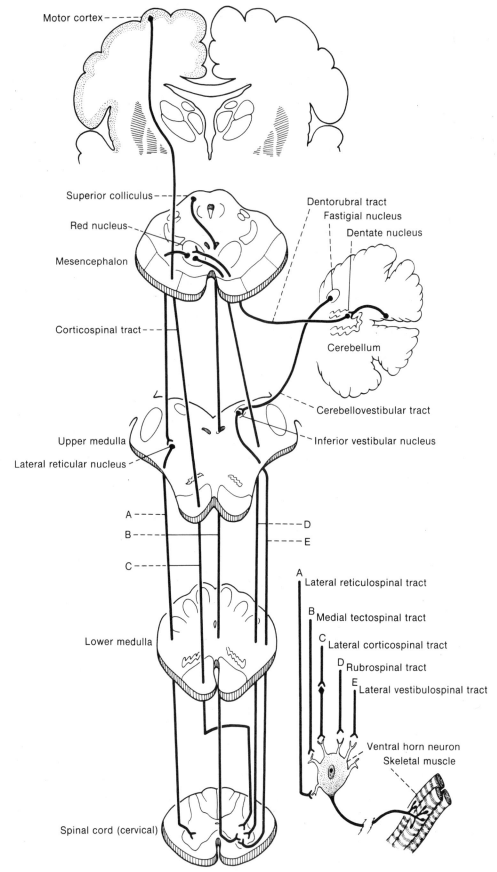

Figure 5–35 • The most important descending motor pathways that act upon the anterior horn cell of the spinal cord (final common pathway). (From Haerer, A. F. [1992]. *DeJong's the neurologic examination* [5th ed.]. Philadelphia: J. B. Lippincott.)

ticulothalamic tracts. These are the major tracts that convey pain and temperature sensation. The afferent impulse enters the cord by way of the **posterolateral tract of Lissauer** and crosses to the opposite side of the spinal cord. Impulses ascend the cord to terminate in the thalamus, with synapsing occurring within the reticular formation of the brain stem.

Proprioception

The posterior funiculus is totally enveloped by two ascending tracts—the **fasciculus gracilis** and **fasciculus cuneatus.** These tracts ascend the cord uncrossed until they reach the area of decussation in the medulla. After the fibers decussate in this area, they proceed initially to the thalamus and then to areas 1 through 3 of the cerebral cortex. These are the major tracts that convey the sensation of **proprioception,** which includes position and movement, vibration, two-point discrimination, deep pressure, and touch.

Coordination of Muscle Contraction

The anterior and posterior spinocerebellar tracts convey impulses of proprioception for the coordination of locomotion in the lower extremities. The fasciculus cuneatus and spinocerebellar tracts convey similar information from the upper half of the body. A summary of the major ascending sensory tracts is found in Table 5-8.

AUTONOMIC NERVOUS SYSTEM

The **autonomic nervous system** (ANS), part of the PNS, is made up of only motor neurons, collectively called the GVE system. The ANS regulates the activities of the viscera, which includes all smooth (involuntary) muscles, cardiac muscles, and glands (Fig. 5-37). The purpose of the ANS is to maintain a relatively stable internal environment for the body. Two major subdivisions of the ANS are the sympathetic and parasympathetic systems.

The **sympathetic system** is activated during stress situations such as fright, fight, or flight phenomena. During these stressful periods, the heart rate and blood pressure increase, and there is vasoconstriction of the peripheral blood vessels.

The **parasympathetic system** stimulates those visceral activities associated with conservation, restoration, and maintenance of a normal functional level. The parasympathetic system decreases heart rate and increases gastrointestinal activity (Table 5-9).

Both divisions of the ANS, which function in an antagonistic relationship, innervate most body organs. The ANS is activated primarily by centers located in the spinal cord, brain stem, and hypothalamus. A two-neuron chain is characteristic of the ANS. The cell bodies and their fibers are classified into the following two categories: (1) the **preganglionic neuron,** which is the primary neuron and is located in the brain stem or cord (intermediolateral gray column in the thoracic cord); and (2) the **postganglionic neuron,** which is the postsynaptic or secondary neuron located in the ganglia and innervating the end-organ.

Sympathetic Nervous System

The sympathetic nervous system is also called the **thoracolumbar system** because its preganglionic fibers emerge from cell bodies in the **intermediolateral nucleus of lamina VII.** The sympathetic nervous system extends through the thoracic and upper two lumbar levels (T-1 through L-2). These preganglionic fibers leave the spinal cord with the motor fibers of the ventral roots. After traveling less than 1 cm, the sympathetic fibers pass into the **white rami communicantes**—a branch of the spinal nerve—which, in turn, enters the **sympathetic chain** or trunk. (The sympathetic chain consists of a chain of ganglia located on either side of the spinal cord that extends from the base of the skull to the coccyx. These ganglia are all interconnected by longitudinal fibers, thus forming a continuous chain). In the sympathetic chain, the fibers may synapse in three possible places. First, the fibers may synapse immediately with postganglionic fibers located in the chain at the level of entry (**paravertebral ganglia**). Second, the fiber may travel up or down the trunk to synapse in one of the chain ganglia above or below the point of entry. Third, the fiber may pass on to synapse with a postganglionic neuron in an outlying sympathetic ganglia (**prevertebral ganglia**).

Some fibers from the postganglionic neuron in the sympathetic chain return to the spinal nerve by way of the **gray rami communicantes** at all levels of the spinal cord. Each spinal nerve receives a gray ramus, which controls the blood vessels, sweat glands, and piloerector muscles of the hairs.

Sympathetic fibers leave the spinal cord to enter the sympathetic chain in only the thoracic and upper lumbar regions; none of the fibers enters the chain in the cervical, lower lumbar, or sacral regions. Sympathetic innervation to the head is supplied by sympathetic fibers extending from the thoracic chain. In this way, the neck and all structures of the head are innervated. Sympathetic fibers also pass downward from the sympathetic chain into the lower abdomen and legs.

The sympathetic outflow is distributed in the following way: T-1 to T-5 innervate the head, creating three ganglia (superior cervical, middle cervical, and cervicothoracic stellate). Of those sympathetic fibers directed to the head, those from T-1 and T-2 innervate the eye for pupillary dilation; T-2 through T-6 innervate the heart and lungs; and T-6 through L-2 innervate the abdominal viscera through the thoracic and lumbar splanchnic nerves. The thoracic splanchnic nerves carry the preganglionic fibers to the prevertebral ganglia of the abdomen. The celiac, superior mesenteric, and aorticorenal ganglia arise in this area. The lumbar splanchnic nerves terminate in the inferior mesenteric and hypogastric ganglia.

The preganglionic sympathetic nerve fibers pass directly to the adrenal medulla without synapsing. These fibers are cholinergic and end directly on the special cells of the medulla that secrete epinephrine and norepinephrine.

Sympathetic Neurotransmitter

The neurotransmitter released by the postganglionic fibers is **norepinephrine** (noradrenaline). This is why the sympathetic system is termed **adrenergic.** Acetylcholine is secreted at the preganglionic terminal and quickly deactivated by cholinesterase. (There are few exceptions in the postganglionic neurons in the sympathetic nervous system.) Some blood vessels in skeletal muscles and most sweat glands in the palms of the hands have adrenergic postganglionic neurons.

▌▌▌▌ **Table 5-8** • MAJOR SPINAL CORD TRACTS

NAME	ORIGIN	TERMINATION	CROSSED	FUNCTION	DYSFUNCTION
Ascending Tracts					
Fasciculus gracilis	Spinal cord at sacral and lumbar level	Medulla → thalamus → cerebral cortex (sensory strip)	Yes	Conscious proprioception, fine touch,* and vibration sense from lower body	Lower body Astereognosis Loss of vibration sense Loss of two-point discrimination Loss of proprioception
Fasciculus cuneatus	Spinal cord at thoracic and cervical levels	Medulla → thalamus → cerebral cortex (sensory strip)	Yes	Conscious proprioception, fine touch,* and vibration sense from upper body	Upper body Astereognosis Loss of vibration sense Loss of two-point discrimination Loss of proprioception
Posterior spinocerebellar	Posterior horn	Cerebellum	No	Conduction of sensory impulses from muscle spindles and tendon organs of the trunk and lower limbs from one side of the body to the same side of cerebellum for the subconscious proprioception necessary for coordinated muscular contractions	Ipsilateral uncoordinated postural movements
Anterior spinocerebellar	Posterior horn	Cerebellum	Some	Conduction of sensory impulses from muscle spindles and tendon organs of the upper and lower limbs from both sides of the body to the cerebellum for the subconscious proprioception necessary for coordinated muscular contractions	Ipsilateral uncoordinated postural movements
Lateral spinothalamic	Posterior horn	Thalamus → cerebral cortex	Yes	Interpretation of pain and temperature	Loss of pain and temperature sensation contralaterally below the level of the lesion
Anterior spinothalamic	Posterior horn	Thalamus → cerebral cortex	Yes	Conduction of sensory impulses for pressure and crude touch† from extremities and trunk	Because one branch of the first neuron immediately synapses with a second, which ascends ipsilaterally for many levels; cord injury rarely results in complete loss of pressure and crude touch sensation

▌▌▌ T a b l e 5 – 8 • MAJOR SPINAL CORD TRACTS (Continued)

NAME	ORIGIN	TERMINATION	CROSSED	FUNCTION	DYSFUNCTION
Descending Tracts					
Lateral corticospinal	Motor cortex (area 4) → internal capsule → midbrain → pons → medulla	Anterior horn; all spinal levels in laminae IV through VII and IX	80%–90% cross at the medulla	Controls voluntary muscle activity	Voluntary muscle paresis/paralysis
Anterior corticospinal	Motor cortex (area 4) → internal capsule → midbrain → medulla → anterior funiculus of the cervical and upper thoracic levels	Anterior horn (at each level of cord, axons cross to other side)	Not at medulla; synapse with cells of lamina VIII	Controls voluntary muscle activity	Voluntary muscle paresis/paralysis
Corticobulbar	Areas 4, 6, and 8 of cortex → internal capsule → brain stem	Brain stem; connects with cranial nerves V, VII, IX, X, XI, and XII	Yes	Controls voluntary head movement and facial expression	Because of bilateral innervation, facial expression is usually not affected
Rubrospinal	Midbrain (red nucleus)	Anterior horn	Yes	Facilitates flexor alpha and gamma motor neurons and inhibits extensor motor neurons; also influences muscle tone and posture, particularly of the arms	Altered muscle tone and posture
Reticulospinals Pontine reticulospinal Medullary reticulospinal	Reticular formation (brain stem)	Anterior horn	No	Facilitates extensor motor neurons, particularly of the legs; input to gamma motor neurons	Altered muscle tone and posture
Vestibulospinals	Reticular formation (brain stem)	Anterior horn	No	Conveys autonomic information from higher levels to preganglionic autonomic nervous system neurons to influence sweating, pupillary dilatation, and circulation	Altered muscle tone and sweat gland activity
Lateral vestibulospinal			No	Facilitates extensor alpha motor neurons and inhibits flexors	Altered muscle tone and postural equilibrium
Medial vestibulospinal			No	Inhibits fibers to upper cervical alpha motor neurons; influences extraocular movements and visual reflexes	Altered muscle tone and equilibrium in response to head movement

* Fine touch is the ability to identify various objects (e.g., a key) that are placed in the hand with the eyes closed.

† Crude touch refers to light touch, which may be tested with a wisp of cotton placed in the hand with the eyes closed.

Parasympathetic Nervous System

The parasympathetic system is also called the **craniosacral system** because its preganglionic fibers emerge with CNs III, VII, IX, and X. The specific parasympathetic innervation to these CNs includes the following:

- Oculomotor (III) supplies the ciliary muscles for accommodation and constrictor sphincter muscles of the pupil.
- Facial (VII) innervates many glands of the head, such as lacrimal, submandibular, sublingual, nasal, oral, and pharyngeal areas.
- Glossopharyngeal (IX) innervates the parotid glands.

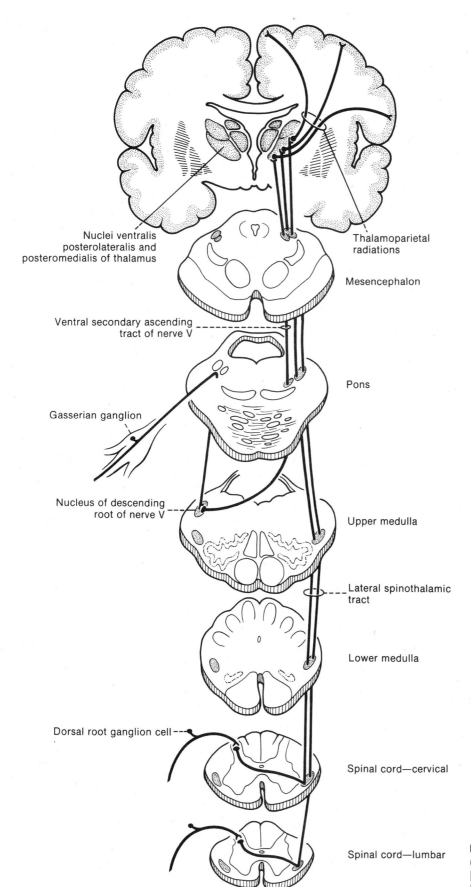

Nuclei ventralis
posterolateralis and
posteromedialis of thalamus

Thalamoparietal
radiations

Mesencephalon

Ventral secondary ascending
tract of nerve V

Pons

Gasserian ganglion

Nucleus of descending
root of nerve V

Upper medulla

Lateral spinothalamic
tract

Lower medulla

Dorsal root ganglion cell

Spinal cord—cervical

Spinal cord—lumbar

Figure 5–36 • The lateral spinothalamic (sensory) tract. (From Haerer, A. F. [1992]. *DeJong's the neurologic examination* [5th ed.]. Philadelphia: J. B. Lippincott.)

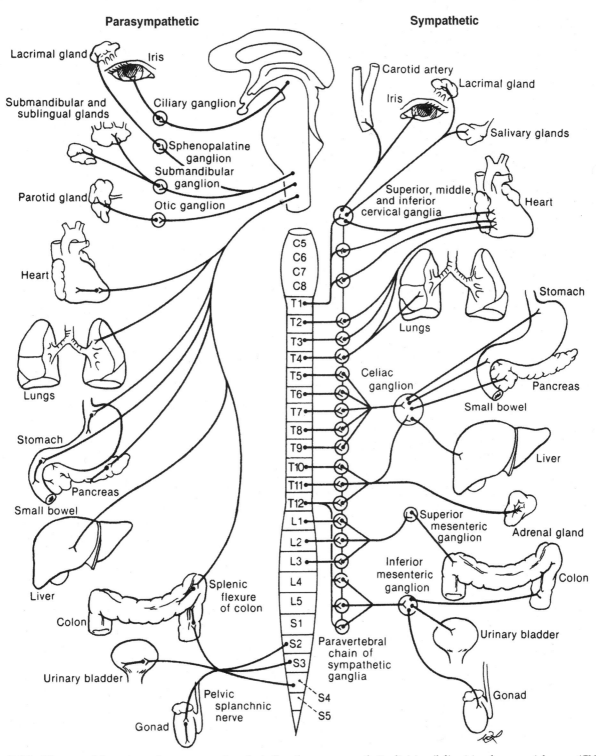

Figure 5–37 • Diagram of the autonomic nervous system, including the parasympathetic division (*left*) arising from cranial nerve (CN) III, CN VII, CN IX, and CN X and from spinal cord segments S2–S4. The sympathetic division (*right*) arises from spinal cord segments T1–T12. (From DeMyer, W. [1998]. *Neuroanatomy* [2nd ed.]. Baltimore: Williams & Wilkins.)

- Vagus (X) synapses with terminal ganglia located adjacent to, or within, the various viscera throughout the body.

The sacral portion of the parasympathetic system arises from cell bodies in the intermediate gray matter of sacral segments S-2 through S-4. These fibers pass through the pelvic splanchnic nerve to synapse in the terminal ganglia with the postganglionic neurons, which innervate the descending colon, rectum, bladder, lower ureters, and external genitalia. The parasympathetic system is involved with the mechanisms of bladder and bowel evacuation and, unlike the sympathetic system, is designed to re-

Table 5–9 • AUTONOMIC EFFECTS OF THE NERVOUS SYSTEM

STRUCTURE OR ACTIVITY	PARASYMPATHETIC EFFECTS	SYMPATHETIC EFFECTS
Pupil of the Eye	Constricted	Dilated
Circulatory System		
Rate and force of heartbeat	Decreased	Increased
Blood vessels		
In heart muscle	Constricted	Dilated
In skeletal muscle	*	Dilated
In abdominal viscera and the skin	*	Constricted
Blood pressure	Decreased	Increased
Respiratory System		
Bronchioles	Constricted	Dilated
Rate of breathing	Decreased	Increased
Digestive System		
Peristaltic movements of digestive tube	Increased	Decreased
Muscular sphincters of digestive tube	Relaxed	Contracted
Secretion of salivary glands	Thin, watery saliva	Thick, viscid saliva
Secretions of stomach, intestine, and pancreas	Increased	*
Conversion of liver glycogen to glucose	*	Increased
Genitourinary System		
Urinary bladder		
Muscular walls	Contracted	Relaxed
Sphincters	Relaxed	Contracted
Muscles of the uterus	Relaxed; variable	Contracted under some conditions; varies with menstrual cycle and pregnancy
Blood vessels of external genitalia	Dilated	*
Integument		
Secretion of sweat	*	Increased
Pilomotor muscles	*	Contracted (gooseflesh)
Medullae of Adrenal Glands	*	Secretion of epinephrine and norepinephrine

* No direct effect.

(From Chaffee, E. E., & Lytle, I. M. [1980]. *Basic physiology and anatomy* [3rd ed]. Philadelphia: J. B. Lippincott.)

spond to a specific stimulus in a localized area for a short period of time.

Parasympathetic Neurotransmitters

The parasympathetic system secretes **acetylcholine** at the postganglionic neuron. This is why the parasympathetic system is termed **cholinergic.** Acetylcholine is also secreted at the preganglionic synapse and is quickly deactivated by **cholinesterase.**

Spinal Reflexes

A **reflex** is a stereotypical response, mediated by the nervous system, to a particular stimulus of sufficient magnitude. The simplest type of stereotypical neural pathway is called a **reflex arc.** There are five components to a reflex arc, including the following (Fig. 5-38):

Receptor – specific sensory fibers that are sensitive to the stimulus
Sensory (afferent) neuron – that relays the impulse through the posterior root to the CNS

Interneuron – an association or connecting neuron located within the CNS
Motor (efferent) neuron – that relays the impulse through the anterior root to the effector organ
Effector – a specific organ that responds

Reflexes can be classified by the extent of the regional involvement of the spinal cord. This classification includes **segmental, intersegmental,** and **suprasegmental reflexes.**

A reflex the arc of which passes through only one anatomic segment is called a **segmental reflex.** A knee-jerk reflex is an example of both a segmental and a simple or monosynaptic reflex. A monosynaptic reflex includes an afferent limb that synapses directly with an efferent limb. Most reflexes, however, are more complex and polysynaptic.

An **intersegmental reflex** involves several spinal segments. A flexor or withdrawal reflex is an example of an intersegmental reflex.

A **suprasegmental reflex** involves interaction between the brain centers that regulate cord activity and the segments of the cord itself. An example of a suprasegmental reflex is extension of the legs in response to movement of the head.

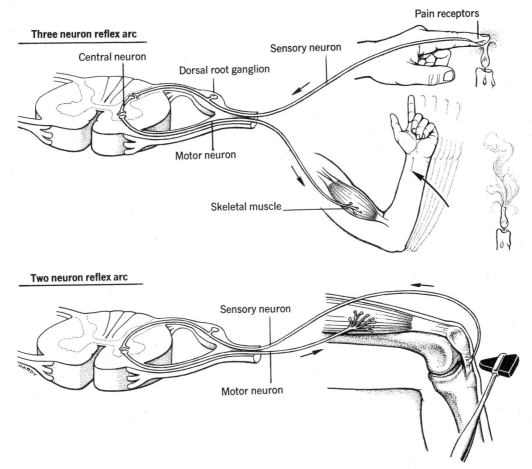

Figure 5–38 • Diagram of a flexor reflex (*top*) and a stretch reflex (*bottom*). (From Chaffee, E. E., & Lytle, I. M. [1980]. *Basic physiology and anatomy.* Philadelphia: J. B. Lippincott.)

Another classification system useful in clinical practice divides reflexes into stretch, cutaneous, and pathologic reflexes.

Muscle stretch reflexes, also called deep tendon reflexes (DTRs), are elicited by striking a tendon that stretches the neuromuscular spindles of the muscle group. The knee-jerk reflex, a stretch reflex, results in contraction of the quadriceps and extension of the leg in response to tapping the patellar tendon. Other common stretch reflexes involve the biceps, triceps, and ankle.

Cutaneous reflexes, also termed superficial reflexes, are initiated when the skin or mucous membrane is stimulated by light stroking or scratching, resulting in a specific response in a muscle or muscle group. The withdrawal reflex, which is a flexor reflex, is an example of a cutaneous reflex that is a protective reflex. In response to a noxious cutaneous stimulus to the fingers, the hand is flexed and withdrawn. Another cutaneous reflex is contraction of the superficial abdominal muscles in response to light, rapid stroking of the skin on the abdomen.

Pathologic reflexes are those reflexes that should not be present and indicate organic interference with CNS function. The method of eliciting these reflexes usually involves stimulation of the skin in a particular area. Presence of a Babinski sign is a common pathologic reflex.

Micturition

Micturition, also called voiding or urination, is the process of evacuating urine from the bladder. In the infant and young child, micturition is a simple reflex initiated by distention of the bladder by urine. Between 2 and 3 years of age, the maturation of spinal cord segments, along with the conscious inhibitory ability of the cerebral cortex, results in voluntary control of micturition. The average capacity of the urinary bladder is 700 to 800 mL. Stimulation of the stretch receptors by a volume of 200 to 300 mL of urine will trigger the micturition reflex and a concurrent conscious desire to void.

Two main anatomic parts constitute the smooth muscle urinary bladder: (1) the body, which is the **detrusor muscle;** and (2) the **trigone,** a small, triangular area at the base of the bladder that includes the bladder-ureter junction, the urethra, and the external sphincter (a voluntary skeletal muscle). The external sphincter is located at the opening of the bladder and is normally contracted to prevent dribbling.

Micturition is primarily a parasympathetic function. The micturition reflex is mediated by S-2, S-3, and S-4 spinal segments, from which the preganglionic parasympathetic fibers synapse within the ganglia located in the bladder wall by way of the pelvic splanchnic nerves (Fig. 5-39). Short postganglionic parasympathetic fibers innervate both the detrusor muscle and

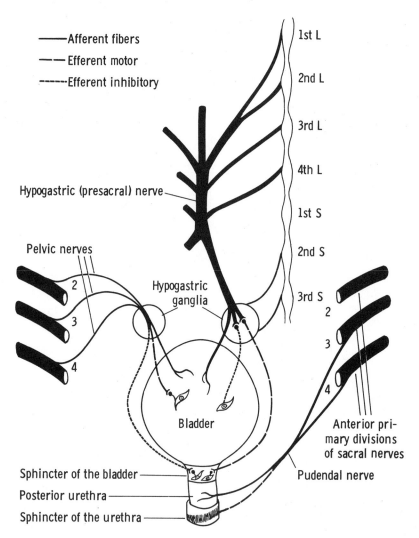

Figure 5–39 • Diagrammatic representation of the innervation of the bladder and urethra. (From Chaffee, E. E., & Lytle, I. M. [1980]. *Basic physiology and anatomy.* Philadelphia: J. B. Lippincott.)

internal sphincter. Parasympathetic stimulation that is caused by the stretching of the bladder wall results in contraction of the detrusor muscle and relaxation of the internal sphincter. Although there is some sympathetic innervation to the bladder, its role is not certain. Micturition is primarily a parasympathetic function.

The external sphincter is under voluntary control and is mediated by the pudendal nerve. It can be voluntarily contracted, but it relaxes by reflex action when urine is released from the internal sphincter.

Defecation

The act of evacuating the large bowel is called **defecation.** Several physiologic mechanisms are involved in defecation. **Peristalsis** is the wavelike movement of smooth muscles within the wall of the large intestines. There are two important reflexes related to defecation. The gastrocolic and duodenocolic reflexes that result from distention of the stomach and duodenum after eating facilitate peristalsis and mass movement along the gastrointestinal tract toward the rectum.

There are also two defecation reflexes. The first, the **intrinsic defecation reflex,** is triggered by feces entering the rectum. Pressure on the rectal wall sends afferent impulses through the **mesenteric plexus** to initiate peristaltic waves in the descending colon, sigmoid, and rectum, forcing feces toward the anus. Peristalsis relaxes the internal anal sphincter, and if the external anal sphincter is also relaxed, defecation occurs. The intrinsic defecation reflex is a weak reflex and must occur in combination with another reflex for defecation to occur.

This second reflex, the **parasympathetic defecation reflex,** involves the sacral segments (S-3, S-4, S-5) of the spinal cord. Stimulated afferent fibers in the rectum send signals to the spinal cord, and signals are sent back to the descending colon, sigmoid, rectum, and anus through the parasympathetic nerve fibers in the pelvic nerves. The parasympathetic signals do three things: intensify peristalsis, relax the internal anal sphincter, and augment the intrinsic defecation reflex. A powerful bowel evacuation can occur if the external anal sphincter is relaxed.

Conscious Control of Defecation

During infancy, defecation is a purely reflex action. However, in early childhood voluntary control is learned so that defecation can be postponed until a socially acceptable place

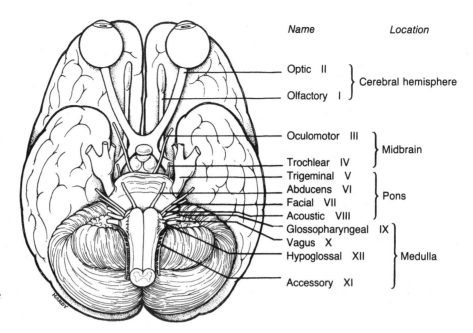

Figure 5-40 • Diagram of the base of the brain showing entrance or exit of the cranial nerves. The eyeballs are shown schematically in relation to the optic nerves. The right column indicates the anatomical location of the connection of each cranial nerve to the central nervous system.

to evacuate the bowel is found. Voluntary consciousness now controls the external anal sphincter. If the sphincter is relaxed, defecation can take place. If contraction of the sphincter prevents defecation, the defecation reflexes soon cease, remaining inactive for several hours until more feces enter the rectum and once again initiate the defecation reflexes. The frequency of defecation among people varies from once per day to two or three times per week.

CRANIAL NERVES

The 12 pairs of CNs are part of the peripheral nervous system. Besides being named, each CN is also identified in Roman numerals. The number is based on the descending order in which the CNs and their nuclei attach to the CNS. CN I connects to the brain in the cerebral hemispheres, whereas CN XII attaches at the lower medulla (Fig. 5-40). There are three pure sensory CNs (I, II, and VIII), five pure motor CNs (III, IV, VI, XI, and XII), and four mixed CNs (V, VII, IX, and X).

The anatomic locations of connection of the CNs are as follows: I and II are in the cerebral hemispheres; III and IV are in the midbrain; V, VI, VII, and VIII are in the pons; and IX, X, XI, and XII are in the medulla. There are a few exceptions to the schemata: CNs VII and VIII have dual citizenship in both the pons and, to a lesser degree, in the medulla. CN V, primarily associated with the pons, also has branches in the midbrain and medulla (Fig. 5-41).

As a rule, CNs do not cross in the brain (with the exception of CN IV). There are three sensory CNs (I, II, and VIII), five motor CNs (III, IV, VI, XI, and XII), and four CNs with mixed functions (V, VII, IX, and X).

Classification of nerve fibers is similar to spinal nerves in some cases and dissimilar in other instances. CNs that have functions similar to those of spinal nerves are categorized as **general**; those with specialized functions (olfactory and gus-

tatory) are **special**. The GSA, GVA, GSE, and GVE fibers are similar to spinal nerves of those categories and have already been discussed with spinal nerves. Fibers that are specific to CNs include **special somatic afferent (SSA)**, **special visceral afferent (SVA)**, and **special visceral efferent (SVE)**. SSA fibers convey sensory impulses from the special sense organs in the eye (vision) and ear (hearing and balance). SVA fibers convey impulses from the olfactory and gustatory receptors. SVE fibers innervate striated skeletal muscles from the brachial arches (jaw muscles, facial expression muscles, and muscles of pharynx and larynx).

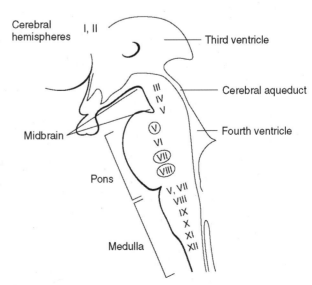

Figure 5-41 • Lateral view of sites of cranial nerves and their nuclei within the cerebral hemispheres and brain stem (midbrain, pons, or medulla).

Olfactory Nerve (Sensory) (CN I)

The olfactory nerve is a pure SVA nerve for the sense of smell. The receptors for smell are located in the superior nasal mucosa of each nostril. The **olfactory** nerve is composed of multiple small fibers from bipolar chemoreceptor cells called olfactory cells. The axons penetrate the skull through the cribriform plate to terminate in the **olfactory bulb.** From the bulb, the **olfactory tract** continues backward to the base of the frontal lobes where the two principal areas—the medial olfactory area and the lateral olfactory area—are located. The **medial olfactory area** is located anteriorly and superiorly to the hypothalamus (septum pellucidum, gyrus subcallosus, paraolfactory area, olfactory trigone, and medial part of the anterior perforated substance). The **lateral olfactory area** is composed of the prepyriform area, the uncus, the lateral part of the anterior perforated substance, and part of the amygdaloid nucleus.

Optic Nerve (Sensory) (CN II)

The **optic nerve,** another pure SSA nerve, arises from the retina of the eyeball and is a part of the visual system. The **fundus** or **optic disc** represents the point where the optic nerve joins the retina and can be visualized by using the ophthalmoscope (it is the only CN that can be visualized). The optic disc is a natural blind spot because it does not contain any rods or cones. The **macula** is a 3-mm circular area on the retina, located near the posterior pole of the orbit, that is the point of clearest vision. The **scotoma** is an expected blind spot on the retina.

Vision is complex not only because many steps are involved in the process, but also because the visual tracts cut through all the lobes of the cerebral hemispheres. Therefore, visual deficits are common with many intracranial problems.

The **rods and cones** of the retina are the photoreceptors that are stimulated by light, thereby initiating nerve impulses that are conducted to the cerebral cortex (Fig. 5-42). Each **optic nerve** (4.5 to 5.0 cm long) runs posteriorly until it meets the optic nerve from the other side at the **optic chiasma.** The **visual pathways** posterior to the retina include a number of structures. The optic nerves come together at the optic chiasma, above the sella turcica. A partial decussation takes place at the chiasma whereby the nasal half of each optic nerve crosses to the other side. The **optic tracts** proceed laterally and posteriorly to terminate in the **lateral geniculate bodies** (a flattened area in the posterolateral surface of the thalamus). Before reaching the lateral geniculate body, a few fibers leave the optic tract to go to the pretectal areas. These fibers become the afferent limb of the light reflex.

The **lateral geniculate body** is the terminal point of the optic tract; the geniculocalcarine tract originates from the cells of the geniculate bodies. The **geniculocalcarine tract** passes through the retrolenticular part of the internal capsule and forms the **optic radiations.** The upper fibers of optic radiations pass posteriorly in the *parietal lobe* and terminate in the superior portion of the calcarine cortex (occipital lobe); the lower fibers (**Meyer's loop**) loop anteriolaterally around the temporal horn of the *temporal lobe* and terminate in the inferior calcarine cortex. The **calcarine cortex,** also called the **primary visual cortex,** is organized such that the upper part of the visual field terminates in the

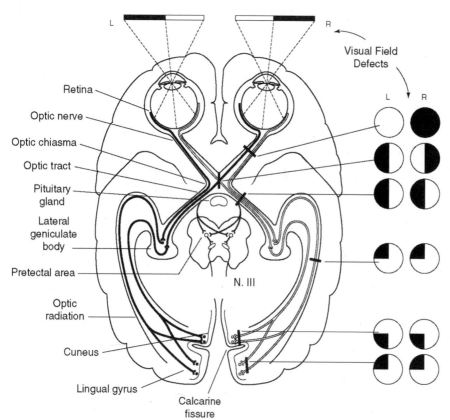

Figure 5–42 • Fields of vision.

inferior calcarine cortex and the lower visual field terminates in the superior cortex. The primary cortex (area 17) is located in the walls of the calcarine fissure and receives primary visual stimuli. The **visual association areas** (areas 18 and 19) are located in the **peristriate cortex** of the temporal and occipital lobes, lateral to the primary cortex. The visual association areas are necessary for visual impressions, recognition of colors and formed objects, and visual memory. In addition, eye movements activated by visual stimuli are controlled by the association areas.

Visual System

When the visual system is considered, it includes not only the optic nerves, visual pathways, and visual cortex but also eye movement itself. Eye movement is addressed here to complete the discussion of the visual system.

Conjugate gaze and eye movement are complex processes for which the following areas have specific functions:

Brain stem for premotor conjugate gaze and vergence eye movement (**vergence** movements are both eyes moving medially to look at a near object or laterally to look into the distance)

Thalamic-midbrain centers for vertical gaze and vergence

Paramedian pontine reticular formation of the pons for horizontal eye movement.

Five subsystems have been identified to enable the fovea to find and fixate on a target, stabilize an image on the retina, and maintain binocular focus during head or target movement.

Saccadic system (a **saccade** is a rapid, refixational eye movement): saccades may be voluntary or involuntary

Pursuit system: provides for eyes to track slowly moving targets

Vestibular system (semicircular canals): maintains a stable image on the retina during head movements

Optokinetic system: enables stabilization of images on the retina during sustained head rotation, such as spinning

Vergence eye movement system: allows the eyes to move convergently and divergently to maintain binocular fixation on a target moving toward or away from the subject

The frontal-parietal gaze center (posterior portion of middle frontal gyrus, area 8; and ventral parietal lobe, area 7a) and the occipital gaze center (areas 18 and 19) are important. The **frontal gaze center** is responsible for rapid (saccadic) voluntary control of conjugate gaze to a point of interest. Its fibers pass through the anterior internal capsule to the pons and connect with the lower centers. The **occipital gaze center** controls involuntary slow-tracking eye movement or visual pursuit. The center is responsible for fixing the eyes on an object and maintaining that visual fixation as the object moves through the visual field. Its fibers pass medially to the optic radiations and down through the posterior portion of the internal capsule, connecting with the conjugate eye movement centers in the midbrain and pons.

The MLF extends from the thalamic-midbrain region to the anterior horn cells of the spinal cord; it coordinates the movement pathways of the eye and neck for gaze. The MLF connects and integrates fibers from the following areas of eye movement: brain-stem oculomotor, trochlear, and abducens nuclei; fibers from the synapse of cerebellar nuclei and the semicircular canals; and the horizontal gaze center of the pons. Convergence of the eyes is not well understood and seems to be mediated by pontine and medullary structures, but not by the MLF. Divergence is controlled by centers located near the abducens nuclei.

The **paramedian pontine reticular formation (PPRF)** is located in the pons and receives fibers from the superior colliculus, the vestibular nuclei, and other parts of the reticular formation. The PPRF is also known as the lateral gaze center. It sends fibers to the ipsilateral abducens nucleus (lateral movement) and through the MLF to cells of the contralateral oculomotor nucleus that supply the medial rectus muscle thus coordinating horizontal. Therefore, the descending pathways for horizontal conjugate gaze include the PPRF and the MLF. Much less is known about vertical movement. The oculomotor and trochlear nuclei, located in the brain stem, are involved in vertical eye movement: vertical and torsional saccadic innervation arise in the midbrain; the vertical gaze-holding impulses are integrated in the midbrain; and the vestibular and pursuit impulses ascend to the midbrain from the lower brainstem.

Oculomotor Nerve (Motor) (CN III)

The oculomotor nerve innervates four of the six extrinsic muscles responsible for movement of the eye. These muscles are the medial, superior, and inferior recti and the inferior oblique; they are controlled by GSE fibers. The eyes are rotated by these muscles in the following manner: medial recti—inward (medially); superior recti—upward and inward; inferior recti—downward and inward; and the inferior oblique—upward and outward (Table 5-10).

The oculomotor nerve has two other functions. First, it innervates the levator palpebrae superioris, which is responsible for elevating the upper eyelid (also GSE fibers). Second, it provides motor innervation to the intrinsic smooth muscles of the iris for pupillary constriction and to the muscles within the ciliary body for lens accommodation (both GVE functions).

The eye is innervated by both parasympathetic and sympathetic fibers to control pupillary size. Parasympathetic innervation is responsible for **pupillary constriction.** The parasympathetic preganglionic fibers arise in the **Edinger-Westphal nucleus** (the visceral nucleus of CN III) and then proceed in CN III to the ciliary ganglion. Here, the preganglionic fibers synapse with postganglionic parasympathetic neurons that send fibers through the ciliary nerves into the eyeball. These nerves excite the ciliary muscles and the pupillary sphincter of the iris, resulting in pupillary constriction.

Pupillary dilation is the result of sympathetic innervation of the pupil originating in the intermediolateral horn cells of the first segment of the spinal cord. Proceeding from here, sympathetic fibers enter the sympathetic chain and pass upward to the superior cervical ganglion, where they synapse with postganglionic neurons. These fibers radiate along the carotid artery and smaller arteries until the eye is

Table 5-10 • CRANIAL NERVE FUNCTION RELATIVE TO EYE MOVEMENT

CRANIAL NERVE	MUSCLE	MOVEMENT OF EYEBALL
Oculomotor (III)*	Medial rectus	Inward or medially on the horizontal plane
	Superior rectus	Upward and outward
	Inferior rectus	Downward and outward
	Inferior oblique	Upward and inward
Trochlear (IV)	Superior oblique	Downward and inward
Abducens (VI)	Lateral rectus	Outward or laterally on the horizontal plane

Inferior oblique (3rd) — Superior rectus (3rd)
Superior rectus (3rd) — Lateral rectus (6th)
Lateral rectus (6th) — Medial rectus (3rd)
Medial rectus (3rd) — Inferior rectus (3rd)
Inferior rectus (3rd) — Superior oblique (4th) — Inferior rectus (3rd)

Note that the eye muscles function in pairs: the superior and inferior recti turn the eye upward and downward when the eye is looking outward (temporally); the inferior and superior obliques turn the eye upward and downward when the eye is looking inward; and the medial and lateral recti turn the eye inward (nasally) and outward (temporally) on the horizontal plane.

* The oculomotor nerve also innervates the levator palpebrae oculoris muscle, which elevates the upper eyelid and the muscles that control the iris and ciliary body.

(Figure from Bates, B. [1980]. *A guide to physical examination.* Philadelphia: J. B. Lippincott.)

reached. Here, the sympathetic fibers excite the radial fibers of the iris and cause pupillary dilation.

Accommodation is the mechanism by which an automatic adjustment or accommodation of the curvature of the lens is made to focus images on the retina for visual acuity. Accommodation results from the contraction or relaxation of the ciliary muscles of the eye. Contraction of the smooth muscle fibers of the ciliary body causes the **suspensory ligaments** to relax and the lens to become thicker. Relaxation of the **ciliary body's** smooth muscle fibers results in tension of the suspensory ligaments and elongation of the lens.

Trochlear Nerve (Motor) (CN IV)

The trochlear nerve, a GSE nerve, supplies the superior oblique muscle. It is responsible for moving the eye downward and inward. The **trochlear nucleus** is located immediately caudal to the oculomotor nucleus at the level of the inferior colliculus in the midbrain. It exits the brain stem dorsally, the only CN to exit from the dorsum (posterior part) of the brain stem. Small bundles of fibers curve around the periaqueductal gray matter and decussate in the superior medullary velum; the trochlear emerges caudal to the inferior colliculus. The superior oblique muscle is supplied by crossed fibers.

Trigeminal Nerve (Mixed) (CN V)

The trigeminal nerve is unique in that its main components are located in the pons with additional components in the midbrain and medulla. The trigeminal nerve has both GSA

and SVE components. Pain, temperature, and light touch are conveyed from the entire face and scalp, the paranasal sinuses, and the nasal and oral cavities by the GSA component. The SVE motor component supplies the muscles of mastication, which arise from the brachial arches.

The GSA fibers arise from the cell bodies in the **trigeminal ganglion.** The sensory components of the trigeminal nerve are divided into three sensory branches: **ophthalmic, maxillary,** and **mandibular** (Fig. 5-43). Axons travel centrally from the ganglion to enter the lateral aspect of the pons. Fibers for touch synapse directly on the **main sensory nucleus of V** that is located in the dorsolateral tegmentum of the pons. Pain and temperature fibers follow a different course. They turn caudally and descend via the dorsolateral medulla and upper three or four segments of the cervical spinal cord as the **spinal tract of the trigeminal nerve.** The peripheral path followed by sensory fibers after the trigeminal ganglion is as follows:

1. The **ophthalmic division (V1)** passes through the superior orbital fissure to innervate the upper face.
2. The **maxillary division (V2)** exits the skull via the foramen rotundum to innervate the midface.
3. The **mandibular division (V3),** joined by the motor root, exits the skull via the foramen ovale to innervate the lower face.

The SVE fibers that innervate the muscles of mastication arise from cell bodies in the **motor nucleus of V,** which is located medial to the main sensory nucleus in the pons. The axons follow a ventrolateral path and exit from the lateral surface of the pons.

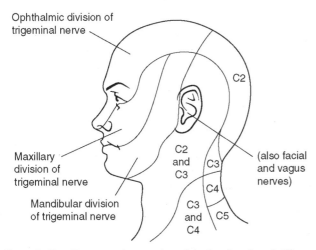

Ophthalmic division of trigeminal nerve

C2

Maxillary division of trigeminal nerve

C2 and C3

C3

(also facial and vagus nerves)

Mandibular division of trigeminal nerve

C4

C3 and C4

C5

Figure 5–43 • Cutaneous innervation of the head and neck. The boundaries between the territories supplied by the three divisions of the trigeminal nerve do not overlap appreciably, as do the boundaries between spinal dermatomes. (From Barr, M. L., & Kiernan, J. A. [1988]. *The human nervous system* [5th ed.]. Philadelphia: J. B. Lippincott.)

Abducens Nerve (Motor) (CN VI)

The abducens is a GSE nerve that innervates the lateral rectus muscle and rotates the eye laterally on the horizontal plane. The abducens nerve arises from the **abducens nuclei** located in the floor of the fourth ventricle of the midpons. Axons follow an anterior course through the tegmentum and basis pontis to the pontomedullary junction. The abducens then ascends to the pontine base through the cavernous sinus and exits the cranium through the superior orbital fissure to the lateral rectus muscle.

Facial Nerve (Mixed) (CN VII)

The facial nerve has its nucleus primarily in the pons, but it also has connections to the medulla. It has SVE, GVE, and SVA components. The **facial nucleus** is located in the pons and has two branches: SVE fibers (arise in one branch and innervate the muscles of facial expression), and GVE and SVA fibers. The SVE branch is responsible for closing the eye, smiling, whistling, showing the teeth, wrinkling the nose, and grimacing. The parasympathetic GVE fibers originate in the superior salivatory nucleus and control tearing and salivation of the lacrimal, sublingual, and submandibular glands. The sensory fibers originate in the **geniculate ganglion**; these SVA components mediate taste to the anterior two thirds of the tongue and sensation from the skin lining the external auditory meatus.

The SVE innervation of the muscles of facial expression can be divided into the muscles of the lower part of the face and the muscles of the upper part of the face. **Crossed fibers** project from the cerebral cortex to the facial nuclei that supply the contralateral lower part of the face (the area below the eye). **Crossed and uncrossed fibers** project to motor cells that innervate the upper part of the face. Movement of the upper face (e.g., wrinkling the brow) comes from bilateral input from the cortex to the facial nerve nucleus.

Because the upper facial muscles receive both crossed and uncrossed fibers, the upper part of the face is spared with central cerebral injury such as in stroke. The upper motor lesion results in a paralysis that is limited to muscles of the contralateral lower face (below the eye). If the facial nerve is injured, the entire side of the face (upper and lower face) would be affected. Therefore, the deficits on the affected side would include an "ironed out" forehead, an inability to close the eye, and a flattening of the nasolabial fold.

Acoustic Nerve (Sensory) (CN VIII)

The acoustic nerve is divided into two branches: the cochlear, which is concerned with hearing, and the vestibular, which influences balance, maintenance of body position, and orientation in space. Because these branches represent two distinct systems, they are discussed separately.

In the **auditory system,** the acoustic nerve has SSA fibers that carry impulses from the cell bodies in the spiral ganglion of the cochlea. Vibrations proceed through the tympanic membrane and activate the three small bones of the middle ear (malleus, incus, and stapes). These vibrations then continue to the cochlea of the inner ear where the basilar membrane with the **organ of Corti** (hairlike mechanoreceptors) send fibers to the spiral ganglion of the cochlea. The spiral ganglion contains the bipolar cells of the cochlea (dorsal and ventral cochlear nuclei) that connect to the brain stem. The primary auditory receptive areas of the cortex are 41 and 42. From here, the impulses proceed to the auditory association area where recognition of the particular sound takes place.

In the **vestibular system,** the **vestibular nerve** has SSA fibers. The vestibular receptor end-organs in the vestibular system include the three cristae ampullares, one located in each of the semicircular canals, and the maculae of the utricle and saccule. All these structures are sensitive to movement in a particular direction. The vestibular ganglion of the vestibular nerve receives input from the vestibular receptors and the cerebellum. The vestibular nuclei have projections into the following areas: spinal cord, by way of the lateral and medial vestibular spinal tracts (inhibitory and facilitory influence to extensor muscle tone and spinal reflexes); cerebellum; reticular formation; and, through the MLF, the nuclei of CNs III, IV, and VI.

Glossopharyngeal Nerve (Mixed) (CN IX)

The glossopharyngeal nerve is a mixed nerve with SVE, GVE, GSA, GVA, and SVE fibers. The vagus nerve is closely related, both anatomically and physiologically, to the glossopharyngeal nerve. The glossopharyngeal nerve has five branches, all of which penetrate the skull through the jugular foramen. The glossopharyngeal nerve innervates the stylopharyngeus of the pharynx (SVE); taste receptors from the posterior third of the tongue (SVA); parasympathetics of the parotid gland (GVE); sensation from the back of the ear (GSA); and sensation from the pharynx, tongue, eustachian tube, carotid sinus, and carotid body (GVA).

The SVE fibers of the stylopharyngeus muscle originate in the nucleus ambiguus. The GVE fibers carry parasympathetic fibers to the parotid gland and terminate in the otic ganglion. The cell bodies for sensory innervation are located in the inferior and superior petrosal ganglia.

Vagus Nerve (Mixed) (CN X)

The vagus nerve is also a mixed nerve with SVE, GVE, GSA, GVA, and SVE fibers. It branches into several segments. The functions include innervation of the striated muscles from the brachial arches (soft palate, pharynx, and larynx [SVE]); the parasympathetic innervation of the thoracic and abdominal organs (GVE); sensory innervation from the external auditory meatus (GSA); sensory innervation from the pharynx, larynx, and thoracic and abdominal viscera (GVA); and sensory innervation from the taste receptors of the posterior pharynx (SVA).

The SVE fibers (soft palate, pharynx, and larynx) come from the nucleus ambiguus found in the lateral medullary region dorsal to the inferior olive. The GVE components include preganglionic parasympathetic fibers coming from the dorsal motor nucleus to supply the thoracic and abdominal viscera. Preganglionic vagal neurons from the nucleus ambiguus innervate the heart. The preganglionic fibers synapse with the postganglionic neurons in the cardiac, pulmonary, esophageal, or celiac plexuses or within the visceral organs. The cell bodies for sensory innervation are dispersed throughout the body in a number of ganglia.

Spinal Accessory Nerve (Motor) (CN XI)

This spinal accessory nerve is an SVE nerve that innervates the sternocleidomastoid and upper portion of the trapezius muscle, allowing one to shrug the shoulders and rotate the head. The two roots of the spinal accessory nerve originate in the lower medulla and the upper five cervical spinal cord segments. It ascends in the spinal canal and enters the skull through the foramen magnum, where it is joined by the minor accessory component originating in the nucleus ambiguus; the spinal nerve leaves the cranial cavity through the jugular foramen to innervate the sternocleidomastoid and trapezius muscles.

Hypoglossal Nerve (Motor) (CN XII)

The hypoglossal nerve is a GSE nerve that innervates the intrinsic muscles of the tongue to permit normal speech and swallowing. The paramedian area of that caudal medulla in the floor of the fourth ventricle is the location of the hypoglossal nucleus. The fibers exit from the ventral medulla, between the medullary pyramids and the olive. The fibers then pass through the hypoglossal canal in the occipital condyle and innervate the striated muscles of the tongue.

RESOURCES
Professional
Published Material

Aird, T. (2000). Functional anatomy of the basal ganglia. *Journal of Neuroscience Nursing, 32*(5), 250–277.

Bear, M. F., Connors, B. W., & Paradiso, M. A. (2001). *Neuroscience: Exploring the brain* (2nd ed.) Philadelphia: Lippincott Williams & Wilkins.

Benarroch, E. E., Westmoreland, B. F., Daube, J. R., Reagan, T. J., & Sandok, B. A. (1999). *Medical neurosciences: An approach to anatomy, pathology, and physiology by systems and levels* (4th ed.). Philadelphia: Lippincott Williams & Wilkins.

Conn, P. M. (Ed.). (1995). *Neuroscience in medicine.* Philadelphia: J. B. Lippincott.

Guarantors of Brain. (2000). *Aids to the examination of the peripheral nervous system* (4th ed.). Edinburgh: W. B. Saunders.

Jennes, L., Traurig, H. H., & Conn, P. M. (1995). *Atlas of the human brain.* Philadelphia: J. B. Lippincott.

Johnson, L. R. (1998). *Essential medical physiology* (2nd ed., Chaps. 48–61). Philadelphia: Lippincott-Raven.

Kandel, E. R., Schwartz, J. H., & Jessell, T. M. (2000). *Principles of neural science* (4th ed.). New York: McGraw-Hill.

Kingsley, R. E. (2000). *Concise text of neuroscience* (2nd ed.). Philadelphia: Lippincott Williams & Wilkins.

Miller, N. R., & Newman, N. J. (1999). *Walsh & Hoyt's Clinical Neuro-ophthalmology* (5th ed.). Philadelphia: Williams & Wilkins.

Minton, M. S., & Hickey, J. V. 1999). A primer of neuroanatomy and neurophysiology. *Nursing Clinics of North America, 34*(3), 555–572.

Robertson, D., Low, P. A., & Polinsky, R. J. (Eds.). (1996). *Primer on the autonomic nervous system.* San Diego: Academic Press.

Snell, R. S. (1997). *Clinical neuroanatomy for medical students* (4th ed.). Philadelphia: Lippincott Williams & Wilkins.

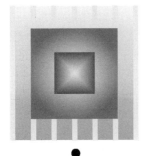

JOANNE V. HICKEY

CHAPTER 6

Diagnostic Procedures and Laboratory Tests for Neuroscience Patients

Diagnostic procedures and laboratory tests for neuroscience patients continue to develop and become more sophisticated and specific. Development of diagnostic technologies has resulted in a cadre of highly specialized health care professionals skilled in the techniques of testing and the interpretation of the findings and providing input to treatment decisions.

More and more diagnostic procedures are scheduled as outpatient procedures in special hospital areas (e.g., radiology departments, special procedures departments) or in facilities dedicated to providing specific diagnostics with results forwarded to referring physicians. These practices have been driven by cost-containment demands, proven safety of outpatient diagnostic procedures, and patient convenience. On the day of the diagnostic procedure, the patient reports to a special hospital area (e.g., 23-hour unit, ambulatory center) or other facility, undergoes the procedure, recovers in a special unit, and is discharged home, usually without an overnight stay. In other instances, diagnostics are ordered during hospitalization.

The variations of entry points for diagnostic procedures create special challenges for patient and family education and preparation. Patient education, a key responsibility of the nurse, has changed (see below). The nurse may not see the patient until arrival for the test, or there may not be a nurse present at all. Nurses need to recognize the realities of how patient teaching is conducted in their environments, a responsibility now shared with others. This sensitivity must be incorporated into interactions with patients and families to ensure patient and family understanding and opportunities for questions. This precludes time for discussion or questions, so that it may be unclear whether the patient reviewed the material.

PATIENT AND FAMILY TEACHING

Focus of Patient Teaching

Patients undergoing a diagnostic procedure need a general explanation of the procedure with special emphasis on what to expect and their role as participants. For example, patients who are about to undergo a brain computed tomography (CT) scan should be told that they must remain very still while the scan is being taken to ensure accuracy and high-quality graphics. For a more thorough briefing, describe the procedure according to the patient's level of understanding and desire for information. Patients should know the exact location of where the procedure will be conducted, who will be there, and where they will be taken on its completion.

If a patient's level of consciousness has been altered sufficiently to affect attention, comprehension, understanding, memory, and appreciation of causal associations, provide a simple explanation. Repetition and reinforcement of information may be necessary because of problems with cognitive deficits (e.g., memory), anxiety, or fear. Patient education and preparation are a collaborative concern of all health care team members involved in the patient's care.

The large number of people undergoing diagnostic procedures on an outpatient ambulatory basis presents special challenges for education and preparation of patients. Education may be provided through a direct patient–nurse conference, a telephone call, mailed written and illustrated material (e.g., instructions and booklets) with or without a videotape or audiocassette, e-mail, or referral to a website. Decisions must be made to match the educational media with the ability, resources, and comfort of the patient. For example, literacy and comprehension level must be assessed and material matched to the patient. Regardless of which media are selected, there is always a need for follow-up to answer questions and clarify information.

OUTPATIENT PROCEDURES

For outpatient procedures, nurses must be knowledgeable about procedures and related protocols and also be sensitive to the anxiety or fear related to the diagnostic process. Patients and families are often aware that the purpose of the procedure is to rule in or rule out certain diagnoses and treatments. As a result, they are often anxious and fearful and need emotional support and education.

HOSPITALIZED PATIENTS AND PROCEDURES

For hospitalized patients, the care nurse assumes responsibility for ensuring the appropriate patient education has been provided. Portions of education may be delegated to other personnel, but the nurse oversees the process and is responsible. Depending on the stability of the patient, unit personnel may accompany the patient to the diagnostic procedure. Sometimes, it is an absolute necessity that a registered nurse accompany the patient, for example, when the patient's condition requires frequent suctioning or the patient is hemodynamically fragile and needs frequent monitoring. A transport protocol, such as one published by the Society of Critical Care Medicine,[1] should be followed to ensure patient safety. For the patient with impaired cognitive function or a high anxiety level, the nurse may make the difference between success or failure of the diagnostic procedure. It is often necessary for the patient to cooperate, lie quietly, or follow instructions. The familiar nurse is often able to gain the patient's cooperation. Judicious use of sedation before and during the procedure is also useful and sometimes necessary.

At other times, the unit care nurse completes certain aspects of preprocedural preparation in the clinical unit. The patient is then taken to the designated area by auxiliary personnel solely responsible for patient transport. After the patient has arrived at the procedure site, technicians and/or the physician are the principal personnel involved. Therefore, it is most important that a proper explanation of the procedure and what to expect be provided to the patient beforehand.

INFORMED CONSENT

Written consent is required for many diagnostic procedures; there may be some variation among institutions. Adhere to institutional policies and procedure manuals. If a patient has an altered level of consciousness, cognitive deficits, or other impairments that will affect ability to give informed consent, a family member must provide written consent and it must be witnessed. It is usually the physician's responsibility to obtain written consent after explaining the procedure, the risks, and answering questions.

X-RAYS OF THE HEAD AND VERTEBRAL COLUMN

Skull/Facial X-rays

Skull films are ordered infrequently because CT and magnetic resonance neuroimaging provide much greater anatomic information including information generally available from skull films. If a CT scan is ordered, the need for skull films is eliminated. One of the most frequent reasons for ordering skull films is to determine whether a skull fracture is present. When skull films are ordered, they usually include anteroposterior and lateral radiographic views (Fig. 6-1). Other angles may be included in the series to provide information about specific areas such as the orbits or paranasal sinuses. Films provide information about the presence of a skull or facial fracture; unusual calcification or presence

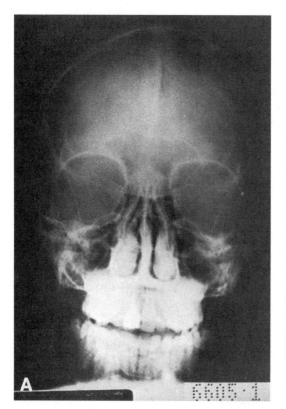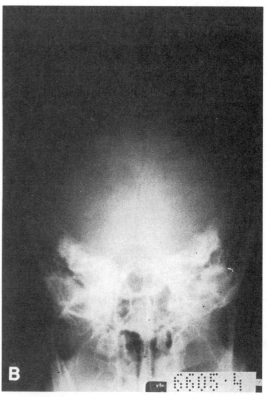

Figure 6–1 • Anterior (*A*) and posterior (*B*) X-ray (radiographic) views of the skull.

of air; the size and shape of skull or facial bones; and bone erosion, particularly of the sella turcica.

When skull films are reviewed, certain landmarks are identified. For example, the pineal body, normally calcified in the adult, is a midline structure. If it appears to be skewed to one side, it suggests that pressure from a space-occupying lesion is responsible for the deviation from the midline. Abnormal calcification raises suspicion of a calcified component located within a tumor; bone erosion suggests the presence of an intracranial lesion close to bone. The following are key points in understanding skull film reports:

- Fractures through the base of the skull or paranasal sinuses may produce pneumocephalus or air pockets in the cranial vault or brain
- A skull fracture with a depression of more than 0.5 cm may result in an underlying contusion.
- Most depressed skull fractures require surgical debridement.

Patient Management

Other than encouraging the patient to lie still for the few moments necessary to take the films, no preparation or postprocedural care is required.

IIII SPINAL X-RAYS

Spinal films are simple radiographs of various regions of the spine: cervical (Fig. 6-2), thoracic, lumbar, or sacral. The most commonly obtained views are the anteroposterior (AP) and the lateral. Because the vertebrae are highly irregular anatomic structures, it is easy to overlook fractures of these bones. This is why lateral films, along with anterior and posterior views, are necessary to rule out the possibility of a fracture. Indications for spinal films include trauma to the back or vertebral column or conditions in which the patient experiences pain or motor or sensory impairment.

In the emergency department, AP and lateral films of the cervical region are taken to rule out cervical fracture. To view the seventh cervical vertebrae, it is often necessary to pull the shoulders downward. To view the odontoid process to determine fracture or instability of C1 and C2 vertebrae, an open-mouth view is necessary. Flexion-extension films are often used to evaluate the presence of spinal injury. When ordered, the patient must be cooperative and cognitively intact to be able to report pain or neurological symptoms. These films are taken under the direct supervision of the physician. A magnetic resonance image (MRI) or CT scan may replace or follow a spinal x-ray for more detailed information.

Abnormal findings found on spinal films may include wedging or compression of a vertebra; bone decalcification (osteoporosis); irregular bone calcification (osteophyte/spur); narrowing of the vertebral canal; vertebral fractures and/or dislocations; and spondylosis.

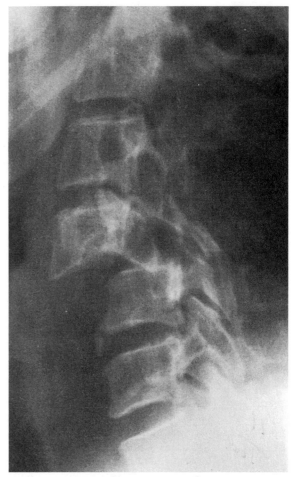

Figure 6–2 • X-ray showing an abnormality of the cervical spine. (From Errico, T. J., Bauer, R. D., & Waugh, T. [1991]. *Spinal trauma.* Philadelphia: J. B. Lippincott.)

Patient Management

Other than encouraging the patient to lie still for the few moments necessary to take the films, there is no preparation or postprocedural care required.

IIII ANATOMIC IMAGING TECHNIQUES OF THE BRAIN

Computed tomography and MRI are the anatomic imaging cornerstones of the diagnostic work-up for neurological and neurosurgical patients and are readily available technologies (Table 6-1). These technologies have made many previously ordered procedures obsolete.

Computed Tomography

Computed tomography, first introduced in 1972 by Hounsfield, is based on use of ionized radiation. CT images are generated by scanning the head in successive layers with

Table 6-1 • COMPARISON OF INDICATIONS FOR COMPUTED TOMOGRAPHY (CT) AND MAGNETIC RESONANCE IMAGING (MRI)*

CT SCAN	MRI
Detection of acute intracranial blood (e.g., subdural, epidural, intracerebral, or subarachnoid hemorrhage)	Lucunar stroke and small ischemic areas
Initial differentiation of acute ischemic stroke from hemorrhagic stroke	Cerebral trauma after initial screening
Cerebral or cerebellar ischemic infarction in first 12–24 hours; after this, MRI used	MRI used after first 12–24 hours with ischemic infarction
Some tumors when enhancement used	Smaller tumors especially of posterior fossa
Arteriovenous malformation or cerebral aneurysm acutely to determine extent of hemorrhage	Dementia (e.g., Alzheimer's disease)
Hydrocephalus	Work-up in epilepsy
Best for detecting abnormal calcification of cranial and vertebral bones	Demyelinating disease (e.g., multiple sclerosis), white matter diseases, and other neurodegenerative conditions
Brain abscess	Spinal cord tumor or trauma
	Intervertebral disk disease

*Note: The choice between CT and MRI for initial evaluation is not always clear; clinical judgment is imperative in selecting the appropriate test at the appropriate time.

x-ray beams that pass through the head from multiple directions. Detectors measure the degree of attenuation of the exiting radiation. Computers integrate this information and construct the images in cross-section.

The thickness of a cross-section, which is called a *cut* or *slice*, can vary from 1.5 to 10 mm. Cuts are taken at a slightly angled horizontal plane. Each cut is subdivided into a grid of tiny cubes or volume elements called *voxels*. The degree of attenuation within each voxel is measured as a numeric value of tissue density. The density number for each voxel is converted to gray scale values with lower numbers coded as black (i.e., cerebrospinal fluid [CSF]) and higher numbers coded as white (i.e., bone). Brain tissue appears in various shades of gray depending on density. The cut is visually displayed as a dot matrix, and filtering techniques improve image quality. Films of the various cuts are then arranged for review. Changes in tissue density, displacement and abnormalities of structures, and calcifications can be noted. CT scans can be done with or without radiocontrast media. Use of a radiopaque medium enhances image sharpness and areas of pathology that resulted from breakdown of the blood–brain barrier.

Procedure

The patient lies on a movable radiographic table with his or her head carefully positioned and immobilized. The head of this table is then rolled several feet into the scanner (Fig. 6-3). A movable circular frame encircles the head and revolves around it, making a clicking sound while taking radiographic readings. Slight, periodic adjustments are made to the machine. The head is scanned numerous times at different angles to collect data.

If contrast enhancement is desired to improve anatomic image clarity, iodinated radiopaque material is administered intravenously. Before administering the medium, consider contraindications, which include pregnancy, allergic reaction to shellfish or iodinated dye, unstable vital signs, and claustrophobia. Some scanning may be done before the con-

trast medium is injected. CT scanning can begin 10 seconds after the beginning of the contrast infusion. When contrast medium is used, a capital "C" will be noted somewhere on the films.

The entire CT scanning procedure takes 10 to 20 minutes. The patient must remain motionless, because movement can cause artifacts that will affect the clarity of the pictures. Agitated or uncooperative patients require sedation or possible anesthesia to ensure the necessary quality of the pictures.

Clinical Applications

The CT scan is most useful to identify hemorrhage (e.g., hematoma, subarachnoid hemorrhage), ventricle size (e.g., enlarged with hydrocephalus, reduced with mass effect), cerebral atrophy, and larger space-occupying lesions. A CT without contrast is ordered to rule out bleeding or a hematoma when a cerebral aneurysm is suspected, and to rule out bleeding to screen candidates for thrombolytic therapy in ischemic stroke. Serial CT scans can be used to follow the resolution of cerebral hemorrhage or edema (Fig. 6-4).

The advantages of CT scans are many. It is a painless, widely available diagnostic tool that requires only minutes to complete, and it can be performed on both conscious and unconscious patients. It is useful in rapidly developing neurological conditions when monitoring and life-support equipment is necessary. CT is sensitive for detection of acute hemorrhage and calcifications and demonstrates the anatomy of skull and vertebral bones well. CT has drastically reduced the need for more dangerous and expensive diagnostic tests. It is also useful when MRI is contraindicated because of metal aneurysm clips, orthopedic prostheses, foreign objects in the eye, pacemakers, and other metal implants. Finally, the cost of a CT scan varies with the type and complexity of the study; generally it is about half the cost of an MRI.[2]

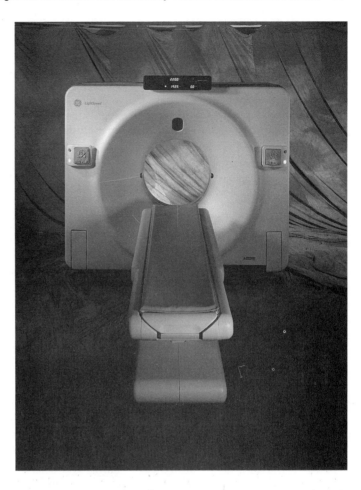

Figure 6–3 • General Electric computed tomography system. (Courtesy of GE Medical Systems, Waukesha, WI.)

Some disadvantages are also noted. CT scans include ionizing radiation exposure whereas MRI does not. CTs have decreased sensitivity for detection of many common neurological diseases, lesions adjacent to bone, small soft-tissue lesions, posterior fossa (cerebellum and brain-stem) lesions, and floor of the middle fossa lesions.[2]

Patient Management

Preparation

All jewelry, eyeglasses, and hair clips or pins should be removed from the head and neck. Unless a contrast medium will be administered, there are no dietary restrictions or

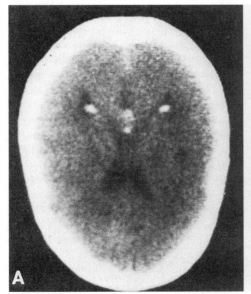
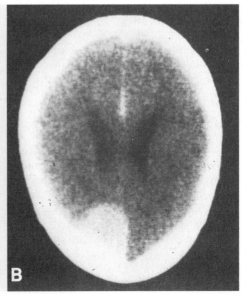

Figure 6–4 • Computed tomography (CT) scan of the brain. (A) Normal scan. (B) Scan showing a large mass in the left frontal lobe.

other screening requirements before the procedure. The amount of time required for conventional MRI had been a drawback for use with rapidly evolving, unstable, and life-threatening conditions. However, development of ultrafast and echoplanar imaging have made MRI as fast as CT.

Premedication such as lorazepam (Ativan) may be ordered before the procedure for anxious patients. For agitated patients, short-acting intravenous sedation may be necessary.

When Contrast Medium Is Used

Before the contrast medium is administered, a skin test is done to check for an allergic reaction. The blood urea nitrogen and creatinine levels are checked for adequate kidney function. Most protocols require the patient to have had nothing by mouth for 4 to 8 hours before the test. Some patients experience flushing or a feeling of warmth, transient headache, a salty taste in the mouth, nausea, or vomiting when the contrast medium is administered; patients should be prepared for these possible reactions.

The procedure and equipment are briefly explained to the patient, and reassurance is given that the procedure is painless. No motion will be felt, and a clicking sound from the equipment is to be expected. Even though the technician and radiologist are outside the room, they can see and maintain voice contact with the patient through an intercom system at all times. The need to remain perfectly still is emphasized.

Postprocedural Care

After the procedure, patients who have received contrast medium should be observed for signs and symptoms of delayed allergic reactions such as hives, skin rash, itching, nausea, or headache. If symptoms are severe, antihistamines may be ordered. Intravenous hydration or oral fluid intake to facilitate clearance of contrast medium is important. Tubular necrosis and acute kidney failure can result from inadequate hydration; older patients are at higher risk because of age-related changes.

Magnetic Resonance Imaging

The second major diagnostic tool for anatomic imaging of the brain and spinal column is the MRI. It is a painless diagnostic procedure used in neuroscience practice that provides images unmatched for exquisitely detailed cross sections of anatomical structures.

Using strong magnetic fields rather than ionized radiation, MRI scanners are located in special, copper-lined rooms that provide shielding from the strong magnetic fields. By applying a strong magnetic field to tissue, certain naturally occurring isotopes (atoms) within the tissue line up within the field, orienting the net tissue magnetization in the longitudinal direction.[2] Although many isotopes are affected, current MRI technology takes advantage of the following unique properties of the hydrogen atom and its differential distribution in tissues of the body:

- Hydrogen atoms have single-proton (i.e., odd number) nuclei.

- These ions resonate under specific conditions.
- Hydrogen atoms are the most abundant isotopes in human tissue.

When the magnetic field is applied, these atoms do not orient precisely in the longitudinal field which are like bipolar magnets, and can wobble a few degrees off center. The atoms are then subjected to computer-programmed transient bursts of radio-frequency (RF) waves perpendicular to the applied magnetic field, reorienting the tissue magnetization from the longitudinal to the transverse plane, thereby increasing the tissue energy level. This effect of rotating the atoms about the axes in a uniform manner is known as **resonance**. When the RF is withdrawn, the net tissue magnetization returns to its original alignment, an effect known as **relaxation**. This results in the generation of MR signals. The signal intensity is detected, stored, and analyzed by computer programs.

The MR signal is produced by the combination of four factors: flow velocity, hydrogen proton density, and T1- and T2-weighted relaxation times. Flow is a measure of flow with a value of 1 in stationary tissue (this is an unimportant parameter in brain imaging). Proton density is a measure of the number of hydrogen nuclei. T1- and T2-relaxation times reflect return of nuclei to their resting state and loss of signal strength, respectively. The contributions of these components to the MR signal can be manipulated by varying the timing of the excitation, called **pulse sequences**. Depending on the weighting of the various components of the signal, images are of three general types: proton density, T1 weighted, or T2 weighted.[3] The pulse sequence variables that are manipulated to produce different types of images are known as **echo time (TE)** and **repetition time (TR)** (Table 6-2). The type of image needed depends on the type of tissue under study and suspected pathology. This ability to manipulate pulse sequence and components enhances the usefulness of MRI.

Some images are based on the amount of time required for the hydrogen protons to relax to their prior magnetic state after they have been tipped 90 or 180 degrees by the RF pulses. This so-called **relaxation parameter** is called "T1." T1 depends on the tissue hydrogen density in specific tissue (e.g., white and gray matter), which differs greatly for various tissue types. A second important relaxation parameter, called "T2," is based on the interaction of the perturbed magnetic fields of hydrogen atoms with each other. The RF pulse pattern causes hydrogen protons to gyrate in unison initially, so that each proton generates its own tiny magnetic field. Because of complex interactions among the magnetic fields, some protons accelerate whereas others decelerate. Various tissues have characteristic differences in their T2 relaxation patterns due to slight differences in tissue biochemistry. These differences can be correlated to the inception of disease processes.

Contrast media may be used in MRI studies; gadolinium-diethylenetriamine pentaacetic acid (gadolinium-DTPA) is the usual non-iodine-based intravascular contrast medium used for enhancement. It alters the magnetic susceptibility of adjacent tissue, thereby providing information about the integrity of the blood–brain barrier. Careful analysis of preenhancement and postenhancement images may help to

▌▌▌▌ Table 6 – 2 • THREE TYPES OF MAGNETIC RESONANCE (MR) IMAGES

MR SIGNAL COMPONENT	DESCRIPTION	IMAGE PRODUCED	BEST USES
Proton density	Short TE and long TR	Has similar color shades for CSF and white matter; gray matter is relatively bright	
T1 weighted	Short TE and short TR	Best tissue discrimination; CSF appears very dark, gray matter is lighter, and white matter is relatively bright	General brain anatomy well visualized (e.g., corpus callosum, cerebral hemispheres)
T2 weighted	Long TE and long TR	Poorest discrimination between gray and white matter; CSF appears very bright	Poor visualization of brain anatomy; very good for identifying areas of tissue pathology (e.g., multiple sclerosis plaques, infarction)

TE, echo time; TR, repetition time; CSF, cerebrospinal fluid.

reveal the precise location of a lesion in situations in which precision is critical.

The interpretation of MRI images depends on the choice of images. Three types of images, which depend on the type of RF pulse sequence employed, are in general use: proton density images, T1-weighted images, and T2-weighted images. Initial evaluations for tumors need to include all three types to be complete. Each type has distinct advantages and disadvantages in its ability to detect the presence of disease at certain tissue interfaces and potential for false-positive information that should be evaluated in light of information obtained from the other sequences. To determine whether an MRI is a T1 or T2 image, look at the color of the CSF. In a T1-weighted image, the CSF appears very dark, gray matter is lighter, and white matter is bright. In a T2-weighted image, the CSF appears very bright and there is poor color discrimination between gray and white matter.

New developments are occurring in MRI technology (Table 6-3).* A MRI technique using fluid-attenuated inversion-recovery (FLAIR) is useful for detecting brain lesions be-

* I would like to thank Nanette Hock, R.N., M.S.N., for her contribution on emerging MRI technology.

cause of its sensitive demonstration of lesions causing T2 prolongation against a suppressed CSF background. The superiority of FLAIR compared with T1-weighted images and T2-weighted images has been shown in many disorders, including stroke, multiple sclerosis, infections, and cerebral hemorrhage.

Procedure

After removing all metal objects and credit cards, the patient lies on a padded stretcher that slides into a tunnel-like chamber. The head is placed in a plastic helmet-like structure; the arms are at the side of the body and are held in place with Velcro straps. The head of the table is then rolled several feet into the scanner. The scanner tube has a restricted opening; it has been compared to the opening of a barrel or large pipe (Fig. 6-5). During the scan, noise, caused by the pulsating RF waves, is heard. The patient must be prepared for this and for the absolute requirement to remain motionless for the scan. Although the patient is alone in the room, voice contact is maintained with the technician through an intercom. If contrast enhancement is desired, gadolinium-DTPA is administered

▌▌▌▌ Table 6 – 3 • DEVELOPMENTS IN MAGNETIC RESONANCE IMAGING (MRI) TECHNOLOGY

NEWER DEVELOPMENTS	USE
Fluid-attenuated inversion recovery image	Gives a high signal for parenchymal lesions and a low signal for CSF
Diffusion-weighted imaging	Detects cytotoxic edema and early ischemic changes
Echoplanar imaging	Includes a technology for ultrafast images that is also used in functional MRI
Functional MRI	Images physiologic function of oxygenation status of hemoglobin to visualize local changes in cerebral blood flow in response to a specific sensory stimulus or motor task
MR angiography	Noninvasive visualization of the cerebral and extracerebral blood vessels; uses various relaxation-time and phase-shifting techniques to enhance appearance of blood and CSF and measure their flow rate through vessels and tissue
MR spectroscopy	Noninvasive and nonradiation method to study cerebral metabolites, brain pH, and some neurotransmitters

CSF, cerebrospinal fluid.

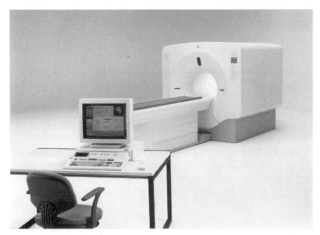

Figure 6–5 • General Electric magnetic resonance system. (Courtesy of GE Medical Systems, Waukesha, WI.)

intravenously. The MRI takes approximately 5 to 50 minutes to complete.

Clinical Applications

Because MRIs are not obscured by bone, the technique is excellent in detecting soft-tissue changes that are insensitive to CT scan. These include ischemic and infarcted areas; degenerative diseases (e.g., multiple sclerosis, Alzheimer's disease); cerebral and spinal cord edema; hemorrhage; arteriovenous malformations; small tumors, particularly in the difficult-to-visualize areas of the brain stem, basal skull, and spinal cord; and congenital anomalies. The superb sharpness and precision of detail are superior for diagnosis and location of lesions.

The following are advantages of MRI:

- Provides detailed sagittal (right-to-left side); axial (top to bottom of the head), and coronal (front to back of the head) images for precise lesion assessment and location
- Does not use ionizing radiation, thus eliminating exposure risk
- Tissue resolution is far superior with MRI with the exception of bone, which cannot be seen with MRI except for bone marrow
- Provides better differentiation than CT for water, iron, fat, and blood using physical and biochemical characteristics of tissues imaged
- Higher level of gray-white matter contrast obtainable compared with CT
- Can detect soft-tissue changes not seen on radiographs such as small tumors along cranial nerves and other tumors as small as 0.3 mm
- Provides higher-resolution detail of the posterior fossa, skull base, and orbits compared with CT scan
- Development of ultrafast and echoplanar imaging have made MRI as fast as CT and thus useful for rapidly evolving, unstable, and life-threatening conditions

Disadvantages of MRI include its higher cost relative to CT scan and the need to exclude a number of patients who could be adversely affected by the procedure because the strong magnetic field can move or dislodge metallic material and cause injury to body tissue. The *contraindications* for MRI include the following:

- Patients with metallic devices, such as artificial pacemakers, cochlear implants, prosthetic devices (e.g., metallic hip replacements, orthopedic pins), artificial limbs, respirators, and other metallic equipment
- Patients with older metal intracranial aneurysm clips or metal bullet fragments in the brain
- Agitated, uncooperative patients or patients with uncontrolled movement disorders (must lie perfectly still)
- Grossly obese patients who cannot fit into the MRI tube
- Claustrophobic patients who cannot tolerate the closeness of the tube to their faces
- Patients who have back pain and cannot lie flat and immobilized, especially when conventional MRI is used

In the last few years, new MRI-friendly materials from the manufacturers of neurological and orthopedic equipment have become available. It is imperative to screen patients accurately for the presence of any devices that are contraindications for MRI *before* scheduling the procedure.

Patient Management

Preparation

Carefully question and screen for the presence of any metal implants. For the patient who is vague about this possibility, radiographic screening may be necessary. The patient should be briefed about the procedure and the necessity to remain still for several minutes in very close quarters. Antianxiety medication may be ordered for some patients. All jewelry, eyeglasses, and hair clips or pins and any other metal objects should be removed. Credit cards should not be in the room because the magnetic field will erase the strip on the card. Unless a contrast medium will be administered, there are no dietary restrictions before the procedure.

Several points need attention if contrast medium is to be used. Adequate kidney function is verified through adequate blood urea nitrogen and creatinine levels. Many protocols require nothing by mouth for 4 to 8 hours before the MRI. Skin testing is done to check for an allergic reaction.

Postprocedural Care

There are no special after-care requirements. When contrast medium is used, adequate hydration is needed.

PHYSIOLOGIC IMAGING TECHNIQUES OF THE BRAIN

The major *physiologic neuroimaging* studies are positron emission tomography (PET) and single-photon emission CT (SPECT). These techniques use nuclear medicine technology to evaluate cerebral metabolism and cerebral blood flow (CBF). PET uses positron-emitting radionuclides, and SPECT uses single photon radioisotopes.

Positron Emission Tomography

Positron emission tomography scanning measures regional physiologic functions such as glucose uptake and metabolism, oxygen uptake, and CBF patterns. The PET scan is the standard criterion against which all other physiologic imaging techniques are measured. Its elegance of detail is unmatched for demonstration of hypometabolic and hypermetabolic regions of the brain. In neuroscience research, PET is a developing technology providing new understanding about epilepsy, dementia (e.g., Alzheimer's disease), cerebrovascular disease, cerebral trauma, and mental illness. It is used clinically in a limited number of patients for diagnostic purposes (Fig. 6-6).

The technology is based on the use of an on-line cyclotron or linear accelerator to create positron-emitting radionuclides. The patient receives an intravenous injection or inhales a compound that has been labeled with the emission of positron "tag" (i.e., F-fluorodeoxyglucose [FDG]). Once inside the body, the tag concentrates in the area of clinical interest and emits positrons. As the positrons decay, they emit photons that move in diametrically opposite directions and are recorded by detectors located on either side of the body. Multiple scanners detect and encode these data into a computerized database that reconstructs cross-sectional images of the tissue.[2]

A major advantage of PET is the clarity of images produced. The major drawbacks of PET are the following:

- An on-line cyclotron or linear accelerator is necessary to manufacture the short-lived isotopes on site; this equipment is found only in major research centers and this thus limits access
- High expense
- Limited availability of PET scan for diagnostic purposes

Procedure

The patient is placed on a stretcher in the imaging center and prepared. An arterial line may be inserted to draw blood samples for measurement of cerebral metabolic rates. No glucose solutions are given. The radiopharmaceutical agent of choice is injected through another venous access. The patient rests quietly in a dimly lit room for about 45 minutes while uptake of the radiopharmaceutical occurs. The head is placed inside the scanner. The scanning portion of the procedure takes about 45 minutes. The patient may be asked to perform cognitive acts such as speaking, mathematical calculations, or reasoning. If blood samples are required, they are drawn quietly by the technician without disturbing the quiet environment created for the study. The entire procedure takes 2 to 3 hours.

Patient Management
Preparation

No caffeine, alcohol, or nicotine should be consumed for 24 hours before the procedure. Maintain NPO status for 6 to 12 hours before the procedure. Glucose solutions should not be used for infusion purposes because they may alter the test results.

Postprocedural Care

After completion of the study, encourage the patient to consume copious fluids to clear the isotope.

Single-Photon Computed Emission Tomography

Single-photon computed emission tomography scans are another physiologic imaging study that measures regional CBF and perfusion. The SPECT scan is based on the same principles as PET technology, but the decay of the radioactive "tags" emits only a single photon and a rotating gamma camera (available in many nuclear medicine departments) is used.

The radioactive tracers used in SPECT scans are commercially prepared and therefore do not require an on-line cyclotron. The most common tracer used is technetium-99m-hexamethyl-propylamine-oxamine. SPECT tracks the single photons resulting from radioactive decay using the gamma camera, which collects data from multiple angles to reconstruct regional blood flow. It is useful to demonstrate hypoperfusion in focal and diffuse cerebral disorders such as dementia, seizures, stroke, and cerebral trauma. It has been useful in confirming brain death.[4]

The major advantage of SPECT is its widespread availability of the technology within many nuclear medicine departments. It detects cerebral perfusion changes and is especially helpful in acute ischemia and monitoring seizure foci. It thus provides excellent perfusion information in stroke, dementia, amnesia, neoplasm, trauma, seizures, brain death, persistent vegetative state, and psychiatric disorders (e.g., schizophrenia and depression). The major disadvantages of SPECT are its cost, about as much as a CT scan, and technical resolution concerns.

Procedure

The patient lies quietly on a padded stretcher and the isotope is administered. The isotope decays in about 1 hour, so the scan must be conducted within that window of time. The patient must lie quietly during the scan. The entire study takes about 1 to 2 hours.

Patient Management
Preparation

No special preparation is required other than the usual explanation of the procedure to the patient.

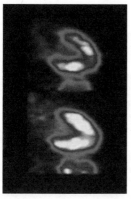

Figure 6–6 • PET scan showing variations in update of isotope.

Postprocedural Care

No special care is required after the procedure.

CEREBROSPINAL FLUID AND SPINAL PROCEDURES

Lumbar Puncture

A lumbar puncture (LP) involves the introduction of a hollow needle with a stylet into the lumbar subarachnoid space of the spinal canal using strict aseptic technique. In the adult, the needle is placed in the interspace between L3–4 or L4–5. This location is a safe distance from the end of the spinal cord, which terminates at L-1. Note that the L3–4 interspace is located at the level of the posterior iliac crests.

The indications for LP can be divided into diagnostic and therapeutic purposes. Diagnostic indications include measurement of CSF pressure; examination of CSF for the presence of blood; collection of CSF for laboratory study; radiologic visualization of parts of the nervous system by injection of air, oxygen, or radiopaque material; and evaluation of spinal dynamics for signs of blockage of CSF flow. Table 6-4 details the characteristics of CSF. Therapeutic indications for LP include the introduction of spinal anesthesia for surgery; intrathecal injection of antibacterial or other drugs; and removal of CSF in benign intracranial hypertension (formerly called pseudotumor cerebri).

Contraindications

The contraindications for LP are relative and require careful medical judgment, weighing benefits against risks. First, when clinical evidence indicates a substantial increase in intracranial pressure (ICP), caution is advised. Increased ICP is found with space-occupying lesions, such as brain tumors. Performing LP in a patient with high increased ICP may result in brain-stem compression, herniation through the foramen magnum, and, ultimately, death. Second, a cutaneous or osseous infection at the proposed puncture site is an absolute contraindication for LP. Additionally, another relative contraindication is patients who are receiving antiplatelet therapy (e.g., aspirin, ticlopidine [Ticlid], clopidogrel [Plavix]) or anticoagulation therapy (heparin, warfarin [Coumadin]) or who have blood dyscrasia because of the high risk of hemorrhage at the puncture site and possible spinal cord compression from perispinal or intraspinal bleeding.

Procedure

The LP is usually done at the patient's bedside or in an outpatient facility. The LP set is prepared. The patient assumes a lateral decubitus position along the edge of the bed, arching the back so that the knees are flexed on the chest with the chin touching the knees (Fig. 6-7). This position allows maximal separation of the vertebrae, thereby facilitating insertion of the lumbar needle and reducing potential trauma. The nurse may be called on to assist the patient if this position cannot be assumed independently. Occasionally, the LP may be performed with the patient seated on the side of the bed. To maximize interspace separation, the patient bends over a pillow that rests on the overbed table.

The lumbar site is aseptically prepared, draped, and locally anesthetized with an intradermal injection of procaine (Novocaine). Strict aseptic technique is essential. The lumbar needle is introduced into the appropriate subarachnoid space, the stylet is removed, and a manometer is affixed to measure and record opening pressure of CSF. The opening

Table 6 – 4 • CHARACTERISTICS OF CEREBROSPINAL FLUID (CSF)

PARAMETER	NORMAL VALUE	ABNORMAL FINDINGS
Volume	About 150 mL	↑ with hydrocephalus
Specific gravity	1.007	↑ with RBCs related to subarachnoid hemorrhage or WBCs related to infection
Pressure	76–200 mm H_2O	↑ with ↑ intracranial pressure
Color	Crystal clear	Xanthochromia (discoloration) of CSF; usually due to breakdown of RBCs from previous intracranial hemorrhage; appears yellow, orange, or brown. (See also Chart 6-3). Turbidity (cloudiness): due to ↑ WBCs or ↑ protein from microorganisms in CSF
Protein count	16–45 mg/dL	Mild ↑ with viral meningitis, subdural hematoma, brain tumor, and multiple sclerosis. Moderate/high ↑ with bacterial or TB meningitis, cerebral hemorrhage, brain and spinal cord tumors, and Guillain-Barré syndrome
White cell count	0–5 cells/mm^3	10–200 cells mostly lymphocytes: viral meningitis, multiple sclerosis, CNS tumor and late neurosyphilis 200–500 cells mostly lymphocytes: TB meningitis, herpes infection of CNS, and meningovascular syphilis >500 cells, mostly granulocytes: acute bacterial meningitis
Glucose	40–80 mg/dL (50%–80% of blood value)	↑ has specific significance; ↓ often seen with all meningitis and subarachnoid hemorrhage
Lactate	10–20 mg/dL	↑ indicates ↑ glucose metabolism often associated with bacterial or fungal meningitis

CSF, cerebrospinal fluid; RBC, red blood cell; WBC, white blood cell; TB, tuberculosis; CNS, central nervous system.

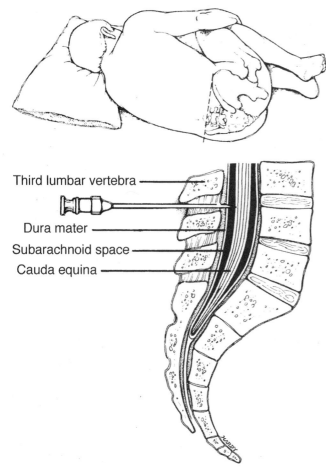

Third lumbar vertebra

Dura mater

Subarachnoid space

Cauda equina

Figure 6–7 • Technique of lumbar puncture. The interspaces between the spines of vertebrae L-3, L-4, and L-5 are just below the line joining the anterosuperior iliac spines. (From Smeltzer, S., & Bare, B. [1996]. *Brunner and Suddarth's textbook of medical-surgical nursing* [8th ed.]. Philadelphia: Lippincott-Raven.)

pressure is approximately the same as ICP in a patient who is reclining if no CSF obstruction is present. After this measurement has been obtained, the manometer is removed and samples of CSF are collected into sterile test tubes for visual and laboratory examination. The physician may choose to record the exit pressure, for which the manometer would again be necessary. When the procedure is completed, the lumbar needle is removed and a Band-Aid is applied over the puncture site. The tubes of CSF should be taken promptly for laboratory analysis.

Complications

It is important to know when a LP has resulted in trauma. A traumatic tap causes trauma to the tissue at the LP site with subsequent bleeding. In this instance, the initial sample of CSF contains blood. Such bleeding could be misinterpreted as evidence of subarachnoid hemorrhage. However, in the case of a traumatic tap, CSF clears progressively in successive samples. If there has been hemorrhage into the subarachnoid space from intracranial bleeding, successive samples of CSF will continue to be as discolored as the first specimen taken.

Patient Management

Preparation

For patient comfort, the bladder should be emptied immediately before the procedure. Usually, no dietary restriction or preprocedural medication is warranted.

Postprocedural Care

Care of a patient who has undergone LP includes the following:

- Have the patient lie flat in bed 6 to 8 hours following the procedure, depending on physician preference, hospital protocol, and continued signs of headache.
- Frequently monitor neurological and vital signs.
- Force fluids after completion of the procedure.
- Administer analgesics (for headache) as needed.

Following LP, mild to severe headache may occur, caused by leakage of CSF at the puncture site or by irritation of the spinal roots. Acetaminophen (Tylenol), 650 mg orally (PO) every 4 hours, is used for mild headaches, whereas methylmorphine (codeine phosphate), 30 mg PO may be ordered for severe headaches. Because headaches are aggravated by an upright position, the patient is advised to lie flat in bed to relieve the pain. An autologous "blood patch" can be used to seal the site of CSF leakage with good results for severe headache. Other possible symptoms that can occur after LP include backache or spasms in the lower back or thighs, transient voiding problems, nuchal rigidity, and a slight rise in temperature. If the LP is done on an outpatient basis, the patient may be discharged 1 to 2 hours after completion. Instruct the patient to lie down in the car and lie flat for 6 to 8 hours at home.

Myelography

Myelography is a diagnostic procedure ordered to visualize the lumbar, thoracic, or cervical subarachnoid space or the entire spinal axis, for diagnosis of a spinal cord compression, spinal cord lesion (e.g., tumor, vascular abnormality), vertebral bone displacement, or intervertebral disc herniation. Any partial or complete obstruction that hinders the flow of CSF and contrast medium will be visualized on the films. Ordering of an MRI has significantly decreased the number of myelograms performed; if an MRI is inconclusive, a myelogram may be ordered.

Procedure

The LP is performed and approximately 10 mL of CSF is removed. A water-soluble contrast medium (e.g., Isovue, Amipaque, Iohexol) is then injected into the subarachnoid space and radiographic films of the spinal cord and vertebral column are taken.

Contrast Media

A few points need to be made about radiopaque media. In the past, oil-based media were used. Since the introduction of water-soluble contrast media, use of oil-based media has ceased. After the water-based contrast medium is injected into the CSF, it diffuses upward through the CSF and penetrates into the nerve root sleeves, nerve rootlets, and narrow areas of the subarachnoid space. Upward diffusion occurs regardless of the position of the patient. The head is kept elevated about 30 degrees at all times, and the patient is kept quiet to reduce the rate of upward dispersion of the contrast medium. Upward dispersion is controlled to prevent the contrast medium from entering the cranial vault, which could result in seizures. The head is maintained elevated in postprocedural care, including transfer, to prevent seizures. In addition, confusion, hallucinations, depression, hyperesthesia, chest pain, and arrhythmias can result from the contrast medium.

Patient Management

Preparation

The patient should be well hydrated. Omit the meal prior to the myelogram. Explain the need to force fluids (3 L) for the first 24 hours after the procedure.

Postprocedural Care

The patient is transported back to his or her room or the recovery area with the head of the stretcher elevated 30 degrees at all times. In addition, the following points should be followed (there may be slight variations among institutional practice guidelines):

- Keep the patient on bedrest for 4 to 8 hours with the head of the bed elevated 30 degrees.
- Keep the patient quiet for few hours after the procedure.
- The patient's head must be elevated (chair or bed) for a total of 12 hours.
- Force fluids to 2400 to 3000 mL per 24 hours.
- Monitor neurological and vital signs.
- Maintain an intake and output record.
- After 4 hours, resume diet as tolerated if there is no nausea or vomiting.
- Do not give any phenothiazine derivatives for 48 hours (because they increase possibility of seizures).
- Monitor for symptoms such as back pain, spasms, elevated temperature, difficulty voiding, nuchal rigidity, nausea, and vomiting.
- Treat nausea with trimethobenzamide hydrochloride (Tigan) 200 mg intramuscularly (IM) every 6 hours as needed or other antiemetic according to physician's order.
- Treat headache with analgesics as needed.

▊▊▊▊ CEREBROVASCULAR STUDIES

Cerebrovascular studies are broadly classified as noninvasive and invasive. The most commonly types of studies used in clinical practice are discussed below.

Transcranial Doppler (TCD)

The TCD uses the principles of Doppler technology to provide information about the patency, flow velocity, turbulence, and directional flow of blood in basal cerebral arteries. Refinement of the technology over the last decade has greatly increased its use in clinical settings to evaluate cerebrovascular flow. It is inexpensive, noninvasive, safe, portable, and can be done at the bedside in a short period of time.

Basics of Ultrasonography and Doppler Ultrasound

Ultrasound technology uses the transmission of ultrasonic pulsed-wave frequency through tissue and the reflection of the sound at tissue interfaces. Christian Doppler built on this knowledge and added the concept of "doppler shift." Doppler shift is the change in the frequency of the pulsed-wave resulting from the movement between the source of sound and the detector. The frequency shift detected is that of the red blood cells traveling through the lumen of the vessel. The application of fast Fourier transform (FFT) to analyze change in frequency of the returning signal further adds precision and additional information. The FFT visually displays the spectral waveform, offers information on direction of flow, and provides a means to establish norm values. In 1982, Aaslid and associates determined that it was possible to send an ultrasound beam through a thinning of the skull and analyze the Doppler signal reflected from basal cerebral arteries through the skull. This concept, which became known as TCD, has been recognized as a breakthrough in evaluating intracranial blood flow.

The TCD does not provide an actual image of the vessel or measure of CBF. Rather, it provides information on vessel patency, flow velocity, turbulence, and directional flow about the moving column of blood in a major artery. With vessel stenosis, there is accelerated flow velocity of red blood cells through the stenosis and concurrent disturbance of blood flow and turbulence distal to the stenosis. The newer models of TCD provide colored printouts and descriptive data about the waveforms of the specific blood vessel (see Fig. 6-8).

Procedure

A Doppler ultrasonic hand-held probe, which sends low-frequency pulsed sound waves, is placed on the skin over the thinned-skull area of the temporal bone or "window." The sound waves reflect back the velocity of the blood flow. These data are amplified, and graphic recordings of the waveforms common to each vessel, as well as sound recordings of the blood flow, are produced. The test takes 10 to 30 minutes.

Uses

Because the TCD is noninvasive and does not use radioactive isotopes or radiation, serial evaluations can be done without potential harm to the patient. For example, serial studies may be conducted to monitor changes over time of the evolution or resolution of vasospasm. Current application of TCD includes the following:

- Detection and monitoring of vasospasm with cerebral aneurysms
- Detection of intracranial stenosis and occlusion (e.g., middle cerebral artery, basilar artery disease)
- Evaluation of impact of extracranial stenosis on intracranial blood flow including collateral blood flow
- Identification of feeder arteries of arteriovenous malformations
- Evaluation and monitoring of intracranial blood flow during surgery (e.g., cardiopulmonary bypass)
- Evaluation of vasomotor tone
- Monitor effect of thrombolytic agents on blood vessel in acute stroke
- Adjunct data in diagnosis of brain death

B-Mode Imaging and Duplex Scanning

Principles of ultrasonography are being used in other ways, including B-mode imaging and duplex scanning. **B-mode (brightness-modulated) imaging**, or real-time ultrasonographic angiography, offers visualization of the structural detail of both the vessel walls and atherosclerotic plaques by recording the reflection of ultrasonic waves introduced through a probe. Two-dimensional images of a pulsating blood vessel in longitudinal and transverse sections allow visualization of most of the vessel's circumference. The image is reflected on a display screen in tones of gray. A photograph of the image can be taken to provide a permanent record. The purpose of the procedure is to detect minimal plaque formation and stenosed carotid vessels. Poor-quality images can result if the patient has a short, thick neck because the carotid bifurcation is high in the neck and difficult to scan. The procedure takes approximately 30 to 45 minutes.

Duplex scanning of the carotids is based on the combination B-mode imaging and pulsed-wave Doppler principles to produce hemodynamic and anatomic information. This dual modality allows evaluation of flow dynamics, the vessel wall, and lumen anywhere along carotid, vertebral, or innominate arteries.[5]

Patient Management

Preparation

Patient management is the same for all noninvasive carotid studies. Regardless of the test to be performed, an explanation of what to expect is necessary. For all these tests, the patient will be asked to remain still. Beyond this, there is no other patient preparation.

Postprocedural Care

Other than washing away any gel used as a conductor in Doppler studies, there is no specific after care required.

Magnetic Resonance Angiography (MRA)

Using MRI technology, MRA is a noninvasive method of visualizing cerebral vessels without the use of radiation. It is useful to visualize areas with blood flow such as aneurysms, arteriovenous malformations, and occlusions. The preparation and after care are similar to those associated with MRI.

Cerebral Blood Flow Studies: Xenon-133

The conceptual basis for the measurement of brain tissue perfusion was developed by the seminal work of Kety and Schmidt in 1945, and current CBF techniques are based on their work. A frequent choice is xenon-133 as a radioactive tracer for cerebral perfusion and CBF either as an inhaled gas or an intra-arterial injection. After administration of the tracer, cerebral washout is followed with external scintillation counters placed over the skull, making it possible to perform regional determination of CBF. The rate of washout is proportional to CBF.

Xenon-enhanced CT may also be used with rapid sequential CT scanning to quantify CBF. CBF studies are useful to determine viability of cerebral tissue globally and regionally and as part of brain death criteria.

Patient Management

Preparation

No special preparation is required.

Postprocedural Care

No special care is required.

Cerebral Angiography

Cerebral angiography is the definitive standard diagnostic procedure for aneurysms, arteriovenous malformations, and other cerebrovascular abnormalities. The lumen of the blood vessels can be visualized to determine patency, narrowing or stenosis, thrombosis, vasospasm, abnormalities such as an aneurysm, and displacement of cerebral vessels. Causes of displacement include space-occupying lesions such as hematomas, cysts, tumors, and abscesses. Cerebral angiography can be performed using local anesthesia or as part of a surgical procedure if the patient is undergoing general anesthesia. For example, cerebral angiography can be obtained during an aneurysm clipping to check the position and integrity of the clip.

Procedure

The patient is placed in a supine position on the radiographic stretcher. A wide area around the puncture site is shaved. A local anesthetic is usually administered; procaine (Novocaine) is often the drug of choice. The puncture site is aseptically cleansed. After local injection with procaine, the contrast medium is either injected directly into the carotid arteries (rarely) or introduced by the indirect route, through catheterization of the carotid or vertebral arteries using the femoral, brachial, subclavian, or axillary artery as a point of entry (the femoral route is the most common). Radiographic films are then taken at various time intervals after injection for visualization of the intracranial and extracranial blood vessels (Fig. 6-9). When the examination is completed, direct manual pressure is applied to the puncture site for 5 to 10 minutes to prevent bleeding into the subcutaneous space.

Possible complications following cerebral angiography include allergic reactions to contrast medium, seizures, stroke, pulmonary emboli, thrombosis, symptoms of carotid sinus sensitivity (hypotension, syncope, and bradycardia), aphasia, and visual deficits.

Patient Management

Preparation

After explaining the procedure and possible risks (e.g., stroke), informed consent is obtained. Preoperative medication is usually administered half an hour before the procedure. The choice of drugs used varies from physician to physician and may include any of the following: pentobarbital (Nembutal); atropine sulfate, IM, to protect against the effect upon the carotid sinus; diazepam (Valium); and meperidine (Demerol), IM. Preparation for the examination is similar to that for any operative procedure. Dentures and eyeglasses are removed. Most physicians prefer that the patient not have anything by mouth for 6 to 8 hours before

the examination. Baseline vital and neurological signs are recorded. The skin is shaved at the puncture site immediately before the procedure, usually in the procedure suite. The patient should be told that, during injection, a burning sensation may be felt for a few (4 to 6) seconds behind the eyes or in the jaw, teeth, tongue, and lips. Even the fillings in the teeth may feel warm. The need to lie still during the procedure is emphasized.

Postprocedural Care

When completed, the patient is returned to his or her room. Nursing responsibilities include the following:

- Maintain the patient on complete bedrest for 8 hours.
- Immobilize the puncture site for 8 hours (a sandbag may be helpful) to prevent bleeding; in most instances, the upper leg is immobilized for a femoral artery puncture.
- Observe the puncture site (pressure dressing) frequently for bleeding.
- Monitor vital signs and neurological signs frequently. After the initial period of monitoring every 15 to 30 minutes, check these signs every 1 to 4 hours for a 24-hour period.
- Check pedal pulses in the affected leg if a femoral puncture was performed; also check the color and temperature of the extremity.
- Maintain an accurate intake and output record.
- Force fluids to clear the contrast medium (a toxic response may include acute kidney failure due to contrast medium).
- Apply an ice bag to the puncture site to promote comfort.

Digital Subtraction Angiography

In evaluating the carotid arteries, invasive digital subtraction angiography (DSA) is a refinement of angiographic technique using digital computer enhancement to produce

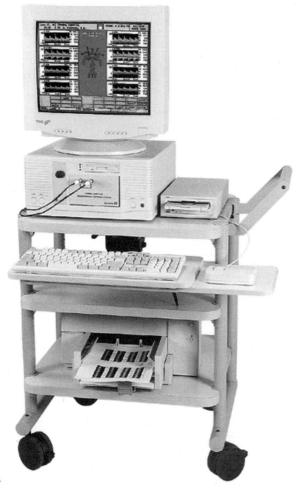

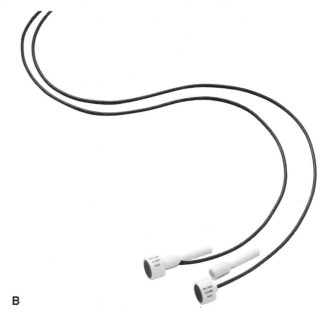

Figure 6–8 • Transcranial Doppler (TCD). (*A*) Neurovision™ instrumentation for transcranial Doppler can be wheeled to the bedside for patient evaluation. The monitor displays the data that are stored in the computer; the display can also be printed. (*B*) These are probes that the technician uses to slide over the areas to be evaluated. (*C*) The basic principle of signal transmission and return through the probe. (*D*) The various data elements that are collected and recorded (*D1* and *D2*). (Photos courtesy of: Multigon Industries Inc, C. R. Gomez M. D., and Emily Stern.)

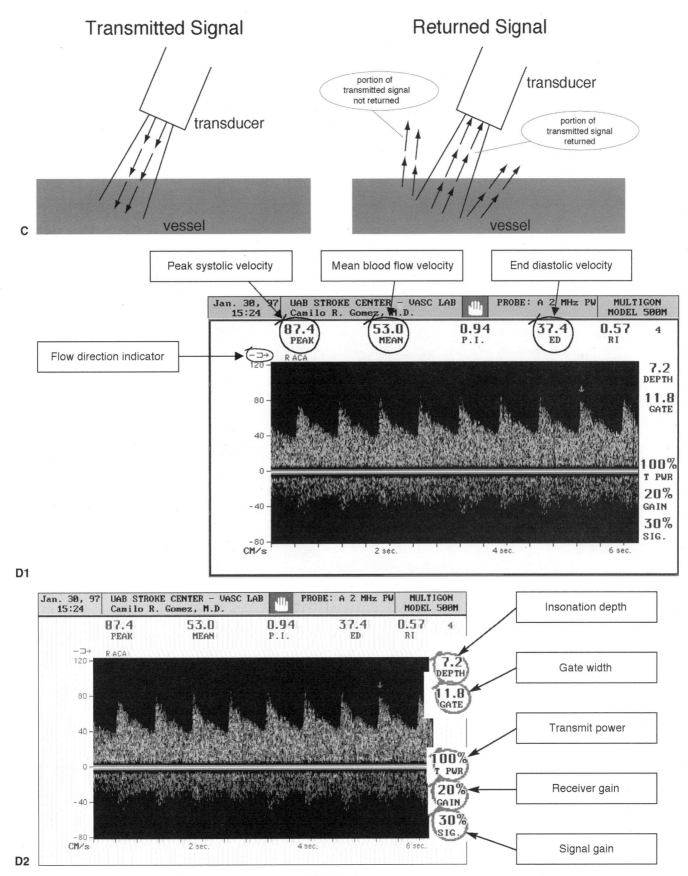

Figure 6–8

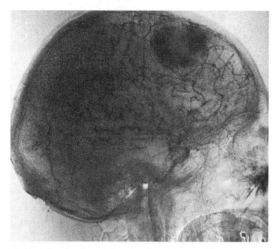

Figure 6–9 • Cerebral arteriogram (angiogram) showing an abnormal, large, space-occupying lesion at one o'clock.

images for visualization of the carotids and other cerebral vessels. The image produced is made more distinct by the elimination of surrounding and interfering anatomical structures. This is accomplished by recording images before and after injection of contrast medium and subtracting the first image from the second.

The purposes of DSA include assistance in the diagnosis of the following conditions:

- Atherosclerotic disease (stenosis, occlusions, large plaques)
- Vascular lesions (arteriovenous malformations, aneurysms, carotid cavernous fistulas)
- Postoperative evaluation of endarterectomy, aneurysm clipping, arteriovenous malformation repair, and anastomosis

Procedure

The antecubital area, usually of the right arm, is cleansed and lidocaine is injected locally so that the antecubital vein (usual approach) or the brachial artery can be incised. A catheter is advanced into the superior vena cava, and contrast medium is injected. Selected vessels are visualized with an image-intensifier video system that displays vessels on a monitor. Images are taken and stored on magnetic tape. The images, which are collected before contrast injection, are received by the computer and are then subtracted from those taken after injection so that the image of the desired area is enhanced. The remaining contrast-enhanced images can be manipulated by the computer to focus on specific problems that might otherwise not be visualized.

On completion of the procedure, which takes from 30 to 45 minutes, the catheter is removed. Pressure is applied to the puncture site for several minutes, and a sterile dressing is applied.

Patient Management

Preparation

Screen patients for any history of allergic reaction to iodine or shellfish. Explain the procedure to the patient. Oral intake is withheld for 2 hours before the procedure. During the procedure, patients are required to hold their breath on command, remain motionless, and lie in the supine position on the x-ray table.

Postprocedural Care

Vital signs and neurological signs are checked and the patient observed for the unlikely occurrence of stroke, allergic reaction, hemorrhage, or hematoma at the injection site. Force fluids to between 2000 to 3000 mL/24 hours to facilitate excretion of the contrast medium. Other possible but rare complications are venous thrombosis and infection.

BIOPSIES

Biopsy of the brain, muscle, nerve, or artery may assist in diagnosis under certain conditions when noninvasive methods such as imaging studies provide inconclusive diagnostic information, when a structure is superficial with easy accessibility, and when the area does not involve a critical area such as the motor strip. **Brain biopsy** may be warranted for diagnosis of brain tumor, infectious disorders such as herpes simplex encephalitis or brain abscess, and certain degenerative diseases such as Creutzfeldt-Jacob disease. **Muscle biopsy** is useful to differentiate underlying weakness of neurogenic or myopathic origin and to diagnose certain inflammatory diseases. Electromyographic findings are not definitive in ruling in or ruling out myopathies or neuropathies. Therefore, a muscle biopsy is complementary to other studies when there is a question about the accuracy of the diagnosis. On rare occasion, **nerve biopsy** may be done to aid in the diagnosis of infection or inflammatory changes, vasculitis, or neoplasms. Finally, for patients who experience facial pain and nonspecific neurological symptoms, a **temporal artery biopsy** may be considered. A small piece of temporal artery is removed and examined for evidence of temporal arteritis.

Patient Management

In preparing the patient, explain the procedure. A surgical permit may need to be signed depending on hospital policy. Medication for sedation may be ordered before the procedure. After the procedure, observe the dressing for bleeding. Vital signs and neurological signs should be monitored.

NERVOUS SYSTEM ELECTRICAL ACTIVITY AND CONDUCTION

Electroencephalography

An electroencephalogram (EEG) is a noninvasive, painless, diagnostic procedure that records the spontaneous electrical activity of the brain (brain waves) using multiple scalp electrodes and records each tracing on graph paper for interpretation (Fig. 6-10). Neuronal electrical signals from

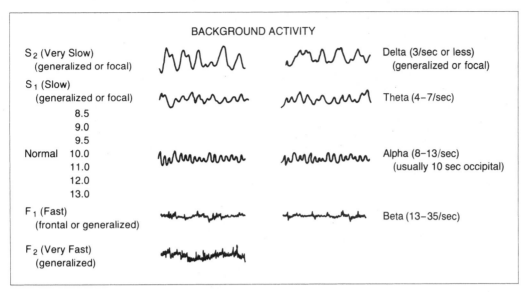

Figure 6–10 • Electroencephalogram classifications.

the cerebral cortex are about 1% as strong as signals from the heart. Signals are picked up from surface cerebral cortex neurons and amplified one million times for an acceptable recording to be made. The EEG provides complementary data to anatomic imaging studies such as CT and MRI. It records the frequency, amplitude, and characteristics of brain waves. The EEG is rarely specific to a cause because a variety of conditions can produce similar EEG changes. Although pattern changes are nonspecific, some changes are highly suggestive of specific conditions such as particular types of epilepsy, herpes simplex encephalitis, and dementia-related disorders. The EEG is useful in follow-up observation of patients with altered states of consciousness and is an important criterion in the determination of brain death.

For patients who have intractable seizures unresponsive to drug therapy, continuous EEG monitoring and videotaping may be helpful. This provides continuous data about cerebral electrical activity and behavioral changes that can be correlated to determine the type and characteristics of the seizure activity. It often helps in identifying epileptogenic areas in the brain. If this is unsuccessful, electrodes can be inserted surgically into the cerebral cortex. This approach allows for better localization of epileptogenic foci amenable to surgical excision for better control of seizures.

Continuous EEG monitoring is also helpful for detection seizure activity in patients with subclinical seizures (without physical manifestations). For example, a comatose patient who appears to be improving but does not awaken may have undiagnosed subclinical seizures that are altering consciousness. Data from the continuous EEG may prompt new treatment to control seizure activity.

Procedure

After a patient has been oriented to the test environment, he or she is made comfortable in an easy chair or on a stretcher. Cooperation is very important to the quality of the test data. A series of small electrodes (16 to 21) are symmetrically affixed to the scalp in standard locations with a paste-like substance. The recording electrodes are interconnected in

chains. Extra electrodes (e.g., nasopharyngeal and sphenoidal) are available to record activity from the undersurface of the temporal lobes. Routinely, brain waves are recorded at rest, after hyperventilation, with photic stimulation, and during drowsiness or sleep. Hyperventilation and photic stimulation are stressors and may precipitate abnormal focal or generalized brain waves changes not detectable under normal circumstances. Wave types vary with activity and specific stimulation.

A baseline of spontaneous brain wave activity at rest is recorded, which takes about 30 minutes. The patient is then asked to hyperventilate for 2 to 3 minutes. The blowing off of CO_2 raises the serum pH to approximately 7.8 from the normal range of 7.35 to 7.45, at which time another recording is obtained. Nerve excitability is increased, which may trigger seizure activity in a susceptible patient. The recording is continued to determine how long it takes to reestablish the baseline. Next, photic stimulation is applied by focusing a flickering light (strobe light) on the closed-eyed patient and a recording is taken. The last recording phase is that of drowsiness or sleep. An EEG takes 45 to 60 minutes and produces about 100 pages of recording paper.

A **sleep deprivation** technique is often used to demonstrate suspected abnormalities that are not evident on routine EEG. The patient is kept awake for most of the night before the EEG. Sleep deprivation stresses the brain and, therefore, may evoke abnormal waves not seen in the normal state. An all-night EEG is useful in studying sleep problems. It takes approximately 45 to 60 minutes to complete the EEG.

Patient Management

Preparation

Explain the procedure and expectations for patient involvement during the EEG. Preparation is very important to allay anxiety and ensure patient cooperation. Anxiety can block alpha waves and produce head and neck muscle tension, resulting in recording artifacts.

Because anticonvulsants, stimulants, tranquilizers, and depressants can alter brain wave activity and mask or suppress abnormal brain waves, the physician may withhold selected medications for 24 to 48 hours before the EEG. Coffee, tea, colas, and chocolate are withheld from the regular diet to exclude dietary stimulants. To promote sleep during the EEG, the patient should go to sleep late and arise early. Napping before the test is discouraged. If a sleep deprivation study is required, the patient should be prevented from sleeping the night before the EEG. The patient's hair should be clean and no oils, sprays, or lotions should be used before the test.

Postprocedural Care

Hair is washed to remove the electrode-affixing paste. Resume drugs withheld specifically for the EEG.

Classification of Brain Waves

Classification of brain waves is based on the number of cycles per second (cps), which are recorded in hertz (Hz) units. Four frequency bands are identified for EEG interpretation:

Alpha rhythms (8 to 12 Hz) are most prominent in the occipital leads. Alpha waves can be blocked by opening of the eyes, mental effort, anxiety, apprehension, and sudden noise or touch.

Beta rhythms (13 to 35 Hz) are most prominent in the frontal and central areas. Beta waves are triggered by opening of the eyes, mental activity, anxiety, or apprehension. They are especially prominent in patients receiving barbiturates and benzodiazepine drugs.

Theta rhythms (4 to 7 Hz) originate from the temporal lobes; there may be a very small amount of delta waves over the temporal regions in normal adults. Theta activity increases slightly in persons over the age of 60 years.

Delta rhythms (1 to 3 Hz) are not normally present in awake adults; normally seen in stages 3 and 4 of sleep (slow wave sleep).

Different areas of the cerebral cortex generate relatively distinctive potential fluctuations, and different patterns also characterize waking and sleep states. In most normal adults, the waking pattern of EEG activity consists primarily of alpha waves occurring mostly over the occipital area and beta waves occurring over the frontal areas. Delta waves are not present in awake adults. Theta and delta waves are seen in sleep; their amount and amplitude correlate with the depth of sleep.

Normal age-related EEG variations are categorized as follows: children and teenagers (younger than 20 years of age); adults (20 to 60 years of age); and older adults (older than 60 years of age). In the older-than-60-years group, EEG patterns are similar to those in the 20- to 60-year group with a few exceptions: alpha waves are slower; beta waves are more prominent; there are more sporadic, generalized slow waves; and intermittent temporal slow waves are evident. Thus, age-related variations must be considered in the interpretation of EEGs.

Common Abnormal Electroencephalographic Abnormalities

An EEG is considered abnormal when it contains epileptiform activities, slowing of normal rhythms, abnormalities of amplitude, or variations from age-specific patterns.

Artifacts

Artifacts are abnormal deflections on the graphic recording that are not caused by cerebral activity but rather by other physiologic activities, such as eye movement, muscle contraction, or heart action.

Findings
Epileptiform Activities

Epileptiform activity appears as single or repetitive focal spikes. These spikes can be divided into focal, multifocal, and generalized events. For example, the patient with temporal lobe seizures will have characteristically abnormal electrical discharges over one anterior temporal lobe, whereas absence epilepsy is evidenced by widespread, bilateral, synchronous 3-Hz discharges. The normal EEG includes a range of variations that must be differentiated from a true form of epilepsy and abnormal activity related to cerebral lesions (Fig. 6-11).

Slow Wave Abnormalities

Slow wave (defined as 1 to 7 Hz) findings are classified as either focal or diffuse abnormalities.

Focal slow waves may be related to gray or white matter dysfunction in a localized area that is secondary to a tumor, hemorrhage, or other space-occupying lesion. Focal lesions directly involve either the cerebral cortex or the thalamocortical projection pathways. The finding of a focal abnormality indicates the need for further diagnostic testing, such as a CT scan or MRI. As the lesion enlarges and affects the diencephalon, slow waves can become diffuse.

Diffuse slow waves are usually seen with toxic (drug toxicity), metabolic (e.g., hepatic), degenerative (e.g., Alzheimer's disease), infectious (e.g., encephalitis), or postictal conditions. Generally, a pattern of diffuse slowing does not point to a specific diagnosis but only provides collaborating diagnostic information. A few forms of dementia, however, do have a characteristic wave pattern.

Flat Electroencephalography or Electrocerebral Silence

The "flat" EEG indicates the absence of brain waves and is one finding seen in brain death (others include absence of brain-stem function and loss of brain-stem reflexes). Brain death is never declared on the basis of a flat EEG only.

Electromyography (EMG) and Nerve Conduction Velocity Studies (NCVS)

Electromyography and NCVS are electrophysiologic studies, known collectively as electromyoneurography, which are usually ordered together. An EMG may be ordered for

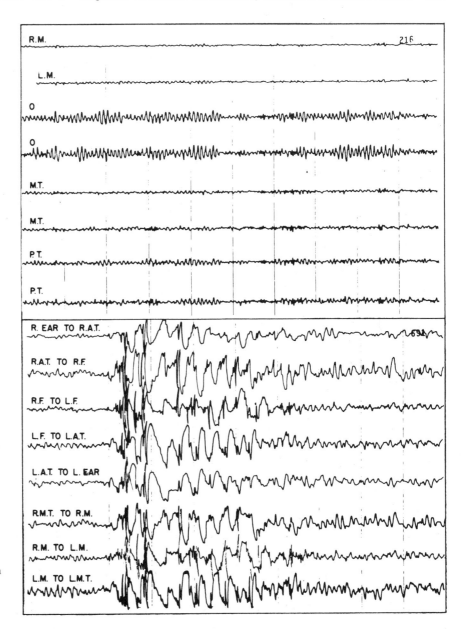

Figure 6–11 • Comparison of a normal electroencephalogram (*top*) with that of an epileptic patient during a tonic–clonic seizure (*bottom*). Note the sharp, spiky waves recorded during the seizure.

patients thought to have myasthenia gravis, Eaton-Lambert syndrome, peripheral nerve injury or neuropathies, or when it is unclear whether the primary problem is a myopathy or neuropathy. It can also differentiate among lesions of the anterior horn cell, root, plexus, and specific nerves and muscles.

NCVS are conducted when nerve damage is suspected because of clinical symptoms of motor weakness or atrophy. They are helpful in the diagnosis of neuropathies (e.g., those induced by diabetes, alcoholism, or nutritional deficiencies and compression of or trauma to the peripheral nerves). Both studies can be used to follow the progression of peripheral nerve disorders and their response to treatment.

Procedures

For an EMG, recordings of muscle activity at rest, during voluntary movement, and with electrical stimulation are made by inserting small needle electrodes into the muscle.

Patterns of muscle activity are displayed on an oscilloscope and compared with standardized norms.

NCVS measure the conduction time and amplitude of electrical stimulation along two or more points of a peripheral nerve using a cathode (negative electrode) and an anode (positive electrode). The recorded response has a simple, biphasic waveform with initial negativity and maximal amplitude. Amplitude, duration, and latency times are measured and compared with standardized norms.

Patient Management

Preparation

Explain the procedure to the patient, emphasizing the importance of cooperation. Some discomfort from the needle electrodes and the electrical stimuli is to be expected.

Postprocedural Care

There is no aftercare required except to cleanse the skin of any contact gel.

Evoked Potentials

Evoked potentials (EPs) are a noninvasive means of applying a specific sensory stimuli and recording the minute electrical potentials that are subsequently created. Using a computerized averaging program, the stimulus is repeated several times, allowing a return to the resting state between stimuli. Each evoked response is measured and the data are stored in the computer. After a number of potentials have been stored (100 to 200), the computer then calculates the average curve.

EPs are used to aid in diagnosing lesions of the cerebral cortex, ascending pathways of the spinal cord, or thalamus; evaluating the extent of central nervous system (CNS) injury; as part of the battery of tests in diagnosing neuromuscular disease; and evaluating comatose patients.[6] EPs are classified into three categories based on the type of stimulus provided and the sensory system stimulated. Each system stimulated produces a characteristic wave formation. The three sensory systems used in EPs are the visual, auditory, and somatosensory pathways.

Visual-Evoked Potentials

In visual evoked potentials (VEPs), checkerboard patterns and flashing lights provide stimuli. The retina is stimulated, allowing the pathways to the occipital cortex to be evaluated. Each eye is tested separately. The response is recorded with electrodes over the occipital region. If the patient wears eyeglasses, they should be worn during the procedure. The cooperation of the patient is necessary during testing. VEPs are used in the diagnosis of optic neuropathies such as optic neuritis often related to multiple sclerosis and optic nerve lesions such as tumors.

Brain-Stem Auditory Evoked Responses

Brain-stem auditory evoked responses (BAERs) are primarily used to evaluate brain-stem function. The stimuli provided, using headphones, include a series of clicks that vary in rate, intensity, and duration. Five wave formations, based on the site of origin, are recorded: wave I from the acoustic nerve, wave II from the cochlear nucleus, wave III from the superior olivary complex, wave IV from the lateral lemniscus, and wave V from the inferior colliculus. BAER testing can be conducted on alert or comatose patients. It is helpful in diagnosing lesions in multiple sclerosis, acoustic neuroma, lesions related to coma, and hearing loss (especially in infants). BAERs are also used intraoperatively to monitor the eighth cranial nerve for surgical injury.

Somatosensory Evoked Responses

Somatosensory evoked responses (SSERs) measure peripheral nerve responses in the upper (median nerve) or lower (posterior tibial nerve) extremities. SSERs are helpful in evaluating spinal cord function, sensory dysfunction associated with multiple sclerosis, and nerve root compression.

TESTING OF THE SPECIAL SENSES

Electronystagmography

Electronystagmography (ENG) measures and graphically records the electrical potentials emitted by eye movements precipitated by spontaneous, positional, or calorically evoked nystagmus. Interpretation of these data can provide information on the frequency, intensity, and maximum speed of the slow and fast components of the nystagmus. The purpose of ENG is to diagnose the underlying etiology of nystagmus or vertigo related to dysfunction of the vestibular branch of the eighth cranial nerve.

Procedure

Electrodes are placed on either side of the eye in the direction of the plane to be recorded. The basic principle underlying ENG is the difference in voltage between two dipole structures, the cornea (+) and retina (−). At least a 1-mV difference normally exists between the two poles. Any changes in potential caused by eye movement are collected, amplified, and recorded. Data are collected during tracking, fixation on points in either plane, and caloric stimulation. The patient is positioned at various angles for data collection. One advantage of ENG is that it enables nystagmus to be recorded behind closed eyelids and in the dark. ENG is contraindicated in a patient with a pacemaker in place.

Patient Management

Preparation

The procedure is explained to the patient, noting that some vertigo may be experienced. Usually, the patient receives nothing by mouth for at least 8 hours before the test. Antivertigo drugs, tranquilizers, depressant drugs, alcohol, and stimulant drugs and foods (e.g., cola, coffee, tea) are usually withheld for 24 to 48 hours before testing. The physician should be consulted about withholding of any medication.

Postprocedural Care

The patient should lie down until any vertigo, dizziness, nausea, or vomiting has subsided. An antiemetic will probably be ordered by the physician. A normal diet is resumed when the patient is able to tolerate it.

Audiometric Studies

Audiometric testing assesses the auditory branch of the eighth cranial nerve for type and cause of hearing loss. Testing is divided into pure-tone audiometry and speech audiometry. The basis for *pure-tone audiometry* is that the louder the sound stimulus (pure or musical tone) necessary before the patient perceives it, the greater the hearing loss.

The decibel (dB) is the unit of measure of loudness. *Speech audiometry* is based on the ability of the patient to understand and discriminate between sounds of the spoken word. In testing, a soundproof room and earphones are used to screen out ambient noise. A graphic representation of testing results is interpreted to differentiate between conduction and sensorineural hearing loss. **Conduction loss** results from outer ear or middle ear dysfunction or impairment to both structures. The inner ear is not involved. In such cases, a hearing aid is helpful. **Sensorineural loss** occurs in diseases of the inner ear or nerve pathways. This type of hearing loss is characterized by loss of sensitivity to and discrimination of sounds. Hearing aids are not very effective with this form of hearing loss.

Hearing loss in the neuroscience patient is usually related to head injury, meningitis, acoustic neuroma, or drug toxicity.

Caloric Testing

Caloric testing is designed to evaluate the vestibular portion of the eighth cranial nerve and the presence or absence of the oculovestibular reflex. The underlying principle of the procedure is that thermal stimulation of the vestibular apparatus (the balance-sensing mechanism in the inner ear) with cold water will elicit the oculovestibular reflex. The test is *contraindicated* in patients with a ruptured tympanic membrane or cervical injury. Patients with diseases involving the vestibular branch of the eighth cranial nerve (e.g., acoustic neuroma or Ménière's disease) will not have the normal eye movements associated with caloric testing; instead, these movements will be diminished or absent.

Procedure

After tympanic membrane intactness is confirmed and the cervical neck is stable, the patient's head is tilted backward at a 60-degree angle from the horizontal plane to allow maximal stimulation of the lateral semicircular canal, the canal that is most responsible for reflex lateral movement. The external auditory canal is slowly irrigated with 10 mL of ice-cold water. The cold irrigation causes convection currents in the endolymph of the labyrinths, resulting in a change in the baseline firing of the vestibular nerve and slow conjugate deviation of the eyes toward the stimulated ear (see Chap. 7, Fig. 7-21). In the normal waking state with an intact oculovestibular reflex, there is an initial conjugate eye movement (lasting about 30 seconds) toward the side being irrigated with the cold water (slow phase). This is controlled by the brain stem. The lateral gaze is corrected shortly by a rapid component of nystagmus that pulls the eyes back to the midline (fast phase). The rapid component is controlled by the cerebral cortex.

As a patient becomes lethargic, the fast component becomes less pronounced. Deterioration into obtundation and coma results in loss of the fast component because the cerebral cortex is depressed. As the patient slips into a deep coma, the lateral deviation toward the side of irrigation (slow component) may be lost. This indicates that the oculovestibular reflex (a reflex controlled by the brain stem) is absent; this is a poor prognostic indicator.

In the emergency department, the oculovestibular reflex may be tested on an unconscious patient. If there is tonic deviation of the eyes toward the side being irrigated, brainstem function is intact. This is considered a positive prognostic sign. With a brain-stem lesion, the caloric reflex is absent. Absence of the reflex is associated with a poor prognosis.

Warm water irrigation produces reversal of endolymphic flow. This results in conjugate eye deviation with the slow phase away from the stimulated ear and normal correction phase toward the irrigated ear. The type of nystagmus is named by the direction of the fast phase. The mnemonic **COWS** (**C**old **O**pposite, **W**arm **S**ame) refers to the **fast phase** of nystagmus. It is also possible to irrigate both ear canals simultaneously with cold water, which results in slow downward deviation; conversely, simultaneous warm water irrigation results in slow upward deviation.

Patient Management

Preparation

In conscious patients, consumption of nothing by mouth should be maintained for at least 8 hours before the procedure. In unconscious patients, this is obviously not a consideration.

Postprocedural Care

Nausea, vomiting, or dizziness can be precipitated by caloric testing in normal patients. Maintain bedrest until nausea, vomiting, vertigo, or dizziness has subsided. A normal diet can be resumed when the patient feels ready.

▌ NEUROPSYCHOLOGICAL EXAMINATION

A neuropsychological examination is a comprehensive assessment of the brain achieved by studying its behavioral products. A licensed neuropsychologist conducts the examination. The purposes of a neuropsychological examination include the following:

- To assist in diagnosis by determining the presence or absence of cognitive deficits
- To determine whether brain dysfunction is localized (focal) or diffuse
- To plan, manage, and evaluate an individualized rehabilitation program
- To determine competency for self-care and decision making
- To document disability for insurance purposes
- To provide information about competency for legal matters such as the need for a guardian
- To conduct research

Lezak[7] conceptualizes behavior as three functional and integrated systems: *cognition*, the information aspect of behavior; *emotionality*, the feelings and motivation of behavior; and *executive functions*, how behavior is expressed. Performance skills are examined in great depth and detail to determine cerebral function. A major benefit of this extensive testing is that subtle changes may be discovered that would not be detected with less refined testing methods or anatomic imaging studies. The comprehensiveness of the examination is reflected in the time required for testing, which is approximately 6 to 10 hours.

Components of a Neuropsychological Evaluation

The examination is tailored to the patient's needs, abilities, and limitations. The specific tests included in a neuropsychological evaluation vary depending on the age of the patient, the nature of the problem, the deficits present, the specific questions asked by the physician in the referral note, and the ability of the person conducting the testing. Information about the type of neurological insult, premorbid function and personality, personal and family history, and data from other diagnostic tests are correlated with data from the neuropsychological examination.

Components of the examination will evaluate the following cognitive functions:

Attention: vigilance (the ability to sustain attention over a period of time, concentration), self-regulation, and screening out of distracting environmental stimuli

Visual perception and visual reasoning: picture completion, picture arrangement, judgment of line orientation, visual search

Memory and learning: short term, immediate, long term; new learning such as remembering word lists; verbal and nonverbal memory. Testing includes sentence repetition, serial digit learning, auditory-verbal learning tests.

Language: understanding of single words and sentences; reading; speaking; and auditory discrimination

General intelligence: verbal and nonverbal; includes information, comprehension, and similarities; naming objects; arithmetic calculations

Constructional ability: drawing to command; drawing to copy; block designs; visual organization of a picture and its parts; right–left orientation; clock setting

Map orientation: being able to read a map

Conceptualization: metaphors and proverbs

Abstraction: verbal and nonverbal abstract reasoning

Perceptual motor speed: ability to plan ahead and shift from one concept to the other

Emotional status: assess for depression, suicidal ideation, anxiety, paranoia, and other abnormal responses

Depression inventory or other inventories of emotional status may be administered in some situations.

IIII COMMON NEUROPSYCHOLOGICAL DEFICITS ASSOCIATED WITH CEREBRAL DYSFUNCTION

Many patients with organic brain dysfunction develop cognitive and behavioral deficits as a result of head trauma, stroke, CNS degenerative disorders (e.g., Alzheimer's disease), and CNS infections (e.g., encephalitis, meningitis). Common deficits include a decreased ability to concentrate, screen irrelevant information, solve problems, sequence complex actions correctly, and learn new tasks. In addition, there may be increased irritability, emotional lability, deficits of memory, logical reasoning, perceptual deficits, and general slowing of all cognitive functions. These cognitive and behavioral deficits cause serious difficulty in activities of daily living, social and vocational readjustment into the family, community, and work setting. Diagnosing the specific deficits and developing a plan for rehabilitation are necessary to help the patient achieve the highest possible level of function and independence.

Because of the focus and time required for neuropsychological evaluation, patient selection is important. The patient must be alert, able to actively participate, and have the physical endurance to complete the examination. The physician should be specific in documenting why neuropsychological evaluation is desired.

Timing of testing is critical. There is some natural recovery that occurs over time after cerebral insult. Seeking neuropsychological evaluation too soon after the insult does not allow sufficient time for spontaneous improvement to be captured. In addition, natural recovery can be so rapid that findings on the examination from one day may be outdated on the next day. Often evaluation is postponed for 3 to 6 months after injury to allow for natural recovery. In some instances, a modified version of the evaluation may be requested.

IIII EMERGING TECHNOLOGIES IN NEUROIMAGING

Magnetic Resonance Spectroscopy

Proton MR spectroscopy (MRS) is a noninvasive method of studying the biochemistry of living tissue. N-acetyl-aspartate (NAA) is a marker of neuronal function, choline marks cell membrane and myelin metabolism, and creatine reflects cellular energy. MRS may reveal a metabolite that is usually present in the brain, and therefore, may be valuable in investigating the pathophysiology of autosomal diseases in the brain and in explaining cellular derangements secondary to apoptosis (programmed cell death). MRS has been used in studies of epilepsy patients.

Functional Magnetic Resonance Imaging

Magnetic resonance imaging can map functional cortical activity during the performance of tasks by detecting cortical regional tissue changes in venous blood oxygenation. This is referred to as blood level–dependent imaging or functional MRI (fMRI) and it relies on the large increase in blood flow and blood oxygenation during brain activation. Applications of fMRI include mapping of brain activation pathways in normal and pathologic states, studying cerebral reorganization, and planning for neurosurgery.

Diffusion and Perfusion Magnetic Resonance Imaging

Magnetic resonance imaging can detect cerebral abnormalities related to ischemia. When MRI uses both the diffusion-weighted imaging (DWI) and perfusion-weighted imaging (PWI), it is possible to identify both metabolically impaired and abnormally perfused brain tissue. Both DWI and PWI provide complementary information about tissue changes in neurological events such as stroke. DWI detects the tiny random movements of water molecules (diffusion) in tissues. This technique allows a map of the average apparent coefficient (ADC) to be calculated. Shortly after an ischemic stroke, the ADC of the brain tissue is significantly reduced because of cytotoxic edema. Over several days, the rapid initial drop in ADC is followed by a return to close to normal values at approximately 1 week. Subsequently, elevated ADC values are seen at chronic timepoints. DWI is remarkably sensitive in detecting and localizing acute ischemic brain lesions and allows differentiation of acute regions of ischemia from chronic infarcts. In addition to ischemic stroke, DWI is also used to study lesions and plaque formation in patients with multiple sclerosis.

PWI assesses the perfusion of the microvasculature after rapid injection of a gadolinium contrast agent. It has been proposed that combined DWI and PWI could determine early extent of brain tissue injury and identify the portions of the brain that are not damaged permanently (i.e., the ischemic penumbra). DWI and PWI could guide acute stroke treatment and potentially identify patients who would benefit from thrombolytic therapy and specific stroke investigational treatments.

Teaching, preparation, and care of a patient who undergoes these emerging MRI techniques are the same as those for a patient who undergoes a standard MRI.

SUMMARY

The major diagnostic procedures commonly used with a neurological patient population have been discussed. Some laboratory studies specific to a condition are included in the pertinent chapter. In caring for patients, the nurse must view the patient holistically and recognize that stabilization and recovery require close monitoring of various laboratory data.

REFERENCES

1. Society of Critical Care Medicine. (1993). Guidelines for the transport of critically ill patients. *Critical Care Medicine, 21*(6), 931–937.
2. Gilman, S. (1998). Imaging of the brain. *New England Journal of Medicine, 338*(12), 812–819.
3. Conn, P. M. (1995). *Neuroscience in medicine* (p. 624). Philadelphia: J. B. Lippincott.
4. Wijdicks, E. F. M. (1997). *The clinical practice of critical care neurology* (p. 126). Philadelphia: Lippincott-Raven.
5. Tegeler, C. H., & Ratanaskorn, D. (1998). Neurosonology. In J. Bogousslavsku & M. Fisher (Eds.). *Textbook of Neurology* (pp. 101–118). Boston: Butterworth-Heinemann.
6. Shpritz, D. W. (1999). Neurodiagnostic studies. *Nursing Clinics of North America, 34*(3), 593–606.
7. Lezak, M. D. (1995). *Neuropsychological assessment* (3rd ed.). New York: Oxford University Press.

RESOURCES

Professional

Published Material

Aaslid, R., Markwalder, T., & Nornes, H. (1982). Noninvasive transcranial Doppler ultrasound recording of flow velocities in the basal cerebral arteries. *Journal of Neurosurgery, 57,* 769–774.

Albers, G. W. (1998). Diffusion-weighted MRI for evaluation of acute stroke. *Neurology, 51,* (Suppl. 3), S47–S49.

Araiza, J. & Araiza, B. (1997). Neuroimaging. *Emergency Medicine Clinics of North America, 24*(3), 507–527.

Bakshi, R., Kamran, S., Kinkel, P. R., et al. (1999). Intraventricular CSF pulsation artifact on fast fluid-attenuated inversion-recovery MR images: analysis of 100 consecutive normal studies. *American Journal of Neuroradiology, 20,* 629–636.

Bell, T. E., LaGrange, K. M., Maier, C. M., & Steinberg, G. K. (1992). Transcranial Doppler: Correlation of blood velocity measurement with clinical status in subarachnoid hemorrhage. *Journal of Neuroscience Nursing, 24*(4), 216–219.

Chestnut, R. M. (1994). Computed tomography of the brain: a guide to understanding and interpreting normal and abnormal images in the critically ill patient. *Critical Care Nursing Quarterly, 17*(1), 33–50.

Fearson, M., & Rusy, K. L. (1996). Transcranial Doppler: Advanced technology for assessing cerebral hemodynamics. *Dimensions of Critical Care Nursing, 13*(5), 241–248.

Gabis, L., Belman, A., Roche, P., et al. (2000). In vivo 1H magnetic resonance spectroscopy study in Cockayne syndrome. *Annals of Neurology, 48,* 489. Poster 277.

Gilman, S. (1998). Imaging the brain. *New England Journal of Medicine, 338*(12), 812–820.

Le Bihan, D., Jezzard, P., Haxby, J., et al. (1995). Functional magnetic resonance imaging of the brain. *Annals of Internal Medicine, 122,* 296–303.

Manno, E. M. (1997). Transcranial Doppler ultrasonography in the neurocritical care unit. *Critical Care Clinics, 13*(1), 79–104.

Marks, M. P., Tong, D. C., Beaulieu, C., et al. (1999). Evaluation of early reperfusion and IV tPA therapy using diffusion- and perfusion-weighted MRI. *Neurology, 52,* 1792–1798.

Simon, R. P., Aminoff, M. J. & Greenberg, D. A. (1999). *Clinical neurology* (4th ed.). Stamford, CT: Appleton & Lange.

Souder, E. & Alavi, A. (1995). A comparison of the neuroimaging modalities for diagnosing dementia. *Nurse Practitioner, 20*(1), 66–74.

Tegeler, C. H., & Ratanaskorn, D. (1998). Neurosonology. In J. Bogousslavsku & M. Fisher (Eds.). *Textbook of neurology* (pp. 101–118). Boston: Butterworth-Heinemann.

Patient and Family

Published Material

Patient information published internally by health care facilities and testing sites and commercially prepared patient education material specific to the diagnostic procedure

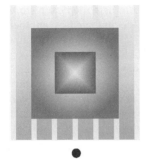

CHAPTER **7**

The Neurological Physical Examination

JOANNE V. HICKEY

PURPOSES

The neurological physical examination is conducted to determine whether nervous system dysfunction is present, to diagnose disease of the nervous system, and to localize disease within the nervous system. Although diagnosis of disease is usually the responsibility of the physician, advanced practice nurses also may conduct the neurological examination. It is the purpose of the data collection that differentiates medical practice from nursing practice. The nursing purposes are to determine whether nervous system dysfunction is present and to determine the human responses to actual or potential health problems precipitated by the dysfunction. Nurse practitioners may overlap with physicians in the purposes of the examination.

The neurological physical examination is included in this text for several reasons. First, the neurological physical examination provides a comprehensive database of critical information about the patient's neurological function. As part of the patient's record, it is available for nurses and other health care providers to review. Second, a review of these data by nurses may be helpful in identifying areas of special consideration in neurological assessment, as well as special observations to be made and documented. These points should be noted in the patient's individualized care plan. Third, potential multidisciplinary collaborative problems may be suggested by the dysfunction identified. For example, a patient with ataxia, a symptom of cerebellar dysfunction, will usually have problems with balance and coordination and needs supervision when ambulating. The potential for falls and injury must be considered by all providers and noted on the care plan or clinical pathway. Finally, although nurses independently establish a nursing database about the patient's neurological function, collaborative practice and relationships suggest a sharing of information so that each participant understands the database on which other participants provide care.

THE NEUROLOGICAL EXAMINATION

Circumstances

The circumstances surrounding the neurological examination can vary greatly. A patient may be seen in the physician's office, in an ambulatory care center, an emergency department, or hospital setting. The patient's overall condition and level of consciousness (LOC) are key factors that control collection of elements of the neurological examination. Many parts of the neurological examination require cooperation and following directions. If a person has periods of confusion but can be reoriented, most aspects of the neurological examination can be completed so long as the examiner takes time to reorient and redirect the patient. However, in the case of a comatose patient, data collection is limited to responses to painful stimuli, reflexes, and a few special techniques for assessment. Other parts of the neurological examination will have to be deferred until the patient's condition improves.

Types

The major components of a neurological examination are listed in Box 7-1. Neurological examinations may be classified as a screening or an extended examination. A **screening examination** refers to a complete medical history and neurological examination for persons who come for a general assessment and may or may not have neurological complaints. An **extended examination** is an extension of the screening examination whereby the examiner follows leads from specific symptoms or abnormal findings and expands the investigation with additional techniques and refinements to determine presence or absence of dysfunction. A **problem-focused examination** is a subset of an extended examination. It is confined to a particular system or region that is related to specific complaints or signs and symptoms. This chapter focuses on an initial neurological *screening examination* (Box 7-2). It also includes components of the extended examination that further explores specific areas of the nervous system that require more refined techniques for evaluation.

Role of the Nurse During the Examination

The nurse may be present during the neurological examination. The role of the nurse is to be supportive of the patient by providing brief explanations, emotional support, physical support, and assistance, as needed. Sometimes, the examiner may prefer to examine the patient alone, particularly

---

Box 7–1 MAJOR COMPONENTS OF THE NEUROLOGICAL EXAMINATION

- Level of consciousness
- Mental status examination
- Cranial nerves
- Motor system
- Sensory system
- Cerebellar system
- Reflexes
- Other signs

---

if the patient is easily distracted by the presence of another person in the room. Additionally, some patients tend to reveal more information to the examiner when the exchange is one-to-one.

Equipment

The usual equipment necessary to conduct a neurological physical examination includes the following:

- Ophthalmoscope
- Pointed/sharp instrument: for instance, picky end of a broken wooden applicator; key
- Stethoscope
- Reflex hammer
- Tongue blade
- Wisp of cotton or fluffed cotton swab (to test corneal reflex and light touch sensation)
- Tuning fork (of the extremities and 512-Hz for evaluating hearing)
- Flashlight
- Tape measure
- Snellen or Rosenbaum eye chart

Approach

The neurological examination is always preceded by a complete medical history and general physical examination. The nervous system is but one system in a body comprising integrated systems. Neurological signs and symptoms may accompany systemic disease and may even be the first evidence of such disease. This may be true in the case of hematologic disorders, vascular disease, heart disease, diabetes mellitus, infections (e.g., human immunodeficiency virus [HIV]), toxemia, neoplasms, metabolic disorders, and many other conditions. In addition, neurological symptoms of either organic or psychogenic origin may include symptoms referable to other systems as a result of central or autonomic nervous system effects on visceral function. Therefore, all signs and symptoms must be adequately investigated within the context of all body systems before a neurological diagnosis is made.

After reviewing the patient's medical record, a history of the neurological problem is obtained. It is advisable to start

at the beginning in collecting the complete medical history even though this has already been documented by another practitioner. An explanation to the patient will help in gaining cooperation. For example, one can say, "I know that you have answered some of these questions before. However, I like to start from the beginning and collect this information without being influenced by what is in your chart so I can make an unbiased assessment of you." Often an examiner with neurological expertise will delve into areas not included in a general screening examination. This information may be critical in making an accurate diagnosis. The examiner may wish to speak with a reliable family member or significant other to collect additional information about the past medical history and chronological development of the neurological problem, especially if the patient's cognitive function is altered.

Medical History

The family history of neurological conditions should be reexamined. Next, ask the patient about a history of hypertension, heart disease, diabetes mellitus, head trauma, alcohol or drug abuse, and exposure to toxins. Any of these conditions as well as many more could have neurological implications. A history of high-risk sexual behavior must be elicited in light of the many neurological complications associated with acquired immune deficiency syndrome (AIDS). A detailed history of all prescribed and over-the-counter medications is imperative because of the high incidence of iatrogenic neurological symptoms or illness.

General Physical Examination

Establish the patient's dominant hand. So-called handedness and cerebral dominance for language are closely aligned. Asking the patient if he or she is left-handed or

---

Box 7–2 COMPONENTS OF THE NEUROLOGICAL SCREENING EXAMINATION

1. Level of consciousness
2. Mental status and cognitive function examination
3. Cranial nerves II to XII
4. Motor tone, muscle bulk, and proximal and distal motor strength in the four extremities; in addition, note any abnormal movements
5. Sensory function of pinprick and light touch in medial and lateral aspects of extremities and face; vibration and position in thumbs and great toes
6. Coordination of rapid alternation movements of hands; finger-nose test; gait; and station
7. Reflexes: biceps, triceps, brachioradialis, quadriceps, Achilles reflexes; check also plantar reflex (i.e., Babinski's sign)
   Note: Abnormal findings or specific symptoms will require an extended evaluation.

right-handed is not sufficient because many left-handed people have been taught to write with their right hand. Helpful questions are "What hand do you use for throwing a ball?" or "What eye do you use to focus a camera?" Next, examine the contour of the skull for bumps, depressions, or malformations. Observe for drainage from the nose or ears. Examine the neck for position, symmetry, and mobility. Auscultate the common carotids for bruits. Examine the facial blood vessels for an edematous, tortuous appearance. The spinal column and vertebrae are investigated for symmetry, full range of movement, muscle atrophy or spasms, and scoliosis. Note any point tenderness. Finally, the heart is auscultated for rate (e.g., atrial fibrillation associated with emboli), murmurs, clicks (e.g., midsystolic click with mitral prolapse), or other abnormalities that could contribute to neurological conditions.

History of Present Illness

A complete accounting of the present illness, including onset, duration, and sequence of symptoms, must be established. Consider the defining characteristics of signs and symptoms, associated symptoms, and relieving/aggravating factors for each symptom.

Every patient with neurological complaints should be directly questioned about each of the following symptoms.[1]

Loss/change in intellectual abilities, onset of memory problems, difficulty with concentration, personality change, depression, or loss of drive
New onset or change in headache patterns
Seizures and loss of consciousness
Dizziness or vertigo
Loss or blurring of vision (one eye or both) or diplopia
Loss of hearing or tinnitus
Incoordination or gait difficulty
Weakness, involuntary movements
Paresthesias, sensory loss, or pain
Speech difficulties
Dysphagia
Urinary difficulties or impotence
Sleep difficulties (insomnia or increased sleep)

The neurological examination is conducted in a systematic, hierarchical, stepwise approach that proceeds from the highest level of function (cerebral cortex) to the lowest (reflexes) and from the general functions to specific functions. It encompasses a review of level of consciousness (LOC), mental status/cognitive function, cranial nerves, motor system, sensory system, cerebellar system, reflexes, and other signs (Table 7-1). By approaching the neurological examination with a conceptual framework in mind, the likelihood of forgetting a part is diminished. The examiner may decide to defer certain parts of the examination. Deciding which parts can be deferred without loss of key data is difficult to say. The judgment and experience of the examiner will guide these decisions. The

 Table 7-1 • MINI-MENTAL STATUS EXAMINATION

The Mini-Mental State Examination is a brief test of cognitive functions used to *screen* for dementia and follow patients over time. The range of scores is 0 to 30. A score of <24 suggests dementia.

ITEMS	MAXIMUM POINTS
Orientation	
Please tell me the year, season, date, month, and day of week (1 point for each)	5
Where are we? state, county, city, building, and floor or room (1 point for each)	5
Registration	
Name three objects slowly and ask the patient to repeat them (1 point per object)	3
Attention and Calculation	
Ask the patient to start at 100 and keep subtracting 7 (serial 7s); an alternate is to ask the patient to spell WORLD backward. The patient should be able to subtract 7 correctly at least 5 times. Subtract 1 point for each error. OR Subtract 1 point for each error in spelling WORLD backward.	5
Recall	
After 3–5 minutes, ask for the names of the objects repeated above.	3
Language	
Show the patient a watch and ask for its name. Repeat with a pencil.	2
Ask the patient to repeat "No ifs, ands, or buts."	1
Follow a three-step command. Give the patient a blank piece of paper and say "Take this paper in your right hand, fold it in half, and put it on the floor."	3
Hold up a piece of paper with the words **CLOSE YOUR EYES** printed on it in large letters. Ask the patient to read it and follow the direction.	1
Ask the patient to write a complete sentence.	1
Construction	
Ask the patient to copy 2 intersecting pentagons onto a blank paper.	1

TOTAL	30

(Adapted from Folstein, M. F., Folstein, S. E., & McHugh, P. R. [1975]. "Mini-Mental State": A practical method for grading the cognitive state of patients for the clinician. *Journal of Psychiatric Research, 12,* 196–198.)

examiner must know the appropriate techniques for testing function, know when further investigation is warranted, and be familiar with the expected range of normal, age-based responses. More information about specific findings in the neurological examination is included in Chapter 8.

This chapter includes the neurological examinations for both the conscious cooperative patient and the comatose patient.

MENTAL STATUS EXAMINATION

Many parts of the **mental status examination** are integrated into the history-taking portion of the interview. This context provides a natural way of collecting information without creating an artificial test setting that could make the patient uncomfortable or anxious. The basic mental processes are the foundation to proceed to complex functions. Higher-level cognitive functions such as memory and abstraction cannot be reliably tested if basic mental functions such as attentiveness or arousal are absent. In appraising mental status the examiner must determine whether there is any dysfunction present, whether the dysfunction is global or focal, and if global, is it a confusional state or dementia.

The mental status examination focusing on three general and often overlapping areas: (1) general impression of awareness and mental function; (2) reception and interpretation of sensory stimuli including awareness and responsiveness to self, to the environment, and to the impressions made by the senses; and (3) cognitive function (Box 7-3). An *extended mental status examination* is warranted if abnormalities are found in the screening examination. Referral for neuropsychological testing may be necessary for some patients.

General Impression of Patient Awareness and Mental Function

Beginning with the interview and history collection, the following areas are evaluated: LOC; general appearance and behavior; mood and emotional state; and thinking processes along with content of thought.

Box 7–3 COMPREHENSIVE MENTAL STATUS EXAMINATION

I. General impression of awareness and mental function
  A. Level of consciousness
  B. General appearance and behavior
  C. Mood and emotional state
  D. General thinking processes
  E. Content of thought

II. Reception and interpretation of sensory stimuli (general cognitive function)
  A. Orientation
  B. Personal identification
  C. Attention
  D. Comprehension

III. Higher-level cognitive functions
  A. Memory (immediate, short-term, long-term)
  B. Calculations
  C. General fund of information
  D. Abstract thinking, reasoning, and judgment
  E. Language and speech
  F. Constructional ability
  G. Motor integrative function

Level of Consciousness

A complete discussion of the various LOCs is found in Chapter 8. What the examiner must determine first is whether the patient is awake or comatose. If the patient is comatose, *proceed to the neurologic examination for the comatose patient later in this chapter*. If awake, is attention sufficiently intact so the patient can cooperate and follow instructions to demonstrate maximum functional ability? If the answer is "yes," you can proceed with the complete neurological examination. If the answer is "no," you will need to limit the neurological examination to what can be collected within the limitations of the LOC and defer other components until the LOC is sufficient to complete the neurological examination.

Two special states of consciousness that will affect the ability to conduct the mental status examination are acute confusional state (delirium) and dementia. **Acute confusional state** and **delirium** (the older term) are used interchangeably, although delirium is most often used when agitation is a major feature. Acute confusional state may initially be mistaken for an acute psychotic reaction. The following is the diagnostic criteria for delirium based on the *Diagnostic and Statistical Manual of Mental Disorders*, 4th ed:[2]

Disturbance of consciousness (reduced clarity of awareness of the environment) in conjunction with reduced ability to focus, sustain, or shift attention

A change in cognition or the development of a perceptual disturbance that cannot be better accounted for by a pre-existing, established, or evolving dementia

Rapid development of syndrome over hours to days, and a course of fluctuation during the day

Evidence from the history, physical examination, or laboratory findings that the disturbance is caused by an underlying disorder: a general medical condition; substance intoxication or side effect; withdrawal from a substance; or multiple factors

Clinically, the most reliable clinical feature that distinguishes acute confusional state from other organic or functional disorders is a clouding of consciousness, a dulling of cognitive processes, and a general impairment of alertness.[3]

Dementia is a progressive and usually irreversible decline in *global* cognitive functions without a reduction in arousal. Memory problems are a prominent symptom. Dementia is a cortical or subcortical disorder in which the person's self-awareness and ability to function independently and assume responsibility for self are seriously impaired or absent. There are many causes of irreversible dementia (see Chapter 31). If dementia is suspected, the Mini-Mental State Examination is a good screening tool (see Table 7-1). Table 7-2 compares acute confusional state and dementia.

Appearance and General Behavior

A patient's attire should be appropriate for the setting and his or her age. A neat and clean appearance reflects good grooming and good personal hygiene habits. An unkempt appearance, conversely, might suggest depression or chronic organic brain disease. **Posture and motor conduct** convey clues about mental state or disease process. A slumped posture coupled with slow movements suggests depression or possibly Parkinson's disease, whereas pacing suggests anxiety.

Table 7-2 • COMPARISON OF ACUTE CONFUSIONAL STATE AND DEMENTIA

KEY CHARACTERISTICS	ACUTE CONFUSIONAL STATE/DELIRIUM	DEMENTIA
Onset	Point in time	Vague
Course	Acute	Chronic
Fluctuation	Hour-to-hour	Day-to-day
Reversible	Yes	Mostly no
Inattention	Yes	No

Facial expression is assessed for appropriateness and variations in expression in relation to topics under discussion. In addition, observe for changes in the characteristics of the skin, features, or hair that is suggestive of other conditions such as hypothyroidism, Cushing's syndrome, vitamin B_{12} deficiency. Finally, **affect and manner** provide a composite of the openness, approachability, and responsiveness of the patient to the environment and other people.

Mood and Emotional State

Ask the patient about his or her perception of his or her mood. Questions that are helpful include "How are your spirits?" "What makes you angry?" and "What makes you sad?" Reactions to the topic being discussed and to the people around should be noted. Abnormal responses might include hostility, evasiveness, anger, tearfulness, or depression. If depression is suspected, a depression screening scale can be administered to further evaluate the patient. Of special concern is any suggestion related to suicide, which must be taken seriously. A direct inquiry can be made. One can ask "Have you ever thought about killing yourself?" or "Do you ever feel that life is not worth living?" Special observation, supervision, and further evaluation are warranted if suicidal tendencies are suspected.

In addition, reports of family or friends can be very helpful in evaluating changes in mood.

Thinking Processes and Content of Thought

The overall characteristics of the thinking processes are evaluated both in response to questions and spontaneous conversation. **Thought processes** refer to the subjective responses to life experiences and how they are verbally expressed. Indicators of intact thought processes are clarity, cohesiveness, relevance, and logical progression and organization of thoughts. Table 7-3 lists disorders of thought processes. **Thought content** refers to themes in expression of ideas. By active listening, reflecting, and exploring the answers offered, the examiner can evaluate the presence of abnormal themes such as compulsive behaviors (i.e., compulsions, obsessions, phobias), anxieties, feelings of unreality, depersonalization, persecution or control by others, delusions, and perceptual deficits (i.e., illusions and hallucinations).

Perception is a person's subjective interpretation of real or perceived stimuli. Illusions and hallucinations are common abnormal perceptual findings. **Illusions** are the misinterpretation of real external stimuli. **Hallucinations** are a subjective sensory perception in the absence of real external stimuli and may be categorized as auditory, visual, olfactory, gustatory, tactile or somatic. Evidence of illusions or hallucinations may indicate depression, mental illness, or organic disease necessitating further evaluation.

Throughout the interview note the characteristics of speech. **Speech** is the motor activity that is the expression of language, and is controlled by the lower cranial nerves and their supranuclear connections. Listen to the **fluency** (i.e., rate, flow, melody of speech, content, use of words) of speech. Note the quality, volume, tone, articulation, inflections, and spontaneity of the speech. Slow monotone speech may be suggestive of depression whereas rapid and loud speech is common in manic states. Problems with *articulation*

Table 7-3 • VARIATIONS/ABNORMALITIES IN THOUGHT PROCESSES

ABNORMALITY	DESCRIPTION OF SPEECH	OBSERVED IN
Circumstantiality	Delay in reaching the point because of unnecessary detail although the content of the descriptions are connected.	Obsessive compulsive disorder and many people without mental illness
Derailment	Shift from one subject to another that is unrelated or marginally related without realizing that the subjects are not connected.	Schizophrenia, manic episodes, and other psychiatric disorders
Flight of ideas	A continuous flow of accelerated speech with abrupt changes from topic to topic; ideas do not progress to sensible conversation.	Most common in manic episodes
Neologisms	Invented or distorted words, or words with new and highly idiosyncratic meanings	Schizophrenics, other psychotic disorders, and aphasics
Incoherence	Largely incomprehensible because of illogic, disconnected, abrupt changes in topic or disordered grammar or word use.	Severely disturbed patients with psychosis (e.g., schizophrenia)
Blocking	Sudden interruption in midsentence or before completion of an idea. Person attributes this to losing the thought.	Normal persons and patients with schizophrenia
Confabulation	Fabrication of facts or events in response to questions to fill in the gaps in an impaired memory	Patients with amnesia
Perseveration	Persistent repetition of words or ideas	Patients with schizophrenia and other psychosis
Echolalia	Repetition of the words and phrases of others	Manic episodes and schizophrenia
Clanging	Words chosen on the basis of sound rather than meaning, as in rhyming and punning speech	Schizophrenia and manic episodes

(Adapted from Bickley, L. S. [1999]. *Bates' guide to physical examination and history taking* [7th ed., p. 114]. Philadelphia: Lippincott.)

(i.e., clarity and distinctness of the spoken word) are associated with dysarthria. **Dysarthria** is a disorder of articulation in which basic language (i.e., grammar, comprehension, and word choice) is intact. The sounds produced are distorted and often nasal and are usually related to deficits in the throat muscles. An interruption of speech inflections and rhythm (i.e., speech melody) is called **dysprosody**. The resulting speech is monotone and halting.

Reception and Interpretation of Sensory Stimuli

The reception and interpretation of sensory stimuli, including awareness and responsiveness of self, the environment, and the impressions made by the senses, are referred to as *sensorium*. The areas included in the evaluation include **orientation; personal identification; attention and concentration;** and **comprehension**. These functions may be clouded by focal or diffuse cerebral conditions, such as a brain tumor, vascular and degenerative disease, or encephalitis.

Orientation

Orientation is the awareness of **time, place,** and **person** and is evaluated by direct questioning.

Time: the time of day, day of the week, month, season, date, and year, as well as any possible upcoming holiday or one in the immediate past may be asked. For some patients, however, a more direct approach, using specific questions (e.g., "What day is it today?") is indicated.

Place: give the present location such as "I am at Mercy Clinic in Detroit, Michigan"

Person: ability of the patient to give his or her own name

Personal Identification

In the context of evaluation, ask the patient's name, address, and background information such as date and place of birth, history of the illness, and specific dates of significant life events will provide insight into awareness of time, place, and person. Note that it should be possible to corroborate this information using the medical record or verification by a family member.

Attention and Concentration

Attention is the ability to focus on a particular sensory stimulus while excluding others; **concentration** is sustained attention. In acute confusional states, attention and concentration are severely impaired. By contrast, both are intact in focal lesions. Attention and concentration can be tested in a number of ways, including number series, serial 7s, and spelling backwards.

Number Series

Read a series of digits to the patient and then asking him or her to repeat the numbers. The series should start with a short list, with each digit being enunciated clearly and paced at 1-second intervals. Number series can begin with two digits, then progress to a maximum of six digits (e.g., 7, 2; 9, 5, 2). Avoid consecutive numbers or digits that form easily recognizable combinations, such as the date 1776. If the patient makes an error in repeating the digits, provide a second chance with another series of digits of similar length. Stop after two consecutive failures in a series of any length. In the second part of this test (beginning with the shortest list of digits), the patient is asked to repeat a series in reverse order. Normally, a person should be able to repeat correctly five to seven digits forward and four in reverse order.

Serial 7s

Another common exercise is to ask the patient to start with 100 and subtract 7s. Normally, one should be able to complete this exercise with few errors in 90 seconds. In practice, if a patient can accurately complete five subtractions, this is usually sufficient. Patients unable to do serial 7s should be instructed to complete serial 3s in a similar manner.

Spelling Backwards

Say a five-letter word and ask the patient to spell it backward. The word commonly used is W-O-R-L-D.

Comprehension

Evidence of the level of comprehension and perception is noted in many components of the examination. **Comprehension** is the ability to grasp and to understand the meaning of visual, auditory, and other stimuli within the context of the total situation accurately. Comprehension, perception, attention, reasoning, and making decisions are complex processes; they contribute to other mental functions such as memory, judgment, general knowledge, and intelligence.

Higher-Level Cognitive Functions

Higher-level cognitive functions include several higher cognitive and integrative functions. In evaluating responses, consider what someone of comparable cultural and educational background would be expected to know. Testing of these higher-level intellectual abilities includes:

- Memory (immediate, short-term, long-term)
- Calculations
- General fund of information
- Abstract thinking, reasoning, and judgment
- Language and speech
- Constructional ability
- Motor integrative function

Memory

Memory is the ability to register, store, and retrieve information. **Registration**, the ability to receive information through the various senses, is closely related to attention. Without the ability to attend, information will not register. **Storage** is the process whereby selected new information is learned; it is mediated by the limbic structures, including the hippocampi, the mamillary bodies, and the dorsal medial nuclei of the thalami. After the sensory input has been received and registered, that information is held temporarily in short-term memory or working memory. Next, the information is stored in a more permanent form (long-term memory). Stored information is reinforced by repetition or by association with other information that is already in storage. **Retrieval**, the final step, is the ability to access previously learned information.

Memory can be subdivided into general time spans and include immediate memory, short-term memory, and long-term memory. The time frame for immediate memory and short-term memory is sometimes imprecise. **Immediate memory** is the retrieval of information within seconds or minutes after presentation as in repeating a series of digits. **Short-term memory**, also referred to as recent memory, is the ability to remember current, day-to-day events such as the date, the name of the health provider, what was eaten for breakfast, or a recent news event. **Long-term memory**, also referred to as remote memory, refers to the recollection of facts or events that occurred several days to years previously, such as family information and historical facts. The clinical significance between short-term memory and long-term memory is that short-term memory requires the *ongoing ability* to learn new information.

In testing immediate memory, give the patient three unrelated words to remember (e.g., lilies, courage, and screwdriver). Ask the patient to repeat each word after you. Then, ask the patient to tell you those three words; this tests immediate memory. Instruct the patient to remember those three words because you will be coming back to them in a few minutes. Go on with the examination. In 3 to 5 minutes, ask the patient to tell you what those three words were. Normally, the patient should be able to remember the three words. In testing long-term memory, the following offers suggestions for typical personal and historical information.

- Date/place of birth: When were you born?
- Where were you born?
- School information: Where did you go to school?
- When did you attend school?
- Where is your school located?
- Vocational history: What do you do for work?
- Where do you work?
- How long have you worked there?
- Family history:
  What are your spouse's and children's names?
  How old are they?
  What was your mother's maiden name?

Memory can be affected by a number of focal and diffuse organic conditions as well as emotional states. **Amnesia** is defined as a defect in memory function and may be an isolated deficit or one component of global cognitive dysfunction. In acute confusional states, attention is impaired resulting in a problem with registration and inability to learn new information. By contrast, attention is usually normal in dementia. Amnesia is classified into specific categories and includes:

Retrograde amnesia: loss of memory for events that occurred *before* a brain insult
Antegrade or posttraumatic amnesia: loss of memory for events *after* a brain insult
Psychogenic amnesia: loss of memory for an emotionally charged event

Calculations

Serial 7s give some indication of subtraction ability. In addition, simple calculations problems should be asked such as:

How much is a quarter, a dime, and a nickel?
How much is 3×9?
How much is $11 + 7$?

General Fund of Information

To evaluate the patient's general knowledge, consider the patient's cultural and educational background. Ask about current events or general information that you would expect an average adult to know who lives in the area. Examples of questions are:

Who is the president of the United States?
Name the last five presidents from the current president back.
What is the capital of England?

Abstract Thinking, Reasoning, and Judgment

An appraisal of abstract thinking, reasoning, and judgment may begin while taking the history, but a closer evaluation is warranted.

Abstract Thinking

To think abstractly is the ability to see subtle relationships and meaning in events and between objects. This can be evaluated through the use of proverbs and similarities. Ask the patient what is meant by the following proverbs:

All that glitters is not gold.
People who live in glass houses should not throw stones.
Rolling stones gather no moss.

A literal, concrete interpretation may indicate organic brain disease, mental illness, mental retardation, or simply limited education.

In evaluating ability to recognize similarities, ask the patient to explain how two given objects are alike, such as:

A rose and a carnation
A piano and a violin
Silk and linen

Reasoning

The ability to use intellectual faculties to discover, formulate, or draw a conclusion is called **reasoning**. This can be evaluated by asking the patient to define or differentiate between combinations such as a mistake and a lie, or sadness and hopelessness.

Judgment

The process of forming an opinion or evaluation about something is called **judgment**. It often includes a component of **insight**, the act of seeing the inner nature of things or of seeing intuitively. The examiner can evaluate a patient's judgment and insight by asking questions such as "What seems to be the problem?" or "Why are you here today?" A person might say that he or she is here to be evaluated because of certain signs and symptoms. Conversely, a patient might say that there is nothing wrong, but his or her spouse insisted on the visit. The latter suggests a lack of insight due to denial, being unaware of the relationship of symptoms to illness, or parietal lobe syndrome. To appraise judgment, ask questions such as "How are you going to manage at home after hospitalization?" or "What activity limitations do you need to follow?" The examiner can de-

IIII **Table 7–4** • TESTING OF LANGUAGE AND SPEECH

ELEMENT OF LANGUAGE	THE FOLLOWING ASSIST QUESTIONS IN DETERMINING ABILITY TO UNDERSTAND THE SPOKEN AND WRITTEN WORD AND TO EXPRESS THOUGHTS ORALLY AND IN WRITING
Fluency	Ask the patient to describe his or her work. Avoid questions that can be answered by "yes" or "no." Another approach is to show the patient a picture and ask what is happening in the picture. Listen to the flow of speech.
Word comprehension	Ask the patient to follow a one-step command such as "point to your hair." If this is successfully completed, give a two-step command such as "point to the door, then tap your knee." Then give a three-step command.
Repetition	Ask the patient to repeat simple words such as "cat"; if successful, increase the complexity to a word such as "moratorium." Finally, pose a more challenging phrase, such as repeat "no ifs, ands, or buts."
Naming	Ask the patient to name objects that you introduce. Include 10–20 objects from a variety of categories (colors; clothing and room objects; body parts; parts of an object). For example, point to the watch stem, watch crystal, shin, or coat lapel.
Reading comprehension	Ask the patient to read a few sentences from a newspaper or magazine. Write a message in large print on a paper such as "Close your eyes." Ask the patient to read the sign and follow the request.
Writing	Ask patient to write a sentence from your dictation. Next, ask the patient to write a sentence about anything of his or her own choosing.

termine how accurate and reasonable judgments are based on the patient's age and education.

Language and Speech

Language is the basic tool of human communication and the basic building block for most cognitive functions.[4] Normally, a person can understand the spoken and written word and also express thoughts verbally and in writing. Disturbances of language and speech are divided into three areas:

1. Disorders of central language processing result in *aphasia*.
2. Disorders of motor programming of language symbols result in *apraxia of speech*.
3. Disorders of the mechanism of speech result in *dysarthria*.

Language and speech are evaluated throughout the patient–provider interaction. If there are deficits in the language system, it will be difficult, if not impossible, to test cognitive skills such as memory, proverb interpretation, or oral calculations. Word comprehension, repetition, naming, fluency, reading, and writing are all essential elements of the language system and all are tested (Table 7-4).

Aphasia is a language disorder due to a dominant hemisphere lesion that produces a defect in the expression or comprehension of any component of language. Aphasia used to be subdivided into nonfluent (expressive) aphasia and fluent (receptive) aphasia, but is now classified on a functional basis. The main types of aphasia include **Broca's aphasia, Wernicke's aphasia,** conduction aphasia, transcortical aphasia, subcortical aphasia, and global aphasia. See Table 7-5 and Figure 7-1 for

IIII **Table 7–5** • TYPES OF APHASIAS WITH ANATOMICAL CORRELATIONS

TYPE	DESCRIPTION/CLINICAL CORRELATION	ANATOMICAL AREA OR LESION
Broca's aphasia	Unable to convert thoughts into meaningful language Agrammatism (inability to organize words into sentences) Telegraphic speech (use of content words without connecting words) Distorted production of speech sounds Impaired repetition Normal reception of language is intact	Broca's area (frontal lobe areas 44 and 45), underlying white matter, or basal ganglia
Wernicke's aphasia	Fluent speech that is unintelligible because of pronunciation errors and use of jargon Impaired comprehension of verbal and written language, but no focal motor deficit Impaired repetition	Wernicke's area (superior temporal gyrus, area 22)
Conduction aphasia	Impaired repetition	Connections between Broca's and Wernicke's areas
Transcortical aphasia	Impaired expression or reception of speech, but *repetition is spared*	Arterial border zones
Subcortical aphasia	Fluent, dysarthric speech and hemiparesis	Left caudate nucleus or the left thalamus
Global aphasia	Combined features of Wernicke's aphasia and Broca's aphasia Impaired comprehension and expression of speech Impaired repetition Commonly associated with a dense contralateral hemiplegia	Perisylvian or central regions; commonly seen with left middle cerebral artery infarction

(Adapted from: Benarroch, E. E., Westmoreland, B. F., Daube, J. R., Reagan, T. J., & Sandok, B. A. [1999]. *Medical neurosciences: An approach to anatomy, pathology, and physiology by systems and levels* (4th ed, p. 567) Philadelphia: Lippincott Williams & Wilkins.)

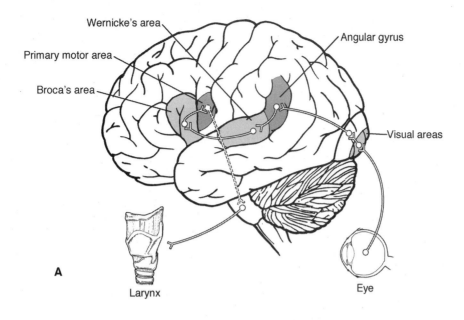

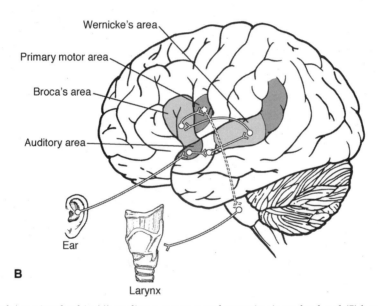

Figure 7–1 • Probable nerve pathways involved in (*A*) reading a sentence and repeating it out loud and (*B*) hearing a question and answering it. Note that Wernicke's area is connected to Broca's area by a bundle of nerve fibers called the *arcuate fasciculus*.

anatomic locations. Most patients have varying degrees of expressive and receptive language deficits, emphasizing the interrelatedness of cortical function.

All aphasias are associated with difficulty naming objects (called **anosmia**). In pure anosmia there is interruption of connections between language and memory resulting in impaired word access. Aphasia must be distinguished from other speech production disorders, including speech apraxia, mutism, and dysarthria. **Motor speech apraxia** results from a focused lesion in Broca's areas (areas 44 and 45). It is characterized by a partial or complete inability to form the articulatory movements of the lips, tongue, and lower jaw to produce individual sounds that constitute words. The patient knows what he or she wants to say but is unable to execute the motor aspects of speech.[5] **Mutism** is a lack of speech production caused by lesions of the prefrontal areas

and cingulate gyrus. **Dysarthria** is a motor speech impairment; it involves difficulty with speech but *not* a deficit with language. Clear speech involves coordinated and modulated activity of muscles supplied by cranial nerves (CNs) V, VII, IX, X, and XII as well as the respiratory muscles. Dysarthria occurs with disorders of the direct and indirect motor pathways, the motor control circuits, and the lower motor neuron system. This is discussed with the section on assessment of the CNs.

Constructional Ability

Construction ability, the ability to reproduce figures or draw a figure on command, can be assessed easily if the patient has motor function in his or her writing hand. This ability can be tested in a number of ways. Draw two five-sided

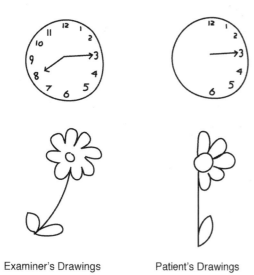

Examiner's Drawings   Patient's Drawings

Figure 7–2 • Examples of impaired performance on a copy test given to a patient with unilateral neglect.

figures that overlap to form a four-sided figure (this figure is included for copying in the Mini Mental State Examination). Ask the patient to copy it. Another option is to ask the patient to draw a clock with all the numbers and to set the clock at a given time. A variation for this drawing is a daisy with petals equally arranged around the center. Abnormalities of visuospatial function and construct abilities are seen in right, but also in left or bilateral, parietal-occipital lesions. Patients with a nondominant parietal lesion may have a hemi-spatial neglect syndrome resulting in nothing being drawn on one half of the clock or flower (Fig. 7-2 shows sample drawings).

Motor Integrative Function: Apraxia

Performing a skilled act on demand requires integrated functions of several areas of the cerebral cortex. Three steps are necessary to execute a purposeful, skilled act successfully, as detailed in Table 7-6. To perform a skilled motor act, a person must understand what the act entails, remember the steps long enough to complete the act, and possess normal motor strength. If a patient is unable to perform a learned skilled motor act (in response to a verbal command) in the absence of paralysis, comprehension deficit, uncooperative behavior, or other obvious reasons, the term **apraxia** is applied. Ask the patient to pantomime activities for you such as brushing the teeth, combing the hair, blowing out a match, and expressing surprise.

CRANIAL NERVE EXAMINATION

The next part of the neurological examination focuses on the CNS. There are twelve pairs of CNs. Each CN has a left and a right nerve; each side must therefore be evaluated separately. There may be dysfunction on one side only or both sides. Findings from each side are compared for symmetry. This chapter is organized to include details of testing, discussion of findings, and abnormal findings. See Chapter 5 for a review of the anatomy and physiology of cranial nerves.

Olfactory Nerve (Sensory) (CN I)

Testing of the olfactory nerve is often deferred unless an anterior fossa mass is suspected. The sense of smell is tested by obstructing one nostril while testing the other. A piece of cotton that has been saturated with a common, odoriferous, nonirritating substance is placed under the unobstructed nostril. Cinnamon, cloves, coffee, or peppermint are possible odors that patients should be able to identify if CN I is intact.

Abnormalities

Anosmia is an inability to smell. It is an early sign in the diagnosis and localization of certain intracranial neoplasms. There are several causes of anosmia, some of which are attributable to neuropathologic conditions such as meningiomas of the sphenoid ridge and olfactory groove, gliomas of the frontal lobe, and parasellar lesions with pressure on the olfactory bulbs or tracts. Common non-neurological causes of anosmia include the common cold, sinusitis, or inflammation of the nasal cavity. The typical syndrome with *sphenoidal ridge meningioma* is one of unilateral optic atrophy or papilledema, exophthalmos, and ipsilateral anosmia. A *meningioma of the olfactory groove or cribriform plate* includes unilateral anosmia with retrobulbar neuritis or optic atrophy with progression to bilateral anosmia. Another possible presentation is the **Foster-Kennedy syndrome**, which includes optic atrophy and anosmia on the side of the lesion and papilledema on the other side.[6]

▌▌▌ **Table 7–6** • PURPOSEFUL MOTOR ACTS AND APRAXIA

STEPS	ACTIVITY	DEFICITS	APRAXIA TYPE
1	Comprehend concept or idea Remember long enough to accomplish the act	General suppression of cerebral function, rather than a lesion in one specific area	Ideational apraxia
2	Formulate an organized plan to accomplish the task Create a mental image of the action	Lesion at the junction of the frontal, temporal, parietal, and occipital lobes	Ideokinetic or ideomotor apraxia
3	Actually execute the detailed plan	Lesion involving premotor frontal cortex The disability is usually limited to one extremity without weakness or loss of movement	Kinetic apraxia

Optic Nerve (Sensory) (CN II)

The optic nerve is the only CN that can be examined directly. Testing encompasses an evaluation of visual acuity, visual fields, and an ophthalmoscopic examination. Each eye is evaluated individually while the other eye is covered.

Visual Acuity

Visual acuity can be evaluated informally by asking the patient to read from printed material, such as a newspaper. A standard Snellen chart is available in office or clinic settings for more formal testing. Each eye is checked individually. The patient is asked to read the line on the chart with the smallest letters that he or she is able to read at a distance of 20 ft. The number beside each line of letters signifies the number of feet at which letters can be read by a person with normal vision. This becomes the denominator in recording vision. Normal vision is 20/20. When vision is defective, the patient may only be able to see the larger letters at 20 feet. For example, persons with 20/40 vision are able to see at 20 feet what those with normal vision can see at 40 feet.

An adaptation of the Snellen chart, the Rosenbaum Pocket Vision Screener, is designed for quick bedside use. The chart is held at a distance of 14 inches from the patient. Normal vision in this instance is 14/14. The ratio is calculated in the same manner as for the Snellen test.

Visual Fields

A **visual field** is the area of vision normally seen with one eye. Each visual field extends 60 degrees on the nasal side, 100 degrees on the temporal side, and 135 degrees vertically

(60 degrees superiorly and 75 degrees). Figure 7-3 displays normal visual fields. The **confrontation test** provides a rough estimate of the scope of each visual field. This is a test in which the examiner "confronts" the patient by sitting 2 feet in front of him or her at eye level. The patient is asked to cover one eye lightly and looks at the examiner's eye directly opposite (i.e., the patient's left eye will be looking at the examiner's right eye). The examiner then closes one eye, the one the visual field of which is *not* being currently used, thus isolating the visual field in the other eye and superimposing it on that of the patient's visual field. A pencil or a moving finger is then introduced from the periphery into the patient's field of vision; each quadrant (upper and lower) is checked individually. The patient is asked to indicate when the object is first seen. The examiner uses his or her own visual field as the norm for comparison to the patient's visual field.

The confrontation test is designed to reveal only gross defects of the visual fields. If any defects are found, the visual fields should be plotted by an ophthalmologist using the standard and more sensitive **perimetric test** or a **tangent screen**. Visual field testing can reveal field cuts related to characteristic deficits along the visual pathway (i.e., optic nerve, optic tract, lateral geniculate body, geniculocalcarine tract, or occipital lobe). Chart 7-1 shows specific field cuts; Figure 7-4 shows field cuts in a person with right homonymous hemianopia.

Cortical blindness with complete or severe loss of vision is called **Anton's syndrome**. Often the patient is unaware or denies the blindness. Normal pupillary responses remain intact. The most common cause of cortical blindness is bilateral occipital lobe infarctions.

Name: **Date:**

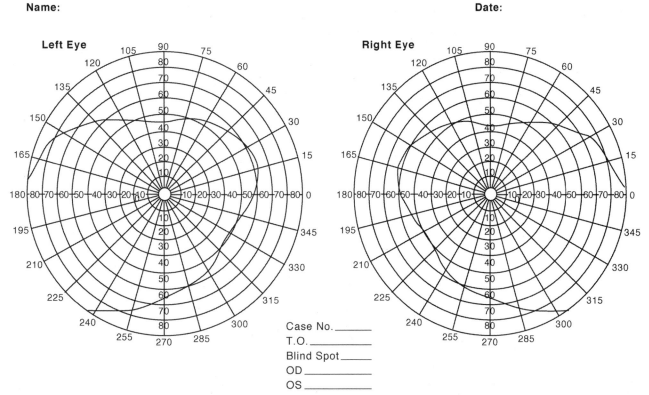

Case No. _____
T.O. _____
Blind Spot _____
OD _____
OS _____

Figure 7–3 • The normal visual fields.

CHART 7 – 1 • **Visual Field Defects Produced by Selected Lesions in the Visual Pathways**

Visual Pathways	Visual Fields	Blackened Field Indicates Area of No Vision

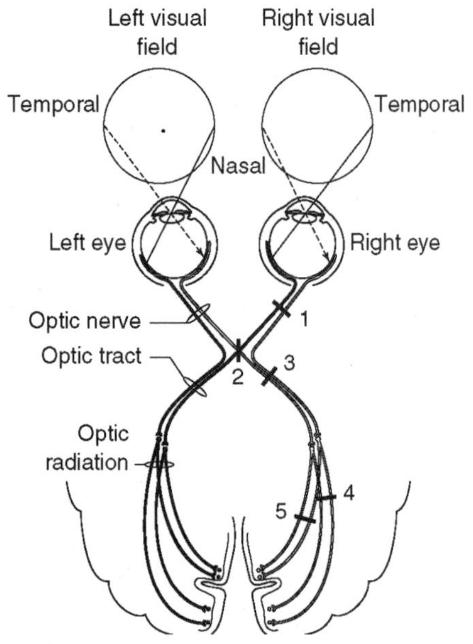

Blind Right Eye (right optic nerve)

A lesion of the optic nerve and, of course, of the eye itself, produces unilateral blindness.

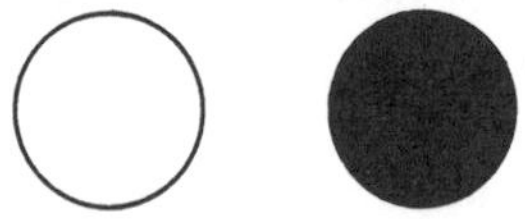

Bitemporal Hemianopia (optic chiasm)

A lesion at the optic chiasm may involve only those fibers that cross over to the opposite side. Because these fibers originate in the nasal half of each retina, visual loss involves the temporal half of each field.

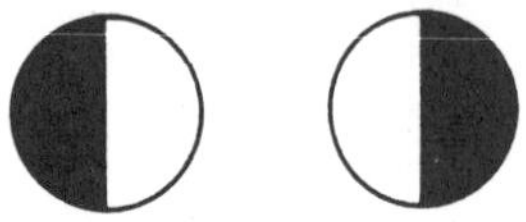

Left Homonymous Hemianopia (right optic tract)

A lesion of the optic tract interrupts fibers originating on the same side of both eyes. Visual loss in the eyes is therefore similar (homonymous) and involves half of each field (hemianopia).

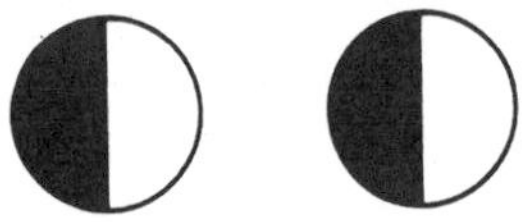

Left Homonymous Quadrantic Defect (optic radiation, partial)

A partial lesion of the optic radiation may involve only a portion of the nerve fibers, producing, for example, a homonymous quadrantic defect.

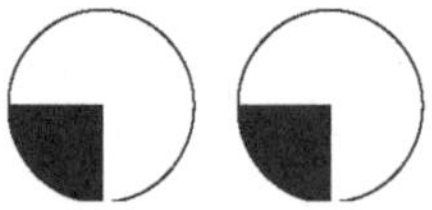

Ophthalmoscopic Examination

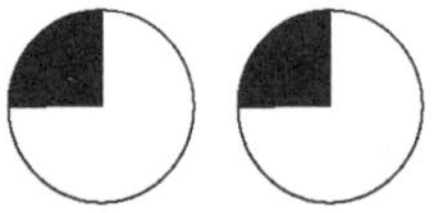

The **ophthalmoscopic examination** is conducted with an ophthalmoscope, which contains a special lens that is used to visualize the retina by shining a beam of light directly into the eye. The room must be darkened and the examiner must sit directly opposite the subject. To examine the patient's right eye, the examiner holds the ophthalmoscope in the right hand and looks through the instrument with the right eye while the patient focuses on an object straight ahead (Fig. 7-5). The diopter is adjusted to visualize the optic disc (fundus), macula, and blood vessels (Fig. 7-6). The termination of the optic nerve, visible as a prominent, tubelike structure at the back of the eyeball, is called the **optic disc**. As one views the optic disc, small blood vessels can be visualized as they exit and enter the eye. The normal disc is round or slightly oval with sharply defined margins. The outer portions of the disc are elevated slightly above the center, or physiologic cup.

The four main pairs of blood vessels exiting and entering the optic disc are examined to compare the diameters of the arteries and veins and to determine whether the veins are tortuous. Normally, the diameter of the veins is about 30% greater than the diameter of arteries in a ratio varying from 2:3 to 4:5. Dilated veins are present with increased intracranial pressure. Another area of the retina is the **macula lutea**, which has the highest density of visual receptors. The center of the macula, called the **fovea**, represents the point of greatest visual acuity. As the retina is examined, any abnormalities, such as hemorrhage, swelling, and exudate, should

Name: Date:

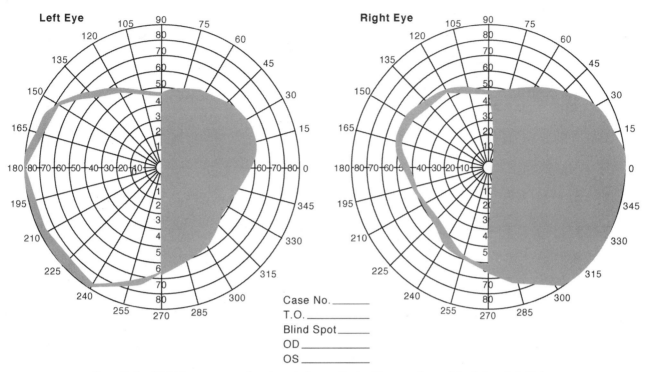

Case No. _____
T.O. _____
Blind Spot_____
OD _____
OS _____

Figure 7–4 • Right homonymous hemianopia in a patient with a neoplasm of the left occipital lobe.

be noted. Table 7-7 summarizes common ophthalmological findings.

Oculomotor (CN III), Trochlear (CN IV), and Abducens (CN VI) Nerves (All Motor)

Cranial nerves III, IV, and VI are tested together because all three supply the extraocular eye muscles (Fig. 7-7). In addition, the oculomotor nerve controls the levator palpebrae

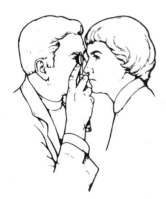

Figure 7–5 • Technique for the proper use of the ophthalmoscope. The examiner holds the ophthalmoscope with the **right** hand and uses the **right** eye to look into the patient's eye. The index finger is used to adjust the lens for proper focus. For a **myopic** (nearsighted) patient, turn the lens control counterclockwise to the minus diopter; for a **hyperopic** (farsighted) patient, turn the lens control clockwise to the plus diopter.

superioris muscle, which raises the upper eyelid, and the parasympathetic innervation to the pupil (which causes constriction of the pupil).

Injury to an extraocular muscle compromises the corresponding extraocular movement (EOM). Injury to the oculomotor nerve can result in an inability to focus the eyes medially on the horizontal plane, upward and outward, downward and outward, and upward and inward. A damaged trochlear nerve results in compromised downward and inward movement of the eye, whereas injury to the abducens nerve causes loss of lateral ocular movement on the horizontal plane. Trochlear nerve dysfunction is rare. The abducens nerve has the longest intracranial course and is frequently involved with neurological disease.

Observations Related to the Eye and Eye Movement

In assessing CNs III, IV, and VI, begin with focused observations on the position of each orbit, upper eyelid, and pupil. Next, examine EOMs for gaze palsy, internuclear ophthalmoplegia, diplopia, and nystagmus. **Gaze** is the act of focusing in a particular direction. It includes coordinated eye and head movements and is the result of complex reflexes of the visual and vestibular systems and the cerebral cortex. Terms related to the eyes are defined in a later section.

Position of Eyes, Eyelids, and Pupils

The **position of the eyes** is noted by looking at the position of the eyeball from frontal and lateral views, as well as by looking down from above the patient's head. Abnormal protrusion of

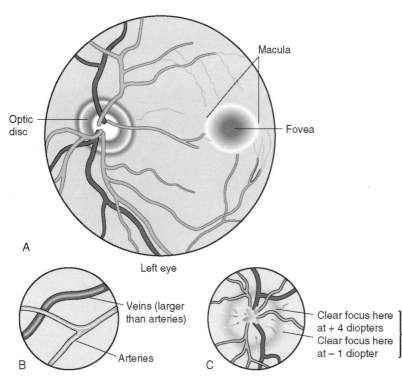

A

Optic disc

Macula

Fovea

Left eye

Veins (larger than arteries)

B

Arteries

C

Clear focus here at + 4 diopters
Clear focus here at – 1 diopter

+ 4 – (–1) = +5
therefore
a disc elevation of 5 diopters

Figure 7–6 • The retina as seen through the ophthalmoscope. The ophthalmoscope is capable of visualizing *only a portion of the retina* at any one time. In examining the retina (*A*) identify the disc; ascertain the sharpness of the disc margins; identify the macula and fovea (bright reflection in the center); (*B*) compare the diameters of the veins to the arteries; follow the vessels in each quadrant from the disc to the periphery; and note any exudate, hemorrhagic areas, or abnormalities present. **Measurements within the eye.** Lesions are recorded in relationship to the optic disc as **disc diameters.** For example, in A, the macula is about 2 disc diameters from the disc. (*C*) For an elevated optic disc due to papilledema, note the **differences in diopters** measurement of the two lenses used to focus clearly on the disc and on the uninvolved retina.

one or both eyeballs is termed **proptosis** or **exophthalmos**. Abnormal recession of an eyeball within the orbit is termed **enophthalmos**. In assessing the **upper eyelid**, the patient is asked to look straight ahead. The width of the palpebral fissure in each eye is noted and a comparison is made. The **palpebral fissure** is the space between the upper and lower eyelids. One lid may droop compared with the other. The term for a drooping upper eyelid is **ptosis**. Note also edema of the eyelid, if present. Edema can result from trauma to the eye or orbit and may occur in the upper eyelid, the lower eyelid, or both. Next, the position of the eyelids in relation to the pupil and the iris in each eye is noted and compared. This also helps the examiner to note a slight ptosis.

EOM Evaluation

The six EOM muscles are evaluated next. Ask the patient to follow the examiner's finger or a pencil through the six cardinal directions of gaze in an "H" sequencing (see Fig.

7-7). Observe for full, symmetrical movement of both eyes. See subsequent section for related terms.

Diplopia. In double vision (**diplopia**), when the eyes move in a particular direction (left or right, or up or down), visual images fall on the retina in different points, rather than on the same point on each retina. The lack of parallelism can cause double vision when the patient focuses in a particular direction. The patient is asked whether diplopia is present. If the answer is yes, is the double image side by side or one on top of the other? If the image is one on top of the other, CN III (oculomotor) or CN VI (trochlear) is involved. If the images are side by side, the examiner needs to determine whether a dysfunction in CN III or VI (abducens) is the cause. Have the patient follow your finger to the left and right on the horizontal plane. Is the diplopia worse when the patient turns to the left or the right? The deficit is on the side where the diplopia is

T a b l e 7–7 • COMMON ABNORMAL OPTIC DISC FINDINGS

TYPE	DESCRIPTION	CAUSES
Papilledema (choked disc)	Margin of the disc is distorted and swollen; the disc has a reddish hue because of congestion	Increased intracranial pressure; pseudotumor cerebri
Optic atrophy	Paleness (the disc is light pink, white, or gray owing to decreased blood supply); visual acuity is decreased	Primary causes: tabes dorsalis and multiple sclerosis Secondary causes: neuritis or prolonged increased intracranial pressure
Retrobulbar neuritis	Inflammatory lesion of the posterior portion of the optic nerve; no swelling of disc	Hemorrhage, diabetes, or retinitis
Optic neuritis	Inflammation of the disc; associated with loss of vision secondary to a central scotoma	Inflammatory process
Cotton wool patches (seen during fundus examination)	Whitish or grayish oval lesions that look like cotton balls; smaller than disc	Hypertension

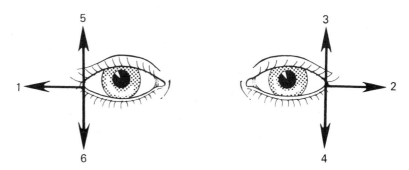

Figure 7–7 • Sequence of eye-testing movements. (*Note:* Numbers indicate the appropriate sequence of movement.)

worse. If the images are one on top of the other, the examiner needs to determine if a dysfunction in CN III or IV is the cause. Have the patient follow your finger up and down both on the inward (inner aspect of the eye) and outward (outer aspect of the eye) on the vertical plane. Is the diplopia worse when the patient looks up down? The deficit is in the direction that is worse. Note that trochlear involvement is uncommon.

Pontine and Frontal Gaze Centers. When considering abnormalities of eye movement, differentiate between pontine and frontal gaze palsy. Acute damage in the **frontal gaze center** causes the eyes to **deviate toward the side of the lesion** (away from an accompanying hemiplegia). The palsy is usually temporary and tends to resolve in minutes to hours. **Pontine gaze palsies** are usually bilateral and symmetrical. They cause eye **deviation away from the side of the lesion** and last much longer than frontal gaze palsies.

Internuclear ophthalmoplegia (INO) is due to a lesion of the medial longitudinal fasciculus resulting in impairment of adduction in the ipsilateral eye and nystagmus in the contralateral eye on gaze away from the side of involvement. The lesion lies between the nuclei of CN VI and opposite CN III. Convergence is intact, thus ruling out a lesion of CN III. There is no diplopia. The most common cause in the elderly is brainstem infarction and multiple sclerosis in younger people. Other causes include trauma and neoplasms. Occasionally INO is associated with metabolic disorders such as hepatic encepha-

lopathy and may be seen in myasthenia gravis. Table 7-8 summarizes other eye movement abnormalities.

Terms Related to Eye Movement

- **Conjugate gaze:** both eyes move in the same direction, at the same speed, and in constant alignment
- **Dysconjugate gaze:** lack of alignment between the two visual axes
- **Strabismus:** deviation of one's eye from its proper direction so that the visual axes of the two eyes cannot both be directed simultaneously on an object (lack of alignment of ocular axes)
- **Oculocephalic reflex** (doll's eye response) and the **oculovestibular reflex** (caloric stimulation) are used in the unconscious patient and provide information about the presence or absence of brainstem reflexes. Both are discussed later in this chapter.
- **Ophthalmoplegia:** paralysis of the eye muscles; Table 7-9 summarizes types of ophthalmoplegias
- **Diplopia:** double vision; seeing two separate images of the same object in visual space, with one of the images displaced from the other; the images can be side by side or one on top of the other; diplopia is usually preceded by blurring of vision.
- **Nystagmus:** a common, involuntary, rhythmic to-and-fro oscillation of the eyes that may be horizontal, vertical, rotary, or mixed in direction. The tempo of the movements can be regular, rhythmic, pendular, or jerky, with a noted fast and slow movement component. True nystag-

▌▌ Table 7–8 • EYE MOVEMENT ABNORMALITIES WITH POSTERIOR FOSSA LESIONS

ABNORMALITY	DESCRIPTION	CAUSE/LESION
Wall-eyed bilateral internuclear ophthalmoplegia (INO)	Bilateral outward eye deviation that occurs with bilateral INO	Pontine infarction or demyelination
"One-and-a-half" syndrome	Impairment of all horizontal conjugate eye movements, except for abduction of the contralateral eye	Parapontine reticular formation (PPRF)
Ocular bobbing	Episodic, intermittent, usually conjugate, downward, brisk eye movement followed by a return to the resting position by a "bobbing action"	Severe destructive lower pontine lesions, pontine hemorrhage, or infection
Skewed deviation	Misalignment of the eyes observed in the vertical plane that is not due to a lesion of the third or fourth cranial nerve. Vertical diplopia results	Pons, usually on side of the higher eye, but may be in the cerebellum
Parinaud's syndrome	Paralysis of conjugate upward gaze; also includes paresis of convergence, convergence-retraction nystagmus, pupillary hyporeactivity, and light-near dissociation	Midbrain tectal area; often caused by a pinealoma, a vascular lesion, or hydrocephalus

Table 7-9 • TYPES OF OPHTHALMOPLEGIAS

TYPE OF OPHTHALMOPLEGIA	DESCRIPTION
External	Paralysis of one or more of the extraocular muscles
Internal	Paralysis of one or more intraocular muscles
Nuclear	Paralysis caused by a lesion involving the nuclei of the motor nerves of the eye (cranial nerve III, IV, or VI)
Internuclear	Paralysis caused by injury or a lesion of the medial longitudinal fasciculus located within the brain stem
Supranuclear	Paralysis caused by injury or a lesion to the conjugate eye movement centers located in the frontal, frontal-parietal, and occipital lobes
Parinaud's syndrome or dorsal midbrain syndrome	A type of supranuclear ophthalmoplegia; conjugate upward gaze paralysis; caused by a lesion in the dorsal midbrain

mus is a pathologic condition caused by a lesion in the central or peripheral vestibular pathways or their cerebellar connections as well as toxic-metabolic disorders, weakness of gaze, and blindness (Table 7-10).

Other Findings

Trauma to the peripheral portion of the CN can result in nerve fiber degeneration, followed by unpredictable regeneration. Because of the proximity of other CNs to each other, the regenerating fibers from one nerve can be misdirected to a nearby cranial nerve, forming connections with adjacent nerves. Such an atypical regeneration is called a **misdirection syndrome**. Two are mentioned—the pseudo-Graefe lid sign and Gunn's syndrome. The **pseudo-Graefe syndrome** is an atypical connection between CNs III and IV. Any attempt to look downward is followed by upper eyelid retraction, medial rotation of the eye, and constriction of the pupil. **Gunn's syndrome** involves CNs III and V. As the mouth is opened and the jaw moves to one side, ptosis of the eyelid changes to lid retraction.

Examination of the Pupils

To assess the pupils, the patient should be directed to focus on a distant object located straight ahead. (With a comatose patient, the pupils are examined however they are found.) The pupils are examined for size, shape, and equality. The normal diameter of a pupil is 2 to 6 mm, with an average diameter of 3.5 mm. When the pupils are compared with each other, their diameters should be equal; however, about 12% to 17% of the normal population has discernibly unequal pupil size (**anisocoria**) in the absence of a pathological condition.

The shape of the pupils is also noted and compared. Normally, the pupils are round; however, in patients who have had cataract surgery, the pupils assume a keyhole shape. An ovoid pupil indicates pupillary dysfunction; it may be seen in early uncal herniation.

Sensitivity to light or **photophobia** may be noted when checking the pupils, or the patient may complain of this problem. The etiology is unclear, but the finding is associated with conditions such as meningitis.

Pupillary Reflexes

A few important reflexes relating to pupillary responses and eye movement can be tested.

Table 7-10 • COMMON TYPES OF NYSTAGMUS

TYPE OF NYSTAGMUS	DESCRIPTION	LOCATION OF LESION	COMMENT
Gaze-evoked nystagmus	With normal eye movement, there may be three or fewer beats at the extremes of eye position; fast phase in direction of gaze	—	Normal finding
Optokinetic nystagmus	Rapid, alternating motion of the eyes normally noted when eyes try to fixate on a moving target; presence indicates physiologic continuity of the optic pathways from the retina to the occipital cortex. Because it is involuntary, a positive response provides reliable verification of intact vision in a patient feigning blindness.	—	Normal finding
Retraction nystagmus	Irregular jerks of the eyes backward into the orbit, precipitated by upward gaze	Midbrain tegmentum	—
Convergence nystagmus	Slow, spontaneous, drifting, ocular divergence with a final quick, convergent jerk	Midbrain	—
See-saw nystagmus	Rapid, pendular, dysconjugate see-saw movement accompanied by deficits of visual fields and visual acuity	Proximal optic chiasm	—
Downbeat nystagmus	Irregular jerks precipitated by downward gaze	Lower medulla	—
Vestibular nystagmus	Mixed nystagmus that can be horizontal, rotational, or both, resulting from vestibular disease	Vestibular pathway	—
Toxic nystagmus	Multidirectional gaze-evoked nystagmus; most often drug induced with toxic levels of phenytoin (Dilantin), barbiturates, and bromides; can also result from cerebellar or central vestibular dysfunction	—	Usually due to drug toxicity

Direct Light Reflex

The sensory receptors for the light reflex are the rods and cones of the retina. Afferent impulses follow the normal visual pathway as far as the lateral geniculate bodies. Rather than entering the geniculate body, sensory impulses enter the pretectal area (near the superior colliculus). Connecting neurons synapse in the **Edinger-Westphal nucleus** (oculomotor nucleus) located in the midbrain. From here, the parasympathetic fibers proceed to the ciliary ganglion to the pupilloconstrictor fibers of the iris, causing the pupil to constrict. When the light is withdrawn, the pupil normally dilates because of sympathetic stimulation. A three-neuron chain begins in the posterior hypothalamus. The first neuron descends dorsally in the brainstem and cervical spinal cord to synapse in the **intermediolateral cells** at the C7 to C12 levels. The second neuron leaves the nervous system through the ventral spinal roots and ascends in the sympathetic chain and synapses in the superior cervical ganglion (at level of carotid bifurcation). The third neuron reaches the iris and Müller's muscles by ascending along the internal carotid artery, then traverses the cavernous sinus and the ciliary ganglion as the long ciliary nerves. The postganglionic sympathetic fibers synapse with the pupillodilator muscles, resulting in pupillary dilation.

The direct light reflex refers to the constriction and dilation of the pupil when a light is shone into that pupil and withdrawn (Fig. 7-8). Each pupil is tested individually and the results are compared. Response to light is recorded as:

- **Brisk:** very rapid constriction when light is introduced
- **Sluggish:** constriction occurs but more slowly than expected
- **Nonreactive or fixed:** no constriction or dilation is noted

Normally, pupillary constriction is brisk, although age may affect the briskness of reaction. Pupils in younger people tend to be larger and more responsive to light than those in older people. In addition to the constriction of the pupil that occurs with direct light stimulation (direct light response), there is a somewhat weaker constriction of the nonstimulated pupil. This is called the **consensual light reflex**, which occurs as a result of fibers crossing from each side that cross both the optic chiasm and the posterior commissure of the midbrain. See Table 7-11 for pupillary abnormalities.

Near-Point Reaction

In testing the near-point reaction, patients are asked to focus on the examiner's finger, which is positioned 2 to 3 feet directly ahead of them, and to follow it with their eyes as it is rapidly moved closer to their face. Three reflex responses normally occur:

- **Convergence:** the medial recti muscles contract, thus directing both eyes toward the midline. This occurs so that the image in each eye will remain focused on the fovea; without this reflex, diplopia would occur.
- **Accommodation:** to sharply focus the image on the fovea, the lenses thicken as a result of tension in the ciliary muscles; the ciliary muscles are innervated by the post-

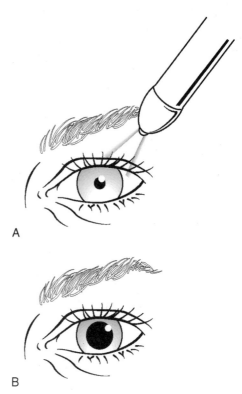

Figure 7–8 • Direct light reflex. (*A*) A bright light is introduced from the temporal area; the pupil normally rapidly constricts when exposed to the light. (*B*) The pupil rapidly dilates when the light is removed.

ganglionic parasympathetic neurons in the ciliary ganglion.
- **Pupillary constriction:** the pupils constrict as an optic adjustment to regulate depth of focus. (This pupillary constriction does not depend on light and is regulated separately from the light reflex.)

Trigeminal Nerve (Mixed) (CN V)

The trigeminal nerve is composed of both sensory and motor components. To assess the sensory component, the three sensory vectors of the face are tested (Fig. 7-9). The **ophthalmic division** innervates the frontal sinuses, the conjunctiva and cornea, the upper lid, the bridge of the nose, the forehead, and the scalp as far as the vertex of the skull. The **maxillary division** innervates the cheek, the maxillary sinus, the lateral aspects of the nose, the upper teeth, the nasal pharynx, the hard palate, and the uvula. The **mandibular division** innervates the chin, the lower jaw, the anterior two thirds of the tongue, the gums and floor of the mouth, and the buccal mucosa of the cheek.

With the patient's eyes closed, ability to appreciate **light touch** is tested by touching the forehead, cheek, and jaw with a wisp of cotton. The patient is instructed to respond every time the skin is touched. **Pain perception** is evaluated with the "picky" (broken) and dull ends of a wooden applicator or by the pinprick method. After demonstrating the difference between sharp and dull, the skin is touched with the sharp end and occasionally with the dull end. The patient is asked to

Table 7-11 • PUPILLARY ABNORMALITIES CLASSIFIED BY AFFERENT AND EFFERENT PUPILLARY DEFECTS

DEFECTS	DESCRIPTION	CAUSE/COMMENT
Afferent defects		
Amaurotic pupil (blind eye) 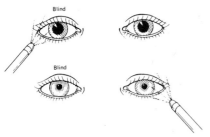	Blindness in one eye results in loss of the sensory limb of the light reflex. If oculomotor nerve (the motor limb) of reflex remains intact, a light directed into the **intact eye** produces normal direct and consensual reactions. In the **blind eye,** you will find • No direct light response • No consensual response • A direct light response in the intact eye • A consensual response in the blind eye (from light shone into the intact eye) • A near pupillary response in both eyes	Disease of the retina or optic nerve
Marcus-Gunn pupil (swinging flashlight sign) 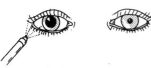	Use a bright light. There is a normal bilateral light response (constriction) when the light is shone into the intact eye, but pupillary dilation occurs when the flashlight is quickly switched to the diseased eye.	Lesions/atrophy of the retina or optic nerve
Argyll-Robertson pupil	Pupils are small and irregularly shaped; react to accommodation but not to direct light.	Seen with neurosyphilis (tabes dorsalis).
Efferent defect: large pupil		
Adie pupil (tonic pupil)	Unilateral dilated pupil that reacts slowly to light after prolonged stimulation; it accommodates slowly. The pupil also dilates slowly in darkness Often associated with diminished knee and ankle reflexes Usually women 20 to 30 years old who are affected Diagnosed by inserting 2.5% methacholine or 0.1% pilocarpine into both eyes; the affected pupil promptly contracts, but the normal pupil does not	Postganglionic denervation of the parasympathetic pupillary innervation Cause unknown, although noted to occur following a viral infection
Mydriatic pupils (large pupils)	Enlarged pupils that result from use of certain drugs, listed in next column; unilateral large pupil in accidental topical ocular application of anticholinergic agents Large pupil can result from direct trauma	Hallucinogens, antihistamines, glutethiamide, anticholinergics, and dopamine Trauma can damage nerve endings of iris sphincter muscle
Efferent defect: small pupil		
Horner's syndrome	Unilateral, small pupil; both pupils react to direct light and accommodation; with a miotic pupil, there is ptosis of the eyelid, and usually loss of sweating on the affected side.	Lesion of descending sympathetic fibers in ipsilateral brainstem or upper cord, or the ascending sympathetic fibers in neck or head; results in unilateral interruption or complete loss of sympathetic innervation to the pupil
Miotic pupils (small pupils)	Small pupils that result from use of certain drugs, listed in next column Also seen in pontine hemorrhage or pontine infarct Direct orbital injury to the eye with destruction of the sympathetic innervation and interruption of the inhibitory pathways to the oculomotor nuclei (Edinger-Westphal nucleus) Miosis following trauma usually results from intraocular inflammation	Miotic drugs (acetylcholine chloride, carbachol, demecarium bromide, echothiophate iodide, isoflurophate, physostigmine, pilocarpine, and others); and narcotics

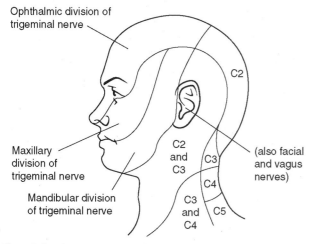

Figure 7–9 • Sensory vectors of the face and neck. Note the three vectors of the trigeminal nerve (CNV): ophthalmic, maxillary, and mandibular divisions.

respond "sharp" or "dull." Accuracy of response and a comparison between findings on each side of the face is made.

Next, the motor component (i.e., the muscles of mastication) is evaluated. The strength of the masseter and temporal muscles is evaluated by palpating them when the jaw is clenched and opened. Differences in muscle tone or atrophy should be noted.

Facial Nerve (Mixed) (CN VII)

The facial nerve has both sensory and motor components. The sensory component includes the sense of taste on the anterior two thirds of the tongue. Testing of this function is often deferred. However, if tested, each side of the protruded tongue is tested separately. There are four basic modalities of taste: sweet (tip of tongue), sour (sides of tongue), salty (over most of tongue but concentrated on the sides), and bitter (back of tongue, controlled by CN IX). The patient is asked to identify the taste of sugar placed on the tip of the tongue, after which a sip of water is given. The same procedure is used with sour and salty substances. If bitter is tested on the posterior third of the tongue, it should be recognized that it is innervated by the glossopharyngeal nerve. Sensation to the external ear is also supplied by the facial nerve.

The motor component is tested by observing the symmetry of the face at rest and during deliberate facial movements, such as smiling, showing the teeth, whistling, pursing the lips, blowing air into the cheeks, wrinkling the nose and forehead, and raising the eyebrows. Note the nasolabial folds for symmetry. In addition, ask the patient to close the eyes tightly. The examiner should not be able to open the patient's eyes. The facial nerve also controls tearing and salivation.

When weakness is noted, it is important to observe whether the entire side of the face or just the lower face (below the eyes) is affected.

There are two types of facial weakness (Fig. 7-10). If the lower portion of one side of the face is involved, the lesion is said to be caused by a central (involves the central nervous system) problem, an **upper motor neuron lesion** (as seen in association with stroke). This involves the corticobulbar tracts, resulting in contralateral weakness of the *lower face*

with normal function of the upper face. Wrinkling of the forehead is left intact because of bilateral innervation of the upper face from the corticobulbar fibers. The lower face, by contrast, has only unilateral contralateral cortical innervation so that retraction of the corner of the mouth to smile is compromised. The second type of facial weakness involves the *total side face* with ipsilateral facial muscle involvement. The lesion is said to be peripheral (involves the peripheral nervous system) or a **lower motor neuron lesion.** Specifically, the condition is called **Bell's palsy**.

In addition to muscle weakness, note any evidence of spasms, atrophy, or tremors of the facial muscles.

Acoustic Nerve (Sensory) (CN VIII)

The acoustic nerve is a pure sensory nerve and is divided into two branches, the **cochlear nerve** for hearing and the **vestibular nerve**, which contributes to equilibrium, coordination, and orientation in space.

Hearing is evaluated in several ways. Much information can be collected in observing the patient. Ability to understand soft and loud tones and low and high pitches is noted. Signs of hearing deficit include inability to hear high or low tones, turning the head toward the speaker when listening, or lip reading. Certain sounds are heard more loudly and at a greater distance. For example, *a*, *e*, and *i* are heard at a greater distance than consonants such as *l*, *m*, and *r* and vowels such as *o* and *u*. "Seventy-six" and "sixty-seven" can be heard at a greater distance than "ninety-nine." To test **hearing**, direct the patient to cover one ear. Standing on the opposite side, 1 to 2 feet away from the ear, whisper a few numbers or a word. An alternative is to rub your fingers

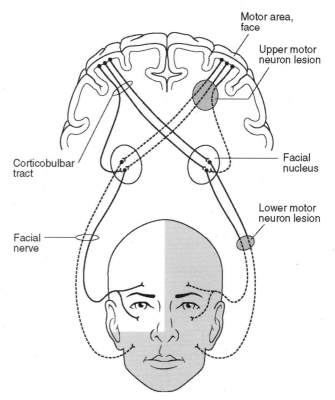

Figure 7–10 • Innervation to the face by the facial nerve.

together. The patient should be able to hear it. Test the other ear. Hearing should be equal in both ears.

Next, check for **lateralization** and **air** and **bone conduction**. **Weber's test** is used to evaluate lateralization, whereas **Rinne's test** evaluates air and bone conduction. Both tests require the use of a 512-Hz tuning fork (Fig. 7-11). For **Weber's test**, place a lightly vibrating tuning fork firmly vertex of the patient's head or in the middle of the forehead. Inquire whether the patient hears the vibration more on the left side, the right side, or in the middle. Normally, the sound is heard in the middle or equally in both ears. If one ear is occluded, the vibration is heard better or more loudly in the occluded ear.

In **Rinne's test**, air conduction and bone conduction are compared. Place the base of a lightly vibrating tuning fork firmly on the mastoid process. Ask the patient to inform you when the vibration is no longer heard. Quickly place the vibrating fork near the ear canal with the vibrating portion toward the ear. Ask the patient to inform you when it can no longer be heard. Normally, the sound should be heard longer through air than through bone (AC greater than BC). In evaluating hearing acuity, it is important to differentiate between **conduction loss** and **sensorineural loss**. The findings for unilateral loss for each are as follows:

TYPE OF DEAFNESS	RINNE	WEBER
Conduction deafness	BC > AC	Lateralizes **to** deafer ear
Sensorineural deafness	AC > BC	Lateralizes **away from** deafer ear

Abnormal findings from either test warrant further investigation with more sensitive testing.

In considering the vestibular nerve, certain tests of vestibular function are closely related to the examination of other portions of the nervous system (i.e. motor system and cerebellar testing). However, all patients with a major complaint of vertigo should receive a **Dix-Hallpike positional test**. It consists of seating the patient on the edge of an examining table and moving him backward rapidly so that the head is hanging backward while the eyes remain open. If no nystagmus or vertigo develops in 20 seconds, the patient is returned to the sitting position. The head is repositioned to the right, and the downward procedure repeated. If no nystagmus or vertigo develops in 20 seconds, return patient to the sitting position. Reposition the head to the left and repeat the procedure (Fig. 7-12). Note the onset, duration, and direction of the nystagmus. In benign paroxysmal positional vertigo (BPPV) nystagmus is noted when the head is turned to either side. The nystagmus beats upward and also has a rotatory component so that the top part of the eye beats toward the down ear. The characteristics of the nystagmus are a latency of 2 to 5 seconds, a duration of 5 to 60 seconds, and it is followed by a downbeating nystagmus when the patient is placed upright in the sitting position.[7] Further evaluation will be required with persistent vertigo.

Glossopharyngeal (CN IX) and Vagus (CN X) Nerves (Both Mixed)

The glossopharyngeal and vagus nerves are tested together because their intimate association of function in the pharynx.

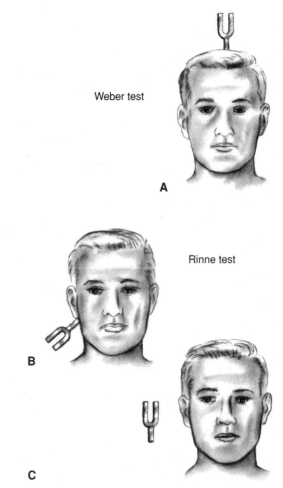

Figure 7–11 • Weber test and Rinne test. Note the placement of a vibrating tuning fork (512 Hz) for each test. (*A*) Weber test for lateralization. Place the vibrating fork firmly on the top of the head or on the middle of the forehead. Normally the sound is perceived midline. Rinne test for comparing bone and air conduction: Place the base of the vibrating tuning fork on the mastoid process until the patient can no longer hear it (*B*); then, quickly place the fork near the external auditory canal, with one side toward the ear (*C*). Normally, the sound can be heard longer through air than through bone (AC > BC).

The glossopharyngeal nerve supplies sensory components to the pharynx, tonsils, soft palate, tympanic membrane, posterior third of the tongue, and secretory fibers of the parotid gland. It also supplies motor fibers to the stylopharyngeal muscle of the pharynx, whose role is to elevate the pharynx. The patient is asked to open the mouth and say "ah." Upward movement of the soft palate and uvula should be noted. The vagus nerve provides parasympathetic fibers to the viscera of the chest and abdomen. Sensory fibers innervate the external ear canal, pharynx, larynx, and viscera of the chest and abdomen. The vagus also provides motor control to the soft palate, larynx, and pharynx.

The soft palate is examined with the patient's mouth open. Normally, when the patient says "ah," the palate elevates and the uvula remains midline. Check to see whether the uvula deviates to one side or the other (Fig. 7-13). The gag reflex is innervated by CNs IX and X. After warning the patient that you are going to check the gag reflex, touch the posterior pharyngeal wall with a tongue blade or applicator first on the left side and next on the right side. A gag response should be stimulated on each side.

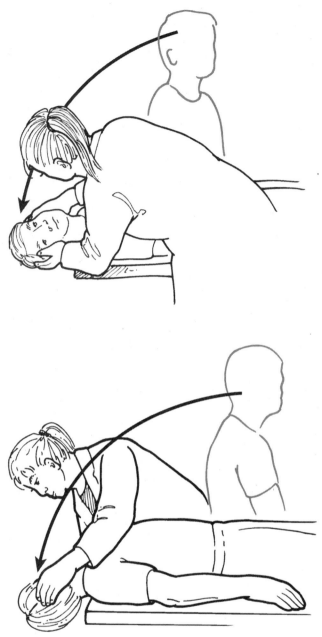

against resistance provided by the examiner's hands. Second, the patient is asked to turn his or her head to one side and push the chin against the examiner's hand, thereby allowing the sternocleidomastoid muscle to be palpated and its strength evaluated. The same procedure is then repeated on the other side. The symmetry of the trapezius and sternocleidomastoid muscles is noted, along with any muscle wasting or spasm.

Hypoglossal Nerve (Motor) (CN XII)

The patient is asked to open his or her mouth. The tongue is first inspected as it lies on the floor of the oral cavity. Note any atrophy or fasciculation of the tongue. Ask the patient to

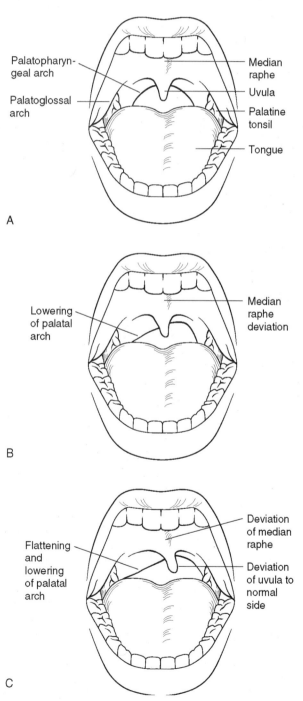

Figure 7–12 • Dix-Hallpike positional test. To precipitate the characteristic nystagmus of benign paroxysmal positional vertigo (BPPV), the patient is rapidly brought into a head position that makes the posterior canal vertical and also brings it through a large angular displacement.

Voice quality is evaluated by listening to the patient speak and noting hoarseness; a soft, whispery voice; or no voice. Difficulty in speaking, such as hoarseness or speaking in a whisper, is termed **dysphonia**. Both are due to paralysis of the soft palate (**palatal paralysis**) and can result in nasal-sounding speech. **Dysarthria** refers to defective articulation that may be caused by a motor deficit of the tongue or speech muscles. Slurred speech should be noted, as should difficulty in pronouncing the letters *m, b, p, t,* and *d* and the number *1.*

Spinal Accessory Nerve (Motor) (CN XI)

The accessory nerve, as it is sometimes called, is tested in two segments. First, the trapezius muscle is palpated and its strength evaluated while the patient shrugs the shoulders

Figure 7–13 • Observing the palate. (*A*) Normal palate with mouth open and at rest. (*B*) Right unilateral vagus paralysis with mouth at rest. (*C*) Right unilateral vagus paralysis when saying "ah."

protrude the tongue. Note asymmetry, atrophy, or deviation from midline. Next, direct the patient to move the tongue from side to side. Note the symmetry of movement. Finally, ask the patient to push the tongue against the inside of each cheek as the examiner palpates externally on the cheek for strength and equality.

A common cause of dysfunction is found in patients who have had a carotid endarterectomy. Surgery under the angle of the jaw can result in stretching or injury to the hypoglossal nerve. On examination, weakness is noted toward the side of the surgery. If the nerve has been stretched, recovery is expected. If the nerve has been cut, no recovery is expected and atrophy of one side of the tongue will occur.[8]

MOTOR SYSTEM EXAMINATION

The motor examination comes next and proceeds from the neck, to the upper limbs, to the trunk and, finally, to the lower extremities. Limb evaluation proceeds from proximal to distal. It is impractical to test all muscles, but major groups are assessed; a more detailed examination can be conducted if deficits are noted in a particular area. The symmetry of each muscle or muscle group is noted. Evaluation muscle size, muscle tone, and muscle strength. Finally, evaluate gait and posture. Throughout the examination, note any involuntary movements.

Muscle Size

Inspect symmetric muscles for both size and contour. When in doubt, a tape measure can be used to measure a muscle and compare it with the same muscle on the opposite side of the body. Measurements must be taken from the same reference point for accuracy. Note muscle wasting, atrophy, or hypertrophy.

Muscle Tone

Tone is the normal state of muscle tension. The muscle is palpated while at rest and during passive stretching. With the patient relaxed, the joints are put through the normal range of motion (e.g., flexion and extension) by the examiner. The systematic evaluation proceeds from the shoulder, elbow, wrist, and fingers in the upper extremities and from the hip, knee, and ankle in the lower extremities. Findings from the left side and the right side are then compared. Abnormalities in muscle tone include spasticity, rigidity, and flaccidity.

Spasticity refers to increased motor tone (**hypertonia**). Tone is greater with rapid passive movement, and less pronounced when the rate is slower. In addition, tone is often greater at the extremes of range of motion. Spasticity results from injury to the upper motor neuron of the corticospinal tract at any point from the cortex to the spinal cord. **Clasp-knife spasticity** is increased tone with a sudden release at the end of extension.

Rigidity is a state of increased resistance that persists throughout the movement. It is due to a lesion in the basal ganglia system. **Cogwheel rigidity** is a series of ratchet-like, small, regular jerks that are felt on passive flexion or exten-

sion. **Lead-pipe rigidity** is resistance that persists throughout extension and flexion.

Flaccidity refers to decrease or loss of muscle tone (**hypotonia**). It is due to a lower motor neuron lesion at any point from the anterior horn cell to the peripheral nerves. The muscle is weak, soft, and floppy.

Muscle Strength

Muscle strength is evaluated by asking the patient to move a muscle actively against gravity and then with resistance provided by the examiner. Muscle strength can be rated using a scale of 0 (no muscle contraction detected) to 5 (active movement against full resistance). Muscle strength is recorded together with the maximum grade achievable on the scale (e.g., 4 out of 5 with 5 being the maximum achievable grade). Compare the functional level of each muscle and compare it to the functional level on the opposite side. See Table 7-12 for grading system. (*Note:* Sometimes an examiner will use a plus [+] or a minus [−] in the "4" category to indicate how strong the patient's muscle strength was against the examiner's resistance. A "4+" indicates that a large amount of resistance by the examiner was necessary for the patient's muscle to be finally overcome.)

Note that the pattern of muscle extremity evaluation includes both proximal and distal muscle groups. When considering patterns of dysfunction, differentiating between proximal and distal deficits is important. Symmetric weakness of the **proximal muscles** suggests **myopathy**, a muscle disorder. By contrast, symmetric weakness of **distal muscles** suggests **polyneuropathy**, a peripheral nerve disorder. Note also that weakness on the same side as a lesion or on both sides simultaneously suggests a spinal cord lesion. Weakness on one side, however, suggests a lesion in the brain on the side opposite to the weakness.

UPPER EXTREMITIES

Table 7-13 summarizes the major muscles, innervating peripheral nerve, and motor action evaluated in the upper extremities. Table 7-14 summarizes the order and method of evaluation of the upper extremity muscles (Fig. 7-14). In evaluating

Table 7-12 • GRADING OF MUSCLE STRENGTH

GRADE	STRENGTH
5	Active movement against gravity and full resistance; normal muscle strength
4	Active movement against gravity and some resistance; the examiner can overcome the muscle resistance
3	Active movement against gravity
2	Active movement of the body part when gravity is eliminated
1	A very weak muscle contraction is palpated; only a trace of a contraction is evident, but no active movement of the body part is noted
0	No muscle contraction is detectable

▌▌▌ **Table 7–13** • SUMMARY OF MAJOR MUSCLES, PERIPHERAL NERVE INNERVATION, AND MUSCLE ACTION OF THE UPPER EXTREMITIES

SPINAL LEVEL	MUSCLE	PERIPHERAL NERVE INNERVATION	ACTION
C5, C6, C7	Serratus anterior	Long thoracic	Movement of shoulder
C5, C6	Deltoid and supraspinatus	Suprascapular and axillary	Abduction of shoulder
C5, C6	Biceps brachii	Musculocutaneous	Flexion of elbow
C5, **C6**	Brachioradialis	Radial	Flexion of elbow
C7, C8	Triceps brachii	Radial	Extension of elbow
C6, **C7**	Extensor carpi radialis longus (C6) and extensor carpi ulnaris (C7)	Radial	Extension of wrist
C7, C8	Flexor carpi radialis (C7) and flexor carpi ulnaris (C8)	Medial and ulnar	Flexion of wrist
C7	Extensor digitorum communis, extensor indicis proprius, and extensor digiti minimi (all C7)	Radial	Extension of fingers
C8, T1	Flexor digitorum superficialis (C8), flexor digitorum profundus (C8), and lumbricals (C8, T1)	Median and ulnar	Flexion of fingers
T1	Dorsal interossei (T1) and abductor digiti quinti (5th finger)	Ulnar	Abduction of fingers
C8, **T1**	Palmar interossei	Ulnar	Adduction of fingers
C8, **T1**	Opponens pollicis	Median	Opposition of thumb

Bold type indicates primary innervation.

▌▌▌ **Table 7–14** • SUMMARY OF EVALUATION OF UPPER EXTREMITIES MOTOR FUNCTION

FUNCTION BEING EVALUATED	LETTER IN FIG. 7-14	DIRECTIONS TO PATIENT	EXAMINER AND OBSERVATIONS
Shoulder movement C5, C6, C7	A	"Extend your arms parallel to the floor and push with your palms against the wall" (Fig. A-1). (*Alternately, you can ask the patient to push against your hands.*)	Observe the scapula for increased prominence of the scapular tip (**winging**). Normally, each scapula is close to the thorax. Winging suggests serratus anterior muscle weakness (Fig. A-2)
Adduction of shoulder C5, C6	B	"Flex your elbow slightly and move your upper arm away from your body." (*Alternately, ask the patient to position his arms like "chicken wings."*)	Try to push the abducted upper arms down against resistance
Flexion of elbow **C5**, C6	C	"Flex your elbow and make a muscle with your palm parallel to the shoulder."	Try to pull the flexed forearm open
Flexion of elbow C5, **C6**	D	"Flex your elbow and make a muscle while your palm is pointed at midline" (midsaggital line)	Try to pull the flexed forearm open
Extension of elbow C7, C8	E	"Push me away with that same arm."	Provide resistance thus trying to prevent extension
Pronator drift	F	(*May examine patient when he or she is standing or sitting.*) "Outstretch both arms in front of you parallel to the floor with hands open and palms up." (*The elbows should be fully extended, the wrists extended also.*) "Now close your eyes (*and stay that way for 20 or 30 seconds*)."	Observe for slow pronation of the wrist, slight flexion of the elbow and fingers, and a downward and lateral drift of the hand; called *pronator drift*. Suggests *mild hemiparesis* and may be noted before any significant weakness noted
Extension of wrist **C6**, C7	G	"Extend your wrist and don't let me straighten it."	The examiner attempts to straighten the wrist. If straightened, it suggests wrist-drop
Flexion of wrist **C7**, C8	H	"Flex your wrist and don't let me straighten it."	The examiner attempts to straighten the wrist
Extension of fingers C7	I	"Put your fingers straight out and don't let me push them down."	Try to push the fingers down
Flexion of fingers **C8**, T1	J	"Flex your fingers and don't let me straighten them."	Try to straighten the fingers
Abduction of fingers (**T1**)	K	"Put your hand on the table and spread your fingers. Try to resist my attempt to bring the fingers together."	Try to push the fingers together
Adduction of fingers (C8, **T1**)	L	"Put your hand on the table with the fingers slightly spread. Try to resist my attempt to pull your fingers outward."	Try to pull the fingers outward
Opposition of thumb C8, T1	M	(*The thumbnail should be parallel to the palm.*) "Touch the tip of your little finger with your thumb."	Try to pull the thumb away from the little finger with your index finger or thumb

Bold type indicates primary innervation.

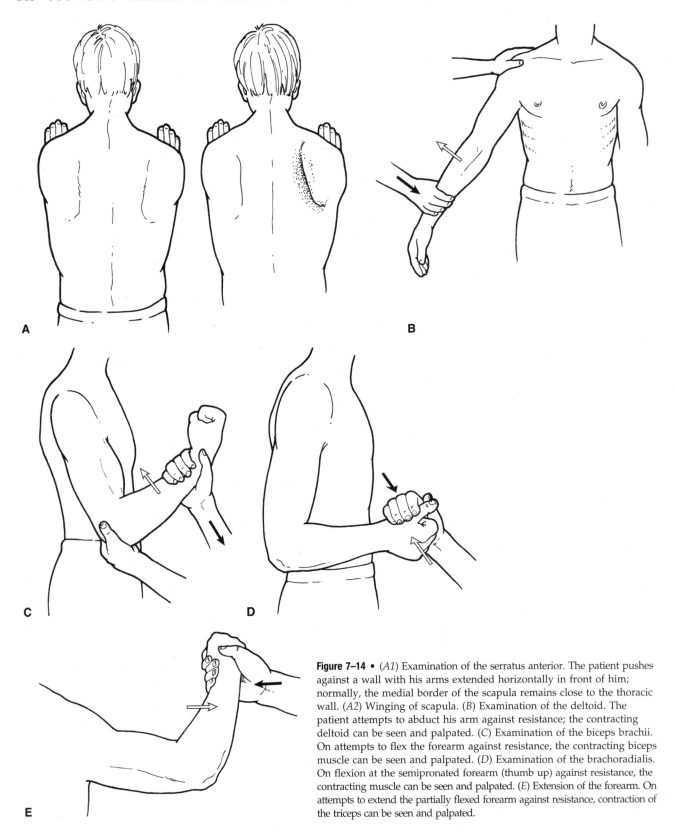

Figure 7–14 • (*A1*) Examination of the serratus anterior. The patient pushes against a wall with his arms extended horizontally in front of him; normally, the medial border of the scapula remains close to the thoracic wall. (*A2*) Winging of scapula. (*B*) Examination of the deltoid. The patient attempts to abduct his arm against resistance; the contracting deltoid can be seen and palpated. (*C*) Examination of the biceps brachii. On attempts to flex the forearm against resistance, the contracting biceps muscle can be seen and palpated. (*D*) Examination of the brachoradialis. On flexion at the semipronated forearm (thumb up) against resistance, the contracting muscle can be seen and palpated. (*E*) Extension of the forearm. On attempts to extend the partially flexed forearm against resistance, contraction of the triceps can be seen and palpated.

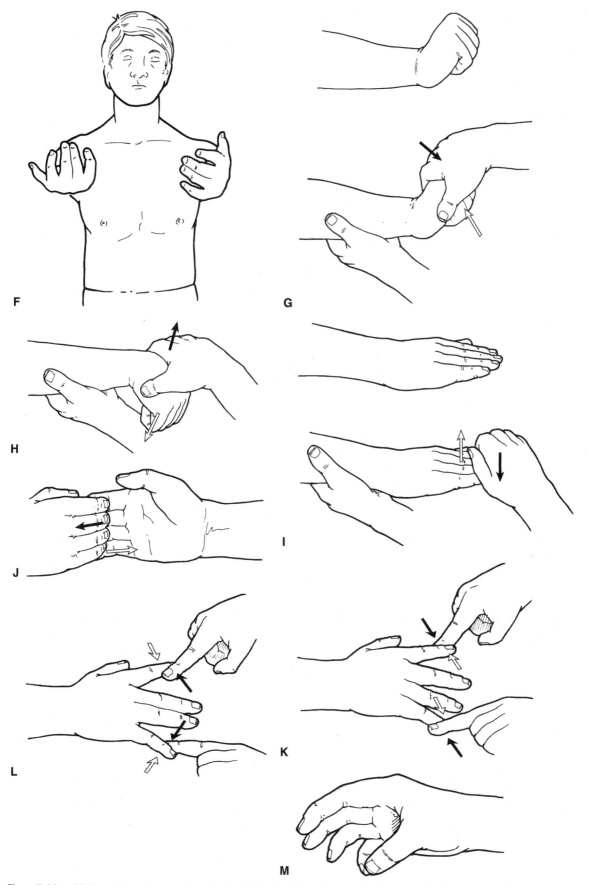

Figure 7–14 • (*F*) Pronation drift-drift in patient with left hemiparesis. (*G*) Examination of wrist extension. On attempts to extend the hand at the wrist against resistance, the bellies of the extensors carpi radialis longus, carpi ulnaris, and digitorum communis can be seen and palpated. (*H*) Examination of the wrist flexors. (*I*) Examination for finger extension. (*J*) Examination of the flexor digitorum profundus. The patient resists attempts to extend the distal phalanges while the middle phalanges are fixed. (*K*) Examination of the abduction of the fingers. The patient resists the examiner's attempt to bring the fingers together. (*L*) Adduction of the fingers. The patient attempts to adduct the fingers against resistance. (*M*) Opposition of the thumb and little finger.

Table 7–15 • SUMMARY OF MAJOR MUSCLES, PERIPHERAL NERVE INNERVATION, AND MUSCLE ACTION OF THE LOWER EXTREMITIES

SPINAL LEVEL	MUSCLE(S)	PERIPHERAL NERVE INNERVATION	MUSCLE ACTION
T12, **L1, L2**, L3	Iliopsoas	Branches from T12, L1, L2, L3	Hip flexion
L2, L3, L4	Adductor brevis, adductor longus, and adductor magnus	Obturator	Hip adduction
L4, **L5**, S1	Gluteus medius	Superior gluteal	Hip abductors
L5, S1, S2	Gluteus maximus	Inferior gluteal	Hip extension
L2, L3, L4	Quadriceps	Femoral	Knee extension
L5, **S1**, S2	Hamstrings	Sciatic	Knee flexion
L4, **L5**	Tibialis anterior, peroneus tertius, extensor digitorum longus, extensor hallucis longus	Deep peroneal	Ankle dorsiflexion
S1, S2	Gastrocnemius and soleus	Tibial	Ankle plantarflexion
L4, L5	Tibialis posterior	Tibial	Foot inversion
L5, **S1**	Peroneus longus and brevis	Superficial peroneal	Foot eversion

Bold type indicates primary innervation.

function, make your directions to the patient clear and succinct. Demonstrate movements and cue as necessary.

LOWER EXTREMITIES

In examining the lower extremities, proceed from the hip to the feet. By positioning the hands appropriately, the examiner provides resistance to movement. Table 7-15 summarizes the major muscles, innervating peripheral nerve, and motor action evaluated in the lower extremities. Table 7-16 summarizes the order and method of evaluating the lower extremity muscles (Fig. 7-15). Make your directions clear and succinct. Demonstrate movements as necessary.

Gait and Posture

Gait is evaluated with the motor examination or at the end of the cerebellar examination. **Gait** is the manner of walking, and **posture** is the position or orientation of the body in space. Any patient able to ambulate, even with assistive devices (cane, walker), should be observed walking, preferably without shoes or stockings. The examiner should be prepared to protect the patient from falls and injury. Observe the patient walking back and forth naturally in the room. The points to note include gait (e.g., smooth or staggering); position of feet (e.g., broad based or normal); symmetry of arm and leg movement (do arms swing naturally?); presence of any uncoordinated movements or tremors; height of step (i.e., shuffling, high, normal); and length of step (i.e., short, long, normal). Note how easily the patient can turn around and how many steps are required to turn. Next, have the patient walk heel to toe (called **tandem walking**), walk on the toes only, and walk on the heels only. An alternative is to ask the patient to hop on one foot and then the other. Chart 7-2 and Table 7-17 list the most common gait disturbances seen with neurological conditions.

Involuntary Movements

Any involuntary movements should be noted. In observing for involuntary movement, consideration is given to rate (cycles per second), distribution (proximal muscles, distal muscles), and relationship to movement (increasing or decreasing with movement). Common abnormalities of movement include tremors, choreiform movements, clonus, myoclonus, athetosis, tics, spasms, and ballism. Table 7-18 summarizes involuntary movements.

SENSORY SYSTEM EXAMINATION

In evaluating the sensory system, the examiner determines the patient's ability to perceive various types of sensations with the **eyes closed**. Each side of the body is compared with the other, as are sensory perceptions at the distal and proximal portions of all extremities. The testing proceeds in an orderly fashion. The body areas commonly evaluated include the face, neck, deltoid regions, forearm, hands (top side), chest, abdomen, thighs, lower legs, and feet (top surface) hands. Compare the left and right sides of the body. The perianal area is assessed only in special circumstances, such as when a sacral injury is suspected. Sensory function is rated according to the following scale:

2: normal
1: present, but diminished (abnormal)
0: absent

A detailed sensory examination is part of the **extended examination** and is undertaken when numbness, pain, trophic changes, or other sensory abnormalities are present. The three main sensory pathways entering the spinal cord are:

• Pain-temperature (anterior and lateral spinothalamic tracts)
• Position and vibration (posterior columns)
• Light touch (involves the anterior and lateral spinothalamic tracts and posterior columns)

Discrimination sensations involve some of the above sensory tracts; it also involves the cerebral cortex, especially the parietal lobe.

The following list shows the sensory modalities with testing methods (Table 7-19). A map of dermatomes (see Chap-

Table 7-16 • SUMMARY OF LOWER EXTREMITY MOTOR EVALUATION

FUNCTION BEING EVALUATED*	LETTER: OF FIG. 7-15	DIRECTIONS TO THE PATIENT	OBSERVED RESPONSE
Hip flexion (iliopsoas) **L1, L2**, L3	A-1 and A-2	(*Position the patient supine*) "Flex your thigh against the resistance provided" (Fig A-1).	*Alternate method:* Have patient sit on the edge of the examining table with legs dangling. Stabilize the pelvis by placing your hand over the iliac crest and the other hand over the distal femoral portion of the knee; apply resistance as the patient attempts to raise knee off the table (Fig. A-2).
Hip adductors **L2**, **L3**, L4	B	"Lie on your back: Extend your legs; now separate them about 6 inches" (*The examiner places both hands firmly between both knees.*) "Try to bring your knees together"	Provide resistance against the inward movement. Determine how much resistance that the patient can overcome
Hip abductors, gluteus medius and minimus L4, **L5**, S1	C	(*The examiner places both hands on the lateral thighs just above the patient's knees.*) "Spread both legs against my hands"	After the legs are abducted, provide resistance and try to push the legs together. Determine how much resistance that the patient can overcome
Hip extension Gluteus maximus **L5, S1**, S2	D	(*One examiner's hand is positioned on the posterior thigh and the other on top; feel for a muscle contraction on the posterior thigh.*) "Push your leg down against the bed"	*Alternate method:* Ask the patient to stand from a sitting position without using the arms.
Knee extension (Quadriceps) L2, **L3, L4**	E-1 and E-2	(*With the patient prone, the examiner supports the partially flexed knee and places his or her other hand on the top of the lower leg about 4 inches above the ankle and provides resistance against extension*) (Fig. E-1.) "Straighten your lower leg"	Stabilize the thigh by placing one hand just above the knee. Place the other hand just above the ankle and provide resistance. Palpate the quadriceps for a contraction with the stabilizing hand. *Alternate method:* Sitting on the side of the examining table: direct the patient to extend the knee (Fig. E-2).
Knee flexion (hamstrings) L5, **S1**, S2	F-1 and F-2	(*The examiner grasps the partially flexed knee about 4 inches above the ankle and stabilizes the hip with the other hand; provides resistance against flexion.*) "Flex your knee"	*Alternate methods:* Have patient sit on the edge of the examining table with legs dangling. Ask patient to bend the knee and keep it bent while you provide resistance (Fig. F-2) *or* ask patient to squat in a deep knee bend (should be able to flex both knees symmetrically)
Dorsiflexion of ankle (tibialis anterior) L4, **L5**	G	(*The examiner positions the ankle in neutral position and then places the other hand on the top of the foot near the fifth metatarsal.*) "Pull your toes toward your nose"	Anchor the ankle by stabilizing the heel; with your flattened fingers on the top of the foot, provide resistance to dorsiflexion. *Alternative method:* ask patient to walk on heels
Plantar flexion of ankle (gastrocnemius) **S1**, S2	H	(*The examiner positions the ankle in neutral position and then places the other hand on the ball of the foot near the fifth metatarsal.*) "Press down like on the gas pedal"	Anchor the ankle by stabilizing the heel; with your palm on the bottom of the foot, provide resistance to plantar flexion. *Alternative method:* ask the patient to walk on toes.
Foot inversion L4, L5	I	(*Position your thumb to dorsiflex and invert the foot.*) "Try to move your foot outward and down"	Try to force the foot into plantar flexion and eversion by pushing against the head and shaft of the first metatarsal; the tendon of the tibialis posterior can be seen and palpated behind the medial malleolus
Foot eversion S1	J	(*Secure ankle by stabilizing the heel and place your other hand that forces plantar flexion and eversion. Provide resistance to the eversion by pushing on the fifth metatarsal with the palm.*) "Turn your foot outward"	*Alternative method:* ask patient to walk on the medial borders of feet.

Bold type indicates primary innervation.

ter 5) should be used to guide the examination or to focus a detailed examination of a particular area. Light touch, pain, and vibration are the modalities tested.

Superficial Sensation

• Light touch: A wisp of cotton is used to lightly touch various areas of the skin.

• Pain: A broken wooden applicator that is "picky" at one end or other "picky" instrument is used to stimulate the skin. A pin-wheel, or a disposable prepacked pin, that can be disposed of safely after use, may be used (never use a needle or anything that will break the skin). To prevent transmission of blood-borne diseases, the instrument for testing should never be used on another patient. The skin is touched arbitrarily with the sharp or dull side. The smooth bottom of the applicator is used

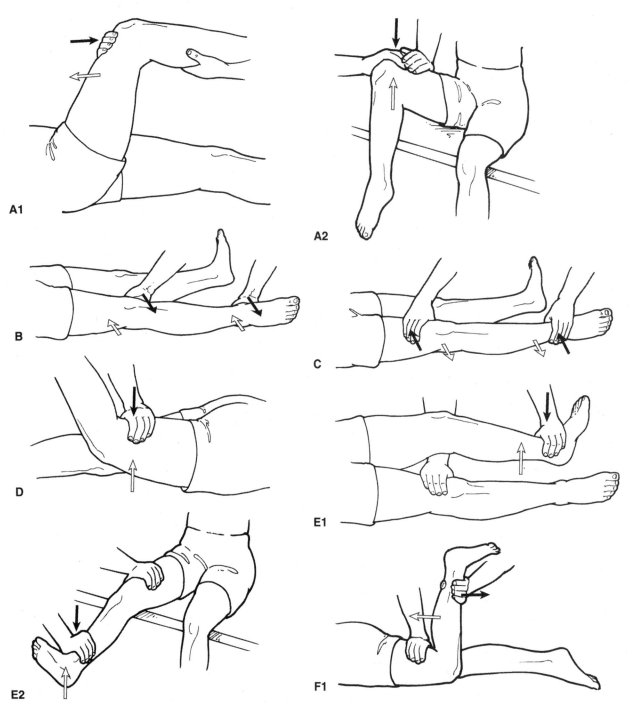

Figure 7–15 • (*A1*) Examination of the flexors of the thigh. The patent attempts to flex the thigh against resistance; the knee is flexed and the leg rests on the examiner's arm. (*A2*) Examination of hip flexion. (*B*) Examination of adduction of the thigh at the hip. The recumbent patient attempts to adduct the extended leg against resistance; contraction of the adductor muscles can be seen and palpated. (*C*) Abduction of the thigh at the hip. The recumbent patient attempts to move the extended leg outward against resistance; contraction of the gluteus medius and tensor fasciae latae can be palpated. (*D*) Examination of the extensors of the thigh at the hip. The patient, lying prone with the leg flexed at the knee, attempts to extend the thigh against resistance; contraction of the gluteus maximus and other extensors can be seen and palpated. (*E1*) Examination of extension of the leg at the knee. The supine patient attempts to extend the leg at the knee against resistance; contraction of the quadriceps femoris can be seen and palpated. (*E2*) Examination of the quadriceps for knee extension. (*F1*) Examination of the hamstring muscle for knee flexion.

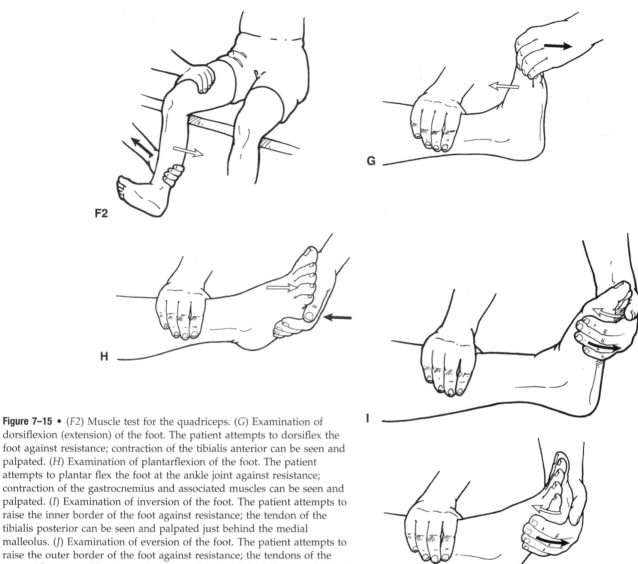

Figure 7–15 • (*F2*) Muscle test for the quadriceps. (*G*) Examination of dorsiflexion (extension) of the foot. The patient attempts to dorsiflex the foot against resistance; contraction of the tibialis anterior can be seen and palpated. (*H*) Examination of plantarflexion of the foot. The patient attempts to plantar flex the foot at the ankle joint against resistance; contraction of the gastrocnemius and associated muscles can be seen and palpated. (*I*) Examination of inversion of the foot. The patient attempts to raise the inner border of the foot against resistance; the tendon of the tibialis posterior can be seen and palpated just behind the medial malleolus. (*J*) Examination of eversion of the foot. The patient attempts to raise the outer border of the foot against resistance; the tendons of the peronei longus and brevis can be seen and palpated just above and behind the lateral malleolus.

for a "dull" source of stimuli. (If pain sensation is intact, testing for temperature sensation is usually omitted.)

• Temperature: A tube of hot water and one of cold water are applied in succession to the same areas used in other tests. The patient is asked to identify "hot" or "cold." A cool tuning fork can also be used; it is placed directly on the skin in a particular location and then moved to the same area on the opposite side of the body. The patient is asked if it feels the same on both sides of the body.

Deep Sensation

• Vibration: A 128-Hz tuning fork is placed on the bony prominence of the big toe and thumb; perception of vibration is a normal finding.

• Deep pressure pain: The Achilles tendon or gastrocnemius muscle belly and forearm muscles are squeezed. The patient should perceive this pressure, and it should feel the same on both sides of the body.

• Proprioception: The thumb and then the large toe are moved up or down. The patient should be able to identify "up" or "down."

Discriminative Sensation (Usually, Not All Modalities Are Tested)

• Two-point discrimination: A part of the body is touched simultaneously with sharp objects to determine if one or two pricks can be felt. (Note: the presence of receptors varies in different parts of the body.)

• **Point discrimination:** The patient is asked to name the location at which he or she was touched with the wooden end of an applicator or the examiner's hand.

• **Recognition of shape and form:** The patient is asked to identify common objects placed in his or her hand such as a key, a pen, or a coin. Inability to recognize objects by touch is called **astereognosis.**

Chart 7–2 • Gait Changes Associated With Anatomic Correlations

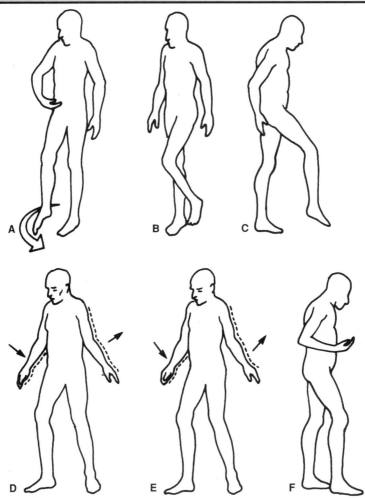

A Spastic hemiparesis is associated with unilateral upper motor neuron disease. One arm is flexed, close to the side, and immobile; the leg is circled stiffly outward and forward (circumducted), often with dragging of the toe.

B Scissors gait is associated with bilateral spastic paresis of the legs. Each leg is advanced slowly and the thighs tend to cross forward on each other at each step. The steps are short. Patients look as if they were walking through water.

C Steppage gait is associated with foot-drop, usually secondary to lower motor neuron disease. The feet are lifted high, with knees flexed, and then brought down with a slap on the floor. Patients look as if they were walking up stairs.

D Sensory ataxia is associated with loss of position sense in the legs. The gait is unsteady and wide-based (the feet are far apart). The feet are lifted high and brought down with a slap. Patients watch the ground to guide their steps. They cannot stand steadily with feet together when the eyes are closed (positive Romberg test).

E Cerebellar ataxia is associated with disease of the cerebellum or associated tracts. The gait is staggering, unsteady, and widely based, with exaggerated difficulty on the turns. The patient cannot stand steadily with feet together, whether eyes are open or closed.

F Parkinsonian gait is associated with the basal ganglia of Parkinson's disease. The posture is stopped, the hips and knees slightly flexed. Steps are short and often shuffling. Arm swings are decreased and the patient turns around stiffly—"all in one piece."

(Adapted from Staab, A. S., & Hodges, L. C. [1996]. *Essentials of gerontological nursing: Adaptation to the aging process.* Philadelphia: J. B. Lippincott.)

- **Texture discrimination:** The patient is asked to differentiate among various textures (e.g., silk, wool).
- **Graphesthesia:** A letter or number is written on the palm with a dull-pointed object; the patient is then asked to identify the symbol.
- **Extension phenomenon:** Touch the patient in the same location on both sides of the body simultaneously; alternate with touching only one side and determine if the patient can tell the difference. If sensation is normal, being touched on the skin on both sides of the body simultaneously should result in both stimuli being perceived.

Table 7–17 • DESCRIPTION OF GAIT DISTURBANCES

NAME	DESCRIPTION	CAUSES
General Gait Disturbances		
• Steppage gait	Associated with foot drop and flaccidity of the leg. To compensate for foot drop, the patient lifts the upper leg high to clear the foot from floor; as a result, the foot slaps the floor	Can be unilateral when caused by a lesion involving the external popliteal nerve. It is bilateral in cases of peroneal muscle atrophy (as in Charcot-Marie-Tooth disease) or bilateral L-5 and S-1 involvement (poliomyelitis or some polyneuropathies)
• Waddling gait	Broad base and lateral jerking movement of the hips and trunk	Weakness of the gluteal, psoas, and truncal muscles
• Hypotonic gait	Hyperextension of the knees, wide-based flail-like movements of the legs accompanied by a high step; the heel touches first, followed by the slap of the foot as the toes touch the floor	Degeneration of the posterior columns (loss of proprioception)
Special Gait Disturbances Classified According to Anatomical Areas		
• Cerebellar gait	Wide-based, staggering, lurching, and uncoordinated gait	Any disease involving the cerebellum (tumor, multiple sclerosis, Friedreich's ataxia)
• Corticospinal gaits		
Hemiplegic	Unilateral; the arm is "semiflexed" with the elbow held close to the waist; fingers are flexed and wristdrop is noted; the extended, spastic, stiff leg is swung in a semicircle when walking; the foot is inverted, and footdrop is evident	Stroke
Spastic	Shuffling, with the legs stiff	Bilateral involvement of the corticospinal tract
Scissor	The legs cross, one in front of the other, with each step; the knees are brought inward; and the person often walks on toes because of the swaying motion. Bilateral condition	Severe spasticity of the adductor muscles of the legs
Basal Ganglia Gaits		
• Parkinsonian	Loss of automatic arm swinging is evident while walking; head and body are flexed forward; the arms are semiflexed and adducted; and the legs are rigid and flexed. A slow, shuffling gait is typical. After walking begins, the person may propel forward with increased momentum	Defect in the basal ganglia
• Athetoid	Sudden, wormlike movements of the arms, head, and legs which make forward progress difficult	Defect in the basal ganglia

CEREBELLAR SYSTEM EXAMINATION

The following outlines the most common methods used to evaluate balance and coordination. (Gait, discussed with the motor examination, may be included at the end of the cerebellar examination.) The patient is instructed to do *one* of the following in each category:

Upper Extremities

- The examiner raises his or her index finger to locate it about 2 feet and central-midface from the patient. The patient is given the instruction, "With your left hand, touch my finger, then touch your nose; do this as fast as you can." Be sure that the upper arm is extended and parallel to the floor. This should be evaluated with the patient's eyes open and then closed. Repeat with other arm.
- Instruct the patient to rapidly pronate and supinate the hand in the other palm; repeat with other hand.
- Instruct the patient to rapidly tap his or her index finger on the thumb; then tap all four fingers, one at a time, against the thumb as rapidly as possible. Repeat with other hand.

If the finger-to-nose test is smooth and on the mark, further evaluation of the upper extremities is not necessary. **Dysmetria** is the inability to control accurately the range of movement in muscle action with resultant overshooting of the mark, especially of hand movement. Overshooting is also called **past-point**.

Lower Extremities

- While lying on the back or sitting, the patient is instructed to slide one heel down the shin of the opposite leg; then repeat the procedure on the opposite side.
- While lying on the back or sitting , the patient is instructed to draw the number 8 with the foot in the air; repeat with the other foot.

Table 7-18 • INVOLUNTARY AND ABNORMAL MOVEMENTS

TYPE	DESCRIPTION	COMMENTS
Tremors	• Involuntary trembling movement of the body or limbs resulting from contraction of opposing muscles; tremors are characterized by rate, distribution, and relationship to movement	• Seen with certain organic diseases; some forms of tremors are psychogenic in origin
• Physiologic	• The occasional tremors seen in healthy people and precipitated by extreme fatigue or stress	
• Essential (familial, senile)	• Tremors occur when muscles are brought into action to support or move an extremity; they may also affect the jaw, lips, and head (head nods from side to side or to and fro) • Absent at rest • Tremor has characteristics similar to those of parkinsonian tremors	• Improvement is usually noted with alcohol ingestion, sedatives, and propranolol
• Toxic	• Tremors are caused by toxic states (e.g., uremia) or ingestion of toxic substances (e.g., drug withdrawal)	
• Cerebellar	• Tremors occur during movement and increase toward the end of the purposeful act	• Caused by cerebellar lesions • May be seen in multiple sclerosis
• Parkinsonian	• These regular, rhythmic tremors are described as "pill-rolling tremors" (alternating flexion-extension of the fingers and adduction-abduction of the thumb) • Observed at rest • Associated with increased muscle tone	• Basal ganglia disorder seen in Parkinson's disease
• Resting tremors	• Tremor occurs when the patient is at rest and is diminished by purposeful activity	
• Intentional tremors	• Tremor is increased or precipitated by purposeful activity	
Choreiform movements	• Characterized by irregular, jerky, uncoordinated movements and abnormal posture • Represent a more generalized condition than tremors • May be evidenced by grimacing and difficulty in chewing, speaking, and swallowing • Increase with purposeful activity, making it difficult to complete the simplest of motor functions	
Clonus/myoclonus	• Sudden, brief, jerking contraction of a muscle or muscle group	
Athetosis	• Involuntary, repetitive, slow gross movements, particularly affecting posture • Arms tend to swing from a widely abducted base	• Movements described as snakelike
Tics	• Involuntary, compulsive, stereotyped movements • Described as "nervous habits" • Repeated at irregular intervals • Often involve the face	• Often psychogenic in origin
Spasms	• Involuntary contraction of large muscle groups (arms, legs, neck)	• Oculogyric spasms, as seen in Parkinson's disease, are an example; these spasms are characterized by a fixed, upward gaze controlled by extraocular muscles
Ballism	• More or less continuous, gross, abrupt contractions of the axial and proximal muscles of the extremities • Violent flail-like movements	• May involve one side of the body (hemiballismus) • Caused by a destructive lesion in or near the contralateral subthalamic nucleus

Table 7–19 • SENSORY SYSTEM ASSESSMENT

SENSORY MODALITIES	DESCRIPTION/TECHNIQUE

Primary sensory modalities
  Superficial sensations
    Superficial tactile (light touch) sensation
	A wisp of cotton is used as the stimulus. Patients are asked to close their eyes and signify with a word, such as "yes," when they feel a light touch. The examiner lightly touches the skin with the cotton wisp, beginning at the head and working downward. Each side of the body is assessed.
	Light touch sensation is often preserved when other sensory modalities are compromised in lesions of the spinal cord. This occurs because of an overlap of innervation.

Superficial pain sensation Within a few segments after entering the cord, fibers conveying pain and temperature synapse and cross the midline through the ventral commissure to the opposite lateral spinothalamic tract. This is important to note because there may be dissociation of pain and temperature loss with preservation of the ability to feel light touch.	A pin or other sharp object is used as the stimulus. Care must be taken to prevent injury to the patient. The same systematic procedure is followed as for light touch.
Temperature sensation Note that the tracts conveying pain and temperature both cross to the opposite side of the spinal cord	Two test tubes, one filled with cold water and the other filled with warm water, are used as stimuli. Alternate: use a cold tuning fork. Following the same procedure as for light touch and pain, the patient is systematically touched and responses are noted.
Deep Sensations Sense of motion and position	Passive motion is tested in the upper extremities on the thumb and in the lower extremities on the big toe. The sides of the toe and thumb are lightly grasped by the examiner's index finger and thumb and moved up or down. Note that the thumb and toe should be touched lightly so that the pressure needed to move the appendage is not apparent to the patient. As the examiner moves the thumb and toe, the patient is asked to identify the direction of movement (up or down).
Deep pain	The Achilles tendon, calf, and forearm muscle are squeezed on each side of the body. Note the patient's sensitivity to this stimulus.
Vibration sensation	Using a vibrating tuning fork, place the instrument on the bony prominences (thumb and big toe). The patient is instructed to signal when the vibration is first felt and when it is no longer present. Compare the sensitivity of the two sides; compare proximal and distal portions of the same extremity. If abnormality is detected, more extensive testing is conducted.
Cortical discrimination (complex somatic sensations requiring cerebral cortex interpretation) Two-point discrimination	A small pair of calipers or another sharp instrument is used as the stimulus. Alternate: touch patient simultaneously or singularly.
Note: Body areas vary in sensitivity in discriminating simultaneous stimuli	The patient, with eyes closed, is simultaneously touched with two sharp objects and then asked whether he or she is being touched by one or two objects. This testing procedure continues over the surface of the body.
Point localization	The patient's skin is lightly touched at a particular point while his or her eyes are closed and is asked to identify where he or she was touched. Compare each side of the body for response.
Stereognosis	With the eyes closed, common objects, such as a pencil, comb, or coin, are placed in the patient's hand. The patient is then asked to identify the object.
Texture discrimination	With eyes closed, the patient is asked to differentiate between materials of varying textures. Each side of the body is tested and compared.
Traced-figure identification	The examiner traces a number or letter on the patient's palm, back, or other part of the body with his or her finger or an applicator stick; the patient is asked to identify the figure traced. Each side of the body is tested.
Double simultaneous stimulation (extinction)	Two corresponding body parts are touched simultaneously. The patient is asked to identify the area touched. The examiner notes whether the patient is aware of being touched on both sides.

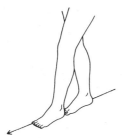

Figure 7–16 • Assessment of cerebellar function. The integrity of the cerebellum can be tested by having the patient walk heel to toe along a line (tandem gait). With cerebellar hemispheric involvement, the patient often falls toward the side of the lesion, and there is ataxia. With midline cerebellar dysfunction, the gait is wide-based and tandem gait walking cannot be performed. (From Weber, J. [1992]. *Nurse's handbook of health assessment* [2nd ed.]. Philadelphia: J. B. Lippincott.)

Balance

Tandem walking is tested (Fig. 7-16). Protect the patient from falls. If the patient sways to one side, it may be an early indicator of cerebellar dysfunction on the side to which he or she sways.

Romberg's test assesses balance in space and is a test of posterior column function (spinal cord tracts). Ask the patient to stand erect with feet together, first with eyes open (visual input) and then with eyes closed (without visual input). To protect the patient from injury, stand beside him or her with your arms positioned to provide support should he or she begin to fall. If the patient loses balance with the eyes opened or can stand with the eyes opened but sways or falls when the eyes are closed, **Romberg's sign** is positive.

▥ REFLEXES

Testing reflexes provides an important indication of the status of the central nervous system in both conscious and unconscious patients. A stimulus is mediated by a definite pathway through the receptor organ, afferent limb, spinal cord or brainstem, efferent limb, and effector organ. The reflex is modified by the simultaneous activity of other pathways, particularly the corticospinal tract. Alterations in reflexes may be the earliest signs of a pathological condition. Reflexes are classified into three categories: (1) muscle-stretch reflexes (also known as deep tendon reflexes or

---

CHART 7 – 3 • Evaluation of Muscle-Stretch Reflexes

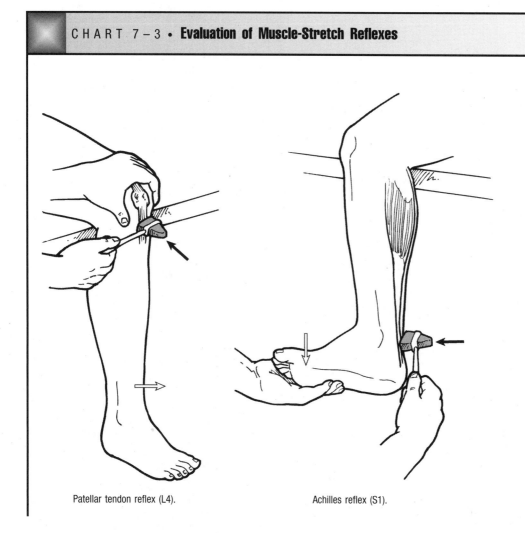

Patellar tendon reflex (L4).   Achilles reflex (S1).

(continued)

CHART 7-3 • Evaluation of Muscle-Stretch Reflexes (Continued)

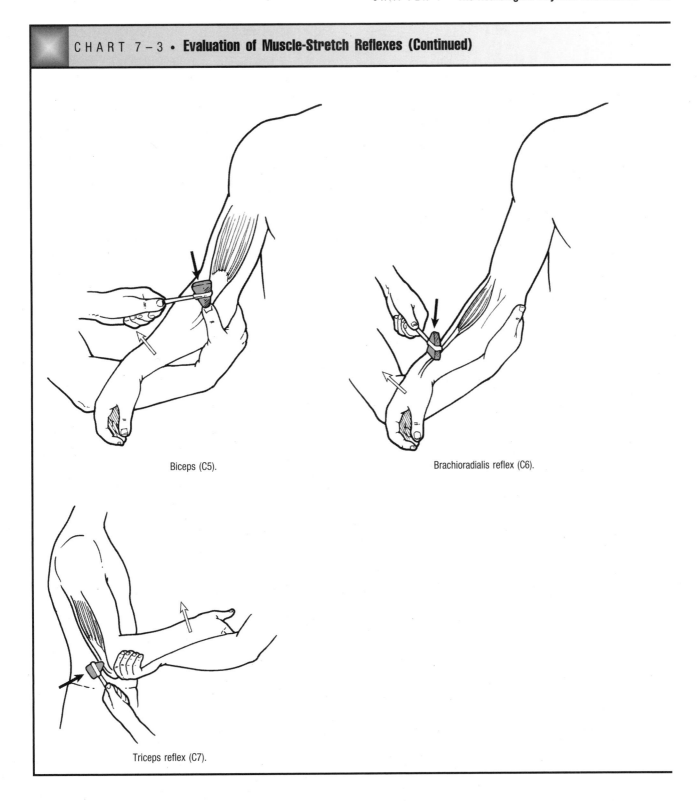

Biceps (C5).

Brachioradialis reflex (C6).

Triceps reflex (C7).

DTRs), (2) superficial or cutaneous reflexes, and (3) pathological reflexes.

Muscle-Stretch Reflexes

The muscle-stretch reflexes are evaluated first. These reflexes occur in response to a sudden stimulus, such as the percussion hammer that causes the muscle to stretch (Chart 7-3). Although there are many muscle-stretch reflexes, the *major* reflexes included in a screening examination are evaluated. It is important to use the proper technique to elicit a particular reflex. With the muscle relaxed and the joint at midposition, the tendon is tapped directly using a percussion or reflex hammer. Normally, contraction of the muscle occurs with a quick movement of the limb or structure innervated by the muscle. Both sides of the body are tested

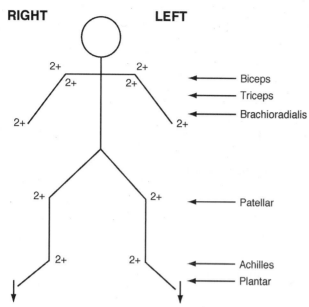

Figure 7–17 • Alternative method of recording the commonly tested muscle stretch reflexes.

and the results are compared. The briskness of the response should also be noted. The muscle-stretch reflex ranges are graded on a scale from 0 to 4, as follows:

4+: Very brisk, hyperactive; muscle undergoes repeated contractions or clonus; often indicative of disease
3+: More brisk than average; may either be normal for that patient or indicative of disease
2+: Average or normal
1+: Minimal or diminished response
0: No response

Note that all reflexes present are indicated by a plus sign; there are no minuses used in reflex grading of DTRs. Findings can be documented using a stick figure on which the magnitude of the reflex is recorded (Fig. 7-17).

Superficial Reflexes

Superficial reflexes are elicited by light, rapid stroking or scratching (depending on the tissue being tested) of a particular area of the skin, cornea, or mucous membrane. Table 7-20 lists the most common superficial reflexes tested (Fig. 7-18). These reflexes are initiated by cutaneous receptors stimulated by stroking. The grading of superficial reflexes differs from the scale used with muscle-stretch reflexes. Superficial reflexes are graded as either present (+) or absent (0). If they are present but weak, they may be recorded as "weak."

Pathological Reflexes

There are several reflexes referred to as *primitive reflexes* because they are seen in the early stages of development and subsequently disappear. If they do reappear, they are evidence of disinhibition resulting from dementia. Table 7-21 lists the most common primitive reflexes. Another primitive reflex is a **flexion reflex**, a general term encompassing various polysynaptic reflexes. Also known as the *withdrawal reflex*, it moves the limb away from the source of stimulation, thus resulting in flexion. Because the stimulus is polysynaptic, there is an afterdischarge in the interneuronal relays, and the motor response outlasts the stimulus. Activation of the flexor motor neurons in the leg is typically widespread, so that flexor muscles at the *ankle, knee,* and *hip* contract to withdraw the whole limb; this triple contraction is sometimes referred to as a **triple flexion** response.

Normally, the toes show plantarflexion in response to stimuli applied to the sole of the foot. Of the pathologic reflexes, the plantar reflexes are very important. **Babinski's reflex** is the most common plantar reflex assessed (Fig. 7-19). Stimulation of the plantar surface of the foot (from heel to toes along lateral aspect of foot) is followed by dorsiflexion of the toes, especially the great toe, and separation or fanning of the toes. A positive plantar reflex is related to disease of the corticospinal tract at any level from the motor cortex through the descending pathways.

Table 7–20 • MAJOR SUPERFICIAL (CUTANEOUS) REFLEXES

REFLEX	INNERVATION	TEST
Corneal	CNs V, VII	Touch cornea lightly with a wisp of cotton; lids should quickly close.
Gag	CNs IX, X	Stimulate the back of the pharynx with a tongue depressor; a retching or gagging response should be elicited.
Swallowing	CNs IX, X	Stimulate one side of the uvula with a cotton applicator; the uvula should elevate.
Upper abdominals	T8–T10	Stroke the outer abdomen toward the umbilicus using a tongue blade; the umbilicus should move up and toward the area being stroked (see Fig. 7-18).
Lower abdominals	T10–T12	Stroke the lower abdomen toward the umbilicus using a tongue blade; the umbilicus should move down and toward the area being stroked (see Fig. 7-18).
Cremasteric (male)	L1–L2	Lightly stroke the inner aspect of the thigh or lower abdomen; elevation of the ipsilateral testicle should occur (see Fig. 7-18).
Bulbocavernous (male)	S3–S4	Apply direct pressure over the bulbocavernous muscle behind the scrotum, or pinch the glans penis; the muscle should contract, raising the scrotum toward the body.
Perianal	S3, S4, S5	Scratch the tissue at the side of the anus with a blunt instrument; there should be a puckering of the anus. Additionally, if a gloved finger is inserted into the rectum, a contraction should be felt.

CN, cranial nerve.

The grading of pathological reflexes involves noting the presence or absence of the pathologic sign. The presence of a pathological sign (+) is abnormal, whereas absence of a pathological sign (−) is normal.

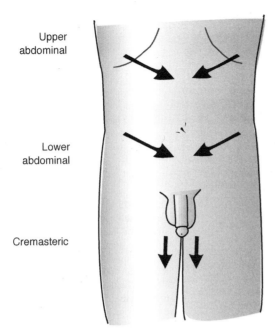

Upper abdominal

Lower abdominal

Cremasteric

Figure 7–18 • The abdominal and cremasteric reflexes. Test the abdominal reflexes by lightly but briskly stroking each side of the abdomen and below the umbilicus in the direction illustrated. Use a key or a tongue blade to stroke the skin. Note the contraction of the abdominal muscles and the deviation of the umbilicus toward the stimulus. Obesity may mask an abdominal reflex. In this situation, use your finger to retract the patient's umbilicus away from the side to be stimulated. Feel with your retracting finger for the muscular contraction. Not routinely done. If tested the cremasteric reflex is assessed by lightly scratching the inner aspect of the upper thigh. Note the elevation of the testicle on that side. Abdominal and cremasteric reflexes may be absent in both upper and lower motor neuron disorders. (From Bates, B. [1983]. *Guide to physical examination* [3rd ed.]. Philadelphia: J. B. Lippincott.)

THE NEUROLOGICAL EXAMINATION OF THE COMATOSE PATIENT

Coma is a pathologic state of unconsciousness characterized by the following: an unarousable sleeplike state; the eyes remain closed at all times; no speech or sound is noted; and there is no spontaneous movement of the extremities. If movement of the extremities occurs, it is a reflex response to painful stimuli such as flexor or extensor posturing (see Chapter 8 for discussion of LOCs). Coma is a *symptom* of a wide variety of disease entities resulting from a cerebral structural lesion or a metabolic condition. For coma to occur there must be bilateral hemispheric dysfunction, brain-stem dysfunction, or both. Sometimes the cause of the coma is obvious (cerebral trauma), and other times it is not (e.g., drug toxicity).

The examiner should think about the underlying cause and pathophysiology. Consciousness has two components, arousal and awareness. Arousal is a state of wakefulness due to activation of the reticular activating system (RAS). The RAS is a diffuse neuronal network located in the cerebral hemispheres and upper portion of the brain stem. Awareness includes self-awareness and cognitive function. Arousal must be intact for awareness to be apparent.

A **supratentorial lesion** (i.e., cerebral hemispheric lesion) that progresses to coma is the result of a *mass effect* of the lesion that expands and effects the bilateral hemisphere and then produces pressure on the rostral brainstem (location of a portion of the RAS). It begins with *asymmetric* signs and symptoms such as a monoplegia or aphasia. As the pathological process proceeds to coma, a rostral-caudal pattern occurs, that is, dysfunction of the hemispheres, then thalamus, then midbrain, then pons, and finally the medulla occurs. An **infratentorial lesion**, that is, a primary lesion in

Table 7-21 • PATHOLOGICAL (PRIMITIVE) REFLEXES

REFLEX	DESCRIPTION	ASSOCIATED CONDITIONS
Grasp reflex	Palmar stimulation results in a grasp response.	Most common in association with dementia and diffuse or bifrontal brain impairment.
Snout reflex	Puckering of lips in response to gentle percussion in the oral region.	As above
Sucking reflex	Sucking movement of the lips in response to light touching, striking, or tapping on the lips, stroking the tongue, or stimulating the palate. Note: may be noticed when the patient is being suctioned or when mouth care is given.	As above
Rooting reflex	Stimulation of the lips result in deviating the head toward the stimuli.	As above
Palmomental reflex	Ipsilateral contraction of the chin (mentalis and perioral muscles) following a scratching stimulation of the palm (thenar area) of the hand.	May be found in unaffected people, but common in dementia
Glabellar reflex (Myerson's sign)	Blinking eyes each time the glabellar area between the eyes is tapped. Normally, the patient blinks only the first few times tapping is initiated.	Seen in Parkinsonism

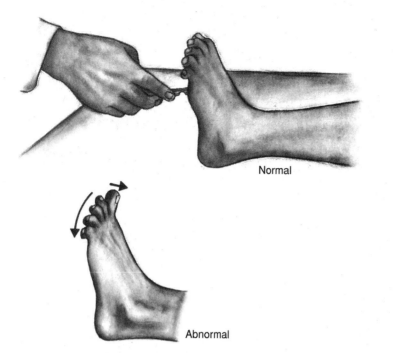
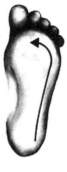

Figure 7–19 • Babinski reflex. With a moderately sharp object, such as a key, stroke the lateral aspect of the sole from the heel to the ball of the foot, curving medially across the ball. Use the lightest stimulus that will provoke a response. Note any movement of the toes, normally flexion. Dorsiflexion of the great toe, with fanning of the other toes, indicates upper motor neuron disease.

the brainstem, affects the RAS directly. Coma occurs without the rostral-caudal pattern of dysfunction. Infratentorial lesions are much less common that supratentorial lesions. In **metabolic conditions,** the brain is affected diffusely through the bloodstream. The progressive rostral-caudal pattern does not occur; instead, *symmetrical* deficits are seen.

Components of the Neurological Examination for a Comatose Patient

The neurological examination of a comatose patient is limited because of the patient's inability to participate in the examination actively. However, a good profile of the nervous system can be constructed by observing the patient and collecting focused data. The purpose of the examination is refocused to identify symmetrical and asymmetrical deficits that will help in determining the underlying problem. The following outlines the areas addressed in the neurological examination:

- Past medical history
- Review of general parameters (e.g., skin, scalp, mouth odor, ears)
- Vital signs, including respiratory pattern
- Level of consciousness
- Pupillary size and response to light
- Eyelids, gaze, and extraocular movement
- Facial symmetry
- Other reflexes (corneal, gag, swallowing reflexes)
- Motor tone and response to pain

Note that CNs I, II, IV, XI, and XII cannot be tested in a comatose patient. The past medical history provided by a family member, if present, can be very helpful in suggesting the underlying cause of coma. For example, a history of diabetes mellitus, cerebral trauma, or drug or alcohol use could be related to the current problem. Knowledge of the circumstances related to the onset of coma as well as length of coma is important.

Begin by examining general components. Look at the skin for color, evidence of a bleeding disorder, needle marks, or bruises. Check the scalp for possible fracture of boggy areas suggestive of trauma. Note the odor from the mouth and any drainage from the nose or mouth. The ears are examined with an otoscope for evidence of trauma, infection, or drainage. Next, assess the vital signs (see Chapter 8 for a discussion of vital signs).

Now move from the general to the specifics of a neurological function. Take a few minutes to look at the patient lying in the bed. Note the predominant position of the extremities, position of the head and neck, presence of spontaneous movement, and the position of the eye when the lids are opened.

Level of Consciousness

The *depth* of the coma is important to ascertain. This is done by providing a verbal stimulus (calling the patient's name or clapping your hands loudly over the patient's head) and observing the response. If there is no response, a noxious stimulus is provided by providing pressure to the nailbeds or pinching the shoulders.

Pupillary Response

Pupillary size and response to direct light are evaluated. Normally, pupils are 3 to 4 mm in diameter (smaller in the elderly) and are equal in size and reaction to light. See Chapter 8 for a discussion of pupillary responses and size.

Eyelashes, Eyelids, Gaze, and Ocular Movement

In association with coma, spontaneous blinking, then loss of blink in response to touching of the eyelashes, and finally the loss of the corneal reflex (see below) are among the most dependable signs of deepening coma.[9]

Observe and stimulate the eyelashes. Raise the eyelids, release them, and observe. In coma, the eyelids close slowly once they are released; in the absence of coma, the lids will close rapidly.

Look at the eyes (with lids held open) for spontaneous movement. **Roving-eye movement** is characterized by spontaneous, slow, and random deviation. It is seen in comatose patients with intact brainstem oculomotor function. Absence of roving-eye movement indicates brainstem dysfunction. Next, look at the eyes for position in the head or a gaze preference. Lesions in the cortex or brainstem above the level of the ocular motor nuclei may impair conjugate movement of the eyes, thus producing one of the following gaze disorders:

CRANIAL NERVE PARALYSIS
- A slight downward deviation of one eye suggests an oculomotor nerve (CN III) palsy, whereas a medial deviation of one eye suggests an abducens (CN VI) palsy.

HEMISPHERIC LESIONS
- With a large **hemispheric lesion**, both **eyes deviate toward** the side of the lesion and away from the hemiparesis; may last several days.
- Seizure discharges involving the frontal gaze centers can result in gaze deviation, so that both **eyes deviate away from** the discharging focus.

MIDBRAIN LESION (UPWARD GAZE DISORDERS)
- Lesions of the dorsal midbrain affect the center for voluntary upward gaze and may therefore produce upward gaze paralysis.
- **Parinaud's syndrome** includes upward gaze paralysis, nystagmus on downward gaze, paralysis of accommodation, midposition pupils, and light-near dissociation.

PONTINE LESIONS (HORIZONTAL GAZE DISORDERS FROM LESION AT PONTINE GAZE CENTERS)
- With a **unilateral pontine lesion**, the **eyes deviate toward hemiparesis** rather than away, unlike hemispheric hemiparesis. Pontine gaze palsies are caused by infarcts, hemorrhages, gliomas, abscesses, Wernicke's encephalopathy, and multiple sclerosis.

In the comatose patient, eye movement is tested by stimulating the vestibular system (semicircular canals of the middle ear) by passive head movement or by ice-water irrigation against the tympanic membrane. These tests are usually performed by the physician. Before moving the patient's neck, be sure that there is no possibility of the existence of a cervical fracture or injury. The **oculocephalic reflex (doll's eye movement)** is elicited by briskly turning the head horizontally from side to side or vertically up and down while holding the eyelids open (Fig. 7-20). Moving the head side to side tests CNs III and VI. Moving the head up and down tests only CN III. If the reflex is intact, the eyes move conjugately in the opposite direction to the head movement. (Note that this reflex is not present in the normal, alert person.) If present, the oculocephalic reflex verifies intact brain-stem gaze centers, the medial longitudinal fasciculus, and ocular motor nerves. If the reflex is absent, the eyes follow the direction of the head movement. Absence of the reflex indicates severe brainstem dysfunction from the pons to the midbrain level. If the eyes do not move, it is a poor

prognostic sign and the patient probably will not regain consciousness.

Cold Caloric Testing

If the oculocephalic response is inconclusive, the **oculovestibular reflex (caloric)** can be assessed (Fig. 7-21). This is a more sensitive test of brainstem function. Before testing, the ear is examined to be sure that there is no perforation of the tympanic membrane, an absolute contraindication to proceeding. Additionally, any major wax deposit in the ear should be removed. Raise the patient's head 30 degrees. In the comatose patient, unilateral irrigation with at least 30 to 50 mL of cold water (33°C) over 30 seconds results in slow eye deviation toward the irrigated ear if the brainstem is intact. Wait at least 5 minutes before testing the other side. Using cold irrigant is the most common method of testing the oculovestibular reflex.

There are other ways of assessing vestibular function. Bilateral irrigation with warm water (44°C) can also be used. If the brainstem is intact, the eyes deviate away from the side of the irrigation. Another possibility is simultaneous bilateral irrigation. Bilateral irrigation with cold water causes downward deviation of the eyes; bilateral irrigation with warm water induces upward deviation if the brain-stem is intact. The response can be remembered by the mnemonic **COWS** (**C**old **O**pposite **W**arm **S**ame).

The importance of the oculocephalic and oculovestibular reflexes is that their presence or absence provides important information on brainstem function that is useful to determine the depth of coma and to predict patient outcome. Full reflex eye movement in the comatose patient is solid evidence of an intact brainstem from the pons to the midbrain level and excludes a mass lesion in the brainstem.[10]

The following are a few abnormal patterns noted in unilateral cold water oculovestibular testing:

- Lesion of the oculomotor nerve or nucleus (e.g., rostral-caudal herniation): no movement toward the side of irrigation on the affected side with unimpaired contralateral abduction.
- Downward deviation of one or both eyes is suggestive of sedative drug intoxication.

Facial Symmetry

Observe for facial symmetry as rest and when the patient is stimulated.

Other Reflexes

The corneal and gag reflexes are two other important brainstem reflexes to assess. These cutaneous reflexes are tested by lightly touching the cornea and mucous membrane. A wisp of cotton from an applicator is used to stimulate the cornea. A complete response is a brisk and immediate blinking of the eye. The response may also be diminished or absent. Assess each eye for response. Asymmetry in corneal responses indicates either an acute lesion of the opposite hemisphere or an ipsilateral lesion in the brainstem. Note that wearers of contact lens may have this reflex abolished. Loss of the corneal reflex is due to a lesion affecting CNs V and VII.

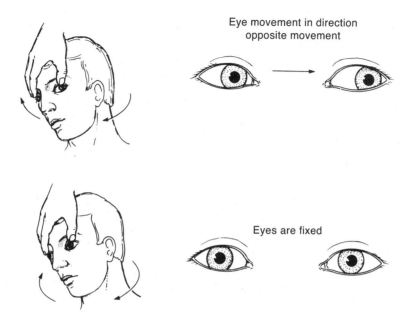

Assessment Technique for the Oculocephalic Reflex

1. Briskly rotate the head from side to side, or
2. Briskly flex and extend the neck.

Eye movement in direction opposite movement

Eyes are fixed

Findings

- When the head is rotated, the eyes should move in the direction opposite to the head movement *(top)*. (If the head is rotated to the left, the eyes appear to move to the right.) Alternative method: When the neck is flexed, the eyes appear to look upward; when the neck is extended, the eyes look downward.
- When the doll's eye reflex is absent, the eyes do not move in the sockets and thus follow the direction of passive rotation. Loss of the oculocephalic reflex in the comatose patient indicates a lesion at the pontine–midbrain level of the brainstem.

Figure 7–20 • Oculocephalic reflex. Eye movement in the unconscious patient can be assessed by the physician by means of the oculocephalic response (doll's eye phenomenon). In the presence or suspicion of a cervical fracture or dislocation, this test is contraindicated. (*Note:* If the presence of the oculocephalic reflex is questioned or the conduction of the test is contraindicated, the oculovestibular reflex is tested. In many hospital emergency departments, the oculovestibular reflex is tested more often than the oculocephalic reflex unless there are contraindications.)

In an intubated patient, the gag and swallowing reflex can be tested by tugging gently on the endotracheal tube. If the reflex is intact, the patient will gag. In a nonintubated patient, the gag reflex can be tested by sequentially stimulating *each side* of the posterior pharynx with a tongue blade or a cotton-tipped applicator. An immediate gag response is noted if the reflex is intact. In an intubated patient, slightly moving the endotracheal tube is sufficient to precipitate a gag response if the reflex is intact. Abnormal findings include a diminished or absent gag reflex and indicate a lesion involving CNs IX and X.

Deep tendon reflexes and the plantar response (Babinski's sign) are included. See previous sections of this chapter for discussion.

Motor Tone and Response to Pain

In the comatose patient, the examiner relies on observing predominant posture, muscle tone, and response to painful stimuli. Note any abnormal posturing (decorticate or decerebrate) as the patient lies in bed (see Chapter 8 for discussion). To assess muscle tone, grasp each forearm a few inches above the wrist and raise the arm to a vertical position. The hand is flexed at almost a right angle in a comatose patient. Lower the arm to 12 to 18 inches from the bed and release the arm. A flaccid arm drops rapidly and flails in a coma compared with a slow descent in a noncomatose patient. To assess the legs, flex both legs so that both heels rest on the bed. Release the legs at the knees. In acute hemiplegia, the flaccid leg drops rapidly, externally rotates at the hip, and the leg extends. A normal leg slowly extends to its original position.

Next, a painful, central stimulus is provided by applying firm pressure to the supraorbital area, pinching the trapezius or pectoralis major at the neck region, or rubbing the sternum. Pressure on the nailbeds may also be used, but because it is peripheral stimulation, it may not be as reliable as central stimulation. Possible responses to painful stimuli are:

- Purposeful: localization/push the painful stimuli away
- Nonpurposeful: movement of the stimulated area, but no attempt to push the stimuli away
- No response: no reaction to painful stimuli

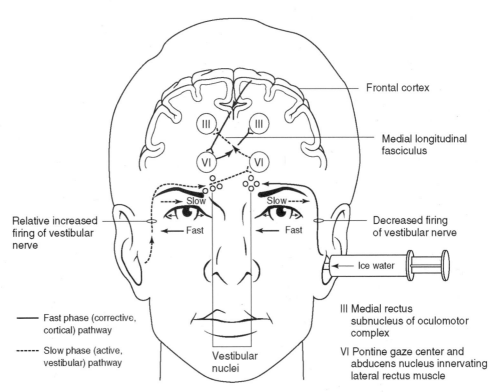

Figure 7–21 • Physiology of the oculovestibular reflex (vestibulo-oculare reflex, cold calorics). Infusion of ice water into the ear of a comatose patient will elicit the oculovestibular reflex if both the cerebral hemisphere and brain stem are intact. With an intact brainstem, a signal passes through pathways from the medulla to the midbrain, generating a slow movement of the eyes to the side of the ice water infusion. This is followed by a rapid corrective movement of the eyes, generated by an intact ipsilateral side of the cerbral hemisphere. The ice water infusion test can be repeated in the other ear of the comatose patient to test the integrity of the other side of the brainstem.

In considering depth of coma on a continuum for prognostic purposes and change over time, a purposeful response suggests moderate severity, a promising response. Abnormal posturing may also be noted. Decortication is associated with a direct lesion of the thalamus or a large hemispheric mass that compresses the thalamus.[10] Decerebration suggests midbrain dysfunction, which is an upper brainstem structure, and is thus considered more ominous than decortication. Finally, flaccid paralysis is seen in the final stages of cerebral demise.

Posturing may follow several patterns. Bilateral symmetrical posturing is seen in both structural and metabolic disorders. Asymmetrical posturing suggests a disorder in the contralateral cerebral hemisphere or brainstem.

Reflexes

Deep tendon reflexes, some cutaneous reflexes, and some pathological reflexes can be tested. The cutaneous reflexes evaluated include the corneal and gag reflexes (see earlier discussion). The patient is also examined for presence of Babinski's reflex (see Fig. 7-19). Table 7-21 provides the most common primitive reflexes, especially the grasping, sucking, and rooting reflexes. Note also triple flexion in the section on pathological reflexes found earlier in this chapter.

▌ SUMMARY

Physical examination of a comatose patient is challenging and requires well-developed clinical reasoning skills that are based on an understanding of anatomy and physiology,

pathophysiology, and patterns of dysfunction. Collection of data from the medical history and physical assessment help the examiner paint a mental picture of intact and lost function that serves to exclude as well as include possible diagnoses so that comprehensive treatment can be instituted by the interdisciplinary collaborative team.

REFERENCES

1. Guberman A. (1994). *An introduction to clinical neurology* (p. 12). Boston: Little, Brown.
2. American Psychiatric Association. (1994). *Diagnostic and statistical manual of mental disorders* (4th ed.). Washington, D. C.: Author.
3. Strub, R. L. (1982). Acute confusional state. In D. F. Benson & D. Blumer (Eds.). *Psychiatric aspects of neurologic disease* (Vol. II, pp. 1–21). New York: Grune & Stratton.
4. Strub, R. L., & Black, F. W. (1993). *The mental status: Examination in neurology* (p. 48). Philadelphia: F. A. Davis.
5. Benarroch, E. E., Westmoreland, B. F., Daube, J. R., Reagan, T. J., & Sandok, B. A. (1999). *Medical neurosciences: An approach to anatomy, pathology, and physiology by systems and levels* (4th ed., p. 568). Philadelphia: Lippincott Williams & Wilkins.
6. Haerer, A. F. (1992). *DeJong's the neurological examination* (5th ed., p. 91). Philadelphia: Lippincott Williams & Wilkins.
7. Goetz, C. G., & Pappert, E. J. (1999). *Textbook of clinical neurology* (pp. 191–192). Philadelphia: W. B. Saunders.
8. Masferrer, R. (2000). Advanced neurological assessments: Clinical and radiographic correlations. Presented at the Eighth International Nurse Practitioner Conference, San Diego, California, September, 28, 2000.
9. Adams, R. D., Victor, M., & Ropper, A. H., (Eds.) (1997). *Principles of neurology* (6th ed., p. 357). New York: McGraw-Hill.
10. Simon, R. P., Aminoff, M. J., & Greenberg, D. A. (Eds.) (1999). *Clinical neurology* (4th ed., pp. 312–314). Stamford, CT: Appleton & Lange.

RESOURCES
Professional

Published Material

Adams, R. D., Victor, M., & Ropper, A. H. (Eds.). (1997). *Principles of neurology* (6th ed.). New York: McGraw-Hill.

Albert, M. S., Levkoff, S. E., Reilly, C. U., Liptzin, B., Pilgrim, D., Cleary, P. D, et al. (1992). The delirium symptom interview: An interview for the detection of delirium symptoms in hospitalized patients. *Journal of Geriatric Psychiatry and Neurology, 5,* 14–21.

Anthony, J. C., Le Resche, L., Niaz, U., Koff, M. R., & Folstein, M. (1982). Limits of the mini-mental state as a screening test for dementia and delirium among hospitalized patients. *Psychological Medicine, 12,* 397–408.

Benarroch, E. E., Westmoreland, B. F., Daube, J. R., Reagan, T. J., & Sandok, B. A. (1999). *Medical neurosciences: An approach to anatomy, pathology, and physiology by systems and levels* (4th ed.). Philadelphia: Lippincott Williams & Wilkins.

Bickley, L. S. (1999). *Bates's guide to physical examination and history taking* (7th ed.). Philadelphia: Lippincott Williams & Wilkins.

Brazis, P. W., Masdeu, J. C., & Biller, J. (1996). *Localization in clinical neurology* (3rd ed.). Boston: Little, Brown.

DeGowin, R. L. (1994). *DeGowin & DeGovin's diagnostic examination* (6th ed). New York: McGraw-Hill.

Fuller, G. (1993). *Neurologic examination made easy.* New York: Churchill Livingstone.

Guarantors of Brain. (2000). *Aids to the examination of the peripheral nervous system* (4th ed.). Edinburgh: W. B. Saunders.

Goldberg, S. (1987). *The four-minute neurologic exam.* Miami, FL: MedMaster, Inc.

Haerer, A. F. (1992). *DeJong's the neurological examination* (5th ed). Philadelphia: Lippincott Williams & Wilkins.

Hoppenfeld, S. (1976). *Physical examination of the spine and extremities.* Norwalk, CT: Appleton & Lange.

Hoppenfeld, S. (1977). *Orthopaedic neurology: A diagnostic guide to neurologic levels.* Philadelphia: J. B. Lippincott.

Miller, N. R., & Newman, N. J. (1999). *Walsh & Hoyt's clinical neuro-ophthalmology—the essentials* (5th ed.). Baltimore: Williams & Wilkins.

Misulis, K. E. (1998). *Disorders of mental status: Dementia, encephalopathy, coma, syncope.* Boston: Butterworth-Heinemann.

Simon, R. P., Aminoff, M. J., & Greenberg, D. A. (Eds.). (1999). *Clinical neurology* (4th ed). Stamford, CT: Appleton & Lange.

Strub, R. L., & Black, F. W. (1993). *The mental status examination in neurology* (3rd ed.). Philadelphia: F. A. Davis.

Swartz, M. H. (1994). *Textbook of physical diagnosis: History and examination* (2nd ed.). Philadelphia: W. B. Saunders.

Wiebers, D. O., Dale, A. J. D., Kokmen, E., & Swanson, J. W. (Eds.). (1998). *Mayo clinic examinations in neurology* (7th ed.). St. Louis: Mosby.

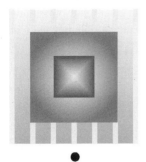

CHAPTER **8**

Neurological Assessment

JOANNE V. HICKEY

The purposes of this chapter are (1) to provide an overview for establishing and updating a database for a hospitalized neuroscience patient, and (2) to provide a framework for understanding the purpose, organization, and interpretation of data from the systematic neurological assessment conducted at the bedside. Some content that appears in Chapter 7 has also been included in this chapter for the convenience of the reader.

ESTABLISHING A NURSING DATABASE

On admission of a patient, the nurse begins to collect a comprehensive database by completing a nursing admission history and general admission assessment before conducting a neurological assessment. Most nursing departments have adopted a specific format for this purpose as part of their documentation system. The data may be entered in a written format or typed into a computerized documentation system. Regardless of how the data are entered or stored, the database is the foundation for ongoing assessment, planning, implementation, and evaluation of care and outcomes. The database is key to maintain continuity of care across levels of care through discharge and follow-up.

One section of the database includes demographics, route and circumstances of admission, vital signs, weight, and other general information (e.g., eyeglasses, hearing aid). The largest section includes a comprehensive systematic assessment often based on body systems or functional patterns. The circumstances of admission affect data collection. Ideally, the nurse has an opportunity to interview the patient and family on admission. The interview is not only a mechanism for gathering data and dispensing information, but also an opportunity to establish rapport with the patient and family. However, if the patient is unable to provide information, a family member may be able to help.

Throughout the interview, the nurse should be alert for any misconceptions or misunderstandings held by the patient or family. Information should be corrected and clarified as necessary and appropriate referrals made. There often is a section to identify high-risk patients and families who have problems that will affect recovery negatively, such as drug abuse or family dysfunction. Early identification can result in timely interventions and referrals.

For a patient with altered consciousness or cognitive deficits, enlist a family member to learn about the patient's personality and behavior before the current illness. This baseline information is useful for future comparison throughout the course of hospitalization. In the event of an emergency admission, some data gathering will be postponed until the patient is stabilized or family can be reached. As soon as possible, the nurse should interview the patient and family to develop a written or computerized plan of care. If care maps are used, the appropriate care map should be reviewed and modified as necessary.

The neurological assessment is the core nursing database for identifying nursing diagnoses and collaborative problems and for planning care. The accuracy of these assessment data and the nurse's critical thinking skills form the foundation of neuroscience nursing practice.

The taxonomy of nursing diagnoses may be a helpful framework to use when analyzing data from neurological assessment. However, there are many collaborative problems that can be identified requiring an interdisciplinary collaborative approach. For example, *increased intracranial pressure* (ICP) is a problem that requires collaboration of the entire health care team. A patient with increased ICP will require supportive and restorative care, along with definitive treatment for the underlying cause. Nurses participate as collaborative team members with physicians, physical therapists, occupational therapists, speech therapists, physiatrists, nutritionists, and social workers to provide for the comprehensive needs of patients. Care includes various supportive, preventive, maintenance, and restorative strategies. Examples of collaborative problems includes safety measure to prevent falls and injury, prevention of the complications of immobility, adaptation of activities of daily living (ADLs), maintenance of a patent airway, maintenance of adequate blood pressure to prevent ischemia or hemorrhagic strokes, and nutritional-hydration support.

OVERVIEW OF NEUROLOGICAL ASSESSMENT

Purposes

The purposes of the care nurse's neurological assessment are different, in some respects, from those conducted by the physician, the advanced practice nurse, and other health care professionals. The care nurse's purposes are to:

- Establish a neurological database
- Identify the presence of nervous system dysfunction
- Determine the effects of nervous system dysfunction on ADLs and independent function
- Detect life-threatening situations
- Compare current data to previous assessment data to determine trends and need for change in interventions
- Provide a database on which nursing diagnoses and collaborative problems will be based

A baseline assessment of neurological signs is made to determine deviations and trends in clinical status. A comparison is made between current assessment data and previously collected data to determine whether neurological signs are stable, deteriorating, or improving. Changes in neurological signs may develop rapidly in a few minutes, or subtly over a period of hours, days, weeks, or even months. There are various sources from which information about the neurological status can be derived, including the nursing admission history and comprehensive assessment, nurses' notes, neurological assessment sheets, and intershift nurses' reports. Other parts of the medical record are also a rich source of data (e.g., comprehensive neurological examination) and should be reviewed.

Nursing management of the neurological patient is based on highly developed nursing assessment and clinical reasoning skills. The nurse must know which parameters to assess, the proper technique for assessment, the appropriate method of documentation, and how to interpret the data to decide what action, if any, should be taken.

In analyzing data from the neurological assessment, the following questions should be asked:

- What do I see?
- What does it mean?
- How does it relate to previous assessments?
- How am I going to proceed?

The third question, "How does it relate to previous assessments?" is critical because data are compared with the previous baseline assessments as well as trends of multiple datapoints over time to denote change. The assessment can reveal no change, subtle change, or dramatic change from previous findings. Generally, a change of any kind is important to note because it usually reflects an intracranial change.

A change in any of the parameters included in the neurological assessment must be considered in conjunction with changes in other areas evaluated in the assessment. For instance, a rapidly developing hematoma or cerebral edema will affect multiple assessment parameters, such as the level of consciousness (LOC) and motor function. If, however, the pupil appears to be dilated and fixed (a new finding from the previous assessment) and the patient continues to be well oriented and maintains motor function, then the pupillary signs should be rechecked and other possible explanations explored.

Critical thinking skills are inherent in this process, both to detect subtle and substantive changes in the neurological assessment data and overall clinical condition, and to incorporate this information within the context of the overall patient profile. Well-developed critical thinking skills are the foundation for all patient management decision making.

Components of the Neurological Assessment

The components included in a neurological assessment depend on the patient's state of consciousness and cooperativeness as well as clinical stability. A comprehensive baseline must be established. A **neurological assessment** is focused on selected critical components that are sensitive to change and that provide an overview of the patient's overall condition. The nurse must decide what other components, if any, should be added to best monitor the patient's condition. An assessment in the intensive care unit for an unconscious patient is quite different than the assessment in an intermediate care unit for a patient who is recovering from a stroke. This neurological assessment at a minimum includes:

- LOC (orientation and cognition)
- Pupillary signs
- Motor tone and strength (e.g., hand grasps, pronator drift, leg movement, motor strength of extremities)

FREQUENCY OF ASSESSMENT AND DOCUMENTATION

The frequency and extent of the neurological assessment will depend on the stability of the patient and the underlying condition. For a stable patient who is doing well, an assessment may be ordered every 4 to 8 hours. However, a patient who is very unstable may warrant assessment every 5 to 15 minutes to monitor changes and the need for intervention. The nurse should use independent clinical judgment to determine the need to assess the patient more frequently or to expand the assessment to include more parameters.

Most facilities use a standardized neurological assessment sheet or computerized assessment template to document neurological parameters. Sometimes, it is necessary to add a narrative description to expand on the data recorded or to add other pertinent information to the data set. Most forms or computer documentation systems allow for these important entries.

CONCEPT OF CONSCIOUSNESS

Consciousness is a state of general awareness of oneself and the environment and includes the ability to orient toward new stimuli. It results from a diffuse yet organized neuronal system located in the brain stem, diencephalon, and cerebral hemispheres.

Consciousness is divided into two components:

- **Arousal** and **wakefulness:** the appearance of wakefulness; reflects activity of the reticular activating system
- **Content of consciousness:** cognitive mental functions; reflects cerebral cortex activity

The content of consciousness is largely a cerebral cortical function, whereas arousal requires both the cerebral hemispheres and the brain stem. Consciousness can be viewed as analogous to a double helix. The difficulties inherent in assessing altered consciousness and underlying pathological states, then, can be compared to the difficulty of trying to separate the strands of a double helix into distinct entities. As a result, consciousness terminology and concepts tend to be somewhat vague. For example, the level of arousal is described by terms such as *clouding of consciousness, drowsiness, obtundation, stupor,* or *coma,* and is assessed by evaluating the content of consciousness, especially as represented by the quality of the patient's perception of self and the environment. Because consciousness cannot be measured directly, it is estimated by observing behavioral indicators in response to stimuli. *Consciousness is the most sensitive indicator of neurological change;* as such, a change in the LOC is usually the first sign to be noted in neurological signs. Consciousness is a dynamic state that is subject to change; it can occur rapidly (within minutes) or very slowly, over a period of hours, days, or weeks. When an assessment is conducted, the patient's arousability and behavior merely provide an estimate of consciousness *at a given point in time.*

Anatomical and Physiological Basis of Consciousness

A centrally positioned neuronal system located in the brainstem, diencephalon, and cerebral hemispheres (i.e., from spinal cord to cerebral cortex) controls consciousness. This system includes portions of the brainstem reticular formation; neurochemically defined nuclear groups of the brain stem; thalamic nuclei; basal forebrain (portions of the ventral and medial cerebral hemispheres); ascending projections to the thalamus and cerebral cortex; and widespread areas of the cerebral cortex (Fig. 8-1).

The **reticular formation** (RF) is a complex network of nuclei and nerve fibers in the central portion of the brainstem, extending from the pyramidal decussation in the medulla to the basal forebrain area and thalamus. The term *reticular* means forming a network. The long radiating dendrites and axons have numerous collaterals that project for long distances centrally with many interconnections and afferent input from various sensory and motor sources.[1] The **reticular activating system** (RAS) is a part of the RF. The multiple ascending pathways, channeled through the RF, receive synaptic input from multiple sensory pathways and send sensory impulses to the thalamus and then to all parts of the cerebral cortex. These impulses, sent to different parts of the cerebral cortex, cause a sleeping person to awaken. Ongoing impulses keep a person alert and awake.

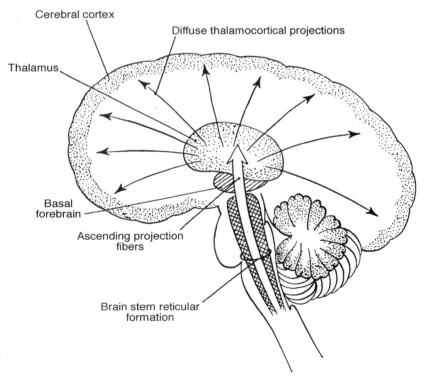

Figure 8–1 • Lateral view of the brain showing the components of the consciousness system.

Alterations in Consciousness

Degree of Dysfunction

Alteration of LOC can vary in severity from slight to severe. An altered LOC indicates brain dysfunction or brain failure. The longer the duration and the more severe the dysfunction, the less chance there is of complete recovery. LOC can change rapidly, as in association with an epidural hematoma, or very slowly over a period of weeks, as noted with a chronic subdural hematoma in an elderly person.

Major Causes

Alterations in the LOC may occur because of

- Direct destruction of the anatomical structures of consciousness by a disease process (structural)
- Toxic effects of endogenous or exogenous substances on the structures (metabolic)
- Alterations in the energy substrates necessary for function of the anatomical structures involved in consciousness (e.g., seizures)

Specifically, use the mnemonics "A-E-I-O-U" and "TIPSS" to recall the major causes of altered consciousness. **A-E-I-O-U** stands for **a**lcohol, **e**pilepsy, **i**nsulin, **o**pium, and **u**remia, whereas **TIPSS** stands for **t**umor, **i**njury, **p**sychiatric, **s**troke, and **s**epsis. A psychiatric cause should be considered only after all other possibilities have been ruled out.[2]

Coma

Various states of altered LOC are discussed in this chapter. However, a few points should be made about coma. Coma is the result of (1) bilateral, diffuse cerebral hemispheric dysfunction, (2) involvement of the brainstem (midbrain and pons, which includes the RAS), or both. A focal hemispheric lesion (e.g., small brain tumor) will not result in coma; only diffuse hemispheric conditions (e.g., diffuse cerebral edema) result in coma. Coma is not a disease itself, but reflects some underlying disease processes involving either (1) primary problems with the central nervous system (CNS) or (2) metabolic or systemic conditions. The following is a summary of the major causes of altered consciousness.[3]

Supratentorial Lesions

A lesion must affect the cerebral hemispheres **directly and widely** to cause diffuse bilateral cerebral hemispheric dysfunction and subsequent coma. Common lesions and associated secondary cerebral edema that can have diffuse effects on the brain include subcortical destructive lesions such as a thalamic lesion, hemorrhagic lesions (intracerebral, epidural, subdural hematomas), infarctions, tumors, abscesses, and head injuries.

Subtentorial (Infratentorial) Lesions

Subtentorial lesions **directly compress or destroy** the neurons of the RAS that lie in the central gray matter of the diencephalon, midbrain, and upper pons. Common compression lesions and associated secondary cerebral edema include basilar artery aneurysms, cerebellar or brainstem hemorrhage, abscess, tumor, or infarction. Common destructive lesions include pontine hemorrhage and brainstem infarction.

Metabolic Disorders

Altered consciousness may also be attributable to metabolic causes and systemic disease, such as deprivation of oxygen and other key metabolic requirements (hypoxia, ischemia hypoglycemia, or vitamin deficiency). It may also be caused by disease of organs excluding the brain, such as the following:

- Nonendocrine organs
  - Kidney (uremic coma)
  - Liver (hepatic coma)
  - Lungs (carbon dioxide narcosis)

- Hypofunction or hyperfunction of endocrine organs
  - Thyroid (myxedema and thyrotoxicosis)
  - Parathyroid (hypoparathyroidism and hyperparathyroidism)
  - Adrenals (Addison's disease, Cushing's disease, pheochromocytoma)
  - Pancreas (diabetes mellitus and hypoglycemia)

- Electrolyte and acid-base imbalance
- Pharmacological agents
  - Sedatives: barbiturates and nonbarbiturates, hypnotics, tranquilizers, ethanol, opiates, and bromides
  - Acidic toxins: paraldehyde, methyl alcohol, ethylene glycol, and ammonium chloride
  - Psychotropic drugs: amphetamines, lithium, tricyclic antidepressants, and others
  - Other drugs: such as steroids, cimetidine, salicylates, anticonvulsants

The most common metabolic causes of altered LOC seen in a hospitalized population are hypoxia, hypoglycemia, and sedative drug overdose. It is routine practice in most emergency departments to draw blood for glucose levels and toxicology screening, as necessary.

In assessing a comatose patient, the nurse should be aware that several problems outside the CNS can cause a decreased LOC. A comparison of the changes that accompany coma caused by metabolic disorders and those occurring with nervous system structural lesions is summarized in Table 8-1.

Level of Consciousness Assessment

The LOC is assessed by applying stimuli and observing the response. The technique used depends on the type of stimuli applied. Auditory and tactile stimuli are the two used to assess consciousness and are considered on a continuum (Fig. 8-2).

Auditory Stimuli

Sound is the stimulus that is applied first. A normal speaking voice is used initially. If the patient responds, then the nurse can talk to him or her and ask questions to assess orientation

Table 8-1 • COMPARISON OF COMA CAUSED BY METABOLIC AND CENTRAL NERVOUS SYSTEM STRUCTURAL LESIONS

OBSERVATION	METABOLIC COMA	CNS STRUCTURAL COMA
Motor system deficits	Diffuse abnormal motor signs (tremors, myoclonus, and, especially, asterixis); symmetrical	Focal abnormal signs that are unilateral; asymmetrical
Motor abnormalities	Coma precedes motor abnormalities	Coma follows motor abnormalities
Pupils	Bilaterally reactive	Unilaterally nonreactive, or later, bilaterally nonreactive
Progression of neurological deterioration	Partial dysfunction affects many levels of the CNS while other functions are retained	Orderly rostral-caudal deterioration with supratentorial lesions
Electroencephalogram	Diffusely but not locally slow	May show slowed activity, but will also show abnormal focal areas

and response to questions (discussed in the next section). If the patient does not respond to a normal voice volume, a louder voice or a loud noise, such as that produced by clapping the hands, is used. If a response is elicited, the nurse can then assess orientation by asking questions.

Tactile Stimuli

If there is no response to auditory stimulation, tactile stimulation is attempted. The patient's arm is gently shaken while calling his or her name. If no response is elicited by this means, painful (or noxious) stimuli are applied.

The most common method of applying painful stimuli is to apply firm pressure to the nail beds (fingernails) or webspaces between the fingers or toes and then observe the motor response (Fig. 8-3). However, this provides a peripheral stimulus; the response elicited *could* be a reflex response. A central stimulus, such as firmly grasping the trapezius or pectoralis major muscle, is another method of providing painful stimuli. The response elicited by a central stimulus is more reliable in comatose patients. Some practitioners suggest using the "sternal rub" (vertically rubbing the tissue along the sternum). However, the soft tissue above the sternum bruises easily in most people. Applying supraorbital pressure is another form of stimulus; it is not recommended if a facial fracture is possible. Motor response to painful stimuli is classified according to the following categories:

Purposeful: withdraws from the painful stimuli and crosses midline; may push the examiner's hand away (seen in light coma)

Nonpurposeful: the stimulated area moves slightly, without any attempt to withdraw from the source of pain; painful

stimuli to the pectoralis or trapezius may result in a contraction of a muscle or muscles, such as the quadriceps or biceps, but the arm does not cross midline

Unresponsive: patient shows no signs of reacting to painful stimuli (seen in deep coma)

IDENTIFYING THE LEVELS OF CONSCIOUSNESS

There is no internationally accepted taxonomy of definitions with which to label LOC, nor is there agreement on the definitive manifestations of the various stages of consciousness. Therefore, no precise terminology exists for conveying information about a patient from one clinician to another. This creates confusion in accurately assessing patients. As a result, the Glasgow Coma Scale is used universally to decrease the subjectivity and confusion associated with assessing LOC in acute situations.

Consciousness can be viewed as a crude continuum, anchored by full consciousness at one end and deep coma on the opposite end (Fig. 8-4). Despite the problems with precise terminology, there are several commonly used terms to describe gradations of consciousness (Table 8-2).

Confusion exists in describing the comatose state because of variations in the definition of coma and the inability to measure consciousness directly. Most texts classify depth of

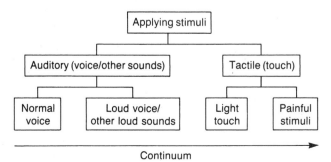

Figure 8-2 • Assessment of consciousness: Applying stimulation.

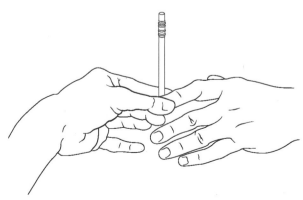

Figure 8-3 • Applying pressure to the fingernails is one kind of stimulus used in assessing the patient's level of consciousness.

Full consciousness	Confusion	Lethargy	Obtundation	Stupor	Coma		
					Light coma	Coma	Deep coma

Figure 8–4 • Continuum of consciousness. Arousal/wakefulness includes a wide range of levels that can be conceptualized as a crude continuum with "full consciousness" as the anchor on one end and "deep coma" as the anchor on the other end.

coma by correlating motor responsiveness (purposeful, non-purposeful, and unresponsive) with painful stimuli with LOC. Clinicians attest that there are gradations of coma, based on motor responsiveness to painful stimuli, which are helpful in evaluating a patient's neurological condition in the clinical setting.

For the purposes of this discussion, **coma** is defined as a sustained pathological state of unconsciousness and unresponsiveness that includes three gradations: light coma (sometimes called semicoma), coma, and deep coma. The critical element that differentiates depth of coma is the response to painful stimuli:

Light coma (semicoma): unarousable; no spontaneous movement noted; withdraws *purposefully* to painful stimuli; usually, the brainstem reflexes, such as the gag, corneal, and pupillary reflexes, are intact.

Coma: unarousable; withdraws *nonpurposefully* to painful stimuli; brainstem reflexes may or may not be intact; decorticate or decerebrate posturing may be present.

Deep coma: unarousable; *unresponsive* to painful stimuli; brainstem reflexes are generally absent; decerebrate posturing or flaccidity is usually present.

THE GLASGOW COMA SCALE

The **Glasgow Coma Scale** (GCS), developed in Glasgow, Scotland, in 1974 is widely used in the United States and internationally for assessment of comatose patients. The scale was developed to standardize observations for the objective and accurate assessment of LOC. The GCS is especially useful for monitoring changes during the first few days after acute injury or in unstable comatose patients.

The scale is divided into three subscales: eye opening, best verbal response, and best motor response (Fig. 8-5). Each subscale has a variety of categories. The information collected can be plotted on a graph to provide a visual record of deterioration, improvement, or stabilization. In interpreting the GCS, the numeric values of each subscale are added for a total score. The range of possible scores is 3 to 15. A score of 15 indicates a fully alert, oriented person, whereas a score of 3, the lowest possible score, indicatives deep coma. Patients with a score of 8 are often unconscious. They require a high standard of nursing care appropriate for an unconscious patient. These patients usually need to be in an intensive care setting.

Table 8–2 • LEVELS OF CONSCIOUSNESS

TERMS	DEFINITIONS	COMMENT
Full consciousness	Awake, alert, and oriented to time, place, and person; comprehends the spoken and written word and is able to express ideas verbally or in writing	Demonstrates reliable and responsible behavior
Confusion	Disoriented in time, place, or person; initially becomes disoriented to time, then to place, and, finally, to person; shortened attention span; memory difficulty is common; becomes bewildered easily; has difficulty following commands; exhibits alterations in perception of stimuli; may have hallucinations; may be agitated, restless, irritable, and increasingly confused at night	High risk for falls and injury Requires frequent observation and supervision High risk for falls and injury
Lethargy	Oriented to time, place, and person; very slow and sluggish in speech, mental processes, and motor activities; responds appropriately to painful stimuli	High risk for falls and injury Pull up side rails Needs frequent observation and supervision
Obtundation	Arousable with stimulation; responds verbally with a word or two; can follow simple commands appropriately when stimulated (e.g., when asked to stick out tongue); otherwise appears very drowsy; responds appropriately to painful stimuli	High risk for injury Unable to assume any responsibility for self; needs complete care
Stupor	Lies quietly with minimal spontaneous movement; generally unresponsive except to vigorous and repeated stimuli; incomprehensible sounds and/or eye opening may be noted; responds appropriately to painful stimuli	High risk for injury Unable to assume any responsibility for self; needs complete care
Coma	Appears to be in a sleeplike state with eyes closed; does not respond appropriately to bodily or environmental stimuli; does not make any verbal sounds; differentiation of coma level is based on motor response to painful stimuli	High risk for injury and aspiration Needs standard of care appropriate for comatose, completely dependent patient Priority of care is maintaining patent airway

Scoring of Eye Opening

- 4 Opens eyes spontaneously when the nurse approaches
- 3 Opens eyes in response to speech (normal or shout)
- 2 Opens eyes only to painful stimuli (*e.g.*, squeezing of nail beds)
- 1 Does not open eyes to painful stimuli

Scoring of Best Motor Response

- 6 Can obey a simple command, such as "Lift your left hand off the bed"
- 5 Localizes to painful stimuli and attempts to remove source
- 4 Purposeless movement in response to pain
- 3 Flexes elbows and wrists while extending lower legs to pain
- 2 Extends upper and lower extremities to pain
- 1 No motor response to pain on any limb

Scoring of Best Verbal Response

- 5 Oriented to time, place, and person
- 4 Converses, although confused
- 3 Speaks only in words or phrases that make little or no sense
- 2 Responds with incomprehensible sounds (*e.g.*, groans)
- 1 No verbal response

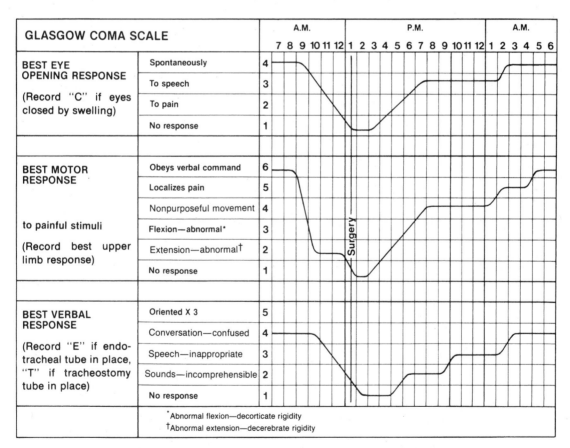

Figure 8–5 • Glasgow coma scale.

CHANGES IN LEVEL OF CONSCIOUSNESS

Changes in the LOC are, to some extent, predictable in that a patient who has been in a coma and now is arousable with repeated stimulation is described as displaying improvement in LOC. Clinicians frequently say "The patient appears to be lighter." What they are actually implying is that the deteriorated LOC appears to have improved since the last examination or the overall trend is one of improvement. The crude continuum of LOC aids the clinician in assessing changes in the patient's condition. It is possible, and indeed probable, that all the levels of consciousness are not observable in a particular patient as he or she recovers from injury.

A few final points about the LOC should be kept in mind:

1. A patient with a head injury who is evaluated during the posttraumatic period may arrive at an extended plateau of consciousness in the recovery process. For example, a patient can be comatose for a period of time and then become restless and agitated. This state may persist for days before it is followed by full consciousness. The pattern of recovery is based on the type, extent, and site of the injury and secondary injuries.
2. If the patient is sedated with very short-acting drugs such as propofol, turn off the drug about 10 minutes before assessing the patient so that the drug's effect will not cloud assessment of LOC.
3. It is important to record the time of observation of postoperative patients who have undergone intracranial surgery. It makes a great difference whether there is a 1-hour or 4-hour interval between observations that indicate how rapidly the neurological status of the patient might be changing following surgery.
4. Recovery from an altered LOC is influenced by age, type of injury, and premorbid health status. Younger patients (especially those under 20 years) have a much better prognosis for recovery than do older patients.
5. As a rule, the longer the coma, the worse the outcome. Absence of corneal, gag, pupillary, or oculocephalic responses initially or during the course of illness indicates a poor outcome. Decortication, decerebration, or flaccidity of the motor system also denotes a poor prognosis.

Special States of Altered Consciousness

According to Plum and Posner, nearly all comatose patients begin to awaken from their comatose state within 2 to 4 weeks after injury, regardless of the severity of brain damage, if they survive at all.[4] After a sleep-wakefulness cycle has been reestablished, the patient is no longer comatose, even though there is no apparent awareness of or interaction with the environment. A few special states of altered consciousness are seen and discussed in the clinical setting and in the literature. These special states include persistent vegetative state and locked-in syndrome. Brain death is also discussed (Chart 8-1). See Chart 8-2 for nursing management of the patient with an altered LOC. It usually requires interdisciplinary collaborative efforts to manage a comatose patient.

Cognition

Assessment

Consciousness has been conceptualized as having two components: arousal and content. Arousal has already been discussed in the previous section. **Content** represents the sum of cognitive and affective function and is controlled by the cerebral cortex. As part of the assessment of LOC, the nurse assesses orientation to time, place, and person. However, this provides limited information about the patient's overall cognitive function. Therefore, in the awake patient, the nurse conducts a cognitive assessment, or mental status examination, to determine the effect of neurological disease on the patient's ability to function in day-to-day living.

There are several areas to address in cognitive assessment (see Chapter 7). The following list includes the major areas covered in a mental status assessment:

- Orientation to time, place, and person
- Attention and vigilance (the ability to sustain attention over a period of time) as well as the ability to focus and concentrate on a task, which requires self-regulation and screening out of distracting environmental stimuli
- Memory (immediate, short-term, long-term)
- General fund of information (e.g., name the presidents starting with current president and going back from the present)
- Language and speech demonstrating an understanding of the written and spoken word, as well as the ability to use language appropriately (e.g., identifying any difficulty with word finding or misuse of words) (see Chapter 7, Table 7-4)
- Calculation
- Abstract thinking, reasoning, problem solving, insight, and judgment
- Special integrative function (skilled motor acts for apraxias, and motor-sensory integration for agnosias)
- Construction ability (ability to draw or copy on command; helpful to identify neglect syndrome)

Assessment of Cognitive Function at the Bedside

In clinical practice, the question of how much of the mental status examination should be conducted and how frequently should particular parameters be assessed is raised. The answer is, "it depends." It depends on the type of clinical setting, the patient's level of consciousness and ability to cooperate, and the purposes of the assessment. In the acute care setting, especially in the intensive care environment, the LOC is usually so depressed that assessing higher-level function is impossible. As the patient begins to regain consciousness, an abbreviated bedside assessment will help the clinician to determine progress. For example, asking the patient to show you two fingers is a simple command that requires understanding of the spoken word and the motor ability to respond to the command. The following is a sample of questions that can be asked at the bedside to assess cognitive and motor function:

- What is the name of this place?
- What is the date?
- Show me two fingers.

CHART 8 – 1 • Special States of Altered Consciousness and Brain Death

PERSISTENT VEGETATIVE STATE

Vegetative state is a term used to describe a subacute or chronic condition that usually occurs following severe cerebral injury. When the condition lasts for a month, it is called **persistent vegetative state (PVS).** Other terms formerly used to describe the vegetative state were *coma vigil* and *irreversible coma.*

Discussion about the definition and clinical course of PVS has been a topic of intense interest in the last few years and has raised many ethical questions about quality of life. In 1989, the American Academy of Neurology published guidelines on the vegetative state.* The Multi-Society Task Force on PVS has built on their work.

The Multi-Society Task Force on PVS defines **vegetative state** as a clinical condition of complete unawareness of the self and the environment, accompanied by sleep-wake cycles, with either complete or partial preservation of hypothalamic and brain-stem autonomic functions. In addition, patients in a vegetative state:†

- Show no evidence of sustained, reproducible, purposeful, or voluntary behavioral responses to visual, auditory, tactile, or noxious stimuli
- Show no evidence of language comprehension or expression
- Show no bowel or bladder control
- Cannot experience pain
- Demonstrate variable patterns of preserved cranial nerve and spinal reflexes (e.g., pupillary light response, corneal, gag); primitive reflexes (e.g., grasping, sucking)
- Maintain vital signs and spontaneous respirations
- Have open eyes and spontaneous eye movement. Sometimes the patient's eyes appear to follow people in the room; however, he or she is unable to follow a command to look in a particular direction.

Further, **PVS** is defined as a vegetative state present 1 month after acute traumatic or nontraumatic brain injury or lasting for at least 1 month in patients with degenerative or metabolic disorders or developmental malformations.

The clinical course and outcome of PVS depend on its cause. The Task Force identifies three categories of disorder that can cause PVS:‡

- Acute traumatic and nontraumatic brain injuries
- Degenerative and metabolic brain disorders
- Severe congenital malformations of the nervous system

Recovery of consciousness is unlikely or rare for both adults and children in the following situations:

- Posttraumatic PVS after 12 months
- Nontraumatic PVS after 3 months
- Degenerative metabolic disorders or congenital malformations after several months

The life expectancy of all PVS patients is substantially reduced; survival ranges from 2 to 5 years; survival beyond 10 years is very unusual.

PVS presents special ethical, moral, and legal issues that will be discussed in Chapter 4.

LOCKED-IN SYNDROME

The term **locked-in syndrome** refers to a state in which full consciousness and cognition are intact but severe paralysis of the voluntary motor system makes movement and communications impossible.†§ Usual cause is the interruption of the descending corticobulbar and corticospinal tracts at or below the pons; however, breathing is left intact. The locked-in syndrome can also be associated with peripheral motor neuron disease or paralysis produced with neuromuscular blocking drugs. Patients with this version of the locked-in syndrome can usually establish simple communications through eye blinking and vertical eye movement. The locked-in syndrome may be seen in certain cerebrovascular diseases with ventral pontine infarction and such conditions as myasthenia gravis and poliomyelitis. The diagnosis is established by clinical examination.

(continued)

CHART 8 – 1 • Special States of Altered Consciousness and Brain Death (Continued)

BRAIN DEATH

Brain death is a state of irreversible loss of both cortical and brain-stem activity.|| It is characterized by irreversible coma and apnea; all brainstem reflexes and cranial nerve function is lost. The diagnosis of brain death is made based on requirements in three areas:¶

- Absence of brainstem reflexes
- Absence of cortical activity
- Demonstration that this state is irreversible

Criteria have been established for the diagnosis of brain death but are still controversial. These criteria and their implications for nurses in managing the patient and family are discussed in Chapter 4.

* American Academy of Neurology. (1989). Position of the American Academy of Neurology on certain aspects of the care and management of the persistent vegetative state patient. *Neurology, 39,* 125–126.

† Multi-Society Task Force on PVS. (1994). Medical aspects of the persistent vegetative state (Part 2). *New England Journal of Medicine, 330*(22), 1572–1579.

‡ Multi-Society Task Force on PVS, p. 1573.

§ Plum & Posner, 1980 (see ref. 4); American Academy, 1989.

|| Barnat, J. L., Culver, C. M., Nelson, J. R., et al. (1981). On the definition of death. *Annals of Internal Medicine, 94,* 389–395.

¶ Barnat et al.: President's Commission for the Study of Ethical Problems in Medicine and Biomedical and Behavioral Research. (1981). *Defining death: Medical, legal, and ethical issues in the determination of death.* Washington, D.C.: U. S. Government Printing Office.

- Stick out your tongue.
- Look toward me.
- Wiggle your thumb or toes.
- How much is a quarter, a dime, and a nickel?

Some cognitive functions are assessed within the context of providing care and observing the patient during ADLs. Deficits may be obvious because of their impact on ADLs. Higher-level deficits may be subtle because the patient may appear to be functional, having devised ways to compensate for deficits. Standardized instruments such as the Mini-Mental Status Examination[5] (see Chapter 7) may also be used to assess cognitive function. The Rancho Los Amigos Scale (see Chapter 13) is another tool used in rehabilitative settings for determining behavioral patterns and includes interventions for various behavioral patterns. The general collaborative problem of **cognitive deficits** may be made. It will require interdisciplinary collaboration to define the particular deficits present and to develop and implement a collaborative plan of care.

RECOVERY AND REHABILITATION

Some improvement in cognitive function is often evident during the course of acute hospitalization due to the natural recovery of the brain. Most natural recovery occurs in the first 3 to 6 months after injury; recovery can still occur after this time, but at a much slower rate. Many patients will have persistent cognitive deficits that will require rehabilitation. In most hospitals, the occupational therapist can perform a short (approximately 30 minutes) cognitive assessment screening to determine areas affected by cognitive deficits. If necessary, a neuropsychologist can conduct a detailed cognitive assessment (several hours) to pinpoint deficits and develop a treatment program. Often, a consultation with the neuropsychologist is postponed to allow for natural recovery. Specific patient management will depend on the overall assessment. Some patients will require only short-term cognitive rehabilitation whereas others will require long-term treatment.

CRANIAL NERVE ASSESSMENT

Occasionally, the nurse may be required to conduct a comprehensive cranial nerve assessment at the time of admission to establish a baseline (see Chapter 7) and at key critical points such as postoperatively. In the real world of clinical practice, however, cranial assessment is often abbreviated. There are two reasons for this. First, the patient may be unable to cooperate and follow specific commands (e.g., smile; stick out the tongue) or to report subjective changes in neurological function (e.g., double vision). The inability to cooperate or to participate is often the result of altered consciousness (e.g., coma) or cognitive-perceptual deficits. Second, after a comprehensive assessment, it is often appropriate to tailor the assessment to the patient's specific condition.

Such tailoring implies an understanding of the pathophysiology of the specific condition and the need to monitor specific functions that are at high risk for dysfunction. For example, a patient who is admitted with a diagnosis of an acoustic neuroma (a tumor involving the eighth cranial

CHART 8-2 • Nursing Management of the Patient With an Altered Level of Consciousness

The following are some basic management points for a patient with altered level of consciousness (LOC):

1. **Maintaining a patient airway is a top priority.** The patient should not be left lying on his or her back because of the increased possibility of aspiration. Position to facilitate drainage of oral secretions.

2. A change in the LOC is the **most sensitive indicator of neurological change** and, therefore, the first neurological sign that changes with altered neurological status. The LOC should be assessed periodically (as often as every 5 to 10 minutes in the acute, unstable patient and every 4 hours in the stable patient). Regardless of all the technological advances in health care, the observations of the nurse who knows the patient are still the most sensitive "sensors" of neurological changes. The nurse who is well acquainted with the personality and behavior pattern of the patient can best evaluate whether behavior changes are caused by pain, fatigue, or neurological deterioration. The nurse has the responsibility of advising the physician of changes in the LOC.

3. When the LOC has deteriorated, the nurse should talk to the patient in a calm, normal, reassuring voice, explaining in simple terms what is being done and orienting him or her to the environment. If the patient normally wears glasses or a hearing aid, they should be worn.

4. When talking to the patient, the nurse should try to screen out external environmental stimuli that might increase confusion. Also, a group of people entering the room and talking to the patient can be both overwhelming and confusing. In essence, it creates a sensory overload for fragile, recovering neurological circuits and can result in confusion and misinterpretation of stimuli.

5. After patients begin to awaken and verbalize, they often recognize a void of time for which they cannot account. This can be very frightening. The nurse should fill the gaps of time by briefly recounting what has happened during the lapse. Also, when the patient begins to make incorrect statements, the nurse should matter-of-factly correct any misconceptions.

6. The nurse is responsible for **protecting the patient from injury.** As the LOC deteriorates, the nurse must assume total responsibility for the patient's safety. The methods employed depend on the availability of staff (usually fewer staff on evenings and nights), the patient's degree of agitation and impulsive behavior, the location of his or her room in relationship to the nurses' station, and the use of supportive equipment (ventilator, CVP and IV lines, ICP monitoring catheter, and others). Regardless of the circumstances, the standard of care for this patient requires much more nursing time and intervention than that required for an alert, oriented patient. The nurse should observe the patient frequently; talk in a calm manner; maintain the bed in low position, unless contraindicated; maintain all siderails in up position; and use restraints as necessary to protect the patient from injury, according to hospital policy.

7. Nighttime and darkness often lead the patient to misinterpretation of environmental and other stimuli. A night light and periodic visits by the nurse can help to control confusion, fear, and hallucinations.

8. The family and other visitors need instruction about how to visit a patient with altered LOC or cognitive functions. The specific guidelines will depend on the particular patient. The nurse should be available to intervene if problems occur during the visit, as well as to evaluate the effects of the visit on the patient and the visitors. If the patient is upset, the possible reasons for the reaction should be explored. Family members may need support after the visit to express their concerns and fears.

---

nerve [CN]) requires assessment of CN VIII function to determine hearing loss and vertigo. Assessment of function would also be required for CN V (sensory loss to the face), CN VII (deficits in motor function of the face), and CNs IX and X (loss of gag reflex or difficulty speaking). The reason for assessment of these cranial nerves is their anatomical proximity in the posterior fossa to CN VIII. As the tumor grows, it may impinge on a number of adjacent cranial nerves, causing dysfunction. Because consciousness is usually not affected by an acoustic neuroma, the patient is able to cooperate with the assessment.

Table 8-3 summarizes the components of cranial nerve assessment as conducted in actual clinical practice (see also Chapter 7). Pupillary signs are of particular importance and can be assessed in all patients regardless of LOC or ability to cooperate. Other CNs can be tested at the bedside only in conscious, responsive patients. Still other cranial nerves can be tested in both conscious and unresponsive patients, using alternative techniques. The following sections describe these practical bedside techniques.

ASSESSMENT OF VISUAL FIELDS (OPTIC NERVE)

The visual field can be easily and quickly assessed for a conscious, cooperative patient at the bedside. This is done by asking the patient to focus on your nose and then introducing a varying number of fingers with both hands simultaneously into the bilateral upper quadrants; repeat in the bilateral lower quadrants (see Chapter 7, Chart 7-1). You can quickly ascertain

Table 8–3 • SUMMARY OF CRANIAL NERVE ASSESSMENT AT THE BEDSIDE

CRANIAL NERVE	ASSESSMENT	COMMENTS
I Olfactory	**Sense of smell** Usually deferred	Deficits noted in only a few cases, usually with lesion in the parasellar area
II Optic	**Vision** Monitor while working with patient; observe for difficulty with ADLs Ask patient to identify how many fingers are being held up or to read menu or newspaper Use Rosenbaum Pocket Vision Screener to assess vision in each eye Monitor for visual field cuts by checking upper and lower quadrants while patient focuses on your nose	Common deficits; deficits can cause blindness in one eye, bitemporal hemianopsia, or homonymous hemianopsia
III Oculomotor	**Pupil constriction; elevation of upper eyelid** Assess size, shape, and direct light reaction of pupils	Changes are common with a number of progressing neurological problems
III Oculomotor, IV Trochlear, & VI Abducens	**Extraocular movement** Tested together in conscious, cooperative patient; ask patient to follow a pencil tip through the six cardinal eye movements	Deficits are common; inability to move the eyes in one or more directions is called strabismus
V Trigeminal	**Sensation to face; mastication muscles** Often deferred If assessed, patient must be cooperative and able to accurately report facial sensation from stimulation **Afferent limb of corneal reflex**	Deficits found in trigeminal neuralgia and sometimes with acoustic neuroma Corneal reflex assessed in trigeminal neuralgia; can assess reflex in unconscious patient
VII Facial	**Muscles for facial expression; efferent limb of corneal reflex** Ask cooperative patient to smile, show teeth, puff cheeks, wrinkle brow; observe for symmetry of face In comatose patient, tickle each nasal passage, one at a time, by inserting a cotton-tipped applicator; observe for facial movement	Total unilateral facial weakness called Bell's palsy Unilateral from below the eye and down, seen in stroke Note the difference between central and peripheral facial involvement
VIII Acoustic	**Hearing and balance** Usually deferred May note deficit while working with patient	Deficits with acoustic neuroma, cerebellar pontine angle tumors, Ménière's disease
IX Glossopharyngeal and X Vagus	**Palate, pharynx, vocal cords, and gag reflex;** tested together because of overlap In conscious patient, have patient open mouth and say "ah"; assess gag reflex Unconscious patient: assess gag reflex	Deficits common in posterior fossa lesions Gag reflex is a brain stem reflex and has prognostic value in unconscious patient
XI Spinal accessory	**Shrug shoulders and move head side to side** Usually deferred	Deficits common in posterior fossa lesions
XII Hypoglossal	**Movement of tongue** In conscious patient, ask him or her to stick out the tongue	Deficits common in posterior fossa lesions

Note: This table summarizes **assessment at the bedside.** Although a baseline assessment of all cranial nerves is recommended, this may not always be possible. In addition, although frequent assessment of particular cranial nerves is critical in certain conditions, it may be safely deferred in other conditions.

whether the patient has full visual fields or gaps in the visual fields such as those that occur with unilateral neglect. If a deficit is noted, further assessment may be necessary.

ASSESSMENT OF PUPILS (OCULOMOTOR NERVE)

Examination of the pupils is an extremely important part of patient assessment that can be carried out in either a conscious or unconscious patient. The general points to note when assessing the pupils include their size, shape, and reaction to light. Accommodation is **not** evaluated in every assessment. The findings in one pupil are always compared with the find-

ings in the other pupil, and differences between the two are noted. Data are documented in the neurological database.

Size

Normally, the pupils are equal in size, measuring about 2 to 6 mm in diameter with an average diameter of 3.5 mm. Two methods are used to record pupillary size: the millimeter scale (most common) and descriptive terms. If the millimeter scale is used, the examiner, using a diagrammatic gauge, estimates the size of each pupil by comparing the gauge with the patient's pupils (Fig. 8-6). The examiner then records a numeric value ranging from 2 to 9 mm to signify the size of each pupil. If descriptive terms are used to

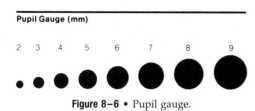

Pupil Gauge (mm)

2   3   4   5   6   7   8   9

Figure 8–6 • Pupil gauge.

evaluate the size of the pupils, the following terms are used: pinpoint, small, midposition, large, and dilated (Chart 8-3).

Shape

Shape is assessed simply by looking at the contour of the pupils. Normally, both pupils are round. Abnormal pupillary shapes are described as ovoid, keyhole, or irregular (Chart 8-4).

Reaction to Light

When light is shone into the eye, the pupil should immediately constrict. Withdrawal of the light should produce an immediate and brisk dilation of the pupil. This is called the **direct light reflex** (Fig. 8-7). Introducing the light into one pupil should cause similar constriction to occur simultaneously in the other pupil. When the light is withdrawn from one eye, the opposite pupil should dilate simultaneously. This response is called the **consensual light reaction.**

Pupillary reaction to light is recorded using descriptive terms or symbols (Chart 8-5). The descriptive terms that are used include brisk, sluggish, and nonreactive or fixed. Plus and minus signs are recorded if a symbol recording system is used. (Common abnormal pupillary responses and findings are found in Chart 8-6. Refer also to Chapter 7 for more information on pupillary assessment.)

CHART 8 – 3 • Nursing Assessment of Pupillary Size

In assessing pupillary size using either descriptive terms or a gauge, each pupil is assessed individually and then the findings for each pupil are compared. This is very important because pupils are normally equal (see note on anisocoria).

Descriptive Term	Definition	Findings
Pinpoint	The pupil is so small that it is barely visible or appears as small as a pinpoint.	Seen with opiate overdose, pontine hemorrhage, ischemia.
Small	The pupil appears smaller than average but larger than pinpoint.	Seen normally if the person is in a brightly lit place; also seen with miotic ophthalmic drops, opiates, pontine hemorrhage, Horner's syndrome, bilateral diencephalic lesions, and metabolic coma.
Midposition	When the pupil and iris are observed, about half of their diameter is iris and half is pupil.	Seen normally; if pupils are midposition and nonreactive, midbrain damage is the cause.
Large	The pupils are larger than average, but there is still an appreciable amount of iris visible.	Seen normally if room is dark; may be seen with some drugs, such as amphetamines; glutethimide (Doriden) overdose; mydriatics; cycloplegic agents; and some orbital injuries.
Dilated	When the pupil and iris are observed, one is struck by the largeness of the pupil with only the slightest ring of iris, which is barely visible.	Abnormal finding; bilateral, fixed, and dilated pupils are seen in the terminal stage of severe anoxia–ischemia or at death.

Note: **Anisocoria** is the term used to describe inequality in size between the pupils. About 17% of the population has slight anisocoria without any related pathological process. It is, therefore, important to make a baseline assessment of pupillary size and compare subsequent assessments with the baseline. If pupillary inequality is a new finding, it should be reported. If the patient is admitted with slight pupillary inequality and no other abnormalities are detected on the neurological assessment, the pupil inequality may not be significant.

CHART 8 – 4 • Nursing Assessment of Pupillary Shape

Descriptive Term	Definition	Findings
Round 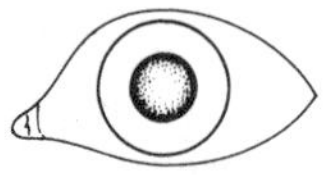	Like a circle	Normal findings
Ovoid 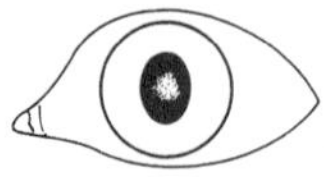	Slightly oval; "ovoid"	Almost always indicates intracranial hypertension and represents an intermediate phase between a normal pupil (round) and a fully dilated fixed pupil; an early sign of transtentorial herniation
Keyhole 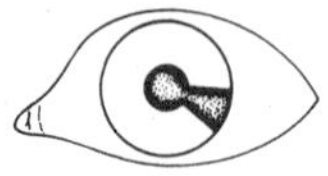	Like a keyhole	Seen in patients who have had an iridectomy (excision of part of the iris). An iridectomy is often part of cataract surgery, a common procedure in the elderly population. (The reaction to light is very slight.)
Irregular 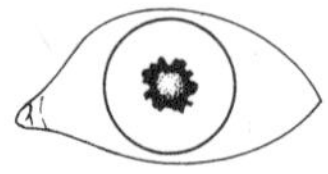	Jagged	Seen in Argyll-Robertson pupils and with traumatic orbital injuries

ASSESSMENT OF EXTRAOCULAR MOVEMENT (OCULOMOTOR, TROCHLEAR, AND ABDUCENS NERVES)

Extraocular movement and the position of the eyeballs are assessed. In the normal healthy person, one would expect the following:

- The eyes move conjugately in the orbital sockets.
- The eyes blink periodically.
- No nystagmus or abnormal eye movement is noted.
- The eyeball neither protrudes nor is sunken in the orbits.
- The upper eyelid does not droop and the palpebral fissures are equal bilaterally.

Some of the data are collected simply through focused observation of the patient for 10 ′ . 15 seconds. Other components require a cooperative patient.

ASSESSMENT OF THE CONSCIOUS, COOPERATIVE PATIENT

The Orbits (Eyeballs)

The position of the orbits within the sockets is assessed by observing the eyes frontally, in profile, and from above the patient's head. If no abnormality is noted, most clinicians will not comment about position in the documentation.

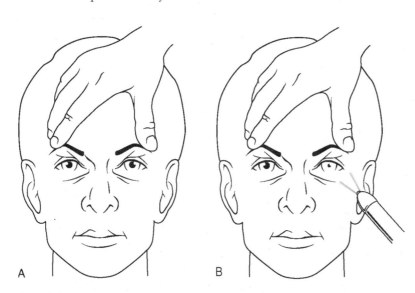

A   B

Figure 8–7 • Evaluating pupillary reactions by checking pupil size (*A*) and reaction to light (*B*).

CHART 8-5 • Nursing Assessment of Pupillary Light Responses

Descriptive Term	Symbol	Findings
Brisk	++	Normal finding
Sluggish	+	Found in conditions that cause some compression of the oculomotor nerve (cranial nerve III); seen in early transtentorial herniation, cerebral edema, and Adie's pupil
Nonreactive or fixed	−	Found in conditions that include compression of the oculomotor nerve; seen with transtentorial herniation syndromes and in severe hypoxia and ischemia (terminal stage just before death)
Swollen closed	c	One or both eyes are tightly closed because of severe periorbital edema; the pupillary light reflex may be difficult to assess.

> One other response—the Hippus phenomenon—is included; this does not usually appear on assessment sheets but may be observed in the clinical area and, therefore, needs to be recorded.

Hippus phenomenon	None	With uniform illumination of the pupil, dilation and contraction are noted. This may be considered normal if pupils are observed under high magnification. The Hippus phenomenon is also observed in patients who are beginning to experience pressure on the third cranial nerve. This is often associated with early transtentorial herniation.

Note: On some pupillary assessment sheets, other symbols are used in place of descriptive terms.

- Abnormal protrusion of one or both eyeballs is termed **proptosis or exophthalmos.**
- Abnormal recession of one or both eyelids is termed **enophthalmos.**

Eyelids

The patient is asked to look straight ahead; observations of each eye are then made and compared. The width of each palpebral fissure is observed. The palpebral fissure is the space between the upper and lower eyelid. Next, the position of the eyelid in relation to the pupil and iris is evaluated. Normally, the lid slightly covers the outer margin of the iris. A narrowed palpebral fissure usually indicates a droopy eyelid, also known as **ptosis.** Ptosis is seen in Horner's syndrome and conditions that affect the oculomotor nerve, such as transtentorial herniation syndromes and myasthenia gravis with ocular involvement.

Note the presence of edema of the eyelids. Edema can result from trauma to the orbit and may occur in the upper eyelid, the lower eyelid, or both.

Movement of the Eyes

Extraocular movement is assessed in conscious patients by asking them to follow a pencil or the examiner's finger through the six cardinal directions of gaze in an "H" sequencing (Fig. 8-8; also see Chapter 7, Fig. 7-7). Inability to move either eye in any direction should be noted. When both eyes move in the same direction, at the same speed, and maintain a constant alignment, the gaze is termed **conjugate gaze.** A lack of parallelism between the two

visual axes or movement in opposite directions is called **dysconjugate gaze.** If the dysfunction is limited to a specific movement or movements, an ophthalmoplegia is present. **Ophthalmoplegia** is defined as paralysis of one or more eye muscles (see Chapter 7, Table 7-9 for a summary of ophthalmoplegias).

The patient is asked whether double vision **(diplopia)** is present. If the answer is yes, is the double image side by side or one on top of the other? This will help determine if the problem is CN III (oculomotor) or CN VI (abducens) on the horizontal plane or CN III or CN IV (trochlear) on the vertical plane. See Chapter 7 for further discussion.

Abnormal Movements

The patient is asked to focus straight ahead and then to follow the examiner's finger (see Fig. 8-8). Any abnormal eye movements should be noted. **Nystagmus** is defined as involuntary movement of an eye, which may be horizontal, vertical, rotary, or mixed in direction. The tempo of the movements can be regular, rhythmical, pendular, or jerky, with the movement having a fast and slow component. Nystagmus can result from several problems. If present, the nurse should document the characteristics of the movement and include any information about related characteristics (e.g., focusing the eye in a certain direction). Specific types of nystagmus are found in Chapter 7, Table 7-10. Periodic blinking is normal and expected. The nurse should assess blinking by observing the patient. In association with some conditions, such as Parkinson's disease, blinking is decreased.

ASSESSMENT OF THE COMATOSE PATIENT

General Observations

The comatose patient appears to be in a sleeplike state, with or without the eyes closed. If the eyes are closed, the eyelids can gently be raised to inspect the position and movement of the eyes. The eyes may assume a prolonged stare without any discernible movement, or they may move slowly from side to side. Absence of any movement suggests that the eye movement center in the brain stem is not functioning. This is a poor prognostic sign. Conversely, slow movement from side to side indicates an intact brain stem. See Chapter 7 for assessment of the unconscious patient.

CHART 8 – 6 • Common Abnormal Pupillary Responses (*Note*: Compare findings with previous assessment data, document, and report new findings to the physician.)

OCULOMOTOR NERVE COMPRESSION

Observation

One pupil (R) is larger than the other (L), which is of normal size. The dilated pupil (R) does not react to light, although the other pupil (L) reacts normally. Ptosis may be seen in the dilated pupil.

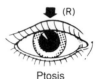

Ptosis

Interpretation

A dilated, nonreactive (fixed) pupil indicates that the control for pupillary constriction is not functioning. The parasympathetic fibers of the oculomotor nerve control pupillary constriction. The most common cause of interruption of this function is compression of the oculomotor nerve, usually against the tentorium or posterior cerebral artery.

Compression of the oculomotor nerve is caused most often by cerebral edema and uncal herniation on the same side of the brain as the dilated pupil.

Action

Compare with data from previous assessments. If the dilated pupil is a new finding, it should immediately be reported to the physician because the process of rostral-caudal downward pressure must be treated without delay. In this situation changes in LOC, motor function, sensory function, and possibly vital signs would be expected.

BILATERAL DIENCEPHALIC DAMAGE

Observation

On examination, the pupils appear small but equal in size, and both react to direct light, contracting when light is introduced and dilating when light is withdrawn.

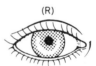

Interpretation

The sympathetic pathway that begins in the hypothalamus is affected. Because both pupils are equal in size and respond equally to light, the damage is bilateral. Therefore, it can be assumed that there is bilateral injury in the diencephalon (thalamus and hypothalamus).

Because metabolic coma can also result in bilaterally small pupils that react to light, this diagnostic possibility must be ruled out.

Action

Compare findings with previous assessments to determine change. Consider metabolic coma by reviewing blood chemistry findings and other data. For example, diabetic acidosis may result in a metabolic coma because of a high blood glucose level.

HORNER'S SYNDROME

Observation

One pupil (L) is smaller than the other (R), although both pupils react to light. The eyelid on the same side as the smaller pupil (L) droops (ptosis). Inability to sweat (anhidrosis) on the same side of the face as the ptosis is common. The symptoms of a small reactive pupil, ptosis, and anhidrosis combine to form Horner's syndrome.

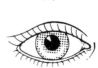

(continued)

CHART 8 – 6 • Common Abnormal Pupillary Responses (*Note*: Compare findings with previous assessment data, document, and report new findings to the physician.) (Continued)

HORNER'S SYNDROME (Continued)

Interpretation

There is an interruption of the ipsilateral sympathetic innervation to the pupil that can be caused by hypothalamic damage, a lesion of the lateral medulla or the ventrolateral cervical spinal cord, and, sometimes, by occlusion of the internal carotid artery.

Action

If this is a new finding, it should be reported.

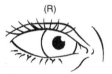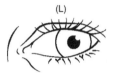

MIDBRAIN DAMAGE

Observation

Both pupils are at midposition and nonreactive to light.

Interpretation

With midposition, nonreactive pupils, neither sympathetic nor parasympathetic innervation is functional. This finding is often associated with midbrain infarction or transtentorial herniation.

Action

Compare findings with previous assessment data. Consider also changes in other components of the assessment. The pupils should be evaluated in conjunction with other neurologic assessments. Report new findings to the physician.

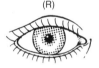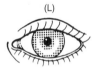

PONTINE DAMAGE

Observation

Very small (pinpoint), nonreactive pupils are seen.

Interpretation

This finding indicates focal damage of the pons often due to hemorrhage or ischemia. *Bilateral* pinpoint pupils may occur from opiate drug overdose, so this possibility should be ruled out.

Action

Compare findings with previous assessment data. Report findings to the physician immediately. Other changes in neurological status, such as a decreased LOC and respiratory abnormalities, would be expected.

BILATERAL DILATED UNREACTIVE PUPILS

Observation

Both pupils are dilated and nonreactive (fixed).

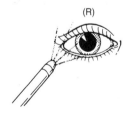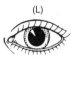

Interpretation

This finding is characteristic of the terminal stages of severe anoxia and death.

Action

Emergency action (code) is necessary to attempt to resuscitate the patient, although the possibility of reversal is low. Oxygen therapy at high concentrations and a patent airway must be ensured to provide oxygen for the ischemic cerebral cells. Other signs and symptoms of neurological deterioration will be present.

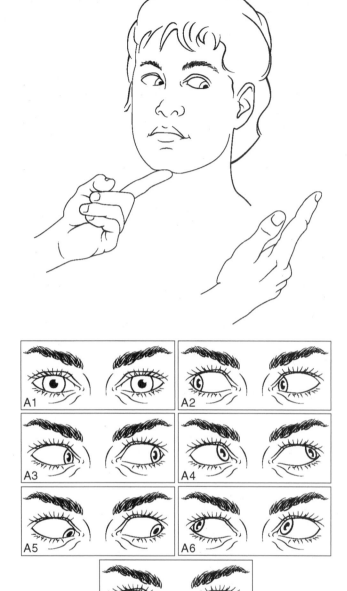

Figure 8−8 • Extraocular movements.

Eyelids

After the eyes are inspected, the eyelids are released. In coma, the lids slowly cover the eyes.

Eye Movement

Because the patient is unconscious and therefore unable to follow commands, voluntary eye movement cannot be assessed. Although not routinely done by the nurse, the physician may wish to evaluate the eye movement brainstem centers to determine if they are intact. For this evaluation, the **oculocephalic reflex (doll's eye response)** (see Fig. 7-20) or **oculovestibular reflex (cold caloric)** can be assessed,

provided there are no contraindications (see Fig. 7-21). (If the eyes do not move, the brainstem is involved and the patient most likely will not awaken.) The physician may choose to evaluate these reflexes in some patients to determine brain-stem function for prognostic purposes or as part of brain death criteria.

Frequency of Assessing Eye Movement

Ocular movement parameters do not change as rapidly as other parameters of the neurologic assessment. The nurse should assess eye movements once during a shift and more often if the patient is unstable.

Assessment of Facial Movement (Facial Nerve)

If the examiner wishes to assess the facial nerve in the conscious, cooperative patient, the patient is asked to smile and show his or her teeth while the examiner observes for symmetrical bilateral facial movements. In the unconscious patient, the easiest and quickest way to assess the facial nerve is to stimulate one nostril and then the other with a cotton-tipped applicator. The patient should respond to the stimulation with a facial contraction. The examiner can determine whether there is symmetrical bilateral facial movement.

Selected Reflexes

The corneal, gag, and swallowing reflexes, all brainstem reflexes, can be assessed in both the conscious and unconscious patient. These brainstem reflexes are helpful in determining the intactness of the brainstem. In the conscious patient or unconscious patient, touch each cornea with a wisp of cotton and observe for a blinking action. Another way to check the corneal reflex in an unconscious patient is to drop a small amount of water or saline (from a plastic ampule used for instillation while suctioning) onto the cornea. If the reflex is intact, the eye will blink. Recall that the corneal reflex is mediated by CNs V and VII.

To assess the gag and swallowing reflexes in the conscious patient, ask the patient to stick out his or her tongue so that a cotton-tipped applicator can be used to touch the posterior pharynx on each side. For an unconscious patient, gentle tugging on an endotracheal tube will cause gagging if the reflex is intact. Alternatively, a cotton-tipped applicator can be used to stimulate each side of the posterior pharynx. In both cases, there should be an immediate retraction of the pharynx or gagging if the reflex is intact. Recall that the gag and swallowing reflexes are mediated by cranial nerves IX and X. Checking these reflexes provides data about intactness of brain stem function.

ASSESSMENT OF MOTOR FUNCTION

The assessment of motor function is conducted in an orderly fashion, beginning with the upper limbs and proceeding to the neck and trunk and, finally, to the lower extremities. Limb evaluation proceeds from proximal to distal.

The purposes of the neurological assessment are a little different from those of the neurological physical examination, which includes a detailed examination of the motor system. The neurological assessment provides a baseline from which to denote change. A sampling of a few key muscles or muscle groups provides a good indicator of function and change. In the neurological assessment, the motor assessment usually focuses on the arms and legs.

Noting motor function helps the nurse to consider the patient's functional level, the effect on independence in ADLs, and the need for adaptation of activities or assistive devices.

The technique used to evaluate motor function depends on the patient's LOC. In the conscious and alert patient, the assessment can be conducted by observing responses to directions such as "Squeeze my hands." The aphasic or apraxic patient may have difficulty following directions and may need cueing.

In an unconscious patient or one who is unable to participate, the nurse must rely on special testing techniques and observations for data. The basic approach to assessment of motor function is detailed in Chart 8-7. A few additional points will help to guide the assessment process. In assessing motor function, the following should be considered: (1) muscle size, (2) muscle tone, (3) muscle strength, (4) presence of involuntary movement, and (5) posture and gait, if appropriate for the patient's condition. When one muscle or muscle group is assessed, it is always compared with the same muscle or group on the opposite side of the body for symmetry.

Muscle Size and Tone

The muscle or muscle group is observed for size. It is also palpated at rest and then during passive movement for tone. Common abnormalities in muscle tone include spasticity, rigidity, and flaccidity.

CHART 8 – 7 • Nursing Assessment of Motor Function at the Bedside

CONSCIOUS PATIENT WHO IS ABLE TO FOLLOW SIMPLE COMMANDS

A sampling of the strength of key muscles in the extremities will provide an overview of motor function. Other muscle groups of interest can be added (see Chap. 7 and Fig. 7-9 for more information).

Upper Extremities

A. Deltoids
B. Biceps
C. Triceps
D. Hand grasps
E. Pronator drift

Lower Extremities:

F. Hamstrings
G. Quadriceps
H. Dorsiflexion
I. Plantar flexion

UNCONSCIOUS PATIENT

Unconscious patients can exhibit abnormal muscle tone or motor responses that appear as stereotyped postures and are initiated by noxious stimuli (see decortication and decerebration).

Upper Extremities: Unconscious Patient

- First observe for spontaneous movement with patient lying in bed.
- Apply a noxious stimulus. *Note:* **Apply a noxious stimulus centrally rather than peripherally. An example of a central stimulus is pinching the pectoralis major muscle. A peripheral stimulus, such as pressing on the nailbed, may result in a reflex response and confuse findings.**

- Observe for withdrawal of the arm on the stimulated side. A purposeful response is present if the arm crossed the midline to noxious stimulus.

Sometimes added to the assessment:

- With the patient lying on his or her back, position the forearms perpendicular to the bed, holding the patient's arms upright by the hands or wrists.
- The movement of both arms is then observed as the extremities are released simultaneously.
- A paralyzed or paretic arm will fall more quickly than an intact arm. The weaker arm may strike the patient's face as it falls.

Lower Extremities: Unconscious Patient

- Observe for spontaneous movements.
- Apply noxious stimuli; observe for motor response.

Sometimes added to the assessment for paralysis or paresis, although often impractical because of abnormal posturing and increased tone:

- Position flat on the back with the knees flexed so both feet are flat on the bed.
- The knees are simultaneously released and the movement of the legs is observed.
- The paralyzed or paretic leg will fall to an extended position with the hip outwardly rotated. The normal leg will maintain the flexed position for a few moments and then gradually assume its previous position.

Spasticity refers to increased resistance to passive movement, often more pronounced at the extremes of range of motion and often followed by a sudden or gradual release of resistance. Spasticity is caused by injury to the corticospinal system. **Clasp-knife spasticity** is increased resistance with a sudden release at the end of extension.

Rigidity is a state of increased resistance. **Cogwheel rigidity** is a series of ratchet-like, small, regular jerks that are perceived on passive flexion or extension. **Lead-pipe rigidity** is resistance that persists throughout extension and flexion.

Flaccidity (hypotonia) refers to decreased muscle tone. The muscle is weak, soft, and flabby and fatigues easily.

Decortication and decerebration, special states of muscle tone seen in some unconscious patients, require more detailed explanation (see next section).

Muscle Tone in the Unconscious Patient

In the unconscious patient, observe the patient lying in the bed for position and abnormal movement. Muscle tone can be assessed by guiding the extremities through passive range of motion. Rigidity, flaccidity, and spasticity can be noted by these simple maneuvers.

Unconscious patients can exhibit abnormal muscle tone or stereotyped postures initiated by noxious stimuli. The particular posture assumed varies according to the anatomical level of injury and motor tract interruption. This response results from rostral-caudal (head to toe) deterioration, which can occur when a hemispheric lesion extends into the midbrain or when a midbrain or upper pons lesion is present.

Decortication and Decerebration

The abnormal postures that may be noted are called *decortication* and *decerebration*, and each can be correlated to structural cerebral dysfunction at a certain level (e.g., hemisphere or upper brain stem). **Decortication** is characterized by adduction of the arm at the shoulder with flexion at the elbow and pronation and flexion at the wrist; the legs extend at the hips and knee. This posture implies a structural lesion of the cerebral hemisphere or diencephalon (*above* the midbrain); the decortication is contralateral to the hemispheric lesion. (Fig. 8-9). **Decerebration** includes extended, adducted, and internally rotated (hyperpronated) of the arm; there is flexion of the wrist and fingers; the legs are extended and the feet are plantarflexed. Decerebration is caused by a structural lesion of the upper brain stem, although severe metabolic disorders may also be the cause. The decerebration is contralateral to the upper brain stem lesion. Decortication and decerebration are the result of rostral-caudal deterioration. **Rostral-caudal deterioration** describes the progressive deterioration in cerebral and brainstem function that occurs with expansion of a supratentorial lesion, thus producing pressure on the brainstem and a pattern of progressive neurological dysfunction (see Chapter 17). Early recognition and reversal of the process are imperative if permanent severe brainstem damage or death is to be prevented.

Intermittent Decortication and Decerebration

If there is a difference in an ischemic response or structural dysfunction between the deep cerebral hemispheric structures and upper brainstem, variations in adequate blood supply to these regions may cause intermittent decortication

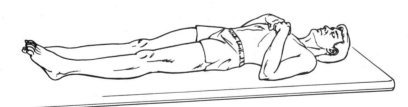

A *Flexor or decorticate posturing response*

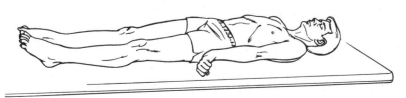

B *Extensor or decerebrate posturing*

Figure 8–9 • Abnormal rigidity. (*A*) Decorticate rigidity. In decorticate rigidity, the upper arms are held tightly to the sides, with elbows, wrists, and fingers flexed. The legs are extended and internally rotated. The feet are plantar flexed. This posture implies a destructive lesion of the corticospinal tracts within or very near the cerebral hemispheres. (*B*) Decerebrate rigidity. In decerebrate rigidity, the jaws are clenched and the neck extended. The arms are adducted and stiffly extended at the elbows with forearms pronated, wrists and fingers flexed. The legs are stiffly extended at the knees, with the feet plantar flexed. Decerebration is caused by a lesion in the diencephalon, midbrain, or pons, although severe metabolic disorders, such as hypoxia or hypoglycemia, may also produce it. (From Fuller, J. & Schaller-Ayers, J. [1994]. *Health assessment: A nursing approach* [2nd ed.]. Philadelphia: J. B. Lippincott.)

or decerebration. Clinically, the patient can change from bilateral decerebration to bilateral decortication (or vice versa), from unilateral decerebration to unilateral decortication, or with decortication on one side and decerebration on the other. Both decerebration and decortication are poor prognostic signs, although decerebration is a more ominous sign than decortication.

ASSESSMENT OF MUSCLE STRENGTH

In the **conscious, cooperative patient**, muscle strength is assessed by active and active resistive movements. What muscle should be assessed as part of the abbreviated neurological assessment at the bedside? Depending on the patient's condition, pronator drift and hand grasps must be tested at the very least. For the lower extremities depending on the patient's condition, asking the patient to move each leg and wiggle his toes and feet provides minimal data on function. A more extensive examination of both upper and lower extremities is found in Tables 7-14 and 7-16. See also Chart 8-7 for a summary of motor function assessment at the bedside. See Chapter 7 for assessment of the unconscious patient.

In the **unconscious patient**, muscle strength is surmised through observing the patient lying in bed and by applying noxious stimuli and noting response. The following responses are possible in response to painful stimuli:

Purposeful: localization/pushes the painful stimuli away
Nonpurposeful: movement of the stimulated area, but no attempt to push the stimuli away
Unresponsive: patient shows no signs of reacting to painful stimuli (seen in deep coma)

Upper Extremities

The unconscious patient is first observed for spontaneous movement as he or she lies in the bed. A noxious stimulus is then applied to elicit a motor response. *Note:* Apply a noxious stimulus centrally rather than peripherally. An example of a central stimulus is squeezing the pectoralis major muscle. A peripheral stimulus, such as pressing on the nailbed, may result in a reflex response. Observe for withdrawal of the arm on the stimulated side. A purposeful response will be evident if the arm crosses the midline as the arm attempts to withdraw from the noxious stimulus. To assess each arm for paresis, place the patient in a neutral supine position. Position the forearms perpendicular to the bed, holding the patient's arms upright by the hands or wrists. The movement of both arms is then observed as the extremities are released simultaneously. A paralyzed or paretic arm will fall more quickly than an intact arm. The weaker arm may strike the patient's face as it falls.

Lower Extremities

Observe for spontaneous movements. Apply a noxious stimulus to observe for any movement. Although often impractical, the legs can be assessed for paralysis or paresis. The patient is positioned flat on the back with the knees flexed so both feet are flat on the bed. The knees are simultaneously released and the movement of the legs is observed. The paralyzed or paretic leg will fall to an extended position with the hip outwardly rotated. The normal leg will maintain the flexed position for a few moments and then gradually assume its previous position.

INVOLUNTARY MOVEMENT, POSTURE, AND GAIT

The presence of involuntary movements, such as tremors, choreiform movements, myoclonus, athetosis, tics, spasms, or ballism, is noted (see Table 7-18). **Posture** is the position or orientation of the body in space; **gait** is the manner of progression in walking. First, the patient's position while he or she is lying in bed is observed. Next, if weight bearing and ambulation are possible, observe the patient's posture while he or she is standing still. The patient is then observed while walking and the following characteristics are noted: erect, stooped, or leaning toward one side; position of the arms in relationship to the body; and quality and amount of movement in the lower extremities. A description of common gait abnormalities appears in Table 7-17 and Chart 7-2.

SENSORY ASSESSMENT

The sensory assessment is usually deferred unless the patient has spinal cord disease (secondary to trauma, neoplasm, infectious processes, or stenosis), intervertebral disc disease, Guillain-Barré syndrome, or other conditions that affect the spinal cord or spinal nerves. The decision to include a sensory assessment is left to the judgment of the clinician. A sensory assessment is conducted in the patient who is conscious, cooperative, and able to respond appropriately. If a sensory assessment is conducted, the sensory modalities that can be assessed include:

- Superficial sensation
- Light touch (cotton-tipped applicator)
- Pain (pin-prick)
- Deep sensation
- Proprioception (the big toe and fingers are moved in various positions)

Pain and **light touch** are the most frequently assessed modalities. The technique for assessment follows these basic principles:

- With the patient's eyes closed, begin either at the face or feet and systematically assess and compare findings on both sides of the body. If you are assessing a patient with spinal cord or spinal nerve deficits, starting at the feet and working upward is helpful to determine the highest level of intact sensory function.
- Ask the patient to tell you when the sensory stimulation is felt.

- Record the highest level of function on each side of the body (there may be unilateral sensory functional loss).

Table 5-6 includes a list of dermatome levels. Table 7-19 discusses sensory assessment in greater detail. Chart 23-4 includes the sensory assessment for spinal cord injury.

FREQUENCY AND DOCUMENTATION OF SENSORY DATA

The frequency of assessment depends on the patient's acuity and stability. Patients with acute spinal cord trauma, acute transverse myelitis, or acute Guillain-Barré syndrome should be assessed for the highest level of function every 1 to 4 hours. In a patient whose condition is stable, assessment once a shift is probably frequent enough to keep the nurse aware of functional level. Documentation of findings can be done in several ways. If a special Spinal Cord Assessment Sheet or dermatome territory map is used, data are entered using a check-mark format. Data may also be recorded in a narrative format, using dermatome landmarks to monitor function (e.g., highest sensory level is one finger above the umbilicus).

ASSESSMENT OF CEREBELLAR FUNCTION

To assess cerebellar function at the bedside, a sample of upper extremity and lower extremity function is acceptable. See Chapter 7 for more details about assessment. For upper extremities assessment, ask the patient to touch your finger and then his or her nose. Continuing doing this movement as fast as possible. Assess first with eyes open then with eyes closed. Note the smoothness of the movement and accuracy of touching the target. An alternative method is to ask the patient to rapidly pronate and supine the hand onto the palm of the other several times.

For the lower extremities, ask the patient to run the heel of one foot down the shin of the other leg. Ataxia and dysmetria are abnormal findings. If the patient is ambulatory, the Romberg test can be used. However, be prepared to support the patient if he or she begins to sway or fall. In addition, observe the patient for any involuntary movements that may be associated with cerebellar dysfunction. Cerebellar function cannot be tested in the unconscious patient. Data that suggest cerebellar dysfunction may be noted by nystagmus (see Table 7-10).

VITAL SIGNS AND CLINICAL IMPLICATIONS

Vital signs are taken on all patients, but in patients with neurological problems there can be special considerations, particularly with increased ICP or brainstem pathophysiology. The relationship between vital signs and neurological function is based on hemodynamics. The brain requires a constant, large volume of oxygen-rich blood to support adequate cerebral perfusion pressure. Without adequate cerebral perfusion pressure, cerebral ischemia develops, affecting cerebral metabolism, and neurological dysfunction occurs.

The following are homeostatic mechanisms important to understanding cerebral hemodynamics.

CNS Ischemic Response

When cerebral blood flow to the brainstem vasomotor center is compromised sufficiently to cause ischemia, the chemosensitive cells within the vasomotor center respond directly by sending efferent commands that strongly stimulate both the vagal and sympathetic nerves. Blood flow to all other tissue, including the kidney, is reduced in favor of maintaining the required flow to the brain and heart. There is a significant rise in arterial pressure. The cerebral ischemic response is interesting in that simultaneous stimulation of both the vagus and the sympathetic nerves results in an increase in myocardial contractility along with slowing of the heart rate because the vagus nerve has the stronger influence on the sinoatrial node. Therefore, the cerebral ischemic response is characterized by profound bradycardia.[6]

Cushing's Response (Reflex)

A special type of CNS ischemic response that results from increased ICP is called Cushing's reflex. When cerebrospinal fluid (CSF) pressure approaches the pressure found within the intracranial cerebral arteries, the cerebral arteries become compressed and begin to collapse, compromising cerebral blood flow. To compensate, Cushing's response is activated, causing the arterial pressure to rise. When the arterial pressure has risen to a higher level than the CSF pressure, cerebral arterial flow is reestablished and the ischemia is relieved. Thus, the arterial pressure is established and maintained at a new, higher level to provide adequate blood flow. Cushing's response is a compensatory response that helps protect the brain from loss of adequate blood flow.

Clinically, the nurse should realize that changes in vital signs are late findings in rostral-caudal deterioration. Therefore, do not wait for changes in vital signs before intervening, because it may be too late to prevent irreversible neurological damage or even death. In the discussion that follows, it is evident that the assessment of vital signs should be both quantitative and qualitative. The numeric value of each vital sign is important, but the characteristic descriptive pattern and rhythm can provide diagnostic indicators of intracranial pathophysiology and neurological progression.

Anatomy and Physiology Related to Vital Signs: Vasomotor Tone, Respirations, and Temperature

The vital sign "centers" are located within the brainstem. Complex networks of neurons in the brainstem reticular formation participate in the regulation of cardiovascular, respiratory, and other visceral functions. Rather than being discrete anatomical centers for a particular function, neurons for autonomic functions are intermingled and functionally related and have reciprocal connections. Observation of a physiological response, such as inspiration, is seen after a particular pattern of the RF is stimulated. The RF receives visceral sensory input polysynaptically through collaterals from ascending spinal cord sensory pathways, through descending fibers from the hypothalamus, and from the limbic system through the dorsal longitudinal fasciculus, medial forebrain bundle, and mamillotegmental tracts.

Vasomotor Tone

The RF neurons that influence cardiovascular function are located primarily in the medulla. The ventrolateral medulla contains a group of **vasomotor neurons** that control blood pressure. Some neurons project directly to preganglionic parasympathetic cranial nerve nuclei (midbrain, CN III; pons, CN VII; and medulla, CNs IX and X). The preganglionic nuclei maintain arterial blood pressure, mediate sympathetic reflexes, and serve as relay stations for sympathetic pathways. The vagus (CN X) is important because its efferent impulses have a major role in control of respiratory, cardiovascular, and gastrointestinal functions. Other neurons in the ventrolateral medulla, the cardiovagal neurons, control heart rate. Finally, portions of the medullary RF coordinate various respiratory and cardiovascular reflexes.

Respirations

Selected neurons within the RF control visceral motor neurons and respiratory motor neurons (Fig. 8-10). Respiratory neurons found in the parabrachial area (pons) are called pontine dorsal or the **pneumotaxic center**, whereas the nucleus tractus solitarius (medulla) and ventrolateral medulla neurons together are called the **ventral respiratory groups**. These excitatory neurons sustain vasomotor tone and respirations. The several respiratory groups include **inspiratory neurons** that project to the spinal phrenic motor neurons and **expiratory neurons** that project to the intercostal respiratory motor neurons. Interneurons located proximal to the ventral respiratory groups are key for the generation of respiratory rhythm.

The **ventral respiratory groups** have a role in controlling inspiration and expiration. The **pneumotaxic center** transmits impulses of varying magnitude for inspirations. The primary function of the center is to limit inspiration; however, by limiting respirations, it exerts a secondary effect on the rate of breathing. Strong pneumotaxic signals can increase the rate of breathing (e.g., 30 to 40 per minute), whereas weak signals will reduce the rate to only a few breaths per minute. The Hering-Breuer reflex also has an effect on turning off respirations.

The **Hering-Breuer reflex** is a protective reflex that prevents excessive lung expansion. Stretch receptors located in the bronchi and bronchioles throughout the lungs transmit signals through the vagus nerve to the dorsal respiratory group when the lungs are overinflated and expiration is initiated. This reflex has a function similar to that of the pneumotaxic center in that it limits the duration of inspiration through a feedback loop that "turns off" inspiratory

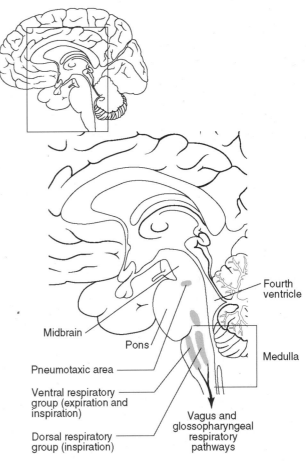

Figure 8–10 • Major brainstem areas for respiratory control.

Labels: Fourth ventricle; Midbrain; Pons; Medulla; Pneumotaxic area; Ventral respiratory group (expiration and inspiration); Dorsal respiratory group (inspiration); Vagus and glossopharyngeal respiratory pathways

effort and reduces the time of inspiration so that the respiratory rate is increased.

Body Temperature

The preoptic nucleus of the anterior hypothalamus is the center for the regulation of body heat and acts by monitoring the temperature of blood. Regulation of heat is accomplished by an integrated response of the sweat glands, peripheral vessels, and skeletal muscles for shivering. Through these structures, the body can conserve or divest itself of body heat.

Assessment of Vital Signs

Respirations

The respiratory pattern has been correlated with dysfunction in specific anatomical brainstem areas in the past, although ataxic breathing is the only one currently thought to have strong localizing significance.[7] However, abnormal respiratory patterns generally suggest brainstem dysfunction and progression of pathophysiology, a prognostic indicator of poor outcome. See Table 8-4 for a discussion of abnormal respiratory patterns and possible site of dysfunction. Clinically, it is not always possible to observe abnormal patterns because the patient may be on a ventilator that is set for a particular mode, rate, and rhythm, thus overriding an inad-

Table 8–4 • ABNORMAL RESPIRATORY PATTERNS ASSOCIATED WITH INTRACRANIAL CONDITIONS

The following abnormal respiratory patterns are seen in conditions that affect the respiratory centers of the brainstem directly and indirectly. *Primary injury* occurs as a result of ischemia, infarction, or a tumor located in the brainstem respiratory centers. Secondary injury may be caused by (1) ↑ intracranial pressure (ICP) pressing on the brainstem secondary to a supratentorial process (e.g., cerebral edema, herniation); or (2) CNS depression from metabolic conditions or drug overdose. However, ↑ ICP with herniation is the major cause of abnormal respiratory patterns.

TYPE AND PATTERN	DESCRIPTION
Cheyne-Strokes respirations 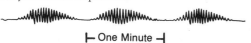 ⊢ One Minute ⊣	Rhythmic waxing and waning in depth and rate of respiration followed by apnea Pattern due to: ↑ sensitivity to CO_2, resulting in change in depth and rate; and ↓ stimulation from respiratory centers, resulting in apnea Respiratory dysfunction attributed to *bilaterally deep* within the cerebral hemispheres, diencephalon, or basal ganglia.
Central neurogenic hyperventilation 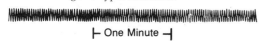 ⊢ One Minute ⊣	↑ Rate and depth of respirations May lead to respiratory alkalosis Pattern thought to be due to release of the reflex mechanisms for respiratory control in the lower brain stem lowers arterial CO_2 and raises pH Unclear level of dysfunction, although midbrain and upper pons considered sites
Apneustic breathing 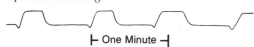 ⊢ One Minute ⊣	A pause of 2 to 3 seconds noted after a full or prolonged inspiration; may alternate with an expiratory pause Lower pons dysfunction

equate respiratory pattern. In some cases, respiratory changes may not be seen until just before death.

Assessment

The rate, rhythm, and characteristics of the inspiratory and expiratory phases of respirations should be noted. In addition to neurological causes of respiratory changes, a number of other etiologies should also be considered, such as acidosis, alkalosis, electrolyte imbalance, congestive heart failure, anxiety, and various respiratory complications (e.g., atelectasis, pneumonia, pulmonary edema). Drugs, particularly narcotic analgesics, sedatives, and anesthetics, may have a depressant effect on the respiratory system. Morphine sulfate depresses the respiratory rate in addition to causing constriction of the pupils. Because it causes respiratory depression and masks the neurological signs of pupillary response, use of morphine sulfate is limited in neurological patients. Small doses of morphine sulfate may be ordered to decrease rapid respirations as long as ongoing monitoring and respiratory support are available.

Changes in Respirations

Regulation of respirations is controlled by many neurologic mechanisms. With cerebral injury, changes can occur in respiratory patterns; documentation by the nurse is important. Table 8-4 describes types of abnormal respiratory patterns. The nurse should consider the complete data set when assessing respiratory function and planning interventions. Metabolic, cardiac, and respiratory conditions can trigger changes in respiratory function. Trauma to the cervical spine

may produce respiratory distress; if the injury is above the phrenic segment (C-4), total arrest will occur.

The role of the nurse in relation to respiratory function includes (1) periodically assess and document the rate, rhythm, and characteristics of respirations; (2) implement interventions to maintain a patent airway and promote respiratory function; (3) assess for secondary conditions that may cause respiratory pattern or rate changes; (4) assess for respiratory complications or insufficiency; and (5) notify the physician if respiratory problems occur.

Pulse and Heart Rate

Assessment

The rate, rhythm, and quality of the pulse and heart rate should be assessed, documented, and compared with previous data. Common changes that may occur in rate and rhythm are tachycardia, bradycardia, and cardiac arrhythmias. A bounding or thready pulse is a common change in pulse quality, and often accompanies rising ICP. A thready pulse is seen in the terminal stages of neurologic demise, or with hemorrhage.

Changes in Heart Rate

Tachycardia in a neurological patient can indicate that a patient is (1) hypoxic, (2) experiencing high ICP, or (3) bleeding internally in the abdominal, thoracic, or pelvic cavity.

Bradycardia can occur in the later stages of progressive increased ICP as part of Cushing's response. The blood is pumped to the edematous brain against great pressure and resistance so that the pulse is decreased to a rate of 40 to 60 per minute and bounding. Additionally, **hypotension and bradycardia** may be secondary to cervical spinal cord injury with interruption of descending sympathetic pathways.

Cardiac arrhythmias are rather common in neurological conditions. Arrhythmias are seen more often in patients who have blood in the CSF (e.g., subarachnoid hemorrhage, severe head injury), have undergone posterior fossa surgery, or have increased ICP. If there is evidence of abnormalities in cardiac rate or rhythm, a rhythm strip should be obtained immediately to document and identify the problem. Treatment should be instituted as necessary. Continuous cardiac monitoring is important in unstable, acute patients.

Blood Pressure

Assessment

In assessing blood pressure, the nurse monitors for hypotension, hypertension, and pulse pressure. A comparison is made with previous assessment data.

Hypertension in the neurological patient may be associated with sympathetic stimulation resulting from massive hypothalamic discharge or a rising ICP. An elevated systolic blood pressure, widening pulse pressure, and bradycardia are seen in the advanced stages of increased ICP and are known as **Cushing's response**.

Hypotension is rarely attributable to cerebral injury. When it is seen with severe neurological injury, it occurs as a terminal event and is accompanied by tachycardia. Inadequate cerebral perfusion denies cerebral tissue of an adequate oxygen supply, and the regulatory mechanisms no longer function. In this stage of decompensation, deterioration is rapid and death results. The suspicion of occult internal hemorrhage (thoracic, abdominal, pelvic, or long bone) should be raised when **hypotension and tachycardia** are seen together. **Hypotension and bradycardia** may be seen in patients with cervical spinal injury as a result of interruption in the descending sympathetic pathways.

Temperature

Assessment

The temperature and the route by which it was taken should be recorded on the flow sheet. If a continuous temperature-monitoring device is being used, this should also be noted on the flow sheet. If the temperature is elevated and the patient has been placed on a hypothermia blanket, the temperature should be monitored frequently, (e.g., every 30 minutes) until it drops to an acceptable level. Shivering increases ICP and should be avoided.

Hypothermia is seen in certain conditions such as spinal shock when autonomic innervation is lost; metabolic or toxic coma of any origin; drug overdose, especially in barbiturate overdose; and destructive brainstem or hypothalamic lesions. Specific treatment depends on the cause. Warm blankets and/or a warming blanket may be applied. Room temperature should also be adjusted.

Hyperthermia is much more common than hypothermia. Fever is a complex, coordinated autonomic, neuroendocrine, and behavioral response that is adaptive and is often part of the acute-phase reaction to immune challenge.[8] Fever can originate from infectious and noninfectious conditions. It is important that this determination is made to save needless diagnostics and inappropriate antimicrobial therapy. Regardless of the cause, the clinical presentation of fever is stereotypical and largely independent of the causative agent. Fever may be associated with any of the following conditions.

Infectious Origins

Various organisms such as *Staphylococcus aureus, Escherichia coli, Pseudomonas aeruginosa,* and others cause infections. Infections can result from open head wounds (meningitis), postoperative wounds or shunts, nosocomial pneumonia, and intravenous lines and tubes (central and peripheral lines, urinary catheters [urosepsis], ventriculostomies). Nonneurological causes of infection should also be considered, such as septicemia, gram-negative sepsis, endocarditis, severe community acquired pneumonia, septic pulmonary emboli, antibiotic-associated diarrhea/colitis, and intra-abdominal or pelvic infection resulting from perforation, trauma, or surgery.

Treatment is based on the selection of a sensitive antimicrobial drug. In addition, strict aseptic dressing technique and line- and tube-change protocols can significantly reduce infections.

Noninfectious Origins

- **Non-neurological,** noninfectious, common causes of fever include acute myocardial infarction, acute pulmonary embolism/infarction, acute pancreatitis, gastrointestinal hemorrhage, phlebitis, hematomas, attacks of acute gout, fevers related to malignancies, and drug hypersensitivity reactions.[9]
- **Drug-induced fever** is caused by an immune response to a drug. Common causative drugs include anticonvulsants such as phenytoin (Dilantin) and carbamazepine (Tegretol); analgesics; phenothiazines; anticholinergic drugs; and antibiotics. The diagnosis is established by withdrawal of the drug and subsequent rechallenge. Cultures of blood, urine, and sputum are negative, and the patient looks better clinically than the temperature would suggest.
- **Posterior fossa syndrome** mimics meningitis with a number of symptoms that include stiff neck. However, unlike meningitis, CSF cultures are negative. Posterior fossa syndrome is seen in patients who have had posterior fossa surgery or blood in the CSF and is often related to subarachnoid hemorrhage.
- **Neuroleptic malignant syndrome** is related to use of antipsychotic drugs and includes muscular rigidity, a catatonic-like state, altered consciousness, and a high fever of up to 41.5°C (107°F). Discontinuing the drug and supporting the patient are the components of a treatment plan.

Central Fever

Central fever is a noninfectious origin of fever. It is caused by a central neurogenic etiology seen with space-occupying lesions, trauma or a lesion that involves the hypothalamus or base of the brain, or traction of the hypothalamus or brain stem. High fever—up to 41.5°C—is the cardinal finding, and perspiration is absent.[10] This is a diagnosis of exclusion and is made only after all other causes of fever have been ruled out.

Effects of Steroids on Temperature

The neurological patient may be treated with large doses of steroids, often dexamethasone (Decadron). Steroids are anti-inflammatory agents that mask the classic clinical signs of infections, such as an elevated temperature and white blood count. Therefore, monitor the patient for signs of infection such as cloudy or foul-smelling urine; yellowish, foul-smelling sputum; or adventitious breath sounds. Cultures and blood counts should be monitored for evidence of infection.

How aggressively should an elevated temperature be treated? Most clinicians who manage neurological patients will treat an elevated temperature when it reaches a certain level (38° or 39° C) because of the effect on the brain. An elevated temperature increases overall body metabolism and cell metabolism of all systems, including the brain, which, in turn, produces an increase in carbon dioxide and lactic acid by-products of cell metabolism. Carbon dioxide, a potent cerebral vasodilator, will cause an increase in ICP in a patient who may already have high ICP. If the oxygen supply to cerebral tissue is insufficient, cerebral ischemia develops. Therefore, treatment of hyperthermia to prevent neurological deterioration is a central concern in management. Usual treatment is acetaminophen and possibly a cooling blanket for high temperatures.

The reason for the elevated temperature should be investigated carefully because there may be a non-neurological cause. The nurse should listen to the patient's chest for breath sounds and rales. The urine and the sputum should be considered for possible culture. Finally, all dressings and drainage, if present, should be assessed.

▍▍▍ SUMMARY

The neurological assessment is the foundational database for the nurse to use in identifying nursing diagnoses and collaborative interdisciplinary problems, planning care, implementing interventions, and evaluating outcomes. It is essential that the nurse develop the skills and knowledge to conduct this assessment competently and engage in the clinical reasoning for patient management.

REFERENCES

1. Benarroch, E. E., Westmoreland, B. F., Danube, J. R., Reagan, T. J., & Sandok, B. A. (1999). *Medical neurosciences: An approach to anatomy, pathology, and physiology by systems and levels* (4th ed., pp. 291–293). Philadelphia: Lippincott Williams & Wilkins.
2. Masferrer, R. (2000). Advanced neurological assessments: Clinical and radiographic correlations. 8th International Nurse Practitioner Conference, San Diego, California, September 28, 2000.
3. Barr, M. L., & Kiernan, J. A. (1993). *The human nervous system: An anatomical viewpoint* (pp. 2, 158–159). Philadelphia: J. B. Lippincott.
4. Plum, F., & Posner, J. (1980). *The diagnosis of stupor and coma* (3rd ed., pp. 178–180). Philadelphia: F. A. Davis.
5. Folstein, M. F., Folstein, S. E., & McHugh, P. R. (1975). Mini-mental state: A practical method for grading the cognitive state of patients for the clinician. *Journal of Psychiatric Research, 12,* 189–198.
6. Johnson, K. R. (Ed.) (1998). *Essential medical physiology* (2nd ed., pp. 212–213). Philadelphia: Lippincott-Raven.
7. Simon, R. P. (1999). Coma. In R. K. Albert & D. J. Dries, *ACCP-SCCM Combined critical care course multidisciplinary board review* (pp. 47–53). Anaheim, CA: Society of Critical Care Medicine.
8. Saper, C. B., & Breder, C. D. (1994). The neurological basis of fever. *New England Journal of Medicine, 330*(26), 1880.
9. Cunha, B. A. (1998). Rash and fever in the critical care unit. *Critical Care Clinics, 14*(1), 35–52.
10. Cunha, B. A., & Tu, R. P. (1988). Fever in the neurosurgical patient. *Heart & Lung, 17*(6, part 1), 611.

RESOURCES
Professional

Published Material

Barr, M. L., & Kiernan, J. A. (1993). *The human nervous system: An anatomical viewpoint* (pp. 364–376). Philadelphia: J. B. Lippincott.

Benarroch, E. E., Westmoreland, B. F., Danube, J. R., Reagan, T. J., & Sandok, B. A. (1999). *Medical neurosciences: An approach to anatomy, pathology, and physiology by systems and levels* (4th ed.). Philadelphia: Lippincott Williams & Wilkins.

Brazis, P. W., Masdeu, J. C., & Biller, J. (1996). *Localization in clinical neurology* (3rd ed.). Boston: Little, Brown, & Company.

Goldberg, S. (1988). *The four-minute neurologic exam.* Miami, FL: MedMaster, Inc.

Guarantors of Brain. (2000). *Aids to the examination of peripheral nervous system* (4th ed.). Edinburgh: W. B. Saunders.

Haerer, A. F. (1992). *DeJong's the neurologic examination* (5th ed.). Philadelphia: Lippincott Williams & Wilkins.

Hoppenfeld, S. (1977). *Orthopedic neurology: A diagnostic guide to neurologic levels.* Philadelphia: J. B. Lippincott.

Saper, C. B., & Breder, C. D. (1994). The neurological basis of fever. *New England Journal of Medicine, 330*(26), 1880–1886.

Strub, R. L., & Black, F. W. (1993). *The mental status examination in neurology* (3rd ed.). Philadelphia: F. A. Davis.

Miller, N. R., & Newman, N. J. (1999). *Walsh & Hoyt's clinical neuro-ophthalmology: The essentials* (5th ed.). Baltimore: Williams & Wilkins.

Wiebers, D. O., Dale, A. J. D., Kokmen, E., & Swanson, J. W. (1998). *Mayo clinical examinations in neurology* (7th ed.). St. Louis: Mosby.

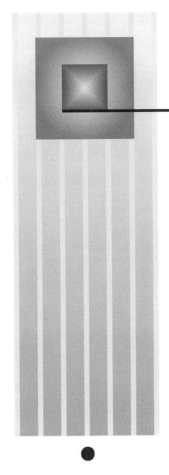

General Considerations in Neuroscience Nursing

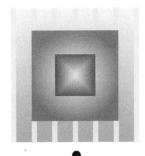

CHAPTER **9**

Nutritional Support for Neuroscience Patients

JOANNE V. HICKEY

A renewed interest in and recognition of the critical importance of meeting energy and nutrient requirements for patients has led to a careful scrutiny of the scientific knowledge base of nutrition and nutritional therapeutics. As a result, evidence-based practice has revised how nutritional therapeutics are provided to hospitalized patients. Many older standards of practice have been revised, based on scientific evidence. New studies have been undertaken to fill the multiple gaps in knowledge and to clarify areas of controversy. The role of the clinical dietitian has emerged as the clinical expert prepared to assume the leadership role in nutritional therapeutics as a member of the interdisciplinary team. For nurses providing holistic comprehensive care for neuroscience patients, meeting nutritional needs is a critical component in the recovery process that requires an appropriate knowledge base. Injury, physiological dysfunction, and stress often change the basic requirements and use of nutrients and water for energy, cellular function, and repair of injured tissue. Additionally, a patient with a neurological condition may have deficits, such as an altered level of consciousness or paresis/paralysis of the muscles for chewing and swallowing, which further complicates ingestion of nutrients. Consideration of these multiple and complex factors, plus the effect of an illness on both the neurological and other body systems, requires the collaborative efforts of the interdisciplinary team. This chapter briefly focuses on nutrition and nutritional therapeutics as applied to a neuroscience population. The reader is referred to other standard texts and periodicals for expansion of knowledge and detailed information.

BASIC NUTRITIONAL REQUIREMENTS

The recommended dietary allowance (RDA) is the most widely recognized definition of nutrient sufficiency. Revised most recently in 1989, the RDA is based on available scientific knowledge and is approved by the Food and Nutrition Board of the National Academy of Sciences Committee on Dietary Allowances. The RDA describes target intake levels of essential nutrients for healthy people. Nutrient requirements include macronutrients (energy, protein, lipids) and micronutrients (vitamins, minerals). Of interest, the RDA is set two standard deviations above the estimated means and therefore exceeds requirements for most people.[1] It is important to keep in mind that the RDA cannot be relied on to precisely calculate the needs of *patients who are ill*, especially if malabsorption is present.[1]

Caloric Intake

The requisite caloric intake depends on a person's age, gender, weight, body size, and activity level, as well as the environment's ambient temperature. According to the National Academy of Science's recommended energy intake, women generally require 1,900 to 2,200 kilocalories (kcal) per day, whereas men need between 2,300 and 2,900 kcal per day. In the general population, a caloric intake of 25 to 35 kcal/kg of body weight is a good rule of thumb for patients who are not edematous or obese. *Note* that calorie and protein requirements should be stated in terms of "amount per kg" rather than "2,300 to 2,900 calories per day."

Caloric requirements increase in any stressful situation, such as physiological trauma, emotional stress, surgery, fever, seizure activity, decorticate or decerebrate rigidity, restlessness, agitation, hypermetabolic states, and sepsis. Although caloric requirements may be significantly increased for patients with ongoing stress or serious illness, typically the most severely stressed neuroscience patients receive some type of treatment that decreases energy expenditure, such as hypothermia therapy, barbiturate coma, and/or neuromuscular paralytics and sedative agents. Septic patients are quickly started on antibiotic therapy that treats infection with concurrent reduction of fever and of elevated white blood counts. Additionally, in recent years there has been a greater understanding of the relationship between overfeeding and complications such as hepatic steatosis (fatty degeneration), hyperglycemia, azotemia, hypertonic dehydration, metabolic acidosis, hypercapnia, hyperlipidemia, and refeeding syndromes. Therefore, it is rare for even the most severely injured neurosurgical patient to require 4,000 or more kilocalories as had been previously recommended based on published reports in the 1980s.[3-5] The rule of 25 to 35 kcal/kg still applies, although the higher end of the recommendation may be appropriate.

Proteins

Proteins are organic substances composed of amino acids, the primary function of which is to build and repair body tissue. When metabolized, 1 g of protein yields 4 calories. Although carbohydrate, fat, and protein all contain carbon, hydrogen, and oxygen, only protein contains nitrogen. Nitrogen is the major component of protein. Almost all nitrogen ingested comes from protein, and most of the nitrogen lost from the body is in the form of nitrogenous end products found in the urine as urea, creatinine, uric acid, and ammonium salts. A small amount of nitrogen loss occurs through the stool and skin. Nitrogen balance indicates whether the patient is **anabolic** (has a positive nitrogen balance) or **catabolic** (has a negative nitrogen balance). The normal healthy adult who is not growing, who consumes an adequate diet, and whose lean body mass remains the same is said to be in nitrogen balance. Nitrogen balance is calculated as follows:

- Nitrogen balance equals nitrogen intake/24 hours minus nitrogen output/24 hours.
- Nitrogen intake is calculated based on protein intake in 24 hours.
- Nitrogen output is calculated from a 24-hour urine urea nitrogen (UUN) excretion study.

A healthy adult requires 0.8 g/kg of protein per day regardless of gender or age. This is approximately 60 to 70g/day. Patients with major injuries or wounds require an increased protein intake.

Classification of Amino Acids and Protein

The amino acids of protein may be classified as either essential or nonessential. **Essential amino acids** are necessary for normal growth and development and cannot be manufactured by the body. **Nonessential amino acids** are defined as amino acids that are not necessary for normal growth and development and can be manufactured by the body.

Protein can also be classified as either complete or incomplete. A **complete protein** is one that contains all the essential amino acids in sufficient quantity and appropriate proportions to supply the body's needs. Proteins of animal origin, such as milk, meat, cheese, and eggs, are examples of complete proteins. An **incomplete protein** is defined as one that is deficient in one or more essential amino acids. Incomplete proteins are of plant origin and include grains, legumes, and nuts.

Carbohydrates

Carbohydrates are defined as starches and sugars that are used by the body for energy. When metabolized, 1 g of carbohydrate yields 4 calories. Carbohydrates are classified as monosaccharides, disaccharides, or polysaccharides. For carbohydrates to be used by the body, they must be broken down into glucose (a monosaccharide), the simplest form of sugar. Glucose is oxidized to release energy and is the source of energy for cerebral cell metabolism. Glucose may also be stored as a reserve in the liver (and in muscle tissue to a lesser degree) in the form of glycogen through a process called **glycogenesis.** Hydrolysis of glycogen to glucose is called **glycolysis** (the anabolic enzymatic conversion of glucose to lactate or pyruvate, resulting in energy stored in the form of adenosine triphosphate (ATP), such as occurs in muscles). In addition, excess glucose can be converted into fat and stored in the body as adipose tissue.

Fats

The purpose of fat in the diet is primarily to produce energy, although it is also important for the manufacture of other fat-related compounds, such as cholesterol, triglycerides, phospholipids, and lecithin. The major sources of fat in the normal diet are butter, margarine, oil, bacon, meat, fats, egg yolks, nuts, and legumes. When 1 g of fat is oxidized, 9 calories are generated.

Fats occurring as organic substances in the body are called lipids. **Fatty acids** are the basic units of structure in lipids; they can be divided into essential fatty acids and nonessential fatty acids. An **essential fatty acid** cannot be manufactured in the body and will cause a specific deficiency disorder if not ingested in an adequate amount. One essential fatty acid, linoleic acid, is important in the maintenance of the skin, hair, nerve lining, and cell membranes as well as being a component of prostaglandins and other body chemicals, such as arachidonic acid. **Nonessential fatty acids** do not cause specific deficiency disorders if not ingested in sufficient amounts because they can be manufactured in the body.

Vitamins, Minerals, and Water

Vitamins, minerals, and water are requisites for basic nutrition. Certain vitamins and minerals cannot be stored in the body, so that deficiencies quickly develop if an adequate diet is not consumed daily. Other vitamins can be stored in the body so that deficiencies are not apparent for weeks to months of inadequate vitamin intake.

Vitamins are classified as either water soluble or fat soluble. **Water-soluble vitamins** are vitamin C and the B-complex vitamins (i.e., thiamine, riboflavin, niacin [nicotinic acid], pyridoxine, pantothenic acid, biotin, folic acid, and cobalamin). The **fat-soluble vitamins** are A, D, E, and K.

Minerals are divided into major minerals and trace minerals. **Major minerals** include calcium, chloride, magnesium, phosphorus, potassium, and sodium. The **trace minerals** include cadmium, chromium, copper, fluoride, iodide, iron, manganese, molybdenum, nickel, selenium, silicon, tin, vanadium, and zinc.

Water requirements for adequate nutrition depend on the temperature of the ambient environment, amount of perspiration, activity, endocrine function, urinary output, and other factors. Under normal conditions, the average person requires approximately 2,600 mL of water per day. Hypermetabolic states, fever, profuse perspiration, significant

▌▌▌▌ Table 9-1 • DIFFERENCES IN EARLY METABOLIC RESPONSES TO FASTING AND INJURY

METABOLIC ACTIVITY	SIMPLE STARVATION	STARVATION SUPERIMPOSED ONTO INJURY OR STRESS
Basal metabolic rate (BMR)	↓ BMR	↓ or normal BMR initially, then ↑
Glucose levels	Low	High (hallmark of stress response)
Glucose utilization	Limited glucose use	↑ Glucose use
Gluconeogenesis	↑ Gluconeogenesis initially, ↓ after 5–7 days	↑ Gluconeogenesis
Protein catabolism	Low	High
Fat catabolism	High	Low/none
Ketone utilization	↑ Ketone use	↓ Ketone use
Ketosis	Present	Absent
Ketosuria	Present	Absent

drainage from wounds, and excessive urinary output are a few situations that warrant an increased fluid intake.

METABOLIC CHANGES FOLLOWING INJURY AND STARVATION

Significant differences accompany the body's metabolic response to starvation superimposed onto injury or acute stress (trauma, surgery, sepsis) and to simple starvation.[6] See Table 9-1 for a comparison. The key difference is that in critical illness, there is an increase in the basal metabolic rate (BMR), glucose use, and gluconeogenesis. Starved, stressed patients do not readily mobilize stored fats; therefore, they do not enter ketoadaptation or conservation phases, and their protein losses are greatly increased as compared to starved patients without injury or illness. Detailed information on simple starvation and starvation superimposed on injury or stress can be found in other references.

NUTRITIONAL ASSESSMENT

Both the Health Care Finance Agency (HCFA) and Joint Commission on Accreditation of Health Care Organization (JCAHO) require multidisciplinary nutritional assessment of patients, including the involvement of a registered dietitian. A registered dietitian (RD) is an expert in the nutritional components of health and illness and is an invaluable member of the health team to guide decision making regarding nutritional assessment, management, and monitoring of nutritional status. The evidence base for practice strongly supports the concept that malnutrition is associated with increased morbidity and mortality. Over 150 studies have been conducted since 1974 on malnutrition in hospitalized patients that collectively report a prevalence rate of between 30% and 55%.[6,7] Other consequences of malnutrition include (1) decreased immunological response to infection; (2) increased risk of complications, including decubitus ulcers and pneumonia; (3) delayed wound healing; (4) difficulty in refeeding; and (5) failure to wean from a ventilator.

Nutritional support is an integral part of care, and therefore it is critical that a nutritional assessment be conducted at hospitalization to identify patients at risk for protein-

energy malnutrition or deficiencies in specific nutrients so that a plan can be developed to support nutritional needs. A nutritional assessment should be a standard of care that occurs soon after a patient is hospitalized (within the first 24 hours). The nutritional assessment includes a thorough history, physical examination, and laboratory studies. The RD assumes responsibility for conducting the nutritional assessment, estimating nutritional requirements, and recommending a nutritional support plan of care. The nurse implements the nutritional plan of care, provides education to patient and family, and monitors both response to therapy and complications. Implementation includes safe administration of nutrients by oral, enteral, or on occasion, parenteral route.

Components of the Nutritional Assessment

History

The history begins with information about recent weight loss, anorexia, nausea, vomiting, and diarrhea. Determine whether there has been unexplained weight loss or weight gain. (An involuntary weight loss of 10% or more in 1 year is significant.) Information on recent dietary changes and what constitutes normal daily dietary intake is noted. This information can be collected from the medical record, a family member, or the patient.

Physical Examination

Physical inspection includes assessment of the following: skin (turgor, dryness, edema, bruising, scaling, dermatitis, seborrhea); mucous membranes (dryness, color, bruising, bleeding, especially gums); tongue (swelling, papillary atrophy); eyes (pale or dry conjunctiva, sunken eyeballs); dry, dull-looking hair or hair loss; and muscles (atrophy, wasting). Note the patient's weight and how it compares with ideal body weight (IBW) recommendations based on gender, age, and height. This is more useful than actual weight because many critically ill patients retain fluid, so that their weight may not correlate with current nutritional status.[8]

Anthropometric measurements such as skin-fold thickness and midarm muscle circumference are not useful in critically ill patients because of frequent presence of fluid retention and edema. Anthropometric measurements are more useful in less severely ill patients. When used, triceps or subscapular skinfold thickness (SFT) estimate body fat, and midarm muscle circumference estimates lean body muscle (protein stores). These data are not helpful if the patient is obese or edematous.[9]

Blood and Urine Chemistries

Some basic serum chemistries intended to indicate nutritional status are indirect measures and of poor validity in the acute care setting. These studies are greatly affected by organ function (especially liver and renal), administration of exogenous fluids, and the acute stress response. Serum *albumin* is often cited as an index of nutritional status. It has a long half-life of approximately 18 days and is a poor marker of the effects of short term feeding in hospitalized patients.[10] *Transferrin*, with a half-life of 8 to 10 days, is also frequently mentioned but is not very helpful with critically ill patients. The most useful chemistries are prealbumin (half-life, 2 to 3 days) and retinol-binding protein (half-life, 10 to 12 hours). Although these tests too are subject to the effects of metabolic response to stress and illness, their shorter half-lives correlate closely with nitrogen balance during nutritional support in hospitalized patients. They are sensitive indicators of the adequacy of nutritional support.[11,12]

Nitrogen represents the end-product of protein metabolism. Nitrogen balance studies, such as 24-hour *urinary urea nitrogen (UUN)* collection, compare nitrogen intake with nitrogen excretion to determine nitrogen balance. The nitrogen intake is determined by a simultaneous 24-hour accurate calorie count. A negative balance reflects protein catabolism. The goal of nutritional support is a positive nitrogen balance. However, a negative nitrogen balance is very common in the acute care setting. It can sometimes be reversed or blunted with abundant protein intake, but it is often intractable until the early phase of injury has passed and healing has begun. Nitrogen equilibrium is not anticipated in spinal cord injury for weeks to months following injury. When calculating nitrogen balance, a correction factor of 2 to 4 g of nitrogen is routinely added to correct for obligatory and insensible protein losses through the skin, lungs, and stool. The results of the study may be unreliable in patients with renal failure or if urine samples for the collection period have been spilled or inadvertently discarded.

Tests of the Immune System

Two tests of the immune system have been employed as nonspecific indicators of malnutrition in nutritional assessment: total circulating lymphocyte count and delayed cutaneous hypersensitivity to skin-test antigens. Most circulating lymphocytes are T cells, which are thymus-dependent immune responses to malnutrition. Reduction in *total circulating lymphocytes* is not specific for any particular nutritional deficiency but is a general indicator of malnutrition. Infections and immunosuppressant drugs alter the number of circulating lymphocytes and thus are not helpful in critically ill patients who most often have infections and may be receiving drugs that are immunosuppressant. The second test mentioned is delayed *cutaneous hypersensitivity skin-testing*. This test is also not helpful in critically ill, malnour-

ished patients because of a decreased cellular immunity response (a decrease in the synthesis of antibodies and the antibody response). Most often, patients fail to react to any of the several skin-test antigens used and are described as "anergic."

ESTIMATING NUTRIENT REQUIREMENTS

Estimating the actual nutrient requirements of a patient is important because there are serious adverse effects from both overfeeding and underfeeding. *Overfeeding* with high glucose infusions can lead to hyperglycemia, hypokalemia, edema, a fatty liver degeneration, and an increased risk of nosocomial infections.[13,14] Overfeeding also increases carbon dioxide production (V_{CO2}), which in turn may lead to difficulty weaning from a ventilator because the minute ventilation cannot be increased.

Estimating Total Daily Requirements (TDRs)

There are a number of ways to make a reasonable estimate of TDRs. Three factors are necessary to calculate TDRs: (1) calculation of the basal metabolic rate (BMR), (2) energy expended during activity (EEA), and (3) the thermogenic effect of food intake (TER). The following formula is useful to determine TDR of energy.[15]

$$TDR = BMR + EEA + TER$$

BMR: a measure of the amount of energy expended in order to maintain a living state while at rest and fasting
REE: a related term to BMR that is sometimes substituted for BMR; it represents the amount of energy expended 2 hours after eating under conditions of rest and thermal neutrality; generally, 10% higher than the BMR
EEA: energy expenditure of activity; a measure of the energy expended by the body to support a variety of physical activity
TER: the thermogenic effect of food is an estimate of the number of calories produced as heat during the ingestion and metabolism of food, which increases the BMR. *Note*: with continuous nutrients, as for hospitalized patients, this negates the need for energy to store and recover nutrients for energy, so that this factor can be ignored.

Direct Methods of Calculating Basal Metabolic Rate

Harris-Benedict Equations

Although there are more than 190 methods to estimate BMR,[16] the Harris-Benedict equation is commonly used when W = weight in kilograms, H = height in centimeters, and A = age in years. The Harris-Benedict equation generally underestimates the BMR by about 20% in malnourished patients,[17] but no constant factor is applied to the formula to adjust the results. It also overestimates the BMR of healthy women greater than 40 Kg by 7% to 14%.[18]

Calculating Basal Metabolic Rate

$$BMR_{men} = 66 + (13.7 \times W) + (5 \times H) - (6.8 \times A)$$

$$BMR_{women} = 665 + (9.6 \times W) + (1.8 \times H) - (4.7 \times A)$$

Calculating the Energy Expended During Activity (EEA)

The EEA provides a correction factor based on the patient's expenditure of energy (Table 9-2). Note that each 1°C increase in body temperature increases the metabolic rate by approximately 5% to 10%; a correction factor is included in Table 9-2 to account for fever.

Calculating the Thermogenic Effect Rate (TER) of Food Intake

The increase in metabolic rate following eating is about 5% to 10% of the daily energy expenditure. The TER is difficult to assess in hospitalized patients. Therefore, using indirect calorimetry during or shortly after feeding infusion eliminates the need to estimate TER.[19]

Formulas for Estimating Resting Energy Expenditure (REE) in Hospitalized Patients

When more precision than the Harris-Benedict equation is needed, and when indirect calorimetry is not available, two newer equations have been developed for hospitalized patients (see below)[20] based on correlations with indirect calorimetry and multivariate regression analysis.[21] Note that equations have been developed for both the ventilator-dependent and spontaneously breathing patients. After the REE has been calculated, a correction factor for activity is made (see Table 9-2). Hospitalized patients who are severely catabolic or malnourished or those with high fever or sepsis require an increase to the REE of 20% to 25%. Care should be taken to prevent overestimating total energy needs to prevent overfeeding syndromes.

Equations

In which *A = age, W = body weight in Kg; S = sex (male = 1, female = 0); T = trauma (present = 1, absent = 0); B = burns (present = 1, absent = 0); O = obesity (present = 1, absent = 0)*

For ventilator-dependent patients:

$$REE = 1925 - 10(A) + 5(W) + 281(S) + 292(T) + 851(B)$$

For spontaneously breathing patients:

$$REE = 629 - 11(A) + 25(W) - 609(O)$$

The above-cited equations are examples of ways to calculate BMR or REE. There are other methods, and it is left to the clinical dietitian to assume the leadership role in setting the standards and specifics for calculations of energy needs within a given service and institution.

Indirect Method of Calculating Basal Metabolic Rate

Indirect Calorimetry (Metabolic Cart)

Another method to measure BMR is by an indirect method called *indirect calorimetry* or *metabolic cart*. This method measures oxygen uptake (V_{O2}) and carbon dioxide output (V_{CO2}) at the mouth.[22] The equipment used includes an open-circuit method with a set of one-way valves to direct expired air into a collection bag. At the end of the collection time, both the volume and the composition of expired air are measured and the rate of oxygen consumption and carbon dioxide production is calculated by the difference between the concentrations of the inspired air and the gas collected.

The data from indirect calorimetry include measurement of V_{O2} and V_{CO2} for 15 to 20 minutes. An estimate of REE and respiratory quotient (RQ) can be calculated and extrapolated to 24 hours. The REE is determined from these data by calculating the RQ, which is V_{CO2}/V_{O2}. The RQ reflects whole body substrate utilization and varies between 0.70 and 1.2. An RQ greater than 1.0 is an indication of excessive carbohydrate calories resulting in fat synthesis, which leads to high CO_2 production, a situation to be avoided.

The advantages of indirect calorimetry are its accuracy and its ability to be used with ventilated patients. Disadvantages include the need for special equipment, skilled personnel, increased cost, and inaccuracy when the inspired FiO_2 is > 0.40. Therefore, the test should be used selectively. Newer technology, with breath-to-breath systems, now allows measurement of REE even in ventilated patients receiving high levels of oxygen (FiO_2 is > 0.40).

Table 9–2 • ENERGY EXPENDITURE CORRECTION FACTOR

CLINICAL CONDITION	CORRECTION FACTOR
Out of bed	1.3
Confined to bed	1.2
Fever	1 + 0.13 per degree, C.
Multiple fractures	1.2–1.4
Soft tissue trauma	1.14–1.37
Sepsis	1.4–1.8
Minor surgery	1.0–1.2
Starvation (in adult)	0.70

(Adapted from Silberman, H. & Eisenberg, D. [1982]. *Parenteral and enteral nutrition for the hospitalized patient* [p. 60]. Norwalk, CT: Appleton-Century-Crofts.)

PROVIDING NUTRIENTS

After a reasonable determination of total daily energy requirements has been made, a series of questions need to be answered.

Does the patient need nutritional support?
If so, what are the energy and protein requirements for this patient?
What route (enteral or parenteral) of administration should be used?
If enteral feeding is used, where should the tube be placed?
When should the feeding begin?
What feeding should be given?

Patients Needing Nutritional Support

The following patients will need nutritional support: those expected to receive nothing by mouth for more than 7 to 10 days, those with hypermetabolic states (sepsis, multitrauma), or those with preexisting undernourishment (loss of 10% or more of usual body weight). In neuroscience populations, comatose, multitrauma, and septic patients are candidates for nutritional support.

Providing Adequate Energy and Protein Requirement

Using the formulas and calculations previously discussed, the *basal caloric requirement* for most hospitalized patients is about 2,100 kcal if the patients do not exceed 200 lb. Even with correction factors for fever and sepsis, patients' total energy requirements are usually less than 3,000 kcal/day. Previous published reports of significantly increased kcal/day have not been substantiated by more recent studies or studies focused on head-injured patients.[23,24] In addition, protein catabolism is high after head injury according to many studies. Reports state that higher levels of protein (2.2 g/kg/day) were needed to reverse a negative nitrogen balance in this population. A general rule of thumb for *caloric requirements* for seriously ill patients is *25 to 35 kcal/kg/day of ideal body weight* and *1.5 g/kg/day for protein* (up to 2.5 g/kg/day is recommended for the sickest patients). These are *initial goals,* which can then be increased, as necessary, based on laboratory data (e.g., prealbumin, UUN balance) and changing clinical condition (e.g., increased fever). Recommendations vary about the allocation of calories from carbohydrate, protein, and lipid sources, but generally about 20% protein, 30% lipid, and 50% carbohydrate is recommended.[8] If hepatic or renal disease is present, special formulas are available.

Route of Administration

Enteral feeding, rather than parenteral nutrition, is clearly the preferred route for administering nutritional support. There are good reasons for preferring enteral nutrition rather than parenteral nutrition. First, nutrients to the intestinal lumen protect the integrity of the gastrointestinal (GI) tract. They preserve optimal gut function, maintain the gut barrier from translocation of microorganisms, and support gut-associated immune system IgA secretion. Second, enteral nutrition is safer, more convenient, and less expensive than parenteral nutrition. Beginning feeding at as low a rate as 10 mL/hour at a continuous rate will maintain the integrity of the endothelial lining of the GI tract and decrease the incidence of sepsis.

The use of the enteral route for feeding is evaluated based on the availability of the GI tract and the adequacy of intestinal function. Conditions to consider when assessing the adequacy of the enteral route include length of intestines (e.g., short from previous surgical procedure), adequate gastric and small bowel motility, and conditions that are potential exclusions for enteral feeding. These conditions include severe diarrhea, bowel disease (e.g., Crohn's disease, inflammatory colon disease), acute GI bleeding, obstructive small bowel or colon lesions, paralytic ileus, and acute inflammation of the pancreas or biliary tract.

Most neurological patients will not require parenteral nutrition (PN). For those patients who need nutritional support but who do not have a usable GI tract for enteral feeding (see discussion above), PN is useful. PN is a method of administering a highly concentrated hypertonic solution of essential macro- and micronutrients intravenously to provide the nutritional needs of the patient over an extended period. Total PN is employed when the GI tract is completely unusable. Partial PN is useful when enteral feeding alone does not meet nutrient requirements. Neuroscience patients who are good candidates for PN include multitrauma patients with GI injuries that interfere with digestion and absorption of nutrients.

Feeding Tubes and Site of Placement

When there is an intact intestinal tract, three possibilities exist for delivering food to the alimentary tract. First, oral feeding is always the preferred method of nutritional support. However, in many hospitalized neurological patients this is not possible for a number of reasons, including coma, high risk for aspiration, and multitrauma. In that case, temporary oral-gastric or nasogastric tubes into the stomach or nasoduodenal tube into the duodenum are available. Because a feeding tube is an extraordinary method of providing nutrition, there are ethical considerations that must be weighed. See Chapter 4 for a discussion of artificial feeding.

The feeding tube is inserted through the nose and into the stomach or upper small bowel. The type and the size of feeding tube chosen vary; each has certain advantages and disadvantages. Larger-bore, rigid feeding tubes can cause erosion of the nasal passages, esophagus, and stomach, but the larger bore of the tube ensures better delivery of the feeding without occlusion. Smaller, more pliable tubes are less likely to erode tissue but are more likely to become occluded. Most continuous infusion enteral feeding is performed through small-bore tubes designed for nasogastric or nasoduodenal placement. The size of these small-bore tubes ranges from about 6- to 12-Fr gauge. *For neuroscience patients with a basal skull fracture, facial fractures, or leakage of cerebrospinal fluid, insertion of a tube nasally is contraindicated.*

There continues to be controversy about the merits of tube placement in the stomach or duodenum. A critical review of the evidence suggests that bypassing the stomach does increase tolerance to feedings, but it does not reduce the risk of aspiration or pneumonia.[25] Further, enteral feeding should not be delayed to establish small-bowel access. Most patients are able to tolerate some gastric feeding early in the course of illness. Small-bowel placement is reserved for those who cannot tolerate gastric feeding, although some physicians prefer the small-bowel site routinely.

Many serious problems can develop from prolonged nasogastric intubation. Possible problems include erosion and/or necrosis of the nares or nasal septum, sinusitis, peptic esophagitis from gastric reflux along the tube, and gastric erosion or ulcers. The need for prolonged tube feeding (i.e., 6 weeks or longer) is an indication for a simple surgical procedure whereby a gastrostomy or jejunostomy tube is sutured into position on the abdominal wall. After the tube is inserted, it is usually left to gravity drainage for the first 24 hours. When bowel sounds have returned, a feeding is begun and advanced as tolerated. The insertion site is treated like any other surgical wound with daily stoma dressing care according to hospital protocol and monitoring of the incision for signs or symptoms of infection.

Another enteral tube placement option for long-term feeding is percutaneous endoscopic gastrostomy (PEG). It involves the placement of a 16- to 18-gauge latex or silicone catheter through the abdominal wall directly into the stomach using an endoscopic approach. This approach does not require anesthesia and has a low complication rate. The tube can be used for feeding within 24 to 48 hours of placement.

Beginning Feedings

Current research-based evidence supports starting enteral feeding as soon as possible following admission to the intensive care unit.[25] Early nutritional support within 12 to 48 hours blunts the hypercatabolic state and sepsis related to serious illness. A common finding in patients with such critical illness is decreased motility of the GI tract that lasts about 5 to 7 days or longer if the patient remains critically ill. Motility and nutrient absorption of the small bowel usually are functional even after severe trauma. Bowel sounds are a poor index of small bowel motility.

After insertion of a nasogastric or nasoduodenal tube, feedings are not begun until an x-ray film of the abdomen confirms appropriate GI placement. Feeding should be started at 25 to 30 mL/hour and increased by 10 to 25 mL/hour every 1 to 4 hours as tolerated until the caloric goal (25 kcal/kg/day) is achieved. Tolerance is evaluated by measurement of gastric residuals (less than 200 mL) and presence of abdominal distention, vomiting, diarrhea. If the gastric residual is greater than 220 mL, the feeding is held for 2 hours and then resumed. Feeding can be increased at a slower rate (e.g., 10 mL every 6 to 12 hours), but this is often not necessary and delays achievement of the caloric intake goal. The goal rate should be achieved by the third day of therapy, if not earlier. Feedings can be administered intermittently a few times a day (running over an hour or two) or continuously with a food pump.

Selection of Feeding Formula

There are at least 150 commercially available enteral nutrition products, which adds to the complexity of the selection process. These products are classified as standard, high protein, very high protein, disease specific, with fiber, elemental, and volume restricted. Table 9-3 provides a summary description of enteral formulas. Examples of commonly used commercially prepared feedings are included in Table 9-4.

Most formulas are complete formulas, that is, they provide recommended daily requirements of micronutrients (vitamins and minerals) in addition to the macronutrients of carbohydrate, protein, and fat. Some patients may need additional vitamin or mineral supplements beyond what is provided in the formula for deficiencies—for example, for patients with a history of alcoholism, thiamine and folate. In some cases thiamine is supplemented to avoid metabolic acidosis.[26] Most enteral formulas, with the exception of elemental formulas, are isotonic at full strength. Dilution of a feeding does not generally enhance tolerance and may delay achievement of caloric intake goals. Feeding formulas, therefore, should *not* be diluted.

In recent years, interest has been increased in the immunomodulating properties of various nutrients such as branch-chained amino acid, nucleotides, arginine, glutamine, and omega-3 fatty acids.[27] There are few randomized control trials evaluating the effect of any of these supplements on clinical outcomes such as infection rates, length of stay, morbidity, or mortality. The few that do exist have insufficient evidence to support routine use of special immunologically enhanced feeding in the critically ill at this time.[25] This may change in the future as new studies are conducted.

PROBLEMS ASSOCIATED WITH TUBE FEEDINGS

Overview of Problems

Infectious and metabolic complications frequently occur in critically ill patients on nutritional support. The most common metabolic complication is undernutrition.[27] The associated major problems are underfeeding and overfeeding. *Underfeeding* is related to starvation, depletion of protein stores, delayed wound healing, high risk for skin breakdown, high risk for nosocomial infections, respiratory muscle weakness and ventilator dependency,[28] and increased mortality and morbidity. The causes of underfeeding are multifactorial, and delay in initiating feeding is common. Diarrhea, vomiting, GI tract dysfunction, and electrolyte imbalance are but a few of the problems that can interfere with adequate nutritional support in the patient receiving enteral feeding. *Overfeeding* is related to complications such as hyperglycemia,[29] azotemia, hypertonic dehydration, electrolyte imbal-

▌▌ Table 9-3 • ENTERAL NUTRITION PRODUCTS

TYPE OF FORMULA	DESCRIPTION	BRAND NAMES AND EXAMPLES
Standard	Complete formulas that provide macronutrients and micronutrients; are recommended daily requirements Lactose free, as are most formulas Provide 1.0 to 1.2 kcal/mL. First choice for most patients	Ensure, Isocal, Magnacal, and Osmolite
High protein	Have a higher protein/nitrogen and a ratio of nonprotein calories to nitrogen of <130:1, but >110:1 For those patients who are severely catabolic and protein deficient, such as severe trauma or patients with large, poorly healing wounds.	Isocal HCN and Isocal HN
Very high protein	Similar to high protein, but with a lower ratio of nonprotein calories to nitrogen of <110:1	Sustacal
Disease-specific	Intact protein designed specifically to meet the protein, electrolyte, and glucose limitations of specific diseases	Glucerna (diabetes mellitus); Hepatic-Aid II (liver disease); Travasorb Renal (renal disease)
With fiber	These formulas produce more fecal residue that increases stool bulk For patients with constipation or diarrhea	Jevity
Elemental	Calories are supplied primarily as free amino acids and oligosaccharides For patients with decreased ability to digest and absorb standard formulas Are hyperosmolar and cause gastric retention and diarrhea	Criticare HN, Stresstein, and Vivonex TEN
Volume-restricted	Caloric density > 1.2 kcal/mL Useful when fluid overload is a problem such as ascites, renal failure, congestive heart failure	Ensure Plus, Ensure Plus HN, and Protain XL

(Adapted from: Alpers, D. H., Stenson, W. F., & Bier, D. M. [1995]. *Manual of nutritional therapeutics* [3rd ed., p. 288, Table 9-4]. Boston: Little, Brown).

ance (especially potassium, magnesium, phosphorous),[30] edema, metabolic acidosis, hypercapnia (related to failure to wean from a ventilator), hyperlipidemia, hepatic steatosis (fatty degeneration), refeeding syndrome,[31] and an increased risk of nosocomial infections.[13,14] The most common cause of overfeeding is overestimating daily caloric needs for the patient. These potential problems and considerations are presented in Table 9-5.

Medications

An important consideration in patients receiving enteral nutrition is that of medications. The size and location of the feeding tube, as well as the specific drug, must be considered.

Tube

The diameter of the tube is important. The smaller the diameter of the tube, the more likely it is to become clogged. Thick liquids such as antacids should not be administered through a tube smaller than 10-Fr. gauge.[30] Determining the location of the tube (stomach, duodenum, jejunum) affects drug metabolism. First, drugs administered beyond the pyloric valve are absorbed more rapidly. Additionally, some drugs, such as antacids and sucralfate, should not be delivered beyond the pylorus. Other drugs with enteric coatings or slow-release drugs (e.g., verapamil hydrochloride [Calan SR] or diltiazem [Cardizem]) should not be crushed, because this may increase the rate of absorption for the slow-release drugs or expose drugs to breakdown in the stomach and cause gastric irritation.

▌▌ Table 9-4 • COMPOSITION OF SELECTED COMMERCIALLY PREPARED TUBE FEEDINGS

PRODUCT	Kcal/mL	CALORIC DISTRIBUTION (%)			mOsm/kg
		Protein	Carbohydrates	Fat	
Ensure	1.06	14	54.5	31.5	470
Ensure Plus	1.5	15	32	53	470
Isocal	1.06	13	50	37	300
Isocal HN	1.06	17	47	36	300
Jevity	1.06	16.7	53.3	30	310
Osmolite	1.06	14	54.6	31.4	300
Osmolite HN	1.06	16.7	53.3	34.8	300
Sustacal	1.0	24	55	23	620
Sustacal Plus	1.5	16	50	34	650

▌▌▌ Table 9-5 • POTENTIAL PROBLEMS WITH ENTERAL TUBE FEEDINGS

PROBLEM	POSSIBLE CAUSES	CONSIDERATIONS
Diarrhea	Multifactorial and common in the acute care setting. Drugs (e.g., antibiotics) Visceral protein depletion (alters oncotic gradient) Stress-associated GI dysfunction (e.g., malabsorption) Infections (*Clostridium difficile*), other infectious disease causes, bacterial overgrowth Impaction GI tract problems: inflammatory bowel, disease, pancreatic insufficiency, short gut syndrome These causes are more common than the tube feeding itself or its administration	Attempt to identify underlying cause Rule out *C. difficile* (stool culture) and other infections (stool smear for ova, parasites) It is rarely necessary to stop enteral feeding
Vomiting	Feeding too soon after intubation or suctioning Too rapid a rate of infusion Underlying GI problems	Allow patient a rest period before beginning feeding Run infusion slowly Explore possibilities
Gastric distention	Decreases lower esophageal sphincter pressure and predisposes to reflex and high risk for aspiration	Observe for distention Monitor gastric residuals; hold if >200 mL for 2 hours Keep head of bed at 30 degree angle
Dehydration	Rapid infusion of hyperosmolar carbohydrates that cause hyperglycemia → osmotic diuresis → dehydration Excessive protein and electrolytes (have an osmotic effect)	Observe for signs and symptoms of dehydration Monitor glucose and acetone levels every 4–6 hours May need regular insulin on sliding scale Adjust/change formula Administer slowly Administer free water Monitor electrolytes
Aspiration	Feeding tube not in stomach/jejunum Vomiting (see under Vomiting for description) *Note:* Aspiration can cause pneumonia or acute respiratory distress syndrome; every precaution should be taken to prevent aspiration.	Check position of tube *before* beginning feeding Elevate head of bed at 30 to 45 degrees Have suction equipment handy
Hyperglycemia	Often seen with dehydration Overnutrition Hyperosmolar condition Precipitates glycosuria that, if untreated, will result in osmotic diuresis and hyperosmolar nonketotic coma Impairs immune response and increases infection rate	Monitor glucose 4–6 hours May need regular insulin on sliding scale Adjust/change formula Administer slowly Administer free water
Electrolyte imbalance	Potassium (K), phosphorous, magnesium are most common Patients with renal, hepatic, or cardiac disease are especially prone to such problems These may decline when nutritional support is beginning due to protein synthesis	Monitor electrolyte blood levels Adjust or change formula to a restrictive formula as necessary (e.g., low K formula) Supplement electrolytes as needed
Other disease related intolerances	Renal or hepatic disease (patient may not tolerate even normal levels of amino acids) Electrolyte imbalances may increase with renal failure	Change feeding to a disease-specific program Monitor renal and liver blood studies
Migrating feeding tube	Can become dislodged during care, pulling by patient, or from effect of tube on GI tract Can cause aspiration or peritonitis	Check position of tube periodically
Refeeding syndrome	Seen when severely malnourished patient begin enteral or parenteral nutrition With refeeding, phosphate and magnesium move from the extracellular to the intracellular space causing hypophosphatemia and hypomagnesemia	Monitor serum magnesium and phosphate If low, replace as necessary
Catheter occlusion	More likely with small bore catheter especially when used to administer medications	Flush tube frequently Do not administer medications through small bore tube

Drug Administration Guidelines

A number of guidelines to provide effective drug administration are outlined by Alpers and coworkers:[32]

Use liquid preparation of a drug, if available.

Crushing or dissolving of tablets is discouraged. If absolutely necessary, dissolve in at least 10 to 15 mL of water.

Hard gelatinous capsules should be opened and dissolved in at least 10 to 15 mL of water.

Drugs irritating to the GI tract should be dissolved in large amounts of water before administration.

Do not add drugs to the enteral feeding.

Stop the feeding before administering the medications.

Flush the feeding tube with water to remove residual formula *before* administering the drug.

Flush the feeding tube with 10 to 30 mL of water *after* administering the drug.

For patients on an intermittent gastric feeding schedule, adjust the timing of medication to the feeding schedule according to the need for drug delivery on a full or empty stomach.

Drugs With Special Administration Requirements With Enteral Feedings

A few drugs commonly administered to neuroscience patients need special mention.

Patients receiving phenytoin (Dilantin) and receiving continuous feedings require increased doses of phenytoin to maintain therapeutic levels because it binds to protein, resulting in decreased absorption of the drug.[33] These patients also tend to develop signs and symptoms of phenytoin toxicity when the nutrition route is switched from tube feedings to oral nutrition if the same dosage is maintained. Because many patients receive both continuous enteral feedings and phenytoin therapy simultaneously, increased doses of phenytoin will be required. The dosage will need to be evaluated and probably decreased when oral nutrition has begun. Patients should have phenytoin levels monitored more frequently when receiving enteral nutrition therapy, and they should be assessed for signs and symptoms of toxicity. If a schedule of intermittent feedings is used, adjust the drug administration schedule to give phenytoin between feedings.

Carbamazepine suspension (Tegretol) is another commonly prescribed anticonvulsant drug. Dilute the suspension so that it will not adhere to the walls of the feeding tube. Flush well after administration.

Monitoring Patients Receiving Enteral Feedings

The following outline suggests laboratory studies helpful in monitoring patients receiving enteral feedings so that abnormalities and deficiencies can be identified and treated appropriately.

Electrolytes: sodium, potassium, chloride, and bicarbonate (baseline and twice per week)

Other chemistries: glucose (baseline until stable, and then 3 times weekly; patients with diabetes will need it more frequently)

Renal function: creatinine levels and blood urea nitrogen (BUN) (baseline and twice per week)

Liver function: as needed based on patient profile

Other laboratory data: calcium, phosphorus, magnesium, albumin, prealbumin (baseline and once per week); triglycerides, cholesterol baseline and as indicated; hematocrit (baseline and twice per week); prothrombin time as needed

Depending on the patient's underlying problems, other laboratory studies may be indicated.

THE NURSE'S ROLE: MEETING THE NUTRITIONAL NEEDS OF PATIENTS

The importance of nutrition in recovery from neurological illness is well established. The nurse works collaboratively with the clinical dietitian and other members of the health care team to meet the nutritional needs of the patients regardless of neurological deficits or acuity of illness. Along the continuum, many hospitalized neuroscience patients require enteral nutritional support. Others may need assistance with reestablishing oral nutrition within the limitations imposed by neurological illness. The nurse begins with conducting a nutritional assessment to establish a baseline and plan of care. The nurse's plan of care is designed to complement the overall nutritional goals for the patient. When nutritional therapeutics have been ordered, the nurse implements the protocol and monitors the patient's response to therapy providing information to the health care team.

Based on a nutritional assessment, various collaborative problems and nursing diagnoses can be made. Because of the complexity of neurological illness that impacts on the nutritional goal, several potential collaborative problems must be kept in mind; they include starvation, paralytic ileus, hypoglycemia, hyperglycemia, negative nitrogen balance, electrolyte imbalance, sepsis, and aspiration pneumonia. Other problems may be added, such as renal or hepatic failure based on complications that may occur as a result of neurological insult. The following nursing diagnoses are often identified for the patient with problems related to nutritional need:

- Nutrition, Altered, More Than Body Requirements
- Nutrition, Altered, Less Than Body Requirement
- Fluid Volume, Deficit or Risk of
- Fluid Volume Excess
- Swallowing, Impaired
- Aspiration, Risk for

Ongoing Nursing Assessment

The nurse can monitor the patient's nutritional status with the following parameters:

- Once stabilized, weigh the patient twice per week, on designated days, and note trends in stability of weight.

- Observe skin turgor, the condition of the tongue and mucous membranes, muscle tone, and muscle bulk daily for evidence of dehydration.
- Record and monitor intake and output and daily balance.
- Maintain a calorie count with the help of the clinical dietitian.
- Monitor tolerance to oral or enteral feeding; use as basis for progress of feeding to caloric goal.
- Monitor appropriate laboratory data (electrolytes, glucose, prealbumin, creatinine, BUN).

Administering Enteral Feedings

Enteral feedings may be administered in one of two ways: continuously with the use of a food pump or intermittently with the use of a gavage bag. The continuous method is recommended for postpyloric feeding, whereas either method can be used for feedings going into the stomach. Most commercial formulas in *open systems* (i.e., bags that are manually filled) are designed to hang for up to 4 hours without refrigeration after being spiked with connecting tubing. Most commercial formulas in *closed systems* (i.e., aseptic 1-L bottles) are designed to hang for 24 hours without refrigeration after they are spiked with the administration tubing.

A few comments about aspiration for residual are warranted. Before initiating a feeding into the stomach (e.g., nasogastric or gastrostomy tube), it is recommended that the tube be aspirated to determine whether retained formula is present. The expectation is that if the GI tract is working properly, there will be minimal or no formula present from the last feeding. Most centers use residual volumes as a guide to monitoring tolerance and subsequent feedings, but

Table 9–6 • COMPARISON OF MANAGEMENT OF A PATIENT RECEIVING ENTERAL FEEDING BY NASOGASTRIC OR GASTROSTOMY TUBE VERSUS NASODUODENAL OR JEJUNOSTOMY TUBE

FOCUS	NASOGASTRIC TUBE OR GASTROSTOMY TUBE FEEDING	NASODUODENAL TUBE OR JEJUNOSTOMY TUBE FEEDING
Site of feeding infusion	Stomach	Small intestines (duodenum or jejunum, both postpyloric valve structures)
Type of formula selected	Appropriate for particular patient	Same
Intermittent/gavage or continuous feeding	Some controversy; either method acceptable, although more support for intermittent method	Continuous Intermittent/gavage *not recommended* because of somatic response of the small bowel to feeding
Initiation of feeding	Follow physician orders A typical order for intermittent method is: Begin with 100–150 mL/q4h of isotonic or slightly hypotonic formula	Follow physician orders A typical order is: Slow constant infusion rate of isotonic or slightly hypotonic formula at 25–50 mL/hour
Advancing infusion rate (based on patient tolerance)	Follow physician orders A typical order for intermittent method is: Advance 50 mL every one or two feedings up to a maximum of about 400 mL q4h	Follow physician orders A typical order is: If after 8–24 hours, rate is tolerated, increase infusion rate by 25–50 mL/hour, until goal is reached Usually tolerated well
Achieving caloric goal (hourly rate set to achieve total calculated daily caloric requirement)	Goal is to achieve calculated daily total caloric requirements within ≤3 days or less Usually achieved with good team collaboration and communications	Goal is the same Usually goal achieved in <3 days
Temperature of material being fed	Follow manufacturer's instructions Most commercially prepared formulas can hang without refrigeration (see previous description) as follows: Open system can hang for up to 4 hours Closed system can hang for up to 24 hours	Same
Elevation of head of bed	At least 30 degrees before beginning feeding, and leave elevated for at least 2 hrs after completion of feeding; designed to decrease aspiration risk	30 degree while feeding
Flushing of feeding tube	Use at least 30 mL of water or dark carbonated soda every feeding and as needed to ensure patency	Use at least 30 mL of water q4h and as needed to maintain patency*
Aspiration for residual	Before each intermittent feeding; if residual exceeds the cut-off point, hold feeding for 2 hours and then recheck before administering another feeding	Do not aspirate tube that is placed beyond the pyloric valve

* Dark carbonated soda and cranberry juice have also been mentioned in the literature; follow facility protocol.

Table 9-7 • POTENTIAL PROBLEMS ASSOCIATED WITH ORAL FEEDINGS

PROBLEM	DESCRIPTION	NURSING ACTIONS
Distractibility/short attention span	Patients become interested in the activity around them and stop eating; patients forget what to do with their food once it is on their eating utensils	Screen patient from the distraction. Take excess dishes off the meal tray. Redirect patient's attention to eating; cue as necessary. Screen patient from excessive environmental stimuli. Break activity of eating into steps and direct the patient in the steps of eating (e.g., pick up the potatoes with your spoon; lift the spoon to your mouth; open your mouth).
Disorientation	Not always aware of time, place, person May think that the food belongs to someone else or that it is poisoned	Provide reality orientation and assist patients in feeding themselves. Give many verbal cues for eating. Correct any misconceptions. Reassure the patient in a calm voice. Be sure the patient is wearing eyeglasses if needed.
Visual deficits		
Diplopia	Double vision	Apply an eye patch to one eye or cover one lens if double vision is present.
Hemianopia	Loss of vision in half of the visual field	If patient eats food from only one side of the dish, turn the dish; remind the patient to turn his or her head to scan the dish.
Dimness of vision	Visual images may be dim or fuzzy	Provision of a good light may help alleviate dimness.
Motor deficits (plegia or paresis)	May involve deficits of cranial nerves V, VII, or XII	Encourage patient to chew food on the unaffected side. Have the patient try to eat with other hand.
Muscles of chewing or of the face or tongue	Associated with hemiparesis or hemiplegia; monoplegia of one extremity may be present	Use built-up eating utensils. Use special equipment, such as a guard around the plate to prevent food from spilling off the dish.
Arm or hand		Consult the occupational therapist for suggestions. Prepare the patient's tray (e.g., cut up meat, pour milk).

there is variation about the cut-off amount to hold a feeding. The range is from 100 mL to 200 mL, although there are few data on which to base any recommendation. One report noted that no patients were intolerant to feeding even when residuals were greater than 300 mL.[34] In most centers, intermittent feeding is held for 2 hours if the amount of residual exceeds the cut-off point set by that facility or by that physician, generally between 100 mL to 200 mL. After the 2-hour delay, the residual is rechecked before administering the next feeding.

Special nursing protocols are followed for safe administration of the feeding to prevent complications (e.g., aspiration, pneumonia). In addition, the previous section offers suggestion for ongoing monitoring. While the feeding is in progress, monitor the patient frequently to detect complications and to assess efficacy of the nutritional support. Because of anatomical considerations, there are some differences in administering enteral feedings into the stomach compared with feeding delivered below the level of the pylorus. These commonalties and differences are included in Table 9-6. The following are a few other nursing responsibilities in managing a patient receiving enteral feeding:

• Check the position of the tube to be sure it has not migrated.
• If the patient has a tracheostomy tube in place, *deflate* the cuff; keep it *deflated* for 1 hour after completion of the feeding. The purpose of this action is to prevent aspiration.
• Addition of a few drops of blue food coloring into the feeding is often recommended as a way to assess pulmo-

nary aspiration of enteral formula in intubated patients. Follow hospital recommendations. If used, observe tracheal secretions to note blue discoloration as an indication of aspiration.[35]
• Intermittent feedings should be administered over a period of 30 to 60 minutes, depending on the amount of the feeding.
• Record the amount and type of feeding on the intake and output record.
• Observe the patient for signs and symptoms of abdominal distention, regurgitation, aspiration, nausea/vomiting, diarrhea, or intolerance to the feeding.

Oral Feeding

Oral feeding is always the first choice for nutritional intake. If enteral feeding is used, the goal is to return the patient to oral feeding as soon as possible. When the patient appears ready to progress to oral feedings, a swallowing study is usually conducted by the speech therapist to assess for dysphagia or silent aspiration. A dysphagia diet and/or the need for thickened liquids are common recommendations (see Chapter 13 for a discussion of dysphagia).

Before beginning to feed the patient by the oral route, the nurse should:

• Assess the gag reflex. Do not initiate oral feedings if the gag reflex is not intact, because of the risk of aspiration.
• Observe for the presence of any facial weakness. The

paresis or paralysis may be confined to only one side of the face. Deficits can cause difficulty in chewing and "pocketing" of food.

- Auscultate the abdomen for the presence of bowel sounds.
- Sit the patient up, if possible. This decreases the risk of aspiration.
- If the patient has a tracheostomy tube in place, the cuff should be *deflated* before beginning to offer oral intake. There is an increased risk of delayed aspiration if food becomes lodged above an inflated cuff, which may, upon deflation, fall into the trachea.

After the preliminary assessment has been conducted and necessary precautions have been taken to prevent aspiration, oral nutrition can be initiated.

Self-Feeding

Assess the patient's ability for self-feeding. Cognitive, motor, and coordination deficits may interfere with this activity. Several problems that interfere with eating may be identified. These problems and appropriate nursing actions are described in Table 9-7. Although it can be time-consuming to supervise a patient, it is an important component in the rehabilitation process and achievement of independence. Every effort should be made to assist the patient in achieving this goal.

REFERENCES

1. Alpers, D. H., Stenson, W. F., & Bier, D. M. (1995). *Manual of nutritional therapeutics* (3rd ed., pp. 3–35). Boston: Little, Brown.
2. Food and Nutrition Board, National Research Council. (1989). *Recommended dietary allowances* (10th ed.). Washington, DC: National Academy Press.
3. Clifton, G. L., Robertson, C. S., & Choi, S. C. (1986). Assessment of nutritional requirements of head-injured patients. *Journal of Neurosurgery, 64,* 895–901.
4. Clifton, G. L., Robertson, C. S., & Constant, C. F. (1985). Enteralhyperalimentation in head injury. *Journal of Neurosurgery, 62,* 186–193.
5. Clifton, G. L., Robertson, C. S., Grossman, R. G., et al. (1984). The metabolic response to severe head injury. *Journal of Neurosurgery, 60,* 687–696.
6. Trujillo, E. B., Robinson, M. K., & Jacobs, D. O. (1999). Nutritional assessment in the critically ill. *Critical Care Nurse, 19*(1), 67–78.
7. Coats, K. G., Morgan, S. L., Bartolucci, A. A., & Weinsier, R. L. (1993). Hospital-associated malnutrition: A reevaluation 12 years later. *Journal of the American Dietetic Association, 93,* 27–33.
8. Roberts, P. R. (1999). Nutrition in the intensive care unit. In D. J. Dries & R. K. Albert (Eds.). *ACCP/SCCM combined critical care course: Multidisciplinary board review* (pp. 425–436). Anaheim, CA: Society of Critical Care Medicine and the American College of Chest Physicians.
9. Alpers, D. H., Stenson, W. F., & Bier, D. M. (1995). *Manual of nutritional therapeutics* (3rd ed., pp. 73–114). Boston: Little, Brown.
10. Doweiko, J. P., & Nompleggi, D. J. (1991). The role of albumin in human physiology and pathophysiology, III: Albumin and disease states. *Journal of Parenteral and Enteral Nutrition, 11,* 476–483.
11. Fletcher, J. P., Little, J. M., & Guest, P. K. (1987). A comparison of serum transferring and serum prealbumin as nutritional parameters. *Journal of Parenteral and Enteral Nutrition, 11,* 144–147.
12. Church, J. M., & Hill, G. L. (1987). Assessing the efficacy of intravenous nutrition in general surgical patients: Dynamic nutritional assessment with plasma proteins. *Journal of Parenteral and Enteral Nutrition, 11,* 135–139.
13. Pomposelli, J. J., Baxter, J. K., & Babineau, T. J. (1998). Early postoperative glucose control predicts nosocomial infection rate in diabetic patients. *Journal of Parenteral and Enteral Nutrition, 22,* 77–81.
14. Pomposelli, J. J. & Bistrian, B. B. (1994). Is total parenteral nutrition immunosuppressive? *New Horizons, 2,* 224–229.
15. Alpers, D. H., Stenson, W. F., & Bier, D. M. (1995). *Manual of nutritional therapeutics* (3rd ed., p. 73). Boston: Little, Brown.
16. Foster, G. D., Knox, L. S., Dempsey, D. T., & Mullen, J. L. (1987). Caloric requirements in total parenteral nutrition. *Journal of the American College of Nutrition, 6*(3), 231–253.
17. Roza, A. M., & Shizgal, H. M. (1984). The Harris Benedict equation reevaluated: Resting energy requirements and health. *American Journal of Clinical Nutrition, 40*(1), 168–182.
18. Owen, O. E., Kavle, E., Owen, R. S., Polansky, M., Caprio, S., Mozzoli, M. A., Kendrick, Z. V., & Bushmen-Boden, G. (1986). A reappraisal of caloric requirements in healthy women. *American Journal of Clinical Nutrition, 44*(1), 1–19.
19. Porte, C., & Cohen, N. H. (1996). Indirect calorimetry in critically ill patients: Role of the clinical dietitian in interpreting results. *Journal of the American Dietetic Association, 96,* 49–54.
20. Ireton-Jones, C. S., Turner, W. W. Jr., Liepa, G. U., & Baxter, C. R. (1992). Equations for estimating energy expenditures in burned patients with special reference to respiratory status. *Journal of Burn Care Rehabilitation, 13*(3), 330–333.
21. Alpers, D. H., Stenson, W. F., & Bier, D. M. (1995). *Manual of nutritional therapeutics* (3rd ed., p. 80). Boston: Little, Brown.
22. Alpers, D. H., Stenson, W. F., & Bier, D. M. (1995). *Manual of nutritional therapeutics* (3rd ed., pp. 81–82). Boston: Little, Brown.
23. Twyman, D. (1997). Nutritional management of the critically ill neurologic patient. *Critical Care Clinics, 23*(1), 39–49.
24. Rapp, R. P., Young, B., & Twyman, D. (1983). The favorable effect of early parenteral feeding on survival in head-injured patients. *Journal of Neurosurgery, 58,* 906–912.
25. Heyland, D. K. (1998). Nutritional support in the critically ill patient: A critical review of the evidence. *Critical Care Clinics, 14*(3), 423–440.
26. Byers, P. M., & Jeejeebhoy, K. N. (1997). Enteral and parenteral nutrition. In J. M. Civetta, R. W. Taylor, & R. R. Kirby. *Critical care* (3rd ed., pp. 457–473). Philadelphia: Lippincott-Raven.
27. Daly, J. M., Lieberman, M. D., Goldfine, J., Shou, J., Weintraub, F., Rosata, E. P., & Lavin, P. (1992). Enteral nutrition with supplemental argentine, RNA, and omega-3 fatty acids in patients after operation: Immunologic, metabolic, and clinical outcome. *Surgery, 112*(1), 56–67.
28. Christman, J. W., & McClain, R. W. (1993). Sensible approach to the nutritional support of mechanically ventilated critically ill patients. *Intensive Care Medicine, 19,* 129.
29. Hennessey, P. J., Black, C. T., & Andrassy, R. J. (1991). Nonenzymatic glycosylation of immunoglobin C impairs complement fixation. *Journal of Parenteral and Enteral Nutrition, 15,* 60.
30. Phelps, S. J., Brown, R. O., Helms, R. A., Christensen, M. L., Kudsk, K., & Cochran, E. B. (1991). Toxicities of parenteral nutrition in the critically ill patient. *Critical Care Clinics, 7*(3), 725–752.
31. Havala, T., & Shronts, E. (1990). Managing the complications associated with refeeding. *Nutrition in Clinical Practice, 5*(1), 23–29.
32. Alpers, D. H., Stenson, W. F., & Bier, D. M. (1995). *Manual of nutritional therapeutics* (3rd ed., pp. 316–317). Boston: Little, Brown.

33. Saklad, J. J., Graves, R., H., & Sharp, W. P. (1986). Interaction of oral phenytoin with enteral feedings. *Journal of Parenteral and Enteral Nutrition, 10*(3), 322–323.

34. McClave, S. A., Snider, H. L., Lower, C. C., McLaughlin, A. J., Greene, L. M., McCombs, R. J., Rodgers, L., Wright, R. A., Roy, T. M., & Schumer, M. O. (1992). Use of residual volume as a marker for enteral feeding intolerance: Prospective blinded comparison with physical examination and radiographic findings. *Journal of Parenteral and Enteral Nutrition, 16*(2), 99–105.

35. Metheny, N. A., Aud, M. A., & Wunderlich, R. J. (1999). A survey of bedside methods used to detect pulmonary aspiration of enteral formula in intubated tube-fed patients. *American Journal of Critical Care, 5*(3), 160–167.

BIBLIOGRAPHY

Anding, R. (1996). Nutrition support for the critically ill older patient. *Critical Care Nurse Quarterly, 19*(2), 13–22.

Bower, R. H. (1993). Nutrition during critical illness and sepsis. *New Horizons, 1*, 348–352.

Bridges, K. J., Trujillo, E. B., & Jacobs, D. O. (1999). Alcohol-related thiamine deficiency and malnutrition. *Critical Care Nurse, 19*(6), 80-85.

Buckley, S., & Kudsk, K. A. (1994). Metabolic response to critical illness and injury. *AACN Clinical Issues in Critical Care Nursing, 5*(4), 443–449.

Cerra, F. B., Benitez, M. R., Blackburn, G. L., Irwin, R. S., Jeejeebhoy, K., Katz, D. P., Pingleton, S. K., Pomposelli, J., Rombeau, J. L., Shronts, E., Wolfe, R. R., & Zaloga, P. (1997). Applied nutrition in ICU patients: A consensus statement of the American College of Chest Physicians. *Chest, 111*(3), 769–778.

Cheever, K. H. (1999). Early enteral feeding of patients with multiple trauma. *Critical Care Nurse, 19*(6), 40–53.

Gora, M. L., Tschampel, M. M., & Visconti, J. A. (1990). Considerations of drug therapy in patients receiving enteral nutrition. *Nutrition in Clinical Practice, 4*, 105–110.

Grant, J. P. (1994). Nutritional support in critically ill patients. *Annals of Surgery, 220*(5), 610–616.

Klien, C. J., Stanek, G. S., & Wiles, C. E. (1998). Overfeeding macronutrients to critically ill adults: Metabolic complication. *Journal of American Dietetic Association, 98*, 785–806.

Lord, L. M, & Sax, H. C. (1994). The role of the gut in critical illness. *AACN Clinical Issues in Critical Care Nursing, 5*(4), 450–458.

Mallampalli, A., McClave, S. A., & Snider, H. L. (2000). Defining tolerance to enteral feeding in the intensive care unit. *Clinical Nutrition, 19*(4), 213–215.

McClave, S. A., Sexton, L. K., Spain, D. A., Adams, J. L., Owens, N. A., Sullins, M. B., Blandford, B. S., & Snider, H. L. (1999). Enteral tube feeding in the intensive care unit: Factors impeding adequate delivery. *Critical Care Medicine, 27*(7), 1252–1256.

Medley, F., Stechmiller, J., & Field, A. (1993). Complications of enteral nutrition in hospitalized patients with artificial airways. *Clinical Nursing Research, 2*(2), 212–213.

Roberts, P. R. (1995). Nutrition in the head injured patient. *New Horizons, 3*, 506–517.

Romito, R. A. (1995). Early administration of enteral nutrients in critically ill patients. *AACN Clinical Issues, 6*(2), 242–256.

Shuster, M. H. (1994). Enteral feeding of the critically ill. *AACN Clinical Issues in Critical Care Nursing, 5*(4), 459–475.

Stanford, G. G. (1994). The stress response to trauma and critical illness. *Critical Care Nursing Clinics of North America, 6*(4), 693–702.

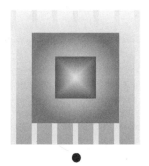

C H A P T E R **10**

Fluid and Electrolyte Management in Neuroscience Patients

JOANNE V. HICKEY

FLUID AND ELECTROLYTE BALANCE

Fluid and electrolyte balance is controlled by several inter-related, complex physiological mechanisms. Metabolic and electrolyte derangements, which are common in neuroscience patients, can be related to non-neurological problems, neurological problems, or a complication of therapeutics. Major electrolyte imbalances, diabetes insipidus (DI), syndrome of inappropriate secretion of antidiuretic hormone (SIADH), cerebral salt wasting, and hyperosmolar nonketotic dehydration syndrome (HONK) are briefly discussed in this chapter.

Distribution of Water in the Body

The major compound in the body is water; it comprises 50% to 60% of the total body weight. **Osmolality** is the concentration of a solution in terms of active particles (osmoles) *per liter* of solution. (**Osmolarity** is, conversely, the concentration of a solution in terms of osmoles of solute expressed *per kilogram* of solution). Osmolality is a useful measure of water balance. Hyperosmolality is a state of depletion of body water whereas hypoosmolality is a state of excess of water. Maintaining a near-constant body fluid osmolality is achieved primarily through a narrow range of regulation of water balance rather than solute balance.[1] Normal values for osmolality are listed in Table 10-1. The following formula is useful to *calculate and estimate* serum osmolality (mOsm/L):

$$2(Na + K) + (glucose \div 18) + (urea \div 2.8)$$

$$= serum\ osmolality\ (mOsm/L)$$

(*Na* is sodium and *K* is potassium; *18* and *2.8* are derived from the conversion of mg/dL to mOsm/L)

Serum osmolality can also be *measured* using the freezing point depression method. Serum osmolality may be increased by contributions from circulating alcohol and other low-molecular weight substances. Because these substances are not included in the calculated osmolality, there will be an osmolar gap directly proportional to their serum concentration and inversely proportional to their molecular weights.

(The *osmolar gap* is determined by subtracting the calculated serum osmolality from the measured serum osmolality.[2] It indicates additional solute osmoles.[3]) If the difference between the calculated and measured serum osmolality is more than 10 mOsm/kg of water, suspect a low-molecular weight toxin (e.g., ethanol, methanol, ethylene glycol, mannitol) or decreased serum water content from hyperlipidemia or hyperproteinemia (if total protein exceeds 10 g/dL).

A related concept is *tonicity*, defined as the force (ability to move water across a semipermeable membrane) exerted by osmotically active particles. Hypotonic solutions lose water to an isotonic solution whereas hypertonic solutions gain water from an isotonic solution. Variation exists in the tonicity of osmoles. For example, urea readily crosses the cell membrane but exerts no tonic force. By contrast, glucose induces movement of water from most cells. Sodium is the major extracellular osmole. It bears most responsibility for variations in serum tonicity and for the volume of extracellular fluid.

HYPOTHALAMIC-NEUROHYPOPHYSEAL SYSTEM

Both the intake and the renal excretion of water are controlled primarily by the hypothalamic-neurohypophyseal system. The hypothalamus-neurohypophysis includes the anatomic structures that control water osmolality. The production, storage, and secretion of **vasopressin**, also called **antidiuretic hormone** (ADH), affect the reabsorption of water by acting on the collecting tubules of the kidney. Within the hypothalamus are two pairs of nuclei cell groupings called the **supraoptic nuclei** and **paraventricular nuclei**, so named for their anatomic locations (Fig. 10-1). Most ADH is synthesized by perikarya of the magnocellular neurons of the supraoptic and paraventricular nuclei. ADH is then loosely bonded with a carrier protein called **neurophysin**. From the supraoptic and paraventricular nuclei, the combined ADH and neurophysin are transported down the **pituitary stalk** or **infundibulum** through terminal nerve fibers and terminal nerve endings. ADH is then stored in large secretory granules in the nerve endings of the posterior

Table 10-1 • TYPES OF HYPOTONIC HYPONATREMIA

TYPES	HYPOVOLEMIC HYPOTONIC HYPONATREMIA	EUVOLEMIC HYPOTONIC HYPONATREMIA	HYPERVOLEMIC HYPOTONIC HYPONATREMIA
ECF	ECF decreased with loss of body water and disproportionate larger sodium deficit	ECF and total body water increased, but the expansion not clinically detectable	ECF and total body water increased with a concurrent decrease in circulating volume
Cause(s)	Suppression of ADH due to: GI loss (vomiting/diarrhea) Skin loss: perspiration or burns Renal loss: overuse of diuretics, renal damage Adrenal insufficiency	SIADH Water intoxication Renal failure Increased secretion of antidiuretic hormone due to CNS or pulmonary disorders, or hemodynamic instability	Congestive heart failure Hepatic failure Renal failure Kidneys retain excessive amounts of salt and water, but the positive balance of water exceeds that of sodium
Clinical picture	Volume depleted patient	Normal volume patient	Patient edematous and hyponatremic
Treatment	Aqueous pitressin in saline or half normal saline continuous infusion	Restrict free water Furosemide Demeclocycline is an antagonist of ADH, but it takes days to become effective. Therefore, furosemide is best choice (increases free water excretion, but unfortunately also causes some salt loss) Concurrent 0.9%–3% saline intravenously	Treat underlying cardiac, renal, or liver disease Induce loss of salt and water with proportionally greater water loss than salt In advanced renal failure, dialysis will be required Restrict fluid intake to 800–1000 mL/day Furosemide for diuresis Monitor potassium balance because it influences sodium balance

ECF, extracellular fluid; ADH, antidiuretic hormone; SIADH, syndrome of inappropriate secretion of antidiuretic hormone; CNS, central nervous system.

pituitary gland (also called the **neurohypophysis**). Secretion of ADH is controlled by electrical impulses generated by the supraoptic and paraventricular nuclei. The impulses travel down the nerve fibers and nerve ending tracts, and ADH is released from the nerve endings. Because of the loose bonding of neurophysin to ADH, the neurophysin immediately separates from ADH. ADH is then absorbed into adjacent capillaries and circulation.

ADH is very potent, and even minute amounts (as little as 2 μg) have an appreciable effect on water balance. The half-life of ADH is 15 to 20 minutes, with metabolic degradation occurring in the liver and kidney. The immediate release and rapid breakdown of ADH account for the quick response time for even minute changes in volume, concentration, and composition of body fluids. The target organ of ADH is the kidney. With ADH, the collecting ducts and tubules become very permeable to water so that fluid is reabsorbed and conserved within the body. Conversely, without ADH, the renal collecting ducts and tubules are almost totally impermeable to water so that fluid is not reabsorbed; therefore, it is excreted in the urine.

Regulation of ADH Secretion

Secretion of ADH is controlled by osmoregulation and baroregulation. These receptors provide negative feedback loops to control secretion of ADH.

Osmoregulation

Changes in the osmolality of body fluids play the most important role in regulating ADH secretion. Changes in osmolality as small as 1% are sufficient to alter ADH secretion significantly.[4] **Osmoreceptors** are specialized cells that sense changes in serum osmolality. The osmoreceptors are located in the hypothalamus near the cells that produce ADH and respond to changes in concentration of **extracellular fluid** (ECF). Concentrated ECF stimulates the supraoptic nuclei to send impulses to release ADH, which will cause reabsorption of water in the kidney. Conversely, dilute ECF around the hypothalamic osmoreceptors inhibits the generation of impulses for the release of ADH. Hypertonic NaCl or sucrose does stimulate ADH release, but hypertonic urea and glucose do not. The ability of osmotic particles to cross the osmoreceptor membrane may account for these differences. Because the osmolality of plasma is determined by the concentration of a number of different solutes, including urea and glucose, the total plasma osmolality alone is not always clearly related to the ADH level.[5]

Baroregulation

Changes in blood volume and blood pressure may also lead to secretion of ADH. **Baroreceptors** are specialized cells that respond to pressure changes. Baroreceptors located in the chest, left atrium, aortic arch, and carotid sinuses sense changes in blood volume and blood pressure. Impulses from the baroreceptors travel via the vagus and glossopharyngeal nerves to the supraoptic and paraventricular nuclei. A decreased blood volume of 5% to 10% results in secretion of ADH. An increased ADH level has important vasopressor, as well as antidiuretic, effects. A decrease in the mean arterial blood pressure of 5% or more also can result in an increased secretion of ADH. This action may mediate the rise in ADH secretion during sleep.[5]

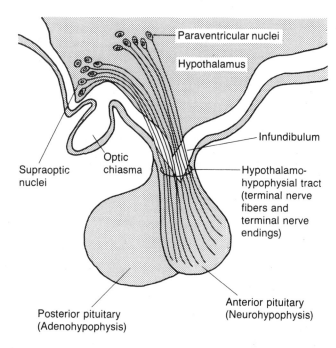

Figure 10–1 • Within the hypothalamus are the supraoptic nuclei and paracentricular nuclei, which produce antidiuretic hormone (ADH). This hormone combines with neurophysin and travels down the terminal nerve fibers and terminal nerve endings to be stored in large secretory granules in the nerve endings of the posterior pituitary gland (neurohypophysis). (The lateral hypothalamic area where the thrist center is located, is not shown.) (From De Graaff, K. M., & Fox, S. I. [1988]. *Concepts of human anatomy and physiology* [2nd ed.]. Dubuque, IA: Wm. C. Brown.)

Under ordinary circumstances, changes in osmolality of body fluids play the most important role in regulating ADH secretion. In certain situations of severe volume depletion, baroreceptors' stimulation of ADH secretion occurs despite significant hypoosmolality. In this case, volume is conserved at the expense of tonicity.

Stimulation, Inhibition, and Enhancement of Antidiuretic Hormone

Stimulates Release of Antidiuretic Hormone

Certain conditions stimulate secretion of ADH, thereby conserving water in the body. They include the upright position, hyperthermia, hypotension, hypovolemia (especially caused by severe blood loss), pain, severe stress, anxiety, nausea, emesis, hypoxia, and trauma. Drugs that increase ADH release include acetaminophen (Tylenol), amitriptyline, anesthetic agents, angiotensin II agents, barbiturates, beta-adrenergic agents, bromocriptine, chlorpromazine (Thorazine), chlorothiazide (Diuril), cholinergic drugs, clofibrate (Atromid S), cyclophosphamide (Cytoxan), haloperidol, histamines, monoamine oxidase inhibitors, meperidine hydrochloride (Demerol), metoclopramide, morphine, nicotine, phenothiazines, prostaglandin E2, and vincristine sulfate (Oncovin).[1,5]

Inhibits Release of Antidiuretic Hormone

Other conditions inhibit release of ADH. They include the recumbent position, hypothermia, hypertension, hypoosmolality, increased blood volume, and sleep. Drugs that decrease ADH secretion include ethanol, alpha-adrenergic agents, anticholinergic agents, demeclocycline (Declomycin), glucocorticosteroids (e.g., dexamethasone), lithium carbonate, narcotic antagonists, phenytoin (Dilantin), tolazamide, and vinblastine.[1,5]

Enhances Release of Antidiuretic Hormone

The following drugs enhance the effect of ADH: chlorpropamide (Diabinese), carbamazepine (Tegretol), nonsteroidal anti-inflammatory drugs (NSAIDs), and tolbutamide.

ADH Action on the Kidney

There are two primary actions of ADH on the kidneys. First, ADH stimulates NaCl reabsorption by the thick ascending limb of Henle's loop. Second, it increases the permeability of the distal convoluted tubule and collecting ducts to water and urea.[4] This process results in the preservation of water and the elaboration of concentrated urine. Reabsorbed water is not excreted and remains in the individual's body, thus lessening the rise in plasma osmolality and assisting in the maintenance of both blood volume and total body water volume. Reabsorption of water completes the feedback loop and tends to decrease the secretion of ADH.[4]

Thirst Center

Within the lateral hypothalamus is the **ventromedian nucleus**, also known as the **thirst center**. The osmoreceptors that stimulate the supraoptic and paraventricular nuclei also stimulate the thirst center. The thirst center, in turn, stimulates the cerebral cortex, signaling the need to drink fluids. So long as the person is able to respond to this impulse, fluid and electrolyte balance can be maintained. However, motor deficits, dysphagia, or a decreased level of consciousness may interfere with the person's ability to respond appropriately to the thirst stimuli.

Fluid and Electrolyte Imbalance

When considering the patient's fluid and electrolyte status, the nurse should be attuned to the various signs and symptoms of electrolyte imbalance. As part of the assessment of patients, a review of the blood chemistry values are included and correlated with the clinical presentation. Some patients can tolerate a wide deviation from the normal range of values, whereas others are sensitive to even slight changes. Note that there may be slight differences in normal values for electrolyte and other chemistries between laboratories.

Hyponatremia

The normal range of serum sodium is 135 to 145 mEq/L. **Hyponatremia**, defined as less than 135 mEq/L, is one of the most common electrolyte disorders seen in neuroscience patients. Hyponatremia may occur with normal, elevated, or low serum osmolality.[6,7] An understanding of the underlying pathophysiology for each form provides a basis for treatment.

Hyponatremia with normal osmolality (pseudohyponatremia) is seen with hyperlipidemia and hyperproteinemia (e.g., multiple myeloma). Lipids and protein normally represent about 7% of the solid components of the blood. A basic assumption in measuring serum sodium is that of a constant solid component of blood. If these components are elevated, normal laboratory techniques for measuring sodium underestimate the true sodium concentration in the serum.[7] *Hyponatremia with high osmolality* is most commonly seen in association with hyperglycemia, toxin injection, and use of mannitol. This solute replaces sodium as the osmotically active particle in the blood. By stimulating water movement into ECF, hyperglycemia, for example, lowers serum sodium (by 1.6 mEq/100 mg/dL glucose), causing hyponatremia with hyperosmolality.[7] This is also true when mannitol is administered. Other molecules that are small and are highly permeable to the cell membrane (e.g., ethanol, urea) do not generally cause hyponatremia. However, high levels of urea, as seen in renal failure, may result in hyponatremia because of impaired water excretion.[7]

The most common type of hyponatremia seen in clinical practice is *hyponatremia with low osmolality* (*hypoosmotic hyponatremia*). There are three types of hypoosmolar hyponatremia categorized based on the clinical assessment of total-body volume[7] (see Table 10-1). Correction of the chronic forms (i.e., those that persist longer than 24 to 36 hours) requires different treatment approaches.[9] Regardless of the hypoosmolar hyponatremia, a slow rate of correction is necessary to allow the brain to adapt.

Hypervolemic Hyponatremia

This is seen in congestive heart failure, cirrhosis, nephrotic syndromes, and renal failure. Patients appear edematous and hyponatremic with a low urine sodium level (less than 20 mEq/L) and a high urine osmolality (more than 300 mOsm/kg; more than 500 mOsm/kg in renal failure).[8] There is an increase in free water with an increase in ECF and extracellular volume (ECV), resulting in a low circulating volume. Low volume is a stimulus for ADH and aldosterone secretion. Treatment is directed at restriction of free water and salt.

Euvolemic Hyponatremia

This condition is seen most often in patients with SIADH, which is discussed later in this chapter. These patients have a high urine osmolality (more than 300 mOsm kg) and a high urine sodium (more than 30 mEq/L). Natriuresis results from an elevated atrial natriuretic hormone, suppressed aldosterone concentrations, and concentrated urine for high ADH levels. Other causes of euvolemic hyponatremia include hypothyroidism, glucocorticoid deficiency, water intoxication, and renal failure. In addition to determining the underlying cause, restriction of free water is the focus of treatment.

Hypovolemic Hyponatremia

There is a loss of ECV and a disproportionate larger sodium deficit. The causes of hypovolemic-hyponatremia are classified into nonrenal sodium loss and renal sodium loss. Nonrenal losses of ECV and sodium are due to gastrointestinal (GI) losses such as vomiting, diarrhea, and fistula drainage; skin losses (burns); dietary sodium loss; and "third spacing" of fluid. Urine's sodium level is less than 15 mEq/L and urine's osmolality more than 400 mOsm/kg of water. Renal losses result from diuretics (most often thiazides that limit free water excretion by inhibiting distal tubular sodium reabsorption)[8]; renal failure; and mineralocorticoid deficiency (e.g., hypoaldosterone). In these cases, urine sodium is more than 30 mEq/L and urine osmolality is less than 300 to 400 mOsm/kg.[7] Concurrently, hypokalemia may be present, especially with GI fluid loss or use of diuretics. Treatment is directed at identifying the underlying cause and administering isotonic saline to correct the moderate-to-severe hyponatremia. Further therapy is directed at potassium replacement, if necessary, and restriction of free water. Table 10-2 includes the major diagnostics used to monitor fluid balance in neuroscience patients.

Clinical Manifestations Associated With Hypoosmolar Hyponatremia

Hypoosmolar hyponatremia can be categorized as *acute* (less than 24 to 36 hours) or *chronic* (more than 24 to 36 hours). Clinical manifestation of acute hypoosmolar hyponatremia covers a broad spectrum of neurological signs and symptoms as well as GI and muscular symptoms (Table 10-3). Most neurological symptoms associated with acute hyponatremia are caused by the osmotic pressure gradient that moves water into the brain, resulting in cerebral edema.[10] Over a finite period of time, the brain adapts to hypoosmolality by losing electrolytes and shedding water, thus creating a new steady state.[8] After the brain has volume-adapted through solute loss and water loss, with subsequent reduction of edema, symptoms are not as prominent. Animal research has demonstrated that morbidity and mortality correlate with the rate of decrease of plasma sodium rather than the actual severity of the sodium deficit.[11] The more rapid the decrease in plasma sodium, the more cerebral edema develops before the brain is able to lose solute and shed water. As a result, patients with acute hyponatremia have more neurological symptoms and mortality than patients with chronic hyponatremia.[10]

The preceding discussion underscores an important principle in correcting severe hyponatremia. That is, *correcting severe hyponatremia too rapidly should be avoided because it can cause pontine and extrapontine myelinolysis, a brain-demyelinating disorder responsible for severe neurological morbidity and mortality.*[12] The increased incidence of central pontine myelinolysis (CPM) is associated with the timeline of correction of hyponatremia, not just the presence of severe hyponatremia.[13,14] CPM is a rare disorder that develops in days to weeks following excessively rapid repair of chronic hyponatremia. The demyelination process causes loss of myelin

Table 10-2 • LABORATORY STUDIES TO MONITOR FLUID IMBALANCE

TEST/NORMAL VALUES	DESCRIPTION	ALTERED LEVELS
Serum sodium 135–145 mEq/L	Sodium accounts for most of the total serum osmolality Serum sodium concentration essentially controlled by the water balance in an individual	Sodium ↑ seen in total body water deprivation Sodium ↓ seen with water overload or water intoxication
Urine sodium 30–70 mEq/L	Helpful in evaluating volume status assuming normal renal, adrenal cortical, and thyroid function	In volume overload, urinary sodium excretion and concentration ↑—**in volume overload >70 mEq/L** In volume depletion, urinary sodium excretion and concentration ↓—**in volume depleted <25 mEq/L**
Plasma osmolality (Osm) 280–295 mOsm/L	Can approximate plasma Osm by doubling the serum sodium concentration More accurate method, see formula on page 201	
Urine Osm 100–800 mOsm/L*	Useful to assess renal function and evaluate abnormalities of water balance Urine Osm may be hypertonic or hypotonic compared to serum Osm	Inability to dilute or concentrate urine can be seen in renal dysfunction or various other causes and in disorders of antidiuretic hormone (ADH) secretion or function
Urine specific gravity 1.010–1.030	An approximate measure of urine Osm if glucose or other chemicals are absent (i.e., they alter specific gravity)	1.001–1.005 in diabetes insipidus
Vasopressin level	Direct measure of ADH Expensive test available in selected laboratories; requires special handling	↑ seen in nephrogenic DI and in states of inappropriate ADH excess ↓ seen in central DI and states of water intoxication
Water deprivation test	Useful for making a differential diagnosis in states of polyuria Both excess water intake and central ADH deficiency are associated with a low level of ADH; this test distinguishes between the two	Lack of response to exogenous ADH after several hours of water deprivation is diagnostic for nephrogenic DI

* On random testing.

DI, diabetes insipidus.

in the central pontine area and extrapontine region. These lesions can be seen on magnetic resonance imaging (MRI) about 3 to 4 weeks after the onset of clinical signs.[15] Possible signs and symptoms include pseudobulbar palsy, quadriparesis, varying behavioral changes, and seizures. Therefore, in all cases of hyponatremia, *care must be taken to prevent too rapid a correction of hyponatremia*. The therapeutic approach to managing a symptomatic chronic hyponatremic patient follows a controlled gradual raising of serum sodium levels. The serum sodium level should not be increased by more than 0.5 to 1 mEq/L/hour and no more than 12 mEq/L in a 24-hour period.[9,16]

Table 10-3 • CLINICAL SIGNS AND SYMPTOMS OF ACUTE HYPONATREMIA

SYSTEM	SIGNS AND SYMPTOMS
	(Note: although significant symptoms do not generally occur until serum sodium is <125 mEq/L, individual thresholds vary widely)
Neurological (hyponatremic encephalopathy)	Headache Disorientation, confusion, irritability, apathy, lethargy, obtundation Neurological deficits Seizures Weakness Cerebral edema Herniation syndromes Respiratory arrest
Gastrointestinal	Nausea and vomiting Anorexia
Muscular	Cramps Muscle weakness Rhabdomyolysis

HYPERNATREMIA

Because thirst provides an excellent protection against hyperosmolality, hypernatremia is unusual unless access to water is impaired. The elderly who have a decreased awareness of thirst, those with impaired consciousness, and incapacitated persons are at high risk for hypernatremia. **Hypernatremia** is defined as a serum sodium level that exceeds 145 mEq/L. It is always associated with hyperosmolality because sodium salts are the main determinants of plasma osmolality. A rise in serum osmolality causes water to shift from the intracellular fluids to the ECF, resulting in cell dehydration and shrinkage. The basic causes are water loss in excess of sodium or sodium gain in excess of water. Specifically, there are three *causes* of hypernatremia: insufficient water intake, excessive water loss, and sodium gain. *Insufficient water intake* may be due to an inability to perceive or respond to thirst (e.g., confused or comatose state), receiving nothing by mouth without sufficient intravenous (IV) fluid replacement, or inability to swallow (e.g., stroke patient). *Excessive water loss* can be due to nonrenal causes (e.g., fever, diaphoresis, burns, hyperventilation, diarrhea) or renal causes such as DI and osmotic diuresis (e.g., glycosuria in hyperglycemia, urea diuresis in high-protein tube feedings, mannitol therapy). *Sodium gain* can occur as a result of sea-water drowning or excessive use of IV sodium solutions (e.g. 3% or 5% hypertonic saline).[17]

Hypernatremia can be subdivided based on ECV into hypovolemic hypernatremia, euvolemic hypernatremia, and hypervolemic hypernatremia (Table 10-4.) The hypovolemic type results from loss of excessive fluids from the GI or renal tract.

Urine

In neuroscience patients, hypernatremia is most often associated with DI, a condition that is discussed later in this chapter. Attention to early feeding and hydration in altered consciousness states (e.g., confusion, coma) and withholding of oral intake because of risk of aspiration have almost eliminated other common causes of hypernatremia.

Signs and symptoms associated with hypernatremia include thirst; dry mucous membranes; dry, rough, and red tongue; and elevated temperature. Early neurological signs and symptoms include lethargy, weakness, and irritability. In severe cases, agitation, delirium, seizures, and coma can occur.

||| OTHER COMMON ELECTROLYTE IMBALANCES

In addition to hyponatremia and hypernatremia, potassium, calcium, magnesium, and phosphorus are other important electrolytes in acute care settings that have been associated with high morbidity and mortality. Relatively small changes in plasma concentrations of potassium, calcium, and magnesium can have significant effects on neuromuscular excitability and cardiac rhythm. Balance of these three cations is maintained largely by regulation of their excretion in the urine.[18] Table 10-5 shows common electrolyte imbalances, causes/related conditions, and signs and symptoms.

Potassium (3.5 to 5.0 mEq/L) is the major intracellular ion. An important determinant of the plasma concentration is the balance between the uptake of potassium into cells and its loss from cells. Potassium uptake into cells is increased by alkalosis, beta-adrenergic agonists, insulin, and aldosterone; it is lost from the cell by acidosis.[18] Potassium is important in cellular metabolism, such as protein and glycogen synthesis, and in maintaining cellular membrane potential.

Calcium (8.5 to 10.5 mg/dL or 4.2 to 5.2 mEq/L) is the most abundant ion in the body, but 99% of it is in bone and does not participate in the regulation of plasma calcium. Calcium is important for blood coagulation, skeletal and cardiac muscle contractility, and several membrane and cellular functions. About one half of the total calcium and magnesium is found as free ions in the plasma. The free form is physiologically active; the other half is bound to albumin and is inactive. When calcium and magnesium levels fall, they usually fall together because both are bound to albumin. Calcium and magnesium are important in neuromuscular conduction and activation.

Magnesium (1.7 to 2.4 mg/dL or 1.4 to 2.0 mEq/L) is the most common intracellular cation after potassium and the fourth most abundant cation in the body overall. Like calcium, magnesium is primarily stored in bone (60%) and muscle (40%). Unlike calcium, no hormones control magnesium balance. Magnesium is a metabolic cofactor in over 300 enzymatic reactions, including the process of energy use and protein and nucleic acid synthesis. It is necessary in cellular phosphated transfer reactions (sodium-potassium adenosine-triphosphatase [Na-K adenosine triphosphatase or ATPase] pump, calcium-ATP pump, proton pump) and participates in the regulation of vascular smooth muscle tone, cellular second messenger systems, and signal transduction.[19] Deficiency of magnesium has been associated with failure to wean from a ventilator.

Phosphorus (2.0 to 4.5 mg/dL or 2.3 to 4.3 mg/dL or 1.5 to 2.8 mEq/L) is a form of a phosphate ion. It is a key component of DNA and RNA and is essential for intracellular storage and conversion of energy (ATP, creatine phosphate), carbohydrate metabolism, regulatory compounds, and dissociation of oxygen. Low phosphorus and magnesium levels are related to failure to wean patients from use of a ventilator.

||| Table 10-4 • THREE TYPES OF HYPERNATREMIA

TYPE	CAUSES	U_{Osm} (mOsm/L)	U_{Na} (mEq/L)	TREATMENT
Hypovolemic	*GI loss:* vomiting, diarrhea, fistula	>800	<20	Combined water and saline
	Renal loss: hyperglycemia, mannitol, high protein feedings	300–800	>30	
Euvolemic	Sweating	>800	<20	Water
	Central diabetes insipidus (DI) or nephrogenic DI	<300	<20	
Hypervolemic	Hypertonic saline, hypertonic sodium bicarbonate, sea water ingestion	>800	>30	Water

Normal values: Urine osmolality (U_{Osm}): 100–800 mOsm/L on random testing. Urine sodium (U_{Na}): in volume depleted <25 mEq/L; in volume overload >70 mEq/L.

▎▎▎▎ **Table 10-5** • OTHER COMMON SERUM ELECTROLYTE IMBALANCES

ELECTROLYTE IMBALANCE	CAUSES/RELATED CONDITIONS	SIGNS AND SYMPTOMS
Hypokalemia (<3.5 mEq/L)	GI loss (diarrhea, fistula, cathartics) Shift into cell from insulin therapy Renal losses related to hypoaldosteronism Urinary diuresis Magnesium depletion	ECG changes or cardiac arrhythmias: U waves, prolonged QT interval, depressed ST segment, low, flat T waves
Hyperkalemia (>5.0 mEq/L)	Cellular shift because of drugs and cell lysis Decreased renal excretion due to decreased tubular secretion Tubulointerstitial nephritis	Mild symptoms if the potassium level is 5–7 mEq/L; severe if the level is >7.0 mEq/L. Symptoms include the following: • *Cardiac:* ECG changes/cardiac arrhythmias (tall peaked T waves, widening QRS complex, shortening of the QT interval); ventricular fibrillations leading to cardiac arrest; bradycardia and hypotension • *Neuromuscular:* weakness, hyporeflexia • *Other:* paresthesia, respiratory paralysis
Hypocalcemia (<4.2 mEq/L)	Most commonly resulting from small-bowel resection or inflammation (e.g., Crohn's disease) Liver or renal disease may also cause vitamin D deficiency	Tingling of fingertips Perioral paresthesia Tetany Abdominal cramps Muscle cramps Carpopedal spasms Seizures Prolonged QT interval
Hypercalcemia (>5.2 mEq/L)	Increased GI absorption Vitamin D intoxication Increased bone absorption related to hyperparathyroidism, osteolytic metastases, multiple myeloma, immobilization Increased renal absorption related to hyperparathyroidism or thiazide diuretics	Anorexia, constipation, and abdominal pain Progressive weakness, lethargy, obtundation, and possible coma Deep bone pain Flank pain from renal calculi Muscle hypotonicity Dehydration
Hypomagnesemia (<1.4 mEq/L)	GI magnesium wasting (malabsorption states, diarrhea, short bowel) Renal magnesium wasting (primary tubular disorders) problems Common in ICU patients Common with long-term diuretic therapy	*Neuromuscular:* hyperexcitability with hyperreflexia *Cardiac:* potentially lethal cardiac conduction disturbances (e.g., PVCs, ventricular fibrillations or tachycardia; torsades de pointes; electrocardiographic changes Deficiency of magnesium associated with failure to wean from a ventilator
Hypermagnesemia (>2.0 mEq/L)	Occurs primarily in patients with renal insufficiency or in those receiving excessive magnesium therapy IV or oral (antacids, laxatives)	Symptoms related to level of elevation and include: • *Cardiovascular:* hypotension progressing to prolonged QRS and PR intervals and finally to heart block • *Neuromuscular:* hyporeflexia, muscle paralysis, and respiratory weakness • *Other:* nausea, vomiting, and skin warmth
Hypophosphatemia (<1.5 mEq/L)	Phosphate binding therapy for renal failure (e.g., antacids, sucralfate, calcium carbonate) Other disease states including hyperparathyroidism, paralytic syndromes, alcoholism, diabetic ketoacidosis, hyperglycemia, hyperosmolar states	*Muscular:* Muscle weakness and myalgia *Respiratory:* Respiratory failure, ventilation dependency, or respiratory muscle fatigue *Renal:* acute tubular necrosis *Neurological:* Paresthesia, weakness, numbness, seizures, and altered mental status
Hyperphosphatemia (>2.8 mEq/L)	Acute and chronic renal failure Hypoparathyroidism Diabetic or alcoholic ketoacidosis	When high phosphorus levels are maintained for an extended time, phosphate deposits may develop in the body

GI, gastrointestinal; ECG, electrocardiographic; ICU, intensive care unit; PVC, premature ventricular contraction.

Correction of Electrolyte Imbalances

A complex interrelatedness exists among electrolytes with overlapping functions and effects. This "big picture" needs to be kept in mind when imbalances are corrected. Several principles guide correction of imbalance and include:

• Estimate the degree of deficit or excess based on laboratory data and clinical signs and symptoms; several formulas are useful to calculate actual deviations.
• Determine underlying cause and correct if possible.
• Consider speed of replacement (most often, slow replacement is advocated).

- Consider what other related electrolytes need to be managed for successful correction.
- Individualize therapy (consider whether acute or chronic problem; choice of drugs).
- Calculate the dosage and time line for correction.
- Monitor the response and other related electrolytes.

Although management and correction of electrolyte imbalances are collaborative problems, the effects of specific imbalances require nursing assessment and monitoring of specific parameters such as vital signs, continuous electro-cardiographic waveforms, and neurological signs. The nurse must be aware of the specific electrolyte imbalance, overall plan for correction, and adverse signs and symptoms to provide comprehensive assessment and monitoring of patients for safe correction of imbalances.

Diabetes Insipidus

Diabetes insipidus is a condition of decreased secretion of ADH. Affected patients void large amounts of dilute urine daily and are at high risk for fluid and electrolyte imbalance and dehydration. The signs and symptoms include the following:

- Polyuria (urine volumes ranging from 4 to 10 L daily; hourly output exceeding 200 mL)
- Low urine specific gravity (1.001 to 1.005)
- Extreme thirst (polydipsia) if the patient is conscious and the thirst center is intact
- High serum osmolality
- Hypovolemia
- Hypernatremia

Pathophysiology

The following summarizes the pathophysiology of DI.[20] Secretion of antidiuretic hormone (ADH) from the posterior pituitary gland is regulated by the paraventricular and supraoptic nuclei (see Fig. 10-1). AVP acts on the target site of the cortical collecting duct of the kidneys. AVP binds to a vasopressin-2 receptor at the basal lateral membrane of the cortical collecting duct. The vasopressin-2 receptor acts with G protein and adenylate cyclase to produce cyclic adenosine monophosphate (AMP). Protein kinase A subsequently is stimulated and acts to promote aquaporin-2 (AQP_2) to recycle vesicles. In the presence of AVP, the exocytic inclusion of AQP_2 protein at the surface of the cortical tubular cells allows water to enter the cell. In the absence of AVP, AQP_2 protein is retrieved by endocytic retrieval mechanisms and returned to the recycling vesicle.

Types of Diabetes Insipidus

Diabetes insipidus (DI) can be classified as central neurogenic DI and nephrogenic DI.

Central neurogenic DI is due to destruction of the posterior pituitary gland by tumors or trauma, resulting in a deficiency of vasopressin. Central neurogenic DI can be subdivided into the following four types:

- **Classical severe DI**, in which there is failure to synthesize or release ADH

- **Defective osmoreceptor DI**, in which very high osmolality fails to trigger secretion of ADH, although the hormone is released in response to hypovolemia
- **Reset osmoreceptor DI**, in which secretion of ADH is not triggered until the plasma osmolality is higher than the usual threshold
- **Partial DI**, in which ADH is released at the usual threshold, but the amount of hormone secreted is decreased

Nephrogenic DI is uncommon and can be acquired through drug toxicity (lithium, demeclocycline, amphotericin B, gentamicin, glyburide, or furosemide). It can be differentiated from neurogenic DI by a lack of response to the administration of ADH.[21] Physiologically, nephrogenic DI arises from end-organ resistance to vasopressin, either from a receptor defect or from medications and other agents that interfere with the AQP_2 transport of water.

Causes and Clinical Presentations

Central neurogenic DI may be neurogenic or idiopathic. Neurogenic causes include primary brain tumor (30%), head trauma (17%), neurosurgery (9%) metastatic carcinoma (8%), intracranial hemorrhage (6%), and granulomatous disease (5%).[20] The presence of CDI is common in brain death, especially when hemodynamic and respiratory support continue to implement an organ donation protocol. Idiopathic DI occurs in 25% of cases.

CDI due to trauma or neurosurgical injury is characterized by polyuria that is often triphasic: an initial period of intense polyuria lasting for hours to several days; followed by a period of normal urinary output; and finally the recurrence of transient or permanent polyuria.

Most DI is transient and resolves spontaneously within a few days or a few weeks. Patients may or may not require treatment, depending on the severity of the condition, their ability to balance intake and output, or adequate treatment and fluid replacement. A condition of permanent DI develops only if 80% to 90% or more of the ADH-producing nuclei of the hypothalamus and the proximal end of the pituitary stalk are destroyed. In this situation, life-long treatment with replacement hormonal therapy is necessary.

Central nervous system (CNS) clinical responses related to hypertonic encephalopathy of DI include irritability, mental dullness, and coma with secondary signs of ataxia, hyperthermia, and hypotension.[1]

Diagnosis and Treatment

The diagnosis of DI is based on a history and the clinical finding of polyuria coupled with low urinary specific gravity levels and high serum osmolality. A water dehydration test may be ordered to determine which type of DI is present when the cause is unclear. If necessary, an MRI is helpful in visualizing the pituitary.

The treatment of DI initially includes the replacement of fluids if the patient is unable to take an adequate amount of fluid orally. Administration of ADH as desmopressin acetate (DDAVP) is used, preferably by the intranasal route at a dosage of 5 to 20 μg daily. Rhinitis and sinusitis may interfere with intranasal absorption of this drug. An oral form of desmopressin is also available, but at a dose 20 times higher than that used for the intranasal route. The increased dosage is necessary because of bioavailability; the recommended starting dose is 0.05 mg twice a day. Aqueous desmopressin can be used IV for acute DI and for brain-death organ protocol. The dosage is 0.5 to 2.0 μg every 3 hours.[21] Drug therapy recommendations are summarized in Table 10-6. For patients with mild DI, drugs known to stimulate production of ADH or to enhance the kidney's response to ADH may be ordered (see Table 10-6). If the DI is a permanent condition, the patient will require education and ongoing medical management.

Nursing Management

Assessment. The nurse caring for a neurosurgical patient should be aware of the possible development of DI and should monitor the patient accordingly. The following parameters should be assessed:

- Urinary output every 1 to 2 hours
- Urinary specific gravity every 1 to 2 hours
- Intake and output balance
- Serum osmolality and electrolytes
- Signs and symptoms of dehydration
- Daily weight, if possible

When assessing the fractional urinary output for a patient with an altered level of consciousness, an indwelling catheter is usually used to measure urinary output on a specific time schedule. The amount of urinary output in just 1 hour can be extraordinary. If the urinary output is 200 mL/hour or more for 2 consecutive hours, this should be reported to the physician because it can quickly lead to dehydration. In most instances, neurosurgical patients and those subject to increased intracranial pressure are maintained in a euvolemic state to control intracranial pressure. The nurse will notice very pale (i.e., straw colored) and dilute urine with a

Table 10-6 • DRUGS USED IN THE TREATMENT OF DIABETES INSIPIDUS (DI)

NAME	USUAL ADULT DOSE	FREQUENCY	COMMENTS
Desmopressin acetate (DDAVP)	5–40 μg intranasally in 1–3 divided doses	Daily; adjustment of morning and evening doses separately for adequate diurnal rhythm of water turnover	Causes minimal nasoconstriction; used for severe permanent, or transient complete, central diabetes insipidus (DI)
Lypressin nasal spray	Spray intranasally three to four times a day	4–6 h	Nasal mucosa must be intact; useful for mild DI; patient may develop nasal congestion, which will interfere with absorption
Aqueous vasopressin	0.5–2.0 μg IV	3 h	Short duration; used for patients who have acute DI who have more than 300 mL/hr for 2 consecutive hours
Desmopressin	Starting doses of 0.05 mg orally with subsequent dose adjustment to achieve optimal water balance	In 2 or 3 divided doses	Adjust individual dosage in increments of 0.1–1.2 mg daily divided into 2 or 3 doses. Optimal dosage range is 0.1–0.8 mg daily in divided doses

In milder forms of DI, (in which antidiuretic hormone (ADH) is secreted in small amounts), the following drugs may be used to enhance the secretion of ADH or to increase the response of the kidney to ADH:

Chloropropamide (Diabinase)	250–750 mg/d PO	Daily	Stimulates release of ADH from the posterior pituitary and enhances its action of small amounts of ADH on renal tubules to augment urine concentrating ability; hypoglycemia in patients taking >500 mg limits its usefulness
Clofibrate (Atromid S)	500 mg orally four times daily	4 times a day	Useful to curtail polyuria in patients with partial central DI by stimulating release of ADH from the hypothalamus
Carbamazepine (Tegretol)	400–600 mg/d	Daily	Same as for clofibrate; in addition, carbamazepine may increase the sensitivity of the kidney to ADH
Hydrochlorothiazide (Hydrodiuril)	50–100 mg/d (or b.i.d.) PO	Daily or in two divided doses	Used in both central and nephrogenic DI

(Johnson, P. H. [Ed.] [1998]. *Nurse practitioner's drug handbook* [2nd ed, pp. 307–308]. Springhouse, PA: Springhouse.)

specific gravity of 1.005 or less. These two concurrent findings are usual signs of DI in the acute care setting. Other findings include a rising serum osmolality, hypernatremia, extreme thirst (if conscious), and dehydration.

Collaborative Problem and Nursing Diagnoses

The major collaborative problem associated with DI is electrolyte imbalance. The major nursing diagnoses include:

- Fluid volume deficit (R/T dehydration)
- Altered cerebral tissue perfusion (R/T hypovolemia, dehydration)

Interventions

The nursing responsibilities for the patient with DI include hourly monitoring of urine output and specific gravity. Blood chemistries such as serum osmolality, electrolytes, and blood urea nitrogen levels should also be monitored carefully. The patient should be weighed daily, and intake and output records should be maintained. The nurse should also observe the patient for signs and symptoms of dehydration, electrolyte imbalance, and hypovolemia.

A major nursing responsibility is managing fluid replacement. The oral route may be used if the patient is conscious and able to swallow adequate amounts of fluid. If this is not possible, an IV route should be used. The rate of infusion should be monitored frequently and the amount of intake compared with the amount of output. In the patient who has triphasic DI, care should be taken to prevent water intoxication during the period of normal urine output. For a patient receiving vasopressin replacement therapy by the intranasal route, monitor for evidence of rhinitis or sinusitis, conditions that would decrease the absorption of the drug. For the patient with permanent DI, a patient teaching plan should be developed and implemented. The following information should be included in the teaching plan:

- Explanation of DI
- Suggestions as to how to adjust the patient's daily schedule to accommodate the care needs associated with DI
- Review the individualized drug protocol (frequency, side effects, overdose)
- Get follow-up care
- Follow recommendations regarding a medical alert bracelet

Syndrome of Inappropriate Secretion of Antidiuretic Hormone

Syndrome of inappropriate secretion of antidiuretic hormone is the single most common cause of hyponatremia in hospitalized and, particularly, postoperative patients. It is characterized by an abnormally high level or continuous secretion of ADH so that water is continually reabsorbed from the kidney tubules, resulting in water intoxication. The continuous release of osmotic or non-osmotic stimuli is a common cause of hyponatremia. The excess of ADH occurs in SIADH or as a consequence of drugs that enhance ADH release or action. Clinically, SIADH is seen in three disease groups: CNS disorders, carcinomas, and pulmonary disorders. SIADH may occur in the following common conditions:

- Almost any CNS disorder, including head trauma, infections (meningitis, encephalitis, abscesses), tumors, cerebrovascular disease, aneurysmal subarachnoid hemorrhage, and Guillain-Barré syndrome
- Carcinoma, especially bronchogenic carcinoma (oat cell carcinoma)
- Pulmonary disorders, such as pneumonia, lung abscess, or tuberculosis

In addition, other conditions may cause temporary SIADH:

- Pain, fear, or major temperature change
- Positive-pressure breathing on a respirator
- Increased secretion of ADH secondary to certain drugs (oral hypoglycemics, general anesthetics, chemotherapeutic agents, sedatives, opiates, and carbamazepine)

Pathophysiology

In SIADH, there is persistent production of ADH or an ADH-like peptide despite body fluid hypotonicity and an expanded effective circulating volume so that the negative feedback mechanisms that normally control the release of ADH fail, and there is continuous release of ADH. As a result, there is excessive retention of water by the kidneys, hyponatremia, and normovolemic or slight expansion of ECF that may cause an increase body weight by 5% to 10%. The volume expansion results in reduced rates of proximal tubular sodium absorption and consequent natriuresis

Diagnosis and Treatment

Diagnosis of SIADH is based on the clinical and laboratory findings associated with the disorder. Associated CNS or respiratory system pathophysiology or drug therapy known to increase ADH secretion can usually be identified as the cause.

The criteria for the diagnosis of SIADH include the following:[21]

- Exclusion of renal, adrenal, or other endocrine disease (hypothyroidism or hypoadrenalism)
- Hyponatremia with low hypoosmolality (usually less than 275 mOsm/L)
- High urine sodium (more than 25 mEq/L)
- High urine osmolality (higher than serum)
- Decreased urinary output (400 to 500 mL/24 hours)
- Possible generalized weight gain (more than 5% of body weight)

In addition, laboratory findings include a normal serum blood urea nitrogen and creatinine, reduced serum uric acid, and fractional excretion of sodium greater than 1%.[1]

The treatment of SIADH depends on its severity and the underlying cause of the problem. The underlying cause should be identified and managed. Usually, SIADH is self-limited in neurological patients. The principles of treatment include the following:

- Restriction of free water (less than 1,000 mL/24 hours). This may be the definitive treatment.
- Slow, judicious replacement of sodium with saline or hypertonic solution (3%) of sodium chloride administered slowly. Correction usually occurs over 3 to 6 days. See discussion of hyponatremia correction for rationale.

Drug therapy for SIADH includes the following:

- Furosemide (Lasix) for diuresis
- In some instances, demeclocycline hydrochloride, 300 mg four times daily, to suppress ADH activity
- Lithium carbonate, 900 to 1,200 mg, to inhibit the renal response to ADH

Nursing Management

Assessment. The patient with SIADH should undergo assessment of the following parameters:

- Intake and output
- Daily weight for gain, if possible
- Urine and serum sodium and osmolalities
- Urine specific gravity
- Blood urea nitrogen
- Signs and symptoms of fluid and electrolyte imbalance (sodium depletion, lethargy, confusion, muscle weakness and cramping, headache, seizures, coma)

Collaborative Problems and Interventions. The major collaborative problem with SIADH, as with DI, is electrolyte imbalance. The nurse caring for the patient with SIADH must monitor the laboratory values for serum and urine sodium and osmolalities. Intake and output must be carefully recorded and monitored. If an intravenous infusion is ordered, it should be administered slowly.

Most patients with SIADH are placed on fluid restriction. The reason for this restriction should be explained to the patient and family. A strict intake and output record is maintained to keep the patient within the prescribed fluid restriction. Frequent mouth care is provided for comfort, because fluid restriction will cause the patient to have a dry mouth.

Because weight gain is common with SIADH, the patient is weighed daily. The accumulation of fluid also predisposes

the bedridden patient to skin breakdown. Frequent skin care, turning, and repositioning should be included in the plan of care.

The hyponatremia associated with SIADH can lead to neurological changes in the sensorium, muscle cramping, headache, seizures, and even coma. The nurse must be aware of the signs and symptoms of sodium depletion and must notify the physician of any such changes so that definitive action can be taken before serious deficits develop.

SPECIAL METABOLIC AND ELECTROLYTE IMBALANCES

Cerebral Salt Wasting

Cerebral salt wasting, a condition characterized by true hyponatremia, primary loss of sodium and concurrent loss of ECF, decreased plasma volume, decreased body weight, increased blood urea nitrogen values, and a negative salt balance, has been discussed in the literature. It challenges the previously held belief that most hyponatremia is caused by SIADH. Table 10-7 presents a comparison of cerebral salt wasting and SIADH. Wijdicks and associates[22] measured plasma volume, fluid, sodium balance, and vasopressin levels in patients with ruptured saccular aneurysms. They found that vasopressin (i.e., ADH) values were elevated at the time of hospitalization and then subsequently declined in the first week, regardless of the presence of hyponatremia. (By definition, SIADH is associated with an increased level of vasopressin.) Thus, they concluded that the natriuresis and hyponatremia were attributable to primary salt wasting rather than SIADH. Further, they recommended that the natriuresis and hyponatremia should be corrected with fluid replacement rather than by fluid restriction, the usual treatment for SIADH.

The role of antinatriuretic factor (ANF) has been considered in cerebral salt wasting. Cells located in the two atria, but especially in the right atrium, produce ANF, a hormone-like substance thought to be secreted in response to stimulation of the stretch receptors in the atrial wall. ANF is a potent hormone that increases renal excretion of sodium. Concomitantly, ECF volume and blood volume decreases slightly. ANF has a role in blood volume regulation, but the

Table 10-7 • COMPARISON OF THE SIGNS AND SYMPTOMS OF SYNDROME OF INAPPROPRIATE SECRETION OF ANTIDIURETIC HORMONE (SIADH) AND CEREBRAL SALT WASTING

SIADH	SALT WASTING
Hyponatremia (dilutional)	Hyponatremia (primary)
Increased extracellular fluid	Decreased extracellular fluid
Serum hypoosmolality (<280 mOsm/L)	Serum hypoosmolality
Increased plasma volume	Decreased plasma volume
Increased body weight	Decreased body weight
Low blood urea nitrogen (BUN)	High BUN
Not necessarily a negative salt balance	Excessive natriuresis
Urine osmolality inappropriately concentrated compared with serum osmolality	Negative salt balance (primary loss of sodium)

specifics of the mechanism are unclear. Hyponatremia and decreased fluid volume are recognized as high-risk factors for development of vasospasm. Vasospasm results in decreased cerebral blood flow to the affected arterial territory, causing ischemia and extension of cerebral deficits. Treatment of symptomatic vasospasm is directed at the primary goal of increasing cerebral perfusion pressure with hypervolemic-hypertensive therapy. Chapter 24 discusses hypervolemic-hypertensive therapy. Because the treatment of SIADH is fluid restriction, compared with fluid volume replacement in cerebral salt wasting, the physician must distinguish the two conditions. Fluid restriction in a patient with cerebral salt wasting places him or her at high risk for the development of vasospasm and cerebral ischemia.

Hyperosmolar Nonketotic Hyperglycemia

Hyperosmolar nonketotic dehydration syndrome (HONK), a serious metabolic complication seen in some neurological patients, is caused by insulin deficiency and is often precipitated by serious illness. The syndrome can develop slowly and is usually seen in older patients (50 to 70 years of age) with a history of non–insulin-dependent diabetes mellitus. However, some patients without a history of diabetes mellitus have developed HONK. A common criteria used to define HONK is hyperglycemia exceeding 800 mg/dL, associated with an abnormal sensorium and the absence of ketoacidosis.[23] Hyperglycemia can exceed 1000 mg/dL and can occasionally reach 2000 mg/dL.

Some conditions appear to place patients at risk for the development of HONK. The most common associated conditions seen in neurological patients are infections (especially those caused by gram-negative organisms, such as certain pneumonias and acute pyelonephritis), enteritis, acute trauma, severe physiological stress, hyperalimentation, and drugs known to interfere with diabetic control (e.g., thiazide diuretics, mannitol, steroids, phenytoin). Most patients who develop HONK have concurrent renal or cardiovascular disease.

Clinically, the patient develops polyuria, which leads to dehydration, marked hypovolemia, high serum osmolality (about 350 mOsm/L), and elevation of serum blood urea nitrogen. Hyponatremia is present. The serum ketone level is negative, and the acetone breath and Kussmaul respiration seen in diabetic coma are usually not present. The skin and mucous membranes are dry, with decreased skin turgor. Neurologically, the level of consciousness deteriorates from confusion to stupor and, finally, to coma. Other neurological findings may include seizures, hemisensory deficits, and visual field cuts.

Treatment of HONK is directed at administration of insulin and replacement of fluids along with electrolyte replacement, as needed. Because of the profound dehydration, vigorous fluid replacement is necessary. According to Kruse,[23] it is important to initiate fluid resuscitation before administering insulin because the hypovolemia is exacerbated and circulatory shock could be precipitated or exacerbated. Hypovolemic shock can occur because insulin drives the glucose intracellularly, decreasing plasma osmolality and causing an osmotic shift of water from the intravascular compartment to the intracellular compartment. Recommended intravenous fluid is normal saline.

The major collaborative problems with HONK are dehydration and hyperglycemia. The major nursing diagnosis related to the care of the patient with HONK is **fluid volume deficit**. The nurse must monitor vital signs, neurological signs, and hemodynamics and provide supportive care to these seriously ill patients. The blood glucose should be monitored every 1 to 2 hours during IV insulin infusion, and electrolytes every 4 to 6 hours until the blood glucose falls below 250 mg/dL. As correction of the hyperglycemia occurs, the hyponatremia can convert to hypernatremia. This is due to the deficit of free water common in HONK. Therefore, close monitoring of the electrolytes is necessary so that the intravenous fluid can be changed accordingly.

REFERENCES

1. Reeves, W. B., & Andreoli, T. E. (1999). The antidiuretic hormone: Physiology and pathophysiology. In A. F. Krisht & G. T. Tindall (Eds.), Pituitary disorders: Comprehensive management (pp. 79–98). Philadelphia: Lippincott Williams & Wilkins.
2. Bakerman, S. (1994). ABC's of interpretive laboratory data (3rd ed., p. 381). Myrtle Beach, SC: Interpretive Laboratory Data.
3. Gennari, F. J. (1984). Serum osmolality: Uses and limitations. New England Journal of Medicine, 312, 310–312.
4. Berne, R. M., & Levy, M. N. (1993). Physiology (3rd ed., pp. 759–767). St. Louis: Mosby.
5. Kettyle, W. M., & Arky, R. A. (1998). Endocrine pathophysiology (pp. 55–57). Philadelphia: Lippincott-Raven.
6. DeFronzo, R. A., & Thier, S. O. (1980). Pathophysiologic approach to hyponatremia. Archives of Internal Medicine, 140(7), 897–902.
7. Civetta, J. M., Taylor, R. W., & Kirby, R. R. (1997). Critical care (3rd ed., pp. 413–441). Philadelphia: Lippincott-Raven.
8. Muther, R. S. (1999). Electrolyte disorders: Disorders of serum sodium, calcium, magnesium, and potassium. In S. Kawada (Ed.). ACCP-SCCM combined critical care course: Multidisciplinary board review (pp. 233–255). Anaheim, CA: Society of Critical Care Medicine and American College of Chest Physicians.
9. Faber, M. D., Kupin, W. L., Heilig, C. W., & Narins, R. G. (1994). Common fluid-electrolyte and acid-base problems in the intensive care unit: Selected issues. Seminars in Nephrology, 14(1), 8–22.
10. Verbalis, J. G. (1998). Adaptation to acute and chronic hyponatremia: Implications for symptomatology, diagnosis, and therapy. Seminars in Nephrology, 18(1), 3–19.
11. Ariedff, A. I., Llach, F., & Massry, S. G. (1976). Neurological manifestations and morbidity of hyponatremia: Correlation with brain water and electrolytes. Medicine, 55, 121–129.
12. Sterns, R. H., Riggs, J. E., & Schochet, S. S. (1986). Osmotic demyelination syndrome following correction of hyponatremia. New England Journal of Medicine, 314, 1535–1542.
13. Wright, D. G., Laureno, R., Victor, M. (1979). Pontine and extrapontine myelinolysis. Brain, 102, 361–385.
14. Laureno, R. (1983). Central pontine myelinolysis following rapid correction of hyponatremia. Annals of Neurology, 13, 232–242.
15. Brunner, J. E., Redmond, J. M., & Haggar, A. M. (1990). Central pontine myelinolysis and pontine lesions after rapid correction of hyponatremia: A prospective magnetic resonance imaging study. Annals of Neurology, 27, 61.
16. Muther, R. S. (1999). Electrolyte disorders: Disorders of serum sodium, calcium, magnesium, and potassium. In D. J. Dries & R. K. Albert, (Eds.). ACCP/SCCM combined critical care course: Multidisciplinary board review (pp. 233–255). Anaheim, CA: Soci-

ety of Critical Care Medicine and the American College of Chest Physicians.

17. Wilson, L. M. (1992). Disorder of fluid volume, osmolality, and electrolytes. In S. A. Price, & L. M. Wilson, (Eds.). *Pathophysiology: Clinical concepts and disease processes* (4th ed., pp. 247–248). St. Louis: Mosby–Year Book.

18. Schafer, J. A. (1998). Renal regulation of potassium, calcium, and magnesium. In L. R. Johnson (Ed.). *Essential medical physiology* (2nd ed., pp. 395–402). Philadelphia: Lippincott-Raven.

19. Salem, M., Munoz, R., & Chernow, B. (1991). Hypomagnesemia in critical illness: A common and clinically important problem. *Critical Care Clinics, 7*(1), 225–252.

20. Saborio, P., Tipton, G. A., & Chan, J. C. M. (2000). Diabetes insipidus. *Pediatrics in Review, 21*(4), 122–129.

21. Wijdicks, E. F. M. (1997). *The clinical practice of critical care neurology* (pp. 363–376). Philadelphia: Lippincott-Raven.

22. Wijdicks, E. F. M., Vermeulen, M., ten Haaf, J. A., Hijdra, A., Bakker, W. H., & van Gijn, J. (1985). Volume depletion and natriuresis in patients with a ruptured intracranial aneurysm. *Annals of Neurology, 18*(2), 211–216.

23. Kruse, J. A. (1999). Endocrine crises. In D. J. Dries & R. K. Albert, (Eds.), *ACCP/SCCM combined critical care course: Multidisciplinary board review* (pp. 187–197). Anaheim, CA: Society of Critical Care Medicine and the American College of Chest Physicians.

RESOURCES

Professional

Published Material

Ahern-Gould, K., & Stark, J. (1998). Quick resource for electrolyte imbalance. *Critical Care Nursing Clinics of North America, 10*(4), 477–490.

Diringer, M. N. (1992). Management of sodium abnormalities in patients with CNS disease. *Clinical Neuropharmacology, 15*(6), 427–447.

Frazier, S. K. (1999). Neurohormonal responses during positive pressure mechanical ventilation. *Heart & Lung, 28*(3), 149–165; quiz 166-7.

Gennari, F. J. (1998). Hypokalemia. *New England Journal of Medicine, 339*(7), 451–458.

Greenberg, A. (1998). Hyperkalemia: Treatment options. *Seminars in Nephrology, 18*(1), 46–57.

Heater, D. W. (1999). If ADH goes out of balance: Diabetes insipidus. *RN, 62*(7), 44–46.

Lord, R. C. (1999). Osmosis, osmometry, and osmoregulation. *Postgraduate Medical Journal, 75*(880), 67–73.

Nickolaus, M. J. (1999). Diabetes insipidus: A current perspective. *Critical Care Nurse, 19*(6), 18–30.

Oster, J. R., & Singer, I. (1999). Hyponatremia, hyposmolality, and hypotonicity: Tables and fables. *Archives of Internal Medicine, 159*, 333–336.

Palevsky, P. M. Hypernatremia. (1998). *Seminars in Nephrology, 18*(1), 20–30.

Service, F. J. (1995). Hypoglycemic disorders. *New England Journal of Medicine, 332*(17), 1144–1152.

Soupart, A., & Decaux, G. (1996). Therapeutic recommendations for management of severe hyponatremia: Current concepts on pathogenesis and prevention of neurologic complications. *Clinical Nephrology, 46*(3), 149–169.

Stark, J. (1998). A comprehensive analysis of the fluid and electrolytes system. An interactive exercise. *Critical Care Nursing Clinics of North America, 10*(4), 471–475

Toto, K. H. (1998). Fluid balance assessment. The total perspective. *Critical Care Nursing Clinics of North America, 10*(4), 383–400.

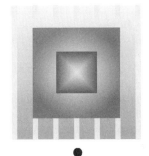

C H A P T E R **11**

Pharmacological Management of Neuroscience Patients

STEPHEN W. JANNING
TIMOTHY F. LASSITER

OVERVIEW

Role of the Pharmacist in Patient Management

Traditionally, the profession of pharmacy has been devoted exclusively to dispensing a high-quality drug product. With advances in technology, pharmacists have been safely able to devote less time to drug distribution services while assuming new roles in multidisciplinary patient management. At the same time, as medical science has advanced, pharmacological management of patients has become increasingly complex. Pharmacists are drug therapy experts whose primary responsibility is preventing and solving drug-related problems and providing drug information to all health care providers and patients. These circumstances have empowered pharmacists to become proactively involved in patient care as part of the multidisciplinary health care team. Pharmacists also develop and implement drug therapy monitoring plans, such as scheduling and reviewing serum drug concentrations, to achieve therapeutic endpoints and avoid toxicity.

Impact of Pharmacotherapy on the Nervous System

Pharmacotherapy has a tremendous impact on the assessment and care of the neuroscience patient. For example, many drugs commonly prescribed in the acute care setting can alter the level of consciousness (LOC). This is an obvious desired endpoint for narcotic analgesics, benzodiazepines, and other sedatives. However, many other drugs can also alter the LOC, either as a side effect (clonidine, H_2 receptor antagonists) or as a symptom of toxicity (relative overdose of imipenem in a patient with renal failure). Toxicity is of particular concern in the elderly and any patient in the intensive care unit (ICU). In both cases, patients may be more sensitive to the pharmacological effects or toxicities of a medication. This sensitivity is frequently compounded by

an impaired ability to eliminate the offending agent because of renal or hepatic insufficiency.

Despite the risks involved, properly managed adjuvant pharmacotherapy can indeed save lives. In addition, drug therapies are being developed that may directly prevent neurological damage or improve recovery. For example, high-dose corticosteroids improve neurological recovery following acute spinal cord trauma. Several distinctly different approaches to limiting secondary brain injury pharmacologically following trauma are under investigation. Neuronal growth factor has been identified and reproduced in the laboratory.

Therapeutic Decision Making

Determining optimal pharmacological management of the neuroscience patient depends on numerous factors. Ultimately, a risk-benefit assessment must be made for each therapeutic decision. Occasionally, this process results in a drug being prescribed that carries with it a high risk of producing a deleterious effect, but it is also potentially life saving. This is frequently the case when amphotericin B or an aminoglycoside is prescribed. Another example is a patient given sedatives and neuromuscular blockers for ventilator compliance at the expense of a reliable neurological examination.

After a careful risk-benefit assessment has been made, a comparable therapy can be selected over another based on relative cost. Such decisions become more difficult when a more expensive drug can potentially shorten a hospitalization or avoid an expensive adverse effect. Unfortunately, studies that comprehensively examine health care costs from a pharmacoeconomic perspective are only beginning to emerge.

COMMONLY USED DRUGS ALONG THE CONTINUUM OF CARE

Discussion of drug therapy in this chapter focuses on practical information necessary to manage the neuroscience patient. Tables are included for a quick reference. Drugs are addressed by body systems. For those who wish more detailed information, pharmacology texts should be consulted.

Hemodynamic Support and Associated Drugs

In addition to proper fluid management, neuroscience patients in the ICU often require therapy with vasoconstrictors, vasodilators, or inotropes. Proper monitoring is essential and typically includes frequent measurement of mean arterial pressure, heart rate, central venous pressure, urine output, and cardiac output as determined by a pulmonary artery catheter. The goal is to meet the oxygen requirements of the body. More definite therapeutic endpoints, such as specifically targeted oxygen delivery values or a minimum acceptable blood pressure, are controversial. Therapy must be individualized for each patient. Hemodynamic regimens often involve multiple drugs, making physical and chemical compatibility an issue with respect to concomitant fluids and intravenous (IV) access. The pharmacist can help solve these complex problems. Never assume compatibility when appropriate data are lacking.

In the neuroscience patient, recent research has focused on cerebral oxygen delivery and consumption optimization, rather than cerebral perfusion pressure, as a therapeutic endpoint for hemodynamic manipulation. This is particularly useful when vasodilators and other antihypertensives are prescribed because of the complex interrelationships between vascular tone and cerebral perfusion in the setting of an acute neurological insult (see Chapter 17).

Vasoconstrictors

Vasoconstrictors are helpful when hypotension is the result of a loss of vascular tone. This is commonly due to either sepsis or spinal shock. They are relatively contraindicated in untreated hypovolemic or cardiogenic shock. A high-dose requirement of vasoconstrictors for a prolonged period is an ominous sign because these drugs preserve blood pressure at the expense of organ perfusion. Extended periods of vital organ hypoperfusion contribute to multiple organ dysfunction syndrome, which carries with it a high mortality rate.

Dopamine is notable in that its pharmacological effects are dose dependent. At low doses ("renal-dose dopamine"), it is thought to increase blood flow to the kidneys and mesentery by selective vasodilatation. As the dose is increased, inotropic (increased cardiac contractility) and chronotropic (increased heart rate) effects predominate. At high doses, it is a potent vasoconstrictor, effectively overriding any selective vasodilatation activity. **Phenylephrine** is a potent vasoconstrictor devoid of direct inotropic or chronotropic activity. Some clinicians consider it the drug of choice for spinal shock, and it is being used more frequently for septic shock. Reflex bradycardia develops occasionally with its use. **Norepinephrine** is a potent vasoconstrictor with concomitant inotropic and chronotropic activity. **Epinephrine** acts as a positive inotropic or chronotropic agent at low doses and a vasoconstrictor with higher infusion rates (Table 11-1).

Regardless of the dose prescribed, great care must be taken to avoid extravasation of these vasoactive substances. This complication can produce extensive skin necrosis due to intense local vasoconstriction. Local instillation of phentolamine is indicated when this occurs.

Inotropic Agents

The inotropic agents are useful when cardiac contractility needs to be increased to optimize cardiac output. Careful titration is necessary because these agents can increase heart rate. Excessive tachycardia can be deleterious due to decreased cardiac output resulting from shortened filling time and diminished stroke volume, or from prolonged excessive myocardial oxygen demand in the setting of ischemic heart

---

▌▌▌▌ **Table 11-1** • VASOCONSTRICTOR AGENTS

DRUG	DOSE	ADVERSE EFFECTS	COMMENTS
Dopamine	2–4 μg/kg/min	Polyuria, tachycardia; skin necrosis with extravasation	"Renal dose" dopamine—may protect kidneys when giving other vasopressors
	4–8 μg/kg/min	Tachycardia compared with equipotent dose of dobutamine; skin necrosis with extravasation	Inotropic dose; may begin to see vasoconstrictor effects
	8–20 μg/kg/min	Tachycardia, hypertension; skin necrosis with extravasation	Prolonged high doses produce organ hypoperfusion and renal dysfunction
Phenylephrine	0.5–5 μg/kg/min	Reflex bradycardia; skin necrosis with extravasation	May be drug of choice for spinal shock; may be useful when other vasoconstrictors cause excessive tachycardia
Norepinephrine	2 μg/min, titrate to effect, titrate to effect (typically <30 μg/minute)	Tachycardia; skin necrosis with extravasation	Useful for patients not responding to dopamine; organ hypoperfusion and renal dysfunction with prolonged high doses
Epinephrine	2–10 μg/min	Tachycardia	Primarily inotropic effect
	10–20 μg/min	Tachycardia	Vasoconstricting dose; preserves coronary and cerebral flow

disease. The inotropic agents can also cause vasodilatation, which is usually tolerated poorly in this setting (Table 11-2).

Dobutamine is the most frequently prescribed positive inotropic agent. It is usually well tolerated and infrequently causes tachycardia. **Amrinone** is a newer agent originally thought to have inotropic activity without direct chronotropic activity. Its ability to raise cardiac output is probably solely due to its vasodilator activity, however, and blood pressure must be monitored closely. Amrinone is associated with a high incidence of thrombocytopenia. **Milrinone** is similar to amrinone but is a much more potent inotropic agent. Milrinone may provide an advantage in right-sided heart failure due to specific effects on the pulmonary vasculature. It is also the most expensive drug in its class. Patients with severely impaired cardiac contractility are sometimes prescribed both milrinone and dobutamine. **Isoproterenol** is used infrequently as an inotropic agent because of its strong concomitant chronotropic activity. It is useful, however, for treating symptomatic bradycardia unresponsive to atropine.

Vasodilators

Vasodilators are routinely prescribed for the neuroscience patient. They can be used in patients with impaired cardiac output to decrease the workload of the heart (afterload) and improve cardiac performance. More typically, they are used to control blood pressure in hypertensive patients with neurological sequelae. Blood pressure goals must be individualized to prevent further damage related to elevated pressures without also worsening cerebral ischemia. As mentioned previously, the most common side effects are hypotension and tachycardia (Table 11-3).

The calcium channel blockers are frequently used. **Nicardipine** is available in IV form and is a smooth-acting vasodilator when given as a continuous infusion. **Nifedipine** given orally or sublingually has been used extensively to treat hypertensive urgencies. It is more potent than nicardipine. Careful monitoring of vital signs and neurological status is required because nifedipine has rarely been associated with worsened ischemic stroke. **Nimodipine**, although an effective antihypertensive, is exclusively used to prevent cerebral vasospasm. In addition to having antihypertensive properties, any calcium-channel blocker may help interrupt

the development of secondary brain injury after trauma. **Verapamil** and **diltiazem** are effective when given as an IV bolus or infusion for supraventricular arrhythmias. They also lower blood pressure but are not routinely used in acute situations. Verapamil and diltiazem are often prescribed chronically to treat hypertension. Sustained-release oral dosage forms are available. They should not be crushed and given through any kind of enteral tube, because this will place the patient at risk for hypotension from the relative overdose. Similarly, immediate-release calcium-channel blockers given once daily are likely to be ineffective unless they have a long half-life like amlodipine.

Nitroglycerin is a vasodilator but is often ineffective in managing severe hypertension. **Sodium nitroprusside** is a potent arterial and venous vasodilator that has been used for many years for hypertensive urgencies and emergencies. It should be avoided in patients with acute neurological injury because it tends to override any remaining vascular protection and expose the brain to excessively high pressures. High doses given for a prolonged period can lead to thiocyanate toxicity, particularly if the risk of renal failure is high. Unexplained acidosis is usually the first sign. Concomitant **sodium thiosulfate** has been advocated to prevent thiocyanate toxicity.

Beta blockers are also useful vasodilators. **Esmolol** is an ultra-short-acting beta blocker that can be given as escalating IV boluses or by a continuous infusion. It is also effective for supraventricular tachycardia. **Labetalol** is a more potent direct vasodilator. Many consider it to be the drug of choice for acutely managing hypertension in the neuroscience population because of its safety record and because it does not cause as much tachycardia as other potent vasodilators. All beta blockers have negative inotropic effects that can limit their use in patients with congestive heart failure. They can also worsen glucose control in patients with diabetes, worsen pulmonary function in asthmatics, and (rarely) cause hyperkalemia. **Metoprolol** and **atenolol** are also alternatives.

Before introduction of labetalol and other newer antihypertensives, **alpha-methyldopa** was frequently used for blood pressure management in the neuroscience ICU. Sedation is a common side effect. Other nonsedating vasodilators are now preferred because they do not affect neurological assessment. The angiotensin-converting enzyme inhibitor, **enalaprilat,** is now available for IV use in the acute care

Table 11-2 • INOTROPIC AGENTS

DRUG	DOSE	ADVERSE EFFECTS	COMMENTS
Dobutamine	2.5 μg/kg/min titrate up to 20 μg/kg/min	Hypotension, ischemia, tachycardia	Wean slowly (1 μg/kg/minute/hour) useful for low cardiac output unresponsive to fluids
Dopamine Epinephrine Norepinephrine			See Table 11-1, Vasoconstrictor Agents, for details
Amrinone	0.75 mg/kg × 1 over 3 minutes, then 5 μg/kg/min titrate up to 15 μg/kg/min	Hypotension, ischemia, thrombocytopenia, tachycardia	Primarily a vasodilator, typically used with dobutamine
Milrinone	50 μg/kg over 10 min × 1, then 0.375–0.75 μg/kg/min	Hypotension, ischemia, tachycardia	More potent than amrinone
Isoproterenol	2–10 μg/min	Tachycardia, hypotension, ischemia	Excessive tachycardia limits use to severe bradycardia only

Table 11-3 • VASODILATORS

DRUG	DOSE	ADVERSE EFFECTS	COMMENTS
Calcium Channel Blockers			
Nicardipine	5 mg/hr IV, titrate q15 minutes up to 15 mg/hour *Onset:* 1–5 minutes	Hypotension, tachycardia	Doses >15 mg/hour not effective, fluid load can be substantial—maximum concentration = 0.2 mg/mL
Nifedipine	PO/SL: 10–30 mg q4–8h. Max daily dose, 180 mg *Onset:* 5–15 minutes	Hypotension, tachycardia, headache, flushing	SL route has been associated with worsened ischemic stroke
Nimodipine	60 mg PO/SL q4h × 21 days	Hypotension, tachycardia	For preventing vasospasm after aneurysm repair only, 30 mg q2h has been used in hypotensive patients
Verapamil	PO: 80 mg q8h up to 480 mg/day	Heart block, worsened CHF, constipation	IV useful for supraventricular arrhythmias, not for acutely elevated BP
Diltiazem	PO: 30 mg q6h up to 360 mg/day IV: 0.25 mg/kg bolus, may repeat × 1 with 0.35 mg/kg. *Infusion range:* 5–15 mg/hour	Similar to those of verapamil, but less pronounced	See verapamil. IV form for SVT or AF only
Nitroglycerin	20–300 μg/minute *Onset:* 1–2 minute	Hypotension, headache, methemaglobinemia	Tachyphylaxis can occur, oral and topical forms available: provide "nitrate free" interval daily to lessen tachyphylaxis
Sodium nitroprusside	0.5–10 μg/kg/minute *Onset:* seconds	Hypotension, cyanide toxicity, especially with concurrent renal failure	Avoid in setting of increased intracranial pressure; some advocate concurrent sodium thiosulfate to minimize risk of cyanide toxicity
Beta Blockers			
Labetolol	IV: 10–20 mg over 2 min, may increase to 40–80 mg and repeat q10 minutes up to total of 300 mg.—see comments *Onset:* 5 minutes	Bradycardia, bronchospasm, worsened glucose control in association with diabetes, worsened CHF	May be the drug of choice for many neuroscience patients; may use continuous infusion starting at 2 mg/minute and titrate to effect
Metoprolol	IV: 5 mg q5 minutes up to 15 mg PO: 25 mg q12h up to 100 mg q6h	See labetolol, cardiac selective up to 200 mg/day	IV maintenance doses up to 20 mg q6h have been tolerated, but are expensive
Esmolol	500 μg/kg × 1, then 25–50 μg/kg/minute up to 400 μg/kg/minute *Onset:* 1–3 minutes	See labetolol	Also useful for SVT, very short acting
Enalaprilat	IV: 0.625–5 mg over 5 minutes q6h *Onset:* 15 minutes PO: 2.5–40 mg/day	Hypotension, hyperkalemia rash, cough, laryngeal edema	Intensity of response depends on fluid status of patient; IV form at least twice as potent as oral.

setting. The relative efficacy of this drug fluctuates depending on the volume status of the patient. Hypovolemic patients tend to have an exaggerated response, whereas fluid-overloaded patients tend to respond poorly. Enalaprilat also can cause hyperkalemia.

Anticonvulsants

Anticonvulsants are a mainstay of therapy for patients with seizure disorders. These agents are effective for control of seizures from various etiologies. Most patients with seizure disorders can be managed with pharmacotherapy alone. More than 20 different drugs are used to control convulsive

episodes, but most patients are effectively managed with four to five agents used alone or in combination. A review of commonly used anticonvulsants is presented in Table 11-4. A more complete discussion of selected agents and nursing implications is offered below.

Phenytoin (Dilantin)

Phenytoin is a member of the hydantoin class of anticonvulsants. It blocks synaptic post-tetanic potentiation and subsequent propagation of electrical discharge in the motor cortex. The drug blocks sodium transport and thereby stabilizes membrane sensitivity to hyperexcitable states. Phenytoin is used for management of tonic-clonic and psychomotor sei-

Table 11-4 • ANTICONVULSANT AGENTS

DRUG	COMMON DOSES	THERAPEUTIC SERUM LEVEL	ADVERSE EFFECTS	COMMENTS
Barbiturates				
Phenobarbital (Luminal)	3–5 mg/kg/day	15–40 mg/L	Sedation, rash, ataxia, hyperactivity, respiratory depression, hypotension (IV)	Induces hepatic metabolism—may increase elimination of drugs
Primidone (Mysoline)	10–25 mg/kg/day	5–20 mg/L	Sedation, ataxia, nausea, dizziness, rash (similar to phenobarbital)	Active metabolites: PEMA and phenobarbital
Hydantoins				
Phenytoin (Dilantin)	4–8 mg/kg/day	10–20 mg/L	Nystagmus, rash, sedation, fever, gingival hyperplasia, ataxia, hypotension and bradycardia, pain on injection (IV)	IV administration: limit 50 mg/min as direct push into running IV line. Enzyme inducer.
Fosphenytoin (Cerebyx)	4–8 mg PE/kg/day	10–20 mg/L	Pruritus, significantly less cardiotoxicity; otherwise similar to phenytoin	150 mg PE/min maximum IV administration
Other Agents				
Carbamazepine (Tegretol, Carbatrol)	10–35 mg/kg/day	4–12 mg/L	Dizziness, ataxia, nystagmus, rash, diplopia, aplastic anemia	Induces own metabolism and metabolism of other drugs
Valproic acid (Depakene, Depakote, Depacon)	15–60 mg/kg/day	50–100 mg/L	Nausea, vomiting, diarrhea, drowsiness, liver toxicity	Hepatic enzyme inhibitor. IV should be divided q6h
Clonazepam (Klonopin)	2–20 mg/day	20–80 ng/mL	Drowsiness, ataxia	Tolerance to anticonvulsant effect may occur
Felbamate (Felbatol)	15–45 mg/kg/day	Not established	Nausea, vomiting, diarrhea, anxiety, insomnia, headache, hypophosphatemia, rash	Risk of fatal aplastic anemia, liver failure; use recommended only if benefits exceed risks
Gabapentin (Neurontin)	900–4,800 mg/day	Not established	Drowsiness, ataxia, dizziness, fatigue	No known interactions with other anticonvulsants; beneficial in pain management
Lamotrigine (Lamictal)	100–500 mg/day	Not established	Dizziness, diplopia, headache, ataxia, nausea, severe skin rash	Slow dosage titration required; approved for monotherapy
Topiramate (Topamax)	200–900 mg/day	Not established	Drowsiness, dizziness, fatigue, parasthesias, impaired cognition	Dosage titration over 8 weeks
Tiagabine (Gabitril)	32–56 mg/day	Not established	Dizziness, somnolence, asthenia, tremor, anxiety, confusion	Rare incidence of serious rash
Oxcarbazepine (Trileptal)	300–1,800 mg/day	Not established	Headache, drowsiness, fatigue, dizziness, hyponatremia	Lacks hematologic toxicity seen with carbamazepine
Zonisamide (Zonegran)	100–400 mg/day	Not established	Impaired memory, drowsiness, ataxia, nystagmus, diplopia, nephrolithiasis	Long plasma half-life of 50–68 hours
Levetiracetam (Keppra)	1,000–3,000 mg/day	Not established	Asthenia, headache, pain, dizziness, somnolence	No titration required; therapy initiated at therapeutic dose
Refractory status epilepticus				
Midazolam (Versed)	0.1–0.2 mg/kg bolus; maintenance IV at 0.04–2 mg/kg/hour	Not established	Hypotension, respiratory depression	Tachyphylaxis may develop rapidly, requiring frequent dose titrations
Propofol (Diprivan)	1–2 mg/kg bolus; maintenance IV at 2–10 mg/kg/hour	Not established	Hypotension, respiratory depression	Cardiac depressant effects at high doses
Pentobarbital (Nembutal)	10–20 mg/kg bolus; maintenance IV at 1–5 mg/kg/hour	Not established	Hypotension, respiratory depression, cardiac depressant	Typically requires fluid and/or pressor support

zures. It may be used alone or in combination with other drugs. When used in combination, it is often possible to reduce the adverse effects of the respective agents and achieve a synergistic effect on controlling seizures. Phenytoin is also used prophylactically in neurosurgical patients to prevent seizures in the postoperative period.

Serum Concentration Monitoring

The accepted therapeutic range for phenytoin is 10 to 20 mg/L. At concentrations above this, side effects such as nystagmus, ataxia, and altered cognition are more apparent. The half-life of phenytoin varies considerably among patients and increases with dosage and plasma level. Steady state levels are normally reached in 7 to 14 days but may take up to 28 days in some patients. Except when patients are loaded with phenytoin, obtaining levels more frequently than every 3 to 4 days is rarely necessary.

Phenytoin is highly protein bound, with about 90% of drug in serum bound to albumin. Only the unbound (free) drug is available to exert a pharmacological effect. Serum phenytoin levels are normally reported as total drug concentrations. Thus, the free concentration is approximately 10% of the total phenytoin concentration, or 1 to 2 mg/L. In patients with hypoalbuminemia, total serum phenytoin levels may appear low when the active free phenytoin component may actually be normal or high. In such patients, measurement of free levels is a better indicator of clinical response. When free phenytoin concentrations are not readily available, total phenytoin levels may be estimated by the following equation:

Adjusted phenytoin level

$$= \text{measured phenytoin} /[(\text{serum albumin}) (0.2) + 0.1]$$

Drug interactions with agents that displace phenytoin from albumin (e.g., valproic acid) will also increase the free concentration and lead to enhanced therapeutic effect or toxicity.

Administration

Phenytoin is available as an IV preparation, chewable tablets, oral suspension, and extended-release capsules. The IV and capsule formulations contain phenytoin sodium, whereas the chewable tablets and suspension contain phenytoin acid. Phenytoin sodium contains 92% phenytoin. In some patients, changing formulations may result in altered serum concentrations due to the different percentages of phenytoin. The extended-release capsule formulation is the only oral form approved for once daily dosing, though daily doses exceeding 400 mg are usually split.

Administration of phenytoin can present problems for patients receiving enteral feedings. The suspension tends to settle out in the bottle, making it difficult to deliver a specific dose consistently. Vigorous shaking is required to re-suspend the drug. When administered concurrently with tube feedings, phenytoin may bind with the feeds, reducing absorption of the drug. Although theoretically possible with all oral forms, this is most frequently reported with the suspension formulation. If serum levels begin declining in patients previously maintained on a fixed dosing regimen, administration may need to be staggered with feedings to allow time for complete absorption. Chewable tablets may be crushed and put down feeding tubes, and the capsules may be emptied and instilled through the tube. The extended phenytoin sodium contained in the capsule formulation retains its delayed release properties even when removed from the capsule shell.

Parenteral formulations of phenytoin are insoluble in water and contain solvents (propylene glycol and alcohol) to produce a solution. These solvents contribute to the problems associated with parenteral administration. Manufacturers recommend direct push into a running IV line at no more than 50 mg/min. Rates exceeding this lead to cardiac toxicity and hypotension. When administering large loading doses, however, this can be inconvenient. Dilution in various fluids can cause precipitation of the drug. Although not recommended by manufacturers, various researchers have studied administration of phenytoin in 0.45% and 0.9% sodium chloride or lactated Ringer's solution with good results. Most studies mixed the drug in 100 to 500 mL of fluid and used an in-line filter to prevent transmission of microcrystals to the patient. This technique may offer an alternative to IV push when large doses of phenytoin are given. Intramuscular administration is not advisable because absorption is highly erratic, and the extreme alkaline pH of the injection causes tissue damage.

Drug Interactions

Phenytoin is subject to interactions with many other drugs. As mentioned previously, any agents that displace phenytoin from binding sites will potentiate its effect. Warfarin, tricyclic antidepressants, and aspirin are examples of agents that cause displacement interactions. Because phenytoin is metabolized in the liver, drugs inhibiting (e.g., fluconazole, valproic acid) or inducing (e.g., phenobarbital, carbamazepine) hepatic metabolism alter serum phenytoin concentrations (pharmacokinetic interaction). Additionally, phenytoin can alter effects of other anticonvulsants by unpredictable complex mechanisms. Phenytoin may increase or decrease the action of phenobarbital and valproic acid and decrease the effect of carbamazepine (pharmacodynamic interaction). Patients should be carefully monitored when adding or discontinuing any medications to their regimen when taking phenytoin. Drug–food interactions may be clinically relevant. Long-term phenytoin administration can lower folic acid levels in patients, whereas folate replacement therapy may decrease its anticonvulsant effects.

Side Effects and Toxicities

With increasing plasma levels, common side effects include nystagmus, drowsiness, ataxia, fatigue, and cognitive impairment. Gastrointestinal (GI) symptoms of nausea, vomiting, or diarrhea are seen frequently. Administering phenytoin with meals can reduce the occurrence of these effects. Some patients may develop a drug-induced fever while on phenytoin. Patients may develop an erythematous morbilliform rash requiring discontinuation of the drug. Gingival hyperplasia is a frequent side effect with long-term phenytoin use. Patients should be counseled on the importance of good oral hygiene to minimize this problem. Rare complications include hepatotoxicity and blood dyscrasias, including thrombocytopenia.

Fosphenytoin (Cerebyx)

Due to the adverse effects associated with parenteral phenytoin, fosphenytoin was developed. It is a water-soluble phosphate ester of phenytoin, which is converted to phenytoin in the blood stream by plasma esterases. Because of molecular weight differences, fosphenytoin is dosed as "phenytoin equivalents" or PEs. Thus, 100 mg PE of fosphenytoin delivers 100 mg of phenytoin. Because it lacks the propylene glycol solvent, fosphenytoin is better tolerated from a cardiovascular standpoint. The maximum rate of administration for fosphenytoin is 150 mg PE per minute, compared with 50 mg per minute for parenteral phenytoin. Due to the time needed for conversion, faster administration does not equate to faster onset of pharmacological effect. The formulation has a less basic pH of 9 (compared with pH 12 for phenytoin), so tissue damage and pain from injection are reduced. As a result, fosphenytoin may be given intramuscularly if necessary. As phenytoin is the active component of fosphenytoin, other side effects noted above with phenytoin are also observed. Pruritus has also been observed in patients receiving fosphenytoin; this is attributed to the phosphate component of the formulation. Although ease of administration and reduced side effects are significant benefits, fosphenytoin is considerably more expensive than phenytoin. Therefore, some health care centers restrict the use of fosphenytoin to patients without central venous access who cannot tolerate enteral phenytoin.

Valproic Acid (Depakene, Depakote, Depacon)

Valproic acid is a carboxylic acid compound that exerts its anticonvulsant activity through increasing brain levels of gamma-aminobutyric acid. There may also be some effect on potassium channels and direct membrane-stabilizing effects. The drug is usually used for treatment of absence seizures or in combination with other agents for control of various convulsive disorders. The enteric-coated formulation, divalproex sodium (Depakote), is metabolized to valproic acid in the gut. An IV formulation, valproate sodium (Depacon), has also been recently introduced. Dosing is the same for all three products. However, the manufacturer currently recommends that Depacon be dosed no less frequently than 6-hour intervals unless trough serum levels are monitored.

Serum Concentration Monitoring

The accepted therapeutic range for valproate is 50 to 100 mg/L. However, some studies have shown that higher levels may be necessary for effective seizure control. Most toxicities associated with valproic acid do not seem to be correlated with serum concentration as much as with total dose administered. Steady state plasma levels are normally achieved in 2 to 4 days.

Drug Interactions

Valproic acid is a potent inhibitor of hepatic microsomal enzymes. As such, drugs that are metabolized in the liver are eliminated more slowly from the body. Phenobarbital clearance is decreased considerably when combined with valproic acid. Valproate is greater than 90% bound to plasma proteins, creating the potential for displacement interactions. These effects may occur simultaneously, leading to unpredictable results when valproic acid is combined with other anticonvulsants. Combinations with phenytoin or carbamazepine are representative of this phenomenon, leading to increased toxicities or loss of seizure control when adding or removing agents from a patient's regimen.

Side Effects and Toxicities

Gastrointestinal complaints are the most frequently reported problem with valproic acid therapy; they include nausea, vomiting, indigestion, diarrhea, and anorexia. These can be reduced by administering the dose with food or by changing to an enteric-coated formulation. Central nervous system (CNS) symptoms of drowsiness, ataxia, and tremor are also reported. Hepatotoxicity may occur, usually within the first 6 months of therapy. This has been most commonly reported in children younger than 2 years on multiple anticonvulsants. Minor elevations in liver function test results are often seen and appear to be dose related. Some physicians recommend L-carnitine treatment to protect against hepatotoxicity, but this has not been clearly proved effective. Valproic acid also affects platelet aggregation and may cause thrombocytopenia and other blood dyscrasias. Reduction in dose usually increases the platelet count.

Carbamazepine (Tegretol)

Carbamazepine is an iminostilbene derivative chemically related to the tricyclic antidepressants. It is believed to reduce polysynaptic responses and block post-tetanic potentiation. The drug is useful in the treatment of tonic-clonic, mixed, and psychomotor seizures.

Serum Concentration Monitoring

Serum levels from 4 to 12 mg/L are considered therapeutic for carbamazepine. Steady state levels are initially reached in 3 to 5 days. Carbamazepine, however, has the unique property of inducing its own metabolism. Initial drug half-life ranges from 25 to 65 hours but decreases to 12 to 17 hours with long-term dosing. This effect is first seen in the first few days of therapy and is normally complete in 3 to 4 weeks. Thus, patients stabilized on a given dose early in the course of therapy may experience decreased levels and loss of seizure control with time. Frequent monitoring and dosage adjustments are necessary in the first few months of treatment to optimize drug therapy.

Drug Interactions

In addition to inducing its own metabolism, carbamazepine can induce the metabolism of other drugs. Interactions have been documented with valproic acid, warfarin, and ethosuximide, resulting in decreased blood levels of these agents. Carbamazepine is 76% bound to plasma proteins; thus, displacement reactions are less a problem than with other anticonvulsants. Other drugs induce (phenobarbital, phenytoin, primidone) or inhibit (valproic acid, cimetidine, erythromycin) the metabolism of carbamazepine and require careful monitoring with concomitant use.

Side Effects and Toxicities

The most common side effects of carbamazepine therapy are drowsiness, dizziness, headache, diplopia, nausea, and vomiting. These may be minimized by slow titration of dose and tend to decrease with time. Serious bone marrow toxicities have been reported, including aplastic anemia, agranulocytosis, and thrombocytopenia; fortunately, these are rare. Leukopenia is the most common blood abnormality seen in about 10% of patients but is usually transient. Skin rashes may occur, ranging from a mildly eczematous form to a Stevens-Johnson syndrome. Carbamazepine may also induce a hyponatremic hypoosmolar condition similar to the syndrome of inappropriate antidiuretic hormone (SIADH).

Phenobarbital

Phenobarbital is a barbiturate that exerts its anticonvulsant effect by depression of post-synaptic excitatory discharge. Therapeutic levels are between 15 and 40 mg/L. The half-life is extremely long (100 hours); thus, steady state levels will not be reached for 3 to 4 weeks after initiating therapy. However, this does allow for convenient once daily dosing in most patients.

Drug Interactions

Phenobarbital is a potent inducer of hepatic microsomal enzymes. Thus, it may reduce blood concentrations of any drug cleared by the liver, including phenytoin, carbamazepine, and valproic acid. Phenobarbital metabolism may be inhibited by valproic acid or ethanol.

Side Effects and Toxicities

The primary side effects of phenobarbital are sedation, fatigue, and depression. Tolerance to these doses develops with long-term use. In children and the elderly, the drug may produce opposite effects, causing insomnia and hyperactivity. Hypotension can occur with IV administration. Intramuscular injections are painful and can produce tissue necrosis. Respiratory depression can be profound after IV injections, especially when combined with benzodiazepines.

Other Agents

Newer anticonvulsants have been marketed for the management of seizure disorders. These include **felbamate (Felbatol), gabapentin (Neurontin), lamotrigine (Lamictal), tiagabine (Gabitril), topiramate (Topamax), oxcarbazepine (Trilepal), levetiracetam (Keppra), and zonisamide (Zonegran).** These agents are indicated for adjunct use in various convulsive disorders. Lamotrigine has demonstrated efficacy as monotherapy in recent trials and has been approved

for use as a single agent for partial seizures. Some patients have developed severe, life-threatening rashes requiring hospitalization while taking lamotrigine, especially when combined with valproic acid. Patients presenting with a rash while on lamotrigine should normally have therapy discontinued.

Gabapentin and the newer agent levetiracetam are unique among the anticonvulsants because they have not been found to interfere with the metabolism of other seizure medications. This is a desirable property when adding these agents to complex medication regimens. Felbamate has been noted to cause aplastic anemia and liver failure in some patients. Given this, the Food and Drug Administration warned that patients should be withdrawn from felbamate treatment when possible. Current recommendations state that felbamate should only be used in patients refractory to other agents. When the risk of uncontrolled seizures outweighs the potential risk of hematological or hepatic problems, physicians are encouraged to obtain informed consent and should perform frequent monitoring for associated symptoms.

Oxcarbazepine is an analogue of carbamazepine that appears to lack the hematological toxicities seen with carbamazepine. Other adverse effects, however, are comparable between the two agents. It also does not appear susceptible to autoinduction as with carbamazepine. In contrast to the classic anticonvulsants, four of the newly available agents are eliminated primarily by the kidney. Dosage reductions are required for patients with renal impairment managed on gabapentin, topiramate, oxcarbazepine or levetiracetam.

Long-Term Management of Anticonvulsants

Patients with epilepsy or other secondary seizure disorders often require long-term therapy with anticonvulsants to keep symptoms under control. Maintaining adherence to their medication regimen is crucial, because the most frequent cause of seizures in this population is abrupt withdrawal from anticonvulsants. Patients will need to be counseled on the importance of maintaining dosing schedules, potential side effects and their management, and the possibility for other drugs to interact with their antiepileptic medications. Frequent blood level monitoring may be necessary, especially when titrating doses of newly added agents. Establishing a relationship with a community pharmacist is essential to ensure safe management of this disease. Pharmacists can help the patient understand the side effects they encounter and provide close monitoring for drug interactions with prescription and nonprescription medications.

Sedation and Neuromuscular Blockade

The decision to give neuroscience patients sedatives is complex. On one hand, untreated agitation can contribute to ventilator noncompliance, self-extubation, and decannulation; can induce or worsen hypertension; and can elevate intracranial pressure (ICP). However, agitation can also be an important symptom of hypoxemia, evolving sepsis, worsening neurological injury, or pain. Potentially reversible causes of agitation must be identified and treated before giving sedatives because the patient's neurological assessment will be compromised once therapy is started.

After the decision to implement sedation has been made, careful monitoring is important. Aspiration precautions should be instituted when appropriate. Respiratory depression and hypotension are common side effects of sedative regimens, so excessive sedation should be avoided. Prolonged sedation from overzealous administration of these drugs can delay extubation and complicate brain-death protocols. Sedation can also mislead clinicians into suspecting acute neurological deterioration and prompt otherwise unnecessary computed tomography scans. For these reasons it is preferable to titrate sedative administration according to a sedation scale, such as the Ramsay, rather than giving an arbitrary amount. Continuous infusions of sedatives are probably more likely to result in excessive sedation than intermittent administration. Either way, the patient must be allowed to recover at regular intervals to allow neurological assessment. Recent research has focused on developing shorter-acting sedatives to minimize these concerns and make them easier to use. Specific details regarding the use of

individual sedatives and neuromuscular blockers can be found in Table 11-5.

Benzodiazepines

Benzodiazepines remain the mainstay for sedation of the neuroscience patient. They can be given as an intermittent IV bolus or a continuous infusion. Benzodiazepines are relatively insoluble in water. This can be an important consideration when fluid limitation is necessary and dose requirements are high. This situation commonly occurs in neuroscience patients with benzodiazepine tolerance for whatever reason (tachyphylaxis) or a history of significant ethanol abuse (accelerated metabolism). The pharmacist should be consulted before dilution when concentrated continuous infusions are required.

Diazepam is the oldest injectable benzodiazepine. It is still frequently used for initial control of seizures. **Lorazepam** has also been available for several years and is particularly useful in patients with hepatic dysfunction because its elimination tends to be preserved under these conditions com-

Table 11-5 • SEDATION AND NEUROMUSCULAR BLOCKADE

DRUG	DOSE*	ADVERSE EFFECTS	COMMENTS
Benzodiazepines			
Diazepam	0.1–0.2 mg/kg q1–2h *Onset:* 1–3 minutes	Excessive sedation, respiratory depression, hypotension	Commonly used for initial control of seizures, active metabolite, vein irritant considerably higher doses may be necessary in patients tolerant to benzodiazepines (see text)
Lorazepam	0.04 mg/kg q2–4h *Onset:* 5–15 minutes	See diazepam	See diazepam, inactive metabolites, predictable response in critically ill
Midazolam	0.025–0.035 mg/kg q1–2h *Onset:* 1–3 minutes *Infusion:* 0.05–5 μg/kg/min	See diazepam, prolonged sedation, especially with continuous infusions	Unpredictable elimination in critically ill patients
Propofol	*Bolus:* 1–2 mg/kg *Infusion:* 5–50 μg/kg/min	Cardiovascular depression, infection risk with long hang times, hypotension	No withdrawal syndrome, quick recovery, expensive, does not directly lower intracranial pressure
Haloperidol	*Initial:* 2–10 mg; may double q30 minutes until symptoms improve *Onset:* 3–5 min *Maintenance:* 5–40 mg	Extrapyramidal side effects; lowers seizure threshold; hypotension (uncommon)	Works particularly well for delirium, up to 100 mg doses and continuous infusions have been tolerated well
Pentobarbital	3–5 mg/kg over 30 minutes, then 1 mg/kg/hr *Onset:* <1 minute	Cardiac depression	Serum concentration of 30–50 μg/mL may produce coma with low risk of cardiac side effects; must have level <10 μg/mL to determine brain death.
Neuromuscular Blockers			
Pancuronium	0.01–0.015 mg/kg q1–2h	Tachycardia	Active metabolite; accumulates in renal failure "train of four" monitoring with nerve stimulator best for monitoring efficacy
Vecuronium	0.01–0.015 mg/kg; repeat q1h or start 1 μg/kg/min infusion	Prolonged paralysis increasingly reported	Partially active metabolite may accumulate in renal failure, expensive, use "train of four" monitoring
Cisatracurium	0.1 mg/kg, then 1–3 μg/kg/minute	Minimal histamine release	Does not accumulate in renal or hepatic failure, expensive, monitor "train of four"

* Sedative doses provided are for parenteral management of acute agitation only. Considerably higher doses are occasionally required with long-term use (see text). Chronic oral dosing (where appropriate) will differ and is highly patient specific.

pared with actions of other benzodiazepines. **Midazolam** is the newest parenteral benzodiazepine, and some clinicians consider it the drug of choice due to its short half-life. However, more recent data have shown that the duration of sedation of all injectable benzodiazepines is roughly equal. In fact, numerous case reports describe long recovery times (i.e., days) after midazolam infusions are stopped in critically ill patients. Midazolam has also been used as a high-dose continuous infusion to control refractory status epilepticus.

Flumazenil is a specific benzodiazepine antagonist that can quickly reverse excessive sedation from these drugs. However, using flumazenil this way is specifically discouraged because it can cause severe withdrawal symptoms and seizures in benzodiazepine-tolerant patients. Patients who receive flumazenil should be monitored closely because it is very short acting. Resedation after it wears off is common.

Other Sedatives

Propofol is a very short-acting sedative that is being used in some ICUs. It is particularly useful when the anticipated duration of sedation is short, because recovery is rapid. Patients with long-term sedation requirements should receive a different agent because the short sedation duration is no longer advantageous. It is the most expensive sedative in routine use. Attempts at using propofol to lower ICP have been disappointing. Individual propofol preparations should not hang for longer than 12 hours because it is provided as a lipid emulsion and is therefore an excellent medium for microbial growth. It is also a significant source of calories that needs to be considered when feeding regimens are titrated. **Haloperidol** is a useful sedative and is particularly effective for patients experiencing delirium. Low doses tend to be prescribed, often with disappointing results; however, a properly titrated dose can be safe and effective. Extremely high doses (in excess of 100 mg per dose) and continuous infusions have been used safely. Haloperidol can lower seizure threshold and is usually not used in patients with known epilepsy. It can also cause hypotension if administered too quickly. The barbiturate **pentobarbital** is usually reserved for inducing pharmacological coma in the setting of status epilepticus or elevated ICP unresponsive to other treatment. High doses can suppress cardiac function. Serum pentobarbital concentrations are monitored, but the correlation with efficacy or toxicity is poor. Low concentrations (less than 10 $\mu g/mL$) need to be documented before declaring brain death in patients who have received high doses of pentobarbital.

Long-Term Management of Sedatives

Long-term sedative use should be reserved for patients in whom agitation secondary to a residual neurological deficit places them or others at risk for harm. Sedatives should be carefully withdrawn at intervals to make sure they are still indicated because excessive or unnecessary sedation can mask or impede neurological recovery. Fall precautions should be observed, even in patients taking these drugs chronically. Aspiration is also a long-term risk. Sudden discontinuation of long-term benzodiazepine therapy can precipitate a withdrawal reaction. Depending on the benzodiazepine, the onset can be delayed for as long as 7 days after cessation of therapy. Extreme agitation with hyperdynamic vital signs is a routine symptom. Seizures are not uncommon. The shorter acting benzodiazepines alprazolam and lorazepam may have a higher risk of seizure with sudden withdrawal.

Neuromuscular Blockade

Occasionally, a patient may be so combative that neuromuscular blockade (NMB) is warranted. Other indications include short-term paralysis for a bedside procedure or elevated ICP unresponsive to other treatments. NMB is also used to decrease the work of breathing in patients with adult respiratory distress syndrome and increase ventilator compliance, particularly when nonphysiological modes, such as inverted inspiratory:expiratory ratio, are used. **Pancuronium**, **vecuronium**, and **cisatracurium** are the most frequently prescribed neuromuscular blockers. Specific details are listed in Table 11-5.

Careful monitoring is important when continuous NMB is prescribed. All neuromuscular blockers are associated with tachyphylaxis. Therefore, as the patient becomes "tolerant" to a drug, higher doses are required. Patients requiring amounts that greatly exceed maximum recommended doses will usually respond to a different agent. Doses should be titrated so that one or two twitches are maintained when a "train of four" is assessed by a nerve stimulator. Failure to do so increases the risk of excessively prolonged NMB after the drug is stopped. Complete blockade lasting several days after drug discontinuation has been reported, particularly with vecuronium, resulting in abnormal neuromuscular weakness lasting several weeks after initial recovery. In addition, excessive doses waste health care dollars because NMB regimens are very expensive. Patients receiving neuromuscular blockers to improve respiratory status may achieve ventilator compliance goals while technically "subtherapeutic" from a train-of-four perspective. Using this as a therapeutic endpoint is appropriate and should limit episodes of prolonged NMB and reduce drug wastage.

NMB should be stopped regularly to allow a full neurological evaluation, because many signs and symptoms of acute deterioration are masked while the patient is paralyzed. Furthermore, the patient must be adequately sedated (and when appropriate, receive adequate analgesia) at all times while the blockade is in effect. These drugs do *not* have sedative or analgesic properties. Hyperdynamic vital signs may be the only clue that sedation or analgesia is ineffective.

ANTIBIOTICS

Indications

Many neuroscience patients require antibiotic therapy at some point during their hospitalization. Antibiotics are often prescribed as prophylaxis in conjunction with neurosurgical procedures. The initial dose should be infused as close to the time of initial incision as possible (within 2 hours is optimal) for maximal efficacy. Therefore, they are best given in preoperative holding, as opposed to "on call to OR," to avoid ineffective prophylaxis due to unanticipated delays. The value of postoperative doses is controversial. The Center for Disease Control and Prevention (CDC) guidelines discourage the routine use of vancomycin for prophylaxis (see below).

Occasionally, patients may have an unrelated preexisting infection, such as a urinary tract infection or community-acquired pneumonia, that requires treatment. In contrast, meningitis and ventricular shunt infections are examples of established CNS infections that require hospitalization for aggressive therapy with antibiotics.

Some patients are admitted with an evolving infection resulting from pre-hospital events. For example, aspiration of gastric contents during an episode of status epilepticus can lead to bacterial pneumonia in addition to a chemical pneumonitis. Presumptive antibiotics are often prescribed under these circumstances. Trauma victims may present with an open skull fracture or other systemic injuries, such as penetrating abdominal trauma, that require presumptive antibiotics for proper management.

Despite strict adherence to aseptic technique and optimal overall management, neuroscience patients are at high risk for developing nosocomial infections. Neurological impairment increases the risk of pneumonia, as a result of continued aspiration, atelectasis, or prolonged mechanical ventilation. Indwelling devices, such as external ventricular drains, all methods of vascular access, and bladder catheters, are associated with infectious complications. Corticosteroid therapy and inadequate nutritional support also increase risk of nosocomial infection in the neuroscience patient.

General Principles

Proper selection of antibiotics depends on numerous factors. These include the presumed site of infection, local antibiotic sensitivity trends, and patient-specific considerations. For example, preexisting conditions, such as drug allergies, a seizure disorder, or renal dysfunction, may preclude use of one antibiotic over another in applicable patients. The selection of an antibiotic regimen for meningitis must take into account the penetration of that drug across the blood–brain barrier.

After a given therapy is selected, the patient is monitored for response and adverse effects. Response is usually determined based on trends in core body temperature, white blood cell count and differential, and results of culture and sensitivity testing. Other tests specific to the infectious source, such as chest radiographs in patients with pneumonia, are also important when grading response. Generally, at least 72 hours are required to gauge the clinical response to a new regimen of antibiotics. Neuroscience patients can be particularly difficult to assess in this capacity. For example, depending on the primary neurological insult, certain patients may remain febrile due to a centrally mediated "resetting" of their core temperature, despite proper treatment of their infection. Corticosteroids can confuse the clinician either by masking an ongoing fever resulting from their antipyretic action or by triggering a sustained leukocytosis. Neuroscience patients may become "colonized" with nosocomial bacteria during a long hospitalization. This results in consistently positive cultures, despite the absence of a clinical infection. Thus, the whole patient must be assessed when determining response to antibiotic therapy.

Compared with other classes of pharmaceuticals, antibiotics (with important exceptions shown in Table 11-6) are remarkably safe to administer. In general, few adverse reactions are related to IV administration. Drug incompatibilities, as always, should be checked before coadministering an antibiotic with another IV fluid or drug infusion. Most IV antibiotics, with the exception of amphotericin B, can be given in reasonable volumes of 0.9% normal saline (NS). See Table 11-6 and later discussion of specific antibiotics for details. Known allergies to antibiotics are common because they are so widely prescribed. Therefore, it is necessary to screen each patient for drug allergies before giving the first dose of any antibiotic. The assistance of a pharmacist can be invaluable in assessing the risk of cross-sensitivity in patients with allergies to certain antibiotics requiring treatment for infection.

All antibiotics can disrupt the normal bacterial flora resulting from their antimicrobial action. Often, this does not cause a detectable problem or may elicit only mild diarrhea. Unfortunately, this can also lead to superinfection by allowing other endogenous microorganisms resistant to the antibiotics to multiply unchecked. One possible outcome, pseudomembranous colitis, is characterized by high-output diarrhea (which is occasionally bloody) and can be life threatening. The diagnosis is usually confirmed by the detection of *Clostridium difficile* toxin in a stool sample. Treatment consists of discontinuing the offending antibiotic(s) whenever possible and starting enterally administered antibiotics, such as metronidazole, to treat the *C. difficile* infection. Antidiarrheals and antimotility agents are contraindicated until the cause of the diarrhea has been identified. Another common example of superinfection is a serious nosocomial infection caused by "selected" multiple-drug-resistant microorganisms that typically develops after a lengthy regimen of broad-spectrum antibiotics. The selection of resistant microorganisms (e.g., *Pseudomonas*) through the prolonged use and misuse of antibiotics ultimately affects the ecology of the entire health care facility. The recent emergence of vancomycin-resistant *Enterococcus faecium* (VRE) as a serious nosocomial pathogen is an example. This unfortunate development has an impact on the neuroscience patient in particular, because the propagation of this new pathogen seems to be related to excessive use of vancomycin, which is commonly prescribed as prophylaxis in neurosurgical patients. Antibiotics that are effective against VRE, such as quinopristin/dalfopristin and linezolid, are just now becoming available.

Specific Antimicrobials

The following is a discussion of specific classes of antibiotics, with special emphasis on nursing implications and application to the neuroscience patient. Specific details regarding dose ranges, clinical use, and adverse effects are listed in Table 11-6.

Beta-Lactam Antibiotics

These antibiotics are the most frequently prescribed class of antimicrobials. This category includes various *penicillins* and *cephalosporins, beta-lactamase inhibitor combinations, monobac-*

Table 11–6 • ANTIBIOTICS*

DRUG	DOSE†	ADVERSE EFFECTS‡	COMMENTS‡
Beta-lactams		Adverse effects common to all beta-lactams and related antibiotics include phlebitis, nausea, diarrhea, pseudomembranous colitis, hypersensitivity reactions (see text), rare disturbances in blood counts	All beta-lactams can cause neurotoxicity, including seizures, with prolonged excessive doses
Penicillins			
Penicillin G	5–30 mU§/day	See above	Particularly useful for streptococcal infections, including Enterococcus; weak activity against *Staphylococcus aureus*
Ampicillin	4–12 g/day		
Antistaphylococcal penicillins		Interstitial nephritis not rare, especially with methicillin, see above	Little activity against anything but S. aureus and certain Streptococcus strains resistant to methicillin resistant to all three agents
Nafcillin	4–12 g/day		
Methicillin	4–12 g/day		
Oxacillin	4–12 g/day		
Extended spectrum		See above, ticarcillin in particular inhibits platelet function	Useful for hospital-acquired gram-negative bacteria; can inactivate aminoglycosides in serum samples, resulting in falsely low values
Piperacillin	8–18 g/day		
Ticarcillin	4–24 g/day		
Mezlocillin	6–18 g/day		
Cephalosporins		See above general adverse effect statement for beta-lactams	Most cephalosporins can falsely elevate creatinine levels
First generation			
Cefazolin	2–6 g/day	See above	Most often used for surgical prophylaxis
Second generation			
Cefuroxime	2.25–4.5 g/day	See above	Cefuroxime particularly useful for community-acquired pneumonia
Cefamandole	2–12 g/day	Hypoprothrombinemia	
Cephamycins			
Cefoxitin	3–8 g/day	See above, can cause hypoprothrombinemia	Expanded spectrum against enterics and anaerobes; good for intra-abdominal infection
Cefotetan	2–4 g/day		
Third generation			
Ceftriaxone	1–4 g/day	See above	All are useful for hospital-acquired pneumonia; ceftazidime and ceftriaxone in particular effective for meningitis
Ceftazidime	1.5–6 g/day		
Ceftizoxime	2–12 g/day		
Cefoperazone	2–4 g/day		
Cefotaxime	2–12 g/day		
Cefepime	2–4 g/day	See above	Better gram-positive coverage than third-generation agents; use 6 g/day in neutropenia
Beta-Lactamase Inhibitor Combinations			
Ampicillin/sulbactam	6–12 g/day	See above	See information on individual drugs; all have expanded spectrum against enterics, *S. aureus,* and anaerobes
Ticarcillin/clavulanate	12.4–18.6 g/day		
Piperacillin/tazobactam	13.5 g/day		
Amoxicillin/clavulanate	1.5–1.75 g/day PO		
Aztreonam	3–8 g/day	See above	Spectrum similar to that of ceftazidime, does not cross-react in penicillin-allergic patients
Imipenem/Cilastatin	1.5–4 g/day	See above; highest incidence of neurological toxicity, including seizures	Very broad spectrum, usually reserved for patients with known resistant bacteria
Meropenem	1.5–3 g/day	See imipenem (may have lower risk of seizures compared with imipenem)	Up to 6 g/day used in meningitis
Aminoglycosides		Nephrotoxicity, possible ototoxicity	Serum concentration monitoring required to ensure efficacy, minimize toxicity (see text), therapeutic amikacin: peak, 25–35; trough, 5–10 µg/mL
Gentamicin	3–5 mg/kg/day		
Tobramycin	3–5 mg/kg/day	Neuromuscular blockade	
Amikacin	15 mg/kg/day		

Table 11–6 • ANTIBIOTICS* (Continued)

DRUG	DOSE†	ADVERSE EFFECTS‡	COMMENTS‡
Vancomycin	*IV:* 2 g/day *PO:* 125 mg q6h *Intrathecal:* 5–10 mg q48–72 h	Red man's syndrome, possible nephrotoxicity, possible ototoxicity	Role of concentration monitoring controversial: peak, 20–40 μg/mL; trough at least 5 μg/mL typical therapeutic goals if measured, oral form only useful against *Clostridium difficile*
Antifungals			
Amphotericin B	0.25–1.0 mg/kg/day	Nephrotoxicity, electrolyte depletion fever, chills, hypotension, anaphylaxis	Drug of choice for the most serious systemic fungal infections, infuse over 4–8 hours, not compatible in saline, 250–500 mL dilution required
Liposomal amphotericin B	5 mg/kg/day	See above; may be milder than regular amphotericin B	Several products; not interchangeable; extremely expensive
Fluconazole	100–800 mg/day	Rash, elevated liver function test results	Excellent enteral absorption, limited antifungal spectrum, drug interactions (see text)
Chloramphenicol	50 mg/kg/day	Aplastic anemia, grey syndrome, fever	Excellent penetration across blood–brain barrier
Fluoroquinolones			
Ciprofloxacin Ofloxacin Levofloxacin	400–1,200 mg/day 400–800 mg/day 500 mg/day	Headache, restlessness, agitation	Significant drug interactions (see text); do not give with antacids, iron, calcium, or sucralfate; several newer agents being released
Acyclovir	15–30 mg/kg/day	Crystalluria, tremors, seizures	Effective for viral meningitis, infuse over at least 1 hour
Trimethoprim/sulfamethoxazole	8–20 mg/kg/day (trimethoprim)	Allergic reactions common, nausea renal failure	Requires dilution in high volumes of dextrose, interacts with warfarin (see text)
Clindamycin	900–2,700 mg/day	Highest risk of pseudomembranous colitis, neuromuscular blockade (rare)	Effective against anaerobes and S. aureus, useful for aspiration pneumonia and intra-abdominal infection
Metronidazole	1–2 g/day	Diarrhea, metallic taste, disulfiram reaction	Active against gram-negative anaerobes only; useful in intra-abdominal infections, oral form is drug of choice for treatment of *C. difficile*, central venous access recommended, active versus vancomycin-resistant enterococci and multidrug-resistant *S. Aureus* (see text); extremely expensive
Quinopristin/dalfopristin	15–22.5 mg/kg/day	Thrombophlebitis, myalgia, arthalgia	
Linezolid	800–1,200 mg/day	Nausea, diarrhea, thrombocytopenia	IV and oral forms equally effective; very expensive

* Antimicrobials listed restricted to those most frequently encountered in neuroscience patients.

† All dosing information refers to intravenous administration except where indicated.

‡ Adverse effects and comments listed for groups of antimicrobials apply to *all* antimicrobials in group unless otherwise specified.

§ mU = million units.

tams, and *carbapenems.* They are effective for a wide variety of clinical infections and prophylaxis. Of particular note in the neuroscience patient are the third-generation cephalosporins, which, unlike most antibiotics, penetrate the blood–brain barrier well. **Ceftazidime** and **ceftriaxone** in particular are useful for gram-negative meningitis and have largely replaced intrathecal instillation of aminoglycosides. Most beta-lactams are eliminated by the kidneys. When high doses of these antibiotics are given to patients with renal failure, subsequent accumulation of the drug can cause neurological side effects, including generalized seizures. Incidence of this adverse drug reaction is probably highest with the carbapenem antibiotic imipenem. A pharmacist can assist with questions regarding the proper dosing of these drugs in patients with renal insufficiency.

A common dilemma encountered in patients prescribed beta-lactam antibiotics is cross sensitivity. When a beta-lactam is ordered for a patient with a history of hypersensitivity to a similar antibiotic, the allergy must first be characterized. A history of a severe reaction, such as anaphylaxis, to any beta-lactam precludes the use of any related antibiotic, with the possible exception of the monobactam aztreonam. Patients with a history of less severe reactions, such as a rash or hives, to a penicillin, for example, should probably not receive another penicillin but will probably tolerate a cephalosporin without incident.

Careful monitoring is required, however. The reported incidence of cross-sensitivity of penicillin-allergic patients to a cephalosporin is probably about 5%. Cross-sensitivity with imipenem is about 10%. Aztreonam does not cross-react in penicillin-allergic patients. Because cephalosporin allergies are relatively uncommon, the incidence of cross-sensitivity with other beta-lactam antibiotics is unknown. Chemically distinct antibiotics should probably be used. It is worth noting that allergic-type adverse drug reactions can occur at any time during a course of antibiotics.

Aminoglycosides

The aminoglycosides are powerful antibiotics that are commonly prescribed for *nosocomial pneumonia, intraabdominal infections,* and *urinary tract infections.* They need to be dosed carefully to maximize efficacy and minimize toxicity. Critically ill neuroscience patients often fail to attain therapeutic peak concentrations with typical doses. Furthermore, impaired renal function can lead to excessive aminoglycoside accumulation and cause nephrotoxicity. Therefore, *peak and trough serum concentration* monitoring is necessary to ensure that the dose selected is safe and effective. These serum samples are usually obtained when the patient has reached a steady state, typically after three to four consecutive, properly timed doses. The recommended time these drug concentrations ("levels") are measured relative to the dose infused varies somewhat. Whatever the strategy, accurate documentation of *actual* infusion times and serum sampling times is critical to allow proper interpretation of aminoglycoside concentrations and prevent inappropriate adjustments. Pharmacists can be of great assistance when questions regarding serum drug concentration sampling arise. Peak concentrations of **gentamicin** or **tobramycin** need to be 6 to 12 μg/mL to treat most infections adequately, whereas trough concentrations should be less than 2 μg/mL to reduce the risk of kidney damage.

Recently, an alternative dosing strategy for the aminoglycosides called single daily dosing (SDD) has gained acceptance in many institutions. With SDD, patients with normal renal function receive their entire daily dose as a single 5 to 7 mg/kg infusion. This dosing strategy may increase efficacy and reduce toxicity. Therapeutic peaks for SDD are 12 to 20 μg/mL, which needs to be considered if an aminoglycoside concentration is reported by the laboratory as toxic. Previously, peaks this high were thought to cause ototoxicity, but this is probably not true. Trough concentrations with SDD are usually undetectable. Therefore, instead of measuring a trough, the second serum level is usually obtained 8 hours after the peak is drawn. Alternatively, the regimen may be evaluated by a single drug concentration measured 6 to 14 hours after a SDD of an aminoglycoside. This number can vary widely and must be compared with a dosing nomogram for proper evaluation. Aminoglycosides should be avoided in patients with myasthenia gravis because they have been shown (rarely) to potentiate neuromuscular junction blockade.

Vancomycin

Vancomycin is a chemically distinct antibiotic that is prescribed for many infections, such as catheter-related sepsis, pneumonia, and meningitis caused by gram-positive bacteria (*Staphylococci, Streptococci*). It is particularly useful in patients with documented allergies to beta-lactam antibiotics. Vancomycin is the drug of choice for the treatment of documented infections with methicillin-resistant *Staphylococcus aureus* (MRSA). Empiric vancomycin prescribing in patients at low risk for MRSA is discouraged by the CDC because of the emergence of *vancomycin-resistant microorganisms.*

An unusual acute flushing or erythematous reaction involving the upper torso and neck, dubbed "red man syndrome," has been associated with the rapid infusion of vancomycin. It resolves spontaneously by slowing down the infusion rate. Hypotension has also been associated with brisk vancomycin administration. To minimize infusion-related adverse effects, each gram of vancomycin should be given over at least 1 hour. Long-standing concerns about the association of excessive vancomycin accumulation with adverse effects, such as ototoxicity and nephrotoxicity, have not been supported in well-designed studies.

Patient-specific vancomycin regimens are calculated based on weight and kidney function. In addition, empiric vancomycin regimens are occasionally monitored with peak and trough serum drug concentrations (see the section Aminoglycosides). This practice has recently been challenged because the relationship between vancomycin concentrations and efficacy or adverse effects is unclear. The need for vancomycin serum concentration monitoring is less controversial in patients with meningitis, in whom high serum concentrations are needed owing to poor penetration of the drug through the blood–brain barrier. In severe cases of meningitis when aggressive vancomycin therapy is indicated, the drug may be given intrathecally to overcome this problem. Patients receiving strictly prophylactic regimens certainly do not benefit from vancomycin concentration monitoring.

Antifungal Therapy

Antifungals are occasionally prescribed in neuroscience patients, usually for meningitis or urinary tract infections. **Amphotericin B** is the drug of choice for most serious systemic fungal infections. It is associated with numerous side effects, including hypotension, fever, nephrotoxicity, hypomagnesemia, and hypokalemia. These adverse drug reactions occur to a greater or lesser extent in virtually every patient who receives amphotericin B. Close monitoring is essential. *Potassium supplementation* requirements in excess of 200 mEq/day are not uncommon. Each dose of amphotericin B should be infused over at least 4 hours in an attempt to minimize these side effects, although it can be given faster in otherwise stable outpatients. Some clinicians advocate giving a 1-mg test dose before the first dose because anaphylaxis has been reported rarely, though this practice is increasingly uncommon. There is some evidence that sodium chloride repletion (500mL of 0.45% NaCl before and/or after the dose) may decrease the risk of nephrotoxicity. Recently, several liposomal amphotericin B products have been marketed. Emerging evidence suggests that the incidence of adverse effects may be lower with these agents. Guidelines regarding their use are still being developed. Proper use is essential because of their high cost ($500.00/day). They all differ and cannot be interchanged. Patients with fungal urinary tract infections may benefit from local treatment with amphotericin B (**not** lipsomal), using either intermittent instillations or a continuous bladder irrigation. No systemic absorption occurs, thus avoiding the many side effects mentioned previously.

Fluconazole is an azole antifungal that is usually well tolerated, but resistance has been reported with selected types of isolates. Its excellent blood–brain barrier penetration makes it particularly useful for cryptococcal meningitis in patients with the acquired immunodeficiency syndrome. Oral absorption is almost complete. Fluconazole interacts with several drugs, including warfarin, phenytoin, and cyclosporin. Reducing the dose of these drugs is usually required to prevent toxicity.

Other Antimicrobials

Information about specific antimicrobials not discussed previously is listed in Table 11-6. Specific issues regarding these antimicrobials in neuroscience patients are discussed next.

Chloramphenicol is a broad-spectrum antibiotic that for years was the drug of choice for meningitis. This is due to its excellent penetration into the CNS. Serious hematological toxicities and the availability of equally effective alternatives limit its use today.

The *fluoroquinolones* (**ciprofloxacin**, others) are useful for many nosocomial and community-acquired infections. Patients with concomitant renal failure require reduced doses to avoid neurological toxicity (see Beta-Lactams). Some fluoroquinolones can interact with several drugs, including warfarin and theophylline. Patients receiving these drugs have an increased risk of toxicity resulting from amplification of their pharmacological effect when the fluoroquinolone is added. Doses of antacids, oral calcium or magnesium supplements, iron, or sucralfate should not be given within 2 hours of an enterally administered dose of a fluoroquinolone, because absorption of the antibiotic will be impaired. Several new fluoroquinolones have been recently marketed.

Acyclovir is an antiviral drug that is indicated for patients with serious viral meningitis. IV doses should be infused over at least 1 hour to avoid kidney damage from crystallization in the nephrons.

Trimethoprim-sulfamethoxazole is routinely prescribed for urinary tract infections. Occasionally, larger IV doses are prescribed for serious systemic infections with resistant microorganisms, such as *Stenotrophomonas maltophilia, Burkholderia cepacia,* or *Pneumocystis carinii*. Large volumes of IV fluid are required for proper administration. Check with a pharmacist before dilution when fluid restriction or isotonic fluids are important. A history of sulfa allergy, which is common, should always be ruled out before giving trimethoprim-sulfamethoxazole. Dermatological allergic reactions can be severe (Stevens-Johnson syndrome). Concomitant trimethoprim-sulfamethoxazole can also interact with warfarin and increase the risk of bleeding complications.

Metronidazole and **clindamycin** are two antibiotics with strong activity against anaerobic bacteria. Clindamycin is particularly useful for treating aspiration pneumonia because it also has activity against *S. aureus*. Diarrhea and, uncommonly, pseudomembranous colitis (see previous discussion) are associated with clindamycin. Metronidazole, in addition to being commonly used for intra-abdominal infections, is the drug of choice for pseudomembranous colitis

(see previous discussion). The beta-lactamase inhibitor combinations (see Table 11-6) also have excellent antianaerobic activity, thus negating the need for concomitant metronidazole or clindamycin.

Long-Term Management of Antimicrobials

Neuroscience patients usually finish antibiotic therapy for serious infections while still hospitalized. However, home-based IV antimicrobials may rarely be encountered in patients finishing long regimens for difficult-to-treat infections such as fungal meningitis. Proper education of the patient and family is crucial for the safety and efficacy of these comparatively complicated therapies.

Unfortunately, patients with incomplete neurological recovery requiring long-term care are still at an increased risk of developing new infections (see Indications). Prophylactic antibiotics have been prescribed under these circumstances. However, this is generally discouraged because prophylactic antibiotics have not been shown to decrease reliably the risk of clinically significant infections. In addition, when infections occur, they tend to be more difficult to treat because of selection of resistant organisms (see General Principles). Furthermore, avoidable drug interactions, adverse drug effects, and increased health care expenditures are associated with these unnecessary antibiotics. When antibiotics become necessary, proper education of the patient and other caregivers is important, because noncompliance contributes directly to therapeutic failure. Having all prescriptions filled at the same pharmacy can decrease the risk of undetected drug interactions.

▌▌▌▌ STEROIDS

Steroids have several potential indications in the neuroscience patient. However, they can also cause significant side effects. Steroids can have either mineralocorticoid activity or glucocorticoid activity, or both. The mineralocorticoid effect causes sodium and water retention, along with potassium wasting. The anti-inflammatory effect of steroids results from glucocorticoid activity, which causes most of the therapeutic and adverse effects of these drugs. The following discussion is limited to systemic applications of these drugs in neuroscience patients.

Dexamethasone

Dexamethasone is a potent steroid that has only glucocorticoid activity. This is advantageous in patients who require limited fluid intake to prevent edema or minimize swelling. It is usually prescribed for patients with vasogenic edema secondary to tumor. Currently available glucocorticoids are ineffective for the cytotoxic edema that commonly accompanies acute head injury, but research on newly discovered steroid derivatives (tirilazad, for example) continues. Dexamethasone is also commonly used to minimize inflammation after spinal cord surgery.

Other Steroids

Methylprednisolone has mineralocorticoid and glucocorticoid activity. Extremely high doses given for 24 to 48 hours have recently been shown to improve recovery after spinal cord injury if started within 8 hours of the initial insult. It has also been used for certain neuromuscular disorders (e.g., multiple sclerosis) but can aggravate others (e.g., myasthenia gravis). Fluid and sodium retention limits the usefulness of methylprednisolone in many neuroscience patients.

Hydrocortisone also possesses mineralocorticoid and glucocorticoid activity and closely resembles the cortisol normally produced by the body. It is routinely used in "stress doses" (200 to 400 mg/day) after trauma or major surgery in patients who take long-term steroid therapy. **Corticotropin** or its synthetic form, **cosyntropin**, triggers cortisol secretion by the adrenal glands. Intermittent therapy has helped some patients with multiple sclerosis. It can also be used as a one-time dose to assess adrenal function.

Fludrocortisone is a pure mineralocorticoid. It is used to reverse the temporary sodium wasting that can occur in neuroscience patients. The drug may also be required chronically after pituitary resection. It usually takes 2 to 3 days to assess the maximum effect of fludrocortisone. In patients with diabetes insipidus, desmopressin or vasopressin is preferred due to their rapid onset of action.

Adverse Effects

Most serious adverse effects of steroids result from glucocorticoid activity. Steroids lower glucose tolerance, leading to hyperglycemia and its complications. White blood cell counts rise, but the result is immunosupression because the cells do not function properly, predisposing the patient to infection. Steroids further confuse the evaluation for infection because they are also antipyretics. They also can prevent or delay wound healing, contribute to muscle atrophy, and cause osteoporosis. Although profound steroid deficiency can make a patient unresponsive to vasopressors, quick IV administration of large doses can cause cardiovascular collapse. An unusual side effect sometimes seen after rapidly infused doses of dexamethasone is anorectal burning. Glucocorticoids can also cause significant GI bleeding. Antacids or H2 antagonists are routinely prescribed concomitantly but have not been effective in preventing this complication. Steroids are appetite stimulants. They can also induce a profound psychological dependence and other neuropsychological changes. Excessive sodium and fluid retention and hypokalemia are common when agents with mineralocorticoid activity are administered. This can be particularly deleterious in patients with underlying heart disease or hypertension.

Long-Term Management of Steroids

Although many neuroscience patients who receive steroids acutely tolerate them fairly well, the incidence of significant adverse effects rises with long-term therapy. Therefore, the risk:benefit ratio needs to be carefully weighed before patients are committed to long-term steroid therapy. After the decision has been made, the minimally effective dose should be used. Drug-free holidays or intermittent ("pulse") therapy should be considered when feasible. However, patients receiving long-term steroid therapy should be instructed never to stop taking it unless instructed to do so by the health care provider. Eventually, the body stops making its own cortisol when high doses of steroids are given for prolonged periods. Abrupt withdrawal can lead to cardiovascular collapse and other complications due to the sudden acute deficiency of this vital hormone. A slow tapering of the dose can minimize these complications. Patients should also be instructed to watch for and report signs of infection (fever, thrush) or GI bleeding (melena, sharp abdominal pain).

DIURETICS

Diuretics are used in neuroscience patients either as part of the hemodynamic management in general or to lower ICP. The osmotic diuretic **mannitol** is preferred for managing intracranial hypertension because it relieves intracellular edema in addition to prompting a diuresis. Patients with pre-existing congestive heart failure should be monitored carefully, because the osmotic load of the drug may shift enough fluid into the intravascular space to cause vascular congestion and pulmonary edema. Serum osmolality should be monitored, especially in patients with renal failure, because the mannitol will accumulate. The drug is ineffective when the serum osmolality exceeds 320 mOsm/kg H_2O. Mannitol is also used to prompt diuresis in an attempt to minimize renal complications after angiography.

Loop diuretics decrease chloride and water reabsorption in the nephron. Therefore, a loop diuretic, such as **furosemide**, may assist in the fluid management of patients with elevated ICPs. However, unlike mannitol, it does nothing to reverse intracellular edema directly. Furosemide is also a vasodilator and can lower blood pressure and relieve pulmonary congestion prior to the onset of diuresis. For this reason, IV doses should be given no faster than 10 mg/minute. Patients with acute renal failure may receive very large doses in an effort to maintain an adequate urine output. Continuous infusions of furosemide have also been used in this setting. Other more expensive diuretics, such as bumetanide or torsemide, have been tried, but they provide no advantage over furosemide when given in equipotent doses.

Hypokalemia and hypomagnesemia occur in virtually 100% of patients who receive a loop diuretic. Monitoring serum values and supplementing when necessary are important to minimize the cardiac sequelae associated with these deficiencies. Some clinicians feel that high doses of loop diuretics may be nephrotoxic, but the effects probably result from excessive diuresis and kidney hypoperfusion from hypovolemia. IV doses need to be doubled when switching to enteral therapy, because absorption is only about 50%. Likewise, patients maintained on oral therapy need to have their dose reduced by 50% when converted to a parenteral regimen unless a more vigorous diuresis is desired.

GASTROINTESTINAL AGENTS

Stress Ulcer Prophylaxis

Neuroscience patients in the ICU are at high risk for developing what is now called stress-related mucosal damage (SRMD). SRMD can result in hemodynamically significant and occasionally life-threatening upper GI hemorrhage. In addition to being "stressed" as are other critically ill populations, neuroscience patients tend to secrete abnormally large amounts of stomach acid. This risk is further compounded when corticosteroids are concomitantly prescribed. Thus, pharmacological prophylaxis is necessary. Whether adequately tolerated upper GI feedings provide acceptable protection against SRMD is controversial. Agents prescribed strictly for SRMD prophylaxis are not typically required as part of the long-term management of neuroscience patients because the risk is only temporary.

Histamine Type 2 Antagonists

Histamine type 2 antagonists (H2 blockers) are effective in preventing SRMD. They act by decreasing stomach acid production. Attempts have been made to correlate a specific targeted gastric aspirate pH with efficacy, but there is no consensus about what that target value should be. A gastric pH that is consistently 3 or lower may need higher doses of H2 antagonists. A continuous infusion that can be titrated according to gastric pH may be indicated. H2 antagonists can also be given enterally in patients with functional GI tracts. Refer to Table 11-7 for specific details.

H2 antagonists are usually well tolerated. They have been associated with acute mental status changes (delirium, sedation), particularly in elderly patients in the ICU. There is

also a potential for drug interactions involving these agents. In the neuroscience patient, **cimetidine** can decrease clearance of phenytoin, resulting in potentially toxic phenytoin concentrations. This is particularly significant when cimetidine is started or stopped in a patient already stabilized on a phenytoin regimen. **Rantidine** and **famotidine** do not appreciably interact with phenytoin. H2 antagonists may also predispose patients to nosocomial pneumonia. The stomach is usually sterile because it is strongly acidic under normal circumstances. Acid suppression allows bacterial overgrowth, which is then available for aspiration and subsequent infection. However, studies to date comparing acid-reducing SRMD prophylaxis regimens with cytoprotective regimens (see following discussion) have not consistently shown a difference in infectious complications.

Sucralfate

Sucralfate has been extensively studied for SRMD prophylaxis. It is as effective as H2 antagonists for preventing SRMD. Sucralfate acts by covering the stomach with a protective coating and stimulating secretion of gastric protective factors. It is not systemically absorbed; therefore, it is ineffective if given through an enteral access tube that empties anywhere but in the stomach. Likewise, suspensions or slurries should not be administered orally, because most of the dose will coat the upper pharynx and esophagus. Because gastric pH is unaffected, it may cause fewer infectious complications. These factors, coupled with sucralfate's being the cheapest SRMD prophylaxis regimen, make it the drug of choice. Sucralfate should not be given at the same time as a fluoroquinolone, because absorption of the antibiotic will be impaired. Separating the administration of these drugs by 2 hours will minimize this effect.

Table 11-7 • STRESS-ULCER PROPHYLAXIS

DRUG	DOSE	ADVERSE EFFECTS	COMMENTS
H$_2$ antagonists			
Ranitidine	*IV:* 50 mg q8h *Infusion:* 6.25 mg/hour *PO:* 150 mg q12h	Altered mental status, elevated liver enzymes, thrombocytopenia	Continuous infusions can be titrated based on gastric pH—see text
Cimetidine	*IV:* 300 mg q8h *Infusion:* 37.5 mg/hour *PO:* 300 mg q6h	See above	See above, interacts with phenytoin, warfarin, theophylline
Famotidine	*IV:* 20 mg q12h *Infusion:* 1.67 mg/hour *PO:* 20 mg q12h	See above	See above, continuous infusion not as well studied as ranitidine and cimetidine
Sucralfate	1 g PO/NG q6h (dissolve in 10–30 mL H$_2$O for NG use)	Constipation, hypophosphatemia	Does not affect gastric pH, do not give through any tube that empties anywhere but the stomach; drug interactions
Antacids	PO/NG: 30 mL q2h	Magnesium-containing: diarrhea, hypermagnesemia in renal failure; aluminum-containing: constipation, hypophosphatemia	Adverse effects depend on antacid used, dose can be titrated if gastric pH remains low; large volumes may be associated with higher risk of aspiration; drug interactions
Omeprazole	PO: 20 mg q24h	Diarrhea, abdominal pain drug interactions increasingly reported	Not well studied for stress ulcer prophylaxis; do not crush capsule contents for administration by tube

Alternative Prophylaxis Regimens for Stress-Related Mucosal Damage

The first SRMD prophylaxis regimen identified used antacids. Large doses have to be given every 1 to 2 hours. This requires considerable nursing time and may predispose to aspiration and subsequent infection (see previous discussion). Proton pump inhibitors such as **omeprazole** are strong inhibitors of gastric acid secretion. They have not been well studied for SRMD prophylaxis and are currently available only in capsule form. The contents of an omeprazole capsule should not be crushed when administering through a tube because this can impair the bioavailability of the drug.

Other GI Agents

Neurological and neurosurgical patients often experience problems related to the GI tract. Many situations contribute to hypoactive bowel function, including surgery, paralysis, inability to ambulate, and medications such as sedatives and narcotic analgesics. In patients receiving enteral feeds, delayed gastric emptying can lead to increased residuals and possible aspiration. The drugs commonly used for treating these conditions are GI prokinetics and stool softeners or laxatives. *GI prokinetics* stimulate the stomach and intestinal tract to improve gastric emptying and shorten intestinal transit time. The two primary agents available are metoclopramide and cisapride.

Metoclopramide (Reglan)

Metoclopramide was first introduced to treat diabetic gastroparesis but is often used in various hypoactive GI conditions. It is also used for gastroesophageal reflux disease and as an antiemetic for cancer chemotherapy. Metoclopramide sensitizes GI receptors to acetylcholine. It primarily affects the upper GI tract, with little effect on colon or gall bladder motility. Doses range from 10 to 20 mg given four times daily, 30 minutes before meals or every 6 hours in patients on continuous feeds. Available formulations include tablets, oral liquid, and injection.

Side effects from metoclopramide are related to its dopaminergic actions. The drug antagonizes central and peripheral dopamine receptors. Extrapyramidal and Parkinson-like symptoms may occur in 1% to 9% of patients, but in doses of 20 mg or less the incidence of these side effects is lower. CNS complaints occur in 12% to 24% of patients and consist of drowsiness, restlessness, fatigue, akathisia, and dizziness. GI symptoms reported include nausea and diarrhea. In patients requiring neurological assessments, metoclopramide's CNS actions may affect examination findings.

Cisapride (Propulsid)

Cisapride was the second prokinetic agent marketed. It promotes the release of acetylcholine from the myenteric plexus in GI smooth muscle by stimulating serotonin receptors. It has promotility effects on gastric, intestinal, and colonic function. Unlike metoclopramide, cisapride has no direct cholinergic effects or significant blocking action on dopaminergic receptors. Thus, it produces a more benign effect on the neurological examination compared with findings for metoclopramide. The dose of cisapride is also 10 to 20 mg four times daily. The drug is available as an oral tablet and suspension. Side effects are primarily limited to the GI tract and consist of abdominal cramping and diarrhea. CNS side effects reported include headache and dizziness. However, increasing reports of cardiac adverse events have occurred, including prolonged QT interval, ventricular arrhythmias, and death. These were more prominent when cisapride was administered with drugs that inhibit hepatic metabolism. Consequently, the manufacturer has withdrawn cisapride from widespread distribution. The drug will only be available directly from the company by physician request after stringent need criteria have been met.

Stool Softeners and Laxatives

These agents are used to promote passage of feces in patients with decreased bowel function. The many available products can be grouped in five primary classes. Bulk-forming laxatives (e.g., psyllium, Metamucil) add fiber to facilitate normal passage of intestinal contents. However, if not given with sufficient fluid, bulk laxatives can have a constipating effect. In fact, these are sometimes given in minimal volume to treat diarrhea. Lubricants (e.g., mineral oil) coat the stool in the intestinal tract to facilitate passage through the colon. Stool softeners (e.g., docusate, Colace) are surfactants that increase the wetting efficiency of intestinal fluid, thus softening fecal mass. Saline laxatives (e.g., milk of magnesia, sodium phosphate) draw water into the bowel through an osmotic process. Finally, stimulant laxatives (e.g., bisacodyl) directly irritate the intestinal wall to promote peristalsis. Overuse of stimulant laxatives can lead to cathartic colon, in which the luminal wall loses tone and functions poorly. Any agent that increases intestinal transit and emptying has the potential to reduce absorption of medications from the gut.

|||| ANTICOAGULANTS AND ANTIPLATELET AGENTS

Drugs that affect coagulation are often encountered in neurological and neurosurgical patients. These may be used to treat primary disease, such as ischemic stroke, or for prophylaxis of embolic complications in immobilized patients. The major anticoagulants used are heparin and warfarin. Antiplatelet agents include dipyridamole, aspirin, ticlopidine, and clopidogrel. (Table 11-8).

Heparin

Heparin is used for the treatment and prevention of venous thromboembolism. It acts by combining with antithrombin III, which inhibits the intrinsic clotting cascade (activated factors XII, XI, IX, X, and thrombin). Thus, by inhibiting coagulation, heparin stops formation and growth of thrombi and allows endogenous thrombolytics to eliminate the clot.

▦ Table 11–8 • ANTICOAGULANT AND ANTIPLATELET AGENTS

DRUG	DOSE	ADVERSE EFFECTS	COMMENTS
Warfarin (Coumadin)	2–10 mg/day	Bleeding, skin necrosis	INR 2.0–3.0 for most indications; INR 2.5–3.5 for prosthetic valve replacement
Heparin	50–100 U/kg bolus, followed by 15–25 U/kg/hour infusion	Bleeding, thrombocytopenia	APTT 1.5–2.0 × control or 40–80 seconds
Enoxaparin (Lovenox)	*Prophylaxis:* 30 mg SC bid or 40 mg SC once daily *Treatment:* 1 mg/kg SC q12h or 1.5 mg/kg SC q24h	Bleeding, pain on injection, thrombocytopenia	Routine laboratory monitoring usually not necessary. Periodic complete blood counts recommended
Aspirin	50–1,500 mg/day	GI upset, bleeding	Typical doses range from 81–325 mg/day
Ticlopidine (Ticlid)	250 mg bid	GI upset, bleeding, neutropenia	Routine complete blood counts recommended
Clopidogrel (Plavix)	75 mg once daily	GI upset, bleeding	Rare incidence of thrombotic thrombocytopenic purpura
Aspirin (ASA)/dipyridamole extended release (Aggrenox)	25 mg ASA/200 mg dipyridamole bid	GI upset, headache	Capsules should be swallowed intact

Dosing

Traditionally, heparin was dosed by giving a 5,000-U bolus intravenously, followed by a 1,000 U/hour continuous infusion. The rate of infusion is titrated to achieve an activated partial thromboplastin time (aPTT) of 1.5 to 2.0 times control. This normally equates to 40 to 80 seconds in most patients. Recent studies have shown reduced bleeding complications by using a weight-based dosing formula. Patients receive a bolus of 50 to 100 U/kg, followed by an infusion of 15 to 25 U/kg per hour. The half-life of heparin ranges from 30 to 150 minutes. Accordingly, serum aPTT measurements should be made 4 to 6 hours after initiation of therapy or any dosage changes. Some institutions are using serum heparin levels or factor X activity levels to guide therapy instead of the aPTT. This is especially useful when other agents such as low-molecular-weight heparin are used in therapeutic doses. For prophylaxis, heparin may also be administered subcutaneously. Common regimens call for 5,000 U given every 8 to 12 hours.

Side Effects

The primary complication of heparin therapy is bleeding. The risk of bleeding is greater when the aPTT is above two times the control value. Given its short half-life, reduction or cessation of the infusion will rapidly reverse the effects. Heparin is a combination of different size polymers, of which only a small portion is believed to cause its anticoagulant effect. Heparin may be reversed by administration of protamine sulfate. A dose of 1 mg of protamine will neutralize approximately 100 U of heparin.

Thrombocytopenia is also a complication of heparin therapy. Two primary effects on platelets are seen. One type presents as a slight fall in the platelet count soon after initiation of therapy. This effect is usually transient, with platelet counts tending to stabilize or return to baseline with continued therapy. The second type (autoimmune-mediated heparin-induced thrombocytopenia or HIT) is normally seen after 3 to 5 days of heparin therapy and is characterized by a continual decline in the platelet count. This form of thrombocytopenia is serious and requires cessation of heparin therapy if counts do not stabilize. Measurement of heparin-induced antibodies may be helpful in establishing the diagnosis. Low-molecular-weight heparin (see next section) may be used when this occurs, although they can also rarely cause HIT.

Low-Molecular-Weight Heparin (LMWH)

Low-molecular-weight heparin provides effective anticoagulation while reducing bleeding complications. One such product, **enoxaparin** (Lovenox), is indicated for both prophylaxis and treatment of thromboembolism. Prophylaxis regimens are either 30 mg subcutaneously twice daily or 40 mg subcutaneously once daily. For treatment of active thromboembolic disease, the recommended dose is 1 mg/kg per dose subcutaneously every 12 hours. Two additional products, **dalteparin** (Fragmin) and **ardeparin** (Normiflo), are dosed in anti-factor Xa units. Doses between LMWHs are not interchangeable and must be individualized for each patient. Although the incidence is lower, adverse effects seen with unfractionated heparin are also possible with the low-molecular-weight products.

Warfarin (Coumadin)

Warfarin (Coumadin) is an anticoagulant that prevents synthesis of vitamin K–dependent clotting factors in the liver (factors II, VII, IX, and X). It is used to treat or prevent complications from venous thrombosis, atrial fibrillation with embolization, or pulmonary embolism. Although the anticoagulant effect occurs within 24 hours of initial treatment, the antithrombotic effect is not present for 4 to 7 days. Because warfarin inhibits the *synthesis* of clotting factors, those in circulation are not affected. For this reason, patients should be maintained on heparin and warfarin for 3 to 5 days to allow for the full antithrombotic effect of warfarin to occur.

Dosing and Therapeutic Monitoring

Normal dosing ranges for warfarin are 2 to 10 mg/day. Doses are titrated to achieve a prothrombin time (PT) of 1.3 to 1.5 times control for deep venous thrombosis or 1.5 to 2.0 times control for prophylaxis in patients with prosthetic heart valves. The World Health Organization now advocates the use of the international normalized ratio (INR) for monitoring warfarin therapy. This method eliminates the variability seen between controls when using the PT. The target INR for most thrombotic conditions is 2.0 to 3.0; for prosthetic heart valves, the desired INR is 2.5 to 3.5.

Side Effects and Drug Interactions

Bleeding is the major concern with warfarin therapy. Warfarin overdoses may be treated by administration of vitamin K, but this will adversely affect continuation of warfarin therapy owing to the synthesis of new clotting factors. Mild bleeding may often be resolved by holding one or more doses. Severe bleeding that is life threatening should be treated with IV fresh frozen plasma. A rare complication of warfarin involves skin necrosis. This occurs within the first 10 days and is due to a hypercoagulable state induced prior to achieving the full antithrombotic effect of the drug. Overlapping heparin administration for the first 5 days of warfarin use helps to minimize this complication. Warfarin is more than 98% bound to albumin, presenting a major bleeding risk from interactions with other highly bound drugs. Because warfarin is eliminated by the liver, enzyme inhibitors can also lead to increased anticoagulant effects.

Antiplatelet Drugs

These drugs prevent platelet aggregation and subsequently reduce formation of arterial thrombi, which could lead to stroke or myocardial infarction. **Aspirin** is the most frequently prescribed antiplatelet agent. It irreversibly acetylates platelet cyclooxygenase, affecting function for the lifespan of the platelet (5 to 7 days). Several studies have shown benefits in neurological conditions, including symptomatic relief of transient ischemic attacks and reduction in incidence of stroke. Doses from these trials ranged from 30 mg to 1.5 gm per day. Most patients, however, are maintained on doses of 81 to 325 mg/day. In myocardial infarction trials, benefits were also seen with doses in this range. Side effects from these doses are minimal and primarily consist of GI complaints.

Ticlopidine (Ticlid) is another irreversible inhibitor of platelet aggregation and is indicated for patients with cerebral ischemic symptoms or for poststroke patients. It blocks the adenosine diphosphate pathway and has no effect on cyclooxygenase. The recommended dose is 250 mg twice daily, taken with food. Because aspirin and ticlopidine act on platelets through different mechanisms, there may be some beneficial effects to using both together. However, this combination potentiates the effects of aspirin and may lead to toxicities. Ticlopidine is associated with severe neutrope-

nia; thus, routine blood counts are necessary to monitor for this complication. Given this finding, it is often reserved for patients intolerant of aspirin therapy. Other ticlopidine side effects include diarrhea, rash, and minor bleeding.

Clopidogrel (Plavix) is an analogue of ticlopidine, which was designed to avoid the blood dyscrasias seen with ticlopidine. Benefits have been shown in both neurology and cardiology populations. The standard dose is 75 mg taken once daily, but higher doses may be used for cardiac catheterization procedures. Side effects consist primarily of GI disturbances and rash. Owing to its more favorable safety profile, clopidogrel has largely replaced ticlopidine in clinical practice. Although no problems were observed during clinical trials, recent cases of thrombotic thrombocytopenic purpura with clopidogrel have been reported.

Aspirin and extended-release dipyridamole (Aggrenox) is the most recent antiplatelet agent introduced for prevention of ischemic stroke. The product consists of 25 mg aspirin plus 200 mg of sustained-release dipyridamole per capsule, given twice daily. Side effects reported are attributable to the individual components and may include gastrointestinal distress, headache, and dizziness.

Long-Term Management of Anticoagulants

Patients with thromboembolic disease often require long-term anticoagulation to prevent further complications. Some conditions in which this may be indicated include deep vein thrombosis, pulmonary embolism, and embolic stroke. The patient must understand the nature of the disease and the need for strict compliance with the medication regimen. Patients should be counseled to watch for any signs or symptoms of bleeding. They should also understand the need for frequent PT monitoring. Dietary counseling is also necessary, because foods rich in vitamin K can blunt the effect of warfarin. Those taking warfarin should be able to identify such foods and maintain consistency in their diet. Patients should be educated about the potential for drug interactions with warfarin. The pharmacist can play a vital role in monitoring the patient's medication regimen for potential problems and offering advice on over-the-counter drugs that may adversely interact with warfarin.

▍▍▍ VOLUME EXPANDERS AND IV FLUIDS

In patients with cerebral ischemic injury from stroke or vasospasm, one cornerstone of treatment involves hypervolemic or hemodilution therapy. This is accomplished by administration of IV fluids (**crystalloids**) or plasma volume expanders (**colloids**). The goal is to increase systemic blood pressure to a level adequate to maintain cerebral perfusion. There is considerable debate among practitioners as to whether colloids or crystalloids are better, so a brief discussion of their respective use follows.

Crystalloids

Crystalloids consist of solutions containing sodium chloride as their osmotic component. When fluids such as 5% dextrose and water (D5W) are infused, the dextrose is rapidly metabolized, leaving free water. This will rapidly equilibrate with extravascular tissues and fluid compartments and can contribute to fluid overload and edema. For this reason, isotonic fluids (0.9% sodium chloride, normal saline or NS) are preferable for hypervolemic therapy. Because the solution is osmotically consistent with body fluids, the solution remains in the vasculature longer. NS will ultimately equilibrate with other body compartments, so the effect is short lived and requires continuous infusion of large volumes to maintain desired pressures. Alternatively, some clinicians choose to use hypertonic saline solutions (1.8% or 3% sodium chloride) for hypervolemic therapy. These solutions draw fluid from other compartments into the intravascular space, allowing for longer effects on blood pressure with lower administered volumes. Caution should be used when infusing hypertonic solutions through peripheral veins due to the potential for irritation and hemolysis. Using central venous catheters for administration avoids this problem. Frequent electrolyte monitoring is also necessary to avoid hypernatremic complications.

Colloids

Colloid solutions contain osmotically active protein or starch molecules that increase plasma oncotic pressure. As with hypertonic solutions, colloids draw fluid from extravascular spaces and provide more sustained hemodynamic effects. Colloid solutions are normally isotonic, minimizing the potential for hemolysis. The effects from colloid administration usually persist for hours, allowing for intermittent dosing and reduction in total fluid given to the patient relative to crystalloids. **Albumin** is the major contributor to plasma oncotic pressure in the body. Commercially, it is available as a 5% or 25% solution. The 5% solution is isotonic and used when the patient is hypovolemic or when fluid status is not an issue. More concentrated 25% solutions are hypertonic, which is beneficial in fluid-restricted patients or those with cerebral edema. **Plasma protein fraction (Plasmanate, PPF)** comes as a 5% solution of plasma proteins, of which 83% to 90% is albumin. Adverse effects from albumin and PPF are rare and usually arise from hypersensitivity reactions to the proteins. Reactions are more common with PPF than albumin and more prevalent when PPF is infused at greater than 10 mL/minute. **Hetastarch** (Hespan, Hextend) is a synthetic colloid used to expand plasma volume. It produces hemodynamic effects much longer than albumin and PPF, ranging from 3 to 12 hours. Recommended doses should not exceed 1,500 mL/day; some patients have tolerated larger doses. The large starch molecule in hetastarch adversely affects coagulation and may precipitate bleeding in various patient populations. Case reports of bleeding and neurological deterioration have been noted in neurosurgical patients treated with hetastarch. In fact, the manufacturer recommends it not be used in patients with subarachnoid hemorrhage or in any neurosurgical patient in whom the possibility of intracranial bleeding exists.

▌▌▌▌ ELECTROLYTE MANAGEMENT

Patients hospitalized with neurological conditions often experience electrolyte abnormalities, especially in the ICU. Surgery, fluid balance, medications, and the patient's own pathophysiology may contribute to imbalances in electrolytes. Without correction, such imbalances may worsen the patient's clinical condition. A discussion of important electrolyte disturbances and treatment follows.

Sodium

This is the main extracellular cation in the body. Sodium performs two principal roles: regulating osmotic pressure and water balance between intracellular and extracellular compartments and maintaining acid-base balance. The normal serum level is 135 to 145 mEq/L. Hypernatremia normally results from some form of dehydration and is treated by fluid replenishment. Hyponatremia may result from several causes, which include fluid overload, cerebral salt-wasting syndrome, SIADH, and medications, such as diuretics. Treatment may include fluid restriction for SIADH or sodium replacement. Replacement may be accomplished with hypertonic saline (1.8% or 3% sodium chloride) or by increasing dietary salt intake. Dietary sodium replacements may be added to enteral feeds or taken by mouth in the form of salt tablets. Fludrocortisone (Florinef) is a mineralocorticoid that produces significant sodium retention and increases urinary potassium excretion. It is useful in patients who remain hyponatremic despite aggressive sodium repletion. Doses range from 0.1 to 0.2 mg twice daily.

Potassium

This is the primary intracellular cation and is important in the regulation of acid-base balance, balance of intracellular volume, and maintenance of electrical conduction in cardiac and skeletal muscle. The normal serum range is 3.5 to 5.0 mEq/L.

Hypokalemia is normally due to net body losses (e.g., nasogastric suctioning, vomiting, diarrhea, and diuretics) or redistribution into cells (e.g., alkalosis). Symptoms include confusion, muscle weakness, diminished reflexes, arrhythmias, hypotension, and electrocardiographic (ECG) changes. Treatment consists of potassium replacement through the oral or parenteral route. Many available oral products may be used interchangeably according to patient acceptance. Enteric-coated potassium tablets should be avoided owing to lesions resulting from dose dumping in the intestines. IV potassium replacement must be done carefully to avoid hyperkalemia secondary to a lag in redistribution into cells. Potassium may be administered safely at a rate of 10 mEq/hour in most patients. Rates of 20 to 40 mEq/hour have been used but should be accompanied by close ECG and serum potassium monitoring, which may not be possible in a non-ICU setting. Peripheral infusions of more than 10 mEq/100 mL are associated with burning during administration. Thus, central venous lines or larger veins should be used whenever possible.

Hyperkalemia usually results from excessive potassium repletion, shifts out of cells as with acidosis, and renal failure. Patients experience irritability, nausea, muscle weakness, and ECG changes. Acute therapy for hyperkalemia includes calcium chloride, which is cardioprotective, and sodium bicarbonate or glucose plus insulin, to shift potassium intracellularly. Follow-up or long-term treatment requires exchange resins such as sodium polystyrene sulfonate (Kayexelate, increase potassium elimination). Severe hyperkalemia may require hemodialysis.

Calcium

The role of calcium in the body is complex and involves various mechanisms, including coagulation, propagation of nerve impulses, insulin release, and cardiac contractility. The accepted normal serum (total) calcium concentration is 8.5 to 10.5 mg/dL. Most laboratories measure total calcium concentrations, but the free or ionized fraction is the active component. Thus, physiological changes can alter ionized calcium levels and make the total level seem abnormally low or high. Acidosis can raise free levels, whereas alkalosis increases calcium binding to albumin. This can cause a clinically relevant hypocalcemia while total calcium levels appear normal. Hypoalbuminemia can also result in lowered calcium levels. Total serum calcium values will decrease 0.8 mg/dL for each 1.0 g/dL deviation of albumin below 4.0 g/dL. When the patient's clinical condition complicates interpretation of total serum levels, ionized calcium concentrations may be necessary.

Hypercalcemia most commonly results from malignancy or hyperparathyroidism. Symptoms include nausea, vomiting, bone pain, renal stones, muscle weakness, coma, and cardiac arrhythmias. Treatment modalities include loop diuretics, calcitonin, gallium nitrate, plicamycin, pamidronate, and oral phosphorus supplementation.

Hypocalcemia may result from a number of causes, including poor nutritional status, low serum albumin levels, pancreatitis, vitamin D deficiency, and hypoparathyroidism. Symptoms consist of tetany, abdominal and skeletal muscle cramping, convulsions, irritability, confusion, and cardiac changes. Correction of symptomatic hypocalcemia requires IV replacement. Calcium chloride or calcium gluconate injections are the most common agents used. Most patients receive 1 to 2 g as a single dose repeated as needed based on findings of measurement of blood chemistries. Administration of a 10% solution (1 g/10 mL) at a rate of 1 mL/minute is considered safe in most patients. The dose may also be added to maintenance IV fluids. Calcium chloride contains more elemental calcium per gram (13.5 mEq) than calcium gluconate (4.5 mEq).

Magnesium

This is the second major intracellular cation and plays a role in nerve conduction, muscular contractility, and activation of multiple enzyme systems. Normal serum values range from 1.6 to 2.4 mEq/L. Hypermagnesemia almost always results from renal insufficiency and is treated by dialysis or aggressive diuresis. Hypomagnesemia is characterized by paresthesias, muscle weakness, tremor, hyperreflexia, nystagmus, ataxia, seizures, and cardiac arrhythmias. Causes include inadequate intake, reduced GI absorption, primary renal diseases, and iatrogenic renal wasting secondary to medications (e.g., amphotericin, diuretics). Magnesium replacement may be accomplished orally or IV; however, oral magnesium absorption is variable, and large doses can in-

duce diarrhea. Examples of oral regimens include milk of magnesia 5 mL or magnesium oxide 400 mg four times daily. Parenteral magnesium sulfate in doses of 1 to 4 g is commonly used to replenish magnesium stores. Solutions more concentrated than 2 g/100 mL are associated with pain during infusion. A 10% solution may be administered as a bolus at a rate of 1.5 mL/minute. As with potassium, a low serum magnesium concentration may indicate a large intracellular deficiency that may require assertive doses over several days to replenish. Follow-up serum measurements are often needed after a "normal" serum level is achieved to ensure intracellular stores are replaced.

Phosphorus

Primarily an intracellular anion, phosphorus is involved in bone formation and is the energy source of adenosine triphosphate to drive numerous physiological processes. The accepted range for serum phosphorus is 2.5 to 5.0 mg/dL. Hyperphosphatemia is normally a condition accompanying renal failure. Treatments involve administration of phosphate binders, such as aluminum hydroxide or calcium acetate. Hypophosphatemia occurs most commonly from insufficient nutritional intake, acid-base disturbances, or phosphate-binding drugs (e.g., antacids, sucralfate, calcium salts). Symptoms include malaise, paresthesias, weakness (including respiratory arrest with severe deficiency), confusion, seizures, and coma. Phosphate salts can be given by the oral or parenteral route. Oral intake for moderately low phosphorus levels should start at 50 to 60 mmol/d in three to four divided doses. Doses for IV administration range from 0.08 to 0.25 mmol/kg of lean body weight, depending on the degree of hypophosphatemia and whether the patient is symptomatic. Infusions should be run slowly over 4 to 6 hours to avoid adverse consequences of intravenous phosphate administration.

▥ RESPIRATORY DRUGS

Occasionally, neurological and neurosurgical patients require medications to improve respiratory function. Conditions such as asthma, chronic obstructive pulmonary disease (COPD), or pneumonia can increase the work of breathing and complicate the patient's recovery. Bronchodilators are often used in this setting to reverse airway obstruction and help mobilize secretions. A brief review of agents used in the hospital setting is presented next. For a more complete coverage of therapeutic management of asthma and COPD, the reader should consult standard references on the subject.

Albuterol (Ventolin, Proventil)

Albuterol is a sympathomimetic that acts on beta-2 receptors in the lung to stimulate bronchodilation. The resultant dilation of the airways is often beneficial to help the patient expectorate pulmonary secretions. Albuterol is available as a metered-dose inhaler, solution for nebulization, and various oral dosage forms. In the ICU patient, dosing usually consists of treatments every 4 hours administered by a respiratory therapist. The nebulizer solution is used most frequently in mechanically ventilated patients, but metered-dose inhalers may be administered as well. In this situation, the normal dose (two puffs) may be exceeded to account for drug loss in the ventilator tubing. Side effects of albuterol include tremor, headache, anxiety, tachycardia, nausea, and hypokalemia. These effects are minimized when the drug is given in an inhalant form but may be encountered more frequently at higher doses. Other sympathomimetics seen in the hospital setting include *metaproterenol (Alupent)*, *isoetharine (Bronkosol)*, and *isoproterenol (Isuprel)*. These agents are less beta-2 specific compared with albuterol and may cause more cardiac effects. In the neurosurgical ICU, these effects may translate to increased ICP in some patients and thus would make such agents less attractive bronchodilators.

Ipratropium (Atrovent)

Ipratropium is a quaternary amine anticholinergic bronchodilator. Its mechanism of action consists of blocking the effect of acetylcholine to maintain bronchial tone. Concomitant use with sympathomimetics provides an additive bronchodilating effect. The drug comes as a metered-dose inhaler and nebulizer solution. Standard doses are two puffs or one nebulizer treatment every 6 hours. Adverse effects from ipratropium are minimal due to its quaternary structure and consist primarily of dry mouth and cough.

RESOURCES

Books

AHFS Drug information 00. (2000). Bethesda, MD: American Society of Health-System Pharmacists.

Boucher, B. A., & Phelps, S. J. (1999). Acute management of the head injury patient. In J. T. DiPiro, R. L. Talbert, G. C. Yee, et al. (Eds.), *Pharmacotherapy: A pathophysiologic approach* (pp. 991–1000). Stamford, CT: Appleton & Lange.

Bradberry, J. C. (1999). Stroke. In J. T. DiPiro, G. L. Talbert, G. C. Yee, et al. (Eds.), *Pharmacotherapy: A pathophysiologic approach* (pp. 327–349). Stamford, CT: Appleton and Lange.

Chernow B. (Ed.) (1995). *Pocket book of critical care pharmacotherapy.* Baltimore: Williams & Wilkins.

Erdman, S. M., Chuck, S. K., & Rodvold, K. A. (1999). Thromboembolic disorders. In J. T. DiPiro, R. L. Talbert, G. C. Yee, et al. (Eds.), *Pharmacotherapy: A pathophysiologic approach* (pp. 295–326). Stamford, CT: Appleton & Lange.

Gahart, B. L., & Nazareno, A. R. (2000). *Intravenous medications* (16th ed.). St. Louis: Mosby.

Graves, N. M., & Garnett, W. R. (1999). Epilepsy. In J. T. DiPiro, R. L. Talbert, G. C. Yee, et al. (Eds.), *Pharmacotherapy: A pathophysiologic approach* (pp. 952–975). Stamford, CT: Appleton & Lange.

Anderson, P. O., Knoben, J. E., & Troutman, W. G. (Eds.) (1999). *Handbook of clinical drug data* (9th ed.). Stamford, CT: Appleton & Lange.

Hebel, S. K. (Ed.) (2000). *Drug facts and comparisons.* St. Louis: Facts and Comparisons.

Samuels, M. A. (Ed.) (1995). *Manual of neurologic therapeutics* (5th ed.). Boston: Little, Brown.

Schultz, N. J., & Slaker, R. A. (1999). Electrolyte homeostasis. In J. T. DiPiro, R. L. Talbert, G. C. Yee, et al. (Eds.), *Pharmacotherapy: A pathophysiologic approach* (pp. 890–917). Stamford, CT: Appleton & Lange.

Susla, G. M., Masur, H., Cunnion, R. E., et al. (Eds.) (1994). *Handbook of critical care drug therapy.* New York: Churchill Livingstone.

Wilson, R. F., & Janning, S. W. (Eds.) (1995). *Handbook of antibiotic therapy for surgery-related infections* (3rd ed.). Springfield, NJ: Scientific Therapeutics Information.

Periodicals

Bennett, C. L., Connors, J. M., Carwile, J. M., et al. (2000). Thrombotic thrombocytopenic purpura associated with clopidogrel. *New England Journal of Medicine, 342,* 1773–1777.

Bracken, M. B., Shepard, M. J., Collins, W. F., et al. (1995). A randomized, controlled trial of methylprednisolone or naloxone in the treatment of acute spinal cord injury. *New England Journal of Medicine, 322,* 1405–1411.

Cully, M. D., Larson, C. P., & Silverberg, G. D. (1987). Hetastarch coagulopathy in a neurosurgical patient [letter]. *Anesthesiology, 66,* 706–707.

Davidson, J. E. (1994). Neuromuscular blockade: Implications, peripheral nerve stimulation, and other concurrent interventions. *New Horizons, 2,* 75–84.

Durbin, C. G. (1994). Sedation in the critically ill patient. *New Horizons, 2,* 64–74.

Fabian, T. C., Boucher, B. A., Croce, M. A., et al. (1993). Pneumonia and stress ulceration in severely injured patients: A prospective evaluation of the effects of stress ulcer prophylaxis. *Archives of Surgery, 128,* 185–192.

Janning, S. W., Stevenson, J. G., & Smolarek, R. T. (1996). Implementing comprehensive pharmaceutical services at an academic tertiary care hospital. *American Journal of Health-Systems Pharmacy, 53,* 542–547.

Lollgen, H., & Drexler, H. (1990). Use of inotropes in the critical care setting. *Critical Care Medicine, 18,* S56–S60.

Pohlman, A. S., Simpson, K. P., & Hall, J. B. (1994). Continuous intravenous infusions of lorazepam versus midazolam for sedation during mechanical ventilatory support: A prospective, randomized study. *Critical Care Medicine, 22,* 1241–1247.

Toole, J. G. (1987). Use of hetastarch for volume expansion-response [letter]. *Journal of Neurosurgery, 66,* 636.

Wagner, B. K. J., & D'Amelio, L. F. (1993). Pharmacologic and clinical considerations in selecting crystalloid, colloidal, and oxygen-carrying resuscitation fluids, part 1. *Clinical Pharmacy, 12,* 335–346.

Wagner, B. K. J., & D'Amelio, L. F. (1993). Pharmacologic and clinical considerations in selecting crystalloid, colloidal, and oxygen-carrying resuscitation fluids, part 2. *Clinical Pharmacy, 12,* 415–428.

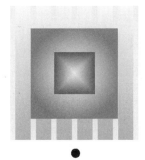

Behavioral and Psychological Responses to Neurological Illness

JOANNE V. HICKEY

The purpose of this chapter is to address the psychosocial aspects of neuroscience nursing practice and to present nursing interventions for the major emotional and behavioral responses to neurological illness. The emotional needs of the patient's family are considered, as are the stresses and responses precipitated in the nursing staff who work with neuroscience patients.

Injury or disease involving the nervous system often has far-reaching effects, not only on the neurological-physiological body system, but also on the cognitive and affective functions, personality, and individual characteristics that give a person uniqueness, individuality, and identity. These compounded deficits and devastating losses create stresses for the patient and family that tax coping and adaptive skills. Because many neurological conditions can alter a person's cognitive abilities, patients often lack an awareness of the change in their behavior and cognitive functions. If these changes in higher-level functions are recognized, patients may not have an insight into the cause, amount or degree, significance, or implications of the behavioral changes in relationship to their lifestyle.

Family members and significant others are better able to accept physiological changes in their loved ones than behavioral, cognitive, or personality changes. Changes in a patient's behavior affect group dynamics and interpersonal relationships as well. The normal patterns of family interactions are altered, and family structure changes accordingly. Changes in patterns of interaction and family structure also alter methods of problem solving and the use of effective coping mechanisms. These factors contribute additional stresses to the already stressful experience of neurological illness.

STRESS AND THE STRESS RESPONSE

The writings of Selye provide a basic foundation for understanding physiological and psychological responses to stress. According to Selye, stress is defined as "the nonspecific response of the body to any type of increased demands upon it."[1] These increased demands on an organism, termed *stressors*, cause stress. Regardless of whether the stressor is associated with a desirable effect *(eustress)* or an undesirable effect *(distress),* the same physiological responses are precipitated.[2] The interaction and integration of physiological and psychological responses to stress were documented by Selye and other writers who preceded him, such as Cannon and Jacobson. Cannon is credited with recognizing that the physiological reactions of the sympathetic system that occur in response to various emotional states are similar to those that occur in response to biological precipitators.[3] Jacobson noted similar reactions in the sympathetic nervous system and skeletal muscles in response to emotional states.[4]

Selye is credited with the introduction of the term *general adaptation syndrome* into the literature. This syndrome comprises the nonspecific reactions of the hypothalamic-pituitary-adrenocortical system to any type of stress. The general endocrine changes associated with the response are enlargement of the adrenal cortex, shrinkage of the thymus gland, and ulceration of the stomach (stress ulcers). These responses are mediated by the pituitary-adrenocortical axis of the neuroendocrine system and cause a multisystemic response. Much interest and numerous research studies have been devoted to understanding the neuroendocrine influence during stress.

When considering the general adaptation syndrome, three phases can be identified: (1) the alarm reaction, in which the sympathetic system is activated and subsequently activates the neuroendocrine system; (2) resistance to stress, a period of adaptation to the stress; and (3) exhaustion from stress, a time when the coping mechanisms are insufficient or ineffective for continuing to deal with the stress. The degree to which the general adaptation syndrome is implemented and the amount of time during which it is operational depend on the intensity and type of stress experienced. Selye suggested that continued intense stimulation from stress would deplete the organism's ability to respond to stress at all, or to respond effectively.

The concept of stress as a psychological phenomenon has evolved from the work of various theorists. The conceptualization of stress has taken on many diverse models. The critical components that contribute to the understanding of stress have been identified as follows: The stimulus (stressor) must be viewed as a threat by the individual; the stimulus, regardless of whether it is positive or negative, must be viewed as being significant or relevant to the individual's welfare; and the organism's capacity for adaptation must have been exceeded. These critical components address the type and intensity of a stimulus, the individual's perception of the stimulus, and the duration of the stimulus that depletes the capacity to cope.

What kinds of stimuli activate the stress response in the neurological patient? Any intense physical or psychological stimuli, such as forced immobilization, trauma, pain, fear, threat of loss, lack of control, or anxiety, can cause a multisystemic stress response. There are degrees of intensity of stimuli that cause a proportional stress response. For example, one would expect a much less intense stress response in a patient who has been admitted for an elective cranioplasty for cosmetic purposes long after an injury occurred than in a patient who has been admitted for a craniotomy for removal of a brain tumor of unidentified histological origin.

HUMAN ADAPTATION AND COPING

Adaptation is the process of change undertaken by an organism in response to a change in the internal or external environment for the purpose of maintaining equilibrium. Physiological adaptation supports survival and homeostasis within the organism. Psychological adaptation is directed toward maintaining a psychological homeostasis and supporting the self-concept and the self-esteem of the person. Adaptation may be positive or negative in that the process either supports or is detrimental to the well-being of that individual. Behaviors that are detrimental to the person are termed *maladaptive behaviors*, whereas those that support the well-being of the person are called *adaptive behaviors*.

Much has been written about how people adapt to changes in their internal and external environments. The conceptualization of adaptation is central to the practice of nursing because much of the nurse's time and energy is directed at supporting healthy adaptation.

The word *coping* refers to the methods, skills, or processes used by an individual in adapting to stresses in the internal or external environment. Coping has been defined in the literature in many different ways to fit the needs of particular models. However, the definition just presented is broad enough to provide a basic conceptual structure. Coping mechanisms are normal—everyone uses them—but some may be effective in dealing with a stressor (problem), whereas others may be ineffective. The choice of coping mechanisms and the manner in which they are applied affect the promotion of health in the health care setting. The roles of the nurse are to help patients identify previously used effective coping mechanisms and to assist and support patients so that they can use effective coping skills and mechanisms to deal with the stresses precipitated by illness. Coping is viewed as the individual's attempt to remove stress and restore physical and emotional equilibrium.

NEUROLOGICAL CONDITIONS AND THEIR PSYCHOLOGICAL EFFECTS

Illness is a stressor that creates physiological and psychological stress for the person involved. Stress responses may be viewed on a scale that varies according to the amount of noxious stimuli, the patient's perception of the significance of the stimuli, and the length of time the stimuli remain. So far, this discussion of stress, adaptation, and coping could be applied to either physiological or psychological stress. The discussion now turns to psychological stresses and psychological responses to neurological illness.

In the case of neurological illness, the psychological stressors and stress response can be particularly taxing in terms of the person's ability to cope and adapt to the illness. Common situations, concerns, and losses precipitated by neurological illness may include the following:

- Threat to survival
- Threat to the quality of life as it was known before the illness—lifestyle, occupation, social and recreational activities, freedom to make changes, and control over one's being and destiny
- Development of neurological deficits:
  - Paresis or paralysis (interferes with mobility, swallowing, self-control, speech)
  - Bowel or bladder dysfunction
  - Communication deficits
  - Sexual dysfunction
  - Emotional deficits and responses (emotional lability, aggression, depression, anxiety)
  - Cognitive deficits (difficulty in reasoning, making judgments, memory)
  - Sensory deficits (hearing loss, loss of visual acuity, diplopia, paresthesias, anesthesia)
  - Autonomic deficits (orthostatic hypotension, loss of ability to perspire, difficulty controlling body temperature)
- Important and significant losses, such as loss of:
  - Independence in the activities of daily living
  - Control over decisions that affect one's destiny
  - The ability to perceive the environment accurately through the senses (stimuli may be perceived as meaningless, confusing, or absent)
  - The ability to understand language and to express oneself verbally and in writing
  - The ability to be responsible for oneself

When assessing the patient's ability to cope and adapt to the emotional and behavioral responses necessitated by the impact of neurological illness, the nurse seeks feedback from the patient to validate perceptions, clarify information, and ascertain whether the patient understands the information provided. The feedback collected is verbal and nonverbal, or it may be only nonverbal in some patients, depending on the type and degree of neurological deficits sustained. For the patient with neurological illness, these interactions may be severely compromised or impossible (e.g., those who are comatose or aphasic).

Many patients' neurological deficits compromise normal interpersonal relationships and the ability to express themselves and to comprehend information. Such situations create additional stress. Stress will cause various emotional and psychological responses that may require the intervention of the nurse.

GENERAL PRINCIPLES FOR CONSIDERING THE PATIENT'S EMOTIONAL AND PSYCHOLOGICAL RESPONSES TO NEUROLOGICAL CONDITIONS

Certain emotional and psychological responses can be expected in patients with any illness. Although the nurse can anticipate responses, patients must be assessed carefully to determine how they have responded to their circumstances. The nurse would expect the person who is alert and well oriented to be fearful of anticipated surgery. However, the specific reasons for or perceptions of the planned events that contribute to the fear can vary from patient to patient. For example, for some patients (particularly adolescents), the most terrifying aspect of undergoing a craniotomy may be having their head shaved. If the nurse recognizes that this issue is the source of greatest fear or stress to these patients, discussing their concerns may help to alleviate some of their fear, especially if they are provided with information and encouraged to participate in problem solving to deal with the temporary loss of hair. Although the shaving of the head will still cause a certain amount of fear, much can be done to dispel some of the underlying concerns, thus modifying the emotional and behavioral response of the patient.

Nursing Assessment and Ongoing Assessment

In assessing the psychological responses of the patient, the nurse should do the following:

1. Observe the patient's behavior when alone and while interacting with others (family members, significant others, staff, other patients); note facial expressions, body language, tone of voice, and reactions to particular individuals.
2. Establish rapport with the patient; provide opportunities for communication in whatever way possible, depending on which communication skills are intact.
3. Focus communication on the patient by using open-ended questions, provided the patient has adequate neurological function to respond.
4. Listen to what the patient has to say and how it is said (e.g., how things are described, use of analogies).
5. Collect information from the patient and family or significant others on:
   Previous adjustment patterns and use of coping mechanisms
   Personality before onset of illness
   Previous emotional and behavioral responses to stress
   Means for dealing with stress (e.g., jogging, withdrawal)
   Support systems
   Family interactions

6. Validate the information collected with the appropriate person(s) (e.g., family, other health care professionals), as necessary.
7. Consult with others to broaden the base of information about the patient.
8. Validate perceptions.

Assessment is an ongoing process involving data collection, analysis, and formulation of nursing diagnoses. After the nursing diagnoses have been established, the nurse must then plan appropriate nursing interventions.

Nursing Diagnoses and Collaborative Problems

The catastrophic and disabling nature of many neurological conditions precipitates many emotional and psychological responses in patients and their families. Various nursing diagnoses, listed in Chart 12-1, may be appropriate. Depending on the nature and severity, there is often need for collaborative interdisciplinary problem identification and treatment. The physician and neuropsychologist may need to be involved in managing the patient effectively.

Nursing Interventions

These nursing interventions, which are necessary for dealing with the many emotional and behavioral responses to the stress of neurological illness, are directed at helping patients maintain their identity, a positive self-concept, and self-esteem. General principles that can guide the nurse to help the patient deal with the many emotional and behavioral responses to the stress of neurological illness include the following:

1. Provide an open, nonjudgmental environment.
2. Be supportive.
3. Develop alternate ways of communication if communication deficits exist.
4. Accept the patient's perceptions and behavior.
5. Correct any inaccurate factual information matter-of-factly.
6. Encourage the patient to express feelings in whatever way possible.
7. Listen empathetically and attentively; reflect the patient's thoughts and perceptions for clarification and validation.
8. Help the patient use positive adaptive coping mechanisms.
9. Allow the patient to make decisions and maintain control to the degree that he or she is able.
10. Allow the patient to be involved in problem solving as much as possible.
11. Provide information and reinforcement as necessary.
12. Make referrals to other health care professionals when appropriate.
13. Help the patient set realistic goals.
14. Support a positive self-concept and self-esteem.
15. Stay calm and relaxed; nurses are role models for the patient and family.

C H A R T   1 2 – 1 • Nursing Diagnoses Related to Emotional and Psychological Responses of Patients or Family to Neurological Conditions

The following nursing diagnoses are often identified for the patient or family with an altered emotional or psychological response to neurological conditions:

Major Nursing Diagnoses	Associated Nursing Diagnoses
• Fear	• Chronic Low Self Esteem
• Personal Identity Disturbance	• Situational Low Self Esteem
• Anxiety	• Anticipatory Grieving
• Hopelessness	• Dysfunctional Grieving
• Powerlessness	• Social Isolation
• Body Image Disturbance	• Risk for Altered Parenting
• Altered Role Performance	• Altered Parenting
• Impaired Social Interaction	• Parental Role Conflict
• Altered Family Processes	• Risk for Violence: Self-directed or directed at others
• Impaired Verbal Communication	• Sleep Pattern Disturbance
• Ineffective Individual Coping	• Decisional Conflict
• Impaired Adjustment	• Post-Trauma Response
• Ineffective Family Coping: Compromised	• Ineffective Family Coping: Disabling
	• Defensive Coping
	• Ineffective Denial
	• Spiritual Distress

COMMON EMOTIONAL AND PSYCHOLOGICAL RESPONSES TO THE STRESS ASSOCIATED WITH NEUROLOGICAL CONDITIONS

The general management principles of assessment and nursing intervention discussed in the previous section can be applied to the management of the common emotional and psychological responses seen in many patients as they face the prospect of acute or chronic neurological disease. The emotional and psychological responses discussed include anxiety, frustration, anger, hostility, fear, regression, denial, guilt, depression, powerlessness, and stigma. Although these common responses are discussed as separate entities, several responses can occur concurrently in the patient.

Anxiety

Anxiety is a feeling of uneasiness, apprehension, or dread that is associated with an unrecognized, subjective source of anticipated danger. It results from the real or perceived conflicts and frustrations of living. For patients who are unable to speak because of neurological disability or a tracheostomy, their ability to express feelings of frustration, anger, and hostility is negated. This causes anxiety for the patient and perhaps for the nurse. Anxiety is often classified as mild, moderate, or severe to convey the notion that the feeling can range from the mild awareness of fear or anticipatory danger to outright panic. Physiological alterations in

the autonomic system, such as an elevated pulse rate and blood pressure, perspiration, tightness in the stomach, or diarrhea, may accompany this mood state. An anxious patient demonstrates various recognizable behaviors associated with the degree of anxiety, including irritability, uneasiness, apprehension, demanding or unreasonable behavior, and often verbal abusiveness. Such a patient is often described as "very difficult." Occasionally, a patient may be charming and agreeable but noncompliant with established treatment protocols. This, too, is a way of dealing with anxiety.

Nursing Interventions

Because anxiety is associated with an unrecognized, subjective source of anticipated danger, time should be spent trying to discover what is generating the anxiety. Often, several concerns are responsible for anxiety, some of which cannot be identified on the conscious level. For the patient who cannot communicate, the nurse must try to anticipate potential sources of anxiety and provide information. Alternative methods of communication should be developed, and the nurse must become very good at reading body language.

Recognizing potential sources of anxiety must be a major concern when caring for the patient. To alleviate anxiety, nurses should explain to the patient what is going to be done before beginning and then keep the patient apprised of what is being done while care is administered. Care should also be explained to the "unresponsive" or "unconscious" patient because there is no way to determine whether sensory stimuli are getting through to the brain and being processed. The caregiver must assume that some verbal stimuli will penetrate the barriers of neurological illness, thus providing information and comfort to the patient.

For patients who are able to follow directions and cooperate, relaxation therapy may reduce anxiety. This is a systematic approach to tightening and relaxing muscle groups to relieve muscle tension. Another relaxation technique is the use of imagery. Patients are encouraged to select an image that is particularly relaxing and pleasing. They are taught to close their eyes, relax, and focus on experiencing all the pleasing sensations of being in this chosen setting. Any type of relaxation technique takes time to learn and must be practiced to achieve optimal results. Appropriate patients must be selected for this therapy.

Frustration

Frustration is the feeling that occurs when a course of action or activity cannot be carried out or brought to a desirable conclusion. Irritability, anxiety, and verbal outbursts often accompany frustration. The amount of frustration experienced will be proportional to the value and desirability the patient places on the thwarted action.

Nursing Interventions

The nurse can help patients identify the basis for their frustration. After being identified, problem solving should be used to determine why the desired result was not achieved. It may be that the patient had set unrealistic goals. In this instance, more realistic goals should be identified. Another possibility may be that an alternate approach is necessary to achieve the desired goal. The patient must be encouraged to examine the situation realistically and to select appropriate strategies or alter the goals. Expressing frustration is helpful in dissipating feelings of frustration.

Anger

Anger is an intense feeling of displeasure and antagonism in response to mounting frustration, conflict, or anxiety. It connotes strong feelings in response to the actual prevention or threat of prevention of achievement or maintenance of a desired goal or state. Anger that is turned inward is called **depression.** The behavioral manifestations of anger may include aggressive or destructive acts, verbal attacks, silence, or depression.

Nursing Interventions

Patients who are angry need the same kind of help and support that anxious or frustrated patients need. If an angry patient is apt to lose self-control and cause injury to another or to herself or himself or if the patient is prone to cause property damage, she or he must be controlled. A quiet environment, drug therapy, or other forms of therapy directed at preventing self-harm may be necessary. The patient must be provided with an appropriate outlet for feelings of anger. If the source of the anger can be identified, it may be possible to alleviate the situation. Verbal de-escalation techniques are useful for managing anger and hostility.

Hostility

Hostility is usually seen in association with anger. It is a feeling of antagonism directed toward another and is associated with a wish to hurt, humiliate, or discredit that person. Hostility is generally thought to be the result of frustrated or unfulfilled needs or wishes. According to Horney, repressed hostility is one of the major sources of anxiety.[5] Kiening describes the development of hostility in the following way:[6]

- A person experiences frustration, loss of self-esteem, or unmet needs for status, prestige, or love.
- Within a given situation, the person has certain expectations for self and for others.
- The expectations are not met.
- The person feels inadequate, hurt, or humiliated.
- The person experiences anxiety, which becomes hostility, causing one of three reactions:
  - The hostility is repressed and the person withdraws.
  - The feeling is disowned and the person behaves in an extremely polite and compliant manner.
  - The person behaves in an overtly hostile manner. This may be manifested verbally or nonverbally.

Nursing Interventions

Patients who are hostile need help in understanding the origin of their feelings. They also need to be able to express their feelings in a safe, nonjudgmental environment. The nurse caring for a hostile patient can use an approach similar to what would be appropriate for an anxious patient.

Fear

Fear is a feeling of extreme apprehension or dread associated with a potential or real threat to the well-being of the individual. Fear may be associated with the unknown, mutilation, loss of control, pain, disability, or other factors. Behavioral manifestations of fear often include excitability, irrational behavior, and irrational and inaccurate beliefs about the feared object. Physiological signs and symptoms of the activated sympathetic nervous system (fight-or-flight response) include pallor, tachycardia, pupillary dilation, dry mouth, and cold, clammy hands.

Nursing Interventions

The nurse should try to identify the basis of the patient's fear. Identifying the source of fear will require exploring concerns with the patient. After the source of the fear has been identified, the nurse may be able to correct any misinformation. The need to verify the patient's understanding and perceptions and to clarify and amplify information is an ongoing, necessary aspect of communication. The nurse may also need to make appropriate referrals to assist the patient in alleviating the fears.

Regression

The person who is subjected to extreme and continued stress may retreat to the use of behavioral patterns that were appropriate during an earlier developmental stage. This response is called **regression.** On a temporary basis, regression can be a protective mechanism that preserves the person's limited ego strength. A certain amount of regression occurs with all serious illness as part of the response to the illness. The behavioral manifestations vary and may include helplessness, crying, temper tantrums, withdrawal from responsibilities, preoccupation with self, dependency, giddiness, and stubbornness.

Nursing Interventions

The patient who demonstrates evidence of regression needs a supportive, safe environment. The regression indicates that the patient is overwhelmed by the current stressors and cannot cope effectively. The nurse needs to implement methods for stress reduction and support effective coping mechanisms.

Denial

Denial is a defense mechanism, sometimes called a temporary protective mechanism, whereby the person refuses to acknowledge the existence or significance of a known fact. The known fact is too painful for the person to deal with, so its existence is denied. The degree of denial varies from person to person. Denial can be an effective, temporary method of dealing with a stress-producing situation until the person is able to muster the ego strength to deal with the problem. Continued denial, however, becomes a negative mechanism, in that the person does not incorporate the known information into reality for problem solving and realistic planning. Rather, the patient behaves as if the situation does not exist or refuses to discuss the topic in relation to himself or herself. Denial is likely to be carried out in fantasy, daydreaming, or games so that reality is temporarily pushed aside.

Nursing Interventions

At some point, denial becomes an ineffective coping mechanism for dealing with stress. The seriousness of the illness or the probable outcome can no longer be denied. An enormous amount of stress is associated with this realization. Patients gradually begin to acknowledge some of the more obvious aspects of their illness. They need the support of the nursing staff to make this adaptation. Questions should be answered honestly and as completely as possible based on the known facts so that patients can gradually face most of the realities of their illness. Depression and grieving are characteristic of this period. Once the painful information is incorporated into reality, the patient is able to make realistic decisions based on an altered and realistic self-concept.

Guilt

The feeling that one has done something wrong and is directly responsible for negative outcomes, pain, or frustration of goals is called **guilt.** The behavioral manifestations of guilt include a feeling of regretful responsibility for negative consequences, self-deprecation, lowered self-esteem, and possibly self-hate.

Nursing Interventions

The nurse should help the patient identify the source of the guilt and deal with the situation realistically and honestly.

Depression

Depression is a feeling of sadness and self-depreciation accompanied by difficulty in thinking and conducting usual activities and responsibilities, a lowered energy level, and self-preoccupation. The depressed person may be unable to express feelings and instead internalizes them. Other patients may be able to express their feelings. Depression has already been defined here as anger turned inward. The characteristic behaviors associated with depression are a sad, expressionless face; flat affect; listlessness; lack of interest in others or the environment; possible crying spells; and a sense of hopelessness. Some people who are depressed see no possible resolution to their situation and may contemplate suicide. Allusions to suicide may be made either directly or indirectly and should be taken seriously.

Nursing Interventions

There are varying degrees of depression. The person who is severely depressed may need psychiatric consultation and help. Drug therapy may be helpful in treating temporary depression. However, the reason(s) for the depression must be sought, identified, addressed, and treated. Suicide precautions may need to be instituted. It is very important to conduct a suicide assessment on all patients. Various helpful instruments are available. All health care agencies must have a method of screening for suicidal potential and a policy and procedure to follow where it is identified. Check for the policy and procedure in your practice site.

Powerlessness

Powerlessness is defined as a perceived or real lack of control over one's body, mind, environment, or life. The typical behavioral characteristics of powerlessness include a feeling of frustration, anger, hopelessness, depression, and apathy.

Nursing Interventions

Patients who perceive themselves as powerless, in the psychological sense, may need to be reminded that they have more power than they believe they do. Because of illness, power is often altered, but it is not lost. Patients need to recognize the power that they have and should be encouraged to use it appropriately.

Neurological illness may have deprived the patient of power over certain physiological functions. Participating in a rehabilitation program may help the patient reclaim his or her altered control and power over body functions. If complete rehabilitation is not possible, the patient may benefit from adaptive devices or altered methods of accomplishing tasks.

Stigma

When a person feels devalued or unable to meet minimum societal norms, this is termed **stigma.** The feeling of stigmatization can result from physical or emotional deficits, behavioral abnormalities, or violation of societal laws or codes. The person who feels stigmatized demonstrates characteristic behaviors that include feelings of shame, alienation, or being devalued; a decreased feeling of self-esteem or social worth; isolation from normal relationships; rejection of attempts by others to reach out to him or her; suspicion; paranoid behavior; loneliness; hostility; and anger.

Nursing Interventions

Dealing with patients who feel stigmatized can be difficult. Their feelings are usually based on deep-seated beliefs and values. These patients need assistance in exploring their feelings so that they can better understand them. The nurse needs to present reality and correct any erroneous information that the patient expresses. It is also important to support and build the patient's self-esteem.

EMOTIONAL AND PSYCHOLOGICAL RESPONSES TO SPECIFIC ASPECTS OF ILLNESS: NURSING IMPLICATIONS

Some emotional and psychological responses associated with certain aspects of neurological illness and hospitalization call for specific nursing interventions in addition to the general nursing approaches discussed previously in this chapter. The following experiences are discussed: loss, grief and bereavement, immobility, dehumanization, change in body image, sensory deprivation, isolation, sensory overload, intensive care unit (ICU) response, and transfer anxiety.

Loss

Loss is defined as a state in which a person experiences deprivation or the complete lack of something that was previously present and available to him or her. The person who has sustained a significant loss will demonstrate behaviors consistent with grieving and bereavement. (See the section that follows on grief and bereavement for specific behavioral manifestations.)

Loss can be sudden or gradual, predictable or unexpected, and temporary or permanent. Paralysis can be used to illustrate sudden and gradual loss. Patients who sustain a spinal cord injury in a motor vehicle accident may experience sudden loss of motor function below the level of injury. By contrast, patients with progressive multiple sclerosis often experience a gradual decline in motor function until paraplegia is complete. In the first instance, paralysis occurs in a split second; in the second, it develops gradually over years.

Some losses are predictable, whereas others are unexpected. The patient diagnosed as having amyotrophic lateral sclerosis will probably develop severe difficulty with speech and swallowing as the illness progresses. Conversely, the patient with a right hemispheric stroke is not expected to develop aphasia.

Some losses are temporary, whereas others are permanent. For example, the patient who has had surgery on the left parietal lobe of the brain may be temporarily aphasic postoperatively because of cerebral edema. Given a few days of treatment of the cerebral edema, speech ability would be expected to return gradually over the next several days. An example of a permanent loss may be seen in the patient who has undergone removal of a large acoustic neuroma that involved the trigeminal (cranial nerve [CN] V) and facial (CN VII) nerve. Unilateral loss of sensation to the face and drooping of the side of the mouth may remain despite surgery.

Significant losses may include loss of spouse, family members, or significant others; body parts; life; possessions; and physical, psychological, or cognitive functions. The individual's response to the loss will depend on the value that is placed on the lost object or body function, the societal and cultural value placed on the loss, and the cultural, economic, and support groups available to assist the individual in dealing with the loss. Each person has a unique value system. How the person values an object, person, or function influences the response to loss. For example, a person who loses the use of the right arm may be devastated if he or she was right-handed and enjoyed activities that require fine motor control of the hands, such as painting. Another patient who is left-handed, retired, and spends his or her leisure time reading or watching television would be inconvenienced by the loss, but it would not alter the basic lifestyle or self-concept to the same degree as the other patient.

Certain body functions, such as continence of the bladder and bowel and sexual function, are highly valued. Loss of these functions may be viewed as major, even catastrophic, losses by the person and society and have a great impact on lifestyle.

Cultural values also dictate an individual's response to loss. If the culture places a high value on the ability or body part lost, then the impact on the individual as a respected member of the culture is significant. When a person sustains a loss, the response and the adjustment to the loss will depend on the cultural, economic, and support groups available. All societies, regardless of whether they are primitive or highly sophisticated, have customs and rituals that are followed when someone dies. However, no such customs exist when there is loss of body function. Often, the loss of body function (disability) renders the person socially unacceptable because other people feel uncomfortable being around that person. For example, the person who has dysphagia may not be a welcome guest at the dinner table. Even if other people were able to accept the patient's difficulty in managing food, the patient may feel humiliated by uncontrolled drooling or food falling from the mouth.

The economic impact resulting from some losses is significant. Life insurance is helpful when a family member dies. Various health insurance policies assist with the cost of health care, and some people elect to purchase policies that provide payments if disability occurs. However, disability often results in an inability to participate in one's occupation, resulting in loss of salary. If the person is able to benefit from a rehabilitation program, he or she may be able to return to work at some job, but it may be at a much lower salary than previously. The resultant decreased financial income lowers the patient's economic status and lifestyle. The spouse or other family member may have to seek employment or, in some cases, may need to leave a job to care for the patient. This decrease in income at a time when extra expenses from loss are incurred has a dramatic effect on the patient's lifestyle and self-concept.

Support groups are available for some patients with particular problems, such as head injuries or multiple sclerosis. The purpose of these support groups is to assist the patient and family members with the loss of health and the disabilities incurred from the illness. The particular services offered vary from organization to organization but may include practical information on how to live with the particular illness, psychological and emotional support, and identification of resources to assist the patient and family.

Nursing Interventions

The nurse must explore with the person the significance of the loss. What does the loss mean to the patient within the context of lifestyle and self-concept? Until the nurse can appreciate the significance of the loss from the patient's point of view, it will be difficult to be supportive. After the nurse understands the significance of the loss, information and assistance can be provided to the patient and family. Referrals to other professionals or organizations may be appropriate.

Grief and Bereavement

According to Engel,[7] the loss of any valued object or function is followed by three stages that lead to healthy resolution: (1) shock and disbelief, (2) development of an awareness (recognition) of the loss, and (3) restitution (reconciliation).

The shock phase immediately follows the loss. Patients are stunned, appear to be out of contact with the environment, and are in a state of disbelief. They may be able to intellectualize the loss but cannot accept it emotionally. They do not believe that this is happening to them and may verbalize that this cannot be true.

During the recognition phase, patients begin to realize that the loss is real. Characteristic behaviors include anger, blaming themselves, depression, and asking, "why me?" These individuals are often preoccupied with the loss and what it means to them. The loss is internalized.

The final stage, restitution, is consistent with a realistic acceptance of what has happened. Gradually, interest in others and the environment returns. Patients begin to see themselves realistically and to integrate the change in body image into a positive self-concept. They are able to make decisions about themselves and the future and to see a realistic future for themselves.

Nursing Interventions

During the shock phase, accept the patient's behavior. Denial may be a protective coping mechanism. Allow patients to deny the loss if they must. Listen to them in an accepting, nonjudgmental manner, and refrain from telling them that you understand how they feel unless you have experienced the same loss.

During the recognition phase, accept the patient's anger. Allow for opportunities to express his or her feelings and to correct any misinformation. Support the patient during depression. Explain the patient's response to the loss to the family. Be supportive of the family. As the period of restitution emerges, encourage the patient to express his or her views and to plan realistically. Help the patient collect necessary information, either personally or by making appropriate referrals. Be supportive, and help the patient adapt and integrate the altered body image into his or her self-concept. Allow the patient to be as independent as possible and to assume self-responsibility.

Immobility

The prescribed, enforced, or unavoidable limitation of movement that occurs over a prolonged period is called **immobility**. Immobility can occur in the physical, psychological, intellectual, or social domains. The person who is physically immobilized may develop psychological immobility. Immobility reduces the quality and quantity of sensory input available to the person. This leads to a reduction in the individual's ability to interact with the environment. The behavioral manifestations of immobility include (1) a sense of confinement and limitation of space, resulting in frustration and anxiety; (2) a lack of control, which can lead to anger and depression; and (3) a forced change in body image and self-concept.

The neurological patient may suffer immobility in all domains. Paresis or paralysis can impose involuntary confinement and immobilization. The patient is not able to move freely; movement is a means of control that is highly cherished as a requisite for independence. Certain types of equipment, such as ventilators, food pumps, urinary catheters, intravenous lines, and orthopedic traction, enforce varying degrees of immobility on the patient. Cognitive and psychological deficits precipitated by neurological disease block or severely compromise psychosocial and intellectual input, making the patient feel confined or immobilized. The patient with an altered level of consciousness may be completely isolated from input in all domains. Social immobility may result from the manner in which other people treat the patient because of physical condition and disabilities.

Nursing Interventions

The goal of the nurse who is caring for immobile patients is to draw them into the mainstream of life, involving them to the extent that the therapeutic plan allows. Provide reality orientation (by using clock, calendar, or radio or telling patients what is happening in their immediate vicinity) so that they will be drawn into the environment. Extend the environment of these patients, if possible, by taking them out of their room, moving them near a window, or providing them with a wheelchair. Encourage social interaction and expression of feelings.

Dehumanization

Viewing patients as disease entities and divesting them of human capacities, qualities, and functions so that they are considered merely objects is called **dehumanization**. When dehumanization exists, the focus of attention is not on the person or unique individual who is experiencing illness, but rather on signs, symptoms, diagnostic data, and equipment. When patients are thus divested of their humanity, they are not consulted on decisions concerning themselves, provided with information, or treated with the respect and consideration normally extended to a person. Instead, the caregivers take over day-to-day decisions affecting the patient.

It is not necessarily the uncaring nurse who treats the patient as less than human. When caring for an unresponsive patient, it is easy to lose sight of the patient as a person. Human relationships are built on interactions between individuals. If this interchange is not ongoing, it is easy to lose sight of the humanity of the other individual.

Nursing Interventions

Address patients by name; think of them by name and as unique individuals rather than as a room number or diagnosis. Treat patients as the unique individuals that they are. Speak to them, and involve them in the environment and in decisions about their care as much as possible. Allow them to assume as much control and responsibility for themselves as possible.

Change in Body Image

A concept basic to one's sense of identity, security, self-esteem, and self-concept is body image. **Body Image** is defined as the conscious and unconscious perceptions (feelings and attitudes) that one has about his or her body as a separate and distinct entity. It is a developmental and social creation that is subject to very slow change in adult life. Illness, disability, and loss of function force a change in body image on the patient. If the change can be integrated realistically within the patient's self-concept without altering self-esteem, then the adaptation and adjustment are positive.

Behavioral manifestations associated with a change in body image often include those that accompany loss, grief, and bereavement. The change is viewed as a threat or sig-

nificant loss, and the patient passes through the characteristic stages of shock, recognition, and reconciliation.

Nursing Interventions

If the nurse views the patient's change in body image within the conceptual framework of loss, grief, and bereavement, the nursing intervention will follow a similar approach. Accept the patient's perception of self. Recognize that changing one's body image is a slow process. Support patients as they begin to recognize the impact of illness on their concept of body image. Help patients to accept and adapt to the change with positive reinforcement.

Sensory Deprivation

Sensory deprivation is defined as a lack of or decreased sensory input from the external or internal environment. There is a lack of or decreased perception of multisensory input of various intensities and meanings to the person. The behavioral manifestations of sensory deprivation vary, depending on the degree of deprivation. They may include abnormalities in feeling states, disorientation, impairment of the ability to think, distortion of perception, and illusions and hallucinations. The patient with neurological illness may experience many neurological deficits that contribute to sensory deprivation, such as an altered level of consciousness, paresis or paralysis, paresthesias, visual deficits, hearing loss, taste or smell deficits, and cognitive or emotional deficits. Head injury, spinal cord injury, cerebrovascular accident, multiple sclerosis, and many other neurological conditions can precipitate sensory deprivation. Therapeutic protocols, such as instituting aneurysm precautions, may also cause sensory deprivation.

Nursing Interventions

The nurse should be aware of the frequency with which sensory deprivation occurs, especially in neurological patients, and should assess patients for its presence. The nurse must identify the causes and the specific types of sensory deficits present. After these questions have been answered, the nurse can develop an approach to provide multisensory stimuli to the patient as a means of compensation. Sensory input can be provided by talking to the patient; playing the radio, television, or tape recordings of family members' voices; providing reality orientation and touch; and positioning. Reality orientation is a process of actively making patients aware of their environment (e.g., describing ongoing activities, weather, date, time, place, people, objects). Sensory deprivation, rather than physiological deficits of the reticular activating system, may be the cause of a patient's disorientation.

Sleep Deprivation

Sleep deprivation is defined as a lack of adequate sleep or dream time in relation to earlier or usual sleep patterns. People who are deprived of sleep for prolonged periods experience behavioral, psychological, and physiological alterations. Behavioral manifestations are similar to those seen in psychosis (alterations in perceptions, cognition, mood, affect). Patients admitted to ICUs, requiring constant care and monitoring, receiving certain medication, and experiencing extreme stress are prime candidates for sleep deprivation. The strange environment and constant activity of the hospital predispose patients to this common phenomenon. Because of injuries to the brain and their need for attention, neurological patients often experience sleep deprivation.

Nursing Interventions

The nurse should assess the patient's 24-hour sleep-wakefulness cycle to determine how much sleep time is actually provided. Nursing care should be planned to provide uninterrupted sleep time. Drug therapy can also have an effect on the quality of sleep and dream time. Certain drugs may alter the depth of sleep and the sleep pattern. Deprivation of the various levels of sleep, such as the rapid eye movement stage, is thought to have a negative effect on the patient. The nurse should be aware of the various factors that influence that patient's ability to sleep and control the environment as much as possible to facilitate sleep.

Sensory Overload

Sudden, excessive, sustained, multisensory experiences that are perceived as confusing, bothersome, meaningless, and extremely stressful to the patient are defined collectively as **sensory overload.** The behavioral manifestations of sensory overload are confusion, disorientation, irritability, restlessness, agitation, anger, panic, and auditory or visual hallucinations.

Neurological patients may experience sensory overload from equipment (e.g., respirator, cardiac monitor), conditions that intensify sensory input (meningitis, encephalitis), or the constant stimuli of nursing care, particularly if they are critically ill.

Nursing Interventions

The nurse should identify the various sensory levels and sources of input in the patient's environment. Every effort should be made to control and moderate the intensity of stimuli. Special situations sometimes exist, such as when subarachnoid precautions are instituted. The purpose of these precautions is to decrease all stimuli so that the patient will not rebleed. In patients with meningitis or encephalitis, tactile stimuli should be minimized, and all other environmental stimuli should be controlled.

Intensive Care Unit Response

Admission to the alien environment of the ICU is stressful for the patient and family for many reasons. The ICU environment is characterized by strange noises, smells, and bright lights, and the open floor plan characteristic of most ICUs offers little privacy. The pervasive atmosphere is one of urgency, danger, and death being held in abeyance by technology and heroic measures of the staff. Ironically, the patient and family can feel profound isolation within this charged environment. Fear, anxiety, depression, and delirium are common responses to the situation, and the patient or family may panic. According to Cassem and Hackett,[8] nothing else distorts personality quite like panic.

Disorientation is common in patients. Sleep deprivation or an altered sleep-wakefulness cycle contributes to disorientation and misinterpretation of reality. Patients may exhibit agitation, hallucinations, delusions, and psychosis. This phenomenon is called **ICU psychosis**. The changes in behavior can be difficult to interpret. When neurological patients exhibit a change in behavior, one often attributes the change to a neurological cause. *However, psychological responses and drug side effects and interactions must also be carefully considered as possible etiologies.*

Nursing Interventions

Institute strategies to provide emotional support, reassurance, and information to the conscious patient, and plan activities to allow for periods of uninterrupted sleep. Provide for the safety needs of agitated patients. In an unconscious patient, provide for "soft stimuli," such as light touch, soft voices, and family visits whereby family members talk quietly to the patient about pleasant topics.

Transfer Anxiety

The increased anxiety and feelings of insecurity experienced by patients when they are moved from one unit or facility to another are collectively called **transfer anxiety.** Patients may be transferred from the ICU to a regular acute care unit. Neurological patients may also be transferred to a rehabilitation facility, chronic care facility, or nursing home. Patients and their families may be concerned that the quality of care and the commitment of the nursing and medical staff will not be as good in the new setting. There may be the underlying feeling that the quality of care will deteriorate and that the person will not be recognized as a unique individual. The unit to which a patient is currently assigned may be perceived as one that offers a higher level of nursing, medical, and technological support than the unit to which the patient is being transferred. Patients may experience fear of the unknown and may view the transfer as a threat to their security and well-being.

The major behavioral manifestation is anxiety that may develop into a panic-like state as the day of transfer approaches. The patient may also experience physiological responses (psychosomatic responses) to the stress of an impending transfer. Common signs and symptoms may include elevation of blood pressure, shortness of breath, tightness in the chest, palpitations, or elevation in body temperature.

Nursing Interventions

Comprehensive discharge planning should include the psychological preparation of the patient and family to ensure a smooth transition from the acute care setting to another facility or home. The liaison nurse from the new facility may need to visit the patient to help facilitate the transition and provide information about the new facility. Questions should be encouraged and complete information provided to dispel the patient's fear of the unknown facility. A visit to the new unit or facility is desirable so that the patient (if possible) or family members can tour the facilities and meet members of the staff.

If the neurological patient is going home, the physical environment should be evaluated, and the delivery of any necessary equipment should be arranged before the day of discharge. Patient and family teaching should be conducted in plenty of time so that they will feel comfortable. If possible, a weekend home visit by the patient should be arranged. In this way, problems can be addressed and resolved before the actual discharge is made. Every attempt should be made to anticipate potential problems so that a smooth transition can occur.

Regardless of the plans after discharge, the patient and family should be given an opportunity to terminate (i.e., say good bye) with the staff.

PSYCHOLOGICAL, EMOTIONAL, AND BEHAVIORAL RESPONSES OF THE FAMILY OR SIGNIFICANT OTHERS

Neurological illness has serious consequences, not only for the patient, but also for family members and significant others. The family structure, relationships, and methods of dealing with stress and crisis become important considerations for the nurse. Family members will react to illness individually across the entire gamut of responses, including anxiety, anger, depression, denial, grieving, and fear. Neurological illness often takes the form of a chronic condition with permanent or progressive disabilities that compel the patient to depend on family or significant others to meet basic needs. The stresses incurred by neurological illness are significant and require the support and assistance of health professionals for the family to make a realistic adjustment. The ability of the family to accept the situation and adapt will directly influence the emotional well-being of every member of the family unit, including the patient. See Chart 12-1 for nursing diagnoses related to the family.

Nursing Interventions

The role of the nurse in supporting the family includes the following:

- Talk to the family to determine their understanding and perception of the patient's illness.
- Determine the schemata of family interactions and support systems.
- Allow the family members to express their feelings.
- Correct misinformation, and provide data as necessary.
- Make referrals as necessary.
- Allow the family to become involved in the care of the patient, if they so wish.
- Promote normality.
- Support the family in their decision about patient's care or plans for posthospital care.
- Be prepared to repeat information.

EMOTIONAL AND PSYCHOLOGICAL RESPONSES OF THE NURSE CARING FOR NEUROLOGICAL PATIENTS

Care of the Caretakers: Secondary Traumatic Stress

Traumatic events affect the lives of many people besides the immediate victims. Working with patients who have suffered neurological illness is challenging and difficult. The literature to date has focused on the patient and family. Some attention should be focused on the nurse and what she or he brings to the therapeutic relationship and how she or he is affected by these relationships. The conscious and the unconscious responses of the nurse need to be examined. These responses include affective, cognitive, and somatic components. Nurses need ongoing and regularly scheduled supportive relationships with their supervisors in the course of which they are able to talk about their feelings and are urged to attend to their own self-care and spiritual renewal.

Common job-related stressors include caring for patients who have the following conditions:

- Neurological injury as a result of trauma (e.g., motor vehicle accidents, assaults, self-inflicted injuries)
- Diagnoses of terminal illness, especially if they are young
- Cognitive and emotional disabilities
- Neurological deficits that render them completely dependent on the nurse
- Tracheostomy tubes, ventilators, and support equipment
- Significant pain that is not alleviated by normal modalities of pain control
- Multiple trauma or a critical illness
- Agreed to become a donor for organ transplant
- Being designated as brain dead
- Being discharged to another facility after a long stay on the unit

Other factors in the work environment that are sources of stress include:

- Experiencing interpersonal conflict with coworkers or administrative personnel
- Dealing with the family of a dying patient

- Dealing with a disoriented, demanding, noisy, or "difficult" patient or family
- Having to assume responsibilities that the nurse is not prepared to manage
- Dealing with physicians, residents, nursing students, and faculty
- Rotating shifts and working double shifts
- Working with insufficient staff
- Working with inadequate supplies or auxiliary staff (e.g., transport and laboratory services)
- Working without effective leadership
- Observing curtailment of programs owing to lack of adequate funding
- Seeing patients who will receive inadequate rehabilitation because of lack of funds
- Receiving no recognition
- Having to channel communications through the bureaucracy to get results
- Downsizing of hospital staffing, which results in rapid turnover of staff
- Being unable to organize staff as a cohesive group owing to rapid changes in staffing patterns
- Feeling devalued with the shift in care from hospitals to outpatient settings

Unless nurses take the time to protect themselves from the acute and chronic stresses of their job, the state of their mental and physical health is at risk. Burnout is the result of chronic stress, and it affects the quality of the care administered to the patient and the professional and personal life of the nurse. Nurses must learn to recognize the signs and symptoms of stress and do something positive to deal with them before serious problems result. Nurses are encouraged to choose appropriate coping mechanisms to deal with stress and to practice good health habits themselves (e.g., eating well, avoiding drug and alcohol abuse, participating in an exercise program or other recreation).

Many articles and continuing education offerings have addressed the needs of the nurse as a person and professional who is subject to significant stress. The concept of burnout is well documented and discussed in the literature. Nurses as caregivers are highly vulnerable to stress, and measures should be taken to protect and support them. Each nurse must assume responsibility for his or her own mental health and practice appropriate methods of stress control.

REFERENCES

1. Selye, H. (1956). *The stress of life.* New York: McGraw-Hill.
2. Selye, H. (1974). *Stress without distress.* Philadelphia: J. B. Lippincott.
3. Cannon, W. B. (1936). *The wisdom of the body.* New York: W. W. Norton.
4. Jacobson, E. (1965). *Anxiety and tension control.* Philadelphia: J. B. Lippincott.
5. Horney, K. (1937). *Collected works of Karen Horney* (Vol. 1, p. 63). New York: W. W. Norton.
6. Kiening, M. M., Sr. (1978). Hostility. In C. E. Carlson & B. Blackwell (Eds.). *Behavioral concepts and nursing interventions* (2nd ed.; p. 131). Philadelphia: J. B. Lippincott.
7. Engel, G. L. (1964). Grief and grieving. *American Journal of Nursing, 64,* 93.
8. Cassem, N., & Hackett, T. (1978). The setting of intensive care. In T. Hackett & N. Cassem (Eds.), *Massachusetts General Hospital handbook of general hospital psychiatry.* St. Louis: C. V. Mosby.

RESOURCES

Professional

Published Material

BOOKS

Aguilera, D. C. (1998). *Crisis intervention: Theory and methodology* (8th ed.). St. Louis: Mosby.
Brooks, N. (Ed.) (1984). *Closed head injury: Psychological, social, and family consequences.* Oxford, U. K.: Oxford University Press.
Dimond, M., & Jones, S. L. (1983). *Chronic illness across the life span.* Norwalk: Appleton-Century-Crofts.
Keltner, N., Palmer, C., & Folks, D. (1998). *Psychobiological foundation of psychiatric care.* St. Louis: Mosby.
Rosenthal, M., Griffith, E. R., Bond, M. R., & Miller, J. D. (1990). *Rehabilitation of the head-injured adult* (2nd ed.). Philadelphia: F. A. Davis.
Shea, C., Stuart, G., Poster, E., Pellitier, L., & Verhey, M. (Eds.). (1999). *Advanced practice nursing in psychiatric and mental health care.* St. Louis: American Psychiatric Nurses Association.

PERIODICALS

Bell, T. (1986). Nurses' attitudes in caring for the comatose head-injured patient. *Journal of Neuroscience Nursing, 18,* 279–283.
Bernstein, L. P. (1990). Family-centered care of the critically ill neurologic patient. *Critical Care Nursing Clinics of North America, 2*(1), 41–50.
Braulin, J. L. D., Rook, J., & Sills, G. M. (1982). Families in crisis: The impact of trauma. *Critical Care Quarterly, 5*(3), 38–46.
Burckhardt, C. S. (1987). Coping strategies of the chronically ill. *Nursing Clinics of North America, 22*(3), 543–550.
Caine, R. M. (1989). Families in crisis: Making the critical difference. *Focus on Critical Care, 16*(3), 184–189.
Campbell, C. H. (1988). Needs of relatives and helpfulness of support groups in severe head injury. *Rehabilitation Medicine, 13,* 320–325.
Clum, M. N., & Ryan, M. (1981). Brain injury and the family. *Journal of Neurosurgical Nursing, 13,* 165–169.
Craig, M. C., Copes, W. S., & Champion, H. R. (1988). Psychosocial considerations in trauma. *Critical Care Quarterly, 11,* 51–58.
Evans, R. L., & Bishop, D. S. (1987). Predicting post-stroke family function: A continuing dilemma. *Psychology Report, 60,* 691–695.
Frye, B. (1987). Head injury and the family: Related literature. *Rehabilitation Nursing, 12,* 135–136.
Grinspun, D. (1987). Teaching families of traumatic brain-injured adults. *Critical Care Quarterly, 10,* 61.
Gull, H. J. (1987). The chronically ill patient's adaptation to hospitalization. *Nursing Clinics of North America, 22*(3), 593–601.
Hegeman, K. M. (1988). A care plan for the family of a brain-trauma client. *Rehabilitation Nursing, 13,* 254–262.
Lambert, C. E., & Lambert, V. A. (1987). Psychological impacts created by chronic illness. *Nursing Clinics of North America, 22*(3), 527–533.

Leske, J. S. (1986). Needs of relatives of critically ill patients: A follow-up. *Heart & Lung, 15,* 189–193.

Lust, B. L. (1984). The patient in the ICU: A family experience. *Critical Care Quarterly, 6*(4), 49–57.

Martin, K. M. (1987). Predicting short-term outcome in comatose head-injured children. *Journal of Neuroscience Nursing, 19*(1), 9–13.

Mathis, M. (1984). Personal needs of the family members of critically ill patients with and without acute brain injury. *Journal of Neurosurgical Nursing, 16*(1), 36–44.

Mauss-Clum, N., & Ryan, M. (1981). Brain injury and the family. *Journal of Neurosurgical Nursing, 13*(4), 165–169.

McCann, I. L., & Pearlman, L. A. (1990). Vicarious traumatization: A contextual model for understanding the effects of trauma on helpers. *Journal of Traumatic Stress, 3*(1), 131–149.

Podrasky, D. L., & Sexton, D. L. (1988). Nurses' reactions to difficult patients. *Image, 20*(1), 16–21.

Pollock, S. E. (1987). Adaptation to chronic illness: Analysis of nursing research. *Nursing Clinics of North America, 22*(3), 631–644.

Pollock, S. E. (1984). The stress response. *Critical Care Quarterly, 6*(4), 1–13.

Printz-Feddersen, V. (1990). Group process effect on caregiver burden. *Journal of Neuroscience Nursing, 22*(3), 164–168.

Soderstrom, S., Fogelsjoo, A., Fugl-Meyer, K. S., & Stensson, S. (1988). I. Head injury. A program for crisis-intervention after traumatic brain injury. *Scandanavian Journal of Rehabilitation Medicine, 17,* (Suppl.), 47–49.

Tilden, V. P., & Weinert, C. (1987). Social support and the chronically ill individual. *Nursing Clinics of North America, 22*(3), 613–620.

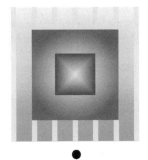

CHAPTER **13**

Rehabilitation of Neuroscience Patients

JOANNE V. HICKEY

This chapter provides nurses caring for neuroscience patients with basic information about the principles and concepts of rehabilitation as they apply to neuroscience patient populations. Rehabilitation nursing is a specialty area of nursing practice with a published scope and standards of practice.[1,2] However, rehabilitation principles and concepts are fundamental components of nursing practice and cut across all practice areas. Understanding of the whole rehabilitation process by neuroscience nurses will facilitate a smooth continuum of care for patients.

FRAMEWORKS FOR DISABILITY

For some years, there have been two widely used conceptual frameworks regarding disability and rehabilitation:[3] the International Classification of Impairments, Disabilities, and Handicaps (ICIDH),[4] and the functional limitations model (also called Nagi's framework).[5] Using these two frameworks as a foundation, the Institute of Medicine proposed a new model in 1991.

The International Classification of Impairments, Disabilities, and Handicaps

The ICIDH[4] was developed by the World Health Organization to organize information about the consequences of disease. In addition to defining disease, it includes three distinct classifications, impairment, disability, and handicap, each related to a different level of response or consequence to disease. Because each level is distinct and independent of the others, a person can be impaired without being disabled and disabled without being handicapped.

- **Disease** is the combination of the underlying diagnosis and the pathological process.
- **Impairment** is an abnormality of a psychological, physiological, or anatomical structure and function; it represents disturbance on the *organ* level.
- **Disability** is the consequences of impairment as it relates to individual functional performance and activity; it represents disturbance on the *person* level.
- **Handicap** refers to the disadvantages experienced by an individual that limit or prevent fulfillment of roles that are normal for the individual as a result of impairment or disability; it represents disturbance on the *societal* level.

Functional Limitations Model[5]

The functional limitations framework consists of four concepts:

- **Pathology** refers to the cellular and tissue alterations occurring from disease, trauma, infection, or congenital problems.
- **Impairment** comprises the specific abnormalities of physical, mental, and biochemical functioning.
- **Functional limitations** occur when there is a decrease in an individual's actual or potential performance.
- **Disability** occurs when conditions interfere with the performance of personal, social, and culturally expected roles.

Institute of Medicine Model[3]

A new model of disability was proposed by the Institute of Medicine (1991) that combined the ICIDH and Nagi's functional limitations framework. The term *handicap* was deleted, and to the Nagi framework was added *risk factors* and *quality of life* to create a new model of the disabling process. The addition of these two dimensions is in line with current thinking about disability. Recommendations were also offered to address prevention and management of disability on a national level.

CONCEPTS OF REHABILITATION

Rehabilitation is a dynamic process through which a person is assisted to achieve optimal physical, emotional, psychological, social, and vocational potential and to maintain dignity, self-respect, and a quality of life that is as self-fulfilling and satisfying as possible. The major goals of rehabilitation are optimizing function; promoting independence, satisfaction, quality of life; and preserving self-esteem. To be effective, rehabilitation must be a philosophy of care and an integral part of health care delivery.

Rehabilitation also comprises the continuum of functional restoration. In some situations, complete functional restoration is possible, as in the situation of a patient who sustains a mild concussion. In this instance, complete recovery is the rule. However, when complete recovery of function is not possible and permanent disability is likely, the patient must be helped to accept, adjust to, and compensate for the existing deficit and to establish an optimal level of function. An example is a paraplegic patient who has sustained a severed spinal cord injury and so is expected to be permanently paralyzed. Present medical technology cannot restore the severed cord to its premorbid condition, although this may be possible sometime in the future. However, a comprehensive rehabilitation program helps the person live a useful, relatively independent life from a wheelchair.

Another aspect of rehabilitation addresses chronic health problems and degenerative diseases, such as multiple sclerosis. Although currently no cure exists for multiple sclerosis, a rehabilitation program can improve quality of life through health promotion, symptom management, prevention of complications, and patient education to promote independence for the longest possible time. As the disease progresses, rehabilitation offers alternate ways of carrying out activities of daily living (ADLs) with adaptive devices and alternate methods of performing skilled acts.

A PHILOSOPHY OF REHABILITATION

A **philosophy** is a set of broad statements about fundamental beliefs and values. The philosophy of rehabilitation offers a framework to shape the overall rehabilitation process and often includes the following premises:

1. *A person with a disability has intrinsic worth that transcends the disability; each person is a unique holistic being who has the right and the responsibility to make informed personal choices regarding health and lifestyle.*[1] Restoring an individual's capacity to a level sufficient to resume roles such as homemaking, parenting, and gainful employment offer many social, emotional, psychological, and financial returns to society.
2. *Rehabilitation is an integral component of all care administered by all health care providers.* Rehabilitation begins the moment a person seeks health care so that prevention is incorporated into the rehabilitation process. A major goal in educating all health care providers is to prepare them to "think rehab" from the moment of initial contact with the patient.
3. *Comprehensive rehabilitation requires the active participation and collaboration of all health care providers through ongoing communication and management.* Scheduled team conferences, informal discussion, written plans of care, and progress notes provide a means of communication. Multidisciplinary collaboration and management mean that all health team members collaborate to achieve specific, identified, mutual goals.

4. *Rehabilitation requires the active participation of the patient to achieve optimal rehabilitative potential.* The patient must be motivated to be actively involved in the rehabilitation process.
5. *Rehabilitation actively involves the patient's family or significant others; they are the patient's potential support systems and assist with the transition back to the home and community.* Family members must be reached at their individual levels of understanding, taking into consideration their educational, socioeconomic, and cultural backgrounds to understand the rehabilitative goals and methods selected to meet these goals. The nurse usually interprets this information for the family, helping them to understand how they can best participate. In addition, the family is a rich source of information about the patient's personality and lifestyle that will be helpful in the transition back to the community.
6. *An individual patient and family evaluation is necessary to determine their ability to contribute to the rehabilitation process.* All families cannot contribute in the same way or to the same degree. Because each family and patient present different problems, individual evaluation is necessary.
7. *The patient experiences illness and disability within the context of her or his previous adjustment patterns.* The strengths and weaknesses of the patient's personality are essentially the same during illness. Team members must recognize the social and cultural influences that affect the patient's adjustment patterns and acceptance of care.
8. *Rehabilitation takes place within the context of the patient's whole life: the sociocultural aspects of life, his or her job or vocation, family, home, place in the community, religion, and relationship to self.* When illness strikes, family life is abruptly interrupted and altered. Illness affects not only the patient, but also the family. Therefore, rehabilitation should also include the needs of the family.
9. *Rehabilitation is a dynamic process with progress, plateaus, and setbacks.* Only through ongoing assessment and problem solving is achievement of patient goals possible.
10. *Transitions in care include plans for continued rehabilitation services. Options include acute or subacute inpatient rehabilitation, community re-entry, outpatient rehabilitation, or home health therapies.* The patient and family should be presented with various care alternatives and helped to evaluate the implications of each choice, including cost and health insurance issues. The patient and family should actively participate in the decision-making process of discharge planning to the degree that they are able and willing to participate for a relatively smooth transition and adjustment.

Terminology of Rehabilitation

The following terms are used consistently in rehabilitative health care:

- **Rehabilitative potential:** dormant power for rehabilitation within a person that exists as a possibility that can eventually become actualized
- **Short-term goals:** goals to be achieved in the immediate future (usually set for 1 week); discrete units or steps involved in the learning of a skill that must be achieved

before more complex skilled acts can be accomplished; the steps through which long-term goals are achieved

- **Long-term goals:** goals projected for completion in the distant future; can be considered the ultimate objectives of a rehabilitation program
- **Optimal goals:** optimal rehabilitation goals that may be expected barring significant setbacks or complications
- **Realistic goals:** goals that reflect a realistic appraisal of the person and achievable outcome
- **Acute disability:** a disability that has a finite duration and is completely resolved in a short period of time; reversible; temporary
- **Chronic disability:** an ongoing disability that limits the person in some way; permanent; irreversible
- **Collaborative model of practice:** representatives from multidisciplines working collaboratively together to achieve measurable functional outcomes for people with disabilities
- **Multidisciplinary team rounds:** activity in which the various health team professionals visit the patient as a group to assess the person's current functional level, problems, and concerns; usually daily or weekly; provide data for further discussion at a team meeting or conference
- **Family meetings:** planned meetings with one or more health care professionals and family members to discuss patient or family education; recognizes the importance of the family in the rehabilitation of the patient, and helps to maintain open communication

Framework for Rehabilitation Decisions

Decisions related to rehabilitation are based primarily on information gathered during a screening examination. The goal is to determine the best possible match between the needs of the patient and capabilities of the rehabilitation programs in the community. In this complex health care environment, decisions regarding health care and expenditure of dollars are scrutinized. One of the key initial decisions regarding rehabilitation is whether the person is a candidate who can benefit from rehabilitation. Figure 13-1 summarizes the process of reaching a rehabilitation decision. This information and figure are taken from the Agency for Health Care Policy and Research (AHCPR) clinical practice guidelines, *Post-Stroke Rehabilitation* (1995), but they are applicable to all initial and subsequent transitional rehabilitation decisions.[6]

Multidisciplinary Team

Several health care disciplines may participate in a multidisciplinary collaborative model of practice to provide a comprehensive rehabilitation program. The central focus of care is the patient and family, and each multidisciplinary team member works with the patient and family to achieve functional outcomes. Although all patients will not require the services of every discipline, they are available for consultation as necessary.

The rehabilitation process begins with a comprehensive functional assessment. The functional independence measure (FIM) is the most widely used standardized instrument to measure severity of disability based on a functional assessment.[7] The FIM assesses self-care, anal sphincter control, transfers, locomotion, communication, and social cognition. In addition, each health care team member can further assess the patient using other instruments specific to the particular discipline.

After a database has been compiled, a comprehensive rehabilitation plan is developed with identified functional outcome measures. Team conferences are one example of a formal communication mode. Informal communications between and among team members are ongoing. These interactions reinforce collaboration among team members by promoting continuity of care and moving the plan forward. Because of the complexity of care and the numbers of people involved, it is easy for communications to break down. Therefore, planned, formal, patient-centered conferences are essential for the vitality of the process.

ASSESSMENT OF ACTIVITIES OF DAILY LIVING

Activities of daily living must be accomplished independently for patients to assume responsibility for their own needs and to participate actively in society. Independence can be measured by the degree of responsibility assumed by the patient for these ADLs that are necessary for successful functioning at home, at work, and in social situations.

Various ADLs focus on different aspects of function:

- **Personal ADLs:** bathing, toileting, grooming, eating, oral hygiene, dressing, ambulating (on various surfaces), and communicating. The ability to perform these activities vastly contributes to independent self-care.
- **Instrumental ADLs:** using the telephone, shopping, using transportation to get around in the community, and walking distances outside the home. Independence in these activities is a key marker for independence in basic activities outside the home.
- **Occupational and role activities:** roles in the home, such as homemaking, parenting, and spousal roles and jobs outside the home. The skills necessary to assume any role or job are identified; the occupational therapist, family counselor, or vocational counselor can assist in assessing critical skills.

Helping the patient relearn ADLs begins with an assessment of the skills that remain intact, those that are lost, and those that cannot be used without some help. The major barriers to relearning ADL skills in the neurological patient are deficits affecting perception, motor activity, communication, vision, and cognitive functions.

The teaching plan is based on the individual needs of the patient and the principles of learning and teaching. For example, an occupational therapist can be helpful in making suggestions for teaching the patient ADLs. If the patient is being seen by the occupational therapist on a regular basis, the nurse should coordinate nursing activities with those of the therapist so that the patient does not become confused.

Each activity that must be relearned must be analyzed to identify the critical components involved in the overall task.

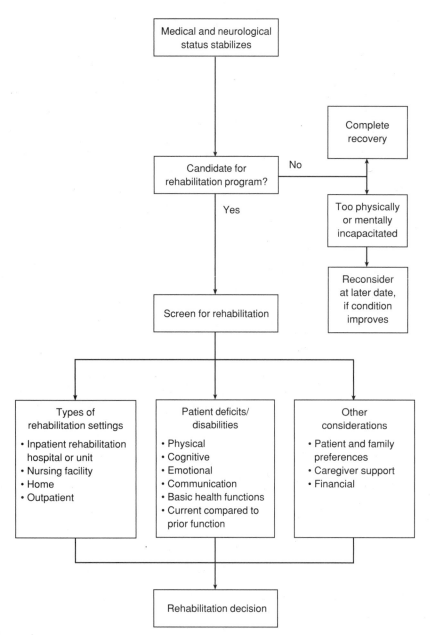

Figure 13–1 • Framework for rehabilitation decisions. (Gresham, G. E., Duncan, P. W., Stason, W. B., et al. [1995] *Post-stroke rehabilitation.* Clinical practice guideline, No. 16. Rockville, MD: U.S. Department of Health and Human Services. Public Health Service, Agency for Health Care Policy and Research. AHCPR Publication No. 95-0662. May.)

Use of adaptive devices may be necessary to compensate for neurological deficits and to allow the patient to perform ADLs independently. For example, a spoon with a bulky stem may allow the patient with contractures of the hand to grasp the spoon, an act that could not be accomplished if the spoon had a regular size or shape. Chart 13-1 details the principles of learning and teaching. The information in Chart 13-2 applies specifically to patients with cerebral injury.

PRINCIPLES OF REHABILITATION NURSING

The principles of rehabilitation are an integral component of independent nursing practice and include the major elements of **prevention, maintenance,** and **restoration.** Many nursing protocols and procedures contain elements of all three components. Preventive measures include special skin care, proper positioning and realignment, frequent turning, and range of motion exercises. The maintenance of intact skills and functions is supported by such activities as getting the patient out of bed to a chair and encouraging the patient to be as independent as possible in ADLs. Instituting exercise programs designed to increase range of motion, teaching ADLs to a patient with a paralyzed limb, and helping a patient relearn names of common objects are examples of restorative nursing activities. This framework can be kept in mind when planning and administering nursing care to address particular deficits.

A fundamental concept of rehabilitation is to do *with* the patient and not do *for* or *to* the patient. According to the American Nurses Association and the Association of Rehabilitation Nurses, the goal of rehabilitation nursing is to assist people who have disability and chronic illness to

CHART 13-1 • Principles of Learning and Teaching

Patient and family education are important components of the rehabilitation process. Effective teaching rests on an understanding of the principles of learning and teaching as applied to the clinical setting.

The following basic principles can serve as a guide in teaching the patient:

- The objectives of the teaching session should be defined clearly; it is wise to write down behavioral objectives to identify the knowledge and skills the patient is expected to learn.
- The skills involved in the activity should be limited to small, critical units to facilitate learning.
- People learn best when they are able to perceive a need or value in the learning.
- Readiness to learn is important if patients are to benefit from the material presented; they must have sufficient physical and mental function to learn successfully.
- The patient should be rested and comfortable before the teaching session begins to enhance concentration.
- The nurse should demonstrate the skill and then have the patient perform the skill under supervision; if the skill is not performed correctly, it should be demonstrated again. The patient may need extensive supervision and opportunity for repetition to master the skill.
- The more senses involved in learning, the more apt the patient is to learn. (For example, the nurse can demonstrate the skill while telling the patient what is being done; gestures may also be used.)
- Reinforcement of learning should be followed through with consistency by all staff members working with the patient. Such reinforcement should be based on a written teaching plan.
- The patient's age, neurological deficits, educational background, fluency, and intelligence should be considered when individualizing a teaching plan that is appropriate for his or her needs.
- The patient should be given positive verbal feedback for accomplishments.
- The patient should be motivated to participate actively in the learning process.
- The patient and family should be encouraged to ask questions.

cloth, but the patient may be able to wash one side of the face. This is a beginning, and it helps to develop the complete skill in the future. Unlike other aspects of nursing, rehabilitation is often a very slow process requiring ongoing dedication and effort. The long-lasting reward is that a human being has been helped to achieve maximal potential.

Rehabilitation is a collaborative interdisciplinary process involving health care professionals working together to achieve mutual goals. As the member of the rehabilitation team who spends the most time with the patient on a daily basis, the nurse provides continuity of care through coordination. The nurse can help coordinate and manipulate the patient's daily schedule so that optimal benefit will be derived from therapy. For example, the patient should be at a high energy level for the strenuous activity of mat work or ambulation in physical therapy. Scheduling these activities when the patient is fatigued is counterproductive to the goals of physical therapy. The nurse also assesses and addresses the patient's physical, emotional, and psychological responses to various therapeutic regimens.

The family often approaches the nurse with questions and concerns about the overall plan of care. In some instances, information and clarification are provided. In other instances, referral of questions to other team members or to initiation of a family-team meeting is most appropriate. Keeping the lines of communication open is a tedious and difficult job that is

CHART 13-2 • Teaching the Patient With Cerebral Injury

Patients with cerebral injury present special problems in learning because of certain cognitive deficits, such as easy distractibility, short attention span, inability to think abstractly, memory deficits, poor judgment, and inability to transfer learning from one situation to another. An assessment to identify deficits and to develop an individualized teaching plan that reflects modifications designed to compensate for deficits is necessary. A few principles should be remembered when teaching such a patient:

- Be realistic in your expectations.
- Assume a calm and positive attitude toward the patient's ability to learn.
- Develop a written teaching plan for use by all nursing staff; be consistent.
- Plan short teaching sessions with specific goals.
- Choose a time when the patient is not tired.
- Use simple, specific instructions.
- Proceed systematically, in a step-by-step fashion.
- Motivate the patient.
- Facilitate learning by repetition and reinforcement.
- For the patient who is easily distracted, structure the environment to minimize distractions.
- Praise any accomplishment.
- Incorporate behavior modification principles.
- Tailor teaching methods to the patient's functional level (e.g., may need visual aids and demonstration rather than explanation).

attain maximum functional ability, maintain optimal health, and adapt to an altered lifestyle.[8] Rehabilitation nurses assist patients to identify goals that are realistic and attainable and consider the patient's continuing accountability for optimal wellness. After a skill has been mastered, it is expected to be maintained, and also to become a skill on which to build to the next functional level. A patient is guided to do any part of a task even if he or she is unable to perform the complete activity. For example, the nurse may soap and squeeze a face compounded by the large number of people involved in the patient's care. The nurse often becomes the clearinghouse for information, concerns, and confrontations.

Patient and family education is key to optimal recovery. Excellent community resources are available through various agencies, such as the American Heart Association and now the American Stroke Association for stroke rehabilitation information through telephone or website. The patient and family need to be aware of these resources and may need assistance in making contact. A list of addresses is provided at the end of this chapter.

Nursing Management of Patients With Impaired Physical Mobility

Assessment

The nurse assesses mobility by conducting a motor function examination and reviewing the data from the FIM. Independence is closely correlated to a person's ability to move individual body parts or the body as a whole. Loss of mobility imposes severe constraints on the individual's freedom and independence.

Nursing management depends on the nursing diagnosis and on collaborative problems. The following are possible nursing diagnoses:

- Impaired Physical Mobility
- Risk for Injury (from falls)
- Risk for Altered Skin Integrity
- Fatigue
- Activity Intolerance

The following are possible collaborative problems although many more preventive focused problems can be cited:

- Pathological fractures
- Joint dislocation
- Falls

The major nursing diagnosis of **Impaired Physical Mobility** is applied to a patient who is experiencing limited physical movement in the environment, including bed mobility, transfers, and ambulating. When considering altered mobility, interventions directed at preventing edema of the extremities, skin breakdown, contractures, subluxation, deconditioning of muscles, pneumonia, and deep vein thrombosis are common collaborative problems in which the nurse plays an important role.

Patients with concurrent cerebral injury and impaired physical mobility may not have sufficient cognitive ability to comprehend fully the extent and implications of their disability or the relationship of prescribed treatment to the maintenance, prevention, and restoration of functional loss. They will need direct supervision. They are at high risk for injury due to falls.

The nursing diagnoses of **Fatigue** and **Activity Intolerance** are related to bed rest reconditioning. Endurance for activity must be developed. As a rule, one day for every day in bed is necessary to build endurance; in elderly patients, it

is longer. The nurse deals with these barriers to help the patient achieve an optimal level of independence.

Interventions

As a member of the multidisciplinary team, the nurse works collaboratively with other team members to assist the patient to regain function. The philosophy of rehabilitation nursing is an integral part of care. The specifics of care depend on the patient's functional deficits and needs as well as expected outcomes

⫿ THE BASIS OF MOVEMENT AND TREATMENT OF MOVEMENT DISORDERS

Normal movement patterns originate in genetically programmed configurations of neurons. Maturation of the central nervous system follows a predetermined pattern of elaboration and refinement of movement. Reflex and voluntary control proceeds in cephalic to caudal and proximal to distal directions. For example, voluntary head movement is learned before voluntary trunk movement. Most motor systems are modifiable within limits, thus providing the basis for developing acquired motor skills.

The maturation and concurrent development of movement and posture follow a deliberate pattern for learning of skilled acts. Mobility develops from synchronized coactivated flexor and extensor muscles that provide the stabilizing forces for posture. Hand and finger control develops from visually directed grasping and releasing of objects.[9] Understanding the underlying physiology and pathophysiology of movement patterns is the basis of treatment.

Neurophysiological and Developmental Treatment Approaches

There are five recognized rehabilitation treatment programs for people with motor control deficits related to cerebral injury: the Root approach; the Bobath neurodevelopmental approach; the Brunnstrom approach; the proprioceptive neuromuscular facilitation; and the Carr and Shepard approach of motor relearning. Because the Bobath neurodevelopmental approach is used by many nurses, it is discussed here in greater detail.

Bobath Neurodevelopmental Treatment Approach

The Bobath approach is used primarily for patients with hemiplegia caused by stroke, brain injury, and cerebral palsy. The major goal is normalization of muscle tone, posture, movement, and function. Underlying premises include the following:[8–10]

- The sensation of movement is learned and not the movement itself.
- Every skilled activity takes place against a backdrop of

basic patterns of postural control, righting, equilibrium, and other protective reactions.

- When cerebral injury occurs, abnormal patterns of posture and movement develop that interfere with the performance of ADLs.
- Abnormal patterns develop because sensation is diverted into the abnormal patterns; this diversion must be stopped to reinstitute control over the motor output in developmental sequence.
- Eliciting the basic patterns of postural control, righting, and equilibrium is necessary, thus providing the normal stimuli while inhibiting abnormal patterns.
- People are allowed to feel, and thus relearn, normal movement patterns and postures.

Nurses can incorporate major principles of treatment into positioning, turning, transferring, and ADLs. These principles include the following:[8]

- Reintegration of function of the two sides of the body is emphasized during movement, ADLs, and bed or chair positioning so that bilateral segmental movement will occur.
- Proximal to distal positioning is recommended (tone in the limbs can be reduced from proximal points, such as the head, shoulder, or pelvic girdle).
- Weight bearing is provided on the affected side to normalize tone. This includes its role in sitting, lying, or rising.
- Tasks should begin from a symmetrical midline position with equal weight bearing on the affected and unaffected sides.
- Movement toward the affected side is encouraged.
- Straightening of the trunk and neck is encouraged to promote symmetry and normalization of tone and posture.
- Hemiplegic patients should be positioned in opposition to the spastic patterns of flexion and adduction in the upper extremity and extension in the lower extremity.

Positioning

Positioning the patient in proper body alignment is necessary to prevent development of musculoskeletal deformities, such as contracture and ankylosis; skin breakdown and pressure ulcers; and decreased vascular supply, thrombosis, and edema.

Positioning of the neuroscience patient may be complicated by nuchal rigidity, spasticity, abnormal posturing (e.g., decerebration), presence of a cast, position restriction secondary to surgery, and lacerations or abrasions associated with multiple trauma. These specific problems encountered in positioning change as the muscles undergo the various phases of recovery (Table 13-1).

A few basic principles are guides for positioning the patient in bed:

- The unconscious patient should be repositioned every 1 to 2 hours around the clock. As consciousness is regained, independent movement in bed and participation in self-care activities are encouraged to maintain muscle strength and tone. Proper positioning should be taught to the patient if he or she has the cognitive ability to participate.
- If spasticity is present, frequent repositioning will be necessary. Splinting and casting to inhibit tone may be applied by a physical therapist.
- Any restrictions of position should be posted conspicuously at the head of the patient's bed and included in the nursing care plan.
- A sufficient number of pillows should be available to maintain body alignment.
- Trochanter rolls, sandbags, and other positioning devices may be used.
- If an arm is weak or paralyzed, it should be positioned to approximate the joint space in the glenoid cavity. The affected arm should not be pulled. A pillow or small wedge in the axillary region will help prevent adduction of the shoulder.
- Special resting hand splints may be ordered to prevent contracture; they should be removed periodically to assess the skin for pressure areas.
- Edema of the extremities, particularly the hands, can be controlled by positioning and elevating the hand higher than the elbow.
- An elastic glove may be ordered to control hand edema.
- Prevention of footdrop is a concern in the lower extremities. Foot positioning devices, such as high-top sneakers or special splints, may be ordered.
- Heels should be kept off the bed to prevent pressure

Table 13-1 • PATTERNS OF MUSCLE RECOVERY IN HEMIPLEGIA

STAGE	NAME	ONSET	DESCRIPTION
I	Flaccidity	From the time of injury to 2 or 3 d after	No tendon reflexes or resistance to passive movement
II	Spasticity (late onset of spasticity indicates a poorer prognosis)	2 d to 5 wk	Hyperactive tendon reflexes and exaggerated response to minimal stimuli
III	Synergy (flexion, then extension)	2–3 wk	Simultaneous flexion of muscle groups in response to flexion of a single muscle (e.g., an attempt to flex the elbow results in contraction of the fingers, elbow, and shoulder)
IV	Near normal, possible weakness or slight incoordination may still be present (late return of tendon reflexes indicates a poor prognosis)	1 wk–6 mo	Control of voluntary movement; recovery occurs predictably from the proximal muscles of the extremity to the distal muscles (i.e., voluntary movement of the hand and foot is last to recover and tends to be weaker)

ulcers from developing. A pillow placed crosswise to elevate the lower legs may be helpful, or heel guards may be applied. (In many instances, the patient will already be wearing elastic stockings and air boots.)

Side-Lying Position

An unconscious patient, or one with a diminished or absent swallowing or gag reflex, should not be positioned supine because of the possible aspiration of secretions or occlusion of the airway by the tongue. Therefore, positioning in the true supine position is reserved only for the conscious patient. The side-lying position with the head of the bed elevated 10 to 30 degrees facilitates drainage of secretions from the mouth. The head should be placed in a neutral position. A soft collar or towel roll can be used to maintain the neutral position and prevent hyperflexion, which would partially obstruct the airway and impede venous drainage from the brain. Proper body alignment is maintained through the use of pillows and positioners.

With a patient for whom long-term bed rest is ordered, a modified position halfway between the supine and side-lying position may be necessary to relieve pressure on body surfaces. This patient can be positioned in good body alignment with the head turned slightly to facilitate drainage of oral secretions and to maintain a patent airway.

Exercise Programs

Voluntary muscles will lose tone and strength if they are not used. Patients with neurological deficits involving paresis and paralysis and those confined to prolonged bed rest are subject to these deleterious muscle effects of immobility (Table 13-2).

Because the flexor and adductor muscles are stronger than the extensors and abductors, contractures of the flexor and adductor muscles will develop quickly if preventive measures are not instituted. An exercise program must be followed aggressively to maintain muscle tone and function, prevent additional disability, and aid in the restoration of motor function.

Range-of-motion exercises include the full range of movement that each joint of the body can *normally* perform. A patient who cannot carry out independent range-of-motion exercises should be assisted in these activities by the nurse. After radiographic studies have been done to rule out fractures and verification has been made that no other medical problems or medical treatments contraindicate movement of a particular body part, range-of-motion exercises should begin.

Exercises can be classified into the following categories:

- **Passive:** motion provided to a body joint by another person or outside force
- **Active:** voluntary motion to a body joint that is independently executed by the individual
- **Active assistive:** motion to a body joint accomplished by the patient with the assistance of another person
- **Active resistive:** motion voluntarily provided to a body joint against resistance
- **Isometric** or **muscle-setting:** exercises accomplished by alternately tightening and relaxing the muscle without joint movement

The exercise program prescribed will depend on the stage of illness and the particular disabilities. In the acute stages of illness, a physical therapist may come to the patient's bedside once or twice daily to administer specific exercises. If only range-of-motion exercises are prescribed, nurses will be the care-provider administering these exercises. After the patient's condition improves, he or she will be taken to the physical medicine department where equipment is available for a more sophisticated, aggressive rehabilitation program. The nurse can reinforce and integrate the skills into other aspects of care. In addition, the patient's family can be taught how to carry out the prescribed exercises.

Passive Range-of-Motion Exercises

When passive range-of-motion exercises are administered, two factors must be considered: the joint being exercised and the placement of the caregiver's hands when carrying out the exercise properly. One hand is placed above the joint to provide support against gravity and any unwanted movement. The other hand gently moves the joint through its normal range of motion.

Passive range-of-motion exercises are usually administered at least four times daily and may be incorporated, in part, with other procedures, such as bathing or repositioning.

- Choose a time when the patient is rested, comfortable, and pain free to gain cooperation.
- Explain what is being done, even if the patient is apparently unconscious.
- Position in proper body alignment, and drape, as necessary, to avoid undue exposure. Drawing the curtains offers privacy and excludes environmental stimuli in the instance of an easily distracted patient.
- Provide a comfortable room temperature to prevent chilling, shivering, and unwanted muscle contractions.
- Maintain good posture to ensure efficient body movement; face the patient to observe facial reaction to the exercises.
- The movements of the exercise should be slow, smooth, and rhythmical.

▌▌▌ **Table 13–2** • EFFECTS OF PROLONGED IMMOBILIZATION ON THE MUSCULOSKELETAL SYSTEM

STRUCTURE	INITIAL CHANGES	ADVANCED CHANGES
Bones	Skeletal malalignment; calcium loss	Skeletal deformities Generalized osteoporosis
Joints	Joint stiffness; mobility limitation; shortening or stretching of ligaments	Ankylosis
Muscles	Muscle weakening; shortening or stretching of tendons	Muscle atrophy Fibrotic changes and muscle contractures

- Move the body part to the point of resistance and stop.
- Move the body part to the point of pain and stop.
- If the patient becomes excessively fatigued, discontinue the exercises.

Although the physiotherapist may move a body part beyond the point of pain or resistance for selected patients, this is not within the scope of nursing practice and should be avoided unless specifically prescribed. As the patient's condition improves, self-care should be encouraged for as many activities as possible. Because return of motor function is a slow process, the patient should be encouraged to carry out the exercises and be reminded of the need to continue with these activities as part of the rehabilitation program.

Other Exercises

Specific exercises, such as lifting hand weights, may be ordered to strengthen a weakened arm. Encourage the patient to engage in these activities. Be sure that the necessary equipment is at hand. Adapt activities to provide movement for specific muscle groups. For example, providing a ball of yarn for a female patient who enjoys knitting can improve motor function of a weakened hand while providing sensory stimulation.

Balancing and Sitting Activities

After the patient's condition has stabilized and range-of-motion exercises have begun, the next skills acquired are balancing and sitting. For patients who have been confined to bed for a long time, it will be necessary to progress slowly. The head of the bed must be raised gradually over days to overcome orthostatic hypotension. Monitor the physiological response by assessing the blood pressure and pulse, skin color and dryness, and asking the patient whether he or she is experiencing dizziness or lightheadedness. Record baseline signs and symptoms. After the head of the bed is raised the prescribed number of degrees, again assess for a drop in blood pressure; a thready, rapid pulse; paleness; diaphoresis; dizziness; or light-headedness. If these signs quickly reverse, no action may be necessary. Sustained symptoms require lowering the head of the bed slightly until symptoms subside. Because many neurological patients are placed at a 30-degree angle while confined to bed, not too much adjustment may be necessary for them to tolerate the change to a vertical position. For those maintained in a flat position or at a 10-degree angle, the adjustment will take longer.

For paraplegic or quadriplegic patients, orthostatic hypotension can be a stubborn problem to manage, because extensive vasomotor paralysis results in a subsequent drop in blood pressure when the vertical position is assumed. Wearing an abdominal binder and thigh-high elastic stockings and elevating the leg rests of the wheelchair help to combat hypotension. These patients, particularly quadriplegics, may require a special program in the physical therapy department in which a tilt table is used to raise the patient gradually over several days.

Balancing

Balancing, the ability to sit or stand erect, can be achieved through consciously using both sides of the body, focusing on the symmetrical midline point, and using support devices that help to steady the patient's center of gravity. Use of a back or neck brace for a cord injury patient can make the difference between success and failure. The hemiplegic patient should be in the sitting position and instructed to support himself or herself with the unaffected arm and hand. The hand should be placed flat on the bed slightly behind or at the side as a means of support. Because there is a tendency to slouch to the affected side, the patient should be reminded to sit straight and erect, focused on a balanced midline. Some conscious patients who have difficulty balancing while sitting in bed do well when they are helped to sit at the side of the bed or in a chair with their feet flat on the floor.

In unconscious patients, the same process for overcoming orthostatic hypotension can be used; however, information regarding the adjustment of these patients must be derived from objective signs. Ability to balance will not be possible until the level of consciousness improves; however, the patient can be propped to the required position.

After balance in the sitting position has been mastered, the patient is ready to begin balancing in the standing position at the bedside.

Sitting

Both conscious and unconscious patients can sit in a chair, although the unconscious patient is not positioned in the sitting position on the side of the bed for obvious safety concerns. The conscious patient may sit on the side of the bed, using the over-bed table and pillows for support. The chair selected should provide firm support and have a high back and arms, especially if the patient has motor weakness or paralysis. For the weak, debilitated patient who cannot hold up the head or neck, a high-back chair that extends to the top of the head is most effective. This patient often has a neck brace, which should be applied for sitting.

A lapboard, pillows, and the overbed table, rolled down to a comfortable height, are helpful for providing added support while positioning a patient in a chair. Pillows or rolls are used to support the arms in the desired position. The feet are positioned flat on the floor. The pressure on the bottom of the feet assists in stretching the heel cord. Footdrop may develop if stretching of the cord is not provided. The head must be positioned carefully so that the airway or tracheostomy is not obstructed. Any equipment that is in place, such as a urinary catheter or feeding tube, should be checked to ensure patency and freedom from traction.

If the patient retains some independent motor function, necessary equipment is placed nearby, possibly on an over-bed table that has been lowered and placed in front of the patient's chair. The call bell is placed closer or attached to the patient's clothing if there are neurological deficits that could interfere with the ability to find the cord easily.

The patient is observed often; tolerance to being out of bed is evaluated. The patient should not be allowed to become overtired. It is best to plan a schedule that allows for periods of bed rest and out-of-bed activity based on an individual assessment of the patient's tolerance and fatigue.

Mobility: Transfer and Ambulation

When considering a patient's mobility, the type(s) of transfer used reflect(s) a continuum from complete dependency to complete independence:

- Two-person lift: physical transfer by at least two nursing staff members; no active patient participation
- Mechanical lift: transfer using a lifting device that is operated by nursing staff members; no active patient participation

After the patient is able to balance and sit, he or she is ready for transfer activities:

- The patient, with assistance from one or more nursing staff members, stands and pivots on the unaffected leg; moderate patient participation is required. A transfer belt is worn around the patient's waist to allow the nurse to grasp it to support the patient. Inspect the transfer belt to be sure it is not worn or defective
- With the assistance of a slide board, the patient is able to transfer from the bed to the chair with or without assistance

- Independent transfer is the patient's ability to transfer without assistance

The degree of assistance necessary for transfer and ambulating can be classified as follows:

- Dependent: maximal, moderate, or minimal
- Contact guard: provision of verbal cues and minimal physical support during the activity, such as holding the arm or waist during ambulation
- Supervision: provision of verbal cues only, as necessary

Transfer Activities

A few basic principles for assisting patients should be kept in mind:

- As a rule, transfer toward the unaffected side.
- Patients should wear properly fitted, sensible shoes rather than slippers, because most slippers offer little support and tend to provide little traction on the floor.
- If a paretic arm is in need of support, it should be supported by gently holding the forearm. The nurse should

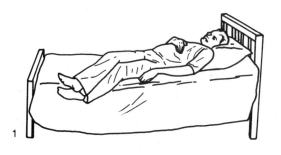

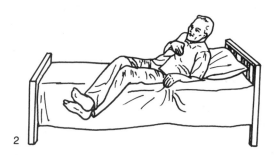

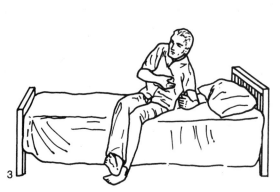

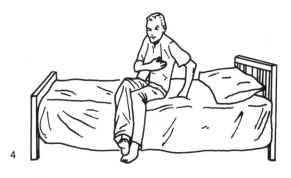

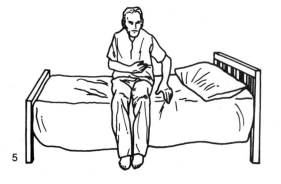

Figure 13–2 • Getting up and sitting on side of the bed. *Clockwise:* (1) Use strong hand to place weak arm across abdomen. Slide strong foot under weak ankle; move both legs to side of the bed on strong side and over side. (2) Grasp edge of mattress as illustrated and push with elbow and forearm against the bed. (3) Come to a half-sitting position, supporting body weight on strong forearm. (4) Move hand to the rear, pushing up to a full sitting position. (5) Move around until sitting securely on side of bed; uncross legs. (*Up and Around.* Reprinted with permission of the American Heart Association.)

never tug on the paretic arm by pulling on the upper arm or shoulder.

- If balance is unsteady, the nurse should stand on the affected side, ready to grasp a belt around the patient's waist (can grasp the top of pants or pajama bottoms, but this is not as secure). A belt is strongly recommended.
- If the patient's knees buckle and additional assistance is required, the nurse stands in front of the patient and pushes with his or her knee against the patient's unaffected knee to lock the knee in position and prevent it from buckling. This action enables the patient to bear some of his or her own body weight.
- A walker or four-point cane may be used for support.
- The patient must learn to stand erect before ambulation training can begin. If difficulty is encountered in raising the affected foot, a special shoe with a plastic foot brace may be helpful.
- Other transfer activities that the patient may need to learn, depending on the permanence of the disability, include transferring from the wheelchair to the toilet, bathtub, or automobile.

Transfer Activity: From Lying in Bed to a Sitting Position

Hemiplegic Patients

For the hemiplegic patient who wants to assume a sitting position from a position lying in bed on the back (Fig. 13-2), these steps are followed:

- Move toward or roll onto the side of the bed on which you intend to sit.
- Slip the unaffected leg under the affected leg at an angle so that the unaffected leg becomes a transfer cradle for the affected limb.
- Place the affected arm on the abdomen or lap.
- Push off the mattress with the unaffected elbow, raising your upper body, while turning your hips toward the side of the bed on which you intend to sit.
- Swing the unaffected leg (on which the affected leg rests) over the side of the bed, and use the unaffected hand to push up.
- Once in the sitting position, lean on the unaffected hand to maintain an erect position.

Paraplegic or Incomplete Quadriplegic Patients

Most transfer activities need to be done for quadriplegic and some incomplete quadriplegic patients. A trapeze over the bed and a sliding board can be used to assist paraplegic patients and some quadriparetic patients.

Transfer Activity: From Sitting on the Side of the Bed to a Back-Lying Position

Returning to the back-lying position from a sitting position on the side of the bed involves the following steps (Fig. 13-3):

- Sit slightly above the center on the side of the bed so that you will be in the proper position on the mattress once the back-lying position is assumed.

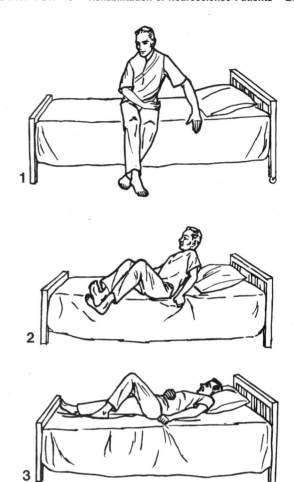

Figure 13–3 • Moving from a sitting position on edge of bed to a back-lying position. (*1*) Place weak arm across the lap. Slide strong foot under weak ankle. (*2*) With strong hand, grasp edge of mattress near the hips and press against bed, lowering body to the bed as the elbow bends. At the same time, swing legs onto bed. (Note: Patient should be seated in the proper spot so that head will be on pillow after lying down.) (*3*) Uncross legs. Bend the strong hip and knee and push against bed with heel to move body up or down in bed to proper position. (*Up and Around.* Reprinted with permission of the American Heart Association)

- Place the affected arm on your lap.
- Slip the unaffected foot under the affected ankle.
- Place the unaffected hand on the edge of the mattress next to the unaffected hip.
- Press the hand into the mattress, lowering your body onto the bed while the elbow bends.
- Simultaneously swing the unaffected leg onto the bed as your body is lowered.
- Uncross the ankle and bend the unaffected knee; push up or pull down on the bed, as necessary, with the bending and pulling action of the knee to position yourself comfortably.

Transfer Activity: From a Sitting Position on the Bed to a Chair

Transferring from the bed into a chair requires planning. If a chair is used, it should provide firm support and have arms. In the case of a wheelchair, the wheels of the chair should be locked with the footrests up.

Hemiplegic Patients

Hemiplegic patients may complete this type of transfer by following these steps (Fig. 13-4):

- Free any catheter or tubes that are secured to the bed.
- Place the chair at a slight angle as close as possible to the bed on the unaffected side.
- With feet close together, the patient leans forward slightly, puts the unaffected hand on the mattress edge, and pushes off to a standing position, bearing weight on the unaffected side.
- Once balance has been maintained and is steady enough for momentary release of support, move the strong hand to the farthest armrest of the chair.
- Keep the body weight well forward; pivot on the unaffected foot, and slowly lower to a sitting position.

Paraplegic or Incomplete Quadriplegic Patients

The paraplegic or quadriplegic patient will need a dependent slide board transfer, which provides less strain on the back than a lift into the chair; the aid of two or three people may be needed, depending on the patient's height and weight. Some paraplegic patients can learn to transfer themselves from the bed to a chair with the use of a slide board.

Transfer Activity: From Chair to Bed

When transferring from a chair to a sitting position on the bed, the following technique is used (Fig. 13-5):

- The chair should be at a slight angle, as close to the bed as possible; the patient's unaffected side should be closest to the bed.
- Place feet firmly on the floor close to the chair, with the unaffected heel slightly in back of the affected heel and directly under the edge of the seat.
- Move forward in the chair, placing the unaffected hand on the front portion of the arm of the chair.
- Lean forward over the unaffected leg; push off to a standing position so that the feet are slightly apart with most of the weight being borne by the unaffected leg.
- After regaining balance with the support of the armrest, lean slightly forward, reach for the edge of the mattress with the unaffected hand, and pivot on the unaffected foot, slowly lowering to a sitting position.

Ambulation

Hemiplegic Patients

Before hemiplegic patients can ambulate, they must first learn to stand and balance themselves in an upright position. Standing exercises can begin at the bedside and proceed to the parallel bars in the physical therapy department. Standing helps to reinforce a positive body image and feeling of wholeness and also improves overall physical fitness.

Once standing has been mastered, an evaluation is conducted to determine whether any special bracing or support equipment is necessary. If the patient is developing footdrop or has a tendency to drag the foot, a short leg plastic brace or a brace with a spring in it can be helpful. These types of

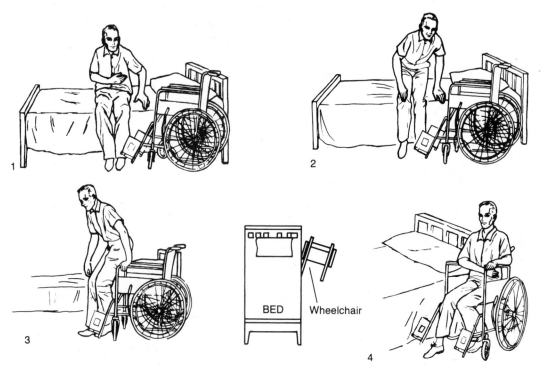

Figure 13–4 • Doing a standing transfer from bed to wheelchair. *Clockwise:* (*1*) Place wheelchair at 45° angle to bed on patient's stronger side; lock brakes and raise footrest; move to the edge of bed. (*2*) Push down on bed with stronger arm; push off bed and stand, keeping weight on the stronger leg. (*3*) Move stronger arm and leg to opposite side of wheelchair. (*4*) Lean forward and sit down while holding on to wheelchair arm. (*Up and Around.* Reprinted with permission of the American Heart Association.)

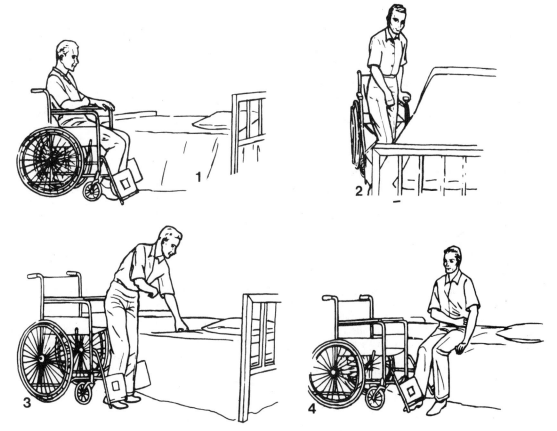

Figure 13–5 • Moving from wheelchair to bed. *Clockwise:* (1) Place wheelchair at 45° angle to the bed on the patient's stronger side; lock brakes and raise footrest; move to edge of chair. (2) Grasp chair arm with stronger arm and push off the chair to a standing position bearing weight on stronger leg. (3) Move strong hand to edge of bed for support. (4) Lean forward, pivot on stronger foot, and slowly sit down. (*Up and Around.* Reprinted with permission of the American Heart Association).

braces are designed to prevent extreme plantar flexion. If the patient is weak, a crutch, four-point cane, or walker may be necessary (Fig. 13-6). A sling may be applied to the affected arm for balance while walking. The sling should be adjusted to approximate the glenoid (shoulder) joint space. The affected arm should not be pulled.

Ambulation or gait training often begins at the parallel bars, where the patient learns to bend a knee and then extend it again. This exercise is alternated from one knee to the other. If the affected knee continues to be weak and tends to buckle, a longer leg brace can be designed to compensate for this disability.

When helping the patient to ambulate, the nurse should walk on the patient's affected side. Added support may be given by grasping the patient's belt or the top of the patient's pants or by applying a safety belt. The patient may feel more secure walking near the wall with the unaffected side nearest the wall. A handrail in the corridor or room is another source of support and security. In the physical therapy department, climbing and descending stairs are taught.

For the patient who is unable to master ambulation, wheelchair mobility may be achieved using the unaffected hand to propel the wheelchair on a level surface. This provides a degree of independence. An electric (i.e., battery-operated) wheelchair is another alternative for providing mobility.

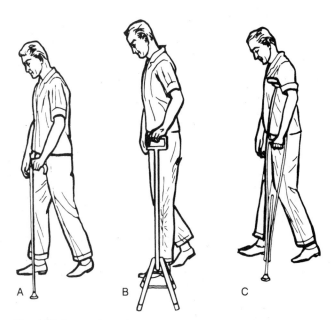

Figure 13–6 • Assistive devices, such as a cane (*A*), a wide-base cane (*B*), or crutches (*C*), may be necessary for ambulation. (*Up and Around.* Reprinted with permission of the American Heart Association.)

It is impossible to state the exact intervals at which balancing, sitting, standing, and walking should be introduced and mastered. Age, severity of illness, other neurological deficits, chronic conditions, endurance, and complications are all factors. Attitude and motivation are important factors in the rehabilitation process. Frequent assessment allows systematic evaluation of the patient's needs so that rehabilitation can progress steadily toward the greatest level of independence.

Paraplegic or Incomplete Quadriplegic Patients

The physiological and psychological benefits of ambulation need to be considered. Research has contributed greatly to ambulation options for spinal injured people. Some paraplegic and a few quadriparetic patients can walk with the help of braces and canes. For others, ambulation is possible using functional electrical stimulation and a walker.

▌▌ **T a b l e 1 3 – 3** • SUMMARY OF MAJOR PERCEPTUAL DEFICITS AND NURSING MANAGEMENT

DEFICIT	ASSESSMENT	INTERVENTION
Perception of Illness		
• Denial of hemiplegia or other motor or sensory deficits • *Anosognosia*—inability to recognize, denial of, or unawareness of a loss of or defect in physical function	• Fails to use the involved side of the body without being reminded to do so • Shows a lack of concern about the disability and fails to understand how paralysis and other deficits will affect lifestyle • Lacks awareness or denies outright the presence of paralysis or other deficits on the involved side • May deny all sensory input on the affected side	• Accept the patient's perception of self, and provide for the safety and cleanliness of the area. • Provide tactile stimuli to the affected side by touching or stroking the affected side by itself, rather than stimulating both sides simultaneously. • Teach the patient to position the affected extremity carefully and to check its position by looking at it; if the patient completely ignores the area, use positioning to improve his or her perception (e.g., position the patient facing the affected side so that the area is in view).
Body Image		

• *Body image*—concept one has of the sum of one's body parts in relationship to the whole
  —Nursing diagnosis: Body Image Disturbance
• *Unilateral neglect*—a condition in which the patient ignores the hemiplegic side
  —Nursing diagnosis: Unilateral Neglect
	• If asked to draw a clock, will not draw the side of the clock same as that on which neglect is present	• Encourage the patient to handle the affected side.
		* Teach visual scanning of the environment to overcome one-sided neglect.
		* Approach the patient from the unaffected side until ready to learn compensatory scanning techniques.
		* Place the food tray toward the unaffected side.
		* Use verbal cues to guide the patient toward the affected side.
		* Provide a mirror, if possible.
		* Position the call light and other equipment on the patient's unaffected side.

Spatial Relationships		
• *Hemianopia*—loss of vision in half of the visual field. —Nursing diagnosis: Sensory/Perceptual Alterations	• Neglects input from the affected side	• See last six interventions listed above (with asterisks). • *Note* visual changes commonly present that change about every 6 months. No ophthalmological check-up is necessary until 6 months have transpired.

• Defects in:
  —Localized objects in space
  —Estimating size
  —Judging distances
  —Remembering arrangement of objects in the environment
  —Finding way to places or back to room
  —Telling time
  —Right-left discrimination
	• Has difficulty walking through a doorway
	• Exhibits impaired recall of the placement of objects in a familiar environment, such as the locations of windows and doors in the room
	• Has difficulty learning the way around the hospital unit (such as how to go from the hospital room to the kitchen and back)
	• Experiences difficulty reading and computing figures because of an inability to move eyes from left to right on a page or to line up numbers accurately to compute figures
	• Is unable to identify left or right
		• Provide verbal cues.
		• Do not allow the patient to wander around the unit alone.
		• Use descriptive terms to identify areas, rather than "left" or "right" directions (e.g., "Lift the unaffected leg" but not "good/bad").
		• Use a mirror to help patients adjust position if they have difficulty maintaining their position.

Table 13-3 • SUMMARY OF MAJOR PERCEPTUAL DEFICITS
AND NURSING MANAGEMENT (Continued)

DEFICIT	ASSESSMENT	INTERVENTION
Agnosia		
• Inability to recognize familiar environmental objects through the senses —Visual agnosia: inability to recognize familiar objects by sight (Nursing diagnosis: Sensory/Perceptual Alterations) —Auditory agnosia: inability to recognize familiar objects through sound (Nursing diagnosis: Sensory/Perceptual Alterations) —Tactile agnosia (astereognosis): inability to recognize familiar objects through the sense of touch (Nursing diagnosis: Sensory/Perceptual Alterations)	• Ask patient to identify common objects by sight. • Observe the patient's response to common sounds, such as a ringing telephone. • With the patient's eye closed, place a common object in his or her hand, and ask the patient to identify the object.	• Use other, intact senses to identify environmental stimuli (e.g., if the patient has visual agnosia, have him or her use voices and sounds to identify familiar objects). • Use the drill method of teaching to help the patient relearn objects that cannot be identified. • Protect the patient from injury • Interpret the patient's behavior for the family.
Apraxia		
• Inability to carry out a learned, voluntary act in the absence of paralysis —Constructional apraxia (Nursing diagnosis: Self-Care Deficit) —Dressing apraxia (Nursing diagnosis: Dressing Self-Care Deficit)	• May exhibit clumsiness or an inability to carry out activities of daily living (ADLs) correctly; may be unable to sequence components of a skilled act • May have difficulty completing the task of drawing a clock and placing the hands at a given time • May have difficulty dressing self (e.g., may put both arms in the same sleeve)	• Encourage patient to participate in ADLs. • Correct any misuse of equipment or incorrect actions; guide the patient's hand, if necessary. • Reteach any forgotten skills. • Protect the patient from injury. • Interpret the patient's behavior for the family.

For a person who needs a wheelchair, the many different types available need to be matched to the needs of the particular patient. Battery-operated wheelchairs that are activated by a breath sensor located near the mouth of the quadriplegic patient provide a degree of independence. Even a quadriplegic patient with an injury at C-5 can use this type of wheelchair. Incomplete quadriplegics with a C-2 to C-5 injury can use chin, eye, or tongue control systems. The paraplegic patient does well in a standard wheelchair or an electric wheelchair operated by hand controls. Wheelchair users can have different chairs for different activities, such as a sports wheelchair for quad rugby, basketball, and others. There is increased awareness of the need to monitor shoulder function in wheelchair users, because shoulder problems increase with age.

Computer-operated equipment programmed to execute many mundane activities, such as closing draperies or turning out lights, has afforded a greater degree of independence to the disabled person. Computer technology for adaptive living is developing rapidly. As the technology improves, the cost decreases, making the equipment more accessible for the patient.

MANAGEMENT OF THE SKIN

The neuroscience patient is at high risk for the development of pressure ulcers because of motor, sensory, and vasomotor deficits related to neurological disease and immobility. Ac-

cording to the AHCPR clinical practice guideline, *Pressure Ulcers in Adults: Prediction and Prevention* (1992),[11] a **pressure ulcer** is any lesion caused by unrelieved pressure resulting in damage of underlying tissue.

Nursing Management of the Patient With Altered Skin Integrity

Assessment

Pressure ulcers are usually over bony prominences and are graded or staged to classify the degree of tissue damage observed. **Impaired Skin Integrity** related to immobility or the effects of pressure, friction, shearing, or maceration is the nursing diagnosis. The AHCPR Pressure Ulcers Guideline (1992)[11] is the standard of practice for prediction, prevention, and early treatment of pressure ulcers in adults. This publication set the standard of evidence-based practice to which all nurses are held; this is the standard of care for neuroscience patients. Numerous research-based publications are available that address implementation and outcomes with use of these standards.

Interventions

Follow the AHCPR pressure ulcer guidelines cited previously.

SENSORY-PERCEPTUAL DEFICITS

Perception is a complex intellectual process of recognizing, interpreting, and integrating sensory stimuli into meaningful information from the internal and external environments. Whereas the left side of the brain is dominant for language, the right side of the brain is dominant for perception of two- and three-dimensional shapes, faces, color, spatial positions, and orientation in space. The parietal lobe is particularly important in perception. Perceptual deficits are often seen in patients with head injury and stroke and may take many forms, including deficits in perception of self, body image, illness, spatial relationships, agnosia, and apraxia.

Nursing Management of Patients With Perceptual Deficits

Assessment

The major perceptual deficits are summarized in Table 13-3. Several nursing diagnoses are applicable; the following are possible nursing diagnoses:

- Sensory/Perceptual Alterations
- Body Image Disturbance
- Impaired Environmental Interpretation Syndrome
- Impaired Memory
- Self-Esteem Disturbance
- Risk for Injury
- Confusion
- Personal Identity Disturbance

Possible collaborative problems include the neglect syndrome and cognitive deficits.

Interventions

Nursing interventions are directed at helping the patient to compensate for any deficits. Patients with perceptual deficits are impulsive and often lack awareness of their deficits. This behavior also places a patient at higher risk for injury.

COMMUNICATION DEFICITS

Aphasia is the loss of ability to use language and to communicate thoughts verbally or in writing. It results from injury to the cortex of the left hemisphere in the posterior frontal or anterior temporal lobes. Aphasia can be subdivided into nonfluent and fluent aphasia. The nursing diagnosis for a patient with aphasia is **Impaired Verbal Communication**. Chart 13-3 summarizes aphasia and the nursing guidelines for working with affected patients. See Chapter 8 for further discussion of aphasia.

Generally, the greatest degree of spontaneous functional return occurs in the first 3 to 6 months following injury, although substantial deficits may persist. Additional improvement can occur for 2 or 3 more years. Each patient must be viewed as an individual in the rehabilitative process. Age, area of injury, presence of other health problems, and motivation are a few factors having a direct bearing on recovery.

Nursing Management of Patients With Altered Communication

Assessment

The nurse will need to assess the patient's communication system to determine which skills are intact or deficient. Assess the following abilities:

- Speaking in response to an open-ended question, such as "tell me about your hobbies"
- Using vocabulary, grammar, and syntax correctly; note spontaneity, hesitancy in pronunciation, and speed of speech
- Responding appropriately to verbal instructions that are one to three steps in complexity
- Responding appropriately to written instructions that are one to three steps in complexity
- Expressing ideas in writing; writing a response to such requests as "Write your name" or "Describe this room"

Note difficulty in expressing thoughts verbally, finding the correct word (word finding), forming words or sentences, following written instructions, and expressing ideas in writing. Other abnormal findings include slurring of speech. As a result of stroke, some patients may be unable to speak the primary language that they had been using and revert to a language spoken in the past.

Several factors associated with neurological illness can mask an accurate assessment of communication skills, such as:

- Altered level of consciousness
- Decreased visual acuity
- Hearing loss
- Dysarthria
- Cognitive deficits (decreased attention or concentration) or short-term memory deficits
- Visual field cuts (hemianopsia)
- Absence of prescription eyeglasses
- Absence of hearing aid normally worn
- Unfamiliarity with the language

A short attention span or inability to concentrate influences the ability to follow verbal or nonverbal cues. Because concentration and attention seem to vary from day to day or even minute to minute, there can be great differences in the patient's ability to communicate at any time.

The following are possible nursing diagnoses:

- Sensory/Perceptual Alterations
- Impaired Verbal Communication
- Impaired Memory
- Collaborative problems include cognitive deficits, aphasia, and neglect syndrome

CHART 13–3 • Deficits In Communications: Descriptions and Nursing Guidelines

Nonfluent Aphasia (Broca's Aphasia)

- The patient will have difficulty expressing thoughts verbally or in writing.
- The degree of difficulty can range from mild word finding difficulty to limitation of expression to "yes" and "no."
- The ability to understand the written and spoken word remains intact.
- The site of injury is Broca's area (in the frontal lobe close to the area of the motor cortex that controls the movement of the lips, jaw, tongue, soft palate, and vocal cords).
- Broca's area contains the memory for motor patterns of speech.

Fluent Aphasia (Wernicke's Aphasia)

- Wernicke's area (in the temporal lobe flanked by Heschl's gyrus on one side and the angular gyrus on the other) is the site of injury.
- Heschl's gyrus is the primary receptor area for auditory and visual fields.
- Wernicke's area provides the connective pathways that bridge the primary auditory cortex and the angular gyrus.
- The patient hears the sounds of speech, but the parts of the brain that give meaning to the sounds of speech are not activated, so that comprehension of speech is impaired.
- Because the control of the musculature for speech is not impaired, the patient can speak but makes many errors when using words.
- Because patients are unaware of their imperfect messages, they may talk at great length.
- The patient's ability to express words in writing may also be compromised.

Global Aphasia

- Results from a massive stroke or lesion involving Broca's and Wernicke's areas of the brain.
- Global aphasia is a combination of expressive and receptive aphasia whereby the patient is left with little, if any, intact communication system.
- Affected patients can neither understand what they hear or read nor convey their thoughts in speech or writing.
- Prognosis is poor.

Mild Nonfluent Aphasia

- Stimulate conversation and ask open-ended questions.
- Allow patients time to search for the words to express themselves.
- Disregard choice of incorrect words.
- Be supportive and accepting of the patient's behavior as he or she deals with the frustration of finding the right words of expression.
- Assure patients that their speech will gradually improve with time.

Severe Nonfluent Aphasia

- Accept self-expression by whatever means possible (e.g., pantomime, pointing).
- Do not pressure the patient into self-expression.
- Be supportive of patients, and accept their behavior if they show frustration (by crying or some other means) because of difficulty encountered in expressing themselves.
- Provide a loose-leaf notebook with pictures of common objects so that the patient can point to the picture when unable to say the word.
- Tell the patient that speech skills can be relearned, given time.
- Anticipate the patient's needs.

Mild Fluent Aphasia

- Stand close to patients (within their line of vision) so that they can also observe lip movements as an added cue to communication.
- Speak slowly and distinctly, using simple sentences and a common vocabulary.
- Use simple gestures as an added cue in speaking.
- Repeat or rephrase any instructions if they are not understood.
- Speak in a normal speaking voice.

Severe Fluent Aphasia

- Use whatever vocabulary the patient can still understand.
- Use very simple sentences or phrases that express only the critical essence of a thought.
- Divide any tasks into small units, working with the individual units to accomplish the task.
- Use pantomime, pointing, touch, and so forth to express ideas.
- Anticipate the patient's needs.

Interventions

To work effectively with the patient, the nurse should assume a calm, reassuring, and supportive manner that conveys acceptance of the patient's behavior. Spending time and assuming an unhurried approach reinforce this message. Guidelines for working with the aphasic patient are included in Chart 13-3. Deficits in the ability to communicate are devastating, frustrating to the patient, and may result in fear and depression.

SWALLOWING DEFICITS

Swallowing is a complex process of ingesting solid or liquid food while protecting the airway (Fig. 13-7). Glenn cites four phases of swallowing:[12]

- **Oral preparatory phase:** Food is taken into the mouth and chewed, forming a bolus.
- **Oral phase:** The bolus of food is centered and moved to the posterior oropharynx.
- **Pharyngeal phase:** The swallowing reflex carries the bolus through the pharynx.

- **Esophageal phase:** Peristalsis carries the bolus to the stomach.

Several cranial nerves are involved in functions related to swallowing (Table 13-4.)

Regardless of whether the food is liquid or solid, protection of the airway is imperative to prevent the most serious of complications—aspiration. Aspiration is serious because it causes a chemical pneumonia. When thinking about aspiration, a picture of someone coughing vigorously comes to mind. This is the case if the gag and cough reflexes are intact. However, there is much discussion about "silent aspiration." A person with diminished or absent gag and cough reflexes can aspirate material without the usual evidence of coughing. In a conscious patient, a moist, wet voice may be noted. Usual symptoms of aspiration are absent. Silent aspiration may first be evident by an elevated temperature or adventitious lung sounds followed by a diagnosis of pneumonia by chest film.

With neurological disease, there can be deficits in the mechanisms controlling swallowing, and aspiration can result. The nursing diagnoses associated with swallowing deficits are **Impaired Swallowing** and **Risk for Aspiration**.

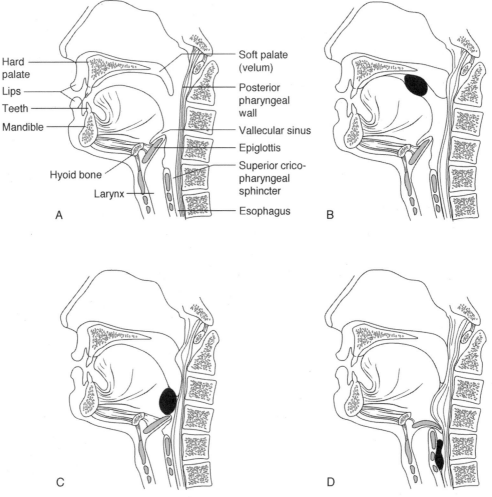

Hard palate
Lips
Teeth
Mandible
Hyoid bone
Larynx

Soft palate (velum)
Posterior pharyngeal wall
Vallecular sinus
Epiglottis
Superior crico-pharyngeal sphincter
Esophagus

A   B   C   D

Figure 13–7 • Components of the swallowing process.

Table 13-4 • CRANIAL NERVES INVOLVED IN SWALLOWING

CRANIAL NERVE (NUMBER)	MOTOR INNERVATION	SENSORY INNERVATION
Trigeminal (V)	Mandibular muscles for chewing and mastication	Two sensory areas of face (maxillary, mandibular)
Facial (VII)	Facial expression, including movement of lips; submandibular and sublingual salivary glands	Taste to anterior two-thirds of tongue
Glossopharyngeal (IX)	Stylopharyngeus muscle to pull up pharynx	Pharynx, tongue, and taste receptors of posterior one-third of tongue
Vagus (X)	Muscles of soft palate, pharynx, and larynx	Pharynx and larynx
Spinal accessory (XI)	Sternocleidomastoid and trapezius to hold head up and rotate head	None
Hypoglossal (XII)	Intrinsic muscle of tongue to move tongue	None

Nursing Management of the Patient With Impaired Swallowing

Assessment

Swallowing is a complex process (see Fig. 13-7 for normal swallowing). The defining characteristics for impaired swallowing are also related to the specific phases of swallowing listed previously (Table 13-5).

Before offering any food or drink orally, the gag and swallowing reflexes are assessed. The gag reflex on each side should be assessed, because an asymmetrical response is possible. The examiner can assess the swallowing reflex by placing her or his index finger on the top of the larynx and asking the patient to swallow. If the reflex is intact, the larynx will elevate (the epiglottis closes over the trachea), displacing the examiner's finger. If the gag or swallowing reflex is not intact, *nothing should be given orally* because the patient cannot protect the airway and will aspirate. Diagnostic tests may be ordered to identify the specific etiology of the dysphasia. Common diagnostic tests include the bedside swallow examination, modified barium swallow with videofluoroscopy, and videoendoscopy. A review of the video film will help to identify the specific portion of the sequence of swallowing that is problematic.

The following are major nursing diagnoses:

- Impaired Swallowing
- Risk for Aspiration

A possible collaborative problem is aspiration pneumonia.

Interventions

Supervise the patient during mealtime and snack time. There are some general interventions to facilitate swallowing. Specific suggestions, based on specific patient needs, may also be made. Consider these general points:

- Feed or eat in the upright, sitting position at a 90-degree angle; avoid slumping.
- The head should be tilted forward and the chin tucked in to prevent food moving to the posterior oropharynx before it has been chewed; if the patient is unable to maintain head position, the nurse can support the head with the palm of the hand against the forehead
- Encourage taking small bites and thorough chewing.
- For patients with hemiplegia or hemiparesis, place food on the unaffected side.
- The nurse should note consistency of food that is troublesome. (Some people have more difficulty with solid foods, and others will have more difficulty with liquids.)
- If "pocketing" of food is a problem, have the patient sweep the mouth with his or her finger after each bite to clear the food.
- The speech therapist can be helpful by suggesting an adaptive cup and special techniques to ensure swallowing.
- Discuss with the physician any persistent problems. If oral feeding is contraindicated, a feeding tube or gastrostomy tube can be considered (see Chapter 9).
- If cognitive deficits are present, the patient may have poor

 Table 13-5 • PHASES OF SWALLOWING

PHASES OF SWALLOWING	CHARACTERISTIC OBSERVATIONS; ALSO OBSERVE FOR EVIDENCE OF ASPIRATION
Oral phase	Drooling or loss of food particles on affected or side of chin Pocketing of food Excessive chewing Facial asymmetry or weakness Tongue weakness or limitation of movement Inability to close lips tightly or move lips Weakness or absence of gag reflex Weakness or absence of swallowing reflex Nasal drainage due to nasal regurgitation Loss of internal or external sensation of the oral cavity or face
Pharyngeal phase	Noted delayed or absence of swallowing Coughing while drinking fluids or eating liquids (e.g., soup) History of aspiration pneumonia Wet, gurgling, moist, or nasal voice, particularly during eating Frequent clearing of throat Complaints of burning (from drugs or other irritating material sticking and irritating tissue) or something sticking in back of throat
Esophageal phase	Burping or substernal distress due to esophageal reflux Coughing or wheezing

impulse control and may stuff the mouth hurriedly with food. If this occurs, the basis of the swallowing problem may be behavioral rather than neurological, and nursing interventions should be directed at managing the behavior and controlling distractions from the focus of eating. This patient requires mealtime supervision and verbal and nonverbal cues.

BLADDER DYSFUNCTION AND RETRAINING

Normal Bladder Function

Bladder control is an integrated function of the brainstem, spinal, and cerebral levels[13] (see Chapter 5).

- **Brain-stem pontine level:** The true micturition centers are located in the dorsal pons. During micturition, the medial pontine region is activated, and the lateral pontine region is inhibited. This activity produces coordinated bladder contraction and sphincter relaxation, resulting in bladder emptying. Disruption in the central nervous system *above* the sacral reflex center usually causes a hyperreflexic bladder and is classified as an upper motor neuron (UMN) injury.
- **Spinal level:** The *sacral reflex control center* of the bladder is located in spinal segments S-2 to S-4. The parasympathetic innervation of the pelvic nerve is responsible for bladder emptying, whereas the sympathetic (hypogastric nerve) and somatic (pudendal nerve) innervations promote retention of urine. Micturition involves a supraspinal-spinopontospinal reflex triggered by stimulation of tension receptors, which result in coordination of the contracted detrusor muscle and relaxation of the sphincter. Interruption of the descending suprasegmental pathways results in micturition through segmental spinospinal sacral reflexes that are triggered by perineal or nociceptive stimulation. The sphincter contractions are not well coordinated. Disruption at the sacral reflex center or in the peripheral nervous system causes an areflexic bladder, which is classified as a lower motor neuron (LMN) injury.
- **Cerebral level:** The micturition centers are controlled by input from the hypothalamus and the medial frontal cortex. Cortical input is responsible for voluntary control of the initiation and cessation of micturition. Lesions of the medial frontal lobes or hypothalamus can interrupt these pathways, resulting in involuntary micturition sometimes called **uninhibited bladder.**

Summary of Effects of Neurological Lesions on Micturition

People with neurological disease or injury may be unable to maintain normal urinary elimination patterns because of dysfunction at the brain-stem, spinal, or cerebral levels. Any disruption of the sensory or motor pathways in the central or peripheral nervous systems that have input to the bladder will cause a disruption in urinary elimination patterns.

Types of Bladder Dysfunction: Alterations in Urinary Elimination Patterns

There are many conceptual frameworks regarding altered urinary elimination, including UMN and LMN injury and a classification of neurogenic bladder types. (A **neurogenic bladder** is defined as any bladder disturbance that is attributable to motor or sensory pathways in the central or peripheral nervous systems that have input to the bladder. See Table 13-6 for a listing of neurogenic bladder types.) From a nursing perspective, nurses focus on assisting people to improve function through a functional health pattern framework; this is the approach taken in this chapter.

Alterations in urinary elimination patterns can be classified generally into urinary incontinence (UI) and urinary retention. Each of these two major classifications can be further subdivided into categories based on cause, characteristics, and pathophysiology to treat the problem effectively. It is important to be able to categorize accurately the type of altered urinary elimination pattern present. The following sections discuss UI and urinary retention with emphasis on altered function in neurological patients.

Urinary Incontinence

Urinary incontinence can be associated with various problems, such as a diminished level of consciousness; cerebral injury, especially to the frontal lobe; or spinal cord injury. The Clinical Practice Guidelines for *Urinary Incontinence in Adults*, published in 1992, is the definitive resource for health professionals in the management of adult UI in ambulatory and non-ambulatory patients in outpatient, inpatient, home care, and long-term care settings.[14]

Classification of Urinary Incontinence

The Clinical Practice Guidelines for *Urinary Incontinence in Adults* have classified UI into four major categories: urge incontinence, stress incontinence, overflow incontinence, and other types of functional incontinence.

- **Urge incontinence** is the involuntary loss of urine associated with an abrupt and strong desire to void (urgency).
- **Stress incontinence** is the involuntary loss of urine during coughing, sneezing, laughing, or other physical activities that increase abdominal pressure.
- **Overflow incontinence** is the involuntary loss of urine associated with overdistension of the bladder.
- **Functional incontinence** is urine loss caused by factors outside the lower urinary tract; this category includes UI not classifiable into the three categories listed previously.

Table 13-7 lists descriptions, related findings, and patient populations associated with each type of UI.

Causes of Urinary Incontinence

The nurse should consider the many common causes of transient UI when assessing the patient for risk factors and related contributing factors for UI. Common causes of UI include altered states of consciousness (e.g., confusion, coma); urinary tract infections; atrophic urethritis or vaginitis; depression; ex-

Table 13-6 • CLASSIFICATION OF NEUROGENIC BLADDER TYPES*†‡

NEUROGENIC BLADDER TYPES	ANATOMICAL LEVEL OF DISRUPTION	CHARACTERISTICS AND DESCRIPTION	ASSOCIATED CLINICAL PROBLEM	MANAGEMENT
Uninhibited neurogenic	Lesion in the frontal brain or pontine micturition centers	• Cortical control of initiation and inhibition to suppress voiding urge diminished • Reduced bladder capacity with little or no residual urine • Urgency, frequency, nocturia, urge incontinence	Stroke, traumatic brain injury, multiple sclerosis (MS), and brain tumor	• Timed voiding • Condom type catheter for male, and "padding" of bed with absorbent pads for female
Reflex neurogenic	Spinal cord lesion above T12–L1	• Upper motor neuron (UMN) lesion with disruption of sensory and motor innervation *above* segments S2–S4 • Control lost from higher brain centers, resulting in uninhibited, involuntary detrusor contractions and uncontrolled voiding; spinal reflex arc takes over • Inability of distal sphincter to relax in coordination with detrusor contraction; results in ↑ bladder pressure with emptying and large amounts of residual urine	Lower spinal cord lesion or patient with blood supply interruption to cord secondary to trauma, tumor, vascular lesion, or MS	• Reflex triggering techniques • Intermittent catheterization • Drugs
Autonomous or areflexic neurogenic	Spinal cord lesion *at or below* T12–L1	• Disruption of sensory and motor innervation of sacral spinal reflex arc (S2–S4), a lower motor neuron (LMN) injury • ↓ sensation of bladder fullness, weak or absent detrusor contractions, and ↑ bladder capacity with high residual urine.† • Loss of voluntary voiding except with straining; overflow incontinence is common	Spina bifida, meningocele, or herniated intervertebral disc with LMN injury	• Intermittent catheterization • Straining using Valsalva's maneuver • Credé's method
Motor paralytic neurogenic	Anterior horn cells of S2–S4 ventral roots	• Partial or complete motor loss of bladder function with intact sensation • Difficulty with starting stream • ↑ bladder capacity; high residual urine; overflow incontinence common	Herniated intervertebral disc, spinal trauma, spinal tumor, and poliomyelitis	• Intermittent catheterization • Straining using Valsalva's maneuver • Credé's method
Sensory paralytic neurogenic	Dorsal roots of sacral reflex center (S2–S4) or in sensory pathways to cerebral cortex	• ↓ or absent sensation of pain or fullness in bladder • Infrequent voiding with large output; ↑ bladder capacity with overflow incontinence common	Diabetic neuropathy, tabes dorsalis, syringomyelia, and MS	• Timed voiding • Intermittent catheterization

* McCourt, A. E. (Ed.) (1993). *Specialty practice of rehabilitation nursing: A core curriculum* (3rd ed., pp. 101–102). Skokie, IL: Rehabilitation Nursing Foundation.

† Hoeman, S. P. (1996). *Rehabilitation nursing: Process and application* (pp. 427–432). St. Louis: C.V. Mosby.

‡ Lapides, J., & Diokno, A. C. (1976). Urine transport, storage, and micturition. In J. Lapides (Ed.), *Fundamentals of urology*. Philadelphia: W.B. Saunders.

cessive urine production related to excess intake; diuresis from drug therapy or endocrine conditions (e.g., hydrochlorothiazide [HydroDIURIL] or diabetes mellitus); restricted mobility related to bed rest; Parkinson's disease; restriction of bed rest; deconditioning (e.g., orthostatic hypotension, weakness, fatigue); and fecal impaction.

In addition, various drugs may contribute to UI secondarily by clouding the sensorium or by directly affecting the organs of micturition. They include sedative hypnotics; diuretics that may overwhelm bladder capacity and lead to polyuria, frequency, and urgency; anticholinergics with related urinary retention and associated urinary frequency and overflow UI; alpha-adrenergic agents (e.g., sphincter tone in the proximal urethra can be decreased with alpha antagonists and increased with alpha agonists); and calcium channel blockers (e.g., can reduce smooth muscle contractility of the bladder, resulting in urinary retention and overflow UI).

Urinary Retention

Urinary retention is often associated with spinal-cord-injured patients. In the acute phase of spinal cord injury, the abrupt interruption of the spinal innervation is lost, which results in spinal shock and an areflexic bladder. The bladder becomes distended, causing overflow UI (Tables 13-6 and 13-7). The bladder gradually converts to a hypersensitive bladder as the spinal shock diminishes over days or weeks. If the spasticity and hypersensitivity of the bladder are severe, any slight stimulus, such as a minimal amount of urine in the bladder (20 to 50 mL) or stroking of the abdomen, thigh, or genitals, will cause the bladder to empty by reflex.

Table 13-7 • TYPES, DESCRIPTIONS, RELATED FINDINGS, AND PATIENT POPULATIONS ASSOCIATED WITH URINARY INCONTINENCE*

TYPES	DIAGNOSIS/DESCRIPTION	RELATED FINDINGS	PATIENTS AFFECTED AND COMMENTS
Urge	• Diagnosed by urodynamics • Usually associated with urodynamic findings of involuntary detrusor contractions • Urodynamic finding of detrusor hyperactivity with impaired bladder contractility (DHIC) • DHIC can mimic other types of urinary incontinence (UI) and result in wrong treatment.	• If associated with neurological disorder, termed detrusor hyperreflexia • If no neurological disorder, called detrusor instability • Patients with DHIC have involuntary detrusor contractions, yet must strain to empty bladder either completely or incompletely; in addition to urge UI with ↑ post-void residual volumes, patients with DHIC may also have obstruction, stress UI, or overflow UI.	• Stroke; in suprasacral spinal cord lesions or multiple sclerosis, detrusor hyperreflexia often accompanied by external sphincter dyssynergia; can cause urinary retention, vesicoureteric reflux, and renal damage[†] • Frail elderly often have DHIC.
Stress	Diagnosed by observed urine loss with an ↑ in abdominal pressure, absence of detrusor contraction, or an overdistended bladder[‡]	Two possible causes: • Hypermobility or significant displacement of urethra and bladder neck during exertion. • Intrinsic urethral sphincter deficiency (ISD); may be related to congenital sphincter weakness	• Patients with myelomeningocele, post-trauma, radiation, or sacral cord lesions; in women may be associated with many surgeries for incontinence • May leak continuously or leak with minimal exertion
Overflow	• Many presentations: constant dribbling, urge UI, or stress UI symptoms	• May be due to: (1) an underactive or acontractile detrusor; or (2) a bladder outlet or urethral obstruction, resulting in overdistention and overflow; and (3) weak detrusor from idiopathic causes	• Underactive detrusor related to certain drugs, fecal impaction, diabetic neuropathy, or low spinal cord injury • Outlet obstruction common in men with prostatic hypertrophy, pelvic prolapse in women, and suprasacral spinal cord injured and multiple sclerosis patients, detrusor external sphincter dyssynergia
Other types of Functional UI	• A diagnosis of exclusion • Caused by factors outside the urinary tract, such as chronic impairments of physical or cognitive functioning • May be caused by ↓ bladder compliance	• May be improved or cured by improving functional level, treating other medical conditions, discontinuing certain drugs, adjusting hydration status, or reducing environmental barriers • May have a combined urge UI and stress UI, which is called **mixed UI** • Severe urgency associated with bladder hypersensitivity without detrusor overactivity called **sensory urgency**	• Immobilized and cognitively impaired may also have other types and causes of UI • Patients with ↓ bladder compliance resulting from inflammatory bladder conditions (chemical or interstitial cystitis) and some patients with myelomeningocele often have **sensory urgency.**

* U.S. Department of Health and Human Services, Agency for Health Care Policy and Research (1992). *Urinary incontinence in adults,* No. 92-0038. Washington, DC: U.S. Department of Health and Human Services, Agency for Health Care Policy and Research.

† McGuire, E. J., Woodside, J. R., Borden, T. A., & Weiss, R. M. (1981). Prognostic value of urodynamic testing in myelodysplastic patients. *Journal of Urology, 132*(2), 205–209.

‡ International Continence Society for the Standardization of Terminology of the Lower Urinary Tract Function (1990). *British Journal of Obstetrics and Gynaecology, 6*(Suppl.), 1–16.

Nursing Management of Patients With Altered Urinary Elimination Patterns

Assessment

The nurse assesses the patient to determine the altered urinary elimination pattern present (Table 13-8). The parameters considered in the assessment include confirming voiding pattern by monitoring the voiding pattern and characteristics over 24 hours, intake and output record, recent urinalysis and culture, and functional level. Factors that may be contributing to or resulting from the altered elimination pattern must be identified, as should the areas in need of further evaluation before therapeutic interventions are begun. The pathophysiology should be considered in relation to normal function. The nurse should discuss with the physician and other team members the need for further evaluation and the best approach to the management of the urinary elimination pattern (Chart 13-4).

Nursing management will depend on the nursing diagnoses. The following are possible nursing diagnoses:

- Altered Urinary Elimination
- Stress Incontinence
- Reflex Incontinence
- Urinary Retention
- Risk for Altered Skin Integrity
- Urge Incontinence
- Functional Incontinence
- Total Incontinence
- Risk for Urinary Tract Infection

The following are possible collaborative problems:

- Acute urinary retention
- Renal insufficiency/renal failure
- Renal calculi

Interventions

Various methods of managing altered urinary elimination patterns are discussed in the next section. Within a collaborative interdisciplinary model of practice, input regarding management of urinary function is provided by the multidisciplinary team. However, the nurse is primarily respon-

Table 13–8 • NURSING ASSESSMENT FOR ALTERED PATTERNS OF URINARY ELIMINATION

Characteristics of Voiding Pattern

- Frequency of voiding and time during day and night
- Amount of voiding each time
- Evidence of dribbling (frequency, amount)
- Urgency
- Ability to delay voiding until in appropriate place
- Awareness of full bladder
- Distended bladder
- Sensation of incomplete bladder emptying
- Difficulty starting stream
- Dysuria
- Foul-smelling urine
- Residual urine greater than 150 mL

Related Factors

Neurological disease or injury
- Cognitive deficits
- Sensory deficits with vision or hearing
- Altered sensorium or consciousness (confusion, coma)
- Neuropathies
- Comorbidity
- Urinary tract infection
- Vaginitis or atrophic urethritis
- Drug therapy that influences urinary output or bladder function
- Depression
- Large amounts of oral or intravenous intake; evaluation of intake and output record
- Environmental barriers to getting to bathroom
- Restricted mobility
- Stool impaction

CHART 13–4 • **Possible Diagnostic and Evaluative Procedures for Patients With Urinary Elimination Problems**

PATIENT DATA

- Medical history
- Physical examination—Abdominal, genital, pelvic, rectal, neurological

ADDITIONAL TESTS RELATED TO VOIDING

- Estimated postvoid residual volume
- Provocation stress test
- Data related to urinary elimination—Voiding diary, voiding pattern, and so forth

LABORATORY TESTS

- Urinalysis
- Blood urea nitrogen, creatinine, protein, complete blood count
- Urine culture

SPECIALIZED TESTS

- Urodynamic tests
- Endoscopic tests
- Imaging tests
  - Upper tract
  - Lower tract with and without voiding

sible for managing the complex multifactorial problem of an altered urinary elimination pattern, integrating all the components of the treatment plan, and preventing complications, such as urinary tract infection and skin breakdown.

To prevent urinary tract infection, remove the indwelling catheter as soon as possible and use alternate methods of emptying and stimulating the bladder on a regular schedule. Follow all the research-based guidelines for maintaining aseptic technique related to catheters, catheterization, and skin care. For example, meatal care is controversial and not recommended.

Maintain an intake and output record, and review it periodically. Fluid intake is an important factor to adjust when trying to establish continence and regular emptying of the bladder. UI is a risk factor for skin breakdown. Provide for meticulous skin care, and keep the patient dry.

Treatment Options for Management of Altered Urinary Elimination Patterns

The three major categories of treatment outlined for UI are behavioral, pharmacological, and surgical.[14] This can be used as a framework for nursing management and is summarized in Table 13-9.

"Acute urinary retention" is a collaborative problem to be addressed with the physician. Management of acute urinary

▌Table 13-9 • MANAGEMENT OF ALTERED URINARY ELIMINATION PATTERNS

URINARY PATTERNS	PATIENT TYPES	TREATMENT
Urge urinary incontinence	Strokes	Timed voiding; bladder training and prompt every 2 hours
Reflex urinary incontinence	Spinal cord injured upper motor neuron (UMN) and lower motor neuron lesions	Anticholinergic drugs and intermittent catheterization Condom catheter for men and "padding" for women
Overflow urinary incontinence	Spinal cord injuries with UMN lesion	Intermittent cauterization
Functional urinary incontinence	Various types of patients with functional deficits	Assistance for toileting and timed voiding • May use condom type catheter for men and "padding" for women
Urinary retention	Spinal cord injuries; some stroke patients	• Intermittent cauterization for life with a goal of 400 mL per catheterization (no voiding on own) • Trigger voiding philosophy for some practitioners

retention is always directed at using some method of evacuating the bladder to prevent reflux and infection. Chronic urinary retention is usually treated with intermittent catheterization.

Whenever possible, the patient should be involved in selecting treatment options from established methods. As a rule, the least invasive and least dangerous procedure should be the first choice. According to the AHCPR guidelines for UI in adults, behavioral techniques are low-risk interventions that decrease the frequency of UI in most individuals when provided by knowledgeable health care professionals. All behavioral techniques involve educating the patient and providing positive reinforcement for effort and progress.[14] Behavioral techniques include bladder training (retraining), habit training (timed voiding), prompted voiding, and pelvic muscle exercises. These are discussed further later. Additional techniques that may be used in conjunction with behavioral methods are biofeedback, vaginal cone retention, and electrical stimulation, which are not discussed further. In addition, the many drugs that can be used to treat urinary elimination problems are not discussed. For those interested in the additional techniques and drug therapy, other references should be consulted.

After the particular type of altered urinary elimination pattern has been identified, treatment options are considered.

Behavioral Techniques

The following behavioral techniques have been effective and are recommended by AHCPR in the adult patient with incontinence.[14]

Bladder Training

Bladder training, also called bladder retraining, includes several variations. The time at which a bladder training program is initiated is critical to the success or failure of the program. Patients must be conscious, alert, and oriented. A bedpan, bedside commode, or access to the bathroom is necessary. The patient should be stable and preferably free from urinary tract infection.

Bladder training includes the three primary components of education, scheduled voiding, and positive reinforcement. The patient needs to be educated to understand the physiology, pathophysiology, technique, and desired outcome. The method of education depends on the patient with consideration for any cognitive or perceptual deficits that may interfere with learning.

A bladder retraining program assists the patient to learn to resist or inhibit the sensation of urgency, postpone voiding, and urinate according to a timetable rather than the urge to void. The strategies of a bladder retraining program vary and may include adjusting the fluid loads and postponing voiding so that progressively larger volumes of urine distend the bladder, and longer intervals between voiding are achieved.[15] Motivating the patient is an important component of bladder training. The initial goal interval may be 2 to 3 hours, although it is not followed during sleep. Bladder retraining may continue for several months, during which time setting realistic goals, reinforcing patient education, and overall health monitoring and supervision are necessary.

Habit Training

Timed voiding is scheduled toileting on a planned basis with the goal of keeping the person dry by asking him or her to void at regular intervals. Unlike bladder training, there is no systematic effort to motivate the patient to delay voiding and resist the urge. An attempt is made to match the timed voiding with the person's usual voiding schedule. The time interval may be from 2 to 4 hours.

Prompted Voiding

Prompted voiding is a technique used primarily with dependent or cognitively impaired people. Prompted voiding attempts to teach the incontinent person awareness of his or her incontinence so that toileting assistance is requested either independently or after being prompted by a caregiver. There are three major elements to prompted voiding:

• **Monitoring:** the person is checked by caregivers on a regular basis and asked to report verbally whether he or she is wet or dry
• **Prompting:** the person is asked (prompted) to try to use the bathroom to void

- **Praising:** the person is praised for maintaining continence and attempting to use the toilet

Pelvic Muscle Exercises

Pelvic muscle exercises, also called Kegel exercises, comprise a behavioral technique that requires repetitive active exercises of the pubococcygeus muscle to improve urethral resistance and urinary control by strengthening the periurethral and pelvic muscles in women. The woman must gain awareness of her pelvic muscles and be taught the correct exercise method of "drawing in" the perivaginal muscles and anal sphincter as if to control urination or defecation without contracting abdominal, buttock, or inner thigh muscles.[16] Muscles are contracted to a count of 10 and then relaxed to a count of 10. About 50 to 100 of these exercises must be done daily to be effective. It takes about 4 to 6 weeks to notice improvement.

Bladder-Triggering Techniques

A few bladder-triggering techniques facilitate bladder emptying. They include suprapubic stimulation, Valsalva's maneuver, and Credé's maneuver.

Suprapubic Stimulation

Suprapubic stimulation activates the sacral-lumbar dermatomes by manually tapping the suprapubic area, pulling pubic hairs, or stroking the medial thighs. This is used for patients with UMN lesions.

Valsalva's Maneuver

Valsalva's maneuver is straining against a closed epiglottis while contracting the abdominal muscles and bearing down on the bladder. The straining is sustained or the breath held until the urine flow ceases. This maneuver is used for patients with LMN lesions.

Credé's Maneuver

Credé's maneuver is placing the hands flat just below the umbilical area and pressing firmly down and inward toward the pelvic arch. The purpose of this maneuver is to express urine from the bladder. It may be repeated as many times as necessary to express all of the urine in the bladder. This method is used only with LMN lesions (sacral reflex arc is not intact). Generally, Credé's maneuver is not used in patients with UMN bladder disorders because it triggers sphincter closure and can cause reflux.

Catheters and Catheterizations

In the acute phase of spinal injury or other acute conditions, an indwelling catheter for continuous urinary drainage may be necessary. However, it should be removed as soon as possible and an intermittent catheterization schedule established.

Intermittent Catheterization

Intermittent catheterization means that the patient is straight catheterized at regular intervals of 2 to 4 hours or more to empty the bladder at regular intervals. Bladder-triggering techniques should be incorporated as a means of emptying the bladder before straight catheterization. After the patient begins to void by reflex, the interval between catheterizations can be extended using postvoid residual urine amount as a guide. Indications for stopping intermittent catheterization include an adequate amount of urine voided, residual urine volume of 100 to 150 mL or less, or genitourinary tract free of pathological changes or infection.[8]

Self-Catheterization

If intermittent catheterization is needed on a long-term basis or in the home setting, many patients can be taught intermittent catheterization using a "clean technique" rather than the "sterile technique" used in care facilities. With the clean technique, the patient starts with a clean catheter rather than sterilized equipment. Warm tap water and soap are used to wash the perineal area. Hands must be meticulously washed with soap and water, but sterile gloves are not worn. If the patient is not able to self-catheterize, use of an external condom type catheter connected to a leg bag may be used by male patients. This method can also be used for continuous drainage during sleep.

Indwelling Suprapubic Catheter

In the past several years, there has been a trend toward placement of indwelling suprapubic urinary catheters for quadriplegics. The rationale for placement has been the excessive burden of intermittent catheterization for both the patient and his or her caregiver. With all of the other care essentials to complete, the suprapubic catheter is attractive. With intermittent catheterization, the patient may be incontinent between catheterizations, which necessitates changing wet bedclothes. Another attractive feature of an indwelling suprapubic catheter is that it frees the patient from trying to pace fluid intake with the timing of intermittent catheterization.

"Padding"

Padding is the placement of absorbent pads in the bed or chair to absorb the urine related to incontinence. Use of padding is preferred to maintaining an indwelling catheter long term for patients who do not respond well to behavioral techniques or are not candidates for behavioral or other techniques.

▌ **BOWEL ELIMINATION AND DYSFUNCTION**

Normal Function

The act of bowel evacuation is called **defecation**. The anus, the terminal end of the large bowel, is controlled by two sphincters: the involuntary proximal anal sphincter (smooth muscle) and the voluntary distal anal sphincter (striated muscle).

Defecation is a coordinated reflex involving sacral segments S-3, S-4, and S-5, which is initiated by stimulated stretch receptors located in the anus that initiate peristaltic waves. These waves propel fecal matter toward the anus and open the proximal sphincter. If the distal sphincter is also open, bowel evacuation will occur.

The sacral reflex for bowel evacuation is weak and is aided by parasympathetic responses (peristalsis caused by ingestion of food and increased pressure within the lower bowel, which opens the proximal sphincter). Additionally, contraction of the abdominal wall aids bowel evacuation by increasing pressure on the bowel. See Chapter 5 for further discussion of defecation.

Types of Altered Bowel Function Patterns

Various neurological conditions and treatment protocols can cause alterations in bowel elimination patterns (constipation, diarrhea, or incontinence). Several risk factors have been identified for these abnormal patterns:

- **Constipation**: fluid restriction, prolonged immobility, nothing by mouth status as a result of swallowing deficits or unconsciousness, decreased bulk in diet, drugs known to decrease peristalsis (e.g., codeine), spinal nerve compression, paralytic ileus, lack of sensation, lack of privacy, interruption of usual bowel routine, failure to respond to defecation stimuli
- **Diarrhea**: intolerance to tube feeding, antibiotic therapy, and fecal impaction
- **Incontinence**: altered consciousness, cognitive deficits (e.g., social disinhibition, lack of impulse control, inability to recognize and respond to defecation impulses), impaired communication, and neurogenic bowel without sensation or control (related to spinal cord injury above T11 or involving sacral reflex arc S2 to S4)

Nursing Management of Patients With Altered Bowel Elimination Pattern

Assessment

The nurse assesses the patient to identify the functional bowel elimination problem present. Parameters to be considered include bowel elimination pattern (frequency, characteristics of stool, presence of discomfort), presence of bowel sounds and abdominal distention, previous elimination pattern, and presence of risk factors (see previous list). Nursing management depends on the nursing diagnosis. The following are possible nursing diagnoses:

- Diarrhea
- Colonic Constipation
- Bowel Incontinence

The following are possible collaborative problems:

- Paralytic ileus/small bowel obstruction
- Gastrointestinal bleeding

Interventions

Nursing management for altered bowel elimination patterns depends on the particular problem identified. However, the goal is for the patient to eliminate a soft, formed stool every 1 to 3 days. An individualized bowel program is developed for each patient following established standards of care and is included in the patient's care plan. Chart 13-5 provides a sample bowel program. Daily documentation should be included in the record.

If the patient is constipated, the following points may need to be considered:

- Determine which risk factors can be controlled or altered.
- Increase fluid intake if not contraindicated.
- Administer any drugs ordered by the physician as part of the bowel program:
  - Bulk-forming agent (e.g., Metamucil, 15 mL daily)
  - Stool softeners (e.g., docusate sodium, 100 mg three times daily)
  - Mild laxatives (e.g., Milk of Magnesia, 30 mL daily)
  - Suppositories (glycerin or Dulcolax as needed)
- Enemas may be ordered.

The nurse should keep in mind the following guidelines when instituting any bowel program:

- Start with an empty lower bowel and then individualize a bowel program to meet needs.

CHART 13-5 • Sample Bowel Program to Establish Normal Elimination

The following protocol includes the basic components of a bowel program, although different physicians may prefer slight variations. Once a normal bowel elimination pattern has been established, an individualized protocol should be followed.

- Make sure the lower bowel is empty; an enema may be necessary before beginning the training program.
- Establish a time of day for a bowel movement based on the patient's previous pattern; adhere to this designated time of day rigidly.
- Encourage a diet high in roughage (whole-grain bread and cereal, fresh fruits, and vegetables); in addition, offer prune juice.
- Unless contraindicated by a fluid restriction, increase fluid intake to 2,000 to 2,500 mL/d.
- Insert a suppository on the first day. If it does not work, you may wait until the next day.
- On the following day, repeat the insertion of the suppository. If it is effective, continue with the protocol every other day, but daily use may be necessary for some patients.
- If at all possible, the patient should be seated on the commode or taken into the bathroom to defecate.
- Administer medications and collaborate with patient and health team members to adjust regimen individualized to the patient.

- Get the patient onto the commode if at all possible.
- Try to establish an evacuation pattern at the same time of day that mimics the patient's preadmission pattern.

In addition to the treatment plan outlined, digital stimulation of the rectum can be used in patients with spinal cord injuries to stimulate defecation. Initiation of Valsalva's maneuver or a push-up on the commode may also aid defecation. (Both hands are placed on the commode seat, and the patient raises himself or herself slightly off the seat.) Autonomic hyperreflexia may be triggered by impaction in patients with high spinal cord injuries (see Chap. 19).

COGNITIVE REHABILITATION

Cognitive deficits are one of the most disabling categories of deficits resulting from brain injury because they have an impact on every aspect of life. Deficits in higher-level cognitive functions can be overlooked without careful assessment of the patient. If they are overlooked, the patient is often set up for failure and will not achieve the highest level of independence and quality of life possible.

Nursing Management of Patients With Cognitive Deficits

Assessment

The patient's cognitive function can be assessed by observing the patient's behavior, interactions, and function in the care setting or by using various assessment techniques and instruments to evaluate cognitive function.

The nurse should observe the patient's reaction to stimuli, ability to perform ADLs, memory, way of dealing with minor stresses, problem-solving abilities, and judgment. The nurse should also identify cognitive deficits that impact on patient safety and implement interventions to protect the patient from injury.

Various instruments may be used to assess specific cognitive functions, such as memory, attention span, affect and general behavior, sequencing skills, problem solving, insight, judgment, and abstract thinking. The Mini-Mental State Examination, Neurobehavioral Cognitive Status Examination, and the Rancho Los Amigos Scale[17] are commonly used in the clinical setting. The Rancho Los Amigos Scale is helpful in clinical practice, because it provides a practical framework for assessment and nursing interventions (Table 13-10).

In many facilities, a short (half-hour) cognitive screening assessment may be conducted by the occupational therapy department. The information derived from this evaluation is helpful to the nurse in planning care if cognitive deficits can be identified. Many physicians prefer this approach rather than a full neuropsychological assessment, which takes many hours, because some recovery is expected during the early weeks after cerebral insult. If problems persist, a complete neuropsychological assessment is reserved for 3 to 6 months after injury.

Interventions

Nurses can provide interventions for many cognitive problems in the acute care setting (see Table 13-10). With knowledge of the patient's cognitive deficits, the nurse can identify realistic goals and expectations for the patient. An important role for the nurse is to explain the patient's behavior to the family and be supportive of their concerns. Family members should be told what kind of behavior to expect and how to interact with the patient.

The patient with severe cognitive deficits will require ongoing treatment following discharge from the acute care setting to a rehabilitation facility or to the patient's home. If a home discharge is planned, referrals for follow-up care should be arranged.

THE HOME-BASED VENTILATOR-DEPENDENT PATIENT

As higher technology becomes possible in the home, more patients are being managed at home on ventilators. These patients need 24-hour care that is provided by professional and family caregivers. Much planning, coordinating, and family teaching are needed to even consider home-care options. For example, the family must be competent in providing manual resuscitation using an Ambu bag, tracheostomy care, and operating of a home ventilator. In addition, provisions must be made for back-up power with a generator if electrical supply is interrupted. See Chapter 19 for further discussion of the care of the spinal-cord—injured patient.

DISCHARGE PLANNING

Some patients will require long-term rehabilitation, which will necessitate the use of community resources if they are living at home or admission to a rehabilitation center or extended care facility. The nurse should evaluate the patient's level of independence in terms of activities of daily living to assess how much help the patient will need. This information, along with evaluations by other health care team members, will provide a database for designing a comprehensive rehabilitation plan.

Family members must also be assessed to determine their ability to participate in the rehabilitation program. Some families are willing and able to care for the patient at home with the help of various community agencies. Other families do not want to care for the patient or are unable to do so because of other family responsibilities. **Caregiver stress** needs to be considered. The decision of how and where to provide for the long-term rehabilitative needs of the patient must be a collaborative one that includes input from the physician, nurse, other health care team members, family, and patient, if possible.

Regardless of whether the patient is going home to be cared for by family or to an extended care facility, the nurse will need to compile a summary assessment of the patient's needs and abilities in performing activities of daily living. Referral forms must be completed and sent to appropriate

▌▌▌▌ Table 13-10 • RANCHO LOS AMIGOS SCALE: LEVELS OF COGNITIVE FUNCTION

COGNITIVE LEVEL	DESCRIPTION	NURSING MANAGEMENT
For levels I–III, the key approach is to provide stimulation.		
I: No response	Completely unresponsive to all stimuli, including painful stimuli	Multiple modalities of sensory input should be used. Examples are listed below, but response should be individualized and expanded based on available materials and patient preferences (determined by obtaining information from the family).
II: Generalized response	Nonpurposeful response; responds to pain, but in a nonpurposeful manner	*Olfactory:* perfumes, flowers, shaving lotion
III: Localized response	Responses more focused: withdraws from pain; turns toward sound; follows moving objects that pass within visual field; pulls on sources of discomfort (e.g., tubes, restraints); may follow simple commands but inconsistently and in a delayed manner	*Visual:* family pictures, card, personal items *Auditory:* radio, television, tapes of family voices or favorite recordings, talking to patient (nurse, family members). The nurse should tell patient what is going to be done, discuss the environment, provide encouragement. *Tactile:* touching skin, rubbing various textures on skin *Movement:* range of motion exercises, turning, repositioning, use of water mattress
For levels IV–VI, the key approach is to provide structure.		
IV: Confused, agitated response	Alert, hyperactive state in which patient responds to internal confusion/agitation; behavior nonpurposeful in relationship to environment; aggressive, bizarre behavior common	For level IV, which lasts 2–4 wk, interventions are directed at decreasing agitation, increasing environmental awareness, and promoting safety. • Approach patient in a calm manner, and use a soft voice. • Screen patient from environmental stimuli (e.g., sounds, sights); provide a quiet, controlled environment. Remove devices that contribute to agitation (e.g., tubes), if possible. • Functional goals cannot be set, because the patient is unable to cooperate.
V: Confused, inappropriate response	When agitation occurs, it is the result of external rather than internal stimuli; focused attention is difficult; memory is severely impaired; responses are fragmented and inappropriate to the situation; there is no carryover of learning from one situation to the other.	For levels V and VI, interventions are directed at decreasing confusion, improving cognitive function, and improving independence in performing ADLs. • Provide supervision. • Use drill method and cues to teach ADLs. Focus the patient's attention and help to increase his or her concentration. • Help the patient organize activity.
VI: Confused, appropriate response	Follows simple directions consistently but is inconsistently oriented to time and place; short-term memory worse than long-term memory; can perform some ADLs	• Clarify misinformation and reorient when confused. Provide a consistent, predictable schedule (e.g., post daily schedule on large poster board).
For levels VII and VIII, the key approach is integration into the community.		
VII: Automatic, appropriate response	Appropriately responsive and oriented within the hospital setting; needs little supervision in ADLs; some carryover of learning; patient has superficial insight into disabilities; has decreased judgment and problem-solving abilities; lacks realistic planning for future	For levels VII and VIII, interventions are directed at increasing the patient's ability to function with minimal or no supervision in the community. • Reduce environmental structure. • Help the patient plan for adapting ADLs for self into the home environment. • Discuss and adapt home living skills (e.g., cleaning, cooking) to patient's ability.
VIII: Purposeful, appropriate response	Alert, oriented, intact memory; has realistic goals for future; judgment and problem-solving skills intact; has realistic plans for community integration	• Discuss integration into the community setting (outside home, church, social activities, possibly the work environment). • Help the patient plan, anticipate concerns, and solve problems.

resources. (See Chap. 2 for information about discharge planning.)

REHABILITATION LEGISLATION AND ENTITLEMENT PROGRAMS

The value of rehabilitation for the individual and society is well appreciated and has been supported through many legislative programs. Information about entitlement programs and rehabilitation can be obtained from a variety of sources, such as the following:

- The social worker
- Local and state health departments through their departments of social service, rehabilitation, or vocational rehabilitation
- Special focus groups, such as the Multiple Sclerosis Society and National Head Injury Foundation

REFERENCES

1. Association of Rehabilitation Nurses (1994). *Standards and scope of rehabilitation nursing practice* (3rd ed). Skokie, IL: Author.
2. Association of Rehabilitation Nurses. (1996). *Scope and standards of advanced clinical practice in rehabilitation nursing.* Skokie, IL: Author.
3. Pope, A. M., & Tarlov, A. R. (Eds.). (1991). *Disability in America: Toward a national agenda for prevention.* Washington, DC: National Academy of Sciences.
4. World Health Organization (1980). *Rehabilitation International classification of impairment, disabilities, and handicaps* (pp. 7–43). Geneva, Switzerland: Author.
5. Nagi, S. Z. (1965). Some conceptual issues in disability and rehabilitation. In M. B. Sussman (Ed.). *Sociology and rehabilitation* (pp. 100–113, 507). Washington, D. C.: American Sociological Association.
6. U.S. Department of Health and Human Services, Agency for Health Care Policy and Research (1995). *Post-stroke rehabilitation* (No. 95-0662). Washington, D. C.: Author.
7. University of Buffalo, The Center for Functional Assessment Research (1997). *Guide for the uniform data set for medical rehabilitation (including the FIM instrument)* (V. 5.1.). Buffalo, NY: Author.
8. McCourt, A. E. (Eds). (1993). *The specialty practice of rehabilitation nursing: A core curriculum* (3rd ed., p. 32). Skokie, IL: The Rehabilitation Nursing Foundation.
9. Borgman-Gainer, M. F. (1996). Independent function: Movement and mobility. In S. P. Hoeman (Ed.). *Rehabilitation nursing: Process and application* (2nd ed., pp. 232–233). St. Louis: C. V. Mosby.
10. Bobath, B. (1990). *Adult hemiplegia: Evaluation and treatment* (3rd ed.). Oxford, U. K.: Butterworth-Heinemann.
11. U. S. Department of Health and Human Services, Agency for Health Care Policy and Research (1992). *Pressure ulcers in adults: Prediction and prevention* (No. 92-0047). Washington, D. C.: Author.
12. Glenn, N. H. (1996). Eating and swallowing. In S. P. Hoeman (Ed.), *Rehabilitation nursing: Process and application* (2nd ed., pp. 347–360). St. Louis: C. V. Mosby.
13. Benarroch, E. E., Westmoreland, B. F., Daube, J. R., Reagan, T. J., & Sandok, B. A. (1999). *Medical neurosciences: An approach to anatomy, pathology, and physiology by systems and levels* (pp. 272–285). Philadelphia: Lippincott Williams & Wilkins.
14. U.S. Department of Health and Human Services, Agency for Health Care Policy and Research (1992). *Urinary incontinence in adults* (No. 92-0038). Washington, D. C.: Author.
15. Keating, J. C., Schulte, E. A., & Miller, E. (1988). Conservative care of urinary incontinence in the elderly. *Journal of Manipulative and Physiological Therapeutics, 11*(4), 463–464.
16. Rose, M. A., Baigis-Smith, J., Smith, D., & Newman, D. (1990). Behavioral management of urinary incontinence in homebound older adults. *Home Healthcare Nurse, 8*(5), 10–15.
17. Rancho Los Amigos Hospital. (1980). *Rehabilitation of the head-injured adult.* Downey, CA: Author.

RESOURCES
Professional

Alexander, T. T., Hiduke, R. J., & Stevens, K. A. (Eds.). (1999). *Rehabilitation nursing procedures manual* (2nd ed.). New York: McGraw-Hill.

Bastable, S. B. (1997). *Nurse as educator: Principles of teaching and learning.* Boston: Jones and Bartlett Publishers.

Chin, D., Finocchiaro, N., & Rosebrough, A. (Eds.) (1998). *Rehabilitation nursing practice.* New York: McGraw-Hill.

Dobkin, B. H. (1996). *Neurologic rehabilitation.* Philadelphia: F. A. Davis.

Harper, C. M., & Lyles, Y. M. (1988). Physiology and complications of bed rest. *Journal of the American Geriatric Society, 36*(11), 1047–1054.

Hoeman, S. P. (1996). *Rehabilitation nursing: Process and application.* St. Louis: C.V. Mosby.

Lezak, M. (1995). *Neuropsychological assessment* (3rd ed.). New York: Oxford University Press.

McCourt, A. E. (Ed.) (1993). *The specialty practice of rehabilitation nursing: A core curriculum* (3rd ed.). Skokie, IL: The Rehabilitation Nursing Foundation.

Sine, R. D. (Ed.) (2000). *Basic rehabilitation techniques: A self-instructional guide* (4th ed.). Gaithersburg, MD: Aspen Publishers.

Smith, M. (Ed.). (1999). *Rehabilitation in adult nursing practice.* Edinburgh and NY: Churchill Livingstone.

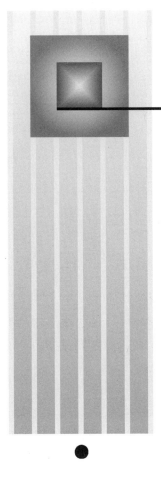

S E C T I O N **4**

Common Management Problems and Approaches to Neuroscience Patients

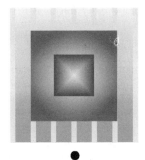

Intracranial Hypertension: Theory and Management of Increased Intracranial Pressure

JOANNE V. HICKEY

Intracranial hypertension is a clinically significant common pathophysiological problem addressed daily by nurses and physicians who care for neuroscience patients. However, the specific sequence of pathophysiological events leading to a sustained or unstable intracranial pressure (ICP) is still poorly understood. This chapter reviews the underlying physiological cerebral hemodynamics and ICP concepts and applies this knowledge to the assessment and interventions for patient management.

CONCEPT OF INTRACRANIAL PRESSURE

Intracranial pressure is the pressure normally exerted by cerebrospinal fluid (CSF) that circulates around the brain and spinal cord and within the cerebral ventricles referenced to the atmosphere on which cardiac and respiratory components are superimposed. The normal range of ICP is generally 0 to 10 mm Hg although 15 mm Hg is considered the upper limit of normal. Monitoring of ICP in the clinical setting provides an average or mean ICP pressure. Abrupt change in ICP from a stable level in response to activity or a sudden change in volume is called *transient increased ICP*. It may be that different physiological mechanisms control steady and transient states of ICP.[1] With cerebral trauma or neurological disease, the normal homeostatic mechanisms controlling ICP may be disrupted, resulting in a sustained high ICP and eventual neurological and clinical death.

Because of the different compartments within the intracranial space, ICP can vary widely within different areas of the brain especially with cerebral trauma or disease. For example, the pressure in the tissue adjacent to an expanding, space-occupying lesion can be elevated, whereas the intraventricular pressure remains within a normal range. Additionally, elevated ICP is not always conveyed to the lumbar subarachnoid space where it would be reflected during a lumbar puncture. It is, therefore, more accurate to think in terms of ICP pressures, rather than a single, uniform ICP pressure.

Physiological Considerations

Monro-Kellie Hypothesis

The average intracranial volume in the adult is approximately 1,700 mL, composed of the brain (1,400 mL), CSF (150 mL), and blood (150 mL). Basic to an understanding of the pathophysiological changes related to ICP is the **Monro-Kellie hypothesis**. It states that the skull, a rigid compartment, is filled to capacity with essentially noncompressible contents—brain and interstitial fluid (80%), intravascular blood (10%), and CSF (in the ventricles and subarachnoid space; 10%). The volume of these three components remains nearly constant in a state of *dynamic equilibrium*. If the volume of any one component increases, another component must decrease reciprocally for the overall volume and dynamic equilibrium to remain constant; otherwise, ICP will rise. This hypothesis applies *only* when the skull is fused (i.e., a closed box). Infants or very young children who have skulls with nonfused suture lines have some space for expansion of the intracranial space in response to increased volume, at least initially.

Volume-Pressure Relationship Within the Intracranial Cavity

According to the Monro-Kellie hypothesis, reciprocal compensation occurs among the three intracranial components—brain tissue, blood, and CSF—to accommodate any alterations within the intracranial contents. The compensatory mechanisms that maintain the intracranial volume in a steady state include the following:

- Displacement of some CSF from the ventricles and cerebral subarachnoid space through the foramen magnum to the spinal subarachnoid space and through the optic foramen to the perioptic subarachnoid space (basal subarachnoid cisterns)
- Compression of the low pressure venous system, especially the dural sinuses
- Decreased production of CSF
- Vasoconstriction of the cerebral vasculature

However, the amount of displacement of the brain, CSF, or blood is limited. After compensatory mechanisms have been exceeded, ICP rises and intracranial hypertension results.

Compliance

Compliance is a measure of the adaptive capacity of the brain to maintain intracranial equilibrium in response to physiological and external challenges to that system. It has been described as a measure of brain "stiffness." Compliance represents the ratio of change in volume to the resulting change in pressure. It is represented by the following formula, in which Δ represents the symbol for change, V volume, and P pressure:

$$C = \Delta V/\Delta P$$

Applying this concept to intracranial dynamics, compliance is the ratio of change in ICP as a result of change in intracranial volume.

The intracranial dynamics are shown in Figure 14-1. The vertical axis represents pressure or ICP (measured in mm Hg). The horizontal axis represents intracranial volume. The shape of the curve demonstrates the effects on ICP when volume is added to the intracranial space. The ICP remains constant from point A to just before point B with the addition of volume. Compensatory mechanisms are adequate, and compliance is high. Point B is a threshold, so that even though the ICP is still within normal limits, compliance is decreased. From points B to C, the slope begins to increase, reflecting a decrease in compensatory mechanisms and low compliance. With even a small increment in volume (points C to D), the compensatory mechanisms are exceeded, compliance is lost, and a disproportionate elevation in ICP is noted.

Factors that influence compliance include the amount of volume increase, the time frame for accommodation of the volume, and the size of the intracranial compartments. Small volume increments made over long periods of time can be accommodated much more easily than a comparable quantity introduced within a short time interval. The size of the intracranial compartments can vary because of cerebral atrophy, craniectomy, or immaturity of the cranium (i.e., suture lines are not fused). For example, an adult with an acute epidural hematoma, a rapidly enlarging lesion, will develop increased ICP much more rapidly than a patient with a large, slowly growing brain tumor, such as a meningioma. In addition, some cerebral atrophy occurs with normal aging, thus creating a little more space in the cranial vault. Because of this extra intracranial space, a subdural hematoma may go unnoticed for weeks or months before there is a rise in ICP. However, a critical point is eventually reached beyond which compensation is exhausted, and there is a dramatic rise in ICP, regardless of how slowly minute-volume increments are added.

Estimating Compliance by Morphological Changes in Intracranial Pressure Waveform

Cerebral compliance can be estimated clinically by examining morphological changes in ICP waveforms in patients with an ICP monitor in place. The ICP wave is observed on a continuous real time display monitor. The pulse wave arises primarily from arterial pulsations and to a lesser degree from the respiratory cycle. Arterial influence comes from arterial sources that pump 10 to 15 mL of blood into the brain per cardiac cycle. In addition, effects from retrovenous pulsation and choroid plexus pulsations also influence the waveform.[2] Observing any variations in waveform during activities, treatments, or environmental changes allows one to determine the effects of these activities on patients and to protect them from risk, if necessary.

The ICP waveform has three peaks that are of clinical importance. Other lesser peaks sometimes occur after P3, but their significance is unknown.[3] The principal waveforms, in order of appearance, are:

- P_1, the percussion wave, which originates from pulsations of the arteries and choroid plexus, is sharply peaked and fairly consistent in amplitude
- P_2, the tidal wave, which is more variable and terminates in the dicrotic notch
- P_3, the dicrotic wave, which immediately follows the dicrotic notch

The pressure tapers down to the diastolic position after P_3 unless retrograde venous pulsation creates additional waves. At low ICP pressure, the pulse wave formation appears as a descending sawtooth pattern (Fig. 14-2). The P_2 wave is a reflection of intracerebral compliance. A rise in ICP is reflected as a progressive rise in P_2. The P_1 and P_3 waves rise to a much lesser degree so that the overall pulse wave has a rounded appearance (Fig. 14-3).

Clinical application of ICP waveform analysis is used to identify patients who exhibit low compliance as evidenced

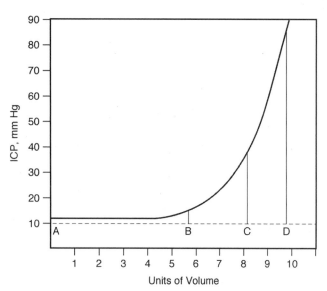

Figure 14–1 • Pressure-volume curve. From point A to just before B, the ICP remains constant, although there is addition of volume (compliance is high). At point B, even though the ICP is within normal limits, compliance begins to change, as evidenced by the slight rise in ICP. From points B to C, the ICP rises with an increase in volume (low compliance). From points C to D, ICP rises significantly with each minute increase in volume (compliance is lost).

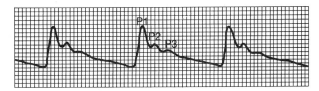

Figure 14–2 • Normal ICP wave form (ICP = 8 mm Hg).

by an elevated P_2 wave. It is unclear whether the height of individual wave components indicates a continuum of compliance compromise from slight to severe. Because it is possible to observe responses to patient activities, treatments, and environmental factors immediately, it may be possible to use this information to develop an individual plan of care based on avoidance of individual risk factors. ICP waveform analysis should be a focus of more clinical research to explore its ramifications for integration into clinical practice.

Cerebral Hemodynamics

Several concepts related to cerebral hemodynamics are important to an understanding of the pathophysiology of increased ICP.

Cerebral Blood Volume

Cerebral blood volume (CBV) refers to the amount of blood in the brain at a given time. Normally, blood occupies about 10% of the intracranial space. Most blood is contained in the low-pressure venous system. CBV is affected by the autoregulatory mechanisms that control cerebral blood flow (CBF). A limited compensatory mechanism is operational when ICP begins to rise. The mechanism responds by decreasing CBV. However, as the compensatory reserve is exhausted, pressure in the venous system rises, CBV increases, and ICP rises. Depending on the rate of decline in CBF and the duration of ischemia, cerebral infarction can occur.

Cerebral Blood Flow

Adequate blood flow and oxygenation are required to maintain normal neural function. The approximate **cerebral blood flow** through the brain is 55 mL/100 gm brain per minute or 750 to 800 mL/minute for the whole brain. Although the brain is only 2% of body weight, it receives 15 to 20% of total cardiac output and uses 20% of the oxygen consumed in the basal state. In normal conditions, the total oxygen consumed by the brain and CBF are almost constant. Local demand for blood can vary depending on different metabolic needs. Cortical gray matter receives about six times the amount of blood as white matter, and changes in blood flow respond to demands of varying neural activity.[4] A basic concept of any hemodynamic system is *the blood flow is directly proportional to the perfusion pressures and inversely proportional to the total resistance of the system.* CBF is represented by the following equation, in which MAP = mean arterial pressure, CVP = central venous pressure, CPP = cerebral perfusion pressure, and CVR = cerebrovascular resistance:

$$CBF = MAP - CVP/CVR \text{ or } CPP/CVR$$

$$\text{Note: } (MAP - CVP = CPP)$$

If the CBF exceeds the amount of blood required for metabolism, a state of hyperemia is said to exist. **Hyperemia,** also called "luxury perfusion," is an excess of blood to a part of the body.

Factors That Modify Cerebral Blood Flow

Cerebral blood flow can be increased or decreased by several extracerebral and intracerebral factors.[5]

Extracerebral Factors

These factors are primarily related to the cardiovascular system and include systemic blood pressure, cardiac function, and blood viscosity.

- **Blood pressure.** *The main force that maintains cerebral circulation is the pressure difference between the arteries and the veins.* In the brain, cerebral venous pressure is low (approximately 5 mm Hg) so that arterial blood pressure is the most important factor in maintaining CBF. Under normal circumstances, intrinsic regulatory mechanisms maintain CBF at a constant level even with systemic arterial blood pressure changes unless the MAP dips to less than 50 to 70 mm Hg.
- **Cardiac function.** Systemic arterial blood pressure is dependent on cardiac output and peripheral vasomotor tone (resistance), which are primarily under autonomic control from the vasomotor center of the medulla. Cardiac arrhythmias, altered myocardial function, and cardiac disease can affect cardiac output, thus influencing CBF. In addition, various carotid sinus and aortic arch reflexes assist in maintaining a constant blood pressure. Advanced age, atherosclerosis, and certain drugs can alter these reflexes, thus affecting arterial blood pressure and CBF secondarily.
- **Blood viscosity.** Anemia may increase blood flow up to 30%, whereas polycythemia may decrease flow by more than 50%.

Intracerebral Factors

The primary intracerebral factors that influence CBF are widespread cerebrovascular artery disease and increased ICP.

Widespread cerebrovascular artery disease can increase cerebrovascular resistance (CVR), resulting in reduced CBF. Processes that rapidly shunt blood from arteries to veins (as in an arteriovenous malformation) can produce an increase in total CBF and a reduction in local tissue perfusion.

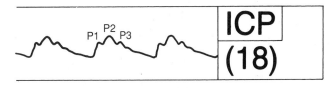

Figure 14–3 • Abnormal ICP wave form (ICP = 18 mm Hg).

When **increased ICP** is present, it is transmitted to the low-pressure venous system, thus increasing cerebral venous pressure and decreasing CBF.

Regulation of Cerebral Blood Flow

Several other intracerebral regulator mechanisms that can modify CBF include autoregulation, chemical-metabolic regulation, and neurogenic regulation.

Autoregulation

The ability of an organ (such as the brain) to maintain a constant blood flow within a broad range despite marked changes in arterial perfusion pressure is called **autoregulation.** Autoregulation operates within limited parameters in healthy people—a mean arterial blood pressure of 60 to 150 mm Hg; below 60 mm Hg, CBF decreases, and above 150 mm Hg, CBF increases. In patients with chronic hypertension, the curve shifts to the right. Autoregulation generally operates with an ICP of less than 40 mm Hg.

Autoregulation is a major homeostatic and protective mechanism occurring in large and small arterioles. Autoregulation is achieved using myogenic, chemical-metabolic, and neurogenic mechanisms. Arterioles contain smooth muscles that respond to stretch receptors and intraluminal pressure causing vasoconstriction to increase intraluminal pressure and vasodilation to decrease intraluminal pressure. Specifically, *autoregulation is primarily a pressure-controlled myogenic mechanism that operates independently, yet synergistically, with other chemical-metabolic and neurogenic autoregulatory mechanisms.* Autoregulation provides a constant CBF, maintained within the normal range by adjusting the diameter of blood vessels.

Compensatory mechanisms are limited. A critical point is reached when other forces overcome autoregulation, thereby causing local or global impairment in an unpredictable pattern. This pattern results from ICP that exceeds 40 to 50 mm Hg, local or diffuse injury, ischemia, or inflammation, or mean blood pressure in excess of 60 to 150 mm Hg. Note that both the upper and lower limits of autoregulation are elevated in patients with chronic hypertension.[5] There is a shift of the autoregulation curve to the right. Without autoregulation, there is reduced cerebrovascular tone, known as **vasomotor paralysis,** and the CBF and CBV become passively dependent on changes in blood pressure.

Chemical-Metabolic Regulation

Chemical and metabolic regulation exert a strong influence on CBF. CO_2, oxygen, and pH are important chemical regulators.

- Carbon dioxide (CO_2), found in the blood and locally in cerebral tissue as an end-product of cell metabolism, is the most potent agent that influences CBF. Cerebral blood vessels respond to changes in local carbon dioxide ($Paco_2$) by vasodilating when $Paco_2$ is high, thus increasing blood flow, and constricting when $Paco_2$ is low, causing a decrease in blood flow. CBF generally changes by 2% to 3% for each change in $Paco_2$ within the range of 20 to 80 mm Hg.

- **Oxygen** (O_2) has the opposite effect: Reduction in local oxygen (Pao_2) produces vasodilation, and an increase in local Pao_2 produces vasoconstriction. The mechanism by which this is achieved is unclear.
- **H+** ions are also powerful agents that influence CBF. In body fluids, CO_2 combines with water to form carbonic acid, with subsequent dissociation of hydrogen ions. Hydrogen ion concentration can also be increased by lactic acid, pyruvic acid, and other acids that result from cell metabolism.
- **pH** changes also have an effect on cerebral arterioles; a low pH (acidosis) results in vasodilation and increased CBF, and a high pH (alkalosis) results in vasoconstriction and a decreased CBF. A buildup of the metabolic end-products of cell metabolism (e.g., lactic acid, pyruvic acid, carbonic acid) causes localized acidosis. An increase in the concentration of these acids will also increase CBF.

Neurogenic Regulation

Neurogenic factors play a lesser role in regulation of CBF than the chemical-metabolic regulators. Neurogenic regulation includes a rich neural network that is extrinsic and intrinsic to the brain.

- **Extrinsic neurogenic control**. Sympathetic innervation comes from postganglionic fibers of the superior cervical sympathetic ganglion that innervate the carotid and vertebral arteries and major intracranial branches. Norepinephrine, a vasoconstrictor, is released from the sympathetic fibers. Parasympathetic fibers come from the facial and superficial petrosal nerves to innervate large- and small-diameter cerebral blood vessels. They use acetylcholine as a neurotransmitter, which causes vasodilation.
- **Intrinsic neurogenic control**. The intrinsic pathways originate in the brain stem and interneurons in the cerebral cortex. Brainstem pathways course from the locus ceruleus (neurons use norepinephrine to produce microcirculatory vasodilation), raphe nuclei (neurons use serotonin, a vasoconstrictor), and fastigial nuclei of the cerebellum. Cortical interneurons contain both vasoconstrictor and vasodilator substances.

Other Factors

An increase in CBF and CBV can also result from pharmacological agents, such as volatile anesthetic agents and some antihypertensives, and from rapid eye movement (REM) sleep, arousal, pain, seizures, elevations in body temperature (about 6% per 1°C), and cerebral trauma.

Cerebral Perfusion Pressure

Cerebral perfusion pressure (CPP) is defined as the blood pressure gradient across the brain. The CPP found in a *normal* adult is in the range of 70 to 100 mm Hg. In the laboratory, ischemia is not seen until the CPP falls below 40 mm Hg.[6] In traumatic brain injury, however, the observations regarding global blood flow and ICP changes may not accurately reflect areas of severe regional ischemia.

Therefore, in cerebral trauma, the lower limits of CPP are probably 70 to 50 mm Hg. Rosner and Daughton recommend a CPP of 70 to 80 mm Hg for patients with cerebral injury and intracranial hypertension.[7] If CPP is inadequate, ischemia develops; if ischemia is not reversed, infarction results.

CPP is calculated as the difference between the incoming MAP and the opposing ICP. It is represented by the following formula:

$$CPP = MAP - ICP$$

CPP is an estimate of the adequacy of cerebral circulation. To calculate CPP, it is first necessary to compute the MAP. This is calculated as follows:

$$MAP = (systolic - diastolic)/3 + diastolic$$

Example: systolic = 130; diastolic = 82; ICP = 15

$$MAP = (130 - 82)/3 + 82 = 98$$

$$MAP - ICP = CPP$$

$$98 - 15 = 83$$

Cerebrovascular Resistance

Cerebrovascular resistance (CVR) is the pressure across the cerebrovascular bed from the arteries to the jugular veins, which is influenced by inflow pressure, outflow pressure, the diameter of the vessels, and ICP. (The cerebral venous system does not have valves as do other veins in the body. Thus, any condition that obstructs or compromises venous outflow may also increase CBV because blood is backed up into the intracranial cavity.) CVR is the amount of resistance created by the cerebral vessels, and it is controlled by the autoregulatory mechanisms of the brain. The CVR increases with vasoconstriction, decreases with vasodilation, and varies inversely with CBV.

Cerebral Metabolism

Under normal circumstances, the brain depends almost exclusively on glucose to obtain its energy needs. The energy needed is supplied from adenosine triphosphate (ATP), which is synthesized through the glycolytic pathway, Krebs' cycle, and respiratory chain. This accounts for the brain's high and critical dependence on oxygen.

Aerobic metabolism is the usual pathway for glucose metabolism. Glucose is metabolized through the previously mentioned pathways to yield 38 moles of ATP per mole of glucose. However, if anaerobic metabolism occurs, Krebs' cycle and the respiratory chain cannot be activated because of lack of oxygen. In these circumstances, pyruvate derived from glycolysis is metabolized to lactate, yielding only 2 moles of ATP per mole of glucose. Therefore, much less ATP is available to fuel the ATP-dependent sodium-potassium pump of cell membranes.

PATHOPHYSIOLOGY

Pathophysiology: Cerebral Ischemia and Cerebral Infarction

Traumatic brain injury (TBI) can cause an immediate primary structural injury as a direct result of the injury. This is termed *primary injury*. *Secondary injury* occurs as a delayed effect of a primary injury or other cerebral pathology and can be caused by ischemia, inflammation, excitotoxicity, metabolic insults, or other pathophysiological processes that affect normal cerebral function. Both primary and secondary injuries can lead to increased ICP.[8]

Ischemia is a state of reversible alteration in cell function caused by decreased oxygen supply. **Infarction** is irreversible alteration in function resulting from lack of oxygen (it is dead tissue). Ischemia becomes infarction if no reversal action is taken. When the brain is deprived of an adequate blood supply, a chain of events occurs called the *ischemic cascade*. The ultimate end-point of this process, unless reversed, is neuronal dysfunction and neuronal death. The ischemic cascade, as outlined, includes the following:

- In the center of the ischemic area is a core of dead or dying cells surrounded by an ischemic area of minimally surviving cells called the **penumbra (halo around the infarction)**. The cells of the penumbra receive marginal blood flow resulting in altered metabolic activities. However, these cells are *still alive and salvageable.*
- Local autoregulation, responsiveness to chemical-metabolic factors, and perfusion pressure are impaired or lost.
- The lack of oxygen and glucose causes a switch to anaerobic metabolism.
- The absence of oxygen and glucose results in failure of ATP production; this, in turn, leads to ineffective cellular function and dysfunction of ATP-dependent neurotransmitter reuptake.
- The release of the excitatory neurotransmitter, glutamate, is increased; this results in increased neuronal necrosis. (Glutamate's neurotoxic effect occurs through activation of N-methyl-D-asparate receptors [NMDA], which cause increased cell permeability to sodium ions, cellular swelling and lysis, and massive entry of calcium ions into the postsynaptic neuron.)
- The increase in intracellular calcium levels activates phospholipases and proteases, which generate oxygen-free radicals and nitric oxide. This leads to membrane, mitochondrial, and microtubular cellular damage and eventual death.

Survival of the penumbral cells depends on successful reestablishment of an adequate circulation, the amount of end-products present, cerebral edema, and the alterations in local blood flow. If the cells of the penumbra die, the core of dead tissue enlarges, and the volume of surrounding tissue at risk increases.

With the breakdown in the blood-brain barrier, water content of the tissue increases, resulting in cerebral edema.

Cerebral Edema

Cerebral edema is an abnormal accumulation of water in the intracellular space, extracellular space, or both that is associated with an increase in brain tissue volume.[9] The edema can be a local or generalized problem, and it is usually associated with increased ICP. It usually peaks 2 to 4 days after TBI.[8] Cerebral edema is serious and can be life threatening because the increase in brain bulk produces pressure on the tissue, resulting in neurological deficit and increased ICP. Severe cerebral edema can produce transtentorial herniation with progressive brainstem compression, herniation, and death. Three types of cerebral edema are recognized: *vasogenic*, *cytotoxic*, and *interstitial* edema.

Vasogenic Edema. **Vasogenic edema** is an extracellular edema of the white matter that results from increased capillary permeability as a result of the widening of tight junctions and increases in pinocytotic vesicles at the level blood-brain barrier. (*Pinocytes* are cells that ingest extracellular fluid and its content. *Pinocytosis* involves the formation of invaginations in the cell membrane, which close and break off to form fluid-filled vacuoles in the cytoplasm.) As a result, a plasma-like filtrate, including large molecules of protein, leaks into the extracellular space. Vasogenic edema is seen locally around brain tumors, although it can develop around a cerebral infarct or a cerebral abscess. Generalized vasogenic edema occurs with cerebral trauma or meningitis. There is disruption of the blood-brain barrier. Magnetic resonance imaging (MRI) or computed tomography (CT) imaging with contrast media can demonstrate parenchymal cerebral enhancement. Use of corticosteroids (dexamethasone) is effective only with brain tumors. An osmotic diuretic (mannitol) may be helpful in the acute phase.

Cytotoxic Edema. **Cytotoxic edema** is an increase in fluid in the neurons, glia and endothelial cells (i.e., intracellular space swelling) as a result of ATP-dependent sodium-potassium pump failure so that fluid and sodium accumulate within the cells, leading to diffuse brain swelling. Both gray and white matter can be involved. Development of cytotoxic edema is associated with a hypoxic or anoxic episode, such as a cardiac arrest or asphyxiation. It is also seen with hypo-osmolarity conditions, such as water intoxication, hyponatremia, and the syndrome of inappropriate secretion of antidiuretic hormone. Corticosteroids (dexamethasone) are not effective in treating cytotoxic edema. Osmotic diuretics may be beneficial in the acute stage when hypo-osmolarity is present.

Interstitial Edema. **Interstitial edema** occurs with hydrocephalus. The edema is found in the periventricular white matter when the intraventricular pressure is greater than the ability of the ependymal cells to contain the CSF within the ventricle. This forces the CSF across the ependymal tissue into the periventricular white matter. It is associated with acute and subacute hydrocephalus and possibly with benign intracranial hypertension (pseudotumor cerebri). Corticosteroids or osmotic diuretics are ineffective; acetazolamide (Diamox) may be administered to decrease CSF production. Treatment options include the temporary drainage of CSF until the condition corrects itself or surgical placement of a shunt.

Summary

Vasogenic and cytotoxic edema may be seen concurrently. Cerebral edema is considered to be proportional to the severity of injury or insult and reaches its maximum level in approximately 2 to 4 days unless secondary injury exacerbates the process. It then gradually begins to subside, although it can persist, depending on the degree of injury and other circumstances such as secondary injury.

Intracranial Hypertension

Intracranial hypertension, more commonly called increased ICP, is a symptom rather than a distinct disease entity. **Intracranial hypertension** is a sustained elevated ICP of 15 mm Hg or higher. The term **malignant hypertension** has been used by some authors to describe a sustained ICP of 20 mm Hg or higher. The underlying cause of increased ICP must be identified and treated to manage the problem effectively. Conditions that can cause intracranial hypertension can be classified as follows:

- Conditions that increase brain volume
  - Space-occupying masses (e.g., hematomas, abscesses, tumors, aneurysms)
  - Cerebral edema (e.g., brain injuries, Reye's syndrome)
- Conditions that increase blood volume
  - Obstruction of venous outflow
  - Hyperemia
  - Hypercapnia
- Conditions that increase CSF
  - Increased production of CSF (e.g., choroid plexus papilloma)
  - Decreased absorption of CSF (e.g., communicating hydrocephalus, subarachnoid hemorrhage)
  - Obstruction to flow of CSF (e.g., communicating hydrocephalus)

The rate of development and extent of involvement of increased ICP and intracranial hypertension are related to cellular dysfunction and its consequences. Several factors influence the process. After cerebral edema and increased ICP are established, a sequence of physiological events contributes to the perpetuation of dysfunction at the cellular level. The sequence of events is as follows:

↓ Regional CBF → ↓ CPP in areas → ↑ CO_2 (hypercapnia) ↓ O_2 (hypoxia) → ↑ acidosis from end-products of cell metabolism → vasodilation → ↑ CBF → → CBV → ↑ ICP → possible impairment of local autoregulation.

Moreover, decreased regional CBF and increased ICP activate the vasopressor ischemic response, resulting in increased MAP and increased CBF. This, in turn, leads to increased edema and ICP.

This circular sequence continues until the autoregulatory mechanisms are inactivated. CBF passively responds to arterial blood pressure. CBF and CPP cannot be maintained in relationship to rising ICP. The CPP approaches zero, and the CBF ceases. Blood vessels and brain tissue are compressed, and herniation and death follow.

Summary of Factors Known to Increase Intracranial Pressure

Various factors known to increase ICP are included in Table 14-1. Many of these factors have been identified as a result of nursing research and are discussed further in the section on nursing management.

HERNIATION SYNDROMES OF THE BRAIN

Increased ICP that continues to develop will result in herniation. **Herniation** is defined as the abnormal protrusion of an organ or other body structure through a defect or natural opening in a covering membrane, muscle, or bone. To understand the pathophysiology of cerebral mass lesions, it is most important to understand the principles that govern herniation. The intracranial cavity is divided into several smaller compartments by folds of the fibrous, relatively rigid dura mater. The most important dural folds are:

- **Falx cerebri** is a double fold of dura mater that drops into the longitudinal fissure and partially divides the supratentorial space into a left and right side.
- **Tentorium cerebelli** is a double fold of dura mater that forms a tent-like partition (higher in the middle) between the cerebrum and cerebellum. The area above the tentorium is the *supratentorial space*, and the area below the tentorium is the *infratentorial space*. To allow the brainstem, blood vessels, and accompanying nerves to pass through the tentorium, there is an oval opening in the tentorium called the **tentorial notch** or **incisura**.

When cerebral edema or a mass lesion occurs within a compartment, the pressure exerted by the lesion is not evenly distributed, resulting in shifting or herniation of the brain from a compartment of high pressure to one of lesser pressure. The shifting of cerebral structures resulting from pressure is called the **mass effect**. With mass effect, there are compression and traction of cerebral tissue that result in ischemia. Ischemia is potentially reversible, but without effective treatment, it will lead to infarction, which is irreversible.

In addition, the **foramen magnum** is the hole at the base of the skull (occipital bone) through which the spinal cord passes. If an elevated ICP resulting from a supratentorial lesion continues to expand unchecked, the uncus of the medial inferior temporal lobe will herniate through the tentorium, with resulting exertion of pressure on the brain stem. This will eventually result in cerebellar tonsillar herniation through the foramen magnum, the only opening in the closed cranial vault. Cerebellar tonsillar herniation is a sure cause of death because of pressure on the vital structures in the medulla.

An expanding mass lesion of the supratentorial space compared with in the infratentorial space behaves differently. The intracranial pathological changes radiate downward and away from the supratentorial lesion in a rostral-caudal pattern. (A **rostral-caudal pattern** means that the deterioration in function proceeds from the head to the tail.)

Of particular importance is the clinical presentation of the Kocher-Cushing signs (more often referred to as *Cushing's response*) of a rising blood pressure, slowing pulse, and a widening pulse pressure that *do not* occur with most supratentorial lesions. Cushing's response is most common with posterior fossa lesions. On rare occasions when these signs are associated with a supratentorial lesion, they usually indicate a rapidly expanding lesion such as an epidural hematoma or a massive hemorrhage that has *suddenly* increased the supratentorial and intraventricular pressure transmitting its pressure effect directly to the posterior fossa and brainstem.[10]

Supratentorial Herniation

Progressive supratentorial lesions develop clinical signs and symptoms in a sequence of ocular, motor, and respiratory function. This pattern indicates the predictable continuum of rostral-caudal failure that proceeds from the diencephalon, to the midbrain, followed by the pons, and finally medullary function. The pattern of deterioration is predictable unless a significant hemorrhage occurs, an abscess ruptures into the ventricles, or a contraindicated lumbar puncture rapidly changes the intracranial dynamics resulting in compression of the medulla.

Three major patterns of herniation, described by Plum and Posner in their classic work, identify syndromes caused by expanding supratentorial lesions: (1) cingulate herniation, (2) central transtentorial herniation, and (3) uncal transtentorial herniation[10] (Fig. 14-4). Cingulate herniation has little clinical significance. A supratentorial developing cerebral lesion results in two distinct clinical syndromes, a *central syndrome* and an *uncal syndrome*. These two syndromes are the major clinical presentations encountered in practice. *Clinically, they are distinct patterns early in their course, but both merge into a singular pattern once the pathophysiology begins to involve the midbrain level and below (brainstem structures).*

Cingulate Herniation

An expanding lesion in one cerebral hemisphere can cause pressure medially so that the cingulate gyrus is forced under the falx cerebri, displacing it toward the opposite side. This displacement of the falx can compress the local blood supply and cerebral tissue, which causes edema and ischemia, which further increase the degree of ICP elevation. Cingulate herniation is common, but little is known about its clinical signs and symptoms.

Central Transtentorial Herniation (Central Syndrome)

The usual causes of rostral-caudal downward displacement of central transtentorial herniation follow:

- A lesion located on the central neural axis
- An extracerebral lesion located around the central apex of the cranium
- Bilaterally positioned lesions in each hemisphere
- Unilateral cingulate herniation

Table 14 – 1 • FACTORS KNOWN TO INCREASE INTRACRANIAL PRESSURE

FACTORS AND DESCRIPTION	MECHANISMS
Hypercapnia $Pco_2 \geq 45$ mm Hg Excessive levels of CO_2 in the blood Potent cerebral vasodilator	Elevated CO_2 results in increased CBF, which leads to increased CBV and ICP Hypercapnia results from underventilation of a patient in such circumstances as: • Sleep • Pulmonary diseases/conditions (e.g., atelectasis, pneumonia, COPD, neurogenic pulmonary edema, ARDS) • Sedation from drugs • Shallow respirations, as seen with anxiety reactions, severe pain, or asynchrony with a respirator • Pressure on brain-stem respiratory centers • Improperly calibrated respirator (e.g., rate, sensitivity)
Hypoxemia $PO_2 < 50$ mm Hg Decreased O_2 in the blood Has a much lesser effect as a vasodilator compared to CO_2	Decreased O_2 does not increase cerebral vasodilation until it is 50 mm Hg or less. Hypoxemia results from: • Insufficient concentration of O_2 administered during O_2 therapy • Insufficient ventilation during and after suctioning • Inadequate ventilation during intubation • Partial or complete airway obstruction
Respiratory Procedures • Suctioning • PEEP • Asynchrony of respiratory rate when Ambu bag is used • Intubation • Increased airway pressure	Suctioning decreases in O_2, increases CO_2, and partially obstructs the airway with a catheter. PEEP increases intrathoracic pressure, which leads to increased central venous pressure, cerebral venous pressure, and ICP. Asynchronous use of the Ambu bag causes a response that is similar to the PEEP response. Same as suctioning
Vasodilating Drugs Anesthetic agents (halothane, enflurane, isoflurane, nitrous oxide) Some antihypertensives Some histamines	Vasodilation causes increased CBF, resulting in increased ICP.
Some Body Positions Trendelenburg's position (always contraindicated in neuroscience patients) Prone position (increased intra-abdominal and intrathoracic pressures; also, neck flexion impedes venous drainage) Extreme hip flexion (increased intra-abdominal pressure) Hip flexion on a pendulous abdomen (increased intraabdominal pressure) Angulation of the neck; neck flexion, even from a small, improperly positioned pillow, or improper lateral positioning when turned (which impedes venous return from the brain) Turning the patient laterally if the head of the bed is up and the knees are flexed on the abdomen (increased intraabdominal pressure)	Obstruction of venous return from the brain increases CBV, which results in increased ICP. The venous cerebrovascular system has no valves; thus, an increase in intraabdominal, intrathoracic, or neck pressure is communicated as increased pressure throughout the open venous system, thus impeding drainage from the brain and increasing ICP. It has been an accepted practice to elevate the head of the bed 30 degrees to facilitate drainage from the brain; current research is inconclusive as to what is the best degree of head elevation for promoting venous drainage from the brain.
Pressure on Neck Snug "track tape," soft collar, or other constricting material	These impede venous drainage from the brain.

Table 14-1 • FACTORS KNOWN TO INCREASE INTRACRANIAL PRESSURE (Continued)

FACTORS AND DESCRIPTION	MECHANISMS
Isometric Muscle Contractions	
Increased muscle tension without lengthening of the muscle Examples: pushing against the bed with one's feet, as in pushing oneself up in bed; pulling on an extremity restraint; shivering; decortication; decerebration; other rigidity	Isometric muscle contractions increase systemic blood pressure and contribute to further elevation of increased ICP in the patient who is on the borderline of brain compliance or who already has increased ICP. Passive range of motion (PROM) exercises do not involve isometric contractions because the length of the muscle does change during contraction. Therefore, PROM exercises should be included in the plan of care. Chlorpromazine (Thorazine) has been used to control shivering; pancuronium bromide (Pavulon) and baclofen (Lioresal) have been used for decerebration in the patient at risk for ICP spikes.
Valsalva's Maneuver	
Exhalation against a closed epiglottis Examples: straining at stool, moving in bed, sneezing	Increased intra-abdominal or increased intrathoracic pressure impede venous return from the brain, thereby increasing ICP. If the patient's ICP is already elevated or brain compliance is borderline, spikes in ICP may occur.
Coughing	
Increases intraabdominal and intrathoracic pressure as a result of muscle visceral contractions	Increased intraabdominal and intrathoracic pressure impede venous drainage from the brain. Also, the increased pressure is transmitted through the spinal subarachnoid space to the intracranial subarachnoid space and through the veins that communicate with the dural venous sinuses and intracranial subarachnoid space. The venous return from the cranial vault is impeded, resulting in increased ICP.
Emotional Upset and Noxious Stimuli	
Upsetting conversations (e.g., about prognosis, legal matters) Noxious stimuli (e.g., invasive procedures, such as lumbar puncture, or painful nursing procedures, such as removal of tape from skin)	Activation of the sympathetic nervous system is probably the major cause of increased blood pressure, increased CBF, and increased ICP, particularly in the patient who already has increased ICP.
Activities That Increase Cerebral Metabolism	
Arousal from sleep REM phase of sleep Seizure activity Hyperthermia	A focal or generalized increase in cerebral metabolism results from these activities. There is regional or generalized increased CBF, which is reflected in increased CBV, which causes an increase in ICP.
Clustering of Activities	
In a patient with already increased ICP, clustering of patient care activities (e.g., bathing, turning) and other activities known to increase ICP can cause dangerous elevations in ICP and plateau waves in the patient at risk. The impact of nursing activities may be compounded after having blood drawn or undergoing an invasive procedure. Note that suctioning is notorious for increasing ICP in the patient at risk.	The compounding effect of activities causes an increase in blood pressure, CBF, and ICP; elevations of ICP can be high enough to cause plateau waves and cerebral ischemia. Spacing of procedures allows the patient's ICP to return to a safe baseline level. Observing the effects and the return to baseline on an ICP monitor provides a guide for delivering safe care to the patient at risk.

CBF, cerebral blood flow; CBV, cerebral blood volume; ICP, intracranial pressure; COPD, chronic obstructive pulmonary disease; ARDS, adult respiratory distress syndrome; PEEP, positive end expiratory pressure; PROM, passive range of motion; REM, rapid eye movement.

The lesion produces a downward displacement of the cerebral hemispheres, basal ganglia, diencephalon, and midbrain through the tentorial incisura. The diencephalon can be compressed tightly against the midbrain with such force that edema and hemorrhage result. Often, anterior choroidal artery depression is noted on the cerebral arteriogram. Central herniation may or may not be accompanied by uncal herniation. The *early* symptoms of the central syndrome include:

- Deterioration in the level of consciousness (LOC) (confusion and restlessness)
- *Bilateral small*, reactive pupils (in early diencephalic stage)
- Gradual loss of upward (vertical) gaze
- Contralateral monoplegia or hemiparesis to hemiplegia

The progression of signs and symptoms with continued pressure is detailed in Table 14-2. There is clinical importance to the signs and symptoms caused by the diencephalic

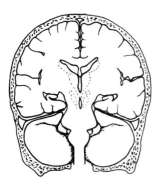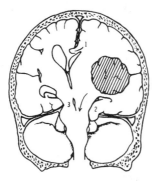

Figure 14–4 • Cross section of a normal brain (*left*) and a brain with intracranial shifts from supratentorial lesions (*right*). (1) Herniation of the cingulate gyrus under the falx. (2) Herniation of the temporal lobe into the tentorial notch. (3) Downward displacement of the brain stem through the notch. (From Plum, F., & Posner, J. [1972]. *Diagnosis of stupor and coma.* [2nd ed.]. Contemporary neurology series. Philadelphia: F.A. Davis.)

stage of progression. If the supratentorial process can be alleviated *before* midbrain signs and symptoms occur, there is a good possibility of complete recovery. However, after the area of pathophysiology has expanded *beyond* the diencephalon and into the brainstem, the process is generally irreversible and prognosis poor. The underlying pathophysiology is that ischemia and compression, both reversible conditions, are the basis for the signs and symptoms of diencephalic involvement. After the midbrain is involved, infarction has begun, an irreversible condition.[10]

Uncal Transtentorial Herniation (Uncal Syndrome)

The most common cerebral herniation syndrome is the *uncal syndrome.* An expanding lesion of the uncus of the hippocampal gyrus of the inferior, medial temporal lobe herniates through the incisura of the tentorium. The diencephalon and midbrain are compressed and displaced to the opposite side by the uncal herniation. With this lateral displacement, the cerebral peduncle (contralateral to the primary uncal herniation) may be compressed against the firm, unyielding edge of the tentorium incisura, producing **Kernohan's notch.** This finding is important because it results in hemiparesis ipsilateral to the expanding supratentorial lesion (Fig. 14-5).[11]

The diencephalon, associated with consciousness, may not be the first anatomical area affected, so that *impaired consciousness is not consistently an early sign of impending uncal herniation.* The oculomotor nerve (cranial nerve [CN] III) and the posterior cerebral artery on the same side of the expanding temporal lobe lesion are frequently caught between the overhanging edematous uncus and the free edge of the tentorium. The entrapment of the oculomotor nerve results in ipsilateral pupillary dilation. *Unilateral pupillary dilation is the earliest and consistent sign of uncal herniation.* The progression of signs and symptoms is outlined in Table 14-3. The signs of uncal herniation include:

- Gradual ipsilateral (to primary lesions) pupillary dilation, sluggish pupillary reaction to light (earliest sign), and possible development of an ovoid pupil

- Paralysis of the oculomotor extraocular muscles
- Restlessness, then LOC deteriorating from stupor to coma
- Contralateral hemiparesis or hemiplegia
- Most often, progression to decerebrate posturing (decorticate posturing is unusual)
- Positive Babinski's signs
- Respiratory changes (e.g., hyperventilation)
- Finally, dilated, fixed pupils; flaccidity; and respiratory arrest

As noted during early development of the uncal syndrome, the unilateral dilating, sluggish pupil is usually the *only sign noted for several hours before other signs occur.* There are no abnormal changes in extraocular movement, motor function, or respirations. Any motor deficits present are those specific to the supratentorial lesion. However, after any signs of herniation or brainstem compression appear, deterioration may proceed rapidly in a time line of only a *few hours* in which a fully conscious patient deteriorates to deep coma. This means that unless uncal herniation is recognized early and interventions effective, after midbrain (upper portion of the brainstem) involvement is noted, the process is most likely irreversible and the outcome poor.

Effects of Supratentorial Herniation

Any supratentorial herniation syndromes can initiate vascular and obstructive complications that can further exaggerate the neurological deterioration. Compression of the aqueducts of the ventricular system can cause CSF circulation to be interrupted. As a result, major spikes in ICP and hydrocephalus can develop. Cingulate herniation can compress both arterial and venous vessels (portions of the anterior cerebral artery and the great cerebral vein), causing exacerbation of already present ischemia and edema.

With uncal herniation, the herniated tissue through the tentorial incisura compresses the posterior cerebral artery, resulting in partial occipital lobe infarction and edema. Brainstem edema, ischemia, and hemorrhage can develop from the diencephalon to the pons-medulla area secondary to the downward displacement from central herniation.

The result of progressive, unresolved downward displacement from any of the supratentorial herniation syndromes is brainstem herniation, in which the medulla herniates into the foramen magnum. Death is immediate and is attributable to medullary compression, ischemia, and infarction. The medulla controls vital functions, such as respiration, blood pressure, cardiac function, and vasomotor tone, all of which are absolutely necessary to sustain life.

Infratentorial Herniation

Lesions of the infratentorial compartment contributing to herniation are much less frequent than those involving the supratentorial region. The infratentorial compartment includes the brainstem and cerebellum. The three possible effects of an expanding lesion in the infratentorial compartment include:

- Direct compression of the brainstem, cerebellum, or their vascular supply
- *Upward transtentorial herniation* of the brainstem and cer-

Table 14-2 • PROGRESSION OF SIGNS AND SYMPTOMS OF THE CENTRAL SYNDROME*

ASSESSMENT	EARLY DIENCEPHALON	LATE DIENCEPHALON	MIDBRAIN UPPER PONS	LOWER PONS/UPPER MEDULLA	MEDULLA
Outcome	Potentially Reversible		Irreversible—Poor Prognosis		
Level of consciousness	Pattern varies from decreased alertness and behavior with difficulty to concentrate Some become agitated, others become drowsy	Stupor to coma	Deep coma	Deep coma	Deep coma
Ocular					
Pupillary size and reaction to light	Small (1–3 mm) reactive, but contraction difficult to see; examine using bright light	Small (1–3 mm), reactive but range of contraction slight; difficult to see	Midpoint (3–5 mm), nonreactive Often irregularly shaped	Midpoint (3–5 mm), nonreactive Often irregularly shaped	Dilated and nonreactive
Extraocular movement Oculocephalic (OC) and oculovestibular (OV) response	Conjugate or slightly dysconjugate at rest; may note roving eyes OC and OV intact	— Brisk lateral OC; impaired upward conjugate on vertical OC Full lateral OV response	— Impaired OC OV difficult to elicit; dysconjugate with limited horizontal movement	Absent OC and OV	— Absent OC and OV
Motor					
Function	Preexisting hemiparesis or hemiplegia develop to *bilateral signs* in early diencephalic stage Hemiparesis or hemiplegia worsens and paratonic rigidity develops homolateral to lesion† Purposeful response to painful stimuli	Decortication first contralateral to primary lesion in response to painful stimuli then bilateral May see a pattern of decortication ipsilateral and decerebration contralateral to primary lesion	Decortication to bilateral decerebration in response to painful stimuli or sometimes spontaneously	Flaccid at rest Occasional flexor response of lower extremities to painful stimuli	Flaccid at rest Occasional flexor response of lower extremities to painful stimuli
Reflexes	Babinski's sign absent	Bilateral Babinski's sign less vigorous ipsilateral to lesion Grasp reflex present	Bilateral Babinski's sign present	Bilateral Babinski's sign present	—
Respirations	Deep sighs, yawns, and occasional pauses	Cheyne-Stokes syndrome	Gradual change to sustained hyperventilation	Normal pattern of respirations, but more rapid (20–40/min) and shallow	Slow and irregular rate and amplitude (ataxic respirations); interrupted by deep sighs, gasps, and periods of apnea
Other			Diabetes insipidus Fluctuation in temperature; hyperthermia	Often hyperthermia Cushing's triad	Often hyperthermia Cushing's triad

* An important point to keep in mind when observing a patient with a possible herniation syndrome is that there is predictable order to the development of signs and symptoms. The neurological deterioration in both central and uncal syndromes proceeds in an orderly rostral-caudal direction; the diencephalon, midbrain, pons, and finally, the medulla are affected from the increasing pressure. Signs and symptoms characteristic of each area can be identified. Notice that the last stages of central and uncal herniation are the same.

† Often there is an original hemispheric lesion that results in contralateral hemiparesis or hemiplegia. With diencephalic involvement, hemiparesis or hemiplegia worsens and extremities ipsilateral to the lesion develop paratonic resistance (an intermittent abnormal increase in resistance to passive movement in a comatose patient).

Table based on classic work of Plum, F., & Posner, J. B. (1982). *The diagnosis of stupor and coma* (3rd ed., pp. 103–108). Philadelphia: FA Davis.

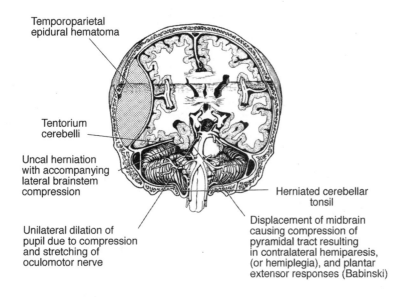

Temporoparietal
epidural hematoma

Tentorium
cerebelli

Uncal herniation
with accompanying
lateral brainstem
compression

Herniated cerebellar
tonsil

Unilateral dilation of
pupil due to compression
and stretching of
oculomotor nerve

Displacement of midbrain
causing compression of
pyramidal tract resulting
in contralateral hemiparesis,
(or hemiplegia), and plantar
extensor responses (Babinski)

Figure 14–5 • Cross-section of the brain showing herniation of part of the temporal lobe through the tentorium as a result of a temporoparietal epidural hematoma. (Kentzel, K. C. [1997]. *Advanced concepts in clinical nursing* [2nd ed.]. Philadelphia: J. B. Lippincott.)

ebellum through the tentorial incisura, resulting in maximal pressure on the midbrain

• *Downward herniation* of both or one cerebellar tonsil through the foramen magnum to the cervical spine with compression of the medulla, an immediate cause of death (Fig. 14-6)

An expanding lesion causes compression and ischemia to selected structures. The increased pressure interferes with the normal function of the involved tissue and causes edema, ischemia, infarction, and necrosis if the process is not reversed. As the lesion continues to enlarge, the only egress from the infratentorial compartment is through the tentorial incisura (above) to the supratentorial compartment or through the larger orifice, the foramen magnum (below), into the cervical spine. In either case, neurological demise is rapid with high mortality.

The brainstem structures, particularly the medulla, contain centers for vital functions. If medullary compression develops, immediate death from respiratory and cardiac arrest occurs. Infratentorial expanding lesions can also encroach on a portion of the ventricular system (third or fourth ventricle) resulting in acute hydrocephalus. The signs and symptoms noted with an infratentorial herniation vary widely depending on the brainstem area most involved. It is unclear whether posterior fossa lesions causing upward transtentorial herniation produce a consistent syndrome.[12] The most prominent signs associated with upward herniation include:

• Immediate onset of deep coma
• Conjugate downward deviation of the eye; to failure of upward voluntary or reflex movement (pretectal compression)
• Small, equal, fixed pupils (pontine compression) to unequal, midpoint fixed pupils
• Decerebration
• Abnormal respiratory patterns (e.g., slow rate with intermittent deep sighs or ataxia)
• Vital sign abnormalities (Cushing's signs)

In summary, herniation syndromes are life-threatening occurrences that can progress rapidly. Early recognition of signs and symptoms (Chart 14-1) is important for prompt intervention to prevent neurological demise.

SIGNS AND SYMPTOMS OF INCREASED INTRACRANIAL PRESSURE

Perspective

Increased ICP is a syndrome with multiple patterns (central syndrome, uncal syndrome), not a specific disease entity. A large percentage of neuroscience patients are at risk for developing ICP. Nursing assessment of neurological signs is directed at detecting *early* signs and symptoms of increased ICP when nursing and medical interventions are still effective. The baseline neurological assessment and ongoing assessments by knowledgeable practitioners are the most sensitive indicators of neurological change. When *late* signs appear (brainstem signs of changes in vital signs or respira-

CHART 14 – 1 • **Signs and Symptoms of Impending Herniation**

• Decreased level of consciousness (coma)
• Pupillary abnormalities
• Motor dysfunction (hemiplegia, decortication, or decerebration)
• Impaired brainstem reflexes (corneal, gag, swallowing)
• Alterations in vital signs, including respiratory irregularities

Table 14-3 • PROGRESSION OF SIGNS AND SYMPTOMS OF THE UNCAL SYNDROME*

ASSESSMENT	EARLY DIENCEPHALON	LATE DIENCEPHALON	MIDBRAIN UPPER PONS	LOWER PONS/ UPPER MEDULLA	MEDULLA
Outcome	**Potentially Reversible**		**Irreversible—Poor Prognosis**		
Level of consciousness	May not be impaired initially	After deterioration begins, quick progression to deep stupor and coma	Deep coma	Deep coma	Deep coma
Ocular					
Pupillary size, reaction to light, and shape	Unilateral dilating pupil ipsilateral to primary lesion Sluggish response Round to ovoid	Fully dilated pupil ipsilateral to lesion Nonreactive Round to ovoid Other pupil dilates	Two possibilities for pupil contralateral to lesion: Fully dilated and fixed *or* Enlarged to midpoint (5–6 mm) and fixed	Bilateral midpoint (5–6 mm) pupils Often irregularly shaped	Bilateral fully dilated and nonreactive
Extraocular movement	Full movement	Paralysis of oculomotor soon after dilated pupil	—	—	—
Oculocephalic (OC) and Oculovestibular (OV) response	OC and OV intact or contralateral eye of OV on cold calorics, may not move medially	OC and OV sluggish, then absent	OC and OV absent	OC and OV absent	OC and OV absent
Motor					
Function	No abnormalities may be present; if present, related to primary supratentorial lesion	• Contralateral intermittent abnormal increase in resistance to passive movement • *Ipsilateral* hemiplegia • Decerebrate posturing of limbs (decortication is uncommon)	Bilateral decerebration	• Flaccid at rest • Occasional flexor response of lower extremities to painful stimuli	• Flaccid at rest • Occasional flexor response of lower extremities to painful stimuli
Reflexes	Babinski's sign	Bilateral positive Babinski's sign	Bilateral positive Babinski's sign	Bilateral positive Babinski's sign	
Respirations	Normal pattern and rate	Most often hyperventilation (20–40/min), rarely Cheyne-Stokes reaction	Hyperventilation (20–40/min)	Normal pattern of respirations, but more rapid (20–40/min) and shallow	Slow and irregular in rate and amplitude (ataxic respirations); interrupted by deep sighs, gasps, and periods of apnea
Other	—	Possible ptosis ipsilateral to primary lesion	—	Often hyperthermia Cushing's triad	Often hyperthermia Cushing's triad

* An important point to keep in mind when observing a patient with a possible herniation syndrome is that there is predictable order to the development of signs and symptoms. Neurological deterioration in both central and uncal syndromes proceeds in an orderly rostral-caudal direction; the diencephalon, midbrain, pons, and finally, the medulla are affected from the increasing pressure. Signs and symptoms characteristic of each area can be identified. Notice that the last stages of central and uncal herniation are the same.

Table based on classic work of Plum, F., & Posner, J. B. (1980). *The diagnosis of stupor and coma* (3rd ed., pp. 109–111). Philadelphia: FA Davis.

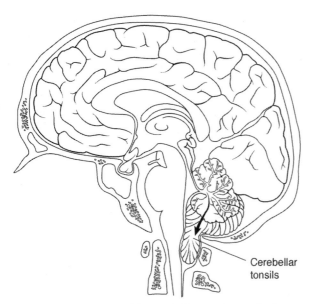

Figure 14–6 • Herniation of the cerebellar tonsils into the foramen magnum is the final outcome of increased intracranial pressure. Respiratory centers within the medulla oblongata are compressed, and apnea leads to cardiac arrest and death.

tory pattern), it may be too late for effective interventions to reverse cerebral deterioration, herniation, or even death. As discussed previously, several cerebral *compensatory mechanisms* provide adequate CBF, CPP, and substrates for cerebral metabolism. These compensatory mechanisms act even when there is evidence of increased ICP. **Cushing's response** is a compensatory response that attempts to provide adequate CPP in the presence of rising ICP. The signs include the following:

• A rising systolic pressure
• A widening pulse pressure
• Bradycardia

These signs profile late brainstem dysfunction resulting from rising ICP and correlate with decreasing brain compliance.

Cushing's triad (also called Cushing's sign) includes the following:

• Hypertension, usually with a widened pulse pressure
• Bradycardia
• Abnormal/irregular respiratory patterns

Cushing's triad/sign is a late finding that in fact may never occur. Cushing's triad is a presentation of brainstem dysfunction and correlates with low or loss of brain compliance. In such cases, cerebral herniation has probably already occurred, resulting in a critically ill patient. Interventions are directed at life-saving measures; cerebral dysfunctions may be irreversible at this point. Therefore, neurological assessment is directed toward *early* identification of neurological alterations so that interventions can be instituted when the chances of control and reversal are good.

Before discussing the traditional signs and symptoms associated with increased ICP, it may be helpful to consider a

few points about ICP and how it can be masked or misinterpreted.

Clinical Variations in Increased Intracranial Pressure

Practitioners rely on clinical assessment for detection of the signs and symptoms of increased ICP and compromised CPP, but these are not necessarily apparent on clinical assessment of neurological signs. The overriding principle in explaining these dynamics is the *degree of compliance in the brain,* as explained by the pressure-volume curve (see Fig. 14-1). One cannot determine by clinical inspection where the patient is in relation to the pressure-volume curve. The patient's brain may be at the high compliance end of the curve or at the *low compliance* end when the slightest increase in ICP will result in decompensation and a significant elevation in ICP.

Direct Brain-Stem Injury

Many of the signs and symptoms of increased ICP often cited (e.g., decerebration, loss of the corneal reflex, changes in vital signs) relate to brainstem dysfunction. Direct primary brain-stem injury can also produce similar signs and symptoms in the absence of increased ICP.

Transient Pressure Signs

The ICP is dynamic rather than constant. Certain activities, such as straining and coughing, can elevate ICP. In a patient at risk who already has an elevated ICP, initiating an activity known to increase ICP can precipitate *transient signs of increased ICP,* also known as *transient pressure signs* or *transient ischemic signs* (Chart 14-2). At the time of such a transient episode, the nurse may observe the onset of new deficits in patients whose previous neurological assessment produced normal results. Reassessment within 5 to 20 minutes may reveal reversal of all symptoms. A transient elevation in ICP caused by a temporary interference with CPP resulting in transient ischemia is responsible for the clinical deterioration noted.

Specific Signs and Symptoms of Increased Intracranial Pressure

The presenting signs and symptoms of increased ICP observed will vary, depending on the following:

• The compartmental location of the lesion (supratentorial or infratentorial)
• The specific location of the mass (e.g., diencephalon, brain stem, or cerebellum)
• The mass effect of the lesion including edema
• The degree of intracranial compensation (compliance)

The following signs and symptoms associated with increased ICP are discussed to clarify their relationship to the cluster of clinical observations found in increased ICP. Guidelines for neurological assessment are found in Chapter 8.

CHART 14-2 • Transient "Pressure Signs"

The following signs and symptoms are associated with transient elevations in ICP and cerebral hypoxia whereby there is temporary interference with CPP, resulting in transient ischemia. The signs and symptoms last a few minutes, occurring most often at the peak of plateau waves and then disappearing as the pressure decreases and CPP is once again reestablished. The signs and symptoms of transient "pressure signs" include:

- Decreased level of consciousness (e.g., confusion, lethargy)
- Pupillary abnormalities
- Visual disturbances
- Motor dysfunction (hemiparesis or hemiplegia)
- Headache
- Aphasia
- Changes in respiratory pattern (e.g., Cheyne-Stokes)
- Changes in vital signs

ICP, intracranial pressure; CPP, cerebral perfusion pressure

Deterioration in Level of Consciousness

As has been noted in the discussion of the uncal syndrome, many patients with early uncal herniation demonstrate near wakefulness. Because LOC may not be affected early in the process, it is *not the earliest sign* of herniation with the uncal syndrome. In the case of the central syndrome, some changes in LOC are part of the constellation of early signs. When LOC is affected, the earliest changes in a deteriorating LOC are confusion, restlessness, and lethargy. Generally, disorientation is noted, first to time, then to place, and finally to person. As the ICP continues to rise, the patient becomes lethargic, stuporous, and finally comatose. In the terminal stages, there is no response to painful stimuli, and the patient is deeply comatose. After the patient becomes comatose, LOC is less useful as a localizing sign and has little value in determining whether the patient is improving or getting worse. The ocular, motor, and respiratory signs become more useful for localization and prognosis.

Pupillary Dysfunction

Pupillary reaction to light is an upper brain-stem function (oculomotor nerve [CN III]) and provides data about brain-stem function that are especially helpful when assessing the unconscious patient. Compression of the oculomotor nerve from mass effect results in changes in pupillary size, shape, and reaction to light. Different pupillary patterns are noted with uncal and central syndromes.

Uncal Syndrome. Unilateral, pupillary dilation is the *most consistent early finding* with uncal herniation. In addition, the pupillary response to light becomes sluggish and the pupil may become slightly ovoid. The hippus response (see Chapter 8) to light may be observed with the beginning of pressure on the oculomotor nerve. Because the source of the rising ICP (e.g., edema, space-occupying lesion) tends to be compartmentalized in the early stages, the pupillary dysfunction is ipsilateral to the lesion. In the later stages of increased ICP, both pupils become dilated to midpoint and nonreactive (fixed) to light. Finally, in the terminal stages with herniation, both pupils become bilaterally maximally dilated and fixed.

Central Syndrome. In contrast, bilateral small (1 to 3 mm) reactive pupils are seen with early central herniation. As the process progresses to involve the midbrain, pupils dilate to 3 to 5 mm. Further pathophysiologic advancement is indistinguishable from that associated with uncal syndrome.

Visual and Extraocular Movement Abnormalities

Visual deficits that can develop in the early stages of increasing ICP include decreased visual acuity, blurred vision, diplopia, and field cuts, all of which are subjective signs. These subjective symptoms require a conscious, conversant patient to provide this information to the examiner. Extraocular motor (EOM) assessment can be conducted with a conscious, cooperative patient or by using the oculocephalic or oculovestibular responses in the unconscious patient.

Decreased acuity and blurring are probably associated with early hemispheric pressure because the visual pathways transect all of the lobes of the cerebral hemisphere. Diplopia is associated with paresis or paralysis of one or more extraocular muscles. With an attempt to focus in one direction, the images from both eyes will not fall on the same point on each retina, resulting in double vision. Visual fields and field cuts can be assessed by confrontation testing, again, requiring a cooperative, conscious patient.

EOM can be tested by directing the patient to follow the examiner's finger through the full range of movement, or in an unconscious patient, the oculocephalic or oculovestibular reflex can be assessed. The oculocephalic reflex provides data on the reflex ability of the eyes to cross midline. Dysfunction may result from pressure from intracranial bulk that affects any EOM. EOM is innervated by CNs nerves III, IV, and VI in the brain stem and provide data about brain-stem function that is especially helpful when assessing the unconscious patient. See Tables 14-2 and 14-3 for variations in uncal and central syndrome patterns.

Deterioration of Motor Function

In the early stages, monoparesis or hemiparesis develops contralateral to the intracranial lesion owing to pressure on the pyramidal tracts. In the later stages, hemiplegia, decortication, or decerebration develops because of increasing pressure on the brain stem. Decortication or decerebration may be unilateral or bilateral. In the terminal stages, the patient becomes bilaterally flaccid.

Clinically, there may be confusion about one of the most primitive flexion reflexes, sometimes called **triple flexion**, seen in the late stages. Flexor motor neuron activation is widespread, and the reflex results in flexor muscle contraction away from the source of the stimuli. This means that the flexor muscles at the ankle, knee, and hip contract to withdraw the whole limb. The clinical significance of this sign is that it is a primitive spinal reflex.

Headache

In the early stages of rising ICP, some patients complain of a slight headache. Headaches are not as common as one might expect. The following hypothesis of headaches and intracranial pathophysiology may be helpful. The intracranial structures that are sensitive to pain are the middle meningeal arteries and branches, the large arteries at the base of the brain, venous sinuses, bridging veins, and the dura at the base of the skull. The brain is normally cushioned by CSF. When the volume of CSF is reduced, the cushion is decreased or eliminated. When the head is in the erect position, the brain sinks. In the horizontal position, the brain shifts to one side. To compensate for the decrease in CSF and to provide an adequate cerebral blood supply, the cerebral vessels dilate, particularly in the venous components. Dilation of the vessels, traction on the bridging veins, and stretching of the arteries at the base of the brain cause pain and headache.

Headache associated with increased ICP is worse on arising in the morning. This can be explained by noting that ICP rises to high levels during the REM phase of sleep, which increases metabolism and produces CO_2 as an end-product. Associated hypercapnia causes vasodilation; this results in traction on proximal venous vessels and arterial stretching at the base of the skull. The result is headache.

Vomiting

Vomiting caused by increasing ICP is associated with infratentorial lesions or direct pressure on the vomiting center, the vagal motor centers located in the floor of the fourth ventricle in the medulla. The vagal motor center also mediates the motility of the gastrointestinal tract. An increase in ventricular pressure transmitted to these centers probably accounts for vomiting. When the vomiting mechanism is directly affected by a neurological lesion, the afferent limb is short circuited to produce vomiting without nausea. Without the warning of nausea, vomitus is ejected with undiminished force because of the suddenness with which the thoracic and abdominal muscles contract.[10] The term *projectile vomiting* is used to describe the forceful character of the vomiting.

Changes in Vital Signs

Blood Pressure

Blood pressure and pulse remain relatively stable in the early stages of rising ICP. In the later stages, when there is pressure on the brainstem, changes in blood pressure occur. An *ischemic reflex* is triggered by ischemia in the medullary vasomotor center, and systemic arterial pressure is increased. The intraluminal arterial pressure must be greater than the ICP for continued blood flow. As ICP rises, the blood pressure rises reflexively to compensate. Cushing's response is activated. The resultant elevation in blood pressure increases cardiac output so that the heart pumps with greater force, thus widening the pulse pressure. Increasing systemic blood pressure with a widening pulse pressure is the compensatory phase of increasing ICP. With deterioration, the decompensation phase begins and blood pressure decreases.

Pulse

In the early stage of increasing ICP, the pulse is relatively stable. Bradycardia probably results from pressure on the vagal control mechanism in the medulla. With a continued rise in pressure, the pulse drops to 60 per minute or less and becomes full and bounding. The decreased rate and bounding quality are compensatory to pump blood upward into vessels on which pressure is being exerted from expanding intracranial bulk. In the decompensatory stage, the pulse becomes irregular, rapid, and thready and then ceases.

Respirations

Alterations in the respiratory pattern are associated with direct pressure on the brainstem respiratory centers of the pons and medulla. The various patterns and associated anatomical levels are discussed in Chapter 8. In addition, an acute increase in ICP can trigger development of acute neurogenic pulmonary edema in the absence of cardiac disease. Other possible acute respiratory complications include adult respiratory distress syndrome and disseminated intravascular coagulopathy.

Temperature

Variations in temperature are usually associated with hypothalamic dysfunction either by direct injury or as a result of traction on connecting tracts. During the compensatory phase of increasing ICP, temperature will probably remain within normal limits. During the decompensatory phase, high temperatures are frequently observed. Elevations in either phase need to be evaluated and differentiated between neurogenic hyperthermia and a temperature elevation due to an infection such as pneumonia.

Loss of Brainstem Reflexes

In the late stages of rising ICP, pressure on the brainstem causes loss or dysfunction of reflexes mediated by the brainstem. These reflexes include the pupillary, corneal, gag, swallowing, oculocephalic, and oculovestibular reflexes. The prognosis is poor for patients who have lost their brainstem reflexes.

Papilledema

Papilledema, discussed in Chapter 8, is a blurring of the optic disc margin as noted during an ophthalmoscopic examination. Because the subdural and subarachnoid spaces continue along the optic nerve, increased pressure within the intracranial cavity is transmitted along the nerve. The result is edema of the head of the optic nerve, which can be seen when viewing the optic disc with an ophthalmoscope.

Depending on circumstances, papilledema may be a late finding with increased ICP. It does not occur until ICP has reached markedly elevated levels. Papilledema is not a universal observation made in all patients with increased ICP. In some patients, this may be the first sign observed if an elevated ICP has developed gradually.

MANAGEMENT OF PATIENTS WITH INTRACRANIAL HYPERTENSION: A COLLABORATIVE PROBLEM

Management of patients with intracranial hypertension is a collaborative problem in which the nurse and physician share responsibilities for patient outcomes. In addition to intracranial hypertension, other possible collaborative problems associated with intracranial hypertension must be kept in mind (Box 14-1).

Medical and nursing management is directed toward early diagnosis and treatment of the underlying cause(s), management of factors known to increase ICP, control and management of intracranial hypertension, support of all body systems, and prevention of complications. Most patients will be admitted to an acute care unit or an intensive care unit (ICU) where technological and other resources are available to support the patient. These are vulnerable patients at high risk for complications and thus need expert assessment, monitoring, and treatment through a collaborative effort of the entire team for optimal patient outcomes. Nurses may also wish to consider nursing diagnoses to guide care. Box 14-2 shows the major nursing diagnoses associated with increased ICP and intracranial hypertension.

BOX 14–1 MAJOR **COLLABORATIVE PROBLEMS**
ASSOCIATED WITH INCREASED ICP
AND INTRACRANIAL HYPERTENSION

- Hypovolemic shock
- Cardiogenic shock
- Dysrhythmias
- Hypotension
- Hypertension
- Deep vein thrombosis/pulmonary embolism
- Disseminated intravascular coagulation
- Neurogenic pulmonary edema
- Atelectasis/pneumonia
- Ventilator dependency
- Electrolyte imbalances
- Hypoglycemia/hyperglycemia
- Diabetes insipidus
- Sepsis
- Acidosis/alkalosis
- Hyperthermia
- Stroke
- Seizures
- Gastric ulcer (Cushing's ulcer) with GI bleeding
- Renal failure

BOX 14–2 MAJOR **NURSING DIAGNOSES**
ASSOCIATED WITH INCREASED ICP
AND INTRACRANIAL HYPERTENSION

- Altered Cerebral Tissue Perfusion
- Ineffective Respiratory Function
- Ineffective Airway Clearance
- Risk for Aspiration
- Risk for Infection
- Risk for Injury
- Hyperthermia
- Total Incontinence
- Constipation

Assessment, Management Strategies, and Interventions for Intracranial Hypertension

Neurological Assessment

Baseline and ongoing neurological assessments are the foundation of patient management. Frequent assessment (every 15 minutes to every 1 hour), depending on stability of neurological signs provides information on changes in neurological status. This includes:

- LOC (i.e., deterioration in LOC)
- Pupillary size and reaction to direct light (unilateral or bilateral pupillary dilation)
- Motor function (weakness, paralysis, or abnormal posturing)
- Respiratory pattern

The most convincing evidence of the development of intracranial hypertension is the evolving presence of one or more of these signs.[14] Changes in findings are often subtle and may be detected only by performing serial assessments and comparing serial data. For example, if the nurse notices that a previously alert and oriented patient is now confused, this is a significant finding. The nurse may need to consider other explanations of confusion, such as response to drugs, but alteration in consciousness is often apparent *before* changes in pupillary size or reaction to light, eye movement, motor or sensory function occur. Vigilant nursing assessment and monitoring are the most sensitive means to detect early change. Early recognition of deterioration allows definitive action to be taken while treatment strategies can still be effective. After pupillary and other signs become apparent, however, the downhill course of events can occur rapidly, and the effectiveness of treatment limited. Noting trends of subtle changes applies not only to the LOC, pupillary size and reaction, and motor function, but also to vital signs. Trends in vital signs must be noted because deterioration in neurological status can herald a change from a compensatory neurological state to one of decompensation. Slowing of the pulse, widening pulse pressure, and an elevating systolic pressure are *late signs* of neurological deterioration. The nurse should not wait until these signs are present before intervening. Therefore, serial neurological assessments are the basis for identifying neurological change.

Management Strategies and Interventions

The integration of brain specific and general supportive strategies and interventions to manage patients with intracranial hypertension are many. This section is divided into brain-specific strategies and interventions for intracranial hypertension and cardiopulmonary supportive strategies and interventions. Evidence-based practice guidelines published in 2000 provide an excellent foundation for patient care and examining the efficacy of specific treatment strategies.[13]

Brain-Specific Strategies and Interventions for Intracranial Hypertension

In this section head elevation, hyperventilation, blood pressure and oxygenation, CPP, CSF drainage, mannitol and corticosteroids, analgesia/sedation, neuromuscular blockade, fluid management, temperature control, seizure control, hypothermia, barbiturate coma, and surgery are discussed.

Elevation of Head of Bed. Elevation of the head of the bed to 30 degrees has been employed to improve jugular venous drainage thereby lowering ICP.[14–18] Venous drainage from the brain has no valves and thus the use of gravity facilitates drainage with concurrent lowering of ICP. This is considered safe so long as the patient is *not hypovolemic*, a condition that could threaten adequate CPP. Therefore, maintaining adequate intravascular volume is necessary to elevate the head of the bed safely.

Chesnut points out one disadvantage of head elevation.[19] Patients must be placed flat for transport, CT scanning, and other procedures. This flat position often results in intracranial hypertension. This effect should be anticipated, so that Chesnut recommends lowering the bed to the flat position 15 to 30 minutes before transport so that alterations in ICP and other physiological parameters can be corrected in the ICU rather than during transport.

Hyperventilation. Use of **hyperventilation** to reduce increased ICP has been controversial, but clearer guidelines are now available.[20] CO_2 is a potent cerebral vasodilator, and lowering cerebral CO_2 can cause rapid cerebral vasoconstriction resulting in decreased CBF and decreased ICP. Change in the pH of the serum and CSF results in alkalosis thus causing cerebral vasoconstriction and a reduced intracranial volume and decreased ICP. In traumatic brain injured (TBI) patients, CBF is lowest in the first day after TBI and slowly increased over the next 3 to 4 days.[21,22] Aggressive lowering of $PaCO_2$ by hyperventilation to levels of 25 mm Hg can rapidly reduce ICP, but the abrupt cerebral vasoconstriction can lead to a decrease in CBF and ischemia.[23]

A prospective study of patients with severe TBI randomized to prophylactic hyperventilation for 5 days after injury with a PCO_2 of 25 mm Hg was compared with findings in a control group without hyperventilation and a PCO_2 of 35 mm Hg. At 3-month and 6-month follow-up, those treated with hyperventilation with a Glasgow Coma Score of 4 or 5 had significantly worse outcomes than the control group.[24]

Monitoring jugular oxygen concentration has demonstrated a relationship between hyperventilation and decreased CBF and decreased cerebral oxygen delivery in two studies.[25,26] In both groups, there was a rapid improvement in jugular venous oxygen concentration following the return to normocapnia, which suggested improved CBF and oxygenation of cerebral tissue.[20] Given these data, which evidence-based guidelines assist the clinician in the use of hyperventilation as a treatment option in managing increased ICP?

Hyperventilation has an important role in rapidly reducing *acute episodes* of increased ICP when a patient has an *acute onset* of "pressure signs" (e.g., deteriorating LOC, dilated or ovoid pupil) and needs rapid reduction of ICP urgently. By inducing hypocarbia, cerebral vasoconstriction and reduced CBF results. As a result, the ICP drops almost immediately. The patient can be hyperventilated using an Ambu bag when a ventilator is not present. This urgent intervention lasts minutes to lower the ICP rapidly so that definitive treatment can be started.

In a ventilated patient, increasing the ventilatory rate while maintaining a tidal volume of 12 to 15 mL/kg provides hyperventilation. The target level of PCO_2 is 30 to 35 mm Hg. The effectiveness of hyperventilation appears to be time limited and thus transient. Hyperventilation is useful as an adjunct to osmotic therapy.[27] Evidence-based guidelines for hyperventilation offer the following recommendations.[13] Neither prophylactic nor prolonged hyperventilation is recommended. *Prophylactic hyperventilation* ($PaCO_2$ of mm Hg or less) during the first 24 hours after severe TBI should be avoided. Hyperventilation may be used for intracranial hypertension for longer periods of time if the ICP does not respond to usual treatment strategies (e.g., sedation, CSF drainage). When hyperventilation is discontinued, it should also be withdrawn gradually over 12 to 24 hours. Hyperventilation is useful and recommended for brief periods to reverse acute neurological deterioration.

To prevent complications from hyperventilation, maintain adequate intravascular volume and systemic blood pressure. A central line is helpful to monitor hemodynamics. End-tidal CO_2 can be used to monitor PCO_2, although arterial gases are more accurate gauges. Review blood gas to determine achievement of target levels. A jugular venous catheter is useful to monitor jugular venous oxygen concentration (Sjo_2) and arterial-jugular venous oxygen content differences ($Avdo_2$) to identify cerebral ischemia. If the patient is agitated or is fighting the ventilator, try to determine the cause and treat it; if the agitation continues, the physician may order sedation or neuromuscular blockade drugs to synchronize the patient with the ventilator. Finally, there is a role for hyperventilation with increased ICP, but specific guidelines must be followed.

Oxygenation and Blood Pressure Control. Managing blood pressure is an important concern because of the serious consequences related to extremes in blood pressure. **Hypotension** is directly related to cerebral ischemia and secondary brain injury, whereas **hypertension** has little effect on CBF and ICP. Maintaining adequate CPP is critical in preventing ischemia; this important point will be further discussed. The guidelines are clear for hypotension (systolic blood pressure below 90 mm Hg). These guidelines state that hypotension or hypoxia (apnea, cyanosis, or a PaO_2 below 60 mm Hg) must be avoided, or if it occurs, must be corrected immediately. The mean arterial blood pressure should be maintained above 90 mm Hg at all times to maintain a CPP above 70 mm Hg.[13] If a hypotensive event occurs, a fluid bolus and a vasoactive drug are indicated (see Chapter 11).

The patient must be carefully monitored to prevent hypotensive episodes. An adequate intravascular volume (euvolemia) must be maintained. In addition to careful clinical assessment, review of arterial blood gases, ongoing data from the pulse oximetry (SpO_2), and invasive monitoring data assist in clinical reasoning. Alarms on the ventilator must be keep on at all times to alert the nurse to any situation that compromises adequate oxygenation.

Cerebral Perfusion Pressure. Cerebral perfusion pressure is the mean arterial blood pressure minus ICP. It is the pressure gradient responsible for CBF and metabolite delivery and is directly related to ischemia. Cerebral ischemia is considered the most important secondary event affecting outcome. Therefore, it is critical to maintain an adequate CPP, a minimum of 70 mm Hg, according to guidelines.[13] Although the exact level is not clear, 70 to 80 mm Hg is considered the critical threshold.

Outcomes and CPP in TBI patients were studied by McGraw.[28] He found that CPP above 80 mm Hg resulted in mortality rates of 35% to 40%. When CPP was reduced below this level, mortality increased by 20% for each 10 mm Hg so that when the CPP was below 60 mm Hg, mortality was about 95%. The rationale for maintaining a CPP of 70 mm Hg or above is also based on evidence that CBF is usually very low after TBI, often near the ischemic threshold.[21,29-32] Further, CBF adjacent to contusions and subdural hematomas is reduced even more than global CBF.[33,34]

Evidence about hypertension has evolved. Concerns have been raised about adverse effects from hypertensive therapy used in some patients with severe TBI to maintain adequate CPP. The concern focuses on an increase in ICP in response to therapy with subsequent poor outcomes.[13] The evidence does not support this concern. For example, the effects on ICP and CBF in response to artificial hypertension were studied by Bouma and Muizelaar in 35 patients with severe TBI.[35] By elevating the mean arterial blood pressure from 92 ± 10 to 123 ± 8 mm Hg resulted in only a slight increase (less than 1%) in ICP in patients with an intact autoregulation. In those with loss of autoregulation, there was a decrease in mean ICP. This study and others demonstrate that ICP usually changes very little when blood pressure is increased by as much as 30 mm Hg in TBI patients regardless of the status of autoregulation (defined as an increase in CBF when the blood pressure is increased). Therefore, there is no direct relationship between CBF and ICP. A moderate increase in blood pressure, such as might be initiated to maintain adequate CPP, should not cause an increase in ICP in most TBI patients.[13] If antihypertensive drugs are indicated, those most often used are intravenous beta blockers or the combined alpha and beta blocker, labetalol (see Chapter 11).

Cerebrospinal Fluid Drainage. The insertion of a catheter into a lateral ventricle through a bur hole made in the skull for CSF drainage is called a **ventriculostomy**. Drainage of CSF from a ventriculostomy is a temporary method to reduce ICP rapidly and can sustain the patient through spikes in ICP or during acute hydrocephalus associated with subarachnoid hemorrhage. A ventriculostomy catheter is connected to a drainage bag. The ventriculostomy can be inserted exclusively for periodic drainage of CSF or the drainage bag can be connected to a system for intraventricular ICP monitoring that has the capability for CSF drainage. See page 310 for a description of one system; see also Figure 14-7. When CSF drainage is desired, the nurse can periodically drain the CSF according to a physician's order. Although there is not an exact target point at which treatment is necessary to decrease ICP, current data support 20 to 25 mm Hg as an upper threshold above which ICP lowering therapy should be initiated.[13] When the ICP reaches or exceeds the given threshold set by the physician (e.g., 20 or 25 mm Hg) the stopcock is opened and CSF drained according to the physician's order (e.g., 5 minutes). There are specific management points that must be followed, such as the stopcock of the drainage system is leveled to the anatomical reference point such as the level of the ear (see pp. 309). Insertion of a ventricular catheter is associated with an increased risk of infection (see page 314 for specifics of management).

Mannitol and Corticosteroids (see also Chapter 11). Mannitol, an osmotic diuretic, works on the principle of establishing a high osmotic gradient to draw water from the extracellular space of the edematous cerebral tissue into the plasma. The extracellular fluid is hypotonic in relation to the hypertonicity of the serum. Water is drawn from the brain, thus reducing the bulk (volume) of the brain. Mannitol is the mainstay of hyperosmolar therapy. Mannitol (Osmitrol) does not cross the blood-brain barrier. Its osmotic effect causes water to be drawn from the extracellular space of the edematous brain into the plasma, thereby reducing brain volume and decreasing ICP. Mannitol (20% to 25%) is considered relatively safe and is administered intravenously through a filter. The filter is necessary because of the risk of crystallization of the drug. The current practice is to give mannitol as a bolus at a dose of 0.25 to 0.5 g/kg or up to 1g/kg every 3 to 6 hours, infused rapidly.[13] The ICP, CPP, and serum osmolality are monitored frequently. Therapy is directed at keeping the serum osmolality at approximately 310 to 315 mOsm. Serum osmolalities above 320 mOsm/L and hypovolemia should be avoided.[13] The maximal effect of mannitol should be noted within 15 to 30 minutes and can last for 1 to 3 hours. In some patients, a rebound effect, observed as a rise in ICP, may occur after administration.

Mannitol can result in dehydration, hypoosmolality, electrolyte imbalance (e.g., hypokalemia, hyponatremia), or renal failure. Serum osmolality, electrolytes, blood-urea-nitrogen, creatinine, and the intake and output record must be monitored. An indwelling catheter is necessary to monitor urinary diuresis. Electrolyte replacement needs replacement (see Chap. 10). Mannitol is not administered to patients with hypovolemic shock, congestive heart failure, dehydration, or kidney disease. Furosemide, a loop diuretic, may be used to manage the rebound effect from mannitol, but it is not a mainstay drug for the primary management of increased ICP.

Corticosteroids have *no* demonstrated benefit for treatment of increased ICP in cerebral infarction with edema or TBI and are, therefore, *not* a standard of care.[36]

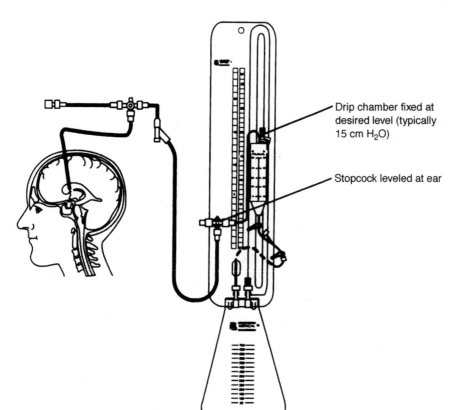

Drip chamber fixed at desired level (typically 15 cm H_2O)

Stopcock leveled at ear

Figure 14-7 • Becker intraventricular external drainage and landmarks for calibration. (Widjicks, E. [1997]. *The clinical practice of critical care neurology.* Philadelphia: Lippincott-Raven.)

Analgesia and Sedation. Pain, restlessness, and agitation are known to exacerbate existing increased ICP. Analgesics with or without sedation can be useful.[19] The Society of Critical Care Medicine has developed and published practice parameters for intravenous analgesia and sedation for adult patient in the ICU. Narcotic analgesics can be effective in controlling pain and providing sedation. These recommendations apply to critically ill adults in the ICU and are summarized in an executive summary.[37] Morphine sulfate is the preferred analgesic agent for critically ill patients. Fentanyl is the best choice if the patient is hemodynamically unstable, demonstrating histamine release with morphine, or allergic to morphine. Hydromorphone can be used as an alternative to morphine. Midazolam (Versed) and propofol (Diprivan)[38] are the preferred choices only for short-term (i.e., less than 24-hour) treatment of anxiety. Lorazepam (Ativan) is the drug of choice for prolonged treatment of anxiety, and haloperidol is preferred for delerium.[37] Pharmacological sedation of this population requires careful consideration of the underlying neurophysiologic disturbances and potential adverse effects introduced by sedative drugs (see Chap. 11).[39]

Neuromuscular Blockade (Paralysis). Paralysis (neuromuscular blockade) and sedation are used as chemical restraints to control restlessness and agitation that increase cerebral metabolism, blood pressure, and ICP. Some motor activities such as dyssynchrony with a ventilator (i.e., "bucking" or fighting the ventilator) or abnormal posturing (e.g., decortication, decerebration) also contribute to increased ICP by increases in intrathoracic pressure and central venous pressure. The Society of Critical Care Medicine has developed

and published practice parameters for sustained neuromuscular blockade in the adult critically ill patient. They are summarized in an executive summary.[37] Three recommendations have been made. Pancuronium is the preferred neuromuscular blockade for most critically ill patients. Vecuronium is preferred for patients with cardiac disease or hemodynamic instability when tachycardia could have a negative effect. All patients receiving neuromuscular blockade should be appropriately assessed for the degree of blockade achieved. Side effects may be minimized by careful monitoring of the degree of muscle blockade and the drug dosage.

Using a peripheral nerve stimulator and monitor of muscle movement are safe ways to periodically monitor the degree of blockade.[40] The peripheral nerve stimulator delivers electrical current to the nerve through electrodes. Before the patch electrodes can be applied, the skin must be hairless, clean, and dry. The terminal outputs of the peripheral nerve stimulator include the positive (anode) and negative (cathode) terminals. The active electrode concentrates the electrical current and is placed near the nerve. The inactive electrode is located farthest from the nerve and is used to complete the circuit (Fig. 14-8). The ulnar, facial, posterior tibial, or peroneal nerve can be used for monitoring. The ulnar nerve is most commonly used because it is superficial and easy to locate. The ulnar nerve innervates the adductor pollicis muscle in the thumb. Various configurations can be used to apply the electrodes. The most accessible part of the ulnar nerve is between the tendon flexor carpi ulnaris medially and the ulnar artery laterally about 2 to 3 inches proximally from the crease of the wrist.[41] Proper positioning of the electrodes along the nerve is necessary for a response (see Fig. 14-8).

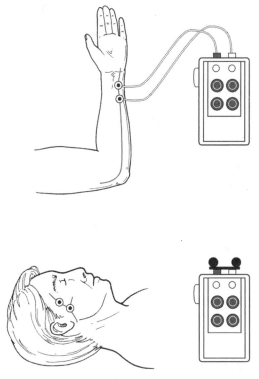

Figure 14–8 • Train of four peripheral stimulator.

The train-of-four (TOF) stimulation is the best and most common method of peripheral nerve stimulator monitoring to assess the level of neuromuscular blockade. Four electrical stimuli of 2 Hz each are delivered at 0.5-second intervals, for a total of four pulses. The number of responses to TOF stimuli indicates the degree of the neuromuscular blockade. As the depth of the blockade increases, the number of elicited responses decreases. The hand on the stimulated limb is positioned palm up. Observe or palpate for thumb adduction with each stimuli. If you see three twitches, it indicates a blockade of 80%, two equal 85%, and one 90%. An absence of twitches is equivalent to 100% blockade.[42] The frequency of TOF depends on whether the drug is being titrated to a set TOF, commonly 2 of 4, or whether an infusion is being maintained. Generally, TOF should be assessed at least every 4 hours. The nurse titrates the drug to a prescribed response such as two adductions out of four stimuli on the TOF.[40] In addition, the level of sedation can be monitored using the Ramsey Scale (Table 14-4).[43]

Fluid Management and Euvolemia. Hypotension and dehydration are dangerous and can result in decreased CPP and cerebral ischemia. The concurrent cerebral hypoxia can result in further increases in ICP. The goal is euvolemia; adequate fluid management with *saline* is used to prevent hypotension and dehydration. Glucose solutions are avoided. Monitoring of serum osmolality, electrolytes, and glucose is necessary to guide clinical decisions regarding electrolyte replacement, selection of saline concentration of fluids, rate of fluid administration, and glucose management. The goal of fluid maintenance is euvolemia.

Hypoglycemia and hyperglycemia can produce neurological changes, so they are to be avoided. Hypotonic glucose intravenous solutions are avoided. Hyperglycemia is controlled with a sliding scale of regular insulin according to periodic finger sticks and, if needed, a regular insulin intravenous drip can be started.

Temperature Control. CBF increases approximately 5% to 6% for each 1°C increase. The cerebral metabolic rate increases 5% to 7% for each 1°C increase.[44] An increased metabolic rate producing more end-products of cellular metabolism (CO_2 and organic acids, such as lactic acid). In the patient with existing cerebral hypertension, the increase in systemic blood pressure and CBF exacerbates the existing increase in ICP. Therefore, it is important to treat hyperthermia aggressively. This is accomplished with antipyretic drugs, such as acetaminophen, used alone or in combination with a hypothermia blanket. If a cooling blanket is used, cool the patient slowly to prevent shivering because this will increase ICP. If shivering does occur, ICP will increase; thus, the patient must be monitored closely to prevent this adverse effect. Thorazine is useful to control shivering.[27] To maintain normothermia, the nurse should:

- Monitor the core body temperature hourly.
- Administer antipyretics as ordered.
- If a cooling blanket is used, turn off the blanket when the temperature is approximately 1°C above the desired level. (Temperature will continue to drift downward because the blanket will remain cool.)
- Lower the temperature gradually to prevent shivering.

Seizure Control. Cerebral metabolic rates are increased with seizures; this results in increased CBF, CBV, and ICP. Posttraumatic seizures are classified as early (occur within 7 days of injury) or late (i.e., 7 days after injury). Seizure prophylaxis should be instituted for patients who are high risk for *early* seizures (e.g., penetrating injury). Routine seizure prophylaxis after 7 days following head injury is not recommended.[13] Both phenytoin (Dilantin) and carbamazepine are effective in preventing early posttraumatic seizures. A loading dose of phenytoin can be given intravenously over 1 hour for the seizing patient. The average maintenance dosage of phenytoin is 100 mg orally or through a nasogastric tube, three to four times daily. See Chapter 11 for further discussion of anticonvulsants. The nursing responsibilities involved in seizure control include:

	Table 14–4 • RAMSEY SCALE FOR ASSESSING LEVEL OF SEDATION

LEVEL OF SEDATION	RESPONSE
1	Patient anxious, agitated, restless, or all three
2	Patient cooperative, accepting ventilation, oriented, and tranquil
3	Patient asleep; brisk response to light glabellar tap or loud auditory stimuli
4	Patient asleep; sluggish response to light glabellar tap or loud auditory stimulus but does respond to painful stimuli
5	Patient does not respond to painful stimulus

- Monitoring serum levels to ensure therapeutic drug levels
- Because phenytoin binds to albumin, monitoring albumin level if serum values drop
- Once tube feedings are started, the protein may decrease a previously therapeutic phenytoin level, thus requiring a bolus dose and higher maintenance dose

Hypothermia. In laboratory animal studies, treatment with moderate, systemic hypothermia reduced the rate of cerebral edema and death after cerebral cortex injury.[45–47] This work was followed by early studies of hypothermia in humans that were inconclusive.[48,49] In two trials of patients with brain injury, moderate hypothermia maintained for 48 and 24 hours resulted in 15% and 18% increases, respectively, in the patients who had a good outcomes compared with others in their cohort group.[50,51] Early use of moderate hypothermia (core temperature 32 to 33°C) for 24 hours was tried to decrease central metabolism and oxygen consumption to preserve neuronal tissue and improve outcomes.[52] Cooling blankets were placed above and below a chemically paralyzed and sedated, mechanically ventilated patient. Side effects of treatment included myocardial suppression, arrhythmias, and renal dysfunction. A large multicenter trial was conducted from 1994 through May 1998. The conclusion of the study was that treatment with hypothermia, with the body temperature reaching 33°C within 8 hours after injury, is *not* effective in improving outcomes in patients with severe brain injury.[53]

High-Dose Barbiturate Coma. High-dose barbiturate therapy has been used for many years. It is a second-tier intervention to manage intractable intracranial hypertension resistant to conventional medical and surgical therapies in hemodynamically stable patients.[13] It has been useful in reducing increased ICP in selected salvageable patients with TBI, Reye's syndrome, encephalitis, and cerebral hemorrhage. The underlying therapeutic of the drug is a vasoconstricting effect and a rapid decrease in cerebral metabolism and CBF, which leads to a decrease in CBV and ICP.

Barbiturate coma therapy consists of administering a loading dose and maintenance doses of a short-acting barbiturate–most often pentobarbital (Nembutal), although some physicians prefer thiopental.[54] After barbiturate coma has been induced, the usual parameters of neurological assessment, such as the pupillary, gag, and swallowing reflexes, are lost. Cortical activity, as measured by electroencephalogram, is depressed, although brain-stem—evoked responses may remain intact. Continuous invasive monitoring of ICP and of cardiac and pulmonary functions is necessary. Peripheral and central lines for fluid and drug administration are required. The patient must remain intubated and mechanically ventilated. Induction of coma is accomplished by administering a loading dose of intravenous pentobarbital, 10 mg/kg, over 30 minutes followed by 5 mg/kg every hour for 3 doses.[6] A maintenance dose of 1 to 3 mg/kg/hour by continuous intravenous infusion is adjusted to maintain control of ICP.[6,20] Control of ICP can generally be achieved with serum barbiturate levels in the range of 30 to 40 mg/dL which will also cause burst suppression on the EEG.

Barbiturate coma should have the almost immediate effect of lowering the ICP. After the patient has maintained an ICP of less than 20 mm Hg pressure (or the level prescribed by protocol) for 24 to 48 hours, the drug is gradually tapered. If there is no response to therapy, the physician must decide how long the trial period should continue before the therapy is declared unsuccessful. The major problems associated with barbiturate coma are hypotension, dehydration, myocardial depression, and erratic dose response. Vasopressors such as phenylephrine hydrochloride or dopamine are administered to maintain blood pressure within targeted ranges. Albumin and other fluids are given to provide adequate volume and to prevent dehydration. Other conventional drugs used in management of increased ICP such as mannitol are also continued.

Barbiturates are stored in body fat. This can create a problem when brain-death criteria are considered because of elevated barbiturate blood levels that could explain loss of spontaneous respirations and brain-stem reflexes. Therefore, brain death criteria cannot be met until the drug is cleared from the body. It can be difficult to wait, especially if organ donation is a consideration. However, there are serious medicolegal implications if all components of brain death criteria are not met (see Chap. 4).

Surgery. If there is a localized mass, such as a hematoma, tumor, or abscess, removal or debulking of the lesion will help reduce intracranial hypertension. In addition, a craniectomy to allow for expansion of the brain due to cerebral edema has gained support to improve control of intracranial hypertension. After the ICP has subsided, the bone flap can be reinserted.

Cardiopulmonary Strategies and Interventions for Increased ICP and Intracranial Hypertension

Although this chapter has addressed increased ICP and intracranial hypertension as a collaborative problem, cardiopulmonary management deserves additional comments especially for the nurse. The brain requires a continuous and adequate supply of oxygen through the cardiac and respiratory systems. The interrelatedness of these systems to cerebral function is critical to patient outcomes.

Cardiac Management

Cardiac dysfunction in acute neurological conditions is common. The negative effects of hypertension and especially hypotension have been addressed in a previous section. Cardiac arrhythmias, left ventricular dysfunction, and cardiac disease or injury are briefly discussed in this section. Cardiac problems associated with specific neurological conditions, such as cerebral aneurysms, are discussed in other chapters.

Cardiac arrhythmias are common and often associated with sympathetic hyperactivity and preponderance, underlying heart disease, pulmonary disease, electrolyte imbalance, hypoxia, and response to therapy (drugs and fluid). Some arrhythmias are life threatening. Left ventricular dysfunction, as a result of various acute neurological conditions, can lead to life threatening arrhythmias and heart failure. The possibility of underlying coronary artery disease that can lead to myocardial infarction (MI) must be kept in mind.

The physiological stress of catastrophic acute neurological illness with sympathetic predominance and side effects of treatments can precipitate a MI. Additionally, in trauma patients, the possibility of direct injury to the heart or major blood vessels can result in various problems such as pericardial effusion or aortic dissection. Therefore, early detection of the cardiac dysfunction, identification of the underlying cause, and prompt treatment are critical to prevention of secondary cerebral injury. Secondary cerebral injury results from hypoxia and cerebral ischemia that can lead to irreversible infarction.

Nursing Management. Patients with acute neurological problems often need common technologies such as electrocardiography (ECG), pulmonary catheter, arterial line, and pulse oximeter for ongoing monitoring. Most continuous ECG monitoring systems are designed to recognize and print tracings of arrhythmias in addition to triggering an alarm. Many systems include an interface of multiple parameters to provide a composite of data.

The focus of nursing management is directed at vigilant ongoing monitoring of cardiac function for early identification of cardiac problems for prompt intervention and treatment. Assessing cardiac function includes:

- Monitoring vital signs, which include heart rate and blood pressure, hourly
- Auscultating for heart sounds (e.g., S_3, S_4, murmurs, clicks)
- Monitoring ongoing ECG leads for sinus rhythm, rate, arrhythmias, and other ECG abnormalities
- Analyzing cardiac waveform components hourly
- Recording periodic 12-lead ECG as necessary
- Maintaining alarms on all systems to alert health care providers that settings have been exceeded
- Monitoring periodic blood gases
- Monitoring hemoglobin for evidence of anemia
- Monitoring cardiac output data (with a pulmonary catheter) for evidence of dysfunction
- Monitoring mean arterial pressure (MAP)
- Calculating CPP hourly for patients with ICP monitors in place
- Monitoring the pulse oximeter (which has been placed on a finger or earlobe)
- Monitoring the jugular venous catheter data for adequacy of cerebral oxygen utilization

Use of technologies requires that the nurse be competent in the use of the equipment and interpretation of the data produced. Target range for physiological parameters must be known and maintained. The physician should be consulted when deviations from normal or targeted ranges occur. Based on abnormal findings, diagnostics such as an echocardiogram or chest radiograph may be ordered.

Interventions. There are often standing orders for treatment of abnormal cardiac findings available to the nurse. Follow the protocol and report unusual findings or trends to the physician.

Respiratory Management

Adequate oxygen and gas exchange, a patent airway, and ability to protect one's airway are necessary for all patients. If a patient is unable to protect his or her airway, an endotracheal tube will need to be inserted and oxygen therapy and possibly ventilatory support will need to be provided. Most patients with intracranial hypertension are intubated and ventilated. If use of a ventilator is indicated, pressure support mode and positive end expiratory pressure (PEEP) may be used within limitations. Many will receive PEEP.[55]

Concerns have been expressed about the effect of PEEP on ventilatory support and the raising of ICP. Positive airway pressure from mechanical ventilation is thought to impede venous return from the brain, thus contributing to an increase in ICP. PEEP elevates the mean airway pressure and thus decreases systemic mean arterial blood pressure by inducing arterial vasodilation. The decrease in systemic arterial pressure can decrease CPP. However, neurogenic pulmonary edema, the chief reason for providing PEEP, decreases pulmonary compliance and attenuates the transmission of positive airway pressure through the lungs to the mediastinal cavity. As a result, PEEP has less of an effect on ICP than previously thought. PEEP of 5 to 15 cm H_2O is well tolerated in patients with increased ICP.[56] Higher levels of PEEP (15 to 20 cm H_2O) may not significantly effect cerebral venous return.[27]

Nursing Management. The focus of nursing management is directed at maintaining a patent airway, supporting adequate ventilation, and preventing complications such as atelectasis, pneumonia, and barotrauma. Assessing the patency of the airway and ventilation adequacy can be determined by:

- Observing the airway for mucus or other drainage
- Auscultating the chest for breath sounds
- Observing the respiratory pattern
- Observing the chest and abdominal movement for evidence of respiratory distress
- Observing synchrony with the ventilator
- Noting presence of restlessness or a change in color of the skin (slight cyanosis)
- Reviewing and monitoring blood gases, hemoglobin, hematocrit, pulse oximetry, and other invasive data
- Determining necessary interventions

Oxygen Therapy. Oxygen therapy is provided to a patient whose airway is often maintained with an endotracheal tube. Suctioning is necessary to maintain patency of the airway. Chest physical therapy should be provided for all patients. The goal is to prevent hypercapnia and hypoxemia, which contribute to increased ICP and cerebral ischemia. The following summarizes respiratory management in the patient with intracranial hypertension. *For ventilated patients,* the following points should be considered:

- Patients who are not synchronized with their ventilator are not being ventilated properly; additionally, their intrathoracic pressure is raised, which impedes venous drainage from the brain and raises ICP.

- Patients who are "bucking" the ventilator (asynchrony) may have to be medicated to decrease the respiratory drive or paralyze the respiratory muscles. See previous discussion on sedation and neuromuscular blockade.
- Maintain mode, pressure support, and PEEP according to physician's orders.

Suctioning. Suctioning can cause elevations in ICP and sometimes plateau waves in patients who already have an elevated ICP. It should be undertaken with great care and gentleness with risk balanced by therapeutic goals. The need to suction is determined by observing the patient's color, chest and abdominal movement, presence of secretions within the upper respiratory pathways, and chest auscultation. Listen for adventitious lung sounds or decreased lung sounds in each lobe, and particularly in the bases of the lungs. The rasping sound of mucus in the upper respiratory tract is obvious to the ear without auscultation. It is critical for the nurse to be alert for the subtle signs of respiratory distress, which can be caused by partial obstruction of the respiratory tract. These subtle symptoms include an increase in pulse rate, perspiration, and restlessness.

Evaluate the patient frequently for any obvious or subtle indications of the need for suctioning. The usual protocol for suctioning includes the following:

- Preoxygenate the patient with 100% oxygen for 20 to 30 seconds before and after suctioning (some ventilators can do this with a manual control) because this helps to maintain levels of oxygen.
- Suction as necessary to remove secretions and maintain a patent airway; suction gently. Limit catheter insertion to **no more than 10 seconds** for each insertion, oxygenate between each catheter insertion, and limit attempts to suction to two insertions.[57,58]

Positioning to Enhance Respiratory Function. In addition to suctioning, respiratory function can be enhanced by changing the patient's position periodically (i.e., by turning patient every 2 hours). Positioning on the side facilitates drainage of oral secretions to promote a patent airway and prevents aspiration. Turn from side to side at least every 2 hours to prevent pooling of secretions. The head of the bed is elevated and the neck maintained in neutral position to facilitate cerebral venous drainage.

Managing Factors Known to Increase Intracranial Pressure

Several nurse researchers have contributed to the body and knowledge for evidence-based practice for patients with increased ICP. These studies have identified relationships between independent nursing activities (e.g., turning, positioning) and changes in ICP. Although many questions are unanswered, the body of knowledge for evidence-based practice continues to grow. Table 14-1 summarizes factors known to cause an increase in ICP. The nurse can apply this knowledge to assist in managing activities that have the potential to increase ICP, some of which are described in the next section.

Positioning and Turning. **Valsalva's maneuver** is the forceful expiration of air against a closed glottis, which increases intra-abdominal and intrathoracic pressure, impedes venous return from the brain, and impedes venous return to the heart. Changing a patient's position may precipitate Valsalva's maneuver. To avoid stimulating Valsalva's maneuver, the patient is turned and positioned in proper body alignment, avoiding angulation of body parts. The proper technique can be compared with rolling a log, which actually facilitates alignment when turning. Special attention must be given to the neck and hips. The neck is maintained in neutral position at all times. A soft collar, towel roll, or small pillow may be helpful if the patient cannot maintain the neutral position independently. The following positions should be avoided:

- Lateral flexion of the neck
- Trendelenburg's or prone position
- Extreme hip flexion or flexion of the upper legs on a pendulous abdomen

The head of the bed is elevated 30 degrees to facilitate cerebral venous drainage. In recent years, there has been discussion about elevation of the head and its effect on CPP. Some physicians prefer to keep the head of the bed flat arguing that this position better facilitates adequate CPP.[59] The flat position is maintained within preset ICP and CPP parameters; after these parameters have been exceeded, the decision may be made to elevate the head of the bed. Elevation of the head of the bed to 30 degrees is the general practice by most physicians. The patient should be positioned in good body alignment in the lateral position. This also facilitates oropharyngeal drainage. Pillows are useful to position the patient properly. If able to follow instructions, the patient should be instructed to exhale when being turned.

Bowel Management. A bowel program should be initiated to prevent constipation, which increases intra-abdominal pressure and causes straining at stool, both of which increase ICP. Stool softeners are usually administered once the patient is stabilized and able to tolerate intake through a feeding tube. Chapter 13 covers the components of a bowel program.

Isometric Muscle Contractions. An **isometric muscle contraction** is characterized by an increase in muscle tension without changes in the length of the muscle. With this in mind, footboards are not used. Canvas or running shoes or other commercially available foot positioners can be applied to maintain foot position. Other activities that cause isometric contractions include:

- Pushing oneself up using the feet or elbows to push against the mattress
- Pulling on arm restraints
- Decortication or decerebration
- Shivering

Emotional Upset and Noxious Stimuli. Conversations that may be emotionally stimulating to the patient, such as a discussion of prognosis, deficits, legal proceedings, restraints, or pain, should not be conducted within the patient's hearing range. Studies have shown that such conversations, when overheard by the patient, cause an elevation in ICP. Families should also be cautioned about refraining from unpleasant or stimulating conversations.

Soft stimuli are useful, such as a soft, soothing voice; pleasant conversation; soft music; the voices of loved ones being played on a tape recorder; or gentle therapeutic touching of the skin. The nurse should guard the patient from emotional upset. Even though certain patients may be classified as comatose, there is no way of knowing whether their hearing is intact or whether they can understand what is being said. The most reasonable approach for the nurse and others to take is to assume that patients can hear and understand.

Noxious stimuli, which are unpleasant or painful stimuli, increase ICP. Common noxious stimuli that the patient might experience include:

- Plugging in a drainage tube (e.g., urinary catheter), which causes pressure and pain from bladder distention
- Painful nursing or medical procedures (e.g., removing tape from the skin)
- Loud noises or sudden jarring of the bed
- Parts of the neurological examination, especially motor response to painful stimuli

Noxious stimuli should be prevented, if possible, or minimized by technique or by avoiding the need to perform multiple uncomfortable procedures. Soft stimuli, such as those mentioned previously, are useful to decrease the input of noxious stimuli when an uncomfortable procedure must be performed. The value of therapeutic touch cannot be overemphasized.

Clustering of Nursing Activities. In patients at risk, clustering of activities and procedures known to increase ICP often has a cumulative effect, causing spikes in ICP that can result in ischemia. For example, bathing, turning, and other common activities involved in routine care when clustered together may increase ICP. Even arousing the patient to assess neurological signs increases ICP. Suctioning and other respiratory procedures that are provided frequently for the acutely ill patient are notorious for their effect of increasing ICP. The nurse should plan care to avoid clustering of activities. In patients who are undergoing continuous ICP monitoring, the nurse should watch the monitor to determine the effect each activity has on ICP. Rest periods between procedures should be planned so that the ICP is allowed to return to the baseline level. If an ICP monitor is in place, it should be observed to determine responses.

MONITORING INTRACRANIAL PRESSURE

Continuous ICP monitoring has become common in neurological ICUs for patients with intracranial hypertension associated with conditions such as severe TBI (Glasgow Coma Scale ratings of 3 to 8), Reye's syndrome, subarachnoid hemorrhage, and herpes encephalitis. A large body of literature and clinical experience identifies the value of ICP monitoring

1. Helps in the earlier detection of intracranial mass lesions
2. Can limit indiscriminate use of therapies to control ICP, which themselves can be potentially harmful
3. Can reduce ICP by CSF drainage and thus improve cerebral perfusion
4. Can help in determining prognosis
5. May improve outcomes

When ICP monitoring is indicated, selection of the type of monitoring device must be made. The optimal ICP monitoring device is one that is accurate, reliable, cost effective, and causes minimal patient discomfort.

There are two types of ICP monitoring devices based on the location of the transducer.[60] The first includes an external strain gauge transducer that use a fluid-filled line to couple the *extracranial transducer* to the patient's intracranial space. Traditional ventricular catheters, subarachnoid bolts, and subdural catheters are included in this group. The ventricular catheter is the most accurate, least expensive, and most reliable method of monitoring ICP; it also allows for therapeutic drainage of CSF. The second type includes a catheter-tip—strain device that directly monitors ICP using an *intracranial transducer* located in the tip of the catheter. Included in this group are fiberoptics and pneumatic systems. Potential sites for placement of an ICP monitoring catheter is the intraventricular space, subarachnoid space, intraparenchyma, epidural space, or subdural space.

Calibration

Regardless of the type of ICP monitoring system used (i.e., external or internal transducer), it is necessary to calibrate or "zero" the system. Calibration is always to an atmospheric reference point called the "zero" point, and the referencing of the transducer to atmospheric pressure is referred to as *"zeroing the transducer."* This process differs for an external and internal transducer.[60]

External Transducer

When an external transducer is used with a fluid-coupled system, the hydrostatic dynamics of the fluid require that transducer must be leveled to a consistent anatomic reference point and zero-balanced to account for variations in the patient's head position. The most common *reference points* used are the top of the ear, external auditory meatus, or outer canthus of the eye. All these points approximate the location of the catheter tip at the foramen of Monro. Regardless of reference point chosen, it is important to *use the same point for all readings consistently* to ensure accuracy. Therefore, whenever there is a change in the position of the patient's head in relation to the transducer, the transducer must be releveled to the consistent anatomical reference point before reading the ICP pressure. For accuracy, a carpenter's level or a laser leveling device is used to level the transducer to the anatomical reference point.[61]

Internal Transducer

Calibrating an ICP monitoring system that uses an intracranial transducer is simpler. A fiberoptic transducer-tipped catheter (FTC) is calibrated by the manufacturer before shipping. Just before insertion, the catheter is zero (atmospherically) balanced. There is no further recalibration possible during use (without an associated ventricular catheter). Therefore, there is no need to level the transducer to an external site, which is a time saver for the nurse. However, if there is drift and if recalibration is not possible, then measurement error will result. With some monitors, in vivo calibration is possible. The advantage of this option is that it allows for in vivo calibration to be performed to counteract the slight drift of the reference point over time that can affect accuracy.[61]

ICP Monitoring Systems: External Transducer and Internal Transducer Systems

External Transducer Systems

Three types of external transducer systems are discussed in this section: the ventricular catheter; the subarachnoid bolt or screw; and subdural catheter (Fig. 14-9). Although epidural placement is possible, it is not often used.

Intraventricular Catheter. The intraventricular catheter (IVC) was pioneered by Lundberg in 1960 and remains the standard criterion with which all other catheters and ICP monitoring systems are compared.[62] The soft, Silastic, radiopaque IVC is inserted through a small bur hole made with a twist drill usually into the anterior horn of the nondominant lateral ventricle (see Fig. 14-9A). The IVC is con-

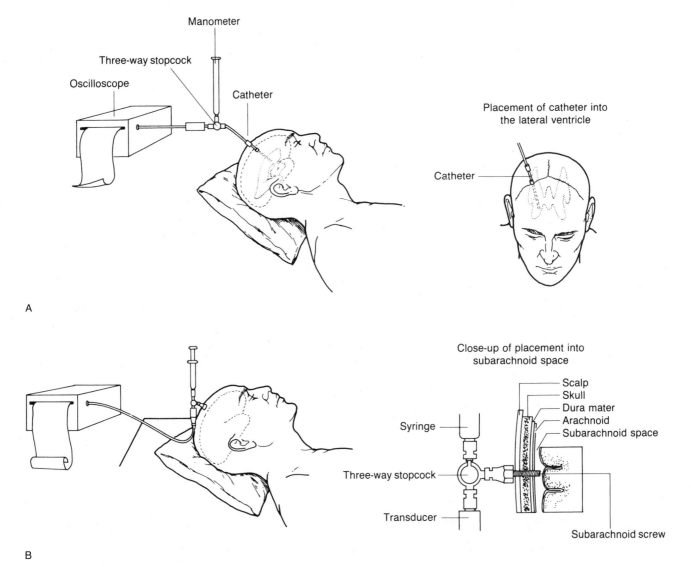

Figure 14–9 • Major intracranial pressure monitoring devices. (*A*) Vetricular catheter monitor. (*B*) Subarachnoid screw or bolt monitor. (From Smeltzer, S., & Bare, B. [1996]. *Brunner and Suddarth's textbook of medical-surgical nursing* [8th ed.]. Philadelphia: Lippincott-Raven Publishers.)

nected to a closed fluid-filled system. Several systems are available, all based on the same principles and components. These components include a proximal stopcock or sampling port and a more distal stopcock that interfaces with either an external transducer for ICP monitoring or a collection system for CSF drainage.[60] For example, the Becker intraventricular external drainage and monitoring system (PS Medical, Goleta, CA) is a commonly used system in many centers (see Fig. 14-7). It consists of a side port that is used for continuous drainage and sampling of CSF. The external pressure transducer can be connected to the main system stopcock, which is leveled to the reference point on the patient's head (e.g., external auditory meatus). The drip chamber can be moved up and down and placed at a desired level against the zero reference level stopcock. The drip chamber at the end of the drain line is typically fixed by a 15-cm length of pressure tubing to secure drainage in the drip chamber when ICP rises above a predetermined level, typically 15 or 20 mm Hg.[27] Using the shortest possible length of tubing between the catheter and the transducer and eliminating air bubbles from the system are necessary for accuracy of ICP readings.

The *advantages* of the IVC are the ability to drain CSF fractionally to reduce ICP; to collect CSF for laboratory analysis; to inject contrast media to visualize the ventricle, as well as its accuracy; and low cost. The *disadvantages* include difficulty of insertion into a small ventricle because of lateral mass shift; CSF leakage around insertion site; plugging of the catheter with blood or cerebral tissue; higher risk of infection; and need to zero and recalibrate frequently.

Subarachnoid Bolt or Screw. The subarachnoid (SA) bolt was developed by Vires in 1973 as an option to decrease infections and insertion limitations associated with IVCs. The insertion is similar to that of an IVC except that there are more options for placement because the brain parenchyma is not penetrated.[63] The bolt consists of a hollow metal shaft or screw that is threaded at one end through a bur hole and dura into the subarachnoid space (see Fig. 14-9B). The bolt is hydrostatically coupled to fluid-filled pressure tubing, a stopcock, and an external transducer. The transducer is leveled to the anatomical reference point. The subarachnoid bolt is only a monitoring device; CSF cannot be readily withdrawn from it, and may lead to bolt occlusion.[63]

The *advantages* of the bolt are the simplicity of the bolt; the ease of rapid insertion; it is usable in patients who fail use of the IVC or are not candidates for IVC placement; and it does not penetrate the brain parenchyma (less invasive), therefore decreasing the possibility of hemorrhage and infection. The *disadvantages* include plugging of the bolt with blood, debris, or obliteration from an edematous brain; that it may underestimate ICP when it is elevated; its inaccurate ICP readings because of a different compartmental pressures; risk of infection, although this is lower than with IVCs; and the need to zero and recalibrate frequently. If plugging is suspected because of a dampened waveform or low ICP pressure, the bolt can be flushed by the physician with 0.1 to 0.2 mL of preservative-free (nonbacteriostatic) saline to restore accurate ICP reading.[64] In most situations, this small amount of saline does not cause dangerous ICP elevations.[63]

Subdural Catheters. Another method of monitoring ICP with an external transducer involves placement of a catheter in the subdural space. Currently this method is not used often because of an underestimation of ICP and dampening of waveforms especially with high ICP pressures.[65] The infection rate and risk of hemorrhage are about the same as with the subarachnoid bolts.

Internal (Intracranial) Transducer Systems

An FTC is available for ICP monitoring and uses a different technology, in part, to overcome some of the disadvantages of external transducer systems. A miniature transducer in the catheter tip is coupled by a long, continuous wire or fiberoptic cable to an external electronic module. One of the better-known fiberoptic systems (Camino Laboratories, San Diego, CA) operates according to the following principle. Light fibers within the catheter convey light impulses created by movement of a mirrored diaphragm, which reflects pressure changes. The light signal is converted into electrical signals in the amplifier connector. Mean pressures are displayed on a digital monitor that can interface with an additional analog monitor for display of continuous waveforms (Fig. 14-10A). The FTC can be inserted easily into the lateral ventricle, subarachnoid space, subdural space, brain parenchyma, or under a bone flap. A scalp stab wound is made, and a small twist drill is used to drill a small bur hole through bone. A housing device (a small bolt) is then screwed into place. The dura is perforated, and the transducer probe is threaded through the housing device to the desired depth and fixed in position by tightening the ring unit over the housing device. Finally, a protective sheath is snapped into position. If the intraventricular monitoring technique is used, it can be configured to both monitor ICP and to drain CSF (see Fig. 14-10B).

This technology is more expensive than fluid-coupled monitoring systems. There is the cost of the disposable catheter and initial expense and maintenance of the cable and compatible monitor. The technology does not interface with the other monitoring systems. It does have its own portable monitor that is transportable so that continuous ICP monitoring is possible during transport. That the catheter is calibrated by the manufacturer and is zero-balanced only once at the time of insertion is both positive and negative. Because the transducer is internal, it does not need to be zero referenced to an anatomical point while in use. Because there is no coupling with fluid, there are no problems of dampening waveforms resulting from catheter occlusion or air bubble entrapment. This is a time saver for the nurse. It is also neither possible to assess for drift that occurs over time, nor to recalibrate if drift is suspected. Drift is a source of measurement error with both external and internal transducer systems,[66–68] but the lack of ability to identify and correct drift with the FTC system is a disadvantage. Finally, nurses who work directly with the fiberoptic cable must take care to prevent bending the cable, which can result from patient movement, transport, or care. After clinicians have become accustomed to working with the equipment, breakage is not a significant problem.[60] In summary, the *advantages* of the FTC are: ease of insertion; options for multiple insertion sites; no need to zero to an anatomical point every time the position of the head changes; decreased risk of

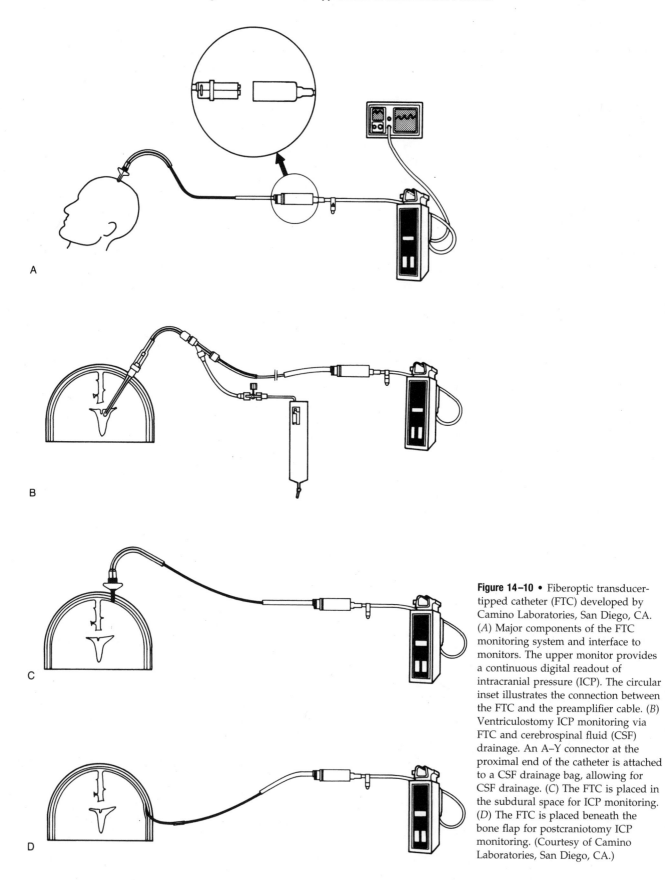

Figure 14-10 • Fiberoptic transducer-tipped catheter (FTC) developed by Camino Laboratories, San Diego, CA. (A) Major components of the FTC monitoring system and interface to monitors. The upper monitor provides a continuous digital readout of intracranial pressure (ICP). The circular inset illustrates the connection between the FTC and the preamplifier cable. (B) Ventriculostomy ICP monitoring via FTC and cerebrospinal fluid (CSF) drainage. An A–Y connector at the proximal end of the catheter is attached to a CSF drainage bag, allowing for CSF drainage. (C) The FTC is placed in the subdural space for ICP monitoring. (D) The FTC is placed beneath the bone flap for postcraniotomy ICP monitoring. (Courtesy of Camino Laboratories, San Diego, CA.)

infection; and continuation of monitoring during transport. Disadvantages include: increased expense as compared to fluid coupled systems; fragile fiberoptic cable that can break; and inability to identify and correct drift.

Pressure Waves

With continuous ICP monitoring, the fluctuations in waveforms correlate with both respirations and the cardiac cycle. Positive deflections of 2 to 10 mm H_2O can be observed in the patient who is not receiving ventilatory support with positive pressure. These deflections are noted immediately after systole and exhalation. Waveforms, which can be examined individually or in trend recordings, are helpful in identifying changes in the patient's condition. The morphology of each waveform has been discussed previously in relation to compliance.

Trend recordings compress continuous ICP recording data into time periods (e.g., 5 to 60 minute blocks) to reflect general trends in ICP over longer periods.

Three distinct pressure waves have been identified by Lundberg:[62] A (plateau) waves, B waves, and C waves (Fig. 14-11). Since their identification over 40 years ago, no new wave patterns have been added, although interpretation of their meaning has evolved. It may be impossible to identify these very low frequency waves unless the sampling frequency is adequate (i.e., more than once per second) to capture these changes.[63] The following sections describe each of the waveforms.

A Waves (Plateau Waves)

These waves derive their name from the "plateau" shape of the trended waveforms. They consist of sudden, transient waves that begin from an *already* elevated ICP from 20 mm Hg or more to levels of 50 to 100 mm Hg, and persist 5 to 20 minutes before terminating with a rapid decline to the level of or below the baseline ICP. Plateau waves are often not accompanied by a corresponding elevation of mean arterial blood pressure so that there is an accompanying low CPP. Therefore, there is sustained low CPP with concurrent cerebral ischemia and transient or paroxysmal symptoms, sometimes called *pressure signs* (see discussion that follows) that are seen in patients with *already* elevated ICP who have *decreased cerebral compliance.*

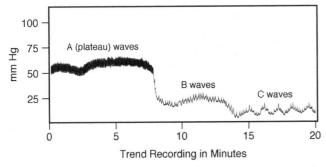

Figure 14–11 • Intracranial pressure waves. Composite diagram of A (plateau) waves, B waves, and C waves.

Plateau waves are precipitated by a chain of physiological and pathophysiological events.[63] A gradual rise from the baseline ICP begins to compromise CPP, causing incomplete ischemia. The ischemia initiates a concurrent vasodilator response and increase in CBV in the cerebral hemispheres.[69-71] Increased CBV rapidly increases ICP, which further reduces CPP and CBF. The plateau waves continue until the intracranial volume is reduced, usually by reduction in the volume of CSF or by reduction of blood volume with hyperventilation. Research has shown that plateau waves are related to poorer outcomes and herniation.[72] Although the patient tolerates the specific event, it suggests a need for expansion of ICP therapies (e.g., CSF drainage, mannitol, hyperventilation). Williams and Hanley call attention to a practical clinical point.[63] They note that the rising phase of a plateau wave (which the patient might conceivably survive) cannot be differentiated clinically *as it is happening* from sudden ICP elevation associated with herniation. Therefore, given the clinical picture, the clinician would treat the patient as herniation and institute expanded ICP therapies. Only on retrospective ICP trend analysis is it apparent that a plateau wave did occur.

B Waves

Sharp, rhythmic spikes occurring every 30 seconds to 2 minutes characterize B waves. The ICP peaks to 20 to 50 mm Hg although these elevated levels are not sustained. In a spontaneously breathing patient, B waves may be seen with Cheyne-Stokes respirations or with brief episodes of decreased respirations or apnea. B waves are probably caused by variations in CVR or reactivity.[62] They indicate a decreased cerebral adaptive capability and may be a warning sign of A waves.[73] It is an indication for initiation of therapy to reduce ICP.

C Waves

These low-amplitude, transient, rhythmic oscillations occur 4 to 8 times per minute, reaching pressures of up to 20 mm Hg.[62] C waves are related to normal changes of the systemic arterial blood pressure and ventilation. The clinical significance of these waves is unknown; therefore there is currently no indication for a change in therapy.

Clinical Implications of Plateau Waves

Plateau waves are clinically significant because they peak to levels of 50 to 100 mm Hg from an **already elevated base ICP**. Plateau waves correlate physiologically with cerebral hypoxia, ischemia, and possible infarction to selected areas. Because cerebral tissue is sensitive to decreased O_2, symptoms of cerebral dysfunction may be evident.

The degree of dysfunction may be subtle (e.g., confusion, restlessness) or pronounced (e.g., hemiplegia, posturing). **Pressure signs** may include deterioration in LOC; decreased pupillary reaction; paresis, paralysis, or decortication or decerebration; aphasia; headache; changes in respiratory pattern (e.g., Cheyne-Stokes); and other changes in vital signs. Although pressure symptoms are paroxysmal transient manifestations, they may last for a prolonged period after the plateau waves have subsided.

Early recognition of a tendency toward plateau waves or the presence of factors that trigger plateau waves should be followed by early intervention to prevent or control these dangerous waves.

Infection Control and the Intracranial Pressure Monitor

Infections are the primary complication encountered with ICP monitoring. The Centers for Disease Control and Prevention have defined CSF infections.[74] The range of CSF infections reported in patients undergoing ICP monitoring was 0% to 40% with an average of 10%.[75–80] In a study by Rebuck and associates, 7.4% of 215 ICP monitored patients developed CSF infection.[81] Risk factors for CSF infection were also examined. They included duration of monitoring longer than 5 days; presence of ventriculostomy; CSF leakage; concurrent systemic infection (e.g., pneumonia, urinary tract infection); and replacement of ICP monitoring device. Patients with intraventricular placement compared with intraparenchymal placement had a higher incidence of infections. Use of prophylactic antibiotics was examined. Although not a standard of practice, antibiotics were administered to 63% of infected and 59% of noninfected patients. Poon and colleagues reported a decreased incidence of infection in patients randomized to prophylaxis for the duration of ICP monitoring.[82] Rebuck and colleagues concluded that duration of prophylaxis has no significant influence on development of infection. When antibiotics were given, vancomycin followed by cefazolin were the drugs of choice.[81]

One can conclude that there are variations in reported incidence and identification of risk factors. More randomized control trials are needed to establish evidence-based practice. Table 14-5 lists the most commonly identified risk factors. However, recommendations do exist to assist the clinician. Ventriculostomy catheters for ICP monitoring should be removed as quickly as possible, and in circumstances in which prolonged monitoring is required, there appears to be no benefit from catheter exchange.[80] With the new onset of fever in a patient with an intracranial device, CSF should be obtained for analysis from the CSF reservoir for a gram stain and culture.[83]

Table 14–5 • RISK FACTORS FOR INFECTIONS IN PATIENTS UNDERGOING ICP MONITORING

- Use of intraventricular catheter
- ICP monitoring longer than 5 days
- Flushing of the system
- CSF leakage
- Concurrent systemic infection
- Serial ICP monitoring catheters (e.g., replacing a catheter)

Nursing Management of the Patient During Intracranial Pressure Monitoring

As outlined earlier in the chapter, ICP monitoring has several well-established purposes. From the nurse's perspective, monitoring of ICP provides data that augments serial neurological assessment data for making treatment decisions, gauging progress, and observing responses to nursing interventions and medical treatment. Most patients who are undergoing ICP monitoring also have central lines for hemodynamic monitoring that supply continuous data on MAP. These data are used to calculate CPP. Normal range is 60 to 90 mm Hg, although the target goal may be set higher than minimum for certain patients, such as those with severe TBI (i.e., 70 mm Hg or above). CPP is a direct indicator of the adequacy of cerebral perfusion, so monitoring the CPP is as important as monitoring ICP. The ability to interpret continuous waveforms, trends in waveforms (previously discussed in this chapter), and CPP accurately assists the nurse in data-based clinical decision making.

The American Association of Neuroscience Nurses has published a clinical guide about ICP monitoring that is helpful.[84] There are several specific considerations in the nursing management of a patient with an ICP monitor.[85] For troubleshooting, follow the manufacturer's specific instructions for use of monitoring system and the treating hospital's policy. The following section outlines key points related to data collection, accuracy of ICP and waveform, and infection prevention:

- Data collection
  - Collect and interpret waveforms.
  - Alert the physician as necessary to evidence of increasing ICP.
  - Monitor waveforms for dampening effect.
  - Calculate CPP hourly (CPP = MAP − ICP).
- Accuracy of ICP and waveforms
  - Re-zero and recalibrate the device according to manufacturer's instruction and hospital policy.
  - Recognize that a certain amount of drift will occur each day that the catheter is in place; take this into consideration in determining the validity and reliability of the data with other clinical data.
- For systems with external transducers
  - Zero to the same anatomical reference point each time.
  - Zero each time the position of the head changes and at least every 2 to 4 hours.
  - If a dampened waveform occurs
    - Observe fluid lines for leakage or disconnection of components; if either occurs, the system is no longer sterile; the physician must be notified; and the system will need to be replaced according to hospital policy.
    - Observe for air bubbles or debris in the tubing; if found, flush the line, being sure to close the stopcock to the catheter and patient (follow hospital policy).
- For systems with internal transducers
  - Recalibrate after insertion is not possible.
  - With FTCs, do not bend the cable as a precaution in preventing breakage.

- Decreasing the risk of infection
  - Maintain an occlusive dry sterile dressing around the insertion site, and change it on a prescribed schedule according to hospital policy (usually every 24 to 72 hours).
  - Monitor the insertion site for signs of infection, drainage, or CSF leakage.
  - Keep all connections tightly connected to maintain the integrity and sterility of the system.
- Ventricular catheter to CSF drainage bag
  - Monitor height of collection chamber and clamps (based on order to open or close) every 2 hours.
  - Adjust height of collection chamber to be level with or above the transducer according to physician's order.
  - **Do not** position the top of the collection chamber **below** the level of the anatomical reference point to prevent siphoning of CSF when the drain is opened.
  - Monitor the color, clarity, and amount of CSF drainage (lack of drainage will occur with obstruction of the catheter or connecting tubing; this should be reported and discussed with the physician).
  - Collection of CSF is done under strict aseptic technique and according to manufacturer's instruction and hospital policy.

SPECIAL SYNDROMES: BENIGN INTRACRANIAL HYPERTENSION AND HYDROCEPHALUS

Two special syndromes associated with increased ICP and CSF flow are benign intracranial hypertension and hydrocephalus.

Benign Intracranial Hypertension (Pseudotumor Cerebri)

Pseudotumor cerebri, now commonly called *benign intracranial hypertension*, is seen most often in obese adolescent girls and young women.[86] The chief complaint is headache and, in some instances, blurred vision, diplopia, slight numbness in the face, or dizziness. On physical examination, the patient is alert, aware, conversant, and seems otherwise well. The only abnormal finding is papilledema. On lumbar puncture, CSF pressure is usually about 250 to 450 mm H_2O. On CT scan or MRI, ventricles are of normal size, and there is no evidence of an intracranial mass or obstruction of CSF. Visual testing may find slight peripheral deficits. The immediate management focus is to reduce the papilledema to prevent visual impairment. Treatment options include:

1. Serial lumbar puncture to remove CSF until normal pressure is maintained (performed daily and then at increasing intervals)
2. Drug therapy if CSF pressure continues to be elevated and papilledema persists
   - Prednisone 40 to 60 mg/day
   - Acetazolamide (Diamox); 750 mg to 1.0 g/day in two to four divided doses; carbonic anhydrase inhibitors that decrease CSF production
3. In the approximately 10% of patients who do not respond to these treatments, a trial of lumbar drainage, followed by placement of a lumbar peritoneal shunt, may be necessary.

Hydrocephalus

Hydrocephalus refers to a progressive dilatation of the ventricular system because the production of CSF exceeds the absorption rate. Hydrocephalus is a clinical syndrome rather than a disease entity. Abnormalities in overproduction, circulation, or reabsorption of CSF can result in hydrocephalus. (See Chap. 5 for a review of CSF and circulation.)

Classification

Hydrocephalus can be subdivided into noncommunicating and communicating hydrocephalus:

- **Noncommunicating hydrocephalus** is a condition in which CSF in the ventricular system does not communicate properly within the subarachnoid space. Obstruction can be caused by a mass, such as a tumor within or adjacent to the ventricular system, a congenital obstruction, or an obliteration from an inflammatory process.
- **Communicating hydrocephalus** is a condition in which too few or nonfunctional arachnoid villi are unable to reabsorb CSF sufficiently. Subarachnoid hemorrhage secondary to aneurysmal rupture or a TBI can produce transient or lasting communicating hydrocephalus. The arachnoid villi become plugged and cannot reabsorb CSF. Plugging can occur from the end-products of blood cell breakdown or the exudate from meningitis.

The signs and symptoms of hydrocephalus depend on the type of hydrocephalus and the age of the patient. For noncommunicating hydrocephalus, treatment of the primary problem is necessary, usually with surgery. In communicating hydrocephalus, CSF drainage may be attempted to clear the arachnoid villi of exudate so that normal function will be resumed in the future. If this is ineffective, a surgical shunting procedure will be necessary. Selection of the particular procedure depends on the age of the patient and any preexisting health problems.

Because the scope of this text is limited to adult problems, no discussion of hydrocephalus in the infant or child is included. The reader is directed to a pediatric text for discussion of this topic.

Normal-Pressure Hydrocephalus

An important type of communicating hydrocephalus seen in older adults is called **normal-pressure hydrocephalus**; it is usually reversible. (This syndrome is also called *occult hydrocephalus*, *low-pressure hydrocephalus*, and *normotensive hydrocephalus*.)

In normal-pressure hydrocephalus, there is ventricular enlargement with compression of the cerebral tissue, but normal CSF pressure is noted on lumbar puncture. Various circumstances have been associated with the development of normal-pressure hydrocephalus:

- Plugging of the arachnoid villi secondary to subarachnoid hemorrhage
- Thrombosis of the superior sagittal sinus
- Injury from brain trauma or related to surgery, in which scarring of the basal cistern is thought to occur
- Bacterial meningitis, in which there is plugging and possible fibrotic changes of the arachnoid villi

After careful evaluation of some patients, particularly those between 60 and 70 years old, if no associated precipitated condition has been found, the diagnosis is **idiopathic normal pressure hydrocephalus.**

Signs and Symptoms

The onset of normal-pressure hydrocephalus is insidious and slow to develop (over weeks or months). Changes occur so slowly so they can easily be overlooked by the patient and family, or they may be attributed to the aging process when an older patient is involved.

The cardinal symptoms include mental changes, urinary incontinence, and disturbances in gait. Mental changes may begin as mild forgetfulness along with a diminished level of generalized cognitive function and progress to severe impairment. In advanced cases, mutism and hypokinesia may be apparent. Gait disturbances begin with a slowed pace that includes wide-based, zigzag steps; subsequently, gait is unsteady, and falling is common. Upper extremity movement may be unaffected or slowed. With progression, the ability to maintain independent ambulation is lost.

Urinary incontinence is not an early sign; it appears later. Lost social inhibition and forgetfulness caused by cerebral atrophy are the probable causes. No headache or papilledema is noted, although unexplained nystagmus is apparent in many patients. Tendon reflexes, particularly in the lower extremities, are increased. In advanced cases, Babinski's, grasping, and sucking reflexes may be present.

Diagnostic Studies

The most common diagnostic studies are CT and MRI. Atrophy and enlarged ventricles are noted. A positive history of a slowly developing progression of symptoms is essential in establishing the diagnosis. Normal CSF pressure is noted on lumbar puncture.

Treatment

The accepted treatment for normal-pressure hydrocephalus is a ventricular shunt. When cerebral atrophy has occurred, reversal of symptoms is minimal. The following describes optimal outcomes from successful ventricular shunting:

- The most dramatic improvement that may be apparent almost immediately is in mental status. The patient will become much more alert, oriented, and manageable. Others, however, will show more gradual improvement.
- Incontinence may be quickly reversed.

- Reversal of gait disturbance takes longer; a permanent residual deficit may result.

▐▐▐ SUMMARY

Management of intracranial hypertension is a fundamental problem in clinical neuroscience practice. A review of the physiological basis for ICP, independent and collaborative nursing roles, and major management concerns has been provided. The current evidence-based practice is growing, and current evidence has been incorporated into this discussion.

REFERENCES

1. Marmarou, A., & Tabaddor, K. (1993). Intracranial pressure: Physiology and pathophysiology. In P. R. Cooper. (Ed.). *Head injury* (3rd ed., pp. 203–224). Baltimore: Williams & Wilkins.
2. Germon, K. (1988). Interpretation of ICP pulse waves to determine intracerebral compliance. *Journal of Neuroscience Nursing, 20*(6), 344–351.
3. Cardosa, E. R., Rowan, J. O., & Galbraith, S. (1983). Analysis of cerebrospinal fluid pulse wave in intracranial pressure. *Journal of Neurosurgery, 59,* 817–821.
4. Benarroch, E. E., Westmoreland, B. F., Daube, J. R., et al. (1999). *Medical neurosciences: An approach to anatomy, pathophysiology, and physiology by systems and level* (4th ed., pp. 136–150, 326–333). Boston: Little, Brown.
5. Ropper, A. H., & Kennedy, S. K. (1993). Physiology and clinical aspects of raised intracranial pressure. In A. H. Ropper, (Ed.). *Neurological and neurosurgical intensive care* (3rd ed., pp. 11–28). New York: Raven Press.
6. Eisenberg, H. M., Frankowski, R. F., Conant, L. P., et al. (1988). High dose barbiturate control of elevated intracranial pressure in patients with severe head injury. *Journal of Neurosurgery, 69,* 15–23.
7. Rosner, M. J., & Daughton, S. (1990). Cerebral perfusion pressure management in head injury. *Journal of Trauma, 30*(8), 933–941.
8. Firlik, A. D., & Marion, D. W. (2000). Intracranial pressure: Physiology and pathophysiology. In P. R. Cooper & J. G. Golfinos (Eds.). *Head injury* (4th ed., pp. 221–228). New York: McGraw-Hill.
9. Klatzo, I. (1967). Neuropathological aspects of brain edema. *Journal of Neuropathology and Experimental Neurology. 20,* 1.
10. Plum, F., & Posner, J. B. (1982). *The diagnosis of stupor and coma* (3rd ed.). Philadelphia: F. A. Davis.
11. Kernohan, J. W., & Woltman, H. W. (1929). Incisura of the crus due to contralateral brain tumor. *Archives of Neurology & Psychiatry, 21,* 274–287.
12. Knupling, R., Fuchs, E. C., Aschenbrenner, C. A., et al. (1979). Chronic and acute transtentorial herniation with tumors of the posterior cranial fossa. *Neurochirurgia, 22,* 9–17.
13. Bullock, R., Chesnut, R. M., Clifton, G., et al. (2000). Guidelines for the management of severe traumatic brain injury. *Journal of Neurotrauma, 17*(6/7), 451–553.
14. Shapiro, H. M. (1973). Intracranial hypertension: Therapeutic and anesthetic considerations. *Anesthesiology, 43,* 445–471.
15. Hulme, A. & Cooper, R. (1976). The effects of head position and jugular vein compression on intracranial pressure. In J. Beks, D. A. Bosch, & M. Brock (Eds.). *Intracranial pressure III* (pp. 259–263). Berlin: Springer-Verlag.
16. Ropper, A. H., Marshall, L. F., & Shapiro, H. M. (1979). High-dose barbiturate therapy in humans: A clinical review of 60 patients. *Annals of Neurology, 6,* 194–199.

17. Durward, Q. J., Amacher, A. L., Delmaestro, R. F., et al. (1983). Cerebral and cardiovascular responses to changes in head elevation with intracranial hypertension. *Journal of Neurosurgery, 59*, 15–23.

18. Feldman, Z., Kanter, M. J., Robertson, C. S. et al. (1992). Effect of head elevation on intracranial pressure, cerebral perfusion pressure, and cerebral blood flow in head injured patients. *Journal of Neurosurgery, 76*, 207–211.

19. Chesnut, R. M. (2000). Medical management of intracranial pressure. In P. F. Cooper & J. G. Golfinos, (Ed.), *Head injury* (4th ed., pp. 259–263). New York: McGraw-Hill.

20. Allen, C. H., & Ward, J. D. (1998). An evidence-based approach to management of increased intracranial pressure. *Critical Care Clinics, 14*(3), 485–495.

21. Bouma, G. J., Muizelaar, J. P, Choi, S. C., et al. (1991). Cerebral circulation and metabolism after severe traumatic brain injury: The elusive role of ischemia. *Journal of Neurosurgery, 75*, 685–693.

22. Robertson, C. S., Constant, C. F., Gokaslan, Z. I., et al. (1992). Cerebral blood flow, arteriovenous oxygen difference, and outcome in head injured patients. *Journal of Neurology, Neurosurgery, and Psychiatry, 55*, 594–603.

23. Raichle, M. E., & Plum, F. (1972). Hyperventilation and cerebral blood flow. *Stroke, 3*, 566–575.

24. Muizlaar, J. P., Marmarou, A., Ward, J. D., et al. (1991). Adverse effects of prolonged hyperventilation in patients with severe head injury: A randomized clinical trial. *Journal of Neurosurgery, 75*, 731–739.

25. Cruz, J., Miner, M. E., Allen, S. J., et al. (1991). Continuous monitoring of cerebral oxygenation in acute brain injury: Assessment of cerebral hemodynamic reserve. *Neurosurgery, 29*, 743–749.

26. Sheinberg, M., Kaner, M. J., Robertson, C. S., et al. (1992). Continuous monitoring of jugular venous oxygen saturation in head-injured patients. *Journal of Neurosurgery, 76*, 212-217.

27. Wijdicks, E. F. M. 1997). *The clinical practice of critical care neurology* (pp. 76-87). Philadelphia: Lippincott-Raven.

28. McGraw, C. P. (1989). A cerebral perfusion pressure greater than 80 mm Hg is more beneficial. In J. T. Hoff & A. L. Betz, (Eds.), *Intracranial pressure*, VII (pp. 839-841). Berlin: Springer-Verlag.

29. Bouma, G. J., Muizelaar, J., Strniger, W., et al. (1992). Ultra early evaluation of regional cerebral blood flow in severely head-injured patients using xenon enhanced computed tomography. *Journal of Neurosurgery, 77*, 360–368.

30. Jaggi, J. L., Obrist, W. D., Gennarelli, T. A., et al. (1990). Relationship of early cerebral blood flow metabolism to outcome in acute head injury. *Journal of Neurosurgery, 72*, 176–182.

31. Marion, D. W., Darby, J., & Yonas, H. (1991). Acute regional cerebral blood flow changes caused by severe head injuries. *Journal of Neurosurgery, 74*, 407–414.

32. Robertson, C. S., Contant, C. F., Narayan, R. K. et al. (1992). Cerebral blood flow, Avdo2, and neurological outcome in head-injured patients. *Journal of Neurotrauma, 9*, S349–S358.

33. McLaughlin, M. R., & Marion, D. W. (1996). Cerebral blood flow and vasoresponsivity within and around cerebral contusions. *Journal of Neurosurgery, 85*(5), 871–876.

34. Salvant, J. B., & Muizellar, J. P. (1993). Changes in cerebral blood flow and metabolism related to the presence of subdural hematoma. *Neurosurgery, 33*, 387–393.

35. Bouma, G. J., Muizelaar, J. P. (1990). Relationship between cardiac output and cerebral blood flow in patients with intact and with impaired autoregulation. *Journal of Neurosurgery, 73*(3), 368–374.

36. Kelley, D. F. (1995). Steroids in head injury. *New Horizons, 3*(3), 453–455.

37. Shapiro, B. A., Warren, J., Egol, A. B., et al. (1995). Practice parameters for intravenous analgesia and sedation for adult patients in the intensive care unit: An executive summary. *Critical Care Medicine, 23*(9), 1596–1600.

38. Covington, H. (1998). Use of propofol for sedation in the ICU. *Critical Care Nurse, 18*(4), 34.

39. Mirski, M. A., Muffelman, B., Ulatowski, J. A., & Hanley, D. F. (1995). Sedation for the critically ill neurologic patient. *Critical Care Medicine, 23*(12), 2038–2053.

40. Ford, E. V. (1995). Monitoring neuromuscular blockade in the adult ICU. *American Journal of Critical Care, 4*(2), 122–130.

41. Muzelaar, J. P., & Obrist, W. D. (1985). Cerebral blood flow and brain metabolism with brain injury. In D. P. Becker & J. T. Povlishock, (Eds.). *Central nervous system trauma report* (p. 123). Washington, DC: NINCDS.

42. Hudes, R., & Lee, L. (1987). Clinical use of peripheral nerve stimulator in anesthesia. *Canadian Journal of Anesthesiology, 34*, 525–534.

43. Ramsey, M. A. E., Savage, T. M., Simpson, B. R. J., et al. (1974). Controlled sedation with alphaxalone/alphadolone. *British Journal of Medicine, 2*, 656–659.

44. Vandam, L. D., & Burnap, T. K. (1959). Hypothermia. *New England Journal of Medicine, 231*, 595–603.

45. Clasen, R. A., Pandolfi, S., Russell, J., Stuart, D., & Hass, G. M. (1968). Hypothermia and hypotension in experimental cerebral edema. *Archives of Neurology, 19*, 472–486.

46. Laskowski, E. J., Klatzo, I., & Baldwin, M. (1960). Experimental study of the effects of hypothermia on local brain injury. *Neurology, 10*, 499–505.

47. Rosomoff, H. L., & Gilbert, R. (1955). Brain volume and cerebrospinal fluid pressure during hypothermia. *American Journal of Physiology, 183*, 19–22.

48. Drake, C. G., & Jory, T. A. (1962). Hypothermia in the treatment of critical head injury. *Canadian Medical Association Journal, 87*, 887–891.

49. Shapiro, H. M., Wyte, S. R., & Loeser, J. (1974). Barbiturate-augmented hypothermia for reduction of persistent intracranial hypertension. *Journal of Neurosurgery, 40*, 90–100.

50. Clifton, G. L., Allen, S. J., Barrodale, P., et al (1993). A phase II study of moderate hypothermia in severe brain injury. *Journal of Neurotrauma, 10*, 263–271.

51. Marion, D. W., Obrist, W. D., Carlier, P. M., Penrod, L. E., & Darby, J. M. (1993). The use of moderate hypothermia for patients with severe head injuries: A preliminary report. *Journal of Neurosurgery, 79*, 354–362.

52. Clifton, G. L. (1995). Hypothermia and hyperbaric oxygen as treatment modalities for severe head injury. *New Horizons, 3*(3), 474–478.

53. Clifton, G. L., Miller, E. R., Sung, C. C., Levin, H. S., et al. (2001). Lack of effect on inductein of hypothermia after acute brain injury. *New England Journal of Medicine, 344*(8), 556–563.

54. Wilberger, J. E., & Cantella, D. (1995). High-dose barbiturates for intracranial pressure control. *New Horizons, 3*(3), 469–473.

55. Borel, C. O., & Guy, J. (1995). Ventilatory management in critical neurologic illness. *Neurologic Clinics, 13*(3), 627–645.

56. Frank, J. (1993). Management of intracranial hypertension. *Medical Clinics of North America, 77*(1), 63.

57. Kerr, M. E., Rudy, E. B., Brucia, J., et al. (1993). Head-injured adults: Recommendations for endotracheal suctioning. *Journal of Neuroscience Nursing, 25*, 86–91.

58. Rudy, E. B., Turner, B. S., Baun, M., et al. (1991). Endotracheal suctioning in adults with head injury. *Heart & Lung, 20*, 667–674.

59. Rosner, M. J., & Coley, I. B. (1986). Cerebral perfusion pressure, intracranial pressure, and head elevation. *Journal of Neurosurgery, 65*, 636–641.

60. McNair, N. D. (1996). Intracranial pressure monitoring. In J M. Clochesy, C. Breu, S. Cardin, A. A. Whittaker, & E. B. Rudy (Eds.). *Critical care nursing* (2nd ed., pp. 289–307). Philadelphia: W. B. Saunders.

61. Bisnaire, D., & Robinson, L. (1997). Accuracy of leveling intraventricular collection drainage systems. *Journal of Neuroscience Nursing 29*(4), 261–268.

62. Lundberg, N. (1960). Continuous recording and control of ventricular fluid pressure in neurosurgical practice. *Acta Psychiatrica et Neurologica Scandinavia, 36*(Suppl 149), 1–193.

63. Williams, M. A., & Hanley, D. F. (1998). Monitoring and interpreting intracranial pressure. In M. J. Tobin (Ed.). *Principles and practice on intensive care monitoring* (pp. 995–1009). New York: McGraw-Hill.

64. Doyle, D. J., & Mark, P. W. S. (1992). Analysis of intracranial pressure. *Journal of Clinical Monitoring, 8,* 81–90.

65. Barlow, P., Mendelow, A. D., Lawrence A. R., et al. (1985). Clinical evaluation of two methods of subdural pressure monitoring. *Journal of Neurosurgery, 63,* 578–582.

66. Piek, J., Beck, W. J. (1990). Continuous monitoring of cerebral tissue pressure in neurosurgical practice-experiences with 100 patients. *Intensive Care Medicine, 16,* 184–188.

67. Piek, J., Kosub, B., Kuch, F., et al. (1987). A practical technique for continuous monitoring of cerebral tissue pressure in neurosurgical patients: Preliminary results. *Acta Neurochirurgica (Wien) 87,* 144–149.

68. Ostrup, R. C., Luerssen, T. G., Marshall, L. F., et al. (1987). Continuous monitoring of intracranial pressure with a miniaturized fiberoptic device. *Journal Neurosurgery, 67,* 206–209.

69. Hayashi, M., Kobayashi, H., Handa, Y., et al. (1985). Brain blood volume and blood flow in patients with plateau waves. *Journal of Neurosurgery, 63,* 556–561.

70. Lundberg, N., Cronqvist, S., & Kjallquist, A. (1968). Clinical investigations on interrelations between intracranial pressure and intracranial hemodynamics. *Progress in Brain Research, 30,* 69–75.

71. Risberg, J., Lundberg, N., & Ingvar, D. H. (1969). Regional cerebral blood volume during acute transient rises of the intracranial pressure (plateau waves). *Journal of Neurosurgery, 31,* 303–310.

72. Tsementzis, S. A., Gordon, A., & Gillingham, F. J. (1979). Prognostic signs during continuous monitoring of the ventricular fluid pressure in patients with severe brain injury. *Acta Neurochirurgica Suppl, 28,* 78–84.

73. McQuillan, K. A., (1991). Intracranial pressure monitoring: Technical imperatives. *AACN Clinical Issues in Critical Care, 2,* 623–639.

74. Garner, J. S., Jarvis, W. R., Emori, T. G., et al. (1988). CDC definitions for nosocomial infections. *American Journal of Infection Control, 16,* 128–140.

75. Aucoin, P. J., Kotilainen, H. R., Gantz, N. M., et al. (1986). Intracranial pressure monitoring: Epidemiological study of risk factors and infections. *American Journal of Medicine, 80,* 369–376.

76. Bader, M. K., Littlejohns, L., & Palmer, S. (1995). Ventriculostomy and intracranial pressure monitoring: In search of a 0% infection rate. *Heart & Lung, 24,* 166–172.

77. Bogdahn, V., Lau, W., Hassel, W., et al. (1992). Continuous pressure controlled external ventriculostomy drainage for treatment of acute hydrocephalus: Evaluation of risk factors. *Neurosurgery, 31,* 898–904.

78. Mayhall, G. C., Archer, N. H., Lamb, V. A., et al. (1984). Ventriculostomy related infections: A prospective epidemiological study. *New England Journal of Medicine, 310,* 553–559.

79. Winfield, J., Rosenthal, P., Kanter, R., et al. (1993). Duration of intracranial pressure monitoring does not predict daily risk of infectious complications. *Neurosurgery, 33,* 424–431.

80. Holloway, K. L., Barnes, T., Choi, S., et al. (1996). Ventriculostomy infections: The effect of monitoring duration and catheter exchange in 584 patients. *Journal of Neurosurgery, 85,* 419–424.

81. Rebuck, J. A., Murry, K. R., Rhoney, D. H., et al. (2000). Infection related to intracranial pressure monitors in adults: Analysis of risk factors and antibiotic prophylaxis. *Journal of Neurology, Neurosurgery, & Psychiatry, 69,* 381–384.

82. Poon, W. S., Ng, S., & Wai, S. (1998). CSF antibiotic prophylaxis for neurosurgical patients with ventriculostomy: A randomized study. *Acta Neurochirurgica Suppl (Wien), 71,* 281–286.

83. O'Grady, N. P., Barie, P. S., Bartlett, J., et al. (1998). Practice parameters for evaluating new fever in critically ill adult patients. *Critical Care Medicine, 26*(2), 392–408.

84. American Association of Neuroscience Nurses. (1997). *Intracranial pressure monitoring.* Chicago, IL: Author.

85. Wisinger, D., & Mest-Beck, L. (1990). Ventriculostomy: A guide to nursing management. *Journal of Neuroscience Nursing, 22,* 365–369.

86. Adams, R. D., Victor, M., & Ropper, A. H. (1997). *Principles of neurology* (6th ed., pp. 634–637). New York: McGraw-Hill.

RESOURCES
Professional

Published Material

BOOKS

Cooper, P. R., & Golfinos, J. G. (Eds.). *Head injury* (4th ed.). New York: McGraw-Hill.

Ropper, A. H. (Ed.) (1993). *Neurological and neurosurgical intensive care* (3rd ed.). New York: Raven Press.

PERIODICALS

Bell, S. D., Guyer, D., Synder, M. A., & Miner, M. (1994). Cerebral hemodynamics: Monitoring arteriojugular oxygen content differences. *Journal of Neuroscience Nursing, 26,* 270–277.

Kerr, M. E., Lovasik, D., & Darby, J. (1995). Evaluating cerebral oxygenation using jugular venous oximetry in head injuries. *AACN Clinical Issues, 6*(1), 11–20.

Mitchell, P. H. (1986). Intracranial hypertension: Influence of nursing care activities. *Nursing Clinics of North America, 21*(4), 563–574.

Parsons, L. C., & Wilson, M. M. (1984). Cerebrovascular status of severe closed head injured patients following passive position changes. *Nursing Research, 33*(2), 68–75.

Parsons, L. C., Peard, A. L., & Page, M. C. (1985). The effects of hygiene interventions on the cerebrovascular status of severe closed head injured persons. *Research in Nursing Health, 8,* 173–181.

Rising, C. J. (1993). The relationship of selected nursing activities to ICP. *Journal of Neuroscience Nursing, 25,* 302–308.

Williams, A., & Coyne, S. M. (1993). Effects of neck position on intracranial pressure. *American Journal of Critical Care, 3,* 68–71.

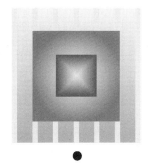

Management of Patients Undergoing Neurosurgical Procedures

JOANNE V. HICKEY

▌ THE PREOPERATIVE PHASE

For the patient undergoing a neurosurgical procedure, the circumstances of admission influence preoperative preparation. Unplanned emergency hospital admissions are usually related to trauma or a sudden, life-threatening event, such as an aneurysmal rupture. Immediate surgery may be necessary as a life-saving measure, and the urgency compresses all preoperative preparation. With planned or postponed surgery, there is time for preoperative teaching. For the patient who is conscious and oriented, the prospect of a neurosurgical procedure is often associated with overwhelming anxiety and fear. Paramount is the fear of loss of life, cognitive and physical abilities, self-control, personality, and independence. In addition, concerns about permanent disability and chronic illness create concerns about their effects on relationships with family and friends and about burden on loved ones. In contrast, patients with an altered level of consciousness or impaired cognitive function may be unable to grasp the seriousness of the situation and appears apathetic.

Informed Consent

In obtaining informed consent, the physician discusses the purpose of surgery, the possibility of alternative treatment, the potential risks, and the expected outcomes. Discussing these points honestly and answering all questions will reduce the possibility of misunderstandings and litigation. Because altered consciousness, impaired cognition, or both can severely influence awareness and comprehension, a responsible family member should be present during the discussion. In some instances, it will be necessary for the next of kin or guardian to give consent for surgery.

Preoperative Teaching and Support

The nurse assumes major responsibility for patient and family preparation and for provision of emotional support throughout the experience. The teaching plan is individual-

ized and is directed toward providing information and anticipatory guidance about activities associated with the neurosurgical procedure (Table 15-1). In addition, printed material is helpful and is a tangible resource that can be reviewed. If slight to moderate cognitive deficits are present, provide a more simplified explanation. With severe deficits, the family assumes a greater decision-making role and often becomes the major focus of teaching. Encourage family members to take care of themselves with adequate rest, nutrition, and support. The expected outcomes of the teaching plan include control of fear and anxiety, and maximization of patient and family coping strategies. Common related nursing diagnoses includes knowledge deficit, anxiety, fear, and family dysfunction.

Before Surgery

In planned admissions, routine tests for any surgical patient are often completed on an outpatient basis. Specific neurological diagnostics have probably been performed to establish a diagnosis that has led to the decision for neurosurgical intervention. Additional tests may be required. Home preparation instructions are provided. Because many patients are now admitted on the day of surgery, any preoperative home preparation must be discussed and expectations clearly specified. Other preoperative activities are completed on admission.

In addition to routine preoperative preparation such as nothing by mouth (NPO) after midnight, other preparation is related to the specific procedure planned and operative site. For intracranial surgery, the hair should be clean and long hair neatly braided. Skin preparation, including shaving, is completed in the operating room (OR). The need to cut some of the hair can be upsetting to some patients. Because neurosurgical procedures are often long, the risk of deep vein thrombosis (DVT) and pulmonary embolus (PE) is high.[1] Therefore, thigh-high support (TED) stockings are applied in conjunction with sequential devices (SCD) that will remain functional during the surgery. The final preoperative neurological assessment and vital signs are recorded and sent with the medical record to the OR with the patient.

Depending on the circumstances, the family may visit briefly before surgery (see Table 15-1 for family support and

Table 15–1 • GENERAL PREOPERATIVE TEACHING PLAN FOR NEUROSURGICAL PROCEDURES

Patient and family*

- Clarify and reinforce information provided by the physician.
- Provide printed material about the specific type of surgery and review it with the patient/family.
- Describe preparatory events before surgery (e.g., blood work, electrocardiogram, chest x-ray, application of thromboembolic (TED) stockings and sequential compression boots, visit from anesthesiologist, NPO before surgery).

Patient

- Teach any special activities, such as leg exercises or deep breathing exercises
- Review what to expect throughout hospitalization and after

Family

Discuss:
- Location of the waiting area and amenities (e.g., telephones, restrooms, food)
- Location of where the neurosurgeon will talk to the family after the surgery
- If not physically present, how can the family be reached by telephone
- Provisions for periodic updates if the surgery time is extended
- Unit to which the patient will go after surgery (e.g., recovery room; intensive care unit [ICU]).
- Visiting hours before surgery and in the ICU
- Length of intracranial surgery (may take several hours and this is not unusual)
- Describe what to expect in the ICU (e.g., tubes, monitors, intravenous lines, change in appearance for dressings or ecchymosis).

* Be prepared to repeat and reinforce information (people under stress often have difficulty retaining information).

needs). Any other special preoperative orders are completed, and the patient is transported to the OR.

THE INTRAOPERATIVE PHASE

Arrival at the Operating Room Suite

Once in the OR suite, monitoring equipment is attached and intravenous (IV) anesthetic induction is begun. Other preparation includes:

- General points
  - If not already present, insert a urinary catheter.
  - To protect the eyes from corneal abrasions, a bland eye ointment is applied and the eyelids taped closed; sterile eye pads are applied.
  - Hair over the operative site is cut and the scalp shaved; the hair is saved and placed in a labeled envelope.
  - Sequential compression boots (SCBs) are connected to prevent pooling of blood in the lower extremities.
  - The anesthesiologist intubates the patient and connects respiratory support equipment.

- Positioning
  - The optimal position to facilitate surgery is selected. Common positions include the sitting, lateral, or prone positions. For example, the sitting position is used for posterior fossa surgery because it affords optimal visualization of the operative field.
  - Various support devices, such as a headrest and armrests, are carefully positioned and adjusted; areas of potential pressure are padded to prevent decubitus ulcer and ischemic pressure injury to peripheral nerves. Positioning is often complex and may take an hour or more to complete.
- General monitoring

Various devices for ongoing intraoperative monitoring are connected. Such equipment includes a device providing for continuous electrocardiograms, esophageal or tympanic temperature probe, arterial line for continual monitoring of arterial blood pressure, central venous catheter, precordial doppler placed over the right atrium (to detect venous air emboli especially if the sitting position is used), pulse oximeter, and other devices as necessary (see below for additional information). In addition, end tidal carbon dioxide ($ETCO_2$) and other respiratory parameters are monitored.

Ongoing Neurophysiological Monitoring

Patients undergoing neurosurgical procedures have an inherent increased risk of ischemic/hypoxic damage or direct injury to the CNS. Intraoperative neurophysiological monitoring may improve patient outcomes in two ways:[2]

1. Allows early diagnosis of ischemia/hypoxia before irreversible damage occurs
2. Facilitates optimal surgical treatment as indicated by the monitoring parameters

The major categories of neurophysiological cerebral monitoring are function, blood flow/pressure, and metabolism. *Functional parameters* include electroencephalography, evoked potentials, and electromyography. *Cerebral blood flow* is monitored by nitrous oxide washing, radioactive xenon clearance, laser Doppler blood flow, and transcranial Doppler studies. *Intracranial pressure* (ICP) data are collected with a catheter placed in the intraventricular, intraparenchymal, subarachnoid, or epidural spaces. *Metabolism* can be monitored invasively and noninvasively. Invasive monitoring is done with a PO_2 electrode, whereas noninvasive monitoring uses transcranial cerebral oximetry (near-infrared spectroscopy) and jugular venous oximetry.[2]

Neuroanesthesia

Preoperative assessment is important to assess the general physical and neurological status of the patient. The American Society of Anesthesiologists developed a five-point grading scale to estimate anesthetic risk based on physical status.[3] Class 1 includes healthy people without any organic disturbances, whereas Class 5 includes moribund patients for whom surgery is a last effort for survival. Physical status and acuity are factors considered in providing anesthesia. Anesthetic management of neurosurgical patients is based on knowledge of how the selected agents influence central nervous system (CNS) physiology. The specific anesthetic regimen is a combination of agents that favorably affects cerebral hemodynamics, cerebral metabolism, and ICP to provide good operating conditions (i.e., hemostasis and adequate brain relaxation) and enhance the probability of optimal outcomes. Of particular interest is the effect on cerebral blood flow (CBF) and cerebral metabolic oxygen consumption (CMO_2) in addition to the ICP (Table 15-2). These criteria are used for evaluating the usefulness and safety of new drugs.[4]

For neurosurgical procedures, a combination of inhalants and IV drugs is used. Common combinations of drugs include:[5,6]

- IV agents
  - Barbiturates (thiopental); hypnotics
  - Benzodiazepines (diazepam, midazolam, lorazepam)
  - Sedatives (etomidate); primarily for induction
  - Sedative hypnotic (propofol)
  - Anesthetics (ketamine)
  - Narcotics (fentanyl, alfentanil, sufentanil)
  - Muscle relaxants (vecuronium, atracurium, pancuronium)
  - Other (e.g., lidocaine; suppresses laryngeal reflexes)
- Inhalational agents
  - Nitrous oxide (potent vasodilator that markedly increased CBF)
  - Halothane
  - Enflurane
  - Isoflurane
  - Desflurane

Table 15-2 • EFFECTS OF ANESTHETIC AGENTS ON CEREBRAL BLOOD FLOW, CEREBRAL METABOLIC OXYGEN CONSUMPTION, AND INTRACRANIAL PRESSURE

ANESTHETIC	CBF	$CMRO_2$	ICP
Thiopental	Decrease	Decrease	Decrease
Etomidate	Decrease	Decrease	Decrease
Propofol	Decrease	Decrease	Decrease
Fentanyl	0/Decrease	0/Decrease	0/Decrease
Alfentanil	0/Decrease/ increase	0/Decrease	0/Decrease/ increase
Sufentanil	0/Decrease/ increase	0/Decrease	0/Decrease/ increase
Ketamine	Increase	0/Increase	Increase
Midazolam	Decrease	Decrease	0/Decrease
Nitrous oxide	Increase	0/Increase	Increase
Halothane	Increase	Decrease	Increase
Enflurane	Increase	Decrease	Increase
Isoflurane	Increase	Decrease	Increase
Desflurane	Increase	Decrease	Increase
Sevoflurane	Increase	Decrease	Increase

CBF, cerebral blood flow; $CMRO_2$, cerebral metabolic oxygen consumption; ICP, intracranial pressure.

From Neufield, P., & Cottrell, J.C. (Eds.) (1999). *Handbook of neuranesthesia.* Philadelphia: Lippincott Williams & Wilkins.

- Sevoflurane
- Oxygen

IV mannitol (20% to 25%) is started to reduce brain volume. Cerebrospinal fluid (CSF) may be removed to facilitate an optimal operative site using a ventricular or lumbar drain.[6] Other drugs administered during the procedure include dexamethasone to control cerebral edema, phenytoin (Dilantin) to control seizure activity, and antibiotics as prophylaxis against infection. Cardiac drugs may be given to control hypotension or hypertension (HPT).

Cerebral Protection

During surgery, the goal is to preserve CBF and avoid hypoxia and hypoxemia. Interventions are directed at maximizing oxygen by increasing oxygen supply (delivery) and decreasing oxygen demand.[7] Controlled hypothermia, hypotension, and hyperventilation are useful to protect cerebral oxygenation.

Hypothermia. Many neurosurgical patients are candidates for hypotensive therapy. They include patients with:[7]

- Space-occupying lesions with or without increased ICP
- Cerebral aneurysm, arteriovenous malformation, or cavernous angioma requiring clipping or excision
- Carotid occlusion requiring extracranial vascular procedures, such as carotid endarterectomy or superficial temporal artery, to middle cerebral artery bypass
- Giant or complex basilar artery aneurysm requiring clipping

Hypothermia is useful to decrease both metabolic and functional activities of the brain by reducing cerebral metabolic rate for oxygen consumption ($CMRO_2$) by 6% to 7% for each 1°C decline. Although the mechanism is not uniformly linear, small decreases in temperature have resulted in significant reductions in the effects of cerebral ischemia. The cerebral protection cascade at the cellular level includes decreased calcium influx, decreased excitatory amino acid (EAA) release, blood-brain barrier preservation, and prevention of lipid peroxidation.[7] The current therapeutic recommendations for hypothermia protection are mild hypothermia with a brain temperature of 32 to 35°C. Tympanic membrane or nasopharyngeal temperature is an accurate reflection of brain temperature. Therefore, either method is useful as a surrogate to monitor brain temperature. If the temperature drops below 28°C (82.4°F), cardiac irritability increases and extracorporeal support of the systemic circulation becomes necessary.

Hypotension. **Induced hypotension** is defined as lowering mean arterial blood pressure (MAP) to a level of 50 to 65 mm Hg in normotensive, anesthetized patients. The purpose is to decrease blood loss during surgery, improve surgical conditions, and decrease the need for blood transfusions.[8] In cerebral aneurysm clipping procedures, induced hypotension is helpful because it lowers intraluminal pressure on the aneurysmal sac, thus decreasing bleeding and rupture and increasing aneurysmal plasticity to facilitate clip application. There are definite risks associated with induced hypotension including myocardial and cerebral ischemia. A uniform safe level of hypotension has not been established and is individual dependent. Close monitoring gauges individual response and optimal level.

Hyperventilation. Controlled hyperventilation is often maintained during neurosurgical procedures to reduce brain bulk and ICP. The reduced PCO_2 blood level results in a reduction in CBF and vasoconstriction, causing a reduction in brain bulk and ICP.

SITTING POSITION

A potentially life-threatening problem associated with the sitting operative position is a venous air embolus (VAE). It is uncommon when the head is raised 20 degrees or less. The head is raised higher than the heart with a person in the sitting position, and a negative pressure (subatmospheric) is created in the dural venous sinuses and veins draining the brain and head. If air is introduced into the venous system, it is quickly carried to the right side of the heart resulting in transient cardiovascular deficits or insufficiencies. Early signs of VAE are precordial Doppler sounds, increased end-tidal nitrogen (ETN_2) and increased $ETCO_2$. Late signs include a rise in CVP, pulmonary artery pressure, and pulse oximetry desaturation. Final signs are hypotension, tachycardia, cyanosis, and a mill-wheel murmur.[6]

When an air embolus is suspected, the surgeon is notified so that an attempt can be made to identify and occlude the possible site of air entry. When the problem site has been occluded, the anesthesiologist aspirates air through the central venous catheter using a 20-mL syringe and an airtight stopcock. If the entry site cannot be located, the patient is placed in the supine position, and the surgery is terminated.

NEUROSURGICAL PROCEDURES AND OTHER RELATED THERAPEUTIC TECHNIQUES

Development of instrumentation, lasers, and radiation therapies has increased the options offered to neurosurgical patients. A craniotomy may be combined with laser treatment for some conditions previously managed by craniotomy alone. Other nonsurgical treatment modalities have been introduced that may decrease the need for surgery in the future.

Definition of Terms and Basic Concepts

Below are explanations of several common terms and neurosurgical procedures:

- **Surgery** can be classified by anatomical location. Two terms differentiate the areas of the brain on which surgery is performed (Fig. 15-1):

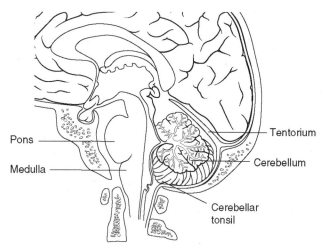

Figure 15–1 • Surgery on the area of the brain above the tentorium is called *supratentorial;* surgery below the tentorium is *infratentorial.*

- **The supratentorial area** is just above the tentorium that includes the cerebral hemispheres. The tentorium cerebelli is a double fold of the dura mater that forms a partition between the cerebral hemispheres and the brain stem and cerebellum. The supratentorial approach is used to gain access to lesions of the frontal, parietal, temporal, and occipital lobes.
- **The infratentorial area** is below the tentorium in the posterior fossa and includes the brain stem (midbrain, pons, medulla) and cerebellum. The infratentorial approach is used to gain access to lesions of the brain stem or cerebellum. Occasionally, temporal or occipital lobe lesions located close to the tentorial margin may be excised through the infratentorial approach.
- A **bur hole** is created in the cranium with a special drill for evacuation of an extracerebral clot or in preparation for craniotomy. In the case of a craniotomy, a series of burr holes are made. The bone between the holes is cut with a special saw, allowing removal of the piece of bone or creation of a flap.
- A **craniotomy** is a surgical opening of the skull to provide access to the intracranial contents for reasons such as removal of a tumor, clipping of an aneurysm, or repair of a cerebral injury. It involves creating a bone flap at the area over the lesion. The flap created is either a free flap or an osteoplastic flap. With a **free flap**, the bone is completely removed and preserved for later replacement. With a **bone flap**, the muscle is left attached to the skull to maintain the vascular supply (Fig. 15-2).
- A **craniectomy** is excision of a portion of the skull without replacement. This procedure may be done to achieve decompression after cerebral debulking or removal of bone fragments from skull fracture. The posterior fossa is a much smaller region than the supratentorial space. The posterior fossa (infratentorial space) is defined by the large transverse venous sinuses superiorly and the foramen magnum inferiorly. Because of the small areas and increased risk of dural tearing, a craniectomy or bone removal without replacement is usually performed for surgical access.[1]
- **Cranioplasty** is repair of the skull to reestablish the con-

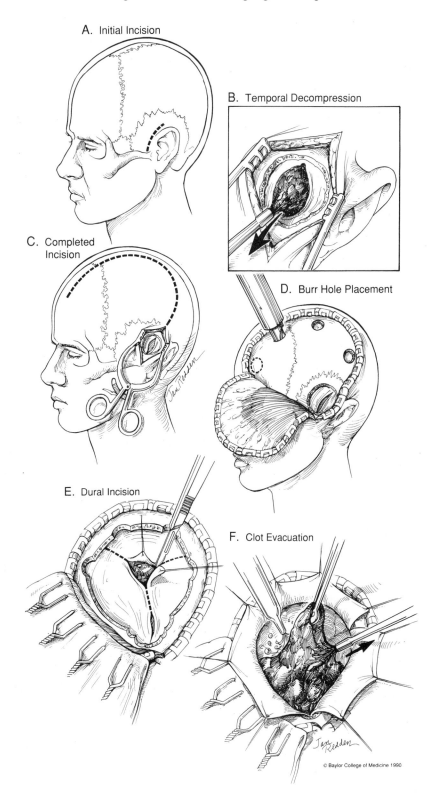

A. Initial Incision

B. Temporal Decompression

C. Completed Incision

D. Burr Hole Placement

E. Dural Incision

F. Clot Evacuation

© Baylor College of Medicine 1990

Figure 15–2 • Craniotomy. The procedure is directed at the removal of an acute subdural hematoma. A number of steps are involved in a craniotomy to gain access to the brain. (*A*) With clinical evidence of rapid neurological deterioration secondary to herniation, temporal decompression is recommended as the first step. An incision is made just anterior to the ear and taken down to the zygoma, which marks the floor of the temporal fossa. (*B*) A burr hole is made, followed by a quick craniectomy. The dura is incised, and as much of the blood clot as possible is aspirated. (*C*) The incision is then extended upward to form a large question mark, the medial extent of which follows the midline. (*D*) Additional burr holes are then made, the medial ones 1.5 cm off the midline to avoid injury to the major venous structures and granulations. A flap is created. The anterior burr hole is placed above the frontal sinus, the size of which can be estimated from preoperative radiographs. (*E*) The dura can be opened with a Y-shaped and X-shaped incision, with a flap being based on the superior sagittal sinus. (*F*) The subdural hematoma is gently evacuated with suction, irrigation, and other mechanical means. Sources of bleeding are identified and cauterized. Contused brain is debrided, and pial edges are carefully cauterized. Ultrasound is used to rule out the presence of occult intracerebral or contralateral hematomas.

tour and integrity of the skull. This procedure involves replacement of part of the cranium with a synthetic material.

• **Microsurgery** is defined as any surgery performed with the assistance of an operating microscope that provides magnification of various intensities. The surgical technique (micro-operative technique), instruments (micro-instrumentation), illumination for visualization, and mag-

nification (operating microscopes), along with a host of other equipment, are specifically designed for this use.

• **Surgical microscopes** have undergone rapid development in the past few years. Advances in optical, electrical, and mechanical technology have made it possible to design microscopes with enhanced precision and usability. Figure 15-3 shows a state-of-the-art surgical microscope with easy maneuverability and precision that also allows the assistant to observe the operative field in three dimensions.

- An **ultrasonic surgical aspirator** is frequently used during a craniotomy. Larger solid lesions with a capsule or pseudocapsular membrane border that are noninfiltrating or surrounding cerebral tissue can be removed with the ultrasonic surgical aspirator. Plastic ultrasonic waves disintegrate the mass into pieces, and gentle concurrent suction "vacuums" the tumor fragments.[9]

Use of Stereotaxis for Precise Positioning and Treatment

Stereotaxis pertains to precise localization of a specific target point based on three-dimensional coordinates derived with the use of a stereotaxis frame and computed tomography (CT) scanner. In this context, "stereo" means three-dimensional in space and "tactic" means touch. It operates according to a target-centered arc principle, which means that all arc paths pass to the target lesion (Fig. 15-4). A stereotactic frame, such as the CRW™, is applied to the patient's head and the target site within the brain is located

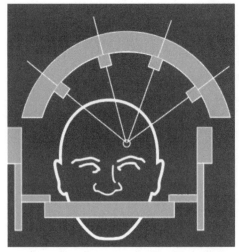

Figure 15–4 • The CRW™ Sterotactic Systems Arc-Center Principle is a target-centered approach, which means all arc paths pass to the target lesion. (Courtesy of Radionics, Burlington, MA.)

by determining the X (anteroposterior), Y (superior-inferior), and Z (left to right) coordinates in relation to the stereotactic frame (Fig. 15-5). The point of intersection of all three coordinates identifies the target tissue. Figure 15-6 illustrates representative stereotactic equipment that can be used to achieve desired results. Various types of stereotactic frames and instruments have already been developed and are constantly being updated. Stereotactic radiosurgery is used in neurosurgery for the precise localization and treatment of deep brain lesions (e.g., thalamic lesions) that were previously surgically inaccessible, with minimal trauma to the adjacent tissue.

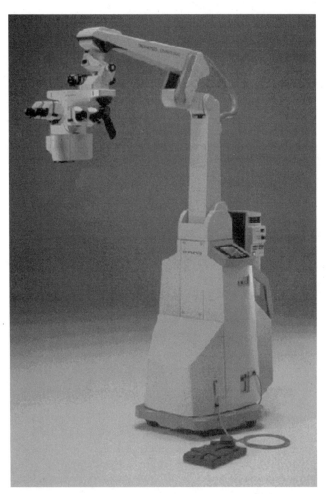

Figure 15–3 • State-of-the-art Olympus OME-8000 surgical microscope with enhanced ease of use and precision. In addition, it provides for three-dimensional viewing by the assistant. (Courtesy of Olympus America, Inc., Melville, NY.)

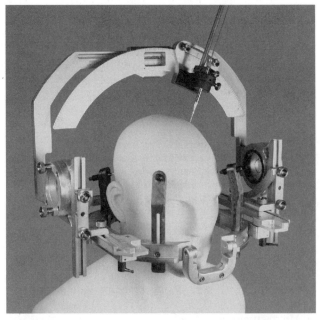

Figure 15–5 • With the CRW™ equipment, all approaches needed to treat various lesions are easily achieved, including transphenoidal, full lateral, posterior fossa, and standard approaches (shown in picture). (Courtesy of Radionics, Burlington, MA.)

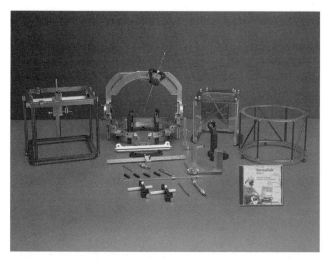

Figure 15–6 • Components of the CRW CT stereotactic system. (Courtesy of Radionics, Burlington, MA.)

After the target area has been identified, the stereotactic electrode or probe is passed through the slide carrier, which is attached to the stereotactic frame, to the target area (Fig. 15-7). Position is verified by a CT scan. Stereotactic surgery is used for various purposes, including:

- Biopsy of deep lesions or those located in the brain stem
- Evacuation of intracerebral hemorrhage
- Catheter placement for drainage of deep lesions, colloid cyst, or abscess
- Ventricular catheter shunt placement
- Implantation of radioactive seeds into brain tumors
- Placement of electrodes for epilepsy
- Ablative procedures for extrapyramidal diseases such as Parkinson's disease (tremors, rigidity, and others)
- Chronic pain control either with placement of a deep brain stimulator or surgical treatment

Recently, a technology has been developed that replaces the head frame with navigational wands, robotic devices, or other frameless systems, some of which locate the tumor by using skin-based markers to fix points in space. Another new development, the Cyberknife, is used in conjunction with a frameless computerized guidance system.[10]

Lasers

Surgical lasers were first introduced in the early 1960s, but it was not until 1979 that laser neurosurgery gained attention in the United States. The word **laser** is an acronym for **l**ight **a**mplification by **s**timulated **e**mission of **r**adiation. A laser is a device that concentrates a single wavelength of light into an intense, narrow beam of coherent monochromatic light energy that can be accurately focused on specific tissue. The selected body tissue absorbs the laser beam. The laser beam is transformed into immense heat energy, and the thermal energy of the laser beam allows simultaneous surgical dissection and coagulation.

Three types of lasers are available: the carbon dioxide, argon, and neodymium:yttrium-aluminum-garnet (Nd: YAG) laser. Each type uses a different light energy and allows different options for controlling and applying the laser beam. The beam can be applied directly to tissue, or it can be used to heat microprobes, which are then applied to tissue.

The value of lasers in neurosurgery is that the surgeon, using microscopic visualization, can dissect a precise structure without causing trauma to surrounding tissue, a consequence of traditional surgical techniques. This technique provides an approach for removing tumors from delicate and formerly inaccessible areas of the brain and spinal cord.

The use of lasers allows accessibility to neurological sites previously inaccessible. Lasers can dissect tissue by vaporization (while leaving adjacent tissue uninjured), coagulate blood vessels, and in some instances, shrink tumors. Because of limited clinical application, patient selection is important. Patients with tumors that are extrinsic to brain tissue but proximal to delicate cerebral tissue are considered good candidates for laser surgery. Acoustic neuromas, craniopharyngiomas, certain brainstem gliomas, pinealomas, ventricular tumors, and me-

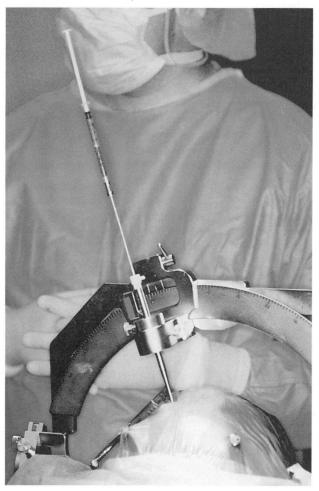

Figure 15–7 • The CRW™ attached to a patient's head with the probe in place. (Courtesy of Radionics, Burlington, MA.)

ningiomas have been removed successfully with laser surgery. Removal of selected intradural and extradural spinal cord tumors has also been successful.

Radiosurgery: The Gamma Knife

The gamma knife, which is not actually a knife at all, was developed at the Karolinska Institute in Stockholm in 1968 (Fig. 15-8). It consists of a heavily shielded helmet containing 201 radially distributed, sealed, radioactive sources containing curies of cobalt-60. These are focused with precision on a central common target for the purpose of delivering high-dose radiation while minimizing damage to surrounding tissue. Stereotaxis is used to focus the point of radiation. Unlike conventional radiation therapy, this stereotactic radiosurgery is capable of destroying deep and inaccessible lesions in a single treatment session.

The gamma knife is used for arteriovenous malformations (AVMs), deep and difficult-to-access brain tumors (e.g., acoustic neuromas), and various other intracranial conditions for which conventional surgery is inappropriate. The patient selection criteria include excessive risk for conventional surgery, previous surgical failure, surgical inaccessibility of the lesion, and refusal to undergo a craniotomy. The cost:benefit ratio associated with the gamma knife is attractive.[11]

A few major concerns relating to use of the gamma knife include:

- The lag time between treatment and result (AVMs take 1 to 3 years for maximal shrinkage; acoustic neuromas can take up to 4 years for maximal shrinkage)
- The lag time before side effects may appear (for example, hearing loss after treatment for an acoustic neuroma may not be noted for a year)

The gamma knife offers a new technology for treatment of patients who previously had no treatment options. Additional uses for the gamma knife will undoubtedly be found as experience is gained.

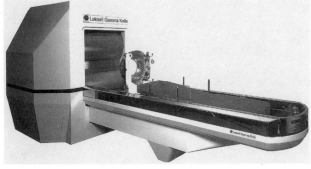

Figure 15-8 • Gamma knife. (Courtesy of Elekta Instruments, Norcross, GA.)

POSTOPERATIVE NURSING MANAGEMENT

After surgery, the patient is taken to the postanesthesia recovery room (PACU) or, at some hospitals, immediately to the neurological intensive care unit (ICU). Regardless of hospital or physician preference, most patients are admitted to an ICU after the PACU, where they remain until well stabilized. The stay in an ICU allows for close observation and extensive physiological monitoring (see Chap. 17 for discussion of critical care management).

Admission to the Intensive Care Unit

During transfer to the ICU, the nurse should expect a complete report, which will include:

- Overview of surgery (reason for surgery, anatomical approach, length of surgery, and specific area of the brain involved)
- History of preoperative neurological deficits
- Pre-existing medical problems
- Current baseline neurological signs
- Information provided to the family
- Review of the postoperative orders

This database is a basis for planning care. The approach to care depends on whether the patient has undergone supratentorial or infratentorial surgery. A comparison of the nursing focus associated with each approach is found in Chart 15-1. The basic maintenance and supportive nursing care provided, regardless of procedure or anatomical location, are summarized in Chart 15-2. See Chapter 11 for information pertinent to postoperative drug therapy.

Assessment and Monitoring in the Intensive Care Unit

Hemodynamic, respiratory, metabolic, and neurological assessment and monitoring are frequent and ongoing. The knowledge that the patient has recently undergone surgical insult is reason enough to draw the conclusion that increased ICP may be present. However, the nurse, when assessing the neurological signs, should identify changes in condition that may be subtle. Current findings are compared with baseline findings to determine trends.

The frequency with which the assessment is conducted will depend on how stable the patient's condition is and how soon after surgery it is performed. Neurological signs should be assessed every 15 to 30 minutes for the first 8 to 12 hours postoperatively, then every hour for the next 12 hours. As the patient stabilizes, the frequency of assessment will eventually be reduced to every 4 hours. Blood chemistries, complete blood counts, and other laboratory monitoring are frequent. Chest radiographs, CT scans, electroencephalogram monitoring, and other diagnostic modalities may be necessary to monitor progress.

(text continues on page 330)

CHART 15-1 • Nursing Management Following Supratentorial and Infratentorial Surgery

Supratentorial	Infratentorial

INCISION

- The scalp incision is made within the boundaries of the hairline, directly over the area to be explored on the cerebral hemisphere. The incision creates a skin flap. The actual location and shape of the skin flap can vary from one that appears horseshoe-shaped to one that follows the hairline in the frontal region.
- Sutures are usually removed within 7–10 d.

- The incision (skin flap) is made above the nape of the neck around the occipital area or posterolaterally in the occipito-temporal region.
- Sutures are usually removed 7–10 d after surgery.

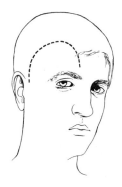

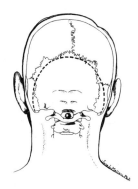

(Figures above are from Smeltzer, S., & Bare, B. [1996]. *Brunner and Suddarth's textbook of medical-surgical nursing* [8th ed.]. Philadelphia: Lippincott-Raven Publishers.)

HEAD DRESSING

- A turban-style dressing is applied initially.
- Many physicians remove the dressing completely after 24 h.
- The dressing is monitored for evidence of blood or cerebrospinal fluid (CSF) drainage.
- The incision is monitored for redness, drainage, or signs of wound infection.

- A turban-style dressing is applied initially.
- Many physicians remove the dressing completely after 24 h.
- The dressing is monitored for evidence of blood or CSF drainage.
- The incision is monitored for redness, drainage, or signs of wound infection.

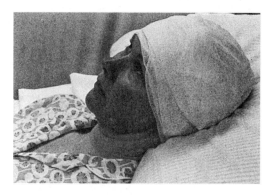

(continued)

C H A R T   1 5 – 1 • **Nursing Management Following Supratentorial and Infratentorial Surgery (Continued)**

POSITIONING OF THE HEAD OF THE BED

The position of the head of the bed (HOB) depends on the specific surgical procedure and the physician's preference. Review the doctor's order sheet for any specific instructions. If there are any position restrictions for the HOB, a sign should be posted conspicuously at the HOB and in the nursing care plan.

Some physicians follow a protocol of gradual elevation of the HOB for postoperative management of ventricular shunts and chronic subdural hematomas to prevent cerebral hemorrhage. An example of a protocol followed for postoperative management of both shunts and evacuation of a chronic subdural hematoma is as follows: keep the HOB flat for 24 h; then elevate the HOB 15 degrees for the next 24 h; then elevate the HOB 30 degrees for the next 24 h; then elevate the HOB 45 degrees for the next 24 h; finally elevate the HOB to 90 degrees.

Supratentorial

- The HOB is elevated 30 degrees. (This position facilitates venous blood return from the brain and promotes a decrease in intracranial pressure [ICP].)
- A pillow may be placed under the patient's head and shoulders. The neck should be maintained in a neutral position.

Infratentorial

- The HOB may be elevated at a 30-degree angle or lowered flat, depending on the preference of the physician.
- *Do not angulate the neck anteriorly or laterally.* A small pillow is placed under the head for comfort.
- For the patient who experiences dizziness or orthostatic hypotension, the HOB is elevated gradually while concurrently monitoring vital signs.

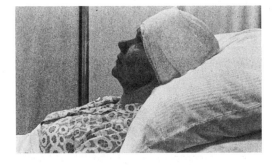

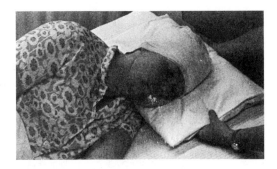

TURNING AND POSITIONING

- There is usually no restriction on turning.
- If a large tumor has been removed from a cerebral hemisphere, the physician may write an order to avoid positioning on the operative site to prevent shifting of cranial contents secondary to gravity.
- Positioning an unconscious patient or one who is recovering from anesthesia on the side facilitates drainage of oral secretions and promotes a patent airway.
- When positioning a patient, avoid extreme flexion of the upper legs or lateral or anterior flexion of the neck. A soft collar may be applied to keep the neck in a neutral position.

- There is usually no restriction on turning.
- If a large tumor has been removed from a cerebral hemisphere, the physician may write an order to avoid positioning on the operative site to prevent shifting of cranial contents secondary to gravity.
- Positioning an unconscious patient or one who is recovering from anesthesia on the side facilitates drainage of oral secretions and promotes a patent airway.
- When positioning a patient, avoid extreme flexion of the upper legs or lateral or anterior flexion of the neck. A soft collar may be applied to keep the neck in a neutral position.

AMBULATION

The patient is allowed out of bed as soon as tolerated, which will depend on general condition and the judgment of the physician and nurse.

The patient is allowed out of bed as soon as the vertical position can be tolerated. Patients undergoing infratentorial procedures are often maintained on bed rest longer than those undergoing supratentorial procedures because of the frequency of dizziness experienced by these patients. This dizziness is caused by transient edema in the area of cranial nerve VIII.

CHART 15-1 • Nursing Management Following Supratentorial and Infratentorial Surgery (Continued)

Supratentorial

NUTRITION

- The patient is given nothing by mouth (NPO) for 24 h; IV fluids are administered slowly.
- If the patient is not experiencing nausea or vomiting and can protect his airway, clear fluids are started.

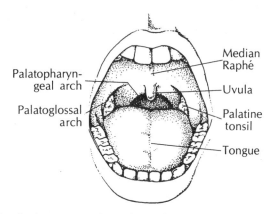

- The diet is progressed as tolerated.
- If fluid restriction is ordered, the daily allowance is strictly maintained.

ELIMINATION

- An indwelling urinary catheter is inserted for most neurosurgical procedures. The catheter is removed as soon as possible. If there is difficulty with voiding, a bladder retraining program is begun.
- Constipation can occur as a result of diuretics and pain medication (e.g., morphine or codeine). Straining at stool initiates the Valsalva's maneuver, which can increase ICP. A bowel program is begun to avoid constipation.

FLUID AND ELECTROLYTE BALANCE

- Most patients are maintained euvolemic. Intake is balanced with output.
- An intake and output record is maintained, and the fluid restriction is adhered to strictly.
- Serum electrolyte and osmolarity levels are monitored.
- If surgery is performed in the area of the pituitary gland or hypothalamus, transient diabetes insipidus may develop. Urinary output and specific gravity are monitored every 1–4 h.

Infratentorial

NUTRITION

- The patient is kept NPO for at least the first 24 h; IV fluids are administered slowly. Nausea tends to be more of a problem with surgery in this region than in the supratentorial area. Presence of the gag reflex and ability to protect the airway must be evident before food and fluids are given.
- Edema of cranial nerves IX and X may affect the swallowing and gag reflexes.
- If no nausea or vomiting is noted, and the gag and swallowing reflexes are present, the patient may sip water using a straw. Ask the patient to take a small sip and swallow it.
- The gag reflex is checked by touching the posterior wall of the pharynx. The normal response is contraction of the pharynx.
- If nausea or vomiting occurs, continue the patient's NPO status and IV therapy; after nausea or vomiting has subsided, ingestion of oral fluids may be attempted again.
- Once the patient is able to tolerate fluids, progress from clear liquids to a diet as tolerated.
- If fluid restriction is ordered, the daily allowance is adhered to strictly.

ELIMINATION

- An indwelling urinary catheter is inserted for most neurosurgical procedures. The catheter is removed as soon as possible. If there is difficulty with voiding, begin a bladder retraining program.
- Constipation can occur as a result of medication (e.g., morphine or codeine). Straining at stool initiates Valsalva's maneuver, which can increase ICP. A bowel program is begun to avoid constipation.

FLUID AND ELECTROLYTE BALANCE

- Most patients are maintained euvolemic. Intake is balanced with output.
- An intake and output record is maintained, and the fluid restriction is adhered to strictly.
- Serum electrolyte and osmolarity levels are monitored.

(continued)

CHART 15-1 • **Nursing Management Following Supratentorial and Infratentorial Surgery (Continued)**

SPECIAL FOCUS OF NEUROLOGICAL ASSESSMENT

The nurse monitors the patient's neurological status, performing an assessment at frequent intervals. Based on an understanding of specific neurological functions controlled by the supratentorial region and infratentorial region, the nurse places special emphasis on the following areas of assessment:

Supratentorial	Infratentorial

• Potential cranial nerve (CN) dysfunction
  Optic nerve (CN II): visual deficits, homonymous hemianopia
  Oculomotor nerve (CN III): ptosis
  Oculomotor, trochlear, abducens (CNs III, IV, VI): deficits in extraocular movement
	• Potential CN dysfunction
	  Oculomotor, trochlear, abducens (CNs III, IV, VI): deficits in extraocular movement
	  Facial (CN VII): lower lid deficit, absent corneal reflex, weakness or paralysis of the facial muscles
	  Acoustic (CN VIII): decreased hearing, dizziness, nystagmus
	  Glossopharyngeal and vagus (CN IX, X): diminished or absent gag or swallowing reflex, orthostatic hypotension
	• Potential cerebellar dysfunction
	  Ataxia, difficulty with fine motor movement, difficulty with coordination

Transfer from the Intensive Care Unit to the Acute Care Unit

After the patient is physiologically stable and discharge criteria have been met, transfer from the ICU occurs. To maintain continuity of care, the ICU nurse communicates with the nurse accepting the patient to ensure a smooth transition. The patient and patient's family need reassurance that the patient is stable and ready for this transfer. If possible, it is helpful for the receiving nurse to meet the patient and family before the transfer to relieve anxiety and fear.

POSTOPERATIVE MANAGEMENT AND PREVENTION OF COMPLICATIONS

Numerous complications can develop after a craniotomy. Some complications are related to the surgical site. For example, patients who undergo posterior fossa surgery are at high risk for lower cranial nerve injury or dysfunction that results in inability to protect the airway. Complications may be time dependent in that some complications have a higher probability of occurring earlier in the postoperative periods, whereas others, such as wound infection, appear later. Other complications can occur at any time, such as pneumonia. The nurse is responsible for providing general management and intensive care with particular attention to the prevention of complications.

Cardiopulmonary Management

The goal of cardiopulmonary monitoring is to assure the adequacy of oxygenation, cardiac output, and tissue perfusion.[12] Oxygenation is monitored in several ways, including the physical examination, pulse oximetry, and arterial blood gases from an arterial line. In a mechanically ventilated patient $ETCO_2$ is helpful. Cardiac function is monitored with ongoing blood pressure monitoring and electrocardiographic monitoring and waveform analysis to detect changes in rate or rhythm and to identify arrhythmias. In addition, hemodynamic monitoring of central venous pressure and hemodynamics derived from the use of a pulmonary artery catheter such as pulmonary wedge pressure, left ventricular end-diastolic pressure, and cardiac output provide ongoing data on cardiac function. Because adequate cerebral oxygenation is a goal in management, a jugular bulb catheter may be used to monitor arteriojugular differences of global cerebrovenous oxygenation (see Chap. 17).

Cardiopulmonary Complications

Hypovolemic Shock. Hypovolemic shock results from general fluid loss (blood, plasma, or water), particularly if osmotic diuretics have been used. Signs and symptoms include decreased CVP, tachycardia; decreasing blood pressure; shallow and rapid respirations; cool, pale skin; low urinary output (10 to 25 mL/hour); and restlessness to coma. Hemodynamics (e.g., CVP, cardiac output), oxygenation (ABGs, SaO_2), and vital signs are monitored frequently. Treatment is directed toward fluid replacement using a bolus of salt solutions; fluid expanders, such as Plasmanate, lactated Ringer's solution; or blood products. Vasopressors (e.g., phenylephrine hydrochloride [Neo-Synephrine], norepinephrine, or dopamine) may be given.

Cardiac Arrhythmias. Cardiac arrhythmias are not unusual, especially after posterior fossa surgery or if blood has entered the CSF. Continuous cardiac monitoring is important for at least the first 24 to 48 hours after surgery. Periodically observe the rate, rhythm, and pattern on the monitor to

CHART 15-2 • Basic Nursing Management Following Cranial Surgery

Nursing Management

- Give basic hygienic care until the patient is able to participate in self-care (e.g., bath, oral hygiene, hair combing, nail cutting).
- Apply thigh-high elastic stockings and sequential compression air boots, and inspect legs daily. Note any signs of thrombophlebitis (redness, tenderness, warmth, swelling).
- Provide skin care every 4 h.

- Turn patient every 2 h, being careful to maintain the patient's body alignment. (It may be necessary to use pillows and other similar devices to maintain good body alignment.)
- Carry out range-of-motion exercises four times daily.

- Provide urinary catheter care daily using soap and water. Pin the catheter to prevent undue traction on the meatus. Remove the catheter as soon as possible.
- Apply warm or cold moist compresses to the eye area.
- Inspect eyes every 4 h for signs of irritation or dryness. Lubricate the eye with normal saline, commercially prepared eye lubricant, or ointment, as prescribed by the physician. To protect the eye from injury (corneal ulcerations or abrasions) if the lids do not tightly cover the eye, use an eye shield, or tape the eye closed.
- Pull up the side rails of the bed, and apply a jacket restraint as necessary.
- Evaluate periods of restlessness for an underlying cause (check for patency of the airway, evidence of pain, or distention of the bladder).

- Administer analgesics as ordered (the drug selected should not mask neurological signs).

- Do not combine nursing activities that are known to increase intracranial pressure (ICP) in the patient at risk.

- Monitor routine vital signs.
- Assess neurological signs at prescribed intervals:
  - Level of consciousness
  - Pupillary reaction
  - Eye movement
  - Motor function
  - Sensory function
- Review laboratory reports. Conventional normal values for some studies are as follows:
  - Hemoglobin: 12.0–16.0 g in females
  - 13.5–18.0 g in males
  - Hematocrit: 37%–48% in females
  - 42%–50% in males
  - BUN: 8–25 mg
  - Potassium: 3.5–5.0 mEq
  - Calcium: 8.5–10.5 mg
  - Sodium: 135–145 mEq
  - Fasting blood sugar: 70–110 mg
  - Creatinine: 0.6–0.9 mg/dL in females
  - 0.8–1.2 mg/dL in males
  - Serum osmolarity: 275–295 mOsm/L

Rationale

- Maintains cleanliness and encourages independence in activities of daily living

- Improves blood return to the heart and decreases the risk of thrombophlebitis

- Cleanses, lubricates, and provides the opportunity for an inspection of the skin to note irritation or skin breakdown
- Prevents prolonged pressure on specific areas of the skin, pooling of secretions, and development of musculoskeletal abnormalities; decreases the risk of pneumonia and atelectasis
- Maintains muscle tone to prevent atrophy and contractures
- Reduces the incidence of urinary tract infection

- Relieves periocular edema
- Decreases the risk of corneal ulceration, eye infections, or injury

- Provides for patient's safety

- In a neurological patient, restlessness may be caused by an obstructed airway, pain, or a distended bladder; the nurse should identify the underlying cause and provide the appropriate intervention.
- Provides for the comfort of the patient and helps to control restlessness

- Prevents dangerous spikes in ICP

- Provides baseline data and data for comparison
- Provides data about the patient's neurological condition and allows comparison with previous signs to detect any change in the patient's condition

- Identifies abnormal levels that signal the need for intervention. Also, some medical orders may set parameters for treatment (e.g., maintain the serum osmolarity at 305–310 mOsm/kg). A review of the laboratory data also provides guidelines for interventions.

determine the presence of an arrhythmia. If a monitor is not available (e.g., after ICU discharge), the apical pulse should be checked during the postoperative period to identify abnormalities in the heart rate or rhythm. Abnormalities should be reported to the physician immediately. In addition, serum potassium levels should be monitored for depletion secondary to diuresis, which can cause arrhythmias.

Airway Obstruction. Partial or complete obstruction of the airway can result from improper positioning or accumulation of mucus or other drainage.

- Unconscious patients should never be positioned on their backs because the tongue can easily slip backward and obstruct the airway.
- Maintain the neck in neutral position.

If an unconscious patient begins to snore, it is most likely attributable to obstruction of the airway. This situation must be corrected immediately to prevent not only respiratory failure, but secondary brain injury from cerebral hypoxia as well. This could easily lead to an increase in ICP. If obstruction is suspected, the jaw is pulled forward and downward to relieve the obstruction and is positioned laterally, with the head elevated to facilitate drainage. Elevating the head of the bed to 30 degrees helps promote a patent airway.

Aspiration. Edema involving the lower cranial nerves following infratentorial surgery can result in inability to protect one's airway. Endotracheal intubation may be necessary to protect the airway. Aspiration can be minimized by properly positioning the patient on the side with the head elevated. Additionally, oral intake should be withheld until the presence of the gag and swallowing reflexes has been verified and the patient is able to protect his or her own airway.

Adult Respiratory Distress Syndrome. Adult respiratory distress syndrome (ARDS) and neurogenic pulmonary edema (NPE) can develop (see Chap. 17 for a discussion of both conditions).

Neurogenic Pulmonary Edema. A sudden, massive increase in ICP can trigger a pressor response, which results in the development of NPE. The signs and symptoms are the same as those associated with acute pulmonary edema caused by cardiac decompensation, although in the neurological patient, there may not be evidence of cardiac disease to which acute pulmonary edema can be attributed.

Neurological Complications

Cerebral Hemorrhage. Hemorrhage is a serious postoperative complication that can occur in the subdural, epidural, intracerebral, or intraventricular space. Unlike bleeding that is visible externally, bleeding within the cranial vault is characterized by signs or symptoms of rapidly increasing ICP that requires early recognition and immediate intervention. Cerebral hemorrhage is diagnosed on a clinical basis and confirmed by CT scan. Treatment depends upon CT findings and may require emergency surgery.

Increased Intracranial Pressure. Although some increase in ICP is expected (with the peak occurring within 72 hours after surgery), great spikes in ICP are life threatening. Great increases in ICP can result from conditions such as cerebral edema, hemorrhage, meningitis, and surgical trauma. Treatment includes management of the underlying cause, judicious use of osmotic diuretics, and possible ventricular drainage. See Chapter 14 for a more detailed discussion of increased ICP.

Tension Pneumocephalus. Pneumocephalus is the entry of air into the subdural, extradural, subarachnoid, intracerebral, or intraventricular compartments. Pneumocephalus is a postoperative complication associated with posterior fossa craniotomy, bur hole for evacuation of a chronic subdural hematoma, and transsphenoidal hypophysectomy. The sitting position assumed during posterior fossa surgery is a risk factor. During hypophysectomy, air enters the subarachnoid space through the pituitary fossa and is gradually absorbed. However, in the presence of CSF rhinorrhea, additional air can enter the intracranial space, creating a pneumocephalus.

The trapped air, when warmed within the body, expands. A small amount of air can usually be reabsorbed and is not problematic. However, if the air pocket is of sufficient volume, it acts as a space-occupying lesion, causing neurological deterioration. The time frame for pneumocephalus to develop is either early (within 24 hours after surgery) or late (1 week following surgery). Signs and symptoms include drowsiness, decreased level of consciousness, and focal or lateral deficits. The diagnosis is established by CT scan. Treatment includes surgical evacuation of the air.

Hydrocephalus. Hydrocephalus can develop at any time during the postoperative course as a result of edema or bleeding into the subarachnoid space. Blood can interfere with the normal absorption of CSF by plugging the arachnoid villi. Such plugging is also associated with a ruptured cerebral aneurysm or head trauma. Scarring or obstruction in the ventricular system can also lead to hydrocephalus. The signs and symptoms of hydrocephalus are outlined in Chapter 14. The usual treatment is a ventriculostomy to drain CSF temporarily. If the hydrocephalus does not resolve, then a surgical shunting procedure is warranted. This is necessary to relieve the brain of excessive CSF and to prevent cerebral atrophy.

Seizures

Seizures following intracranial surgery may take the form of generalized convulsions or focal seizure activity. Seizures can occur at any time although seizures within the first 7 days after surgery are more common. Focal seizures in the form of twitching of selected muscles, particularly of the face or hand, are also common. Focal seizures in these two areas are common because both occupy large areas on the motor strip of the cerebral cortex; therefore, irritation from surgery or cerebral edema can easily initiate such seizure activity.

Because seizures are common after intracranial surgery, patients undergoing craniotomy usually receive prophylactic anticonvulsants, most commonly phenytoin, to prevent seizure activity. Drug blood levels must be monitored to maintain a therapeutic range.

Cerebrospinal Fluid Leakage. Leakage of CSF can occur at any time in the postoperative course and is caused by an opening in dura to the subarachnoid space. It is seen most often as CSF leakage from the operative site, but it may be noted as it drains from the ears or nose. A CSF leak can also be associated with head trauma, especially a basal skull fracture. To determine whether the drainage is CSF, a Dextrostix can be used to test the fluid. If the drainage is CSF, the fluid will test positive for glucose. Mucus does not contain glucose, although blood does contain glucose. If more conclusive evidence is required and CSF can be collected, it should be sent to the laboratory to be checked for chloride. CSF will show a glucose level that is approximately 60% to 80% of that of the blood level, and a chloride level greater than the serum level.

If CSF is present in nasal drainage, nasal suctioning or blowing of the nose is prohibited. The physician should be notified at once if there is evidence of a CSF leak. A CSF leak will often seal spontaneously. Serial lumbar punctures or a CSF lumbar drain may be necessary to keep CSF pressure low. If these measures are not successful, surgical repair may be indicated. Prophylactic antibiotics are ordered to prevent infection when a CSF leak is discovered.

Meningitis. Microorganisms that cause meningitis can be introduced into the meninges or CSF by spreading from a wound infection, from a head injury in which the dura mater has been punctured, by contamination during surgery, or by a contaminated dressing on a head wound. Presence of a dural tear, which is a prime site for entrance of microorganisms, is a risk factor for meningitis. Meningitis is treated with antibiotics and a quiet environment.

Prevention measures such as strict aseptic technique should be followed in the management of the surgical site. Most neurosurgeons routinely order prophylactic antibiotics during and after all intracranial surgery and continue antibiotic therapy for a few days to prevent meningitis. Part of the nursing responsibility is checking for drainage on the dressing and observing its character. A wet dressing should be reinforced immediately and the physician notified. Because moisture provides organisms with a transport system, a wet dressing is an ideal medium on which organisms can grow. The gauze used in most dressings absorbs drainage by capillary attraction. The wicking action helps to remove drainage from the skin. If a wet dressing is allowed to remain on the incision, the incision will be contaminated by organisms in the air or on the bedclothes by the wicking action of the moist dressing.

When head dressings are changed, a strictly aseptic technique must be followed. Usually, the initial dressing is not touched until the sutures have been removed or unless it has become wet. The wound should be kept dry until stitches or staples are removed. Some physicians remove the dressing completely after 24 hours. The policy of the treating hospital and physician preference should be followed.

Wound Infection. Wound infections can result from poor aseptic technique during surgery or dressing changes or because of the patient's touching the incision. To avoid this, patients must be cautioned against such action and restrained if necessary. The most frequent causative organisms for wound infections are the various staphylococcal organisms. Redness and drainage from the wound are the usual early symptoms. Observe the incision and dressing for evidence of drainage. A foul odor from the wound or an elevated white blood cell count raise suspicion of a wound infection. Strict aseptic technique should be followed in the management of the wound or dressing.

Other Complications

Gastric Ulceration/Hemorrhage. Gastric ulcerations accompanied by GI hemorrhage is not uncommon. Neurological procedures and acute and chronic CNS disease (e.g., craniocerebral trauma, tumors) have been associated with symptoms of active gastric bleeding. An increased incidence of gastric ulcers is associated with posterior fossa injury or surgery. Some of the drugs used in neurological treatment protocols (dexamethasone [Decadron], phenytoin, and certain antibiotics) also contribute to gastric irritation. For this reason, acetaminophen (Tylenol) is preferred over aspirin for the treatment of mild discomfort or as an antipyretic drug. When dexamethasone is administered, magnesium hydroxide (Maalox) is often given to reduce gastric irritation.

Monitor the hematocrit and hemoglobin levels. Stools should be monitored daily for occult blood, an indicator of bleeding somewhere in the GI tract. A histamine H_2-blocker is administered to reduce gastric secretions and protect against gastric hemorrhage.

Deep Vein Thrombosis. Neurosurgical patients are at high risk for deep vein thrombosis (DVT) and pulmonary embolus because of the longer surgery, positioning during surgery, and therapies during surgery such as hypothermia. In addition, bed rest adds to the risk. As mentioned earlier, elastic TED stockings and SCDs are applied before surgery, and the SCDs remain operational during surgery. TEDs and SCDs should be used on a continuous basis in the postoperative period.

Metabolic Imbalances

The most common metabolic and fluid imbalances result from diabetes insipidus (DI), cerebral salt wasting, hyperglycemia, and electrolyte imbalances (see Chap. 10 for detailed discussion).

Diabetes Insipidus. Supratentorial surgery, particularly in and around the pituitary fossa, can lead to temporary DI. DI is caused by a disturbance of the posterior lobe of the pituitary gland, which produces antidiuretic hormone (ADH). If this hormone is not secreted in sufficient quantity, the patient excretes large amounts of urine with a low specific gravity. The danger is fluid and electrolyte imbalance with dehydration, a serious concern.

Development of DI is often a transient problem requiring

no specific treatment other than adjusting IV therapy to correlate with urinary output. An accurate intake and output record must be kept and fractional urinary output must be monitored. An indwelling urinary catheter is placed in the early postoperative period when DI is most apt to appear. The specific gravity of the urine is monitored every 1 to 4 hours. A reading of 1.005 or less is considered low. If the condition does not correct itself, desmopressin acetate is the drug of choice for DI.

Cerebral Salt Wasting. Hyponatremia is common and may result from cerebral salt wasting (see Chap. 10). Treatment is saline solution to slowly correct the low sodium level.

Hyperglycemia. Hyperglycemia is related to poorer outcomes and should be avoided. Monitor glucose periodically and treat with regular insulin.

NEUROLOGICAL DEFICITS IN THE POSTOPERATIVE PERIOD

As a result of surgery, various transient neurological deficits may be noted. The particular deficits depend on preoperative deficits, the type of surgical procedure, and the amount of edema present. Many of these deficits resolve completely in the postoperative period. Others may require rehabilitation. The nurse assesses and monitors the patient for changes. Independent nursing and collaborative interventions may be implemented to manage the various problems.

Diminished Level of Consciousness. As cerebral edema subsides postoperatively, ICP decreases and the level of consciousness (LOC) improves. It is often surprising to find a patient who is fully alert and well oriented after surgery. Debulking of a mass, such as a brain tumor, can make a significant difference. For other patients, improvement in the LOC occurs slowly as cerebral edema gradually subsides.

Communication Deficits. The ability to express oneself verbally and to understand the spoken word depends on which deficits were present before surgery and which part of the brain was subject to surgery. If deficits are associated with cerebral edema, they will most likely improve as cerebral edema subsides. If the deficit was prominent before surgery or if surgical dissection was close to the language area, recovery will be slower, perhaps requiring referral to a speech therapist. Evaluate the type of communication deficit present and develop an alternative method of communication. The care plan should include a notation describing which alterations in communication patterns are necessary. If these adjustments are made by all personnel, it will greatly reduce the frustration of the patient and staff when communicating. An evaluation by speech therapy may also be helpful.

Motor and Sensory Deficits. As with other deficits, a decrease in cerebral edema results in improved motor and sensory function. For patients with motor deficits, a physical therapy evaluation and treatment plan are implemented to facilitate return of motor function. The nurse must be aware of specific deficits experienced by the patient and should participate in and support the principles of the physiotherapeutic program, thereby promoting continuity of care. Adaptations of nursing care may be necessary to meet the needs of the patient.

The nurse can participate by encouraging the patient to use a weak limb in the activities of daily living (ADLs), administering range-of-motion exercises, ensuring proper positioning, applying prescribed braces and splints, and helping the patient ambulate. In addition, the nurse should enlist the family's help and participation in physiotherapy. Most of all, the nurse provides emotional support as the patient deals with loss of body function and alterations in body image.

Headache. Postoperatively, headache is expected in the first few days, and it may be moderate to severe. Much of the pain originates from surgical stretching or irritation of the nerves of the scalp. Pain can also result from traction on the dura or large blood vessels within the intracranial space. A headache can be intensified by a head dressing that has been applied too tightly. The snugness of the dressing should be assessed for comfort. Codeine sulfate and acetaminophen are the drugs most commonly ordered to alleviate headache, often in a combination such as Tylenol #3. A quiet environment with limited direct light or a dimly lit room is soothing.

Elevation in Temperature. A modest elevation in temperature is common in the early postoperative period. Fever may indicate the presence of infection or irritation of the hypothalamus, the area of the brain responsible for regulation of the body temperature. The specific cause of the fever must be determined. Traction or petechial hemorrhage of the hypothalamus or pons can cause major elevations in body temperature (105°F; 40.6°C). Surgery in or around the third or fourth ventricle can also cause spikes in body temperature because of the proximity to the hypothalamus. Along with temperature elevation is an increase in blood pressure, cerebral blood flow, and cerebral metabolic rate. As cerebral metabolism increases, production of the metabolic by-products (carbon dioxide and lactic acid) increases. Both carbon dioxide and lactic acid are potent vasodilating agents that contribute to increased ICP.

An elevation in temperature is treated with antipyretic drugs, such as acetaminophen, administered by mouth, feeding tube, or rectally. Drug therapy may be used in conjunction with other adjunct therapies such as a hypothermia blanket, control of the environmental temperature, removal of excess bedclothes, or cool water sponging. Lower the temperature gradually to prevent shivering that can increase ICP. If shivering occurs, chlorpromazine (Thorazine) may be ordered.

Periocular Edema. Swelling around the eyes (periocular edema) is common after cranial surgery because of the manipulation of scalp, skull, and intracranial contents. It is usually accompanied by discoloration and ecchymosis, and peaks about 48 to 72 hours postoperatively.

Cold compresses help reduce edema. Cleanse the eyes to prevent crusting and lubricate with saline eye drops. Periocular edema disappears within 5 to 6 days. Discoloration and ecchymosis will take 10 to 14 days to resolve.

Diminished Gag/Swallowing Reflexes. The gag and swallowing reflexes are controlled by cranial nerves (CNs) IX and X. Both nerves are located in the lower brain stem at the medulla. Surgery in the posterior fossa (infratentorial area) may cause edema to the CNs proximal to the operative site, resulting in temporary loss or diminished response of both reflexes. As edema subsides, the reflexes will return. The danger of a temporary loss of either reflex is inability to protect the airway that can lead to aspiration and aspiration pneumonia. Therefore, oral intake should not be started unless the patient is able to protect his or her airway. Suction equipment should be readily available for use should the need arise.

Visual Disturbances. Diplopia and field cuts can be assessed in the patient who is sufficiently conscious to provide information. If diplopia is present, an eye patch can be worn.

Even in noncommunicative patients, the nurse can often draw a presumptive conclusion about visual deficits by observation. For example, the patient may not notice objects on one side of the bed or may react only when someone approaches from a particular side. Both situations suggest visual deficits.

Loss of Corneal Reflex. If the corneal reflex is absent, the affected eye must be protected from injury. Corneal abrasion and ulceration can develop from direct injury or from depriving the eye of proper lubrication. Blindness can be the unfortunate and permanent consequence of corneal ulceration. Applying an eye shield or taping the lids closed can prevent corneal abrasion. Periodic inspection and administration of artificial tears or saline solution (four times per day) can moisten the eye and prevent drying of the cornea.

Personality Changes. Changes in the baseline personality may be temporary or permanent. Permanent changes can occur from cerebral anoxia or surgery in the frontal area, whereas temporary personality changes can result from cerebral edema, surgery, drugs, or emotional stress. Temporary changes resolve in the postoperative period. Personality changes, although common after cranial surgery, are most disturbing sequelae for the patient and the family.

NURSE'S ROLE IN REHABILITATION AND DISCHARGE PLANNING

Although a craniotomy is a conventional neurosurgical treatment for many underlying problems, the degree and time of recovery and the need for further treatment and rehabilitation are individual. For example, the discharge planning for a young patient who has had a craniotomy for a benign pituitary tumor will be different from the plan for an elderly person undergoing craniotomy for a malignant tumor. The neurological deficits in these two patients will be different, as is the impact of surgery on the patients and their

families. The need for individual planning thus becomes apparent. As cerebral edema subsides, a more accurate profile of neurological deficits emerges. Some deficits recover spontaneously with time, whereas other deficits need treatment and rehabilitation to achieve the optimal level of recovery. The human impact is assessed by talking to the patient and family and assessing their responses.

Independent Nursing Role

As part of the independent nursing role, the nurse assesses the patient's functional level and collects the following data, which will be used for planning nursing care and for discharge planning:

- Level of consciousness and cognitive function (important for patient teaching)
- Presence of neurological deficits
- Verbal communication skills (ability to participate in a conversation, any word-finding difficulty)
- Independence in performing ADLs
- Emotional response to surgery and the underlying problems (e.g., depression)
- Safety concerns (Is the patient at risk for injury or falls?)
- Previous family role and responsibilities
- Support systems and living situation (Could the patient manage at home safely? If the patient needs assistance, will a family member be available to assist the patient?)

Integration of the principles of rehabilitation into the plan of nursing care is directed at helping the patient achieve the highest level of independence possible. Involve the patient with the environment and ADLs as much as possible. Many patients are easily fatigued after surgery. Plan rest to prevent exhaustion and increase endurance. Support the patient and family throughout the hospitalization and prepare them for discharge. Patient and family teaching begun earlier in the course of hospitalization is now expanded. The family is encouraged to participate in basic care and ADL routines to develop skill and confidence in post-hospital care.

Anxiety, ambivalence, hostility, and depression are common in the postoperative period and continue even after transition to the home. One interesting cause of depression relates to the degree of progress made postoperatively. During the hospital stay and initially after discharge, recovery and improvement are often rapid. If one were to chart this on a graph, it would be represented initially by a steeply ascending line; a plateau would then be reached, marking a period of small improvements or no apparent improvement. If patients are unable to perform activities that they believe are realistic and feasible, they may become upset. Discouragement is further augmented by fatigue, which causes these patients to abandon certain activities. This sequence of events reinforces discouragement, depression, and complaints of constant fatigue. In these circumstances, the patient needs to be helped to set more realistic goals. A sympathetic approach and explanation of the postoperative course is helpful.

Collaborative Role

Early in the postoperative period, the nurse and physician collaboratively identify neurological deficits that need further evaluation by other health care professionals. Although the needs of each patient vary, the most frequent referrals are made to physical therapy, occupational therapy, speech therapy, social services, and sometimes psychiatry. The physician may also make a referral to another physician, such as the neuro-oncologist or neuroradiologist. After the patient has been evaluated and patient needs are identified in concrete terms, a discharge plan is formalized and implemented.

It is impossible to generalize about typical responses to a craniotomy. For some patients, a craniotomy provides a cure for a treatable condition, such as a subdural hematoma. For others, intracranial surgery ameliorates symptoms of cerebral compression so that an extension of time can be offered for patients with a disorder with a terminal prognosis. The implications of the craniotomy in terms of the patient's life can only be assessed individually. Depending on the reason for surgery and the prognosis, the patient or family may need to make major decisions about postacute care facilities and choice of treatment.

SELECTED NEUROSURGICAL PROCEDURES

Three surgical procedures are discussed in this section: transsphenoidal hypophysectomy, carotid endarterectomy, and placement of a ventricular shunt.

Transsphenoidal Hypophysectomy

Description

The transsphenoidal approach is possible because of the development of microsurgical techniques and equipment (Fig. 15-9). Pituitary adenomas, craniopharyngiomas, and a complete hypophysectomy for control of bone pain in metastatic cancer are the usual conditions for which a transsphenoidal surgical approach is used. The transsphenoidal surgical approach affords access to the pituitary gland by means of an incision made inside the superior upper lip, in front of the hard palate. After the sphenoid sinus floor is dissected, the sella turcica is visible. A portion of the sella floor is removed, and the dura incised. With the aid of a surgical microscope, the pituitary is partially or completely removed or the impinging tumor is excised. A graft of muscle taken from the anterior surface of the thigh or a fat pad (taken from the abdomen or thigh) is then applied to the surgical site as a patch to prevent CSF leakage. Nasal Vaseline packings are inserted to control bleeding and to replace the septal mucosa. A dry, sterile dressing is firmly applied to the donor site (abdomen or thigh).

The specific tissue that is surgically excised depends on the reason for surgery. If surgery was scheduled for removal of a pituitary adenoma, the pituitary gland would be left

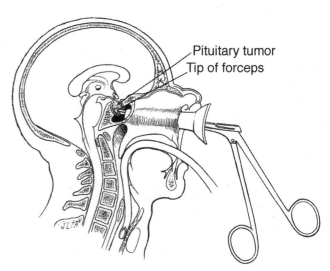

Figure 15–9 • Transsphenoidal approach in pituitary surgery. (From Smeltzer, S. C. & Bare, B. G. [1996]. *Brunner and Suddarth's textbook of medical-surgical nursing* [8th ed.] [p. 1738]. Philadelphia: Lippincott-Raven Publishers.)

intact, if possible, and the tumor excised. In a patient who undergoes craniopharyngioma surgery, only the tumor would be excised.

Palliative Surgery for Pain Secondary to Cancer

Palliative hypophysectomy for cancer necessitates total removal of the pituitary. The surgeon attempts to excise the pituitary in one piece, because cells left at the surgical site continue to secrete hormones and decrease the anticipated relief of pain. It is unclear why a hypophysectomy can alleviate pain or further slow metastasis. Removal of the anterior lobe, with the resultant cessation of prolactin and the growth-stimulating hormone, helps to control breast and prostate cancer. Preoperative preparation begins with patient and family teaching. The patient needs realistic expectations of outcome and the need for drug replacement therapy.

Postoperative Complications

The major complications associated with transsphenoidal hypophysectomy include CSF leakage (rhinorrhea), DI, sinusitis, and delayed epistaxis. The patient should be monitored for the development of these complications. Of these complications, only DI is discussed.

Postsurgical Diabetes Insipidus

Central DI is defined as the cessation of ADH secretion by the pituitary gland as a result of damage from disease or injury of the hypothalamus, the supraoptic hypophyseal tract, or the posterior pituitary. The most common cause of central DI is neurosurgery. Postsurgical DI can occur up to 2 weeks postoperatively.

Monitoring for the development of DI is a major postoperative nursing responsibility (see Chap. 10 for further discussion). The symptoms of DI are copious amounts of pale urine (more than 250 mL/hour for 2 consecutive hours) and a low urinary specific gravity (less than 1.005). Therefore, fractional urinary output, specific gravity, and serum osmolality need to be checked every 1 to 2 hours.

Other patients may experience a pattern of transient copious urinary output and low specific gravity. If the patient is able to drink enough fluid to quench thirst and maintain fluid and electrolyte balance, no medical treatment is indicated. Some patients may also experience a period of low urinary output 2 or 3 days postoperatively before permanent DI develops.

In the case of a total hypophysectomy, permanent DI is expected and replacement therapy is begun. With partial resection, DI is not permanent. In the immediate postoperative period, aqueous vasopressin (Pitressin) intramuscularly (IM), subcutaneously, or IV *or* DDAVP subcutaneously or IV titrated to output (see Chap. 11) should be instituted. After the nasal packings have been removed, intranasal DDAVP can be used.[13] The patient must be instructed in the safe use of the drug.

- Nasal mucosa irritation may occur; this will interfere with absorption of the drug.
- Overuse of the drug will cause water intoxication (mental confusion, drowsiness). For some patients, it may be more convenient and safer to use vasopressin in oil, 2.5 to 5.0 mg IM every 2 to 3 days, to control DI.
- Daily weight must be monitored.
- Oral intake must be balanced with daily output.

Hormonal Replacement

In the case of total hypophysectomy, other hormonal replacement is necessary. The usual drugs ordered include:

- Adrenocorticotropic hormone (ACTH), 25 mg IM in the morning and 12.5 mg IM at night, beginning immediately after surgery.
- Thyroxin, 0.2 to 0.3 mg daily. Thyroid replacement therapy is delayed for 3 to 4 weeks following surgery.
- Cortisone acetate, 100 mg/d IM, beginning 2 days *before* surgery to prevent adrenal insufficiency. The drug is continued postoperatively but at a lower dose than that indicated previously.

Patient Teaching for Drug Replacement

If lifelong replacement drug therapy is necessary, it is most important that the patient and family understand the purposes of drug therapy. The nurse should begin with a basic overview of the pituitary gland to foster an understanding of the rationale for drug replacement therapy. The degree of sophistication with which this information is presented will depend on the learner's level of understanding. To reinforce the verbal explanation, written and visual aids are helpful. The teaching plan should include:

- Specific information to record and submit to the physician, such as daily weight
- Signs and symptoms of undermedication or overmedication
- Side effects of drugs

- Lifestyle alterations necessitated as a result of drug therapy

Adrenocorticotropic Hormone

Certain cells of the anterior pituitary gland produce ACTH, which is stored until the hypothalamus secretes corticotropin-releasing hormone (CRH), which signals the pituitary gland to release ACTH. The target of ACTH is the cortex of the adrenal glands by way of the bloodstream. The following hormones are secreted by the adrenal cortex:

- The glucocorticoids, such as cortisol (hydrocortisone) and cortisone, are the major secretions and are necessary for carbohydrate, protein, and fat metabolism. They also help the body cope with physical and emotional environmental stresses. Cortisone is a hormone that requires daily replacement for survival.
- The mineralocorticoids (particularly aldosterone) control salt and water metabolism by reabsorbing sodium ions in exchange for potassium in the kidney. This hormone does not require replacement on a daily basis.
- Certain male and female hormones play a minor role in comparison with the secretions of the ovaries and the testes. Replacement therapy is contraindicated if a hypophysectomy was done to control breast or prostate cancer. In other patients, replacement therapy may be necessary on a monthly basis, depending on age and other considerations. This determination will be made by the physician.

High blood levels of corticotropic hormone inhibit secretion of CRH so that no additional ACTH is secreted by the pituitary gland. The body normally produces the largest amount of ACTH in the early morning hours so that the glucocorticoids necessary for carbohydrate, protein, and fat metabolism are available when needed.

During times of physical and emotional stress, individuals require large amounts of cortisol. ACTH is continually produced to meet this need. Under severe stress, ten times the normal amount of cortisol may be required; approximately 25 mg is the daily requirement under normal circumstances.

Following hypophysectomy, the adrenal gland is deprived of stimulation because ACTH that is normally produced by the pituitary gland is absent. The patient will require ACTH replacement or administration of hydrocortisone, the natural glucocorticoid secreted by the adrenal cortex. This drug has some of the mineralocorticoid properties that are provided by adrenal secretion.

The patient receiving **cortisone therapy** should know the following:

- The drug must be taken daily as ordered; failure to take the drug can be life threatening.
- The dosage must be increased during periods of emotional stress, illness, excessive exercise, major changes in daily routine, exposure to high altitudes, tooth extraction, fever, or infection.
- Gastric irritation, a side effect of steroid therapy, can be minimized by taking an antacid (30 mL of magnesium hydroxide) with each dose of the drug.
- The presence of tarry stools indicates gastrointestinal

hemorrhage, which should be reported to the physician immediately.

- Check blood pressure periodically for HPT (an elevation in blood pressure is common with cortisone therapy); if the patient is taking antihypertensives, adjustments in the dosage may be necessary.
- Check for hyperglycemia; ACTH is associated with diabetes mellitus.
- Behavioral changes, such as euphoria, restlessness, sleeplessness, agitation, and depression are common with cortisone therapy.
- The following are signs and symptoms of *undermedication* (addisonian crisis):
  - Weakness, dizziness, orthostatic hypotension
  - Nausea and vomiting
  - Sodium and water retention
  - Decreased blood pressure
- Management of cortisone insufficiency requires parenteral hydrocortisone sodium succinate (Solu-Cortef). Failure to treat will lead to circulatory collapse.
- The following are signs and symptoms of *overmedication*:
  - Cushingoid signs (moon face, fat pads, buffalo hump, acne, hirsutism, and weight gain)
  - Psychic disturbances
  - Peptic ulcers
  - Headache, vertigo, cataracts, and increased ICP and intraocular pressure
- A medical alert bracelet must be worn at all times.
- An emergency kit of hydrocortisone sodium succinate must be carried at all times.

Postoperative Nursing Management After Transsphenoidal Surgery

Specific points regarding the nursing management of the patient undergoing surgery by the transsphenoidal approach are outlined in Chart 15-3. After surgery, minimal pain is noted at the oronasal suture line because the pain receptor fibers have been cut, resulting in loss of pain perception. Nasal mucosa requires at least 1 month to heal satisfactorily. Nasal packings are removed in 3 to 4 days. The senses of smell and taste return in 2 or 3 weeks. Headache, as a result of sinus congestion or ear discomfort related to the nasal packings, is common.

If the hypophysectomy was performed to control metastasis and bone pain, relief may be evident within hours after surgery; in other patients, it may take days to a few weeks. The surgery is a "last chance" effort to control severe pain that has made ADLs impossible. Many patients express a desire for their families to see them comfortable without the use of drugs and to fulfill certain life goals before death. The nurse's role in such cases is supportive. Clarifying and providing necessary information are vital.

Carotid Artery Surgery

Cerebrovascular insufficiency can result from occlusion of the carotid artery secondary to atherosclerosis. If untreated, this can lead to transient ischemic attacks (TIAs) or stroke. In some instances, even though the internal carotid artery is occluded, the external carotid artery will remain patent as a result of collateral blood flow from the contralateral external carotid artery. In this event, the external carotid artery becomes extremely important in maintaining an adequate blood supply to the brain. Thus, a patient with occlusion of a carotid artery may be asymptomatic because of continued collateral circulation.

Carotid Atherosclerosis

For reasons unknown, atheromas (atherosclerotic plaques) commonly form in the larger cerebral arteries such as the common carotid artery, especially at the bifurcation of the internal and external carotid arteries. The atheroma gradual narrows the blood vessel, which impinges on adequate cerebral blood flow. The atheroma can become the site for the formation of a thrombus, or it can break off and act as an embolus. Both processes can lead to cerebral ischemia and stroke (cerebral infarction).

Diagnosis and Treatment

Diagnosis of cerebral vascular insufficiency is made on the basis of a history of TIAs, CT scan, transcranial Doppler studies, or a possible cerebral arteriogram. The most common cerebral revascularization surgical procedure is the carotid endarterectomy (CEA). Superior temporal artery–middle cerebral artery (STA-MCA) anastomosis is ineffective.[14]

Carotid Endarterectomy

Carotid endarterectomy is the most frequently performed noncardiac vascular procedure today (Fig. 15-10).[15] The first successful CEA dates back to 1953, when it was performed by DeBakey.[16] In the United States, the number of CEAs rose from 15,000 in 1971 to 107,000 in 1985.[17] However, there was much controversy about the appropriateness and effectiveness of the procedure in light of declining stroke rates, new emphasis on risk factor management, and new antiplatelet pharmacological therapies. Early randomized trials to evaluate results of CEA were disappointing.[18,19] By 1989, the number of CEAs performed had declined to 70,000 owing to confusion about efficacy, patient selection, and outcomes.[17] Concurrently, a randomized trial to evaluate extracranial-intracranial bypass to prevent stroke found that the procedure was ineffective in preventing stroke.[14] Renewed interest in the CEA resulted in new studies.

The results of a landmark study, the North American Symptomatic Carotid Endarterectomy Trial (NASCET), were reported in 1991.[20,21] Patients were randomized to either medical or surgical therapy for TIA or mild disabling stroke ipsilateral to a 70% to 90% narrowing of the internal carotid artery. The CEA group had a clear benefit in reducing the overall risk of fatal and nonfatal ipsilateral stroke, despite any preoperative risk of stroke or death from any cause. Over 26% of the medical group and 9% of the CEA group had a fatal or nonfatal ipsilateral stroke at 24 months. These findings report an absolute risk reduction from CEA of 17% and a relative risk reduction of 65%. Other analysis examined the role of risk factors present (e.g., age, gender, systolic and/or diastolic HPT). It was found that the benefit

CHART 15-3 • Nursing Management After Transsphenoidal Surgery

Nursing Management	Rationale
EARLY POSTOPERATIVE MANAGEMENT	
• Frequently monitor vital and neurological signs.	• Provides information for baseline comparisons to indicate trends, deterioration, or complications
• Maintain the head of bed at 30 degrees.	• Promotes venous drainage from the brain, controls intracranial pressure, and prevents hemorrhage at the operative site
• Check the dressing at the donor site on the thigh for evidence of bleeding.	• Detects bleeding for early intervention
• Frequently check nasal drains and packing; observe for hemorrhage or cerebrospinal fluid (CSF) drainage from the operative site; the mustache dressing should be observed and changed as necessary.	• Promotes early detection of hemorrhage or CSF and subsequent early intervention
PREVENTION OF COMPLICATIONS	
• Monitor urinary output and specific gravity frequently.	• Monitor for evidence of diabetes insipidus

• Monitor electrolyte and osmolarity laboratory values for abnormally high or low readings (serum and urine osmolarity, serum sodium). Normal values are as follows:
    Serum osmolarity: 280–295 mOsm/L
    Urine osmolarity: 500–800 mOsm/L
    Serum sodium: 135–145 mEq/L
	• In diabetes insipidus, the serum sodium level is increased, serum osmolarity is increased, and urine osmolarity is decreased; also, serum electrolyte testing can indicate an electrolyte imbalance

• Give frequent mouth care, but do not allow the patient to brush teeth if the oral approach was used.	• Prevents injury at the suture line, yet allows the mouth to be refreshed and cleansed
• Progress diet from liquid to soft as necessary.	• Prevents injury to the suture line
• After packings are removed, caution the patient against blowing the nose or sneezing for at least 1 mo.	• Prevents hemorrhage from fragile nasal tissue at operative site
SUPPORTIVE CARE	
• Provide for routine hygienic care, such as bathing, hair combing, and nail cutting.	• Maintains general well-being
• Offer fluids frequently, as ordered.	• Maintains hydration and moistens the oral mucous membrane, which becomes dry from mouth breathing (required when nasal packings are in place)
• Provide eye care (clean and lubricate).	• Prevents infection, inflammation, and drying of the cornea
• Apply compresses to the periocular region if periocular edema occurs.	• Controls and alleviates periocular edema
PATIENT TEACHING	
• Prepare and implement a patient teaching plan to outline any adjustments in lifestyle, precautions necessary with the drug protocol, and general information about the patient's health problem.	• Provides for the safety and well-being of the patient and includes the patient as an involved, informed participant in health management
• Provide written material to summarize the major points of home management for the patient.	• Reinforces the major points of the teaching plan and reduces the possibility of confusion or questions about home protocol
• Include the family in the teaching plan.	• Includes the family in the plan of care so that they can become a knowledgeable support system for the patient

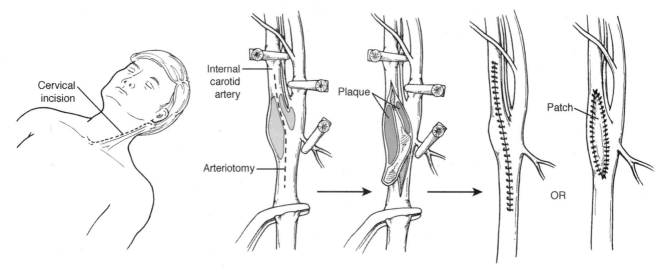

Figure 15–10 • Carotid endarterectomy. An oblique cervical incision allows dissection of the carotid bifurcation. Following heparinization, the arteries of the bifurcation are cross-clamped and an arteriotomy is performed. The plaque is dissected precisely in the subintimal plane, with a subsequent closure (primary or via patch reconstruction) of the arteriotomy. Other aspects of the surgery include intraoperative monitoring during cross-clamping, microsurgical technique allowing optimal lighting and magnification, patch angioplasty, shunting, and verification of patency.

derived from CEA was directly proportional to the risk faced without surgery, and that those with the highest risks at entry gained the most benefit.[17] Finally, it was found that patients with 70% stenosis or more benefited from a CEA, whereas it remained unclear about benefit in those with a stenosis of less than 70%. The large European Carotid Surgery Trial (ECST) also demonstrated a clear benefit for CEA for patients with advanced stenosis.[22]

The NASCET focused on symptomatic patients. In 1992, CEA practice guidelines[23] were published followed by American Heart Association (AHA) guidelines in 1995.[25] The next question was how best to manage asymptomatic patients with carotid stenosis. Further randomized studies have clarified the indication for surgery in asymptomatic patients. This was addressed in the Asymptomatic Carotid Atherosclerosis Study (ACAS).[15]

Asymptomatic Carotid Artery Disease

In the ACAS trial, patients were randomly assigned to a surgical group ($n = 825$) or medical group ($n = 834$). All patients received aspirin (325 mg/day) and risk factor–reduction counseling. Follow-up occurred after 1 month and every 3 months thereafter. Doppler ultrasound was ordered at the initial 3-month follow-up, then every 6 months for 2 years, and annually up to 5 years or until endpoints were reached. Endpoints were defined as death or stroke. The medical group had a lower risk (0.4%) in the 42-day perioperative period, but higher risk (11%) for endpoint criteria after 5 years. Surgery reduced absolute risk by 5.9% and relative risk by 53% at 5 years. The knowledge gained from the ACAS study is reflected in the updated AHA 1998 guidelines for CEA.[15] Note that the recommendations are organized around surgical risk. Surgical risk is based on neurological stability, comorbidity, angiographic risk, and is graded from I to IV. Grade I includes patients who are neurologically stable with no medical or angiographic risks,

whereas grade IV comprises neurologically unstable patients with or without medical or angiographic risks.[26] In addition, ulcerations are classified from type A to C (Table 15-3).[27] Guidelines for proven and acceptable indications for CEA for patients with asymptomatic carotid artery disease are found in Table 15-4.

Update on CEA for Symptomatic Patients

Further analysis of NASCET and the ECST data helps clarify CEA benefits supported by Grade A recommendations that are based on well-designed randomized control trials. The Grade A recommendations support CEA as beneficial for symptomatic patients with recent nondisabling carotid artery ischemic events and ipsilateral 70% to 99% carotid artery stenosis. CEA is not beneficial for symptomatic patients with 0% to 29% stenosis. Uncertainty remains about the potential benefit of CEA for symptomatic patients with 30% to 69% stenosis. ECST data do not support CEA for patients with less than 50% stenosis.[22] CEA is *three times* as effective as medical therapy alone in reducing incidence of stroke in patients with symptomatic stenosis of 70% to 99%.[22,28,29] However, CEA is not without preoperative risks and complications. To justify CEA, the significant complica-

Table 15–3 • CLASSIFICATION OF CAROTID ULCERATIONS

TYPE	DESCRIPTION	ANNUAL STROKE RATE
A	Small, smooth, shallow	0.5%
B	Large, deep	0.5–4.5%
C	Complex, cavitated	5–7%

From Martin, N. A., Hadley, M. N., Spetzler, R. F., et al. (1986). Management of asymptomatic carotid arteriosclerosis. *Neurosurgery, 18,* 505–512.

Table 15-4 • RECOMMENDATIONS FOR PATIENTS WITH ASYMPTOMATIC CAROTID ARTERY DISEASE BASED ON SURGICAL RISK

INDICATIONS/ RISK	PROVEN	ACCEPTABLE/NOT PROVEN	UNCERTAIN
Surgical risk: <3% and life expectancy of at least 5 years	Ipsilateral carotid endarterectomy (CEA) for stenotic lesions (≥60% diameter reduction of distal outflow tract with or without ulceration and with or without antiplatelet therapy, irrespective of contralateral artery status, ranging from no disease to occlusion).	Unilateral CEA simultaneous with coronary artery bypass graft for stenotic lesions (≥60% diameter reduction with or without ulcerations with or without antiplatelet therapy, irrespective of contralateral artery status).	Unilateral CEA for stenosis >50% with B or C ulcer irrespective of contralateral internal carotid artery status
Surgical risk: 3% to 5%	None	Ipsilateral CEA for stenosis ≥75% with or without ulcerations but in the presence of contralateral internal carotid artery stenosis ranging from 75% to total occlusion	See guidelines
Surgical risk: 5% to 10%	None	None	See guidelines

From Biller, J., Feinberg, W. M., Castoldo, J. E., et al. (1998). Guidelines for carotid endarterectomy: A statement for healthcare professionals from a special writing group of the Stroke Council, American Heart Association. *Circulation, 97,* 501–509.

tion rate should be 3% or lower, according to the above-mentioned studies. Patient selection and the skill of the surgeon and surgical team are important factors in maintaining low surgical complications. In addition, the quality of nursing care is critical in prevention and early recognition of complications and in supporting optimal outcomes.

Preoperative Concerns

Many patients who have cerebrovascular atherosclerosis also have other concurrent conditions and risk factors, such as coronary artery disease, peripheral vascular disease, renal disease, diabetes mellitus, hyperlipidemia, and HPT. Treatment and stabilization of these and other medical conditions and attention to risk factors are necessary before surgery. In particular, HPT must be controlled before surgery. Table 15-5 lists these risk factors.

Perioperative and Postoperative Complications

Perioperative complications of CEA include stroke, myocardial infarction, and death. Postoperative complications include HPT, hypotension, hyperperfusion syndrome, intracerebral hemorrhage, seizures, nerve injury, cranial nerve injury, and wound hematoma.

Postoperative Hypertension (HPT). Preoperative HPT is the single most important determinant for the development of postoperative HPT. Poorly controlled HPT increases the risk of wound hematoma and hyperperfusion syndrome. In addition, neurological deficits, intracerebral hemorrhage, and death were more common in those patients who developed postoperative HPT. The first 48 hours after the CEA is the peak time for postoperative HPT. About 21% of normotensive patients may have increased blood pressure after

CEA.[30] The pathophysiology of postoperative HPT is probably related to surgically induced changes in carotid body baroreceptor sensitivity. Prevention of injury to the vagus nerve and carotid sinus during surgery is important to avoid baroreceptor dysfunction. Unstable blood pressure is common during the first 24-hours after CEA, which occurs in about 73% of patients.[31] It is a temporary problem that resolves in most instances. Therefore, frequent monitoring of blood pressure is very important in the postoperative period. Blood pressure must be maintained within a target range to prevent complications previously mentioned.

Postoperative Hypotension. Postoperative hypotension (i.e., systolic blood pressure less than 120 mm Hg) occurs in approximately 5% of patients.[32] A fluid bolus and low-dose phenylephrine infusion are usually effective. It usually resolves in 24 to 48 hours. If significant hypotension persists, a myocardial infarction must be ruled out through serial electrocardiograms and cardiac enzyme measurements. Possible consequences of hypotension include cerebral hypoxia and ischemic stroke; therefore, adequate blood pressure within a targeted range must be maintained. Monitoring central venous pressure in the early postoperative period is helpful.

Hyperperfusion Syndrome. Patients at risk for hyperperfusion syndrome are those with high-grade stenosis of the internal carotid and those with chronic HPT. The risk is further compounded if a severe contralateral stenosis is present.[15] Impairment of autoregulation is the basis for the syndrome. The cerebral hemodynamics are thought to be similar to that of normal perfusion breakthrough as seen after AVM resection.[32,33] As a result of the high-grade stenosis, a chronic state of hypoperfusion exists in the hemisphere distal to the stenosis. The smaller blood vessels are in a chronic state of maximal dilation to provide adequate blood flow that results in a loss of autoregulation. After the stenosis has been

Table 15-5 • STROKE RISK FACTORS, MANAGEMENT, AND RELATIONSHIP TO OUTCOMES AFTER CAROTID ENDARTERECTOMY (CEA)

RISK FACTOR FOR STROKE	EFFECT AFTER CEA	TREATMENT
Hypertension (HPT)	↑ risk of hyperperfusion syndrome ↑ risk of intracerebral bleeding	Control blood pressure according to JNC VI standards*
Cigarette smoking	Risk factor for restenosis	Smoking cessation program
Hyperlipidemia	Risk factor for restenosis Drug Rx ↓ stroke by 30%†	Follow NCEP guidelines‡
Alcohol consumption	High consumption = ↑ risk of stroke Moderate consumption = no effect or slight protection	Avoid high consumption of alcohol
Postmenopausal estrogen	No effect or slight ↓ risk	Unclear; individual decision at this time
Antiplatelet drugs	23% ↓ for non-fatal stroke 22% ↓ for all vascular events (nonfatal stroke, nonfatal myocardial infarction, and vascular death)§	? dose of aspirin; guidelines recommend 325 mg/dy‖

* The Sixth Report of the Joint National Committee on Prevention, Detection, Evaluation, and Treatment of High Blood Pressure. (1997). *Archives of Internal Medicine, 157,* 2413–2446.

† Scandinavian Simvastatin Survival Study Group. (1994). Randomized trial of cholesterol lowering in 4444 patients with coronary heart disease: The Scandinavian Simvastatin Survival Study (4S). *Lancet, 344,* 1383–1389.

‡ National Cholesterol Education Program (NCEP) Expert Panel. (1993). Summary of the second report of the National Cholesterol Education Program (NCEP) Expert Panel on detection, evacuation and treatment of high blood cholesterol in adults. *JAMA, 269,* 3015–3023.

§ Antiplatelet Trialists' Collaboration. Collaborative overview of randomized trials of antiplatelet therapy I: Prevention of death, myocardial infarction, and stroke by prolonged antiplatelet therapy in various categories of patients. *BMJ, 308,* 81–106.

‖ Ad Hoc Committee on Guidelines for the Management of Transient Ischemic Attacks of the Stroke Council of the American Heart Association. (1994). Guidelines for the management of transient ischemic stroke. *Stroke, 25,* 1320–1335.

corrected, the hypoperfused hemisphere receives blood at a normal or elevated perfusion pressure. If autoregulation is impaired, vasoconstriction cannot occur to protect the capillaries. This results in edema and hemorrhage.[15] Clinically, hyperperfusion syndrome is characterized by a severe unilateral headache, seizures, and altered mental status or focal neurological deficits. Raising the head of the bed will often improve the headache. Strict control of blood pressure is key to prevent or to limit the severity of hyperperfusion syndrome.

Intracerebral Hemorrhage. Secondary to a hyperperfusion syndrome, the potential exists for intracerebral hemorrhage. This is often fatal (60%); less frequently, it results in poor patient outcomes (25%).[34] The risk factors for hemorrhage are the same as for hyperperfusion syndrome, with the addition of advanced age and poor collateral flow on angiography. Control of blood pressure is critical to avoid or control hemorrhage.

Seizures. The occurrence of seizures is reported at 3%.[35] They are related to hyperperfusion syndrome and hypertensive encephalopathy unless infarction or hemorrhage has occurred.

Nerve Injury. The transverse cervical nerve and the greater auricular nerve are frequently severed or injured during the course of CEA. What results is a permanent ipsilateral numbness of the upper neck, lower face, and lower ear that is generally well tolerated.[17] Damage to the cervical sympathetic chain can result in a complete or incomplete Horner's syndrome.

Cranial Nerve Injury. Injury to the cranial nerves is a potential problem, although it is infrequent. The cranial nerves that are most vulnerable are the facial, glossopharyngeal, vagus, spinal accessory, and hypoglossal.[17,26] The surgeon's skill is critical to a good outcome. Postoperative neurological assessment is important for early identification of potential deficits.

Wound Hematoma. In the NASCET study, a wound hematoma occurred in about 5.5% of patients.[29] Most hematomas are small and are not uncomfortable. Larger hematomas can expand quickly and may necessitate emergency surgical evacuation. If the airway has been compromised, the physician may need to open the wound at the bedside during an emergency procedure. Meticulous attention to hemostasis is important to prevention. Therefore, frequent monitoring of the incision for the development of a hematoma is important.

Postoperative Management

Many potentially life-threatening cardiovascular and cerebrovascular complications exist. Thus, frequent neurological and vital sign monitoring and close medical management of these patients are critical for optimal outcomes. Throughout the country, patients are admitted to areas offering various levels of care after postoperative discharge from the ICU: an intermediate unit or general floor care (after a few hours in a PACU). In the last few years, questions have been raised about the need for ICU admission. Few studies have been conducted. One study reported that only a few patients benefit from ICU care.[36] One must recognize that these patients are at high risk for complications. Within this population are those patients identified as being at particularly high risk because of characteristics already mentioned as representing a pre-existing comorbidity (e.g., HPT). Appropriate monitoring and care must be provided regardless of clinical setting selected.

Ongoing Nursing Assessment and Monitoring

Frequent vital sign, neurological, and wound assessment should be conducted. Some physicians insert a Jackson-Pratt drain at the operative site to manage drainage. The purpose of the drain is to prevent development of a hematoma, which could compress the airway. If a venous graft is used, the donor site is also monitored. The physician sets the target parameters for maintenance of systolic and diastolic blood pressure, based on a reasonable baseline before surgery. Vasopressors or antihypertensives may be ordered to maintain the desired blood pressure levels.

Frequent monitoring of neurological signs is necessary to determine any neurological changes associated with cerebral ischemia or stroke. In addition, the cranial nerves, especially V, VII, IX, X, XI, and XII, are assessed for deficits (facial drooping, hoarseness, diminished/lost gag and/or swallowing reflexes, and weakness of the tongue). Note presence of a small unilateral pupil with flushing of the skin, which may suggest development of Horner's syndrome. In the immediate postoperative period, the head of the bed may be flat or elevated, depending on the preference of the physician. The patient is positioned off the operative site. A central venous line, peripheral IV line, urinary catheter, cardiac monitor, and oxygen therapy are usually used. After protection of the airway has been established, items may be added to the patient's diet.

Most patients are discharged from the hospital in a day or two with a prescription for lifetime aspirin therapy (325 mg/day), unless a contraindication is found. Patient education should include what to report immediately to the physician. This includes new onset of unilateral headache, neurological deficits, or seizure activity. The importance of maintaining good blood pressure control and monitoring of blood pressure is stressed. Other risk modification, with the assistance of the primary care provider, is also discussed.

Other Cerebral Vascular Procedures

Carotid Stenting and Angioplasty

Although carotid stenting and angioplasty are available, experience and understanding are limited about their potential use. Currently, their clinical applications are being explored and evaluated.[37]

Ventricular Shunts

A ventricular shunt is used to treat hydrocephalus. It consists of a primary catheter, a reservoir, a one-way valve, and a terminal catheter. It is implanted surgically to provide for drainage of excessive CSF from the brain to decrease or prevent increased ICP. The primary catheter is implanted into the lateral ventricle through a bur hole. An incision is

made under the scalp, and the catheter is pulled through so that the reservoir rests on the mastoid bone. CSF flows from the catheter to the reservoir, in which the CSF collects. A one-way valve on the reservoir prevents CSF reflux. A special instrument is used to pull the terminal catheter under the skin to the terminal point, which is the subarachnoid space or another body cavity (peritoneum, vena cava). The terminal catheter is then secured into position. In the adult, the peritoneal cavity is often used. The shunt is left in place permanently unless it becomes dislodged, plugged, or infected. In these situations, the shunt would be removed surgically and replaced.

Depending on the type of shunt placed, the physician may write an order to pump the shunt a given number of times at prescribed intervals (e.g., 10 times every 6 hours). The purpose of pumping a shunt is to flush the system of exudate that could plug the small tubing. To pump the shunt, lightly palpate the mastoid process with the index and middle fingers until the reservoir is palpated. It will feel bouncy to the touch. Next, with the index or middle finger, compress and gently release the reservoir the prescribed number of times. Documentation and any changes in neurological function are recorded in the patient's chart.

REFERENCES

1. Hamilton, M. G., Hull, R. D., & Pineo, G. F. (1994). Venous thromboembolism in neurosurgery and neurology patients: A review. *Neurosurgery, 34,* 280–296.
2. Lam. A. M. (1999). Neurophysiological monitoring. In P. Newfield & J. C. Cottrell (Eds.). *Handbook of neuroanesthesia* (3rd ed., pp. 34-52). Philadelphia: Lippincott Williams & Wilkins.
3. American Society of Anesthesiologists. (1963). New classification of physical status. *Anesthesiology, 24,* 111.
4. Hickey, R. (1999). Effects of anesthesia on cerebral and spinal cord physiology. In P. Newfield & J. C. Cottrell (Eds.), *Handbook of neuroanesthesia* (3rd ed., pp. 20–33). Philadelphia: Lippincott Williams & Wilkins.
5. Greenberg, M. S. (1997). *Handbook of neurosurgery* (4th ed., pp. 460–465). Lakeland, FL: Greenberg Graphics.
6. Carras, D., Farrell, S. & Todd, M. M. (1999). Neuroanesthesia. In R. G. Grossman & C. M. Loftus (Eds.), *Principles of neurosurgery* (2nd ed., pp. 15–30). Philadelphia: Lippincott-Raven.
7. Pittman, J. & Cottrell, J. E. (1999). Cerebral protection and resuscitation. In P. Newfield & J. C. Cottrell (Eds.). *Handbook of neuroanesthesia* (3rd ed., pp. 53–73). Philadelphia: Lippincott Williams & Wilkins.
8. Gorarten, W., & Van Aken, H. (1999). Induced hypotension. In P. Newfield & J. C. Cottrell (Eds.). *Handbook of neuroanesthesia* (3rd ed., pp. 299–309). Philadelphia: Lippincott Williams & Wilkins.
9. Walker, M. L., Emadian, S. M., & Honeycutt, Jr., J. H. (1999). Diagnosis and management of primary pediatric brain tumors. In R. G. Grossman & C. M. Loftus (Eds.). *Principles of neurosurgery* (2nd ed., pp. 33–46). Philadelphia: Lippincott-Raven.
10. Brain Tumor Society. (2000). Available treatments. http://www.tbts.org/treatment.htm.
11. Somaza, A., Lunsford, L. D., Kondziolka, D., Flickinger, J. C., & Maitz, A. (1999). Gamma knife radiosurgery. In R. G. Grossman & C. M. Loftus (Eds.). *Principles of neurosurgery* (2nd ed., pp. 721–736). Philadelphia: Lippincott-Raven.
12. Andrews, B. T. (1999). General management and intensive care of the neurosurgical patient. In R. G. Grossman & C. M. Loftus (Eds.). *Principles of neurosurgery* (2nd ed., pp. 3–14). Philadelphia: Lippincott-Raven.

13. Greenberg, M. S. (1997). *Handbook of neurosurgery* (4th ed., pp. 271–287). Lakeland, FL: Greenberg Graphics.

14. The EC/IC Bypass Study Group. (1985). Failure of extracranial-intracranial arterial bypass to reduce the risk of ischemic stroke: Results of an international randomized trial. *New England Journal of Medicine, 313*(19), 1191–2000.

15. Biller, J., Feinberg, W. M., Castoldo, J. E., et al. (1998). Guidelines for carotid endarterectomy: A statement for healthcare professionals from a special writing group of the Stroke Council, American Heart Association. *Circulation, 97*, 501–509.

16. DeBakey, M. E. (1975). Successful carotid endarterectomy for cerebrovascular insufficiency. *JAMA, 233*(10), 1083–1085.

17. Clagett, G. P., & Robertson, J. T. (1998). Surgical considerations in symptomatic disease. In H. J. M. Barnett, J. P. Mohr, B. M. Stein, & F. M. Yatsu (Eds.). *Stroke: Pathophysiology, diagnosis, and management* (pp. 1209–1228). New York: Churchill Livingstone.

18. Fields, W. S., Lemak, N. A, Frankowski, R. F., et al. (1978). Controlled trial of aspirin in cerebral ischemia. *Stroke, 9*, 309–319.

19. Shaw, D. A. M., Venables, G. S., Cartlidge, N. E. F., et al. (1984). Carotid endarterectomy in patients with transient cerebral ischemia. *Journal of Neurological Science, 64*(1), 45–53.

20. NINDS. (1991). Clinical alert: Benefit of endarterectomy for patients with high-grade stenosis of the internal carotid artery. *NINDS News Release*, February 27.

21. Steering Committee of NASCET. (1991). North American Symptomatic Carotid Endarterectomy trial: Methods, patients' characteristics and progress. *Stroke, 22*, 711–720.

22. European Carotid Surgery Trialists' Collaborative Group. (1991). MRC European Surgery Trial: Interim results for symptomatic patients with server (70–99%) or with mild (0–29%) carotid stenosis. *Lancet, 337*, 1235–1243.

23. Moore, W. S., Mohr, J. P., Najafi, H., et al. (1992). Carotid endarterectomy: Practice guidelines. Report of the ad hoc Committee to the Joint Council of the Society for Vascular Surgery and the North American Chapter of the International Society of Cardiovascular surgery. *Journal of Vascular Surgery, 15*, 469-479.

24. Moore, W. S., Barnett, H. J., Beebe, H. G., et al. (1995). Guidelines for carotid endarterectomy: A multidisciplinary consensus statement from the Ad Hoc Committee, American Heart Association. *Circulation, 91*, 566–579.

25. Executive Committee for the Asymptomatic Carotid Atherosclerosis Study. (1995). Endarterectomy for asymptomatic carotid artery stenosis. *JAMA, 273*, 1421–1428.

26. Greenberg, M. S. (1997). *Handbook of neurosurgery* (4th ed., pp. 901–926). Lakeland, FL: Greenberg Graphics, Inc.

27. Martin, N. A., Hadley, M. N., Spetzler, R. F., et al. (1986). Management of asymptomatic carotid arteriosclerosis. *Neurosurgery, 18*, 505–512.

28. European Carotid Surgery Trialists' Collaborative Group. (1996). Endarterectomy for moderate symptomatic carotid stenosis: interim results form the MRC European Surgery Trial. *Lancet, 347*, 1591–1593.

29. North American Symptomatic Carotid Endarterectomy Trial Collaborators. (1991). Beneficial effect of carotid endarterectomy in symptomatic patients with high-grade carotid stenosis. *New England Journal of Medicine, 325*, 445–453.

30. Benzel, E. C., & Hoppens, K. D. (1991). Factors associated with postoperative hypertension complicating carotid endarterectomy. *Acta Neurochirurgica (Wien), 112*, 8–12.

31. Fein, J. M. (1985). Carotid endarterectomy. In J. M. Fein & E. S. Flamm (Eds.). *Cerebrovascular surgery* (Vol. 2, pp. 399–427). New York: Springer-Verlag.

32. Zabramski, J. M., Greene, K. A., Marciano, F. F., & Spetzler, R. F. (1994). Carotid endarterectomy. In L. P. Carter, R. F. Spetzler, & M. G. Hamilton (Eds.). *Neurovascular surgery* (pp. 325–357). New York: McGraw-Hill.

33. Bernstein, M., Fleming, J. F. R., & Deck, J. H. N. (1984). Cerebral hyperperfusion after carotid endarterectomy: A cause of cerebral hemorrhage. *Neurosurgery, 15*, 50–56.

34. Piepgras, D. G., Morgan, M. K., Sundt, T. M., Yanagihara, T., & Mussman, L. M. (1988). Intracerebral hemorrhage after carotid endarterectomy. *Journal of Neurosurgery, 68*, 532–536.

35. Nielsen, T. G., Sillesen, H., & Schroeder, T. V. (1995). Seizures following carotid endarterectomy in patients with severely compromised cerebral circulation. *European Journal of Vascular Endovascular Surgery, 9*, 53–57.

36. O'Brien, M. S., & Ricotta, J. J. (1991). Conserving resources after carotid endarterectomy: Selective use of the intensive care unit. *Journal of Vascular Surgery, 14*, 796–800.

37. Bettmann, M. A., Katzen, B. T., Whisnamt, J., et al. (1998). Carotid stenting and angioplasty: A statement for healthcare professionals from the Councils on Cardiovascular Radiology, Stroke, Cardio-Thoracic and Vascular Surgery, Epidemiology and Prevention, and Clinical Cardiology, American Heart Association. *Circulation, 97*, 121–123.

RESOURCES

Professional

Published Material

Greenberg, M. S. (1997). *Handbook of neurosurgery* (4th ed). Lakeland, FL: Greenberg Graphics.

Grossman, R. G., & Loftus, C. M. (Eds.). (1999). *Principles of neurosurgery* (2nd ed.). Philadelphia: Lippincott-Raven.

Ojemann, R. G., Ogilvy, C. G., Crowell, R. M., & Heros, R. C. (1995). *Surgical management of cerebrovascular disease* (3rd ed.). Baltimore: Williams & Wilkins.

Rengachary, S. S., & Wilkins, R. H., (Eds.). (1994). *Principles of neurosurgery*. New York: Wolfe.

Patient and Family

Published Material

StayWell Company. (1999). *Craniotomy: Understanding your care*. San Bruno, CA: Author (Telephone: 1-800-333-3032).

Websites

See website specific to primary problem for surgery.

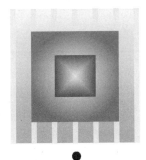

C H A P T E R **16**

Management of the Unconscious Neurological Patient

JOANNE V. HICKEY

Unconsciousness is a physiological state in which the patient is unresponsive to sensory stimuli and lacks awareness of self and the environment. Myriad central nervous system conditions and dysfunction of other body organs can result in unconsciousness. The depth and duration of unconsciousness span a broad spectrum of presentations from fainting, with momentary loss of consciousness, to prolonged coma lasting weeks or months. The term *coma* is reserved for a clinical presentation in which the state of unconsciousness is maintained for a prolonged period, from hours to months. The pathophysiological basis for coma is damage or dysfunction in *both* cerebral hemispheres, the brain stem, or both hemispheres and brain stem. (See Chap. 8 for discussion of coma.) In addition, metabolic disorders can lead to coma by interfering with the normal cellular metabolic environment of neurons.

In neuroscience nursing practice, the nurse often cares for patients who are unconscious for prolonged periods of time. Unconscious patients lack voluntary movement and are bedridden. The physiological consequences of short- and long-term immobilization contribute to poor outcome. Not only does patient survival directly depend on the quality of care provided, but also the realization of optimal rehabilitation potential hinges on the quality of nursing care. In addition to managing the primary neurological problem, the nurse must also incorporate a rehabilitation framework to maintain intact function, prevent complications and disabilities, and restore lost function to the degree possible.

The purpose of this chapter is to provide a basic nursing care framework for the unconscious, neurological patient designed to achieve optimal outcomes and to include specific points of care relative to the management of the neuroscience patient. *Because unconsciousness is caused by many neurological problems, there may be variations in care related to the primary diagnosis.* The basic standard of care for an unconscious patient is outlined in this chapter. (Chart 16-1 gives a sample nursing care plan.)

IMMOBILITY

Kinesis, a word of Greek origin, means motion or to move. The human body is designed for physical activity and movement. Even at rest, the normal healthy adult changes position on average every 11.6 minutes during sleep; this phys-

iological requirement for movement is termed the **minimal physiological mobility requirement.**[1]

Exercise contributes to health, whereas lack of exercise, regardless of reason, leads to a continuum of multisystem deconditioning and anatomical and physiological changes. Bed rest was first recognized as a therapeutic modality in the 1860s. The therapeutic value of bed rest includes decreased oxygen consumption, prevention or reduction of trauma to a body part, and redirection of energy resources toward healing.[2] Immobility has also been described as the most potentially dangerous treatment prescribed today.[3]

Immobility is a *disuse phenomenon* that results in physiological as well as psychosocial effects. The morbidity of immobility is directly associated with the length of time of immobilization and patient-specific risk factors. Some physiological effects occur almost immediately on institution of bed rest, whereas other physiological and pathophysiological changes occur over a longer period of time. Therefore, although there are physiological changes with short periods (e.g., 1–3 days) of immobility, they are less severe and may be reversible. Prolonged periods of immobility, which often occur with coma, spinal cord injury, or Guillain-Barré syndrome, result in pathophysiological changes associated with serious morbidity and permanent disabilities. Risk factors that increase the probability of complications from immobility include length and degree of immobility, incontinence, poor nutrition, hypotension, infection, altered motor or sensory function, multiorgan failure, underweight or obesity, advanced age, and comorbidity. Elderly people are particularly vulnerable to the deleterious effects of immobility resulting from concurrent age-related factors.[4] Immobility and its consequences to each body system are well known. Efforts to prevent the ravages of immobility have resulted in varying degrees of success.

SUPPORT SURFACES AND SPECIALTY BEDS

Various types of support surfaces and specialty beds are used to prevent decubitus ulcers in high-risk patients and other complications of immobility. A wide range of mattress

(text continues on page 349)

CHART 16-1 • Nursing Care Plan for the Unconscious Patient

Nursing Diagnosis/Expected Outcomes	Nursing Interventions
SELF-CARE DEFICIT: R/T IMMOBILITY AND UNCONSCIOUSNESS*	
• Basic self-care needs will be provided by the nursing staff. • Self-care deficit syndrome: Bathing/hygiene Dressing/grooming Feeding Toileting	• Provide basic hygiene care. • Dress and groom patient. • Provide nutritional support by alternate means, as ordered. • Provide for the elimination needs of the patient.
RESPIRATORY FUNCTION	
Risk for Altered Respiratory Function: R/T immobility	
• Adequate respiratory function will be maintained.	• Conduct a risk assessment of respiratory function. • Apply preventive strategies to prevent complications.
Risk for Aspiration	
• Patient will not aspirate.	• Keep NPO until a risk assessment is completed. • Do not feed if airway protection or swallowing is compromised. • Position to facilitate oral drainage. • Follow precautions to prevent enteral feeding aspiration.
Ineffective Airway Clearance: R/T immobility and ineffective cough reflex	
• A patent airway will be maintained. • Drainage of secretions from the oropharynx will be facilitated.	• Keep the neck in a neutral position. • Limit suctioning to 10 seconds or less and one insertion per attempt. • If a tracheostomy tube in place, administer tracheostomy care every 4 hours. • Position in the lateral recumbent position; reposition every 1 to 2 hours. • Elevate the head of the bed 30 degrees, unless contraindicated.
Ineffective Breathing Pattern: R/T immobility and underlying neurological problem(s)	
• An effective breathing pattern will be maintained.	• Monitor the rate, depth, and pattern of respirations frequently. • Monitor tidal volume and blood gas levels. • Observe frequently for signs and symptoms of respiratory distress. • Auscultate the chest frequently. • Elevate the head of the bed 30 degrees unless contraindicated. • Position to facilitate respirations. • For patients maintained on a ventilator, monitor for synchrony with the ventilator; report asynchrony to the physician.
Impaired Gas Exchange: R/T immobility	
• Adequate gas exchange will be facilitated.	• Auscultate the chest every 2 hours for adventitious sounds. • Monitor period blood gases and continue pulse oximetry. • Monitor for cyanosis and respiratory distress. • Turn patient side to side at least every 2 hours. • Provide for periodic chest physiotherapy. • Preoxygenate with 100% oxygen before and after suctioning (with approval of the physician). • Administer oxygen as ordered.

CHART 16-1 • Nursing Care Plan for the Unconscious Patient (Continued)

Nursing Diagnosis/Expected Outcomes	Nursing Interventions
CARDIOVASCULAR FUNCTION	
Cardiac Output, Altered: R/T immobility	
• Cardiac output will be maintained within targeted limits.	• Monitor vital signs frequently. • Monitor the rate, rhythm, and quality of the radial and apical pulses. • Document any arrhythmias. • Observe monitor every 30 minutes–1 hour; maintain alarms at all times.
Altered Peripheral Tissue Perfusion: R/T immobility	
• Adequate peripheral perfusion will be maintained. • Dependent edema will not develop in the arms.	• Apply thigh-high elastic stockings and sequential compression air boots. • When placing patient in the lateral recumbent position, position upper leg so that it does not cause pressure on the lower leg. • Do not use the foot gatch under the patient's knees or place constricting objects to the backs of the knees. • Position so that each joint is higher than the previous joint so that the distal joints are highest. • Monitor for signs of deep vein thrombosis.
Altered Cerebral Tissue Perfusion: R/T immobility	
• Adequate cerebral perfusion pressure will be maintained.	• Maintain patient's head and neck in a neutral position. • Elevate the head of the bed at 30 degrees unless contraindicated. • Avoid positions known to increase intracranial pressure (e.g., hip flexion, prone; see Chapter 14). • If an intracranial pressure monitor is being used, observe monitor periodically for a rise in pressure. • Do not cluster nursing activities; allow pressure fall before beginning another procedure. • Maintain normothermia. • Provide "soft" stimuli (e.g., soft music, family voices).
INTEGUMENTARY SYSTEM	
Risk for Impaired Skin Integrity: R/T immobility	
• Skin will remain intact.	• Provide skin care frequently (daily baths; mouth, back, and perineal care). • Lubricate dry lips with balm and skin with cream or lanolin. • Monitor skin for redness and decubitus ulcers frequently. • Do not position patient on reddened areas of skin. • Provide clean tape for securing of nasogastric or endotracheal tube daily, wash the skin, and do not apply new tape in the same place. • Keep the heels off the bed at all times. • Cut and file fingernails and toenails. • Turn and reposition at least every 2 hours.
Risk for Impaired Tissue Integrity (corneal): R/T immobility	
• The eye will be maintained infection and injury free.	• Inspect the eyes for signs of irritation and cleanse them every 4 hours. • Position patient to protect the eyes; apply shield or tape eyelids as ordered. • Instill methylcellulose drops, as ordered.

(continued)

CHART 16-1 • Nursing Care Plan for the Unconscious Patient (Continued)

Nursing Diagnosis/Expected Outcomes	Nursing Interventions
Altered Oral Mucous Membrane: R/T dryness, decreased saliva	
• The oral mucosa will remain intact and free of dryness, lesions, and exudate.	• Provide oral hygiene frequently. • Brush patient's teeth once every shift. • Monitor patient's mouth for lesions, dryness, or bleeding.
MUSCULOSKELETAL FUNCTION	
Impaired Physical Mobility: R/T immobility and underlying neurological problem(s) causing paresis, paralysis, or rigidity	
• Intact function will be maintained and deformities/contractures prevented.	• Administer passive range-of-motion exercises at least four times daily. • Position in proper body alignment; reposition every 2 hours. Use trochanter roll, splints, slings, pillows, foot positioners/athletic shoes, as needed. • Reposition decorticate or decerebrate patients every hour; control noxious stimuli that may affect abnormal positioning. • Collaborate with the physical therapist.
Risk for Trauma: Stress fracture and joint dislocation	
• No stress fractures or joint dislocations will occur.	• Administer passive range-of-motion exercises at least four times daily. • Position in proper body alignment. • Provide rolls and pillows to maintain desired position. • Do not pull or tug on joints.
Altered Urinary Elimination: R/T immobility: incontinence, retention, or large residual urine	
• Adequate urinary elimination will be maintained.	• Monitor intake and output. • Remove the catheter as soon as possible. • Consider an intermittent catheterization program. • Provide perineal care. • Palpate the bladder to check for distention.
Risk for Infection: R/T immobility: urinary tract infection	
• Factors contributing to infection will be controlled.	• Follow strict aseptic technique in the care of the patient's catheter. • Remove the catheter as soon as possible. • Monitor urinalysis and urine culture and sensitivity as appropriate. • Monitor urinary output for signs and symptoms of infection.
GASTROINTESTINAL FUNCTION	
Altered Bowel Elimination: R/T immobility	
• Stool will be soft and formed. • The bowel will be evacuated every 1–3 days.	• Monitor and record character and frequency of bowel movements. • Auscultate abdomen for bowel sounds. • Initiate a bowel program.
NEUROLOGICAL FUNCTION	
Hyperthermia: R/T underlying neurological problem(s) or infection	
• Normothermia will be achieved and maintained.	• Monitor patient's temperature periodically. • If temperature elevated, remove excess clothing and top linen; provide a sponge bath, as necessary. • Consider the underlying reasons for hyperthermia; implement appropriate interventions. • Administer antipyretics and other cooling interventions (e.g., cooling blanket) as indicated.

CHART 16 – 1 • Nursing Care Plan for the Unconscious Patient (Continued)

Nursing Diagnosis/Expected Outcomes	Nursing Interventions
Sensory/Perceptual Alterations: R/T unconsciousness	
• Multisensory stimuli will be provided throughout the day.	• Provide sensory stimuli by talking to the patient; describe surroundings, treatments, etc. • Stimulate as many senses as possible. • Turn on the radio, TV, or tape recorder when no one is with the patient. • Encourage family to touch and talk to the patient. • After patient begins to awaken, use orientation instruments, such as a clock, calendar, window, favorite objects, or family pictures.
NUTRITION AND HYDRATION	
Altered Nutrition: Less than Body Requirements: R/T unconsciousness	
• Adequate nutrition will be provided. • An appropriate weight level will be maintained.	• Monitor the patient's weight at least twice weekly. • Request a nutritional consultation. • Collaborate with the clinical dietician for a nutrition consultation and orders. • Maintain an accurate intake and output record; include a daily calorie count.
Fluid Volume Deficit: R/T unconsciousness	
• Adequate fluid volume will be maintained.	• Maintain accurate intake and output record. • Monitor skin turgor and mucous membranes for dryness. • Monitor vital signs, specific gravity of urine, and serum osmolarity values. • Provide hydration as ordered.

overlays and mattresses are available, and each manufacturer offers special features that may be of particular value to patients depending on their individual needs. On admission, a risk assessment for pressure ulcers is conducted, most often using the Braden Scale. Based on this score, there are usually wound-care protocols and algorithms that guide surface or bed selection as well as other treatment. Risk assessment using the Braden Scale is conducted periodically to determine changes in risk or treatment needs. The cost effectiveness of ordering a special bed must be considered. Managed care plans and heath care facilities have established criteria for identifying high-risk patients for whom special beds will be helpful and cost effective. Institutional guidelines should be followed in the selection and use of such beds.

THE CONSEQUENCES OF IMMOBILITY: NURSING MANAGEMENT OF THE UNCONSCIOUS PATIENT

Meticulous nursing care has a direct impact on patient outcomes. Clinical reasoning, based on a systematic ongoing assessment of all body systems, alerts the nurse to evidence of complications. The nurse should implement preventive strategies as well as treatment protocols related to optimal outcomes. Ongoing assessment is the basis for identifying collaborative problems and nursing diagnoses. Several *collaborative problems* that are common to most unconscious patients are listed in Chart 16-2. Because the patient is immobilized and multiple body systems are threatened, the *nursing diagnoses* of **Disuse Syndrome** encompassing all systems and **Total Self-Care Deficit Syndrome** addressing the total dependency are prominent for the nurse to provide care. The remaining content of this chapter is organized according to body systems and related treatment implications.

Respiratory Function

Assuming the supine position causes physiological changes in the mechanics of breathing and in lung volumes. Mechanical restriction results from decreased overall respiratory muscle strength and from reduced intercostal, diaphragmatic, and abdominal muscle excursion with a consequent decrease in thoracic volume. Normally, tidal breathing in the upright position predominantly results from rib cage movement, whereas in the supine position, abdominal muscles predominate. Maximal in-

CHART 16-2 • Common Collaborative Problems for the Unconscious Patient

- Atelectasis/pneumonia (aspiration, bacterial pneumonia)
- Deep vein thrombosis/pulmonary embolism
- Ventilator dependency
- Tracheal necrosis
- Anemia
- Pressure ulcers (decubitus ulcers)
- Acute urinary retention
- Paralytic ileus
- Gastric ulcer
- Electrolyte imbalance
- Negative nitrogen balance
- Peripheral nerve impairment/neuropathies
- Corneal ulceration
- Stress fractures
- Osteoporosis
- Joint dislocation

spiration capacity is decreased, resulting in decreased vital and functional respiratory capacities.[5]

All lung volumes decrease except for tidal volume. The decrease in thoracic size and increase in intrathoracic blood volume associated with the supine position cause a decrease in residual volume and functional residual capacity (FRC).[2] Normally, FRC exceeds closing volume through maintaining an open airway. When the FRC is exceeded by the closing volume, the partial or complete collapse of lung units causes atelectasis, regional differences in ventilation-perfusion ratio (V/Q mismatch), poorly ventilated and overly perfused areas, and arteriovenous shunts. If increased metabolic demands occur, hypoxia results.[6] In addition, impaired mucociliary function causes mucous secretions to accumulate in the dependent respiratory bronchiole, which contributes to the development of atelectasis and hypostatic pneumonia.

Assessment

Respiratory function is assessed using a number of parameters: airway patency; rate, quality, and pattern of respirations; chest auscultation; and objective signs of oxygenation (pulse oximetry). The highest priority in managing a patient is assigned to **airway patency**, which is the openness of the upper airway (nose, mouth, pharynx, and trachea, bronchi) that provides the route for air exchange. Obstruction of the airway may be caused by injury, edema, mucus, or other drainage. Airway patency is assessed frequently.

Clinical evidence of an ineffective breathing pattern includes apnea, dyspnea, shortness of breath, stridor, rapid or shallow respirations, a prolonged expiration or inspiration phase, nasal flaring, pursed lips, intercostal or substernal retraction, abdominal breathing, and altered chest expansion.

Assess and monitor the following:

- Airway patency
- Rate, quality, and pattern of respirations
- Adventitious breath sounds by chest auscultation
- Correlation of findings of recent chest radiograph with clinical findings
- Amount and characteristics of airway secretions (for infection)
- Capillary refill and subtle cyanosis or dustiness in periorbital area, ear lobes, and fingernails
- Oxygen saturation with pulse oximetry
- Periodic blood gases
- Lung volumes and respiratory mechanics

Respiratory Problems

The unconscious patient is at high risk for developing respiratory problems. The secondary effect of compromised respiratory function is cerebral hypoxia, which leads to secondary brain injury unless the early signs and symptoms of respiratory insufficiency are recognized and interventions initiated expeditiously. Respiratory problems to be considered include airway obstruction, aspiration, atelectasis, and pneumonia. Other conditions seen in relation to trauma and intracranial hemorrhage are neurogenic pulmonary edema, adult respiratory distress syndrome, and disseminated intravascular coagulation; these conditions are discussed in other chapters.

Airway Obstruction. In the unconscious patient, a partially or completely obstructed airway can occur because of mucus accumulation or plugging by other foreign materials or through posterior displacement of oropharyngeal soft-tissue structures, particularly the tongue, as a result of improper positioning of the head and neck.[7] A comatose patient is unable to reposition his or her head and neck to maintain airway patency. Other mechanical deficits that affect respiratory structures include postanesthesia recovery, airway edema following extubation, and diaphragmatic or intercostal muscle paralysis related to spinal cord injury or neuromuscular diseases. Results of partial airway obstruction include alveolar hypoventilation, hypoxia, hypercarbia, increased respiratory rate, and atelectasis. The early signs and symptoms observed are shallow and noisy respirations, increased secretions, and restlessness.

Aspiration. The unconscious patient is unable to protect the airway and therefore is at high risk for aspiration. Regurgitation and microaspiration, rather than actual vomiting of gastric contents, may occur, resulting in a chemical pneumonitis. Aspiration of tube feedings from a dislodged feeding tube or vomiting from a distended stomach can also lead to aspiration pneumonia.

Atelectasis and Pneumonia. Atelectasis, a state of alveolar collapse in a segment or lobe, has long been known to be a consequence of prolonged bed rest and immobility. The concurrent stasis and pooling of secretions collected in the dependent position leads to hypostatic pneumonia and a medium ripe for bacterial growth. If the patient is dehydrated or receiving drugs that affect the tenacity of the secretions, bacteria can rapidly develop. In addition, patients are at high risk for nosocomial infections as a result of a compromised immunological state and potential for colonization of the endotracheal tube.

Common related nursing diagnoses include Ineffective Airway Clearance, Risk for Aspiration, Ineffective Breathing Pattern, Impaired Gas Exchange, Risk for Altered Respiratory Function, Dysfunctional Ventilatory Weaning Response, and Risk for Infection.

Nursing Interventions

Nursing interventions are aimed at maintaining a patent airway and facilitating adequate respirations.

Airway Patency. A patent airway is the highest priority. The unconscious patient is defenseless against threats to a patent airway, particularly if the cough reflex is absent. In these patients and in conscious patients who do not have an intact cough reflex and are therefore at high risk for aspiration, suctioning will be necessary (see below). If there is evidence of inability to protect the airway, the physician may insert an endotracheal tube on an emergency basis to prevent aspiration and the risk of aspiration-related infection. If unconsciousness is prolonged and the patient continues to need an artificial airway, a tracheotomy tube will be needed.

Positioning. The lateral recumbent position promotes drainage of secretions, facilitates respirations, prevents pooling of secretions, and prevents the tongue from obstructing the airway. Turn the patient from side to side every 2 hours to prevent pooling of secretions. Unconscious patients are cautiously positioned on their backs because of the risk of soft-tissue obstruction of the airway and the threat of aspiration. Unless contraindicated, the head should be elevated and turned to the side to facilitate drainage of secretions when lying in bed.

Suctioning. Periodic oropharyngeal or tracheal suctioning may be necessary to clear the airway of mucus, blood, or other drainage. Do not suction nasally if there is any possibility of a basal skull fracture or cerebrospinal fluid drainage from the nose or ear. With increased intracranial pressure (ICP), suctioning is limited to 10 seconds or less and cather insertion is limited to only two times to prevent hypoxia. The lungs are oxygenated (using an Ambu bag) with 100% oxygen with a few breaths before and after suctioning to control hypoxemia. (A patient with chronic obstructive lung disease should not receive 100% oxygen; a lower concentration must be used.) Suction equipment is checked at the beginning of every shift and maintained in a ready state for immediate use.

Other. A consultation with the respiratory therapist is helpful. Chest physical therapy may be recommended. Chest physical therapy consists of percussion and vibration, oropharyngeal stimulation of coughing, suctioning, and possible use of bronchodilators or mucolytic agents to facilitate movement of secretions. Managing a patient on a ventilator and ventilator weaning are discussed in Chapter 17.

Cardiovascular Function

Physiological changes in cardiovascular function associated with immobility include increased cardiac workload and heart rate, decreased cardiac output, decreased stroke volume, increased peripheral vascular resistance, and decreased blood pressure.

Cardiac workload is affected by Valsalva's maneuver. **Valsalva's maneuver** is defined as a forced expiration against a closed epiglottis. Physiological alterations include a period of thoracic fixation without expiration, which elevates intrathoracic pressure, thereby impeding venous blood from entering the large veins. When the patient exhales, there is a significant decrease in intrathoracic pressure, and a surge of blood is injected into the heart, thus increasing the workload of the heart. Neuroscience nurses are well aware of the effect of ICP spikes that result from Valsalva's maneuver. Spikes are potentially dangerous to patients with already elevated ICP.

Assessment

Assessment of cardiovascular function in the unconscious patient includes:

- Rate, rhythm, and quality of the apical and radial pulses
- Chest auscultation of heart sounds
- Blood pressure, including ranges of systolic and diastolic over time
- Evidence of orthostatic hypotension with head elevation
- Periodic review of electrolytes to maintain normal ranges
- Complete blood count, including hematocrit and hemoglobin
- Other hemodynamic parameters, such as cardiac output, peripheral vascular resistance, and pulmonary artery wedge pressure, if centrally monitored

Cardiovascular Problems

Various cardiovascular problems result from cardiac deconditioning, deep vein thrombosis, pulmonary emboli, and orthostatic hypotension. Deconditioning of the cardiovascular system occurs within days; fluid shift, fluid loss, decreased cardiac output, decreased peak oxygen uptake, and increased resting heart rate result.[8]

Cardiac Deconditioning. Central fluid shifts occur with immobilization from the upright to supine position. The physiological effect is an 11% total blood volume shift from the legs to other parts or the body, of which 80% moves to the thorax and 20% to the head.[9] The result is an increased central venous pressure (CVP), left ventricular end-diastolic pressure, and stroke volume. In a patient with increased ICP, elevation of the head to 30 degrees is directed at decreasing the impact of fluid shift and increased CVP. In response to the supine position, volume receptors are stimulated and diuresis occurs. As a result there is a reduction of plasma volume, total blood volume, and end-diastolic filling pressures and volumes; this is independent of total fluid intake.[2] With prolonged bed rest, there is an initial decrease in interstitial volume, although plasma volume remains low.[9]

Alterations in blood pressure and pulse may be the result of cardiac reconditioning or may be related to the primary neurological problem. A brief discussion is included here for the nurse to consider when evaluating the patient. Hypotension or hypertension should be viewed in relation to the patient's pulse rate, pulse quality, and pulse pressure.

- **Hypotension and pulse variations.** Hypotension is rarely attributable to brain injury. In these rare instances, hypotension is associated with severe cerebral injury and occurs only as a terminal event. The concurrent findings of hypotension and tachycardia should raise suspicion of occult internal hemorrhage (intra-abdominal, intrathoracic, pelvic, or long bone injury) or hypovolemic shock. Other signs of hypovolemic shock include restlessness, ashen skin color, cold and clammy skin, and a rapid, thready pulse. The combination of hypotension and bradycardia may be secondary to cervical spinal cord injury because of interruption of descending sympathetic pathways. Hypotension and tachycardia can also be a hemodynamic response to prolonged bed rest.
- **Hypertension and pulse variations.** Hypertension may occur with increases in intracranial pressure related to various problems, such as hypertensive stroke or subarachnoid hemorrhage. The combination of an elevated blood pressure, widening pulse pressure, and bradycardia is called Cushing's response (see Chap. 8). Hypertension may also be attributable to preexisting hypertension or pain. Drug therapy may be instituted to control and maintain the blood pressure within a target range. These parameters may be set in a hypertensive range to maintain cerebral perfusion pressure if increased intracranial pressure is present.

Deep Vein Thrombosis or Pulmonary Emboli. Immobilization is a risk factor for the formation of a deep venous thrombus with the potential for pulmonary emboli. Thrombus formation is caused by venous stasis, decreased vasomotor tone, pressure on the blood vessels, and hypercoagulable state. Several factors put the patient at higher risk for the development of thrombi:

- Muscle contraction of the legs ordinarily promotes venous return to the heart, but in the case of the immobilized unconscious patient, the blood pools and venous stasis results.
- Hypercoagulability is a common finding. Immobility is often associated with dehydration and resulting hemoconcentration. Dehydration and a state of hypercoagulability, common in these patients, contribute to venous thrombosis.[10] In addition, increased serum calcium contributes to hypercoagulation. (Calcium is liberated from the bones of any non—weight-bearing person.)
- Prolonged external pressure leads to intimal layer injury of blood vessels. Platelets collect at the injured intimal site, forming a layer that can become the foundation for clot formation. External pressure can result from pillow placement under the knees, from the upper leg resting on the lower leg in the lateral recumbent position, and from continual resting of the heels on the bed.

Orthostatic Hypotension. The third major effect of immobility on cardiovascular function is **orthostatic hypotension**, which is the inability of the autonomic nervous system to maintain an adequate blood supply to the upper regions of the body when the patient is placed upright in bed. In the immobilized patient, orthostatic hypotension is attributable to a loss of general motor tone and decreased efficiency of the orthostatic neurovascular reflexes (which normally cause contraction of the blood vessels so that blood can flow upward against gravity). Common related nursing diagnoses include Decreased Cardiac Output, Peripheral Neurovascular Dysfunction, Altered Peripheral Tissue Perfusion, Altered Cerebral Tissue Perfusion, and Activity Intolerance.

Interventions

Appropriate nursing interventions and nursing management designed to support cardiovascular function in the unconscious immobilized patient include the following:

- Turn and reposition the patient frequently, usually every 2 hours.
- When positioning the patient in the lateral recumbent position, position the upper leg to prevent pressure on the lower leg. Use a pillow to separate the legs.
- Apply thigh-high elastic stockings and sequential compression air boots to improve blood return to the heart and minimize venous stasis.
- Monitor the patient for signs and symptoms of deep vein thrombosis or thrombophlebitis.
- Sit the patient in a chair, if at all possible; this alters intravascular pressure and stimulates the orthostatic neurovascular reflexes.
- Review the hemodynamic profile and trends over time.
- Maintain blood pressure within targeted range.

The Skin and Related Structures

The skin is an important barrier to infection; it assists in heat regulation through sweating in the heat and piloerection in the cold and cushions bony prominences. Sustained pressure from immobilization is the most important cause of skin breakdown. Pressure transmitted to the skin, subcutaneous tissue, and muscles, particularly over bony prominences, can result in ischemia and necrosis. Shearing forces and friction related to moving patients can cause direct injury to the skin that results in pressure ulcers. In addition, incontinence, profuse perspiration, poor nutrition, and obesity are factors related to pressure ulcer development. Immobilized unconscious patients are at high risk for developing pressure ulcers.

Assessment

The skin and related structures (hair, fingernails, toenails, scalp, hair, eyes, and oral cavity) should be assessed according to the following guidelines:

SKIN
- Identify all risk factors present for skin breakdown. Use the *Clinical Practice Guideline, Pressure Ulcers in Adults: Prediction and Prevention for Assessment and Management of Patients.*[11]

- Assess the skin using the Braden Scale or Norton Scale.
- Assess the skin for color, temperature, dryness, redness, abrasions, and pressure ulcers.
- Every square inch of skin should be observed every shift (many areas are observed more frequently).
- Bony prominences, such as the elbows, iliac crest, or outer aspect of the ankle, can become irritated and red; assess all bony prominences for redness, irritated, or broken tissue.
- Do not position the patient on an area with reddened or broken skin.
- Assess fingernails and toenails for length and cleanliness.
- Assess the nose for signs of skin breakdown resulting from irritation caused by a nasogastric tube.

OTHER
- Assess the mucous membranes of the oral cavity for dryness, irritation, signs of oral infections (yeast and others), and broken areas; the tongue may be coated.
- Assess eyes for edema, redness, and drainage.
- Assess scalp and hair for reddened areas (especially at occiput), abrasions, and pediculosis.

Abnormal findings may include redness of the skin, broken skin, pressure ulcers, dry lips and oral cavity, cracked lips, oral infection, eye infection, dryness of the eye, inability to close the eye, matted hair, pediculosis, long fingernails that cut into the palms of hand, and long toenails that scratch the skin. Common related nursing diagnoses include Risk for Impaired Skin Integrity, Altered Oral Mucous Membrane, Risk for Infection, and Risk for Impaired Tissue Integrity (Corneal).

Nursing Interventions

Evidence-based practice guidelines are available to predict, prevent, and treat pressure ulcers. These are outlined in the *Clinical Practice Guideline, Pressure Ulcers in Adults: Prediction and Prevention*.[11] This resource is the standard to which all nurses are held when providing care. Refer to it for the specifics of care.

The following section lists additional points for nursing care.

SKIN CARE
- Keep the skin clean and dry; provide frequent skin care.
- Male patients should be shaved daily. If the patient is receiving anticoagulation therapy, an electric razor should be used.
- Trophic skin changes, such as dryness, can occur with some neurological conditions; lubricate the skin with lotion to prevent skin breakdown.
- Provide frequent skin care.
- Turn and reposition the patient every 2 hours; be sure the heels are off the bed and other vulnerable areas are positioned and protected to prevent pressure.
- When moving the patient, turn and lift rather than pull, which results in shearing and friction on skin.
- Consider using a special bed to prevent skin breakdown in high-risk patients.

- Retape and reposition the nasogastric tube daily to prevent traction on the tube.

MOUTH CARE
- Cleanse and lubricate the mouth, gingiva, and tongue frequently (e.g., q4h) to prevent dryness, oral infections, and gum disease.
- Brush the teeth three to four times daily with the aid of a suction catheter.
- Lubricate the lips to prevent dryness and cracking.

EYE CARE
- Inspect eyes for signs of edema, ecchymosis, eye drainage, irritation, or abrasions.
- Cleanse eyes to remove exudate with cotton balls and saline; the eyes should then be lubricated with methylcellulose or normal saline drops four times daily. The unconscious patient cannot blink periodically to cleanse and lubricate the eyes. Corneal drying or injury to the eye can lead to corneal ulceration and blindness. Many physicians order taping of the eyelids to reduce corneal abrasions. Application of an eye patch or eye shield may be helpful to protect the eye from injury.

SCALP AND HAIR CARE
The scalp and hair require attention:

- Examine the scalp for abrasions, pressure ulcers (especially in the occiput region), and edema. Treat any bruised or broken area.
- Patients with head trauma may have hair that is matted with blood, dirt, or glass; remove by combing and washing the hair, if not contraindicated, according to hospital procedure.
- Comb the hair; long hair can be braided or pulled to the side with an elastic band.

FINGERNAILS AND TOENAILS
An unconscious patient may clench the fists, thereby digging the nails into the hands and causing injury. File and clip fingernails and toenails to protect the patient from injury

Musculoskeletal Function

Immobility has a profound effect on the musculoskeletal system, including decreased muscle strength, shortening of muscles, increased muscle weakness and atrophy, contractures, and osteoporosis. At the cellular level, intracellular adenosine triphosphate (ATP) and glycogen concentrations decrease, rates of protein degradation increase, and contractility declines.[8]

- **Decreased muscle strength:** The degree of loss varies with the particular muscle groups and the degree of immobility. The antigravitational muscles of the legs lose strength twice as fast as the arm muscles, and recovery is longer.
- **Muscle atrophy:** Muscle atrophy means loss of muscle mass. When a muscle is relaxed, it atrophies about twice as fast as one held in a stretched position. Because increased muscle tone prevents complete atrophy, patients

with upper motor neuron disease and spastic paralysis lose less muscle mass. In contrast, with lower motor neuron disease and flaccid paralysis, muscle bulk lost is much more rapid. Muscle fibers are replaced by connective tissue with disuse.

- **Contractures:** A contracture is a loss of full range of motion, usually of a joint. When a muscle is maintained in a relaxed, shortened position for even 5 to 7 days, the muscle shortens. Prolonged immobility results in loss of muscle mass. Joints change to dense connective tissue characteristic of a contracture.
- **Osteoporosis:** Weight bearing and movement are critical to maintain bone formation and calcium balance. Immobilization results in significant bone loss. Hypercalcemia and hypercalciuria, which reflect loss of total body calcium, occur with bed rest. The high level of calcium in the urinary tract contributes to urinary calculus formation. Osteoporosis predisposes the patient to vertebral compression, long bone, and hip fractures.

Assessment

The muscles of the upper and lower extremities, neck, and shoulders should be assessed for tone, bulk, and range of motion, and both sides of the body should be compared

Musculoskeletal Problems

Abnormal findings include decreased muscle tone (flaccidity, paresis, paralysis), increased muscle tone (rigidity, decortication, decerebration, tremors), muscle atrophy, contractures, ankylosis, and joint dislocation. Common related nursing diagnoses include Impaired Physical Mobility and Risk for Trauma (e.g., contractures, stress fractures, and joint dislocation).

Nursing Interventions

The following nursing interventions are useful for preserving musculoskeletal function in the unconscious patient:

- Position the patient in a neutral side-lying position in body alignment using pillows, rolls, and other equipment (e.g., positioning boots, splints, and trochanter rolls) as needed (see Chap. 13).
- Although the side-lying position is most often used, the dorsal position with the patient lying on his or her back is also useful. The same principles apply for alignment.
  - The head is in neutral position aligned with the spine.
  - The arms are slightly flexed at the elbows with the hands resting at the sides on pillows with the fingers extended over the pillows.
  - The hips are aligned with the head. Place a pillow between the legs to prevent internal rotation, adduction, and inversion of the upper leg.
  - The knees are extended in slight flexion, often supported by a pillow for each leg. Care must be taken to prevent pressure on the peroneal nerve at the fibula head.
  - The feet should be flexed at the ankles with the feet close to parallel with the wall. The heels should be elevated to prevent pressure and potential decubitus

ulcer formation on the heels. Athletic shoes or positioning boots are useful to maintain the position of the feet.

- Variations in positioning are noted for *flaccid paralysis* and *extensor posturing* (decortication or decerebration).
  - **Flaccid paralysis:** Positioning boots, splints to prevent a contracture, and trochanter towel rolls to prevent entrapment neuropathy of the peroneal nerve. Avoid compression at the elbows to prevent injury to the ulnar nerve.[12]
  - **Extensor posturing:** These patients are difficult to position because of the rigidity, and splints are not useful. Application of athletic shoe assist in proper positioning of the feet.
- Points of positioning vary for *hemiplegia*. Whether on the back or side-lying position, align the head, neck, and spine in neutral position.
- In the side-lying position, position the patient on the unaffected side. The affected arm is slightly flexed, on a pillow that extends just below the axillary region. The pillow placement counteracts arm and shoulder adduction and internal rotation.
  - To prevent dependent edema, position each joint higher than the preceding joint, moving from the proximal to the terminal joints.
  - Flex the lower leg and place a pillow between the legs to align the legs properly.
  - For patients with a hemi-neglect syndrome, positioning the patient facing toward the affected side is useful.
  - Use a trochanter roll to prevent external rotation of the hip.
- In the dorsal position, lying on the back, use the pillow, as already described, to position the arms, hips, and legs.
- Reposition in proper body alignment every 2 hours or more frequently if reddened areas are present. Do not position the patient on reddened areas.
- If splints are used, take them off periodically and monitor skin for redness or breakdown.
- Administer passive range-of-motion exercises every 4 hours.
- Involve physical therapy in the plan of care immediately and collaborate with them on the care. (An order is usually written for a physical therapy consultation with admission orders.)

Genitourinary Function

Assuming the supine position with immobility results in urinary stasis in the renal pelvis and urinary bladder, which provides a medium for bacterial growth. In addition, urinary retention and bladder distention are common. An unconscious patient will be incontinent because of an altered level of consciousness and the effects of the supine position.

The unconscious patient is at risk for two major problems: urinary tract infections and kidney and bladder stones (calculi). The causes of infection are the indwelling catheter and the stasis of urine. The stasis of urine in the bladder promotes bladder infections and ascending infections, which can involve the kidneys. The stasis of urine in the renal pelvis and bladder encourages formation of calculi. The increased levels of calcium being excreted from demineralized bones, another effect of immobilization, result in hypercalciuria and contribute to the formation of urinary calculi. In addition, acute renal failure can develop.

Assessment

- Monitor 24-hour intake and output record.
- Identify the characteristics of the urine (e.g., color, cloudiness).
- Monitor urinalysis, urine cultures, creatinine, and blood urea nitrogen.

Common related nursing diagnoses include Altered Urinary Elimination, Incontinence, and Risk for Infection.

Nursing Interventions

In an unconscious patient, methods of managing urine must be considered. On admission, an indwelling catheter is usually inserted. This may be necessary to monitor fractional urinary output for patients receiving diuretic therapy (e.g., mannitol), those with diabetes insipidus, or other patients in whom careful and frequent monitoring of output is necessary. Another reason for catheter insertion is to keep the patient dry to prevent skin breakdown. The catheter itself is a foreign body and thus an irritant to the urinary tract. The literature supports a direct relationship between urinary catheters and urinary tract infection. There are some special considerations when weighing the benefits and risks of inserting and maintaining an indwelling catheter.

- If an indwelling catheter is necessary temporarily, remove it as soon as possible.
- For the male patient, a condom catheter is a possible choice.
- An alternative to continuous urinary drainage is an intermittent catheterization program, useful in both genders.
- For some patients, absorbent incontinence pads that are changed frequently may be chosen to avoid the risk of infection from a catheter.
- Consider the condition of the skin. If areas of skin breakdown already exist, being wet for even a short time could increase that breakdown. (See Chap. 13 for further discussion, which includes *Urinary Incontinence in Adults, Clinical Practice Guideline.*[13])
- The indwelling catheter should be removed as early as possible.

Gastrointestinal Function

Gastric ulcers, gastrointestinal bleeding, constipation, and fecal impaction are common in immobilized and unconscious patients. Gastric irritation can develop from drug therapy or hypersympathetic activity related to the primary neurological problems. Normal stimulants to peristalsis, such as physical activity and a high-fiber diet, are absent. Nutrition is commonly provided by enteral tube feeding, which does not generally stimulate peristalsis.

Some components of the therapeutic plan, such as drugs, contribute to constipation. Loose stools or diarrhea are also common in the unconscious immobilized patient, most often in response to poorly tolerated enteral feeding or drugs, especially antibiotics.

Assessment

- Auscultate the abdomen for bowel sounds.
- Note and record the consistency, color, size, and frequency of stools.
- Review the intake and output record and 24-hour balance for the last several days to determine the hydration status of the patient.
- Review the medication sheet to identify drugs that can affect peristalsis and bowel evacuation.
- Ascertain the amount of fiber in the tube feeding.
- Test each stool for occult blood.
- If possible, monitor gastric aspiration for occult blood.

Gastrointestinal Problems

Abnormal findings may include a distended abdomen with decreased or absent bowel sounds, paralytic ileus, hyperactive bowel sounds, or positive hemo-occult gastric aspirant or stools. Common related nursing diagnoses include Bowel Incontinence, Diarrhea (related to intolerance of tube feeding or effects of drugs), and Colonic Constipation.

Nursing Interventions

A hospital-approved bowel program (e.g., stool softeners, bulk former, mild laxatives) should be instituted and followed. These drugs can be given through a feeding tube, gastrostomy, or jejunostomy tube. (See Chap. 13 for a sample protocol.) If constipation is a problem, a few points should be kept in mind.

- Constipation increases intra-abdominal pressure, which in turn increases intracranial pressure.
- A drug to stimulate peristalsis may be added, such as metoclopramide (Reglan).
- In the case of diarrhea, the following should be kept in mind:
  - Review the type and rate of enteral feeding ordered; feeding intolerance, especially to lactose, may be present.
  - Consult with the clinical dietitian to determine dietary options (e.g., change the feeding to one of increased bulk or slow the rate of administration).
- Concurrent drug therapy, especially antibiotics, can cause diarrhea. Discuss discontinuing a highly suspected drug or changing it to another drug.
- Consider adjusting the dosage and frequency of the drug.
- Add drug therapy to decrease peristalsis and control diarrhea.

Gastric aspirations and stool should be monitored for occult blood. This is necessary because gastrointestinal bleeding in the neurological patient is common, especially if a head injury or intracranial insult has occurred. A gastric ulcer associated with neurological problems is called Cushing's ulcer. Another risk factor for gastrointestinal bleeding is concurrent drug therapy, such as dexamethasone, which is irritating to the gastrointestinal tract.

Nosocomial Infections

Unconsciousness is related to high risk for infection for several reasons. Serious illnesses, often involving multiple body systems, challenge the body's immune system. Invasive procedures (e.g., surgery) and invasive equipment (e.g., central lines and urinary catheters) can lead to infection. Moreover, the use of antibiotics may result in opportunistic infections. Follow Centers for Disease Control and Prevention (CDC) standards for body substance isolation. Body substance isolation means that gloves should be worn for anticipated contact with blood, secretions, and any moist body substances. Gloves are re-

moved and properly disposed of between procedures and patients. When it is anticipated that contact with a patient could result in splashing of clothing, the skin, or face of the care giver with secretions, blood, or body fluids, protective gear that includes gloves, a plastic apron, a mask, and goggles is worn. Proper disposal of contaminated material will isolate infectious material. The most effective method to prevent spread of infectious agents continues to be hand washing. Follow CDC guidelines for hand washing. Table 16-1 lists major causes of infections.

Other Considerations

A nutrition consultation within the first 24 hours is necessary. See Chapter 9 for discussion of nutrition. Promote comfort and rest. Analgesics and sedatives are useful for restless patients. Create an environment that supports rest with decreased stimuli, especially at night. In intensive care

---

▊▊▊ **T a b l e   1 6 – 1** • CAUSES AND PREVENTION OF COMMON NOSOCOMIAL INFECTIONS

TYPE OF INFECTIONS	PREDISPOSING FACTORS	COMMON CAUSATIVE ORGANISMS*	PREVENTIVE MEASURES
Urinary tract infections	Indwelling catheters Straight catheterization	Gram-negative bacilli such as *Escherichia coli, Proteus mirabili, Enterococci faecali,* and *yeast;* in patients who had received an earlier course of antibiotic therapy *Pseudomonas aeruginosa, Serratia marcescens,* or *Enterobacter species* may be the causative organism.[†]	• Maintain a sterile closed urinary drainage system; no breaks in system when collecting urine samples. • Maintain dependent drainage. • Remove indwelling catheter as soon as possible. • Provide perineal care. • Prevent cross-contamination by strict adherence to handwashing protocol and wearing of gloves.
Respiratory infections (pneumonia)	Ventilatory assistance devices Dehydration Presence of tracheostomy or endotracheal tube Microaspiration	*Pseudomonas aeruginosa, Acinetobacter, Staphylococcus aureus, Haemophilus influenzae, Pneumococcus, Aspergillus* (chronic obstructive pulmonary disease patients with steroid use), multidrug-resistant *S. aureus, Legionella,* anaerobes (aspiration)	• Change ventilation equipment according to hospital policy. • Follow aseptic suctioning procedure. • Administer tracheostomy care every 4 hours. • Adhere to strict handwashing technique and principles of aseptic technique.
Vascular infections	Intravenous, arterial, and central catheters (phlebitis is the most common catheter-related infection) Hyperalimentation	Coagulase-negative *Staphylococci (Staphylococcus epidermidis* most common followed by *S. aureus, Enterococci, P. aeruginosa, Candida* organisms, *Enterobacter* organisms, *Acinetobacter* organisms, and *Serratia* organisms[†]	• Change tubing according to hospital policy. • Inspect wound site for evidence of redness or infection. • Follow strict aseptic technique on insertion. • Change dressings according to hospital policy, using strict aseptic technique.
Intracranial; ventriculitis, other central nervous system infections	Intracranial pressure monitors or catheters Contamination of craniotomy or spinal surgery incision Leakage of cerebrospinal fluid due to basal skull fractures	Ventriculitis: *S. epidermidis, S. aureus* Other infections: *S. aureus, Streptococcus, Neisseria meningitidis, H. influenzae, E. coli*	• Maintain a closed system. • Use strict aseptic technique for insertion and dressing change according to hospital policy. • Monitor insertion site and incision for evidence of infection.

* O'Grady, N. P., Barie, P. S., Bartlett, J., et al. (1998). Practice parameters for evaluating new fever in critically ill adult patients. *Critical Care Medicine, 26*(2), 392–408.

[†] Wijdicks, E. F. M. (1997). *The clinical practice of critical care neurology* (pp. 386–398). Philadelphia: Lippincott-Raven.

units there are numerous environmental stimuli from lights, technological monitoring equipment, ventilators, and providers that can cause overstimulation. Sensory deprivation is also possible.

Although unconscious patients appear to be completely unaware of their environment, it is impossible to determine whether they are aware of any stimulus in the immediate environment. Many patients have regained consciousness and given accurate accounts of what happened and what was said to them when they were supposedly unconscious; therefore, it is important to maintain a positive attitude in the presence of these patients and assume that some stimuli do penetrate the complexities of unconsciousness.[14,15] Stimuli can be provided by playing the radio, touching the patient, and talking. In providing care, patients should be told what you will be doing. In addition, orient the patient to person, place, time, and the environment (weather and so forth).

REGAINING CONSCIOUSNESS

Awakening from unconsciousness is usually a gradual process that varies, to some degree, among patients. The amount of reconditioning and retraining needed to achieve optimal rehabilitation potential will depend on the length of unconsciousness, comorbidity, complications, and age. See Chapter 13 for rehabilitation of patients.

REFERENCES

1. Milazzo, V., & Resh, C. (1981). Kinetic nursing–a new approach to the problems of immobility. *Journal of Neurosurgical Nursing, 14*, 120–124.
2. Szaflarski, N. L. (1996). Immobility phenomena in critically ill adults. In J. M. Clochesy, C. Breu, S. Cardin, A. A. Whitaker, & E. B. Rudy (Eds). *Critical care nursing* (2nd ed., pp. 1313–1334). Philadelphia: W. B. Saunders.
3. Brouse, N. L. (1965). *The physiology and pathology of bedrest.* Springfield IL: Charles C Thomas.
4. Mobily, P., & Kelley, L. (1991). Iatrogenesis in the elderly: Factors of immobility. *Journal of Gerontological Nursing, 17*(9), 5–10.
5. Sharp, J. T. Goldberg, N. B., & Druz, W. S. (1975). Relative contributions of rib cage and abdomen to breathing in normal subjects. *Journal of Applied Physiology, 39*, 608.
6. Harper, C. M., & Lyles, Y. M. (1988). Physiology and complications of bed rest. *Journal of the American Geriatric Society, 36*, 1047–1054.
7. Kennecy, S. K. (1993). Airway management and respiratory support. In A. H. Ropper (Ed.). *Neurological and neurosurgical intensive care* (3rd ed., pp. 69–95). New York: Raven Press.
8. Resnick, N. M. (1998). Geriatric medicine. In A. Fauci, E. Braunwald, K. J. Isselbacher et al. (Eds.). *Harrison's principles of internal medicine* (14th ed., pp. 37–46). New York: McGraw-Hill.
9. Rubin, M. (1988). The physiology of bedrest. *American Journal of Nursing, 88*, 50–56.
10. Saleem, S., & Vallbona, C. (1995). Immobilization. In S. J. Garrison (Ed.). *Handbook of medicine and rehabilitation basics* (pp. 185–196). Philadelphia: J. B. Lippincott.
11. Panel for the Prediction and Prevention of Pressure Ulcers in Adults. (1992). *Pressure ulcers in adults: Prediction and prevention for assessment and management of patients.* Clinical Practice Guideline, No. 3. AHCPR Publication No. 92-0047. Rockville, MD: Agency for Health Care Policy and Research, U. S. Department of Health and Human Services.
12. Wijdicks, E. F. M. (1997). *The clinical practice of critical care neurology* (pp. 4–14). Philadelphia: Lippincott-Raven.
13. Urinary Incontinence Guideline Panel. (1992). *Urinary incontinence in adults: Clinical practice guideline.* AHCPR Publication No. 92-0038. Rockville, MD: Agency for Health Care Policy and Research, Public Health Service. U.S. Department of Health and Human Services.
14. Jacobson, A. F. (2000). Caring for unconscious patients: Do they really remember? *American Journal of Nursing, 100*(1), 69.
15. Stein-Parbury, J., & McKinley, S. (2000). Patients' experiences of being in an intensive care unit: A select literature review. *American Journal of Critical Care, 9*(1), 20–27.

RESOURCES
Professional

Published Material

See also medical-surgical and critical care nursing texts for basic care of the unconscious patient.

Bohachick, P. A. (1987). Pulmonary embolism in neurological and neurosurgical patients. *Journal of Neuroscience Nursing, 19*(4), 191–197.

Creditor, M. C. (1993). Hazards of hospitalization of the elderly. *Annals of Internal Medicine, 118*(3), 219–223.

Dittmer, D. K., & Teasell, R. (1993). Complications of immobilization and bed rest. Part 1: Musculoskeletal and cardiovascular complications. *Canadian Family Physician, 39*, 1428–1432, 1435–1437.

Gradon, J. (1995). Immobility and infection: A practical review for the neurologist. *The Neurologist, 1*, 115–124.

Olson, E. V. (1990). The hazards of immobility. *American Journal of Nursing, 90*(3), 43–48.

Puma, J. L., Schiedermayer, D. L., Gulyas, A. E., & Siegler, M. (1988). Talking to comatose patients. *Archives of Neurology, 45*, 20–22.

Rousseau, P. (1993). Immobility in the aged. *Archives of Family Medicine, 2*(2), 169–177.

Szaflarski, N. L. (1996). Immobility phenomena in critically ill adults. In J. M. Clochesy, C. Breu, S. Cardin, A. A. Whittaker, & E. B. Rudy (Eds.). *Critical care nursing* (2nd ed., pp. 1313–1334). Philadelphia: W. B. Saunders.

Teasell, R., & Dittmer, D. K. (1993). Complications of immobilization and bed rest. Part 2: Other complications. *Canadian Family Physician, 39*, 1440–1442, 1445–1446.

Von Rueden, K. T., & Harris, J. R. (1995). Pulmonary dysfunction related to immobility in the trauma patient. *AACN Clinical Issues, 6*(2), 212–228.

Whitney, J. D., Stotts, N. A., Goodson, W. H., & Janson-Bjerklie, S. (1993). The effects of activity and bed rest on tissue oxygen tension, perfusion, and plasma volume. *Nursing Research, 42*(6), 349–355.

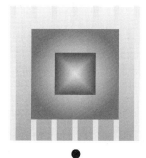

C H A P T E R **17**

Neuroscience Critical Care

MELANIE S. MINTON
JOANNE V. HICKEY

COMPONENTS OF INTENSIVE CARE ENVIRONMENTS

This chapter provides an overview of the environments and the care available for critically ill neuroscience patients. Specific aspects of the current intensive care unit (ICU) environment to be covered include technology, patient characteristics, diagnosis, and care criteria. Additionally, emphasis is placed on structure, process, and outcome to provide a context for discussion of quality care. To enhance understanding of patient needs, information is included on physiological instability, technological dependence, and high risk for development of complications. Clinical decision models are presented to assist in correlating clinical conditions with technological interventions.

Nurses are increasingly challenged by the demands of greater patient acuity, shortened lengths of stay, decreasing patient resources, and intense scrutiny of resource utilization. To respond to these challenges, nurses must be clinically competent, clinically confident, and focused on delivering quality care. The key to clinical competence is through critical reasoning skills, supported by personal experience.[1]

Quality

Quality is a concept that is difficult to define and measure. Outcomes research seeks to address this difficulty by tying quality to optimal patient outcomes. ICUs are designed to improve outcomes of critically ill patients through care delivery that uses advanced structures and processes. To achieve optimal outcomes in the ICU and provide high-quality care, certain structures and processes must be in place. The structure-process-outcome model first described by Donabedian[2,3] and outcomes management introduced by Ellwood,[4] provide a framework for discussion of ICU care. The following terms are used in this model:

- **Structure:** the setting for health care and the materials and resources to provide that care. Structure includes:

- **System:** type of organization; specialty mix of providers; workloads of providers; access and convenience for patients
  - **Provider:** specialty training and certification; preferences; job satisfaction
  - **Patient:** diagnosis or condition; severity; comorbidity; health habits
- **Processes:** a set of activities that functions within and between the patient and practitioner. Process types include:[2]
  - **Technical:** encounters with practitioner; medications; therapies and treatment; diagnostics; hospitalization; intensive care
  - **Interpersonal:** practitioner's communication skills; empathic counseling; interpersonal skills
- **Outcomes:** results of the interaction of structure and process that encompass:
  - **Clinical endpoints:** morbidity/mortality; physiological and/or psychological targets; signs and symptoms; quality of life; functional outcomes; patient/family satisfaction; and cost factors
  - **Health-related quality of life (HRQL):** physical, mental, and social function as well as role execution
  - **Satisfaction with care:** convenience; access; quality; general satisfaction with overall care, medical care, and nursing care; focused satisfaction (with educational information, symptom relief, pain management, control of adverse treatment effects)

Application of the Model to ICU Care for Neuroscience Patients

The following important characteristics of structural components and processes provide a context for creating quality and influencing outcomes for neuroscience ICU patients.

Structure

Various *structural components* must be considered in providing ICU care for patients with neurological problems. The first structural consideration relates to the *system* characteristics of the facility to which the critically ill neuroscience patient is admitted. The following questions address important system characteristics. Is the facility rural or urban? Is it part of a health care system, or is it a free-standing facility? If it is part of a system, how does the flow of patients in the system for both inpatient and outpatient care affect continuity of care? If it is a free-standing facility, how are patients managed after ICU and general hospitalization? Is referral made back to the primary care provider who coordinates all care, or to specialists for particular problems? Is the ICU care for neuroscience patients provided in a specialty neuroscience ICU or a general medical, surgical, or trauma ICU? Where is the ICU located physically in relationship to the emergency department (ED), computed tomography (CT) and magnetic resonance imaging (MRI) scanners, and operating rooms? How is the ICU equipped (i.e., specialty beds, physiological monitoring systems, information technology systems, e.g., electronic charting and clinical management databases, bar-code patient identification technology for charges and procedures)?

Another important component of structure is financing. Although 42 million Americans are without health care insurance, the other 200 million are covered by various types of health plans. Medicare provides health care for older Americans. Other age groups receive health care coverage through various payers, including managed care organizations. How health care is financed and reimbursed has a powerful impact on how a facility conducts business and which services it offers.

The second structural consideration relates to the levels of expertise of all intensivist team members (e.g., physicians, nurses, respiratory therapists). Expertise is needed in general ICU management, as well as neuroscience critical care. Board certification and other credentialing such as advanced cardiac life support (ACLS) and advanced trauma life support (ATLS) are necessary for all those participating in the care of the critically ill neuroscience patient. The model for intensivist practice incorporates an interdisciplinary team, each of whom is expert in an aspect of managing neuroscience patients and who all work collaboratively to provide care within the ICU environment. Closely linked to the model of practice is the integration into direct practice of evidence-based standards, guidelines, and protocols. Admission and discharge protocols should reflect criteria contained in accrediting body standards. In general, these practice guidelines and/or protocols are essential to the care of the critically ill neuroscience patient because they assist in decision making regarding patient selection (e.g., which patients are most appropriate for ICU care and when it is safe to transfer a stable patient to another level of care). Some guidelines are directed at prevention, such as those for deep vein thrombosis, skin breakdown, and aspiration pneumonia. All guidelines provide a standard of care, which incorporates scientific evidence for management of specific patient populations. Examples of neuroscience patient populations include patients with severe brain trauma, intracranial aneurysmal rupture, and ischemic stroke. Many practice guidelines are computerized and available at the bedside for point of care support to make clinical decisions.[5]

The third structural consideration relates to the characteristics of patient groupings as admitted to the hospital, which shape patients' needs. Such patient characteristics include demographics (e.g., age groups, socioeconomic factors, education, occupation), comorbidity, and categories of neuroscience problems. As people live longer, the presence and severity of other illnesses concomitant with neurological problems increase the complexity of managing neuroscience patients. These patients are more vulnerable for complications. With attention to patients' characteristics, the health care provider can better plan for the services needed along the continuum of care, better provide for special needs of population subsets, and make better postacute placement decisions.

Processes

Processes include technical and interpersonal activities. *Technical* activities determine how patient care is managed and delivered, that is, who does what, and how they do it. It includes implementation of evidence-based practice and best-practice standards, guidelines, algorithms, and protocols tailored for the care of specific subsets of neuroscience patients, such as the severely brain injured, stroke, and cerebral aneurysm patients already mentioned. Clinical reasoning guides patient-care decision making and thus actualizes the processes. Often, clinical reasoning is anticipatory and is reflected in established criteria, such as when a patient's feeding should begin. One goal of clinical reasoning is to strike a balance between the need for information and the cost of obtaining that information. Most clinical reasoning involves the application of evidence-based knowledge at the bedside of a given patient to support an optimal outcome through appropriate assessments, drug therapies, invasive and noninvasive monitoring, treatments, and consultations.

Interpersonal activities of care involve person-to-person linkage through communications that are open, honest, and empathetic. Because ICU care entails such a high level of technology, alienation between patient and caregiver can become a serious issue. In caring for critically ill neuroscience patients, who are surrounded by the latest technological advancements and who may have significant cognitive deficits, the nurse may find little time for interpersonal activities unless such activities are deemed a priority. Caring is a moral imperative; caring for patients is the core of nursing. Caring for patients in an ICU environment is stressful not only for the patient but also for the nurse. Through this journey, both patient and nurse are vulnerable to many human emotions, whether hope, joy, pain, or despair. Health care providers must establish trust and rapport with the patient and family in a partnership to meet the needs of the patient. Providing information on treatment, care options, and outcomes helps the patient and family to make critical decisions that influence care. This communication can be fostered in numerous ways, such as liberal visiting hours, frequent contact with the family, patient conferences, and ongoing updates. The nurse is in a prime position to serve as the mediator between technology and care for the patient and family as they experience this often-unknown territory.

Outcomes

Outcomes are the result of the interaction of structure with processes. Although there is agreement on the desire to achieve optimal patient outcomes, there are questions about which elements of care contribute to a sense of high-quality care, and how to measure these elements. Further, how does one use outcomes data to guide practice? Categories of data elements useful in establishing a database for determination of outcomes are presented in Table 17-1. Data can be collected about severity of illness, complications, use of resources, functionality, discharge status, length of stay, and cost of care. The neuroscience nurse should have a working knowledge of standardized scales and be able to incorporate them into the care of critically ill neuroscience patients. For example, knowledge of a patient's severity of illness at admission, compared with information about other similar patients, can assist in predicting use of resources, length of stay, and outcome. Advanced age, comorbidity, or a severe neurological/neurosurgical problem places patients at risk from the time they are admitted. Therefore, determining severity of illness is important when comparing individual patients and examining outcomes.

Information systems help collect, store, and analyze data for large data sets and are needed to support clinical management. When the system is tied to electronic charting, data can be extracted from patients' records automatically. This facilitates storage and accessing of data and saves considerable time in collecting and analyzing data.[6,7] With an electronic system, data can also be stored and analysis can be based on individual specifications and needs, which fosters *knowledge-based decision making*. Electronic data system capability is useful for developing new clinical programs for patients; providing support for expensive protocols that result in better outcomes in a shorter period of time; improving productivity of providers; controlling cost of services; better using resources; and shortening length of stay. This capability also helps with benchmarking, that is, comparing a facility's performance and outcomes with those of other similar facilities that have outstanding practices. The database becomes the foundation for continuous quality improvement. Therefore, the ICU of the 21st century must invest time and resources in creating and maintaining a database for knowledge-based decision making and continuous quality improvement.[8]

ALTERATIONS IN CEREBRAL OXYGEN: A BASIS FOR PHYSIOLOGICAL INSTABILITY

The framework for managing critically ill neuroscience patients in the ICU encompasses a triad of concerns: physiological instability, technological dependence, and high risk for complications. The basis for physiological instability in critically ill neuroscience patients is alteration in cerebral blood flow and cerebral perfusion. At the core of many neuroscience problems, these alterations lead directly to

Table 17-1 • EXAMPLES OF DATA ELEMENTS FOR A NEUROSCIENCE INTENSIVE CARE UNIT (NICU) DATABASE THAT ARE USEFUL IN DETERMINING OUTCOMES

Demographics
  Age, gender, ethnicity, income
Severity of illness
  APACHE II score, Glasgow Coma score, Hunt-Hess score
Comorbidity
  Hypertension, coronary artery disease, diabetes mellitus, alcohol abuse, obesity
Origin
  Emergency department, step-down unit, general care unit, transfer from outside hospital
Resuscitation status
  Full code
  No CPR
  Limited intensiveness
  Advanced directive
Complications
  Pneumonia
  Arrhythmia
  Hypoxic events
  Falls
  ICP Spikes (≥20 mm H_2O)
Consultations
  Physical therapy
  Occupational therapy
  Speech therapy
  Nutrition
  Pastoral support

Medical treatment
  Drugs: inotropes, vasoactives, morphine drip; antibiotics (list drug used); low-dose heparin; full anticoagulation heparin; full oral anticoagulation; low molecular heparin
  Neuromuscular blockade
  Stress prophylaxis
  Enteral feeding (begun when?)
  Sequential compression boots
  Oxygen therapy
  Specialty bed (list type)
Procedures
  Arterial line
  Pulmonary catheter
  Jugular catheter
  Ventriculostomy
  Intubation
  Extubation
  Ventilator support
  Feeding tube placement
Diagnostics
  CT scan
  MRI
  Transcranial doppler
  Cerebral angiography
  Electroencephalography

Intensity/use of resources:
  Therapeutic Intervention Severity Score
Functionality at discharge
  Barthel Index
  National Institutes of Health Stroke Scale
  Mini-Mental Status Examination
  Rankin score
Length of stay
  In NICU
  In hospital
Discharge status
  Died
  Transfer to other ICU
  Transfer to step-down unit
  Transfer to general care unit
  Transfer to other facility
  Transfer to rehabilitation facility
Cost
  Drugs
  Medical treatments
  Procedures
  Overall cost for NICU stay

hypoxia and ischemia, each of which can trigger multiple pathological consequences potentially lethal to the patient. Hypoxia occurs when there is a lowered partial pressure of oxygen. Ischemia is a mismatch between oxygen supply and demand. Cerebral ischemia in the vulnerable brain is defined as cerebral blood flow of less than 20 mL/100g per minute. When the rate of oxygen use is not matched by the supply of oxygen delivered in the blood, irreversible cellular injury occurs and toxic metabolites build up in the blood.[9]

When blood flow is reduced, neurons extract increased oxygen from the surrounding tissues. This increased extraction is an attempt to maintain adequate metabolic function. If the ability of neurons to increase oxygen extraction is exceeded, ischemia occurs. The normal brain commands a cerebral blood flow (CBF) of 15% to 20% of resting cardiac output, with gray matter (the cell bodies of neurons) receiving 300% to 400% more than white matter (the tracts and processes of the neurons). If blood flow to the brain and spinal cord is inadequate or if the oxygen in the blood is inadequate, or if both occur simultaneously, clinical manifestations will become apparent within a short time. These manifestations include alterations in the level of consciousness, motor impairments, and ultimately coma. Cerebral perfusion pressure (CPP), which must be calculated because it cannot actually be measured, is the driving force in maintaining CBF.[9–11] Through autoregulation, the normal brain can modify cerebral vascular resistance (CVR) and maintain constant CBF.

Several physiological stressors have an impact on CBF and cerebral perfusion. For example, a decrease in blood pressure due to blood loss, shock, heart disease, or increased intracranial pressure (ICP) (see Chap. 14), from whatever cause, will impede CBF and cerebral perfusion. Ongoing research that is investigating the effect of time element on cerebral hypoxia indicates that damage to the central nervous system (CNS) can occur within minutes of a CBF reduction and thus compromise the patient's clinical status. In addition to oxygen depletion, other serious implications of an alteration in CBF and cerebral perfusion include disruptions of neurotransmitter activity, glucose transport, protein synthesis, and internal membrane stability. Because the critically ill neuroscience patient is always at risk for hypoxemia and ischemia, all nursing interventions must be directed at maintaining adequate blood flow and perfusion to the CNS.[12]

IMPLICATIONS OF TECHNOLOGICAL DEPENDENCE AND HIGH RISK OF COMPLICATIONS

When derangement of intracranial physiology results in hypoxemia and ischemia, the critically ill neuroscience patient becomes technologically dependent on monitoring of various physiological parameters. This multidimensional monitoring is required both to protect the patient and to obtain valuable information necessary to diagnose, treat, manage, and provide nursing care for the patient. (See Chart 17-1 for common physiological monitoring.)

CHART 17–1 • Common Technological Modalities Used in the Care of Critically Ill Neuroscience Patients

- Continuous EKG monitoring
- Continuous BP monitoring (arterial catheter and/or noninvasive cuff pressure)
- Hemodynamic monitoring (subclavian catheter and/or pulmonary artery catheter)
- Respiratory and ventilator monitoring
- Pulse oximetry
- Continuous intracranial pressure monitoring
- Jugular venous oxygen monitoring
- Continuous electroencephalographic monitoring

The neuroscience ICU patient who is physiologically unstable and technologically dependent is at high risk for complications. Such complications may occur from the primary diagnosis, from comorbid conditions, or from complications resulting from management and treatment. It is the responsibility of the nurse to have a working knowledge of various neuroscience conditions, recommended treatments, and potential complications.[9,11]

USE OF TECHNOLOGY FOR MONITORING OF NEUROSCIENCE PATIENTS IN INTENSIVE CARE UNITS

The following are typical technical data available at the bedside of a critically ill neuroscience patient on an ICU:

GCS8, PERRLA 6 MM, BP 180/100, ABGs pH 7.52, pCO2 40, pO2 89, SVR 1100 dynes/sec., ICP 12, CPP 68, T-max 100.8, K+ 3.0, PAP 20/8 mm Hg, Wedge 9 mmHg, CO 5.4L/min, CI 3.2L/min/m2, CVP 5 mmHg, and INR 1.3.

A technological marvel of the 21st century, continuous exchange of such real-time data is essential to the care of the neuroscience patient in the high-technology environment of an ICU.[13] Multimodality monitoring using the instrumentation and computers commonly available in ICUs[14] provides multiple sets of data that help create a dynamic picture of the patient's physiological status. Large-capacity storage and compression of data allow caregivers to examine trends over time. From the clinician's perspective, technology for monitoring must be safe, accurate, reliable, valid, easy to collect, and displayed in an easily understandable format. Reliability is the degree of consistency or dependability with which an instrument measures the attribute it is designed to measure.[15] Validity is the degree to which an instrument measures what it is intended to measure.[16] Validity and reliability of data are critical if treatment decisions are going to be based on collected data. Unfortunately, there are no known perfect technological monitoring systems currently available. Therefore, to use technology competently, the nurse must be able to understand its purpose; know the technique to collect data accurately; interpret data; identify possible inaccuracies; troubleshoot the equipment; and integrate data from various sources to provide a comprehensive clinical picture of the patient.

On admission to the ICU, the patient may be placed on a special therapeutic bed and will be connected to a physiological monitoring system. Several invasive monitoring lines may be inserted, including an arterial line, pulmonary artery catheter, ventriculostomy, ICP monitor, and possibly a retrograde jugular catheter. The nurse is responsible for knowing how to use and troubleshoot this equipment, interpret the data collected, and use this information in clinical reasoning and decision making. Some patients may be connected to a mechanical ventilator through an endotracheal tube, end-tidal CO_2, cardiac monitoring leads, sequential compression boots, pulse oximetry, and rectal temperature probe. A nasogastric (NG) tube for gastric decompression, a feeding tube for nutritional support, and Foley catheter for continuous urinary drainage are inserted. The NG tube is inserted after the endotracheal tube is in position because the insertion of a NG tube may cause vomiting and aspiration.

With *primary* injury or insult to the brain already present, the focus of ICU care when the patient arrives is prevention of secondary injury. Cerebral hypoxia and cerebral ischemia are two of the most important causes of secondary brain injury. Whether the patient has undergone a neurosurgical intervention or had traumatic brain injury, stroke, or cardiac or respiratory dysfunction, delivery of oxygen-rich blood to the brain is in danger of being compromised. Early detection and treatment of cerebral ischemia may prevent additional damage to the brain and prevent injury to an otherwise intact brain.

One of the principal duties of the nurse is to monitor the patient for signs and symptoms of a change in condition. Monitoring, within the ICU context of nursing practice, means closely observing the patient using physical assessment and technologically produced data. Using clinical reasoning skills, the competent nurse can attach meaning and relevance to the data and form a comprehensive picture of the patient.[17]

The following section discusses the use of technology for monitoring neuroscience patients in the ICU. Addressed are specific monitoring technologies for the neurological, cardiovascular, and respiratory systems. The commonly used technologies discussed provide information on direct and indirect oxygen delivery to the brain and the adequacy of the supply of oxygen to the brain. The goal of treatment is to provide a continuous and adequate oxygen supply to meet cerebral metabolic needs so that cerebral hypoxia and ischemia are avoided.

Neurological Monitoring With Technology

The following modalities targeted to the neurological system are addressed in this section: jugular venous oxygen saturation, transcranial Doppler, continuous electroencephalogram, and ICP monitoring.

Jugular Bulb Venous Oxygen Saturation

A retrograde catheter is inserted into the bulb of the internal jugular vein for continuous measurement of jugular venous oxygen saturation (SjO_2). This assists in identifying existing or impending cerebral ischemia by providing a *global* measure of the oxygen saturation of the venous blood leaving the brain and a measure of the difference in arterial-jugular oxygen content.[18] The oximetric catheter may be inserted into the jugular bulb on the dominant side, the side of injury, or bilaterally. The jugular bulb receives venous blood from the brain with minimal contamination from extracerebral origins.[19] The retrograde jugular catheter provides a means to assess oxygen consumption and delivery by monitoring oxygen extraction in three ways:

1. Calculating cerebral oxygen extraction
2. Calculating arteriovenous difference in oxygen ($AVDO_2$)
3. Monitoring SjO_2 on an ongoing basis

Continuous monitoring of jugular venous oxygen saturation has as its goal early identification of cerebral hypoxia or ischemia.[20–22] Normal values for SjO_2 are 60% to 80%; values less than 54% are considered desaturation and consistent with the development of ischemia.[23–25] A high $SjO2$ (i.e., more than 90%) is an indication of cerebral hyperemia or high flow states (i.e., supply exceeds demand) such as hypertensive states, increased $PaCO_2$, early sepsis, and brain tissue death.[26] Low SjO_2 saturation (less than 54%) indicates ischemia or low flow states (i.e., demand exceeds supply). A strong correlation between the incidence of jugular venous desaturation and poor long-term neurological outcomes has been reported.[27]

Investigation of the reliability of the catheter revealed that up to 50% of SjO_2 oximetric catheter readings were unreliable.[28] Such factors as the positioning of the catheter, migration of the catheter, positioning of the patient, variation in light intensity levels of the technology, and system calibration issues were common causes of unreliability.[29,30] The oximetric catheter readings provide a *global index* and are, therefore, unable to provide information about regional cerebral tissue oxygenation and metabolism. This factor is a major limitation of SjO_2. Therefore, making clinical decisions based solely on SjO_2 data requires caution and further evaluation.

Transcranial Doppler Studies

Transcranial Doppler (TCD) is a noninvasive technique to examine the flow of cerebral blood through the major cerebral arteries, such as the middle cerebral artery. It measures flow velocities and the pulse index. TCD technology is described and discussed in Chapter 6. TCD serial data are used to determine the adequacy of cerebral blood flow, the patency of major cerebral blood vessels, response to therapy (e.g., carotid endarterectomy), and to identify vasospasm (e.g., after subarachnoid hemorrhage).

Continuous Electroencephalogram

Continuous electrophysiological monitoring has gained acceptance at the bedside. Several electroencephalographic (EEG) patterns have been described that correlate with distinct levels of coma and prognosis (see Chap. 6). Using compressed spectral array technology, continuous EEG data are compressed into tracings that illustrate a spectrum of frequencies and power. Compression of data makes it easier to manage and analyze voluminous data that would otherwise be unmanageable. In neuroscience patients, particularly those who are sedated or receiving neuromuscular blockade, seizure activity may be present without accompanying motor activity (nonconvulsive seizures).[31] Note that patients who are not sedated or receiving neuromuscular blockade may also experience nonconvulsive seizures.

ICP Monitoring

Use of continuous ICP monitoring is common in the ICU for patients with intracranial hypertension. The types, uses, validity, reliability, and limitations are described in detail in Chapter 14. ICP monitoring provides data on mean ICP; this is subtracted from mean arterial pressure (MAP) to calculate CPP. It is generally accepted that CPP must be kept *above* 70 mm Hg to sustain an adequate supply of blood and oxygen to the brain. Targeted therapy is often directed at maintaining the CPP above 70 mm Hg.

Cardiovascular Monitoring With Technology

The common cardiovascular monitoring conducted on neuroscience patients in the ICU includes electrocardiography, arterial pressure, pulmonary artery catheterization, and cardiac output.

Electrocardiography (ECG)

From the beginning of ICU care, continuous ECG monitoring has been a cornerstone. Leads selected for monitoring may vary, depending on the area of myocardial interest.[32] Life-threatening cardiac arrhythmias and abnormal patterns are common in neuroscience patients because of autonomic nervous system stimulation from cerebral injury and compromise. Myocardial ischemia and infarction are also common. Therefore, continuous ECG monitoring provides important information in the overall management of neuroscience patients.

Arterial Pressure

Invasive monitoring of arterial pressure provides continuous moment-to-moment arterial waveforms that can be analyzed for pathological and diagnostic patterns. Arterial monitoring is indicated for patients with severe hypertension, shock syndromes, or labile blood pressure. It is also helpful to monitor patients receiving intravenous vasoactive and cardioactive agents. Reasons for arterial cannulation other than for monitoring arterial pressure include the need for frequent measurement of arterial blood gases. Additional indications may include administration of intra-arterial infusion of certain drugs and placement of intra-aortic counterpulsation balloon pumps.[33] The radial artery is the most common site of arterial cannulation. As with any invasive

procedure, patient selection is important. The most serious complication is catheter-related infection.

Pulmonary Artery Catheterization

Since introduction of the flotation pulmonary artery catheter (PAC) in 1970,[34] right-heart catheterization has been the accepted method for directly measuring cardiac pressures on the right side of the heart (e.g., preload) and for indirectly measuring left ventricular filling pressures with the use of a wedging technique. Thermodilution cardiac output is used to quantify ventricular energy output intermittently and to calculate oxygen delivery and consumption.[35] Nurses are usually responsible to monitor and collect data using the PAC. To collect accurate data, certain procedures, for example, referencing and zeroing of the hemodynamic system, must be followed.[36]

PAC patterns help the clinician diagnose and monitor hypovolemia, cardiac dysfunction, adult respiratory distress syndrome (ARDS), pulmonary edema, and sepsis, all common findings in critically ill neuroscience patients. PAC is used to measure cardiac output, usually with a thermodilution method. Cold saline is injected through the proximal port of the PAC. The saline mixes with the blood in the right heart chamber and lowers the temperature of the blood. This temperature change is recorded by a thermistor at the distal end of the PAC and is used to calculate cardiac output. Although the efficacy and safety of the PAC were recently questioned and reviewed, it continues to be a valuable monitoring resource in the ICU and is helpful in guiding treatment decisions with critically ill neurological patients.[37]

Respiratory Monitoring With Technology

Many neuroscience patients require ventilatory support of respirations. Ventilators are now sophisticated pieces of equipment with multiple modes and settings to meet the varying needs of patients (Figs. 17-1 and 17-2). The most common respiratory monitoring conducted with critically ill neuroscience patients includes blood gases and work of breathing. The work of breathing provides information that helps determine when patients are ready for rapid weaning from ventilatory support and/or extubation.[38] Prolonged respiratory dependency increases complication rates, resource use, and cost, and has an adverse impact on overall patient outcomes. Therefore, any method that can reliably identify readiness for weaning is important.

Pulse Oximetry

Pulse oximetry (SpO_2) is a noninvasive technology that continuously measures arterial oxygenation. Operating on spectrophotometric principles, it senses specific wavelengths of light emitted by the hemoglobin in blood through a probe that is most often attached to finger.[39] Pulse oximetry is a useful guide for clinical reasoning and decision making regarding the need to increase oxygen concentration administration and the need for intubation. Patients with acute ischemic or hemorrhagic stroke, cerebral aneurysm bleeding, increased ICP, Guillain-Barré syndrome, and those being weaned from a ventilator require pulse oximetry. Factors

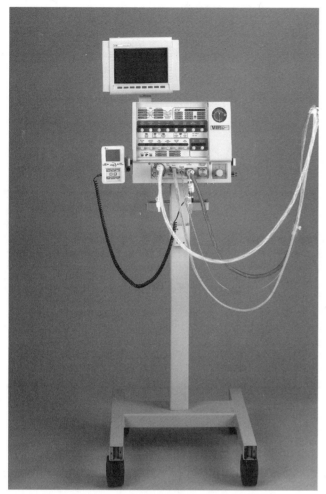

Figure 17–1 • Full view of the Bird (VIP Gold) ventilator. (Courtesy Thermo Respiratory Group, Palm Springs, CA.)

that affect accuracy include anemia, nail polish, cardiac arrhythmias, skin pigmentation, and low perfusion states.

Summary

Managing neuroscience patients within an ICU setting requires that nurses employ multiple high-technology systems to monitor a patient's physiological responses to injury, illness, and specific elements of care. Much of the monitoring is directed at prevention of hypoxic and ischemic episodes known to cause secondary brain injury. Critical reasoning skills guide the nurse in identifying patterns and trends in monitoring data so that serious problems, such as cerebral hypoxia and ischemia, can be immediately addressed and prevented.

VULNERABILITY TO COMPLICATIONS

Critically ill patients are highly vulnerable to complications related to the primary neurological problem (e.g., ARDS with severe brain trauma),[40] comorbid conditions, immobil-

ity, nosocomial infections/sepsis,[41,42] and stressors related to ICU hospitalization. The most common complications found in neuroscience patients, listed in Table 17-2, are either related to treatment itself or result from pathophysiological events. These potential complications are collaborative problems that are addressed by the intensivist team. The nurse's role is to monitor for the detection of the onset or status of these problems and, in collaboration with other team members, to provide definitive treatment. Early identification of patients who are at high risk for particular complications provides an opportunity to institute preventive measures. After complications occur, appropriate treatment is provided based on evidence-based practice. Complications contribute to prolonged length of stay, increased cost, and poorer patient outcomes.

MEDICAL TREATMENT AND MANAGEMENT IN THE INTENSIVE CARE UNIT

After a comprehensive assessment, a specific treatment plan should be developed for each patient that addresses each of the patient's problems and needs. The plan of care should incorporate clinical guidelines and protocols based on the best evidence-based practice. Specific evidence-based practice guidelines for various neurological problems are found in designated chapters of this text. However, clinicians must be

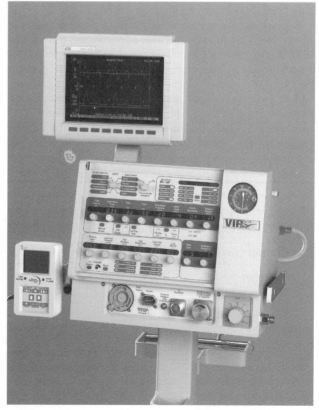

Figure 17–2 • Close-up of the Bird (VIP Gold) ventilator. (Courtesy Thermo Respiratory Group, Palm Springs, CA.)

Table 17-2 • POTENTIAL COMPLICATIONS FREQUENTLY SEEN IN CRITICALLY ILL NEUROSCIENCE PATIENTS

Cardiac
Arrhythmias
Cardiogenic shock
Deep vein thrombosis (DVT)
Hypovolemic shock
Hypotension
Hypertension
Ischemic heart disease including acute myocardial infarction
Anemia
Disseminated intravascular coagulation (DIC)

Metabolic/Immune
Hyperglycemia
Negative nitrogen balance
Electrolyte imbalance
Hyperthermia
Acidosis/alkalosis
Diabetes insipidus (DI)
Syndrome of inappropriate secretion of antidiuretic hormone (SIADH)
Cerebral salt wasting
Sepsis

Respiratory
Atelectasis
Pneumonia (aspiration, bacterial, other)
Neurogenic pulmonary edema
Pulmonary embolism (PE)
Ventilator dependency

Integumentary/Mucus Membrane
Corneal ulceration
Skin breakdown (decubitus ulcer)
Laryngeal edema

Gastrointestinal
Gastric ulcer
Hemorrhage
Small bowel obstruction

Neurological
Increased intracranial pressure
Herniation syndromes
Stroke
Seizures
Hydrocephalus
Meningitis
Cranial nerve impairment
Paresis/paralysis
Paresthesia
Peripheral nerve impairment

Musculoskeletal
Contractures
Spasticity

Other
Multiorgan dysfunction syndrome (MODS)

aware that application of new knowledge to clinical practice is an ongoing process and that breakthroughs, provided they have a rigorous scientific basis, should be integrated into practice. Updating and revising practice guidelines to incorporate new knowledge is an ongoing responsibility (Table 17-3).

Through the use of various therapeutic interventions, *collaborative* efforts among providers are often directed toward controlling physiological parameters to target values. The targeted values include a range, such as maintaining the MAP between 90 and 100 mm Hg, or a critical threshold, such as maintaining CPP at more than 70 mm Hg. To maintain physiological parameters in accordance with targeted goals, the nurse may need to titrate drugs (e.g., dopamine to a set cardiac output), suction in response to a declining systemic arterial oxygen

saturation (SaO_2), or reposition the patient's neck in response to noisy respirations (partially obstructed airway). The setting and maintaining of physiological targets are intended to optimize physiological function, prevent complications, and minimize secondary brain injury.

TRANSFER OF CRITICALLY ILL PATIENTS

Every nurse in clinical practice can relate stories of patients "going bad" during transport for procedures within a facility or during transport between facilities. The risks of trans-

 Table 17-3 • EXAMPLES OF COMMON STANDARDS, PRACTICE GUIDELINES, AND PROTOCOLS USED TO DELIVER COST-EFFECTIVE QUALITY CARE FOR NEUROSCIENCE PATIENTS REQUIRING ICU CARE

STANDARDS/CRITERIA	PRACTICE GUIDELINES	PROTOCOLS
• Admission to and discharge from the ICU • Need for computed tomography scan or magnetic resonance imaging • Nutrition consultation • Hemodynamic monitoring • Intubation criteria • Extubation criteria • PEG feeding tube criteria • Tracheostomy criteria • Drug level monitoring • Beginning oral feeding	• Severe traumatic brain injury guidelines • Hemorrhagic stroke guidelines • Prophylaxis for cerebral vasospasm after cerebral aneurysm bleed • Transport of critically ill patients • Rapid therapeutic anticonvulsant therapy	• Weaning from ventilator support • Management of ventriculostomy dressing • Dressing change for central lines • Gastrointestinal prophylaxis • Deep vein thrombosis prophylaxis • Ventriculostomy drainage • Potassium replacement • Status epilepticus • Neuromuscular blockade

porting a critically ill neuroscience patient include partial or complete airway obstruction, hypotensive episodes, spikes in ICP, and cardiac pump failure. Any of these events can lead to hypoxia or ischemia and result in secondary brain injury. These significant risks associated with a decision to transport must be balanced by carefully reasoned benefits to the patient. The primary reason for moving a patient is to provide additional technological or specialist care that is not available in the current care setting.[43] Risk to the patient during transport can be minimized through careful planning, excellent communications, well-prepared and qualified personnel, and use of appropriate equipment. There should be no cessation of monitoring or maintenance of the patient's vital functions during transport. Patients who are not physiologically stable should not be transported until they are stabilized. The *Guidelines for the Transfer of Critically Ill Patients*[37] have been published by the American College of Critical Care Medicine and American Association of Critical-Care Nurses to guide safe transfer of patients. The *Guidelines* have been adapted to the specific needs of neuroscience patients.[44] Each facility should have a procedure and guideline for the safe transfer and transport of critically ill patients.

FUTURE TRENDS IN ICU CARE

Intensive care services are being reorganized to better meet the needs of patients in a cost-effective way.[45,46] The ICU of the 21st century must encompass a synergy between technological advances and humanistic caring components that will support a healing environment. Multidisciplinary intensivist teams are being challenged by the difficulties of integrating technology while recognizing the needs of the vulnerable patient connected to the technology. Critical care clinicians must carefully and methodically assess new technologies. The goal of this assessment is to adopt only those technologies that are obtainable at a reasonable cost and that improve unit operation and staff efficiency, support educational programs, and, most important, enhance patient outcomes.[47] The following provides a glimpse of what will be the ICU practice setting of the 21st century.

Miniature biosensors and computers will collect and process multimodal monitoring data noninvasively while providing greater freedom of movement for patients. With improved understanding of critical illnesses at the molecular level will come the development of a new generation of monitors capable of sensing disturbances in homeostasis before clinical manifestations are evident.[48] Clinical information systems will move from mere documentation system to a new plateau. Capable of analyzing data online, integrating data with knowledge systems, and providing linkages to support efficient workflow management, the new systems will become valuable tools for clinical decision making.[49]

The current usefulness of point-of-care testing (POCT) will be rapidly upgraded. New technology will miniaturize POCT devices while simultaneously incorporating advances in function, automation, testing profiles, and quality control.[50] The awesome strides already made in diagnostic imaging and interventional therapies guided by imaging will continue and lead to improvement in the quality of information and improved patient outcomes. Continued developments in computer processing technology will make POCT available in multidimensional forms at the bedside.[51]

Nursing practice, as well as the overall delivery of care, will become ever more dependent on evidence-based guidelines, protocols, and standards. Pharmacological advances will provide new therapies for neuroprotection and reperfusion of cerebral tissue. One can expect to see new pharmacological therapies to improve neurological recovery from global ischemia after cardiac arrest, to address regional ischemia after cerebral brain trauma, to mitigate cerebral herniation syndromes, and to ameliorate the consequences of other cerebral insults.[52] Some additional exciting trends herald such future technological advances as ongoing monitoring of continuous partial pressure of oxygen in brain tissue ($PtiO_2$), further expansion and incorporation of cerebral microdialysis, and laser Doppler flowmetry (LDF).[9]

The concept of an interdisciplinary collaborative intensivist team will become the norm in the ICU, and the roles of both the bedside nurse and the advanced practice nurse will be expanded and clarified. The 24-hour, interdisciplinary care may be provided by a team hundreds or thousands of miles away off-site through telemedicine and telenursing. The sophistication of the technology will support physical assessment such as the ability to assess patients' pupils and other parameters. This information, along with the ongoing review of the computerized patient medical record, will take clinical decision making from the actual patient bedside to the computer-based bedside of the expert intensivist team located miles away.

High-quality care at a reasonable cost will become more dependent on audio-video links for accessing physical assessment and other relevant data. Early experience with telemedicine in ICUs reports decreased mortality, decreased complications, and decreased costs.[53] The advent of telemedicine and telenursing on a large scale will require new models for educating clinicians and for collaborative partnerships among practitioners. This revolution in health care delivery will also challenge those involved with state licensure and credentialing of providers. Amid all these technology-based advances, a major problem looms–further patient—practitioner alienation. Creating a humanistic caring environment in which healing may occur will continue to be challenging.[54]

The general ICU paradigm just described reflects a 21st century environment that is possible for critically ill neuroscience patients. Although one cannot precisely predict the future course of ICU practice, certain realities are evident. There will be enormous growth of knowledge in the neurosciences and in its clinical applications. Whether these innovations will be quickly adapted into routine practice is a function of available resources. However, in an environment of limited resources, we must maintain a balance among science, technology, and humanism to create a healing environment that supports the body, the psyche, and the soul of our patients.

REFERENCES

1. Chinn, P. (1995). *Exemplars in criticism* (pp. 88–102, 201–212). Gaithersburg, MD: Aspen Publications.
2. Donabedian, A. (1966). Evaluating the quality of medical care. *Milbank Memorial Fund Quarterly, 44*, 166–206.

3. Donabedian, A. (1980). *The definition of quality and approaches to its assessment, Vol. I: Explorations in quality assessment and monitoring.* Ann Arbor, MI: Health Administration Press.

4. Ellwood, P. M. (1988). Outcome management. A technology of patient experience. *New England Journal of Medicine, 318,* 1549–1556.

5. Morris, A. H. (1999). Computerized protocols and bedside decision support. *Critical Care Clinics, 15*(3), 523–545.

6. Marik, P.E., & Varon, J. (1999). Severity scoring and outcome assessment: Computerized predictive models and scoring systems. *Critical Care Clinics.* 15(3), 633–646.

7. Cowen, J. S., & Matchett, S. C. (1999). The clinical management database. *Critical Care Clinics, 15*(3), 481–497.

8. Rainey, T. G., & Shapiro, M. J. (2001). Critical care medicine for the 21st century. *Critical Care Medicine, 29*(2), 436–437.

9. Schell, H. A., & Puntillo, K. A. (1992). *Critical care nursing secrets* (pp. 231–265). Philadelphia: Hanley & Belfus.

10. Chulay, M., Guzzetta, C., & Dossey, B. (1997). *AANN handbook of critical care nursing.* Stanford: Appleton & Lange.

11. Lewis, A. J. (1976). *Mechanisms of neurological disease* (pp. 235–255). Boston: Little, Brown & Company.

12. Oyesiku, N. M., & Amacher, L. A. (1990). *Patient care in neurosurgery* (3rd ed., pp. 3–15). Boston: Little, Brown & Company.

13. Helfaer, M. (1998). *ICU care* (pp. 65–93). Baltimore: Williams & Wilkins.

14. Booth, F. V. (1999). Computerized physiological monitoring. *Critical Care Clinics, 15*(3), 547–561.

15. Polit, D. F., & Hungler, B. P. (1999). *Nursing research: Principles and methods* (6th ed., p. 613). Philadelphia: Lippincott-Raven.

16. Polit, D. F., & Hungler, B. P. (1999). *Nursing research: Principles and methods* (6th ed., p. 717) Philadelphia: Lippincott-Raven.

17. Booth, F. V. (1999). Computerized physiologic monitoring. *Critical Care Clinics, 15*(3), 547–562.

18. Nakajima, T., Ohsumi, H., & Kuro. M. (1993). Accuracy of continuous jugular venous oximetry during cardiopulmonary bypass. *Anesthesia & Analgesia, 77,* 1111–1115.

19. Eisenhart, K. (1994). New perspective in the management of adults with severe head injury. *Critical Care Quarterly, 17*(2), 1–12.

20. Bell, S. D., Guyer, D., Snyder, M. A., & Miner, M. (1994). Cerebral hemodynamics: Monitoring arteriojugular oxygen, content differences. *Journal of Neuroscience Nursing* 26(5), 270–277.

21. Kerr, M. E., Lovasik, D., & Darby, J. (1995). Evaluating cerebral oxygenation using jugular venous oximetry in head injuries. *AACN Clinical Issues, 6*(1), 11–20.

22. March, K. (1994). Retrograde jugular catheter: Monitoring SjO_2. *Journal of Neuroscience Nursing, 26*(1), 48–51.

23. Brain Trauma Foundation, American Association of Neurological Surgeons, Joint Section on Neurotrauma and Critical Care. (1996). Guidelines for the management of severe head injury. *Journal of Neurotrauma, 13,* 641–734.

24. Chan, K. H., Dearden, N. M., Miller, J. D., et al. (1993). Multimodality monitoring as a guide to treatment of intracranial hypertension after severe brain injury. *Neurosurgery, 32,* 547–553.

25. Sheinberg, M., Kanter, M. J., Robertson, C. S., et al. (1992). Continuous monitoring of jugular venous oxygen saturation in head-injured patients. *Journal of Neurosurgery, 76,* 212–217.

26. De Deyne, C., Vandekerckhove, T., Decruyenaere, J., & Colardyn, F. (1996). Analysis of abnormal jugular bulb oxygen saturation data in patients with severe head injury. *Acta Neurochirurgica 138,* 1409–1415.

27. Robertson, C. S., Narayan, R. K., Gokaslan, Z. L., et al. (1989). Cerebral arteriovenous oxygen difference as an estimate of cerebral blood glow in comatose patients. *Journal of Neurosurgery, 70,* 222–230.

28. Clay, H. D. (2000). Validity and reliability of the SjO2 catheter in neurologically impaired patients: A critical review of the literature. *Journal of Neuroscience Nursing, 32*(4), 194–203.

29. Bullock, R., Stewart, L., Rafferty, C, & Teasdale, G. M. (1993). Continuous monitoring of jugular bulb oxygen saturation and the effects of drugs acting on cerebral metabolism. *Acta Neurochirurgica, 59*(Suppl.), 86–90.

30. Cruz, J., Miner, M. E., Allen, S. J., et al. (1991). Continuous monitoring of cerebral oxygenation in acute brain, injury: Assessment of cerebral hemodynamic reserve. *Neurosurgery, 29,* 743–749.

31. Young, G. B., Jordon, K. G., & Doig, G. S. (1996). An assessment of nonconvulsive seizures in the intensive care unit using continuous EEG monitoring: An investigation of variables associated with mortality. *Neurology, 47,* 83–89.

32. Jacobson, C. (1998). Bedside cardiac monitoring. *Critical Care Nurse, 18*(3), 82–85.

33. Lodato, R. F. Arterial pressure monitoring. (1998). In M. J. Tobin, (Ed.). *Principles and practice of intensive care monitoring* (pp. 733–749). New York: McGraw-Hill.

34. Swan, H. J. C., Ganz, W., Forrester, J. S., et al. (1970). Catheterization of the heart in man with use of a flow-directed balloon-tipped catheter. *New England Journal of Medicine, 283,* 447–451.

35. Chang, C. Monitoring of critically ill patients. (1999). *New Horizons, 7*(1), 35–45.

36. Keckeisen, M. (1999). Monitoring pulmonary artery pressure. *Critical Care Nurse, 19*(6), 88–91.

37. Bernard, G. R., Sopko, G., Cerra, F., et al. (2000). Pulmonary artery catheterization and clinical outcomes. *JAMA, 283,* 2568–2572.

38. Kirton, O. C., DeHaven, B., Morgan, J. P., et al. (1995). Elevated imposed work of breathing masquerading as ventilator weaning intolerance. *Chest, 108,* 1021–1025.

39. Jubran, A. (1998). Pulse oximetry. In M. J. Tobin (Ed.). *Principles and practice of intensive care monitoring* (pp. 261–287). New York: McGraw-Hill.

40. Van Soeren, M. H., Diehl-Jones, W., Maykut, R. J., Haddara, W. M. R. (2000). Pathophysiology and implications for treatment of acute respiratory distress syndrome. *AACN Clinical Issues, 11*(2), 179–197.

41. Harris, J. R., Joshi, M., Morton, P. G., & Socken, K. L. (2000). Risk factors for nosocomial pneumonia in critically ill trauma patients. *AACN Clinical Issues, 11*(2), 198–231.

42. Wheeler, A. P., & Bernard, G. R. (2000). Treating patients with severe sepsis. *New England Journal of Medicine, 340*(3), 207–214.

43. American College of Critical Care Medicine and American Association of Critical-Care Nurses. (1993). Guidelines for the transfer of critically ill patients. *Critical Care Medicine, 21,* 931–937.

44. Kalisch, B. J., Kalisch, P. A., Burns, S. M., Kocan, M. J., & Presdergast, V. (1995). Intrahospital transport of neuro ICU patients. *Journal of Neuroscience Nursing, 27*(2), 69–77.

45. Bryan-Brown, C. W., & Dracup, K. (1999). The critical care trajectory. *American Journal of Critical Care, 5*(3), 137–139.

46. Randolph, A. G. (1999). Reorganizing the delivery of intensive care may improve patient outcomes. *JAMA, 281*(14), 1330–1331.

47. Pastores, S. A., & Halpern, N. A. (2000). Acquisition strategies for critical care technology. *Critical Care Clinics, 16*(4), 545–556.

48. Kohlo-Seth, R., & Oropello, J. M. (2000). The future of bedside monitoring. *Critical Care Clinics, 16*(4),557–578.

49. Seiver, A. (2000). Critical care computing: past, present and future. *Critical Care Clinics, 16*(4), 601–622.

50. Halpern, N. A. (2000). Point of care diagnostics and networks. *Critical Care Clinics, 16*(4), 623–640.

51. Henry, D. A. (2000). Imaging in the new millennium. *Critical Care Clinics, 16*(4), 579–600.

52. Manning, J. E., Katz, L. M. (2000). Cardiopulmonary and cerebral resuscitation. *Critical Care Clinics, 16*(4), 659–680.

53. Breslow, M. J. (2000). Telemedicine: Organization and communication. *Critical Care Clinics, 16*(4), 707–722.
54. Jastremski, C. A. (2000). ICU bedside environment: A nursing perspective. *Critical Care Clinics, 16*(4), 723–734.

RESOURCES

Professional

Published Material

Burns, S. M. (2001). Ventilatory management: Volume and pressure modes. In D. J. Lynn-McHale & K. K. Carlson (Eds.). *AACN procedure manual for critical care* (4th ed., pp. 178–189). Philadephia: W. B. Saunders.

Burns, S. M. (2001). Standard weaning criteria: Negative inspiratory pressure, positive expiratory pressure, spontaneous tidal volume, and vital capacity. In D. J. Lynn-McHale & K. K. Carlson (Eds.). *AACN procedure manual for critical care* (4th ed., pp. 191–204). Philadelphia: W. B. Saunders.

Burns, S. M. (2001). Arterial-venous oxygen difference calculation. In D. J. Lynn-McHale & K. K. Carlson (Eds.). *AACN procedure manual for critical care* (4th ed., pp. 155–157). Philadelphia: W. B. Saunders.

Tobin, M. J. (2001). Advances in mechanical ventilation. *New England Journal of Medicine, 344*(26), 1986–1996.

Tobin, M. J. (Ed.). (1998). *Principles and practice of intensive care monitoring.* New York: McGraw-Hill.

Sundrani, S. (1995). Neurologic intensive care unit management and economic issues. *Neurologic Clinics 13*(3), 679–693.

Sullivan, J. (2001). Jugular venous oxygen saturation monitoring: Insertion (assist), care troubleshooting and removal. In D. J. Lynn-McHale & K. K. Carlson (Eds.). *AACN procedure manual for critical care* (4th ed., pp. 570–579). Philadephia: W. B. Saunders.

Wijdicks, E. F. M. (1997). *The clinical practice of critical care neurology.* Philadelphia: Lippincott-Raven.

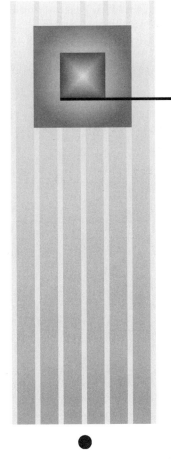

Nursing Management of Patients With Injury to the Neurological System

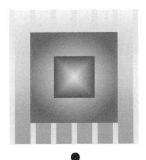

C H A P T E R **18**

Craniocerebral Trauma

JOANNE V. HICKEY

SCOPE OF THE PROBLEM

In 1998, approximately 500,000 people in the United States suffered traumatic brain injury (TBI), 50,000 of whom died before reaching a medical facility. Of the remaining 450,000 TBIs, 80% (360,000) were mild, 10% (45,000) were moderate, and 10% (45,000) were severe.[1] Another 1.6 million people were reported with craniocerebral trauma, but they were not admitted to the hospital for medical care. Incidence of TBI is highest in younger people (15 to 44 years), although peaks are noted in infants, children, and the elderly. Motor vehicle accidents (50%), falls (21%,), assaults and violence, (12%), and sports and recreational activities (10%) are the major causes of TBI. Of the major reasons for motor vehicle accidents (MVA)s, lack of helmets for motorcyclists, lack of restraints for automobile occupants, and consumption of alcohol before driving are the most common.

Disability after craniocerebral trauma has significance for the brain-injured person, the family, and society. Conservative estimates for permanent disability in brain-injured people are 10% in mild, 66% in moderate, and 100% in severe. Based on these estimates, there are 82,814 new patients with long-term residual disabilities secondary to brain injury. This number includes 2,000 who remain in a permanent vegetative state.[2] The loss of human potential and the physical, emotional, psychosocial and vocational impacts on the patient and family function are immeasurable and devastating. These impacts create the need for many health-related and community services.

OVERVIEW OF CRANIOCEREBRAL TRAUMA

Definitions and Classification

Traumatic brain injury refers to any injury to the scalp, skull (cranium or facial bones), or brain. That term and **craniocerebral trauma** are general designations to denote injury to the skull, brain, or both, that is of sufficient magnitude to interfere with normal function and to require treatment. The more accurate term to describe the major traumatic event, however, is **traumatic brain injury**. Classification criteria presented in this chapter include descriptors of location and types of injuries (Chart 18-1); mechanisms of injury; and a severity of injury index, the Glasgow Coma Scale (GCS) (Chart 18-2).

Anatomical Considerations

The cranial vault can be imagined as a closed box with one major opening at the base of the skull, the foramen magnum. The three compartments (i.e., fossae) within the cranial vault (anterior, middle, and posterior fossae) are separated by irregularly shaped, bony buttresses (see Chap. 5). The contour of the intracranial vault is smooth in some areas (e.g., occipital area) and highly irregular in other areas (e.g., frontal-orbital and temporal areas). Within the bones are etched tracts for some major blood vessels. An example is the middle meningeal artery located on the inside plate of the temporal bone in an area where the skull is the thinnest. With temporal bone fractures, this artery may be torn, causing an epidural hematoma.

PRIMARY AND SECONDARY INJURIES

There are two main stages in the development of brain damage after TBI: primary injury and secondary injury (Fig. 18-1).[3] **Primary injury** comes through direct contact to the head and brain as an immediate result of the initial insult at the moment of injury. The cerebral injury may be focal (contusion or laceration) or diffuse (concussion or diffuse axonal injury). **Secondary injury** results from complicating processes initiated at the moment of injury, which present later in the clinical course. These processes include intracranial hemorrhage, cerebral edema, increased intracranial pressure (ICP), hypoxic (ischemic) brain damage, and infection.[4] Flow-metabolism mismatch results in cerebral *ischemia*, unleashing the ischemic cascade and other biochemical changes on the cellular level that can lead to neuronal injury

CHART 18–1 • Classification of Head Injuries by Location and Type

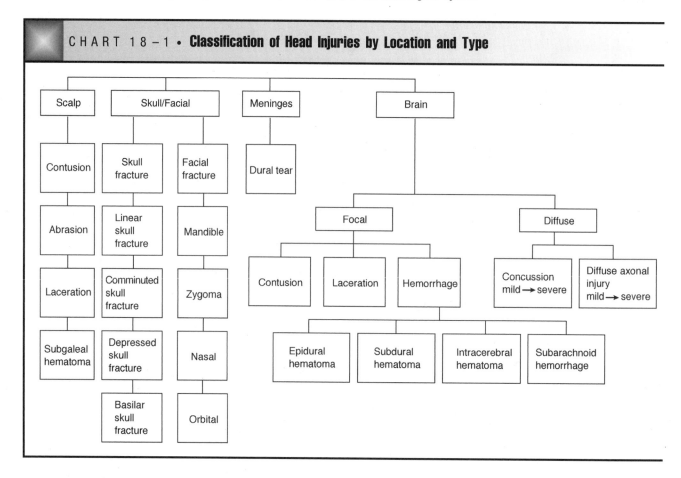

and cell death. Other later causes of secondary injury can result from a single event, series of events, or multisystem complications. For example, episodes of hypoxemia, systemic hypotension, sustained increased ICP, respiratory complications, electrolyte imbalance, and infections can precipitate additional pathophysiological effects on the brain. Secondary injuries contribute to poor outcomes.

Experimental Models for Understanding Traumatic Brain Injury

Most of what is known about primary TBI comes from biomechanically induced acute brain trauma in animal experimental studies.[5] Extrapolation of knowledge from animal studies (of-

ten small animals) to clinical application in humans has limitations.[6] Models of TBI have been classified according to the method of production of the injury and include:

- *Percussion concussion,* which includes fluid-percussion (F-P) models
- *Acceleration concussion,* which includes inertial and impact acceleration injury models.

The F-P model produces variable and relatively small contusion in the vicinity of the fluid pulse with some axonal damage. Varying severities of injury (e.g., mild, moderate, or severe) can be reproduced for study. The acceleration model is used to produce acute subdural hematoma (SDH) and diffuse axonal injury. Tissue-tear hemorrhages of central white matter and gliding contusions occur at the parasagittal junctions of gray and white matter. These models produce prolonged coma and widespread axonal damage.[7] The acceleration model is more closely associated with human pathology.

CHART 18–2 • Classification of Brain Injury According to Glasgow Coma Scale

```
              Glasgow Coma Scale (GCS)
        ┌────────────────┼────────────────┐
     Mild            Moderate           Severe
  brain injury     brain injury       brain injury
  GCS: 13–15       GCS: 9–12          GCS: 3–8
```

MECHANISMS, PATHOPHYSIOLOGY, AND PATHOLOGY ASSOCIATED WITH TRAUMATIC BRAIN INJURY

Multiple complex factors and interrelated mechanical, pathophysiological, and pathological processes underlie primary and secondary brain injuries.

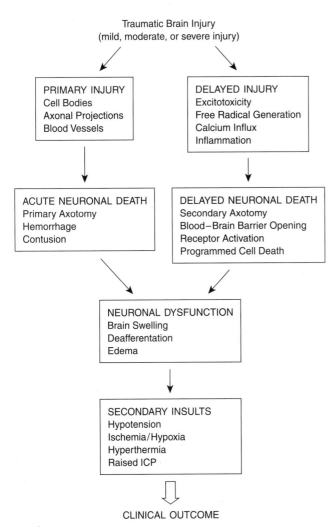

Figure 18–1 • Key primary and secondary pathological events with traumatic brain injury. (Dietrich, W. D. [2000]. Trauma of the nervous system A. Basic neuroscience of neurotrauma. In W. G. Bradley, R. B. Daroff, G. M. Fenichel, & C. D. Marsden [Eds.]. *Neurology in clinical practice* [3rd ed., pp. 1045–1054]. Boston: Butterworth & Heinemann.)

Primary Brain Injury

Classification of the major mechanisms of craniocerebral injury includes (1) *contact phenomena* and (2) *head motions of acceleration and deceleration* (Fig. 18-2).[8]

- **Contact phenomena injuries** are the direct result of an object's striking the head and include local effects such as scalp laceration, skull fracture, extradural hematoma, contusions, lacerations, and intracerebral hemorrhage (ICH).[9] The velocity (low or high) of the impact determines whether the injury is restricted to the scalp or skull (low velocity) or includes the brain (high velocity) (Fig. 18-3).
- **Acceleration-deceleration** injuries are caused by the abrupt changes in the velocity of the brain's principally rapid forward movement followed by abrupt stop (inertia) within the cranial vault. Acceleration-deceleration is produced by head motion at the instant after injury[5] and causes strain on cerebral tissue. These strains often operate simultaneously or in rapid succession to produce injury by:
  - **Compression** (pushing together of tissue)
  - **Tension** (traction on tissue)
  - **Shearing** (opposite but parallel sliding motion of the planes of an object)

A special type of acceleration-deceleration motion is **rotation** (sometimes called **angular acceleration**); it is common at sites where the brain tissue hits bony buttresses in the cranial vault. The effects of linear acceleration of the head are much less significant than those resulting from rotation. The acceleration-deceleration mechanism is responsible for two important types of injury encountered in blunt TBI: acute subdural hematoma and diffuse axonal injury.

Whether the head is fixed or free, a certain amount of acceleration-deceleration always occurs at the time of impact to the skull. The difference in density between the skull (a solid substance) and the brain (a semisolid substance) causes the skull to move faster than its intracranial contents. The brain, which is located within the rigid skull and compart-

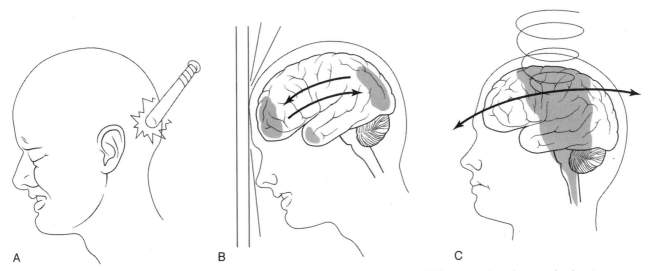

Figure 18–2 • Mechanisms of injury: (*A*) contact, (*B*) acceleration-deceleration, and (*C*) rotational acceleration-deceleration.

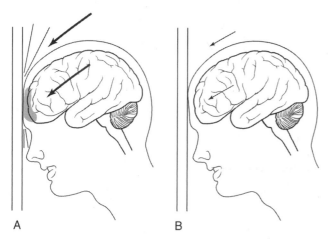

Figure 18–3 • (*A*) High-velocity contact impact on the brain and skull. (*B*) A low-velocity contact impact damages only the skull.

mentalized by the dura and bony buttresses, responds to force exerted on the skull by gliding forward and then rotating within the compartment. The rotational force produces distortion of the brain as well as tension, stretching, and shearing of involved tissue.

The maximal amount of injury is usually found at the frontal and temporal poles and on the inferior surfaces of the frontal and temporal lobes where brain tissue comes in contact with bony protuberances at the base of the skull. Shearing or sliding of cerebral tissue over another portion implies stresses on two different planes. With rotational acceleration, the stress of shearing is directed toward areas where tough, fibrous tissue and cerebral tissue meet. These high-risk areas include the crista galli, the sphenoid wing, the margins of the tentorium or falx, and the foramen magnum. The degree of injury will depend on the extent and direction of the angular acceleration. Rotational movement in the brain can cause damage to axons even without gross visible lesions.[10]

Secondary Brain Injury

Secondary injury is produced by various events and changes, which can lead to cellular injury and/or cellular death. They include biochemical changes, intracranial hemorrhage, brain swelling, increased ICP, and hypoxic (ischemic) brain damage.

Pathophysiological and Biochemical Changes Associated With TBI

In animal models, the initial cellular responses to TBI may be a consequence of both primary and secondary events initiated by a complex cascade of cellular interactions (see Fig. 18-1).

Primary Injury. Because of the contact phenomena, two types of injury occur. First, superficial or contusional hemorrhage occurs through coup and contrecoup mechanisms. Second, an acceleration mechanism produces diffuse axonal injury with axonal shearing (*primary axotomy*) alone or together

with tearing of blood vessels that cause microscopic petechial hemorrhage. In animal models, primary axotomy in which axons are sheared, severed, or disconnected, is uncommon.[11,12] In transected axons, axoplasmic transport from the cell body to the axon terminal continues. However, the transported material cannot pass the damaged area, where it accumulates, causing the axon to swell.[13] Most axons undergo a series of changes that result in *secondary axotomy*. Although the timeline for neuronal death varies, primary axotomy usual occurs in approximately an hour whereas secondary axotomy is more protracted.

The postulated sequence of axotomy is summarized as follows:[7]

- **Primary axotomy** (<1 hour)
  - Axolemma permeability increases ⎫
  - An influx of calcium occurs ⎬ Axotomy
  - Microtubules are lost ⎭
  - Mitochondria swell
  - Focal loss of axonal transport occurs

Axonal injury is a dynamic, established, sequential pathophysiological cascade of events that result in secondary axotomy.[14]

- **Secondary axotomy** (>4 hours)
  - Activation of intracellular leukocytic and proteolytic enzymes, including protein kinase ⎫
  - Changes occur in phosphorylation ⎬ Axotomy
  - Change occurs in the structure of neurofilament ⎭
  - Loss of axonal transport occurs
  - Axonal swelling occurs in 2 to 4 hours
  - Neurofilament proteolysis occurs

During the first 12 hours after injury, axonal damage can only be seen with an electron microscope.[15] Between 3 to 6 hours postinjury, axon abnormalities can be noted. Damaged axons are seen in increasing numbers during the first several days after injury, during which they undergo changes until they finally appear as so-called retraction balls, the hallmark of diffuse axonal injury.[16]

Secondary Injury. Experimental models suggest that there are a number of biochemical changes associated with TBI. Excitotoxicity, the release of excitatory amino acids such as glutamate and aspartate, is widespread after trauma, resulting in cell swelling, vacuolization, and cell death.[17] Through activation of excitatory amino acid receptors (e.g., glutamate and aspartate), there is an abnormal intracellular calcium influx. In addition, extensive membrane depolarization, induced by trauma, allows for a nonselective opening of the voltage-sensitive calcium channels and an abnormal accumulation of calcium within neurons and glia. The calcium shifts are associated with activation of intracellular lipolytic and proteolytic enzymes, protein kinases (calpains), protein phosphatases, dissolution of microtubules, expression of neurotropic factors, altered gene expression, and activation of cell death genes.[18–21] Concurrent free radical generation includes superoxide, hydroxyl, hydrogen peroxide, singlet oxygen, and nitrous oxide. The free radicals can damage proteins, the phospholipid components of cells, and organelle membranes, which results in membrane hydrolysis. All these biochemical events result in secondary neural injury.

Axons first respond to injury by failure of aerobic glycolysis, phosphocreatine production, activation of high-energy cellular functions, and production of adenosine triphosphate (ATP). Failure of aerobic glycolysis increases lactate production and decreases intracellular pH, resulting in cellular acidosis. With failure of ATP production, the sodium-potassium pump can no longer maintain the homeostatic balance of intracellular ions (higher intracellular concentrations of K^+ and higher extracellular concentrations of Na^+). The result is that extracellular K^+ increases as K^+ leaks out of the cell, and Na^+, Ca^{2+}, and water move into the cell from the extracellular space.[4]

A major final common pathway for cell death is loss of *calcium homeostasis*.[6] Loss of calcium homeostasis inhibits cellular metabolism. This, in turn, leads to increased breakdown of protein and lipids, increased breakdown of cell membrane from phospholipids hydrolysis, and the production of toxins (eicosanoid, platelet-activating factor, and free radicals). Concurrently, following trauma, there is immediate severe cellular energy failure causing a strikingly increased level of extracellular excitatory neurotransmitters (EEN). These EENs include the excitatory amino acids (EAA) glutamate and aspartate and the amine acetylcholine. The source of EAA is believed to be injured, energy-depleted, and depolarized neural cells (neurons and glia) that release their glutamate. Escalating levels of glutamate and aspartate stimulate specific EAA receptors that normally mediate excitatory synaptic transmission between neurons.

There are two subclasses of glutamate receptors: (1) metabotropic receptors that act by G protein and second messenger; and (2) inotropic receptors that are ligand-gated ion channels. Three ion channels are known to be activated by glutamate and are named for the pharmacologic congeners of glutamate to which they respond maximally. These ion channels are kainate receptor ($\uparrow$ Na^+ influx and K^+ efflux), adenosine monophosphate (AMP) A receptor (α-amino-3-hydroxy-5-methyl-4-isoxazole propionic acid) ($\uparrow$ Na^+ influx and K^+ efflux), and N-methyl-D-aspartate (NMDA) receptor ($\uparrow$ Na^{+}, Ca^{++}). Excessive stimulation of glutamate receptors opens ionic channels, which causes sodium-mediated cellular swelling and calcium-mediated neuronal disintegration from membrane lipid hydrolysis and protease activation.[7] Thus, overstimulated EAA receptors have been implicated as a final common pathway of neurotoxicity in numerous central nervous system problems, including traumatic injury.[8]

Free radicals disrupt the cellular membrane. Various pathophysiological processes lead to the formation of free radicals. Three free oxygen radicals, superoxide, hyperoxyl, and hydroxyl, occur with injury. Their activity varies with tissue pH and the availability of superoxide dismutase (SOD). SOD converts superoxide to hydrogen peroxide, which in turn is converted to water by catalase. Free radicals disrupt cellular membranes creating a vicious cycle of further generation of free radicals and ongoing cellular damage.[9]

The blood and breakdown products within the brain following tissue injury become another source of oxygen free radicals. Free iron from hemoglobin breakdown can transfer an electron to oxygen-forming superoxide molecules or to hydrogen peroxide to form hydroxyl. These free radicals can overwhelm cytoplasm defenses and begin to oxidize cellular membrane by *lipid peroxidation*. Through lipid peroxidation, electrons are transferred to unsaturated fatty acids, which form free radicals called lipid peroxyl or alkoxyl moieties.[10] Ongoing lipid peroxidation causes breakdown of the cellular membrane and oxidation of membrane lipoproteins. The process also spreads to adjacent cells and perpetuates cell death and edema.[11]

Research has focused on attempts to identify neuroprotective agents to ameliorate secondary injury and thus improve outcomes. Two large randomized trials have examined the free radical scavengers, tirilazad mesylate and polyethylene glycol-superoxide dismutase (PEG-SOD). Neither trial has shown an effect on reduction in mortality or improved outcome.[22] Other studies continue.

Intracranial Hemorrhage. Although hemorrhage often begins at the time of injury, there is usually a time lag between the onset of hemorrhage and the clinical presentation associated with the signs and symptoms of an intracranial expanding lesion. The hemorrhage can occur in the epidural space, resulting in an **epidural hematoma** (EDH); in the subdural space, resulting in a **subdural hematoma;** or within the brain parenchyma as an **intracerebral hematoma** or **intracerebellar hematoma**. A final classification of hemorrhage is the **burst lobe,** which is an intracerebral or intracerebellar hematoma in continuity with a related SDH.[9] All forms of hemorrhage are discussed later in this chapter.

Some hemorrhages are clinically apparent soon after injury, and others are not clinically evident for 24 hours or more even though they may have been noted on an earlier CT scan. Secondary brain injury associated with the delayed recognition of an expanding hematoma or the late development of a hematoma after 24 hours has important clinical considerations. In a study of patients who "talked but then died," the fact that they talked at all is evidence that the primary injury was not catastrophic.[23] Death resulted from a secondary expanding hematoma, a situation that might have been prevented with early diagnosis and treatment.[24] After a hematoma becomes large enough, it can cause a mass effect, an increase in ICP, and possible herniation.

Brain Swelling. Brain swelling is an increase in volume of all or part of the brain. It can occur in a localized or global pattern and can result in increased ICP, mass effect, and herniation syndromes. The cause is generally an increase in cerebral blood volume (congestive brain swelling) or an increase in water content of the brain itself (cerebral edema).[9] Chapter 14 discusses types of cerebral edema. In adults, swelling is common adjacent (localized pattern) to a contusion from direct damage to the tissue. In a direct injury, the blood-brain barrier is disrupted, normal arteriole autoregulation is lost, and vasogenic edema of the white matter occurs.[25] A global pattern of brain swelling is most often seen when an acute SDH is evacuated.[9,26] On evacuation, there is vasodilation of the involved brain tissue and a breakdown of the blood-brain barrier. The brain expands to fill the void and cerebral edema occurs. These events lead to increased ICP, mass effect, and possible herniation syndromes.

Increased ICP. Brain injury can occur secondary to increased ICP in patients who have sustained a blunt TBI. The usual causes of increased ICP in TBI are intracranial hematoma or brain swelling. The effects of increased ICP are mass effect and herniation syndromes. Increased ICP can lead to neurological deterioration and coma, resulting in a poor outcome.

Ischemic Brain Damage. Ischemic brain damage is brain injury caused by an insufficient supply of oxygen to the brain. Cerebral ischemia has a profound effect on cerebral function. Two groups of patients are more apt to sustain secondary ischemic brain damage after blunt TBI: (1) patients known to have sustained a clinical episode of hypoxia (systolic blood pressure of less than 80 mm Hg for at least 15 minutes *or* a PaO$_2$ of less than 50 mm Hg at some time postinjury); and (2) patients who have experienced a high ICP.[9] Ischemic brain injury, a cause of coma, is related to vegetative state and poor outcomes after TBI.

PRIMARY INJURY: BLUNT TRAUMATIC BRAIN INJURY

Scalp Lacerations

The scalp is composed of five layers covering the bone of the top of the skull (calvarium):

- **Dermal (skin) layer**: has hair and protects the scalp from injury.
- **Subcutaneous fascia**: a tough fibrotic tissue with a vascular fatty layer that can bleed profusely when the scalp is lacerated.
- **Galea aponeurotica**: a sheet-like tendon layer that connects the frontalis and occipitalis muscles.
- **Subgaleal areolar space**: below the galea is the subgaleal space that contains emissary veins that empty into the venous sinus. It is a potential area for the development of a hematoma. If an infection develops in this space, it can spread to the brain.
- **Periosteum**: located below the subgaleal space, is a very thin layer of tissue that can be stripped away from the skull.

The velocity and characteristics of the impacting contact object determine the extent of scalp injury. Injuries to the scalp can be classified as follows:

- **Abrasion**: The top layer of the scalp is scraped away; this is a minor injury that may cause slight bleeding. The area is cleaned and possibly dressed, and no other treatment is required.
- **Contusion**: The scalp is bruised with possible effusion of blood into the subcutaneous layer without a break in the integrity of the skin; there is no specific treatment.
- **Laceration**: The scalp is torn and may bleed profusely; suturing may be necessary.
- **Subgaleal hematoma**: A hematoma in the subgaleal layer of the scalp occurs and will usually absorb on its own.

Skull Fractures

The skull is the bony framework of the head. The **cranium (calvarium)** is that part of the skull that encloses the brain; it is composed of the frontal, parietal, temporal, occipital, sphenoid, and ethmoid bones. Although not part of the cranium, the **facial bones** provide a framework for the face and include the maxillary, zygomatic, nasal, lacrimal, and palatine bones and the inferior nasal concha, vomer, mandible, and part of the ethmoid and sphenoid bones (see Fig. 5-5). The mandible is the only movable bone in the facial portion of the skull. Facial bones can be fractured during TBI, especially with vehicular occupants who are not wearing seatbelts.

The mechanism of skull injury is direct contact. Factors that determine the degree of injury include the skull's thickness at the point of impact and the weight, velocity, and angle of impact of the intruding object. At impact, several actions are set in motion in split-second sequence. At the point of impact, there is a relative indentation that may be temporary or permanent, depending on velocity. Stress waves are set into motion, radiating throughout the entire skull. With *high-velocity impact*, a depressed skull fracture with or without a dual tear and cerebral laceration can occur. With *low-velocity impact*, the area of indentation rebounds outward and may result in no fracture, a linear fracture, or comminuted fracture (see Fig. 18-2). The fracture line extends from the point of impact and is directed by bony buttresses toward the base of the skull.

Classification

Skull fractures are classified as follows:

- **Linear**: a singular fracture line occurring to the skull
- **Comminuted**: the skull is splintered or shattered into pieces
- **Depressed**: a fracture of the skull in which a fragment is depressed; the scalp and/or dura may or may not be torn
- **Open depressed fracture**: an opening of the skull as a result of comminuted depressed skull fractures and tearing of the dura mater and the scalp
- **Basal skull fracture**: a fracture involving the base of the skull that may be a linear or a depressed fracture

Basal Skull Fracture. A basal skull fracture often arises from extension of a linear fracture into the base of the skull. The frontal and temporal bones are usually affected so that the fracture involves the anterior or middle fossae. It is important to distinguish between fractures of the cranial vault and those of the base of the skull. Although the mechanism by which the fractures arise is similar, the consequences of basilar fractures are more serious than those of cranial vault fractures. A feature of basal skull fractures is the frequency with which they traverse the paranasal air sinuses (frontal, maxillary, or ethmoid) of the frontal bone or the air sinuses located in the petrous portion of the temporal bone. The fragility of the bones in these areas and the intimate adherence of delicate dura account for the frequency of lesions in these areas and the consequent leakage of cerebrospinal fluid (CSF) through the dural tear.

Drainage of CSF from the nose is called **rhinorrhea,** whereas drainage of CSF from the ear is called **otorrhea.** When CSF drains from the paranasal sinuses, it drains into the postnasal area and is felt as a postnasal drip. The appearance of blood encircled by a yellowish stain on the dressing or bed linen is called the **halo sign** and is highly suggestive of blood encircled by CSF. Continued leakage of CSF can lead to serious infection-related complications. Such patients are at high risk for meningitis, abscess formation, and osteomyelitis from organisms gaining entry by way of the ear, nose, or paranasal sinuses through the dural tear.

Two additional categories of complications associated with basal skull fractures deserve mention. The *first* is cerebrovascular injury, including injury to the internal carotid artery injury at the point of entrance to the cranial vault through the foramen at the base of the skull. Fracture in or around the foramen can result in cerebral hemorrhage from laceration, thrombosis, development of a traumatic aneurysm, a carotid-cavernous sinus fistula, or carotid-cavernous sinus compression. A *carotid-cavernous sinus fistula* is characterized by chemosis, bruit, and pulsating exophthalmos. The oculomotor, trochlear, trigeminal, and abducens cranial nerves pass through the cavernous sinus. Compression of the sinus may be evident because of ophthalmoplegia or trigeminal dysfunction.

The *second* potential complication is trapping portions of the frontal arachnoid and dura between the fracture edges, thus creating a permanent route for leakage of CSF. Radiographic and surgical identification of the exact area of the dural tear is extremely difficult, yet such identification is necessary to facilitate surgical repair.

Meningeal Tears

A tear of the dura mater can result from a basal skull fracture, depressed fracture involving the temporal or frontal bones, or some facial fractures. As a result of a dural tear, CSF may leak from the ear, the nose, or postnasally. There may also be blood behind the tympanic membrane (hemotympanum).

Traumatic Brain Injuries

Injuries to the brain can be focal or diffuse. *Focal injuries* include contusion, lacerations, and ICHs. Concussions and diffuse axonal injuries are the major *diffuse injuries.*

Focal Cerebral Injuries: Contusions, Lacerations, and Hematomas

Contusions and Lacerations. The following anatomical considerations help to explain focal injuries to the brain.

The anterior and middle fossae at the base of the skull have irregular, bony buttresses that are capable of contusing or lacerating the brain on impact. The distribution of *contusions* in these particular areas is explained by the movement of the brain within the skull (Fig. 18-4). The frontal and temporal poles are vulnerable because of the relative restraint created by the sphenoidal ridges and other bony irregularities of the base of the skull. Less common sites of

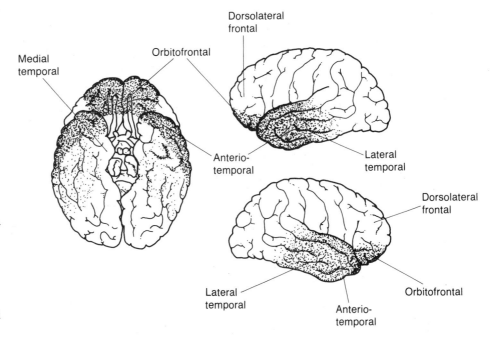

Figure 18-4 • Cerebral contusions. The most frequently involved areas of the brain in cerebral contusions are the orbitofrontal and anterior-temporal regions. These are the areas that come in direct contact with the irregular bony surfaces in the inside frontal skull area.

injury are the inferolateral angles of the occipital lobes, the medial surfaces of the hemispheres, and the corpus callosum. The firm falx cerebri and tentorium cerebelli not only restrict movement of the brain, but also contribute to contusion or laceration during impact as cerebral tissue impacts on these hard surfaces. This is particularly true when the rotational force of acceleration-deceleration is applied to the frontal-temporal area. Injury to the inferolateral angles of the occipital lobe and, less commonly, the inferior surface of the cerebellar and cerebral peduncles can result from impact by the tentorium. A blow to the vertex of the head may cause cerebellar, cerebellar-tonsillar, and brain-stem contusions initiated by the downward thrust of the brain toward the foramen magnum.

A **cerebral contusion** is a bruising of the surface of the brain (cerebral parenchyma). Contusions may occur from blunt trauma (direct contact), a depressed skull fracture, a penetrating wound, or an acceleration-deceleration closed injury. With acceleration-deceleration, the sites of injury are generally predictable and are located where the brain has an impact on the bony protuberances within the skull (see Fig. 18-4). These areas include the frontal poles, frontal-orbital areas, the frontal-temporal junction around the Sylvian fissure (where the brain is close to the lesser sphenoidal wings), and the temporal poles (the inferior and lateral surfaces of the temporal lobes where there is a shelf-like separation between the anterior and middle fossae).

The clinical effect of a contusion depends on its size and related cerebral edema. Small, unilateral, frontal lesions may be asymptomatic, whereas larger lesions may result in a frontal lobe syndrome of inappropriate behavior and cognitive deficits. Contusions can cause secondary mass effect from edema resulting in increased ICP, and possible herniation syndromes.

Classification. The categories of contusions include the following:[9]

- **Fracture contusions** occur at the sites of fractures and are particularly severe in the frontal lobes when associated with fractures in the anterior fossa.
- **Coup contusions** are found directly under the areas of impact (contact).
- **Contrecoup contusions**, by contrast, are cerebral injuries at the opposite pole of direct contact. A contrecoup injury is most often a contusion, but occasionally it may be a laceration. Both coup and contrecoup injuries are caused by the rapid acceleration-deceleration of the semisolid brain within the rigid cranial vault.
- **Herniation contusions** occur at the time of injury at the point of contact where the medial part of the temporal lobe produces an impact at the edge of the tentorium or the cerebellar tonsils against the foramen magnum.

One final distinction is made between *surface contusions* and gliding contusions. **Gliding contusions**, common with diffuse axonal injuries, are focal hemorrhages in the cortex and adjacent white matter or the superior margins of the cerebral hemispheres.

A **cerebral laceration** refers to a traumatic tearing of the cortical surface of the brain. The difference between a contusion and laceration is that the pia-arachnoid is intact over a contusion but torn over a laceration.[9] Both contusions and lacerations are surface injuries.

Intracranial Hemorrhage. Traumatic intracranial hemorrhage is a common complication of TBI. Although bleeding may begin immediately after injury, its presence may not be clinically apparent until sufficient blood accumulates to cause signs and symptoms of a space-occupying lesion and mass effect. The interval between bleeding and the appearance of clinical symptoms may be minutes or weeks, depending on the site and rate of bleeding. Intracranial hemorrhage may be an occult development in a patient who has sustained a seemingly minor TBI in which consciousness has been maintained or quickly restored. Other patients with hemorrhage may be unconscious from the moment of impact.

The major types of bleeding associated with head trauma are EDH, SDH, and ICH. Each lesion is a distinct clinical entity, but two or more types of hemorrhagic lesions can coexist.

Epidural Hematoma. An **EDH**, also known as an extradural hematoma, refers to bleeding into the potential space between the inner table of the skull (inner periosteum) and the dura mater (Fig. 18-5A).

Most (85%) EDHs are arterial in origin, occurring from a tear of a branch of the middle meningeal artery in a patient who has sustained a skull fracture to the thin, squamous portion of the temporal bone, under which is located the middle meningeal artery. The hematoma is therefore located in the temporal-parietal region. Occasionally an EDH may be venous, the result of torn dural venous sinuses particularly in the parieto-occipital region or posterior fossa. As the hematoma enlarges, it gradually strips away the dura from the inner table of the skull, and a large, ovoid mass develops, creating pressure on the underlying brain and causing a mass effect. EDHs are seen most often in children and young people because their dura is less firmly attached to the bone table than it is in older people. EDHs are relatively uncommon and account for about 0.5% to 6% of posttraumatic intracranial lesions.

Clinically, the "classic" description of an EDH was that of momentary unconsciousness followed by a lucid period lasting for minutes to several hours. The lucid period was followed by rapid deterioration in the level of consciousness (LOC) from drowsiness, to lethargy, and to coma as a mass effect and herniation developed. Other findings included pupillary signs (ipsilateral dilated, sluggish, fixed), headache, possible seizures, hemiparesis or hemiplegia, decortication or decerebration, respiratory distress, and death. *Few patients follow this profile.* The most common presentation is headache, vomiting, seizures, unilateral hyperreflexia with a positive Babinski sign, and elevated CSF pressure.[27] In 60% of patients, a unilateral dilated ipsilateral pupil is found. The same percentage of patients have no initial loss of consciousness. After the LOC begins to deteriorate, coma occurs rapidly. Bradycardia and respiratory distress are late findings.

Subdural Hematoma. SDH refers to bleeding between the dura mater and arachnoid or pial layer (see Fig. 18-5B). Approximately 30% of patients with post-traumatic intracranial le-

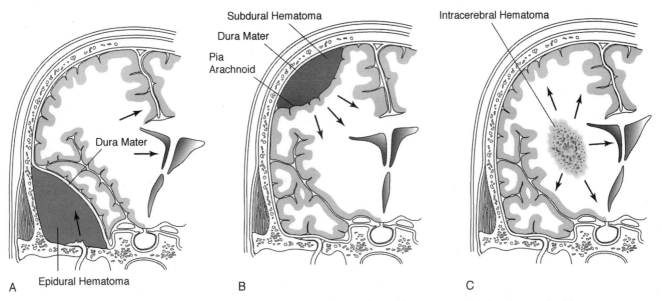

Figure 18–5 • Cerebral hematomas: (A) an epidural hematoma, (B) a subdural hemotoma, and (C) an intracerebral hematoma.

sions have SDHs. Most SDHs are caused by tearing of the bridging veins located over the convexity of the brain. Other causes include tearing of small cortical arteries, cerebral contusions, and acute bleeding into chronic SDHs. Bilateral SDHs are not uncommon. SDHs are categorized based on the interval between injury and the appearance of signs and symptoms. Although there are no uniform definitions, three classes with approximate time intervals are recognized:

- *Acute:* Up to 48 hours. This consists of clotted blood that is hypodense on computed tomography (CT).
- *Subacute:* 2 days to about 2 to 3 weeks. The clot now lyses, and blood products and fluid are present.
- *Chronic:* Longer than 3 weeks to several months. The clot is a fluid mass and is hypodense on CT.

SDHs are also classified according to appearance of blood and fluid composition. The *acute* SDH is composed of clotted blood, the *subacute* is a mixture of clotted and fluid blood, and the *chronic* is composed of fluid only.[28]

Common signs and symptoms associated with an *acute SDH* include gradual or rapid deterioration of the LOC from drowsiness, slow cerebration, and confusion to coma; pupillary changes; and hemiparesis or hemiplegia. *Subacute SDHs* are associated with less severe underlying contusions. Failure of a patient to regain consciousness raises the suspicion of an SDH. Signs and symptoms of subacute SDHs correspond closely to those of the acute SDH.

Chronic SDHs can develop from seemingly minor TBIs. The time elapsed between injury and the development of symptoms may be months, so the initial injury itself may not be recalled. The lesion becomes encased within a membrane that is easily separated from the arachnoid and dura. The SDH slowly enlarges, probably because of repeated small bleeding, until a mass effect occurs. The most common symptoms of a chronic SDH include headache (progressing in severity), slow cerebration, confusion, drowsiness, and possibly seizure. Papilledema, sluggish ipsilateral pupillary response, and finally hemiparesis may develop.

Elderly patients with cerebral atrophy associated with the normal aging process are prone to develop SDHs because of traction on fragile bridging veins. This is particularly true with tear and rupture in the elderly with cerebral trauma. Atrophy also provides more free space into which bleeding can occur before symptoms are evident from a mass effect. With chronic SDHs, the development of symptoms can be subtle because of gradual spatial compensation. Patients who have had long term alcohol abuse with related cerebral atrophy and impaired blood clotting resulting from deteriorated liver function, are also especially prone to SDHs.

Intracerebral Hemorrhage. An ICH refers to bleeding into the cerebral parenchyma, a complication seen in 4% to 15% of brain-injured patients[27] (see Fig. 18-5C). Most ICHs are related to contusions and therefore tend to be found in the frontal and temporal lobes. They occur through the same mechanisms as contusions. Clinically, ICHs behave as expanding, space-occupying lesions. Serial CT scanning has demonstrated delayed traumatic ICHs in about 1% to 7% of patients. **Delayed traumatic ICHs** occur hours to days after TBI following an interval during which no hematoma is present.[28] Although the pathogenesis of these lesions is uncertain, bleeding into existing traumatized areas, such as a contusion, is generally accepted. ICHs are associated with poor outcomes and increased mortality. Signs and symptoms of ICH include headache, deteriorating consciousness progressing to deep coma, hemiplegia on the contralateral side, and a dilated ipsilateral pupil. As ICP increases, there is evidence of developing transtentorial herniation.

Other Focal Bleeding: Subarachnoid/Intraventricular Hemorrhages and Torn Blood Vessels. A traumatic subarachnoid hematoma may be found with severe TBI. Intraventricular hemorrhage occurs secondary to subarachnoid hemorrhage or as an extension from an ICH. Signs and symptoms are related to increased ICP and irritation of the meninges. Nuchal rigidity, an ipsilateral dilated pupil, a deteriorating LOC, hemiparesis or hemiplegia, and abnormal posturing are the signs commonly seen.

Injury to and tears of cerebral blood vessels can cause vasospasm, resulting in focal ischemia. Subsequent to an intracranial hematoma, vessels can also be compressed by the traumatic mass or by localized cerebral edema. In addition, cerebral blood vessels may become thrombosed or occluded, or a traumatic aneurysm may develop when vessels are stretched or torn at the time of injury.

Diffuse Cerebral Injuries: Concussions and Diffuse Axonal Injuries

Concussions. The word **concussion** means a violent shaking. A **cerebral concussion** is defined as a transient, temporary, neurogenic dysfunction caused by mechanical force to the brain. Signs and symptoms may include immediate unconsciousness lasting a few seconds, minutes, or hours; momentary loss of reflexes; and momentary (few seconds) and possible retrograde or antegrade amnesia (loss of memory for events immediately before and after the injury, respectively). Other common signs and symptoms include headache, drowsiness, confusion, dizziness, irritability, giddiness, visual disturbances (seeing stars), and gait disturbances.

Acceleration-deceleration (with shearing stress on the reticular formation) is the mechanism of injury. Patients who have sustained other TBIs, such as contusions, lacerations, and hematomas, have also sustained a concussion in most instances. Concussions are classified as mild or classic, based on the degree of symptoms, particularly those of unconsciousness and memory loss. **Mild concussion** is defined as temporary neurological dysfunction without loss of consciousness or memory. By contrast, a **classic concussion** includes temporary neurological dysfunction, unconsciousness, and memory loss. Recovery of consciousness usually takes minutes to hours. Some patients will develop a postconcussion syndrome (described later in this section).

Diffuse Axonal Injury. Diffuse axonal injury (DAI) is a primary TBI associated with acceleration-deceleration during which shearing forces damage nerve fibers at the moment of injury (Fig. 18-6). Because of the difference in acceleration gradient on certain areas of the brain during primary impact, shearing forces at the white-gray junction, corpus callosum, brain stem, and sometimes cerebellum produce diffuse tearing of axons and small blood vessels.[29,30] DAI accounts for approximately 50% of primary brain injuries and 35% of deaths from all TBI.[9,31] It is characterized by distinct gross and microscopic findings including axonal swellings that are widely distributed in the cerebral hemispheric white matter, corpus collasum, and upper brain stem; gross hemorrhagic lesions of the corpus callosum; and gross hemorrhagic lesions involving one or both dorsolateral quadrants of the rostral brain stem.[32]

A grading system based on the distribution of *pathological findings* includes:[32]

- **DAI Grade 1:** histological evidence of axonal damage in the white matter of the cerebral hemispheres, corpus callosum, brain stem, and less commonly cerebellum.
- **DAI Grade 2:** in addition to evidence of axonal injury, there are also focal lesions of the corpus callosum.
- **DAI Grade 3:** in addition to findings of grades 1 and 2, there are lesions of the dorsolateral quadrant of the rostral brain stem.

Substantial recent research has increased our understanding of DAI. Diffuse injury to axons, which are apparent microscopically throughout the white matter of the cerebral hemispheres, the cerebellum, and the brainstem, has three presentation forms related to the length of the patient's survival.[9] In short-term survival (days), there are a large

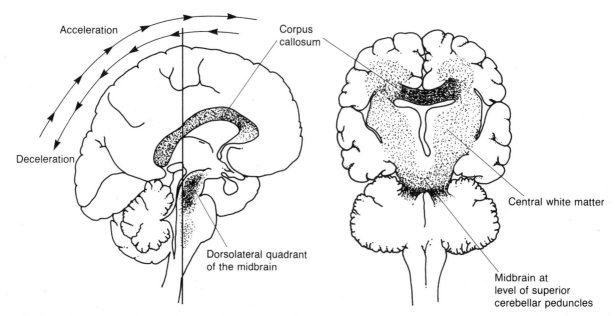

Figure 18-6 • Diffuse axonal injury. Diffuse axonal injury results from acceleration-deceleration and shearing force on the brain. Depending on the severity of the injury, the areas of the brain most often affected are the corpus callosum, the dorsolateral area of the midbrain, and the parasagittal white matter.

number of axonal bulbs throughout the white matter. It takes about 15 to 18 hours for the axonal bulbs to appear in humans.[33] In intermediate survival (weeks), there are large numbers of microglia clusters throughout the white matter. In long-term survival (e.g., vegetative state), there is long tract degeneration of the wallerian type in these areas. In these survivors, the degenerative effects are finally replaced by diffuse white matter gliosis. Gliosis is the chief finding in long-term survivors and is related to severe and permanent disabilities.[34,35]

Clinically, DAI is characterized by a sequence of events beginning with immediate unconsciousness, leading to a longer period of confusion and associated post-traumatic amnesia, and followed by a prolonged recovery period. The immediate coma is found without accompanying intracranial mass lesions. DAI can be classified clinically as mild, moderate, or severe based on coma duration and brainstem signs.[36,37]

- **Mild DAI:** coma lasting 6 to 24 hours with the patient beginning to follow commands by 24 hours. Outcome: death is uncommon, but cognitive and neurological deficits are common.
- **Moderate DAI:** coma lasting longer than 24 hours, but without prominent brainstem signs. This is a common presentation (about 45% of all patients). Outcome: incomplete recovery in those who survive.
- **Severe DAI:** coma is prolonged and associated with prominent brainstem signs (e.g., decortication, decerebration). This presentation is seen in about 36% of all DAI patients. Outcome: death or severe disability.

Penetrating Injuries

Brain Injuries Caused by Gunshots and Impalement

Gunshot wounds to the head are responsible for most penetrating brain injuries, and they account for approximately 35% of deaths from brain injury in people younger than 45 years of age.[38] The wound created by the bullet depends on ballistics, that is, the size, shape, velocity, and direction of the bullet. As the bullet propels forward and penetrates the skull, it compresses the air in front of it, thereby increasing the destruction of brain tissue locally and remotely.[39] Missile injuries are classified as follows:

- **Tangential injuries,** in which the missile does not enter the cranial cavity but produces a scalp laceration, facial injury, comminuted skull fracture, meningeal tear, or cerebral contusion-laceration.
- **Penetrating injuries,** in which the missile enters the cranial cavity but does not pass through it, resulting in the presence of metal, bone fragments, hair, and skin within the brain. There is direct injury to cerebral tissue in the path of the bullet as well as injury to tissue from the high-pressure waves created by the high velocity bullet. This high pressure can cause coup and contrecoup injuries, spikes in ICP, and herniation.
- **Through-and-through injuries,** in which the missile perforates the cranial contents and leaves through an exit wound. Possible cerebral injuries are the same as for penetrating injuries. There is one tract created from a missile entering the brain, although several tracts are possible intracranially if the bullet ricochets off bony structures within the cranial vault.

The major effects of missile injuries are cerebral contusions and lacerations, focal tissue necrosis, hemorrhage from tearing of blood vessels, and focal or generalized cerebral edema. Hemorrhage and edema may produce increased ICP and possible herniation associated with rapid expansion during impact and in response to a space-occupying lesion. The severity of injury sustained depends on the structures involved and herniation. Cerebral abscesses are postinjury concerns because of the microorganisms that have been carried into the brain from surface debris of skin, hair, and bone fragments. Other late complications include traumatic aneurysms, seizures, and fragment migration.[27]

Summary

The major types of primary TBI have been discussed. There is still much to be learned about these injuries and the effect on the brain. Evidence-based practice and best practice continues to evolve as more is learned about the mechanical and biochemical effects of TBI. In the next section of this chapter, diagnosis and treatment of primary TBI are discussed.

DIAGNOSIS AND TREATMENT

This section addresses the diagnosis and treatment of traumatic scalp, skull, and brain injuries.

Scalp Lacerations

Scalp injury is diagnosed by physical inspection. Abrasions require no specific treatment. A scalp contusion may benefit from the application of ice initially to prevent a hematoma from forming. Skull films may be ordered to rule out a skull fracture. Depending on other signs and symptoms, a CT scan rather than a skull film may be ordered, to rule out underlying skull or brain injury.

All scalp lacerations are irrigated with saline and explored with a sterile gloved finger to determine whether a fracture or a foreign body is present. Severely contused tissue may need to be debrided. The subgaleal area is examined for evidence of a hematoma. Small fractures are not always seen on radiographic studies but may be found by visualization and palpation. Evidence of bone fragments or a depressed skull fracture warrants surgical exploration. Scalp lacerations often require suturing and aseptic management.

Skull Fractures

A plain CT of the brain or plain skull films are used to diagnose a skull fracture. The ease with which a diagnosis of skull fracture is made depends on the site of the fracture. If a fracture is found on x-ray, there is always the question of associated brain injury and the need for a plain CT. Most basal skull fractures are extensions of fractures of the cranial vault. CT is often poor for directly demonstrating a basal skull fracture. Plain skull films and clinical criteria are usually more sensitive.[27] For example, a linear fracture of the parietal bone may be readily evident on a plain x-ray, whereas thin-slice CT may be necessary to find a basal skull fracture. If the paranasal sinuses are fractured, air may be evident in the frontal and maxillary sinuses on x-ray studies. With fracture of the temporal bone, the mastoid sinuses may be opaque. Common findings of **anterior fossa fractures** (fractures of the paranasal sinuses) include the following:

- Rhinorrhea (drainage of CSF, blood, or both from the nose)
- Subconjunctival hemorrhage of the eye
- Periorbital ecchymosis (raccoon's eyes)

With **middle fossa fractures** (fractures associated with fracture of the temporal petrous bone) common findings include:

- Otorrhea (drainage of CSF, blood, or both from the ear)
- Hemotympanum (blood behind the tympanic membrane)
- Battle's sign (ecchymosis over mastoid bone that develops for 12 to 24 hours after injury)
- Conductive hearing loss (may be associated with signs of vestibular dysfunction, such as vertigo, nausea, and nystagmus)
- Possibly facial nerve palsy (Bell's palsy) that appears 5 to 7 days after injury

Treatment of skull fractures depends on the type of fracture. Generally, linear skull fractures do not require special medical management other than observation for underlying cerebral injury. A depressed skull fracture with an open scalp, skull, and dura mater requires surgery to debride, elevate, and remove bone fragments from the wound. If the fragments are extensive, a craniectomy may be necessary. For cosmetic and brain protective purposes, a cranioplasty with insertion of a bone or artificial graft may follow immediately or be postponed for a few months (approximately 3 to 6 months) if brain swelling is present.

Use of prophylactic antibiotics with basal skull fractures is controversial; many argue that prophylactic use allows for proliferation of other virulent organisms. Most CSF leaks resolve spontaneously within 7 to 10 days. To aid resolution of leakage lasting more than 4 to 5 days, a lumbar catheter for continual drainage of CSF may be inserted.[40] If leakage of CSF continues, a craniotomy may be necessary to repair the tear surgically or to repair the leakage with grafts.

Traumatic Brain Injuries

In all cases, the diagnosis of TBI (contusion, laceration, and hematoma) is made with a noncontrast CT scan. In some cases, a contrast CT or magnetic resonance image (MRI) may be requested after a noncontrast CT scan, but neither a contrast CT nor MRI is required on an emergency basis. The major emergency conditions to rule out with CT are hemorrhage or hematoma, cerebral edema, and cerebral anoxia (i.e., loss of gray-white matter interface, midline shift, pneumocephalus, or hydrocephalus).[27] In severe TBI, a follow-up CT is often ordered 3 to 5 days post injury or as necessary to follow progress.

Recent bleeding appears as bright white on noncontrast CT scan. The scan also demonstrates differences in appearance of hematoma. An *EDH* most often appears as a high-density biconvex (lens)—shaped object adjacent to the skull. An *acute SDH* appears as a crescent mass of increased brightness adjacent to the inner table of bone. With *chronic SDHs*, a membrane forms around the blood, which is now dark, thick fluid. Bilateral chronic SDHs are present 25% of the time, so careful review of films for bilateral hematomas is necessary.

Treatment of hematoma depends on the type, size, and effect (e.g., increased ICP, mass effect) of the lesion on the brain. Bur holes are primarily a diagnostic tool. Most acute hematomas are composed of congealed blood that is too thick to be removed through a bur hole.[27] Surgical evacuation of a hematoma is generally through a craniotomy. In the case of intracerebral hematoma, surgical evacuation remains very controversial. Most patients are managed medically unless there is significant mass effect. Poor outcomes are associated with surgical evacuation of intracerebral hematomas.

Contusions and Lacerations. For patients with a cerebral contusion or laceration, no surgical intervention is indicated and patients are managed medically. Cerebral edema, elevation of ICP, and possible herniation can occur and require treatment. Depending on the degree of injury and location of a contusion or laceration, some patients have an uneventful recovery, whereas others develop post-traumatic seizures or functional deficits.

Hematomas. Small hematomas may reabsorb without surgical intervention. Larger lesions often cause mass effect and increased ICP, threatening herniation, which requires a craniotomy for evacuation. Most EDHs require surgery because bleeding is usually arterial and deterioration is rapid. The rapidly expanding lesion is treated as a neurosurgical emergency with a craniotomy.[30] All SDHs accompanied by signs and symptoms require surgical evacuation. The elderly and people with long-term alcohol abuse, who have had a chronic SDH evacuation, tend to rebleed after surgical evacuation and need careful observation.

Intracerebral Hemorrhage. As is true with EDH and SDH, the size of the ICH determines the best treatment approach. Considerable controversy exists regarding the indications for surgery in ICH. This is a complex decision based on the patient's neurological condition, size and location of the hematoma, patient's age, and patient/family wishes. Surgery rarely improves neurological outcome.[27] As a result, many patients are managed medically with supportive care and management of increased ICP.

Subarachnoid and Intraventricular Hemorrhages. Treatment includes drainage of CSF with a ventriculostomy.

Concussions. The diagnosis of concussion is based on the patient's history, neurological examination, and absence of any focal lesion on a CT scan, if a CT scan is done. The patient is supported and observed to ensure that no other focal lesion, such as an SDH, has been overlooked. Depending on the severity of the concussion, a short-stay admission may be chosen to observe for other developing lesions. In other cases, a patient may be discharged home with verbal and written instructions about what signs and symptoms to look for and report immediately to the physician.

Diffuse Axonal Injury. Clinical diagnosis of DAI is based on immediate onset of unconsciousness in a patient who has significant cerebral trauma and no intracranial lesion by CT scan. In some cases, an MRI may demonstrate small lesions not evident on CT.

Treatment is supportive care provided for an unconscious patient who has sustained TBI. This is discussed further later in the chapter.

Gunshot Injuries. The history and evidence of entrance and possible exit gunshot wounds indicate injury. A CT scan determines amount of injury, identifies bone fragments and the site of bullets not exiting, and determines the surgical approach if contemplated. Emergency surgical intervention is common for salvageable patients to evacuate hematomas, such as EDH or SDH; to debride the wound and remove the bullet and necrotic tissue; and to treat other system injuries caused by bullets or trauma. Secondary brain injury can result from hypoxia and hypotension related to hemorrhage in other body systems. Survivors usually require ICU management for intracranial hypertension and systems complications associated with severe TBI as well of injuries to other body systems.

OTHER INJURIES RELATED TO TRAUMATIC BRAIN INJURY

Facial Fractures

Facial fracture is common with vehicular trauma, especially if the patient was a driver or passenger who was not using a seatbelt. Injuries may involve the soft tissue (contusions, lacerations), the facial bones (fractures), or both. The facial bones include most of the paranasal sinuses and the primary receptor organs for the senses of vision, hearing, taste, and smell. Facial injuries can result in disfigurement, motor and sensory dysfunction, and deficits in communication. Table 18-1 summarizes common facial fractures.

Cranial Nerve Injuries Associated With Skull Fractures

Specific cranial nerves tend to be compressed or injured because of anatomical location, transection, and attachments. *Frontal bone fractures* are associated with olfactory nerve (most vulnerable) and sometimes optic nerve injury. Cribriform plate fractures often produce anosmia because of

injury of the olfactory nerve. Orbital plate fractures may affect the optic and oculomotor nerves, resulting in loss of vision and impaired eye movement. The orbits are created by the fusion of many bones. Any of these bones may become fractured in a TBI. Isolated lesions of the trochlear or abducens nerves are rare. *Temporal bone fractures* often result in facial nerve paralysis, the most commonly injured motor cranial nerve. Auditory nerve dysfunction of the cochlear or vestibular branches is seen with less frequency.

Treatment

Many facial fractures require surgical repair and reconstruction for cosmetic effects. A series of surgical procedures may be necessary to achieve the desired outcome. Timing of surgery depends on stabilization and management of other higher priority needs. Some studies have shown that early craniofacial repair can be performed safely with appropriate general surgical and neurosurgical support in selected patients, thus avoiding costly delay and complications.[41]

MANAGEMENT OF THE TBI PATIENT: THE CONTINUUM OF CARE

A landmark contribution to TBI literature was made in 1996 with the publication of the *Guidelines for the Management of Severe Brain Injury*.[42] These guidelines are based on a stringent review of the scientific basis for management of TBI and set forth guidelines. It was recognized that updating and expanding the document would be an ongoing process, and in 2000 *Guidelines for the Management of Severe Traumatic Brain Injury* was published.[43] Laboratory and clinical research has remarkably increased our understanding of the pathophysiology of neurological damage that occurs not only at the moment of impact, but also over the following hours and days. This delayed evolution of brain injury occurs at both the clinical and biochemical levels.[43] An understanding of these processes has led to management strategies that can positively affect patient outcomes, so that evidence-based care can be directed not only at treatment of immediate injuries but also at prevention of secondary brain injury.

The recent *Guidelines*[43] define evidence-based care and best practices for severe TBI and are the foundation for the care discussed in this chapter. The methodology used to develop the Guidelines began with a thorough review of the evidence, followed by a classification into one of three categories:

- **Class I evidence:** prospective randomized controlled trials
- **Class II evidence:** prospective clinical studies (e.g., observational, cohort, or prevalence studies)
- **Class III evidence:** studies based on retrospectively collected data (e.g., registries, case review)

The overall degree of certainty of the evidence was further evaluated. As a result, the following three categories of recommendations were developed:

Table 18–1 • COMMON FACIAL FRACTURES

BONE	FRACTURE	SIGNS AND SYMPTOMS
Mandible • Only movable bone of the face • Composed of lower jaw and ramus • Lower jaw or chin, portion that contains the teeth • Ramus portion vertical with condyloid processes that fit into the temporomandibular joint	• Most frequently fractured facial bone • Because of its arched shape, fractures common in two places	• Malalignment of the teeth • Pain • Bruising and laceration over the fracture site • Ecchymosis in floor of the mouth • Palpation of a "shelf" defect in the inferior border • Inability to palpate condylar movement when the little finger is placed in the external ear canal and the jaw is opened

Maxilla
• Holds upper teeth
• Includes the palate
• Forms a portion of the floor of the orbits
• Forms part of floor and outer wall of the nasal fossa
• Meets temporal and zygoma bones laterally
• Contains maxillary sinus
	• Involved in midface fractures (involves the maxillae, nasoorbital bones, and the zygomatic bones)
	• Midface fractures classified using the system devised by René Le Fort:
	  Le Fort I fracture: horizontal detachment of the maxilla at the nasal floor; leaves maxillary alveolar ridge of the hard palate mobile
	  Le Fort II fracture: pyramid-shaped fracture of the central part of the face; includes transverse fractures across the medial maxillae and nasal bones, medial half of the infraorbital rim, and the medial part of the orbit and orbital floor
	  Le Fort III fracture: separates the cranial and facial bones; includes a Le Fort II fracture along with fractures of both zygomatic bones so that the fracture line cuts through both orbits transversely
		Midface fractures
		• Distortion of facial symmetry (elongated face, flattened nasoorbital area)
		• Possible pushing of the upper and lower molar teeth together
		• Inability to close jaw
		• Pain
		• Edema
		• Ecchymosis of buccal mucosa in the lateral portions
		• Abnormal movement (free-floating maxillary segment)
		• Possible respiratory obstruction
		• Hemorrhage

Zygoma • Forms the prominence of cheekbone • Forms part of outer wall and floor of orbit • Part of temporal and zygomatic fossa	• Often involved in midface fractures • Fractures of the zygoma often called tripod fractures because of their shape • Fracture of the zygoma always involves the orbits	• Flatness of the cheek • Loss of sensation on the side of the face of the fracture • Diplopia • Ophthalmoplegia
Nasal • Forms bridge of nose • Forms part of upper inner orbit	• May occur alone or in conjunction with orbital or Le Fort fractures	• Ecchymosis and edema of the dorsum of the nose • Nosebleed • Laceration
Orbital • Seven facial and cranial bones that form the orbits (frontal, maxillary, zygomatic, lacrimal, sphenoid, ethmoid, and palatine)	• Fracture as Le Fort fractures or, less frequently, as orbital blow-out fracture • Blow-out fractures, result from spike in intraorbital pressure caused by a blunt object (fist, baseball) directed at the globe; spike in pressure, fracture at the weakest point—the orbital floor or medial wall; the orbital contents may protrude into the maxillary sinus	*Blow-out fractures* • Sinking of globe • Diplopia (secondary to injury of the extraocular muscles) • Ophthalmoplegia • Possible blindness (secondary to detached retina) • Edema • Ecchymosis of the eyelid • Conjunctival hemorrhage • Paresthesia

(Data from Bertz, J. [1981]. Maxillofacial injuries. *Clinical Symposia 33*[4], 1–32; Black, J., & Arnold, P. G. [1982]. Facial fractures. *American Journal of Nursing, 82*[7], 1086; and Lower, J. [1986]. Maxillofacial trauma. *Nursing Clinics of North America, 21*[4], 611–28.)

- **Standards:** represent principles of patient management that reflect a *high* degree of clinical certainty (strong Class I evidence)
- **Guidelines:** represent a particular strategy or range of management strategies that reflect a *moderate* clinical certainty (mostly Class II evidence)
- **Options:** include the remaining strategies for patient management based on *unclear* clinical certainty (Class III evidence)

The *Guidelines for the Management of Severe Traumatic Brain Injury* is an important resource and should be consulted for a more thorough discussion of the methodology, grading of evidence, degree of certainty, and literature reviewed.

The continuum of care begins at the trauma scene and continues throughout the various levels and settings of care. Continuity between settings and transitions is critical for obtaining optimal, cost-effective patient outcomes. This section addresses the essential components along the continuum and the evidence-based care needed to support optimal outcomes along the continuum.

Trauma Systems and Prehospital Management

All regions of the country should have an organized trauma care system in place. *The American College of Surgeons Committee on Trauma Resources for Optimal Care of the Injured Patient: 1999* has determined that neurosurgeons should have an organized and responsive system of care for patients with neurotrauma. This system should include planning of care, prehospital management and triage, direct trauma center transport, maintaining appropriate call schedules, reviewing trauma care records for quality improvement, and participating in trauma education programs.[44] Based on case reports and before-and-after comparison studies, mortality is reduced after major trauma in patients treated in an organized trauma system.[43]

Prehospital management refers to the initial resuscitation and interventions to stabilize the patient at the injury scene and en route to the hospital. This care has a profound impact on the subsequent course of events and outcomes. Timely and effective brain resuscitation is critical because the brain has minimal reserves to meet ongoing metabolic needs. When insufficient substrates are available to the brain because of reduced CBF and cerebral oxygen delivery, ischemia and hypoxia develop, precipitating the pathophysiological processes described earlier in this chapter. This inevitably leads to secondary brain injury and negatively affects patients' outcomes.

The American College of Surgeons has set national standards and developed Advanced Trauma Life Support (ATLS) training programs to prepare health care professionals to manage trauma victims effectively. Emergency medical services systems are designed to provide timely resuscitation and stabilization by well-trained personnel who can rapidly triage and transport victims to the *appropriate* health care facility. The emergency medical system includes telecommunication linkages with personnel at the health care facility where collaborative data analysis and clinical decision making occur through consultation that guide patient management at the trauma site and during transport. Because many TBI patients sustain multisystem trauma, primary and secondary trauma survey (see following section) is instituted to assess patients for evidence of these injuries systematically. Chart 18-3 provides a primary and secondary survey outline.

Initial Management

Owing to insufficient data, neither standards nor guidelines are recommended for initial management. However, options (class III evidence) for initial management are discussed in the *Guidelines*. The first priority for the **initial management** for TBI patients is complete and rapid physiological resuscitation.

According to one study, raising blood pressure in hypotensive, severe TBI patients improves outcomes in proportion to the efficacy of the resuscitation.[45] Several solid studies report that early episodes of hypotension or hypoxia greatly increase morbidity and mortality for severe TBI patients. Early hypotension, defined as a single episode of systolic blood pressure of 90 mm Hg or less, or hypoxia resulting from apnea or cyanosis in the field, or a PaO_2 of less than 60 mm Hg by arterial blood gas analysis, are all associated with increased mortality and morbidity.[46-48] Therefore,[43]

- Maintain a mean arterial blood pressure at more than 90 mm Hg through the infusion of fluids throughout the care cycles. This intervention is designed to support a cerebral perfusion pressure (CPP) of more than 70 mm Hg.
- Note that *mean arterial blood pressure*, a component in calculating CPP, is the important parameter. However, until an arterial line is in place, the focus will be on maintaining *systolic blood pressure*. Because of intracranial hypertension during the prehospital and resuscitation phases, it will probably be necessary to maintained systolic blood pressure significantly higher than 90 mm Hg to maintain a CPP above 70 mm Hg.
- Maintain a patent airway and adequate oxygen supply. Patients with a GCS below 9, who are unable to maintain their airway, or who remain hypoxemic despite supplemental oxygen, will require airway support, preferably by endotracheal intubation.

The fluid of choice is hypertonic saline because it also reduces intracranial hypertension. Maneuvers to maintain airway patency must be modified to prevent cervical injuries. One cannot overemphasize the importance of treating all TBI patients for possible cervical fractures or spinal injury by immediately immobilizing the head and neck. All emergency medical personnel must be mindful of the disastrous consequences (cord transection, quadriplegia, death) associated with neck manipulation.

No specific treatment should be directed at intracranial hypertension without clinical evidence of transtentorial herniation or progressive neurological deterioration that are *not* attributable to extracranial causes. When there is clinical

CHART 18 – 3 • Primary and Secondary Survey

Primary and secondary surveys are conducted according to standards of Advanced Trauma Life Support course. The following cautions must be considered with patients with traumatic brain injury (TBI) when conducting a *primary survey:*

AIRWAY MAINTENANCE

Patency of the airway must be maintained. The following points address airway patency:

- All *unconscious* TBI patients are intubated to prevent aspiration. Note: Tracheal intubation may be contraindicated in patients with midface trauma and sometimes with basal skull fractures.
- Intubation technique reflects consideration of potential cervical fracture or spinal cord injury and should only be executed by trained personnel.
- The nose and mouth are suctioned to remove blood, mucus, and drainage to ensure airway patency; nasal suctioning is *contraindicated* if a basal skull fracture is suspected.
- The airway is suctioned as necessary; suctioning is limited to **10 seconds** or less per pass after intubation.
- Aspiration related to trauma is common and assumed present. It may be present even with negative early chest x-rays.

BREATHING

After a patent airway is established, breathing is assessed, and measures are instituted to support respirations and adequate oxygenation. Oxygen therapy is implemented, and often a ventilator is needed.

CIRCULATION

Pulses, capillary refill, and blood pressure are assessed. Hypotension is disastrous to the brain and must be aggressively treated. The underlying cause must be determined, such as occult bleeding. If hypertension is present, it is usually related to the TBI and is managed with an increased ICP protocol.

After the patient is stabilized, the *secondary survey* is conducted.

ASSESSMENT FOR TBI

Key elements for assessment of TBI include:

- History and circumstances of injury
- Initial assessment **ABC** (**a**irway with cervical spine control, **b**reathing, and **c**irculation)
- Assessment of vital signs (hypotension, often related to other system injuries, is disastrous); note patterns such as Cushing's response associated with increased ICP (see Chart 18–4)
- **AVPU** (the level of consciousness: **A**, alert; **V**, response to **v**ocal stimuli; **P**, response to **p**ainful stimuli; and **U**, **u**nresponsive)
- Mini-neurological examination

GLASGOW COMA SCALE

(see Chart 18–2 for severity of injury)

- Pupillary size and response
- Motor function (lateralization suggests focal lesion)

Committee on Trauma. (1993). *Advanced trauma life support: Course for physicians* (5th ed., pp. 161–183). Chicago: American College of Surgeons.

---

evidence of transtentorial herniation or progressive neurological deterioration not attributable to extracranial causes, the patient must be aggressively treated for intracranial hypertension. These interventions include:[43]

- Hyperventilation.
- Mannitol, but *only* if adequate volume resuscitation has occurred.
- Sedation and neuromuscular blockade are useful to optimize transport, but both interfere with the neurological examination. Sedation should be tried first, and short-acting neuromuscular blockade is provided only if sedation is inadequate.

Emergency Department or Trauma Center Management

On arrival at the Emergency Department (ED), multiple and concurrent activities are initiated by a well-trained team of health care professionals. Activity includes inserting arterial and central lines, inserting an indwelling urinary catheter, attaching monitoring equipment such as continuous electrocardiography, and conducting primary and secondary trauma surveys. The history and circumstances of injury and previous treatment are verified and clarified. The following are examples of important information to consider:

- Circumstances of injury (e.g., direct blow to head, thrown from car, fell off bar stool)
- Seat belt or helmet worn (e.g., type of seat belt: lap or shoulder)
- How patient was found (e.g., lying face down)
- Unconsciousness (immediate; lucid period)
- Documented apnea or cyanosis and length of time
- Significant blood loss at the scene of accident

Resuscitation and stabilization treatment continue; diagnostic testing is conducted. A decision is made concerning the need for emergency neurosurgery.

Laboratory Studies and Other Diagnostics

The following lists laboratory studies for the initial resuscitation and treatment of severe TBI (GCS 8 or lower):

- Complete blood count (CBC), arterial blood gases, electrolytes, glucose, creatinine, and blood urea nitrogen
- Drug screen
- Chest radiograph
- Cervical spine films (to rule out cervical fractures or unstable vertebral column)
- CT scan without contrast, as soon as possible, to rule out intracranial bleeding
- Peritoneal lavage (to rule out abdominal bleeding)
- Other emergency diagnostic studies

The CT scan is the gold standard for diagnosis of TBI. It is done immediately on admission or may be postponed until the patient's condition has stabilized. The CT scan can identify a depressed skull fracture, EDH, SDH, ICH, contusion, and most DAIs. If an operable lesion is found, the patient is transferred to the operating room on an emergency basis. If there is no lesion requiring surgery, transfer is to the intensive care unit (ICU).

Resuscitation

The initial brain resuscitation[49] for severe TBI is directed at controlling the intracranial hypertension. As mentioned above, mannitol and controlled hyperventilation are the key interventions available for *emergency* management of intracranial hypertension. Endotracheal intubation protects the airway and facilitates controlled hyperventilation. Use of oxygen, sedation or neuromuscular blockade, seizure management, and hyperthermia control are all designed to optimize oxygen supply by controlling activities known to increase cerebral metabolic rate of oxygen consumption ($CMRO_2$) and therefore increase the demand for oxygen. In the ED, a ventriculostomy may be necessary to reduce increased ICP by periodic CSF drainage.

In summary, management of the TBI patient in the ED is directed at resuscitation, stabilization, and establishment of a diagnosis. After these steps have been completed, a decision is made regarding immediate surgical intervention for life-threatening injuries or transfer to the ICU for medical management.

ICU Management of Severe Traumatic Brain Injury

Severe TBI patients are admitted directly to the ICU from the ED or after emergency neurosurgery for close monitoring and technology interface. The goals of ICU care are to manage intracranial hypertension, maintain adequate cerebral oxygen delivery to meet cerebral metabolic needs, prevent secondary brain injury, and prevent or manage other systemic problems that can contribute to morbidity, mortality, and increased costs. Care maps for severe TBI are useful to guide care and address interdisciplinary care needs. The case manager, nurse, physician, physical therapist, speech therapist, occupational therapist, pharmacist, clinical nutritionist, and other health care professionals must work closely together to move the patient along in the continuum of care (see Chap. 17, Neurological Critical Care).

Monitoring and Technology

On admission to the ICU, the patient may be placed on a special therapeutic bed and will be connected to a physiological monitoring system. Several invasive monitoring lines are inserted, including an arterial line, central venous pressure catheter, pulmonary catheter, ventriculostomy, ICP monitor, and, possibly, a retrograde jugular catheter. The patient may be connected to a mechanical ventilator through the endotracheal tube; end-tidal CO_2; cardiac monitoring leads; sequential compression boots; pulse oximetry; and a rectal temperature probe. Use of ICP monitoring is appropriate for severe TBI patients with an abnormal CT scan on admission and a GCS of 3 to 8 after cardiopulmonary resuscitation. It is also recommended for patients with a severe TBI if two or more of the following are present at admission: age older than 40 years, unilateral or bilateral motor posturing, or systolic blood pressure less than 90 mm Hg.[43] See Chapter 14 for a discussion of ICP monitoring. ICP monitoring is not recommended for mild or moderate TBI.

If not already done, the cervical spine must be cleared as soon as possible. (Patients must be treated as if a cervical spinal injury is present until a negative x-ray is obtained.) A nasogastric (NG) tube is inserted unless there is an anterior fossa basilar skull or midface fracture. With an anterior fossa basilar skull fracture, an NG tube can be inserted through the mouth and guided by a laryngoscope to avoid passing the tube through the fracture area into the brain. The NG tube should be inserted after the endotracheal tube is in position because the insertion of a NG tube may cause vomiting and aspiration.

Setting and maintaining physiological targets are directed at optimizing physiological function and preventing complications that can lead to secondary brain injury. Each physiological targeted goal is set as either a range, such as maintaining the MAP between 90 and 100 mm Hg, or as a critical threshold, such as maintaining CPP at 70 mm Hg or more. To maintain the targeted goals, the nurse may need to titrate drugs (e.g., dopamine to a set cardiac output), suction in response to a declining pulse oximetry reading, or reposition the patient's neck in response to noisy respirations (partial obstructed airway). See Table 17-1 for common values.

Management of Intracranial Hypertension

Although no absolute ICP threshold exists above which treatment to lower ICP should begin, current data support a threshold of 20 to 25 mm Hg.[43,50] The basic treatment strategies for intracranial hypertension management are summarized in Table 18-2. Figure 18-7 provides an algorithm for the treatment of intracranial hypertension.

Two categories of medical management strategies for intracranial hypertension are recognized: conventional treatments and treatments for intracranial hypertension refractory to conventional therapies. The conventional therapies are organized in a sequence based on a risk:benefit ratio as suggested by Chesnut.[51] The following section briefly discusses the management of intracranial hypertension and maintenance of ade-

Table 18–2 • EARLY MANAGEMENT OF SEVERE BRAIN INJURY (GCS ≤ 8) FOCUS ON INCREASED ICP MANAGEMENT

MEDICAL THERAPEUTICS: MEDICAL MANAGEMENT	MAINTAIN PHYSIOLOGICAL PARAMETERS: COLLABORATIVE EFFORT	NURSING INTERVENTIONS: INDEPENDENT NURSING PRACTICE
• Mechanical ventilatory support • Oxygen 20%–40% • Hyperventilation: $PaCO_2$ 30–35 • Mannitol (0.25–1.0 g/kg) bolus • Indwelling urinary catheter • Sedation • Analgesics • Neuromuscular blockage • Treat seizures or prophylaxis for high risk for seizures • Fluid replacement with saline • Intracranial pressure (ICP) monitoring • Possible ventriculostomy for drainage if ICP >20 mm Hg	• PaO_2: 90–100 mm Hg • $PaCO_2$: 27–30 mm Hg • SaO_2: 92–100 • MAP: 90–100 mm Hg; to support CPP >70 mm Hg • Maintain systolic 140–160 mm Hg • CPP: >70 mm Hg • ICP: <20 mm Hg • CO: 4–6 L/min • CI: >3.0 L/min • SVR: 900–1400 dynes • CVP: 8–10 mm Hg • PWCP: 14–16 • Serum osmolality: <320 mOsm • Hct: <32% • Normal glucose (<150 mg/dL) • Normal electrolytes • Hgb: >10 g • Normothermia • Normal range urine-specific gravity • Adequate urinary output/hour • Tightly controlled intake and output balance for euvolemia • Monitor arterial blood gases	• Elevate head of bed to 30 degrees • Maintain neutral head position • Maintain patent airway: suction prn (<10 sec/insertion) • Turn q2h from side to side • Control noxious stimuli • Oxygenate before and after suctioning • Perform chest PT q2h • Prevent Valsalva's maneuver • Do not hyperventilate when suction; maintain normal $PaCO_2$ • Possible blockade when suctioning if ICP spikes • Frequently monitor vital neurological signs; look for deviation trends • Treat elevated temperature aggressively • Control coughing • Control asynchrony with vent • Prevent shivering

Second-Line: Refractory to Conventional Therapy

• Hyperventilation: $PaCO_2$ 27–30
• Barbiturate coma
• Hypothermia
• Decompression craniectomy
• Hypertensive therapy

quate cerebral oxygen delivery. A thorough discussion of intracranial hypertension management is found in Chapter 14.

Cerebrospinal Fluid Drainage

Many patients with severe TBI will have a ventriculostomy inserted for periodic drainage of CSF, an effective method of lowering elevated ICP. The ventriculostomy may incorporate an ICP monitoring device, or there may be separate devices. However, continuous ICP monitoring will be operational. The physician will determine the threshold at which CSF will be drained. The order to drain CSF is set to a mean ICP threshold, most often 20 mm Hg. Unit protocol for draining should be followed. The protocol should identify the duration of drainage (e.g., 5 minutes) and the points to be documented. The color of the drainage should be monitored (e.g., very bloody, pinkish) along with the amount of drainage. During drainage, the ICP waveform is lost with some types of ventriculostomy systems.

Sedation, Analgesics, and Neuromuscular Blockade

The following must be considered when evaluating potential drugs: effect on $CMRO_2$, CBF, ICP, cardiovascular function, and respiratory function; toxicity; side effects; time to awaken-

ing after discontinuation; incidence of prolonged weakness after discontinuation; efficacy; effect on outcome; and cost.[52]

Sedation. Many therapeutic protocols for severely TBI patients include sedatives and analgesics to ameliorate intracranial hypertension related to agitation; restlessness; posturing; asynchrony with the mechanical ventilator; and painful interventions that increase $CMRO_2$ and oxygen needs.

Benzodiazepines are the most commonly used sedatives and do not affect $CMRO_2$, CBF, or ICP. Lorazepam (Ativan) and midazolam (Versed) are frequently used. Propofol (Diprivan), a sedative-hypnotic agent that is supplied in an intralipid emulsion for intravenous (IV) use, decreases $CMRO_2$, CBF, ICP, and CPP. An ultra-short-acting drug, it has a major advantage in that an IV infusion can be weaned and a neurological assessment conducted in about 5 to 10 minutes without masking from the drug. The disadvantages are cost, dose-dependent hypotension, potential for bacterial or fungal infection associated with use of a preservative-free emulsion, and muscle weakness with prolonged use. Because propofol is a lipid emulsion, triglycerides need to be monitored and intralipid nutrition adjusted.

CRITICAL PATHWAY FOR TREATMENT OF INTRACRANIAL HYPERTENSION

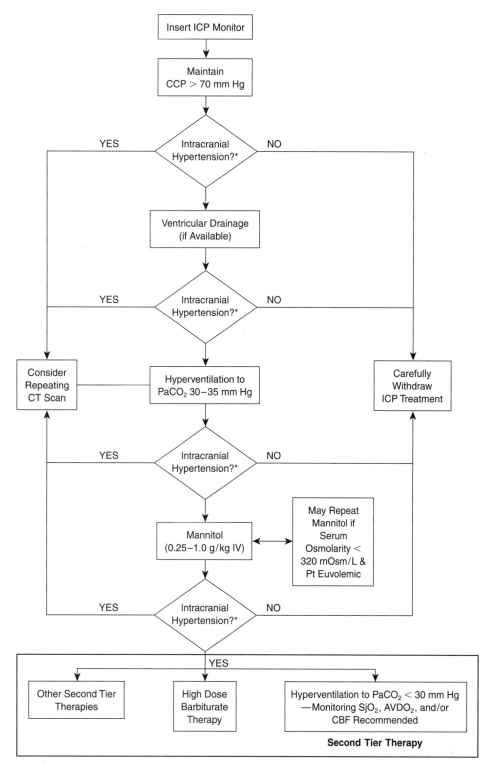

Figure 18–7 • Algorithm for the treatment of intracranial hypertension. (Bullock, K. H., Chestnut, R. H., & Clifton, G. L. [2000]. Guidelines for the treatment of severe TBI. *Journal of Neurotrauma, 17*[6/7], 538.)

* Threshold of 20–25 mm Hg may be used. Other variable may be substituted in individual conditions.

Analgesics. Sedatives do not possess analgesic properties. Without administration of analgesia, sedation of patients with pain may lead to increased agitation and combativeness. Therefore, need for analgesics must be considered.[52] Parenteral narcotics, such as fentanyl or morphine, are frequently used for analgesia. These drugs do not increase $CMRO_2$, CBF, or ICP in conventional doses. A low-dose continuous infusion of morphine is a frequently used method of administration. Respiratory depression is the major side effect of morphine and is a concern only if the patient is not intubated, which is unlikely in a severe TBI patient.

Neuromuscular Blockade. From 1% to 10% of ICU patients now receive continuous administration of neuromuscular blockade drugs for more than 24 hours.[53] Selected drugs in a neuromuscular blockade protocol induce paralysis to counteract the increase in ICP that occurs with interventions such as suctioning and ventilation. Drugs commonly used include pancuronium, vecuronium, pipecuronium, and atracurium. The depth of paralysis is routinely monitored at the bedside using a peripheral nerve stimulator and an assessment method known as the train-of-four.[54,55] A series of four low-voltage electrical stimulation (i.e., train-of-four) are applied to a peripheral nerve, such as the ulnar nerve, and the twitch response is noted. A complete blockade (0 of 4) response is related to deep paralysis. The major complication of paralysis in patients is prolonged weakness or myopathy after extended use (i.e., longer than 24 hours). If it is difficult to obtain a response, such as in a patient with edema of the arms, other sites such as the facial nerve may be used.

Steroids. Based on strong evidence from prospective randomized controlled trials,[56,57] steroids do not reduce ICP or improve outcomes[43] and therefore are *not recommended for managing severe TBI.*

Seizure Management

Post-traumatic seizures (PTS) are classified according to the time of occurrence. Early PTS occur within 7 days following injury, whereas late PTS occur after 7 days after injury.[58,59]

Studies have shown that prophylactic anticonvulsants are effective in preventing early PTS[60] but are not useful for prevention of delayed PTS.[61,62] Based on Class I evidence, a seizure management standard is recommendations in the *Guidelines for Management of Severe Traumatic Brain Injury.* Prophylactic use of phenytoin, carbamazepine, phenobarbital, or valproate is *not* recommended for prevention of *late PTS.*[43] In one study, phenytoin was found to exert a temporary beneficial effect by reducing seizures during the first week after severe TBI.[60] Seizures need to be controlled because they greatly increase $CMRO_2$ and ICP. In patients receiving neuromuscular blockade, seizure activity or status epilepticus, if either occurs, may not exhibit the usual motor activity typical of a seizure. Tachycardia, blood pressure instability, and intracranial hypertension may be the only evidence of seizure activity.[30] The rationale for seizure prophylaxis is based on the high risk of secondary injury from clinically undetected seizures. Patients who do not "wake up" despite other clinical data suggesting improved neurological status may be engulfed in subclinical seizures. Use of compressed spectral array EEG bedside monitoring is becoming common in ICUs to detect subclinical seizures. Nurses can expect to be required to assess and monitor these data more frequently as part of their ongoing assessment.

If seizures do occur, aggressive treatment is necessary to control the seizure and the concurrent cerebral hypoxia. Phenytoin is the most common drug used for acute seizure management. A loading dose of 1 g IV phenytoin, with subsequent maintenance doses, is given to maintain a therapeutic level. Phenytoin IV should not be given any faster than 50 mg/min because of the possibility of hypotension and cardiac arrhythmias. It must be administered in normal saline and with a filter. For maintenance, phenytoin can be administered through a nasogastric tube. The usual dose of phenytoin is 300 to 400 mg daily. It is necessary to monitor blood levels of phenytoin to maintain a therapeutic range (10 to 20 mg/mL). Adjustment in dosage may be necessary when a tube feeding is started, because phenytoin binds to the protein within the feeding. Therefore, a patient who has been in a therapeutic range may now be subtherapeutic and need dose adjustment. When administering the phenytoin IV, the manufacturer's instructions should be followed. Fosphenytoin rather than phenytoin may be administered to manage seizures. See Chapter 11 for further discussion of anticonvulsant drugs.

Nursing responsibilities related to seizures include maintaining seizure precautions, observing for seizure activity, and monitoring anticonvulsant drug blood level. As mentioned previously, motor signs of seizure activity may not be evident in a sedated patient or one receiving neuromuscular blockade. The only clinical evidence may be tachycardia, blood pressure instability, and intracranial hypertension. If there is suspicion of seizure activity, continuous EEG monitoring is diagnostic.

In the ICU environment, seizure precautions are integrated into care. The patient's airway is maintained with an endotracheal tube or other airway, and suctioning equipment is readily available. Padded side rails are usually left up when the nurse is not at the bedside. Padding can easily be added to the side rails. Protection from injury is a consideration for an awake and ambulatory patient.

Hyperthermia Management

Hyperthermia can result from local or systemic infections, central injury to the hypothalamus, cerebral irritation from hemorrhage, or drug response, particularly to anticonvulsants. With hyperthermia, cerebral metabolic rate increases 5% to 7% per degree centigrade.[63] This puts the patient at high risk for inadequate oxygen supply at the cellular level and secondary injury. Therefore, frequent monitoring and aggressive management of an elevated temperature are critical. It is important to identify the cause of the elevated temperature and treat the primary cause. The patient should be pan-cultured (screening for the sites of infection) to determine the cause of the elevation. Treatment includes acetaminophen (650 mg every 4 to 6 hours, as needed) and other cooling measures (e.g., cooling blanket, removal of excess bed covers, environmental control). The goal is to maintain normothermia while preventing shivering.

Mannitol

Osmotic diuretics are recommended in the *Guidelines* for control of acute increased ICP caused by cerebral edema.[43] The osmotic diuretic of choice is mannitol, 0.25 to 1.0 g/kg through IV bolus (usual adult dose is 25 to 50 g) every 3 to 6 hours. The goal is to reduce extracellular fluid and cerebral edema. *Before* ICP, monitoring the administration of mannitol is triggered in a patient exhibiting signs of transtentorial herniation or progressive neurological deterioration not attributable to extracranial causes. With mannitol administration, euvolemia must always be maintained through adequate fluid replacement. An indwelling urinary catheter is necessary to monitor urinary output and diuresis. Serum osmolarity should be maintained at less than 320 mOsm to counter renal failure. Blood pressure and electrolytes should be monitored carefully, because one danger associated with diuresis is hypotension, which results in cerebral hypoperfusion and ischemia. Electrolyte imbalance, also common, must be monitored and treated as necessary.

Hyperventilation

Cerebral physiology and cerebral blood flow (CBF) after TBI are well understood, and this information forms the basis for both a recommended standard and a guideline for management of TBI.[43] It is well established that CBF is lowest in the 24-hour period after TBI and remains low for approximately 3 more days except in patients who do not survive because of uncontrolled intracranial hypertension.[64–68] CBF averages about 30 mL/100 g per minute during the first 8 hours after injury, and may be as low as 20 mL/100 g/minute in the first 4 hours for the most critically ill patients.[43] Although the CBF threshold for irreversible ischemia or infarction is not clearly delineated, it is thought to be around the <15 mL/100 g/minute level. Normal CBF is about 55 mL/100 g/minute. Interestingly, in severe TBI patients CBF is lowest in patients with SDH, diffuse injuries, and hypotension; it is highest in patients with an epidural hematoma with normal CT results.[68–72]

Hyperventilation involves serious risks and its use should closely conform to the *Guidelines*. The *purported* therapeutic effect of hyperventilation is that hypocapnia (lowered $PaCO_2$) causes vasoconstriction and decreases ICP. However, what in fact happens is that hyperventilation reduces CBF, does not consistently reduce ICP, and may cause loss of autoregulation. Additionally, there is wide local variability of perfusion and vasoconstriction.[43,73] Accordingly, the *Guidelines*[43] recommend that chronic prophylactic hyperventilation therapy ($PaCO_2$ of 25 mm Hg or less) be avoided after severe TBI in the absence of increased ICP. *The use of prophylactic hyperventilation ($PaCO_2$ 35 mm Hg or lower) should be avoided for the first 5 days after severe TBI, but especially during the first 24 hours when CBF is lowest, because it compromises cerebral perfusion.*

So when is hyperventilation a useful option? As an emergency measure, it can be helpful for *brief* periods when there is acute neurological deterioration. For *longer* periods, it may be useful when intracranial hypertension is nonresponsive to the usual treatment strategies of sedation, paralysis, drainage of CSF through a ventriculostomy, and osmotic diuretics. In this circumstance, hyperventilation becomes a second-tier strategy for a gravely ill patient. Abrupt cessation can cause a rebound effect of ICP. The effect on cerebral and CSF acidosis is short lived.

The following is recommended for monitoring $PaCO_2$ values for evidence of cerebral ischemia during hyperventilation: jugular venous oxygen saturation (SjO_2), arterial-jugular venous oxygen ($AVDO_2$) content differences, brain tissue oxygen monitoring, and cerebral blood extraction (CBE) monitoring. Currently, there is no direct way to monitor for focal ischemia in the brain. It should be kept in mind that, although SjO_2 monitoring is helpful, it provides a global value of cerebral oxygenation and does not provide information on the injured area only.

Fluid Management

Fluid restriction can be harmful after TBI, causing hypotension and vasoconstriction secondary to decreased volume. *It has been abandoned in favor of euvolemia.* Movement of water between the brain and the intravascular space is controlled by osmotic gradients. Hypertonic saline solutions decrease brain water and ICP while temporarily increasing systolic blood pressure and cardiac output.[74] Saline solutions in strengths from 0.9% to 3.0% are commonly used. The higher saline concentration is used when concurrent hyponatremia is present.

Hypotonic glucose and other hypotonic solutions (0.45 saline) should not be given rapidly or in large volumes to patients with intracranial hypertension. Excess free water from these solutions lowers plasma osmolality and drives water across the blood-brain barrier, thus increasing cerebral water content and ICP. With ischemia and brain injury, plasma glucose is metabolized to lactic acid, thereby lowering tissue pH (acidosis).[75] An elevated serum glucose level may aggravate ischemic insult in TBI patients and worsen neurological outcome; therefore, glucose solutions should be avoided.[76] A glucose serum level below 150 mg/dL should be maintained.

Colloids Used as Volume Expanders

Human albumin solutions are available either as 5% or 25% concentrations. Albumin (Plasmanate) is an effective volume expander and has no intrinsic effects on clotting. There are also synthetic colloid volume expanders, including hetastarch, pentastarch, and pentafraction. Of these, hetastarch is used most frequently, although its use is limited owing to its effect of prolonging clotting time.[77] Packed red blood cells may also be given to expand volume if the hematocrit or hemoglobin level is low.

Other Therapies for Intractable ICP

The intracranial hypertension associated with severe TBI may not respond (i.e., be intractable) to the usual treatment strategies. In these circumstances, second-tier treatment strategies may be employed such as hyperventilation to a $PaCO_2$ below 30 mm Hg or high-dose barbiturate therapy.

Hyperventilation has been addressed previously. If this is used, concurrent SjO_2 and $AVDO_2$ monitoring is recommended.

Barbiturates assist with intractable ICP by protecting the cerebrum and lowering ICP through the mechanisms of alterations in vascular tone, suppression of metabolism, and inhibition of free radical mediated lipid peroxidation.[78,79] As a result, CBF is better matched to regional metabolic demands, and metabolic needs are lowered. The effect of these physiological alterations is that ICP decreases and global cerebral perfusion improves.

The *Guidelines* make the following recommendation: "High-dose barbiturate therapy may be considered in hemodynamically stable salvageable severe head injured patients with intracranial hypertension refractory to maximal medical and surgical intracranial ICP lowering therapy."[43] See Chapter 14 for further discussion of barbiturate therapy.

With regard to the role of hypothermia in the management of TBI patients, a large, multi-site trial concluded that treatment with hypothermia, with the body temperature reaching 33° C within 8 hours after injury, is *not effective* in improving outcomes in patients with severe TBI.[80]

Gastric Prophylaxis

In severe head trauma there is an increased risk of gastric irritation, gastric ulcers, and gastrointestinal (GI) hemorrhage, a syndrome called Cushing's ulcer. The common prophylactic GI drug protocols include H_2 receptor antagonists, such as ranitidine (Zantac)—150 mg twice daily through an NG tube, or 50 mg every 6 to 8 hours IV, or famotidine (Pepcid)—20 mg twice daily through an NG tube or 20 mg every 12 hours IV; and antacids, such as Maalox—30 mL every 3 to 4 hours through a NG tube as a standing order or in response to assessment of gastric contents for pH. The goal is to maintain the pH above 5.0. Stools should be monitored for occult blood. A drop in hemoglobin levels may suggest bleeding and, therefore, should be monitored.

Bowel Management

To prevent constipation and stimulation of Valsalva's maneuver, a bowel program is instituted. A stool softener, such as docusate (Colace), 150 mg twice a day through a NG tube, is useful. A laxative of choice, often Milk of Magnesia, 30 mL through a NG tube at hour of sleep, is helpful. The frequency and consistency of bowel movements are monitored. The abdomen should be assessed for distension and peristalsis.

Summary of the Management of Severe TBI

Evidence-based practice guidelines for the management of severe TBI are discussed in this chapter. These guidelines will continue to evolve as new evidence is added to the repository of knowledge. One final point deserves comment. The proper approach to intracranial hypertension management in TBI is the subject of ongoing debate. Should therapy be directed at control of ICP or maintenance of adequate CPP? These are properly major components of the larger discussion of maintaining optimal cerebral function. A body of knowledge addresses CPP management protocols.[81] According to the *Guidelines,*[43] there is insufficient evidence with the required degree of certainty to recommend either standards or guidelines for CPP. However, maintaining CPP at a minimum of 70 mm Hg is "suggested" in the management of severe TBI. As more evidence becomes available, a stronger recommendation may be included in future guidelines. For the time being, maintaining CPP at a level of at least 70 mm Hg is considered good practice and thought to improve patient outcomes.

▌ ASSESSMENT AND CLINICAL REASONING: KEY ROLE OF THE NEUROSCIENCE NURSE

The following reviews key points of assessment and clinical reasoning as they apply to TBI patients.

Vital Signs

Chart 18-4 reviews the significance of vital signs as they relate to neurological function and other body systems. The frequency for monitoring vital signs depends on the stability of the patient's condition. In the ICU setting, monitoring should occur at least every hour.

Neurological Signs

After an initial baseline assessment, frequent subsequent assessments should be conducted to determine trends in neurological status (stability, deterioration, or improvement). Impending cerebral herniation and onset of new intracranial hemorrhage are major problems of acute deterioration that are life threatening; therefore, the importance of frequent serial assessments cannot be overstated. The frequency with which a serial neurological assessment is conducted depends on the patient's condition and degree of stability. In the unstable patient, neurological signs may be monitored as frequently as every 5 to 15 minutes. After the patient has been well stabilized, monitoring every 2 to 4 hours may be sufficient. However, this is the standard on regular care units and not in the ICU. The following are specific areas of the neurological assessment:

- Level of consciousness and cognition (if responding verbally); if comatose, GCS is used
- Size, shape, and reaction of pupils to light (asymmetry seen with a focal lesion)
- Brainstem function, as evidenced by corneal and gag reflexes and extraocular movement
- Motor function (focal mass indicated by asymmetry or lateralization)

Level of Consciousness

Level of consciousness is the most sensitive indicator of neurological change. If the patient is able to respond verbally, orientation to time, place, and person is assessed. Cognition is assessed by asking simple questions and requests, such as "Show me two fingers." "Show me your left thumb." "Raise your left arm." "Why are you here?" If comatose, the GCS is used.

Brainstem Reflexes

Assessing and monitoring brainstem function begin with the pupils. Pupils are normally equal in size and midposition, round, and briskly reactive to direct light. Any *new* change in the size or reaction of one or both of the pupils needs to be evaluated. With lateral transtentorial herniation caused by localized cerebral edema (peaks about 72 hours after injury) or a focal lesion, one pupil will become dilated and progressively unresponsive to light. This is attributable to unilateral compression of the oculomotor nerve by the edematous herniating brain. An oval or ovoid pupil is also an early sign of transtentorial herniation. Immediate intervention may be necessary to prevent herniation and irreversible neurological deterioration. In

CHART 18 – 4 • Vital Signs and Their Significance in a Head-Injured Patient

RESPIRATIONS

- Brain injuries can result in abnormal respiratory patterns that roughly correlate with the level of neurological dysfunction (see Chap. 8 for a discussion of abnormal patterns and level of injury).
- In general, an initial increase in intracranial pressure (ICP) results in slowing of respirations. If ICP continues to increase, the pattern becomes rapid and noisy until the terminal stage, when respirations cease.
- A few conditions can affect respirations:
  —Complications of metabolic disorders, such as diabetic acidosis, can change respiratory patterns (Kussmaul's respirations)
  —Injuries to the cervical spine below C-4 can cause respiratory difficulty, whereas injuries above C-4, the site of phrenic nerve innervation, can cause total arrest

BLOOD PRESSURE

- Hypotension is rarely attributable to cerebral injury
  —*Hypotension and tachycardia* are seen as terminal events in head injury.
  —*Hypotension and tachycardia* in a patient who is not terminal is usually related to occult bleeding, most likely in the abdominal, pelvic, or thoracic cavity.
  —*Note:* The inherent risk of hypotension involves its relationship to CBF, CPP, and subsequent hypoperfusion and ischemia CCP. Hypoperfusion is associated with CPP.
  —*Hypotension and bradycardia* may be a secondary response to cervical cord injury if the descending sympathetic pathways have been interrupted.
- Hypertension is commonly associated with ↑ ICP; it may also be associated with pain, fear, or anxiety.
  —*Hypertension and bradycardia* are associated with ↑ ICP; they are late signs that correlate with pressure on the brain stem.
  > *Cushing's response* is an ischemic response of the body that maintains cerebral blood flow in the presence of rising ICP. Cushing's response includes hypertension, bradycardia, and a widening pulse pressure.

Cushing's triad includes hypertension, bradycardia, and an irregular respiratory pattern; it reflects a rising ICP in which there is direct pressure on the medullary center of the brain stem. It is often seen in the terminal stage and is associated with irreversible brainstem damage.

PULSE

- Pulse has been discussed in conjunction with blood pressure.
- *Bradycardia* is associated with increasing ICP or cervical injury.
- *Tachycardia* is associated with the following:
  —Occult (nonneurological) hemorrhage or hypovolemic shock
  —An autonomic response to injury of the hypothalamus or its connections
  —A terminal event in severe brain injury

TEMPERATURE

- *Hypothermia* can occur as a result of hypothalamic injury, because the hypothalamus is the heat regulatory center of the brain. The patient will assume the temperature of the ambient room air; if it is cold, body temperature will drop. Hypothermia (96°–97°F) is also seen early in cervical cord injuries.
- *Hyperthermia* in the brain-injured patient can be associated with direct injury to the hypothalamus or petechial bleeding into the hypothalamus or pons. Hyperthermia must be controlled because it *increases* the metabolic rate of all body cells, including those in the brain.
  —Oxygen consumption rises approximately 10% for every 1°C rise in temperature
  A rise from 37°C (98.6°F) to 40.5°C (105°F) results in a 35% increase in oxygen consumption.
  This can result in ischemia for the injured brain that was barely meeting metabolic needs when the temperature was within normal range.

CBF, cerebral blood flow; CPP, cerebral perfusion pressure.

addition, when looking into the eyes, observe their position in terms of spontaneous asynchronous movement (nystagmus) or extraocular movements (EOM) deviation.

The corneal and gag reflexes can be assessed easily at the bedside. The absence of either of these reflexes is a poor prognostic sign. Special protective eye care and lubrication should be applied if the corneal reflex is absent. Symmetry of the facial nerve can be checked by inserting a cotton-tipped applicator first in one nostril and then the other. By observing each side for grimacing, one can determine if a facial nerve deficit is present.

Without a gag reflex, the patient is at high risk for aspiration pneumonia. The ability to protect the airway and an intact gag reflex are criteria for consideration before removing an endotracheal tube. Provided there is no cervical fracture or dislocation, confirmed by cervical spine films, the eyes can be checked for doll's eye reflex (oculocephalic reflex) by the physician in the unconscious patient to provide information on severity of coma and prognosis.

Motor Function

Observe the patient for spontaneous movement. Asymmetry of movement or lateralization suggests a focal mass lesion on one side of the brain. Hemiparesis and hemiplegia, which involve only one side of the body, are signs of lateralization, with the lesion located in the hemisphere opposite the side of motor weakness. Decortication (flexor) or decerebration (extensor) posturing is observed in comatose patients who have suffered severe TBI. Additionally, bilateral or unilateral flaccidity may be associated with spinal injuries.

Other Observations

The patient's face and scalp should be examined for signs of injury, such as abrasions or contusions that may have been missed. Note the presence of ecchymosis on the mastoid bone (Battle's sign), periorbital ecchymosis (raccoon's eye), conjunctival hemorrhage, or clear or bloody drainage from the ear, nose, or postnasal area. These signs indicate a basal skull fracture. Assess the neck for evidence of nuchal rigidity, a sign of meningeal irritation. Nuchal rigidity can be caused by meningitis or blood in the CSF from subarachnoid hemorrhage.

If an ICP monitor is in place, observe for elevations in pressure and the shape of the P1, P2, and P3 components (see Chap. 14). Often, standing orders are in place for interventions to be implemented at a certain level of pressure elevation. The monitor also helps the nurse observe the effect of various nursing interventions on ICP. If the ICP is elevated, planned activities may be postponed until the pressure decreases.

IIII NURSING MANAGEMENT OF MULTISYSTEM COMPLICATIONS OF TRAUMATIC BRAIN INJURY

A management focus for TBI patients is prevention of secondary brain injury by optimizing cerebral perfusion, early recognition of complications, and management of multisystem problems (Table 18-3). To achieve optimal outcomes for the patient, a collaborative interdisciplinary effort is needed. Some complications are more apt to occur in the first few days after injury; others are delayed. As a member of the collaborative interdisciplinary team, the nurse has both independent and interdependent roles. Evidence-based nursing practice, or best practice, should be provided.[82] For example, research findings, such as for positioning of patients with severe TBI, can guide nursing practice.[83] The following addresses collaborative problems as they relate to TBI organized by body system.

Respiratory Complications

The area of respiratory management of the patient with a severe TBI has undergone rapid development in the last few years. Newer mechanical ventilators with positive end-expiratory pressure (PEEP) and pressure support have become standard in the management of TBI patients. PEEP increases PaO_2 in patients suffering from *decreased* functional residual capacity (FRC) resulting from interstitial edema or alveolar collapse, such as occurs with adult respiratory distress syndrome (ARDS). PEEP is ineffective in conditions with a high FRC, such as emphysema. PEEP elevates ICP only when mean airway pressures are increased, causing transmission pressure to the mediastinum. Complications associated with high PEEP are barotrauma and cardiovascular decompensation. PEEP must be withdrawn gradually. Oxygen therapy is often delivered at an FIO_2 between 20% and 40%, although higher levels may be necessary.

Monitoring of SaO_2 saturation, blood gases, CBC, sputum cultures, and chest x-rays assists in evaluating respiratory function. Chest auscultation and quality of respirations are the major clinical parameters for assessment.

Airway Patency

Maintaining a patent airway, the common pathway to the respiratory system, is the top priority in TBI management. In the acute phase of TBI, patients are neither able to manage their own secretions nor able to position themselves in the most expeditious way for adequate drainage of secretions. Meeting the patient's needs in these regards is a nursing care objective of the highest priority. Suction as needed to prevent an increase in carbon dioxide and subsequent hypercapnia, which contributes to cerebral vasodilation, cerebral edema, and increased ICP.

- Position the patient on the side to facilitate drainage of secretions and prevent aspiration, if not intubated.
- Preoxygenate with 100% oxygen before suctioning (with physician's approval).
- Limit the catheter insertion to 10 seconds or less to prevent an increase of CO_2.
- If a tracheostomy is present, provide tracheostomy care frequently to prevent crusting and build-up of secretions that can obstruct the airway.
- Do not hyperextend or hyperflex the neck, because such maneuvers create a partial obstruction of the airway.

Hypoxemia is an early systemic condition commonly found in TBI patients. Defined as less than 85 to 100 mm Hg, the normal range of arterial blood oxygen, hypoxemia is probably a direct result of TBI. A short period of apnea occurs at the time of injury, followed by spontaneous respirations. However, spotty atelectasis may result from incomplete alveolar *expansion*. For this reason, supplemental oxygen should be provided as soon as possible.

Hypoxia, defined as diminished tissue oxygen, results from pathophysiological changes in cerebral autoregulation and in neuronal metabolism. Hypoxia of the cerebral tissue, that is, cerebral ischemia, leads to death of the involved neurons, if not corrected.

Atelectasis, a collapsed or airless state that may involve any part of the lung, is a respiratory problem that can develop rapidly. It is, therefore, important to be sure that all areas of the lungs are expanded. To assess the lungs for atelectasis, the nurse auscultates the chest for breath sounds, making sure to listen to the entire chest, especially the bases of the lungs. Nursing management directed at preventing atelectasis includes:

- **Adjust for sighs** on ventilator if this is an option.
- **Perform pulmonary percussion** if the patient is on a bed specially designed for this procedure.
- **Encourage deep breathing exercises and use the incen-

T a b l e 18–3 • MAJOR COLLABORATIVE PROBLEMS IN THE MANAGEMENT OF ACUTE, SEVERE TRAUMATIC BRAIN INJURY

SYSTEM	COLLABORATIVE PROBLEMS	ASSESS AND MONITOR	INTERVENTIONS/MANAGEMENT
Neurological	Increased ICP Herniation syndromes Seizures Cerebral ischemia	Monitor frequent neurological assessments Assess frequently for signs and symptoms of ↑ ICP Monitor anticonvulsant blood level (if anticonvulsants ordered) Monitor mean ICP with ICP monitor Monitor jugular venous oxygen saturation	Institute severe TBI protocol based on published *Guidelines for the Management of Severe Traumatic Brain Injury*, Table 18–2 and pp. 390–394 Maintain seizure precautions
Respiratory	Atelectasis Pneumonia (aspiration and bacterial) Hypoxemia Ventilator dependency Neurogenic pulmonary edema ARDS Pulmonary embolus	Auscultate chest for breath sounds Monitor rate, rhythm, and pattern of respirations Monitor periodic arterial blood gases Monitor pulse oximetry Review periodic chest x-rays Monitor sputum cultures Monitor vital signs Monitor CBC	Administer oxygen Provide ventilatory support Oxygenate before suctioning Limit suctioning to no longer than 10 sec Turn patient periodically Provide chest physical therapy
Cardiovascular	Hypotension Hypertension Dysrhythmias Cardiogenic shock Deep vein thrombosis (DVT) Anemia DIC	Assess frequently vital signs Observe legs for DVTs Monitor CPP Monitor for dysrhythmias Monitor cardiac dynamics with arterial line and central line on ongoing basis Ongoing EKG patterns Monitor hemodynamic data Monitor CBC, Hgb, Hct, electrolytes, and coagulation studies	Maintain systolic >90 mm Hg Maintain CPP >70 mm Hg Insertion of arterial and central line for hemodynamic monitoring Maintain thigh-high elastic hose and sequential compression boots Use appropriate drug therapy to maintain blood pressure to targeted range
Gastrointestinal (GI)	GI hemorrhage Curling's ulcer Constipation Paralytic ileus Small bowel obstruction	Auscultate abdomen for bowel sounds and distension Monitor for GI bleeding Monitor for occult blood in stools Monitor serial Hgb and Hct	Administer prophylactic H_2 blockers Institute bowel program to prevent constipation
Genitourinary	Urinary tract infection (UTI) Acute renal failure Acute urinary retention	Monitor for evidence of UTI Monitor periodic urinalysis Monitor prn urine culture Monitor intake and output record Monitor periodic BUN, creatinine	Remove indwelling catheter as soon as possible Institute bladder retraining as soon as possible Maintain adequate fluid volume Treat UTI and acute renal failure
Skin/mucous membranes	Decubitus ulcer Laryngeal ulceration Oral thrush Corneal ulceration	Frequently inspect skin for redness/breakdown Inspect mouth for evidence of oral infection Inspect eyes for evidence of corneal ulceration Monitor oral-tracheal secretions for evidence of bleeding	Consider use of a special bed Turn and reposition patient frequently Insert artificial tears to each eye QID Maintain eye shields Secure endotracheal tube to prevent unnecessary movement Treat oral infection as needed Institute special skin treatment protocol for evidence of redness or decubitus
Metabolic	Electrolyte imbalance SIADH Cerebral salt wasting Diabetes insipidus Hyperglycemia Sepsis	Monitor frequent electrolytes, glucose, calcium, phosphorus, magnesium Monitor serum and urine osmolality Monitor urine specific gravity Monitor ongoing core temperature Monitor for evidence of sepsis	Determine underlying fluid or electrolyte problem and treat Replace depleted electrolytes Maintain euvolemia Maintain tight control of glucose with regular insulin as necessary Administer mannitol as needed Maintain normothermia Treat sepsis as needed

(continued)

Table 18–3 • MAJOR COLLABORATIVE PROBLEMS IN THE MANAGEMENT OF ACUTE, SEVERE TRAUMATIC BRAIN INJURY (Continued)

SYSTEM	COLLABORATIVE PROBLEMS	ASSESS AND MONITOR	INTERVENTIONS/MANAGEMENT
Musculoskeletal	Contracture Spasticity	Monitor range of motion of joints Observe for spasticity	Request physical therapy consult and therapy Provide range of motion exercises QID Apply splints, casting, etc. as ordered
Nutrition	Weight loss Dehydration Negative nitrogen balance	Monitor daily weight Monitor intake and output record Monitor daily caloric intake Monitor for need to adjust daily caloric goals Monitor blood chemistries	Consult with clinical dietician to calculate caloric/dietary needs, nutrition source, and frequency of feeding Insert enteral feeding tube Request metabolic cart, as needed
Psychosocial	Agitation Family stress/dysfunction	Assess family function Assess family's understanding of patient status and prognosis Assess for any special needs of family	Provide information at a scheduled time Provide compassionate support Offer counseling services Identify family spokesperson and contact

tive spirometer in the conscious patient to expand the lungs and loosen secretions.

Pneumonia

In the ICU environment, there are many opportunities for a patient to develop pneumonia. *Aspiration pneumonia* from aspiration at the time of injury or thereafter, *bacterial pneumonia* from bacterial invasion, and *hypostatic pneumonia* from stasis of fluid in the lungs are common types. *Nosocomial pneumonias* are also common and are usually caused by gram-positive organisms (*Staphylococcus aureus, Streptococcus pneumonia,* and *Haemophilus influenzae*) and sometimes gram-negative organisms (enteric bacteria or *Pseudomonas*).

The nurse should assess for the signs and symptoms of pneumonia by auscultating the chest for breath sounds and adventitious sounds, monitoring the character of the sputum for color and foul odor, as well as the temperature and white blood cell count for elevation. Nursing management to prevent pneumonia should incorporate the following:

- Maintain a patent airway.
- Turn from side to side every 2 hours to prevent stasis of fluid in the lungs.
- Do not position on the back, because this increases the possibility of aspiration.
- Administer chest physiotherapy to loosen and drain pulmonary secretions.
- Use meticulous aseptic technique when delivering care. The intubated or tracheotomized patient is at high risk for infection.
- Be sure to clear secretions from the back of the throat when suctioning.
- Elevate the head of the bed to 30 degrees.
- Maintain an inflated cuff on the tracheostomy tube to prevent aspiration.
- Confirm that the gag reflex is intact before feeding a patient.

Neurogenic pulmonary edema is a complication seen commonly in severe TBI patients with increased ICP and is sometimes seen in these patients after a major generalized seizure. This acute pulmonary edema is noncardiogenic, not related to injured alveolar epithelium or capillary endothelium, and occurs minutes to days after injury. Although poorly understood, the pathophysiology probably relates to a combination of hydrostatic forces and permeability changes. At the time of impact, an abrupt rise in ICP and sympathetic discharge shunts blood into the lungs, causing a rise in fluid in the extracapillary spaces (alveoli). Clinical findings are nonspecific (dyspnea, tachypnea, tachycardia, hypoxemia, and mild elevation in leukocytes). On a chest x-ray, "fluffy" infiltrates are seen. Neurogenic pulmonary edema can progress to respiratory failure and a condition similar to ARDS, or it can be self-limiting, resolving in hours to days. Treatment consists of normalizing the underlying increased ICP with medical and nursing strategies and providing ventilatory support with PEEP.

Pulmonary emboli develop in the immobilized TBI patient from deep vein thromboses (DVTs). Signs and symptoms include cough, often with hemoptysis; dyspnea and tachypnea; and chest pain. In the comatose patient the only signs may be tachypnea and tachycardia. Nursing management directed at the prevention of DVT includes the application of elastic stockings and sequential compression boots to improve blood return to the heart and, possibly, the administration of subcutaneous heparin.

Cardiovascular Complications

Cardiac arrhythmias are often reported in conjunction with TBI. Some are associated with myocardial ischemia and can be life threatening. Others are more common when there is bleeding into the subarachnoid space. The cause of these cardiac problems is thought to be autonomic discharge at injury with an ensuing hyperdynamic state.

To assess cardiovascular function, the patient's vital signs should be monitored frequently, and the continuous pattern on a cardiac monitor should be observed for arrhythmias. In addition, the following may be ordered:

electrolytes; coagulation studies; CBC; creatine kinase isoenzyme for myocardial infarction; perhaps an echocardiogram if cardiac mechanics are questioned; and a 12-lead EKG. Any abnormality should be analyzed promptly for its underlying cause, and the appropriate treatment should be aggressively instituted.

Nursing management is directed toward detecting and correcting arrhythmias and other cardiac-related abnormalities. Patient monitoring should include chest auscultation, pulse and blood pressure, and observation of the EKG pattern on the cardiac monitor. Treatment, usually pharmacological, is guided by targeted physiological values for hemodynamic variables, such as cardiac output and MAP. Drug administration is titrated to obtain the targeted range.

Many drug options are available to maintain higher blood pressure for patients with intracranial pathology. Alpha- and beta-adrenergic blockers do not directly affect CBF and have no effect on ICP in patients with intracranial hypertension; therefore, they may be preferred for control of blood pressure in brain-injured people.[84] Adequate MAP is facilitated with vasopressor drugs progressing from dopamine (Intropin) to phenylephrine (Neo-Synephrine). *Dopamine*, the precursor of norepinephrine, increases kidney perfusion at lower doses (2 to 5 μg/kg/minute) and causes alpha effects at 10 to 20 μg/kg/minute with peripheral vasoconstriction and increased cerebral perfusion. It is often titrated to cardiac output. *Phenylephrine* is a vasopressor, which acts by stimulating alpha-adrenergic receptors. Levophed may also be used.

Hypertensive crisis requires immediate attention to prevent a stroke. Although there is no ideal drug, a nitroprusside drip is often the drug of choice for hypertensive crisis. *Sodium nitroprusside* (Nipride) has a rapid onset (within seconds) and lasts 1 to 3 minutes. It decreases cerebral vascular resistance and increases ICP by dilating arterial and venous smooth muscles so that CPP falls by as much as 50%. With *nitroglycerin,* the fall in CPP and rise in ICP are even worse than they are with nitroprusside. Nimodipine and verapamil are the major calcium channel blockers used in hypertensive crisis. *Nimodipine* has an unpredictable effect on ICP, CBF, and CPP, but it is useful for cerebral vasospasm. *Verapamil* lowers systemic blood pressure and CPP significantly (about 33%) and increases ICP by up to 67%.

Hematological Complications

Many TBI patients develop a problem with clotting in the absence of evidence of excessive bleeding. Some develop disseminated intravascular coagulation (DIC), a catastrophic insult in brain injury. This condition results from a combination of the release of large amounts of thromboplastin and the presence of tissue emboli. The tissue emboli are produced by circulating factor XII from the vascular endothelial lining.[85]

Abnormal findings on the activated partial thromboplastin time (PTT), prothrombin time (PT), platelet count, and plasma fibrinogen level do not present a complete picture. Therefore, careful and accurate diagnostic reasoning is important. High titer of fibrin degradation products (FDPs) and prolonged PT and PTT are highly suggestive of DIC. The double-D-dimer degradation product is used to confirm the diagnosis. Other useful analyses include PT, ethanol gelatin tests, and fibrinopeptide-A level. If the patient survives, DIC corrects within hours. The mainstay of treatment is replacement of clotting factors and maintenance of adequate blood volume. Fresh frozen plasma is used to replace the fibrinogen and clotting factor VIII. Cryoprecipitate is used to replace clotting factor V.

Clotting Abnormalities Without Bleeding

Abnormalities in the aPTT, PT, platelet count, or plasma fibrinogen levels should be treated only when the underlying correctable cause has been identified (e.g., an anticonvulsant drug causing thrombocytopenia).

Deep Vein Thrombosis

About 40% of patients with TBI develop DVT.[86] For neurosurgical patients in general, the incidence of DVT in the calves is 29% to 43%. The development of DVT is related to surgery, immobility, motor deficits, lower-extremity trauma, and gram-negative sepsis, which are all common in TBI patients. Contrast venogram, an invasive procedure, provides a definitive diagnosis. Clinical evidence in the presence of DVT is found in only a small number of patients. Because DVT can lead to pulmonary embolus, it needs to be treated when suspected. Treatment includes heparin therapy and possibly the insertion of a filter into the vena cava. However, prevention is the better alternative. Prophylaxis includes antiembolic elastic stockings and sequential compression boots. If not contraindicated, minidoses of heparin, 5,000 U subcutaneously every 12 hours, are helpful.

Gastrointestinal Complications

In the early acute phase of serious TBI, two major concerns for the nurse are gastric hemorrhage and gastric atony. Cushing's ulcer, common in TBI patients, occurs in the upper GI tract, whereas stress-related ulcerations usually occur in the duodenum. The use of H_2 blockers has decreased the incidence of Cushing's ulcers. If present, gastric atony, another common problem, delays beginning of feeding and may increase the risk of aspiration.[87] See the previous section on GI prophylaxis.

Metabolic Complications

Electrolyte and neuroendocrine disturbances are common in TBI patients. The most common electrolyte problem is hyponatremia often associated with either syndrome of inappropriate secretion of antidiuretic hormone (SIADH) or cerebral salt wasting. Hypernatremia is associated with diabetes insipidus. When potassium is affected, the more common condition involves hypokalemia rather than hyperkalemia. Hypokalemia is associated with an imbalance of aldosterone, hyperventilation, and the use of diuretics. Common neuroendocrine problems include diabetes insipidus, SIADH, cerebral salt wasting, and sometimes nonketotic hyperosmolar hyperglycemia. Some of these problems correct with supportive therapy, for example, maintaining fluid and electrolyte balance and volume replacement. See Chapter 10 for a detailed discussion and treatment.

Hyponatremia. Early recognition of hyponatremia is important so that early corrective measures can be instituted. IV solutions with higher concentrations of saline, extra salt added to the tube feeding, and drug therapy, such as fludrocortisone acetate (Florinef), are used. Fludrocortisone, a mineralocorticoid, increases sodium reabsorption in renal tubules and increases excretion of potassium and hydrogen. Dosage is 0.1 to 0.2 mg/day. To counter hypokalemia, potassium chloride is given in either a separate 20 to 40 mEq/ 1,000 mL IV unit or through a 20 mEq IV piggyback.

Hyperglycemia. In patients with TBI, an elevated serum glucose may be due to a stress response to head trauma or may be related to borderline or documented diabetes. As discussed previously in this chapter (see fluid management), an elevated serum glucose may aggravate ischemic insult in TBI patients and worsen neurological outcome. Therefore, glucose solutions should be avoided.[88] If serum glucose is elevated, a normal range can be established and maintained by starting a regular insulin drip. If the glucose remains high, a divided schedule of regular insulin and NPH insulin given subcutaneously should be started. Glucose must be aggressively controlled.

Fluid Replacement. The goal of fluid balance is euvolemia. (See the section on fluid replacement in this chapter.) Nursing management is directed toward monitoring serum electrolytes, glucose, osmolality, urine-specific gravity, fractional urinary output, and overall intake and output balance. Negative fluid balance contributes to hypotension and can lead to secondary brain injury.

Nutritional Support

Undernutrition or outright starvation is a common problem in patients with severe TBI. Starved patients lose sufficient nitrogen to reduce body weight by 15% each week. It is recommended that 140% of the resting metabolism level be replaced in nonparalyzed patients and that 100% be replaced in paralyzed patients.[43] The recommended route is by jejunal feeding because it avoids gastric intolerance and is easy to administer. By day 7 after injury, at least 15% of the calories in the feeding formula should be from protein.

A nutrition consultation should be obtained with the clinical dietitian within 24 hours of admission. Feeding should begin as soon as possible (within 24 hours of admission). Insertion of a Dobbhoff feeding tube into the jejunum of the small intestines is common because it avoids the problem of gastric intolerance, regurgitation, and aspiration common with a NG tube. Early feeding is important to maintain the integrity of the mucosal lining of the intestines; a beginning rate of 10 to 20 mL is reasonable. The clinical dietitian recommends the type of feeding and daily nutritional goals

until the patient is at the desired nutritional level. Feeding rate is gradually increased to the intended level, with the rate based on the patient's tolerance and response. Because the gut may trigger the development of multiple organ failure syndrome, postponement of feeding will increase this risk.

Nursing management is directed toward immediately addressing nutritional needs and beginning feeding expeditiously. Serum calcium, potassium, phosphorus, blood urea nitrogen, creatinine, and other laboratory values related to nutrition should be monitored. Interruptions in the feeding schedule should be avoided when possible as they can decrease the daily intake.[89] (See Chap. 9 for a discussion of nutritional needs.)

Sepsis and Sepsis Syndromes

Patients with TBI can develop sepsis from infection of initial injury sites (e.g., gunshot and other open head wounds), from infections associated with invasive procedures (e.g., ICP monitor, indwelling urinary catheter, pulmonary catheter, surgery), or from nosocomial infections. Universal precautions, strict aseptic technique, and adherence to culture and dressing protocols are critical for prevention. See the previous section on hyperthermia management and respiratory complications for additional information on prevention. The ICU nurse needs to be familiar with signs and symptoms of septic syndromes (e.g., decreased systemic vascular resistance and increased cardiac index) for early identification and management.

▌▌ NURSING MANAGEMENT FOR SPECIAL PROBLEMS

Basal Skull Fractures

The types of clinical evidence presented by a patient with a basal skull fracture depend on the particular basal skull fossa involved. Signs and symptoms may include ecchymosis of the mastoid process (Battle's sign), periorbital hemorrhage (raccoon's eyes) and ecchymosis, blood behind the eardrum (hemotympanum), decreased hearing, drainage from the nose (rhinorrhea) or ear (otorrhea), and postnasal drainage (postnasal drip). Nursing management addresses the risk of meningitis through the following strategies:

- Never suction through the nose if there is question of a basal skull fracture; the catheter could slip into the dural tear and become a source of contamination.
- In a conscious patient, caution against blowing the nose; this act could introduce microorganisms into the meninges or brain through a dural tear.
- Do not introduce any foreign body into the orifice (nares or ear) or irrigate the area; sterile cotton or other absorbent material should be placed loosely around the orifice and changed frequently.

If there is any question whether the drainage is CSF, laboratory analysis of a test tube specimen for chloride concentration is helpful. CSF's chloride concentration is greater than that of serum. Glucose testing for the presence of CSF is unreliable because nasal secretions can yield a positive reaction. The presence of drainage from the nose or ear is highly suggestive of CSF leakage. In clinical practice, drainage is often a combination of CSF and blood. A characteristic stain with a dark center and a lighter outer area (halo sign) is often seen. Most CSF leaks heal spontaneously within days. In rare instances, surgery is necessary to find and patch the tear. Use of prophylactic antibiotics for basal skull fractures is controversial.

A basal skull fracture can be very serious if rapidly developing local edema is close to vital brainstem structures. It can lead to life-threatening respiratory problems, including respiratory arrest. Nursing management includes monitoring for deterioration in vital or neurological signs as well as for signs of meningeal irritation.

Carotid-Cavernous Fistula

A carotid-cavernous fistula is a rare complication of TBI in which a laceration of the carotid artery results in direct communication between the high-pressure arterial blood of the internal carotid artery (ICA) and the low-pressure venous blood of the cavernous sinus. The cavernous sinuses are located at the basal skull on either side of the sphenoid body. The ICA, several of its branches, and the oculomotor, the trochlear, two divisions of the trigeminal, and the abducens nerves pass through the cavernous sinus. A patient with a carotid-cavernous fistula may present with one or more of the following signs: a bruit over the affected orbit; pulsating proptosis; conjunctival edema; orbital pain and chemosis; facial pain; limitation of extraocular movement; headache; diplopia; photophobia; and visual deficits (decreased visual acuity that can lead to blindness). The definitive diagnostic procedure is carotid angiography. Although spontaneous resolution may occur in a few patients, surgery is necessary for most. Surgical procedures include ligation of the ICA above and below the fistula or embolization. Nursing management includes neurological assessment, including all cranial nerves; auscultation of the bruit; assessment of pain; and monitoring for the presence of conjunctival edema. Special care is needed to prevent corneal ulceration and other injuries to the eyes.

Hygroma

A **hygroma,** which is an encapsulated collection of CSF, is caused by a tear in the arachnoid, which allows fluid to escape into the subdural space. Concurrent cerebral edema locks the fluid into the space and creates pressure on the brain. The total accumulation of fluid may range from a few milliliters to, in rare cases, as much as 50 mL. A subdural hygroma is unilateral but may extend over the entire hemisphere or become encapsulated. The fluid's high protein content may account for its occasional coagulation. Symptoms corresponding to a slowly developing SDH occur, beginning with headache, which becomes severe and persistent. The only effective treatment is surgical removal.

Nursing Management During the Intermediate Phase of Severe Traumatic Brain Injury

After the patient has been physiologically stabilized and no longer needs continuous monitoring, the collaborative team, working closely with the case manager, makes the decision to transfer the patient to an intermediate unit. The interdisciplinary care map that guided care in the ICU environment now continues in this next phase. Although the goals of nursing management remain much the same, the major focus now becomes rehabilitation and discharge planning.

Assessment and Ongoing Monitoring

Vital signs and neurological signs are assessed every 4 to 8 hours, depending on the patient's condition. If the patient is awake and able to follow commands, a much more complete assessment, especially with regard to cognitive status, is possible. Ability to respond to questions and participate in higher-level skills (e.g., doing calculations, identifying similarities between concepts, memory retrieval and problem solving) should be evaluated.

General nursing management principles include the following:

- Assess level of consciousness frequently to note any changes.
- If consciousness is altered, consider new neurological-related causes or causes other than neurological for the change.
- Reorient the patient to time, place, and person; use the patient's name.
- For patients who are classified as Level I to III on the Rancho Los Amigos Scale (RLAS), provide environmental stimuli or a sensory stimulation program;[90] talk to the patient, turn on the radio, open the shades, place family pictures in their visual field, and so forth.
- For patients who are at level IV to VI on the RLAS, provide structure and control stimulation.
- For patients who are at level VII to VIII on the RLAS, provide for practice in higher cognitive skills needed to integrate back into the community.

See Chapter 13 for a discussion of cognitive rehabilitation and the RLAS.

Cranial nerve, motor, sensory, and cerebellar function are assessed to determine functional deficits and their effect on activities of daily living. Collaboration with the case manager, social worker, physical therapist, occupational therapist, speech therapist, and others will refine the discharge plan. In the managed care environment, patients move through the system rapidly. Any education and teaching of the patient or family must be done in a compressed time frame.

The patient is monitored for evidence of medical complications and risks associated with secondary injury.

Minor and Moderate Traumatic Brain Injuries

The incidence of mild and moderate TBI is difficult to determine for several reasons, including the fact that many of these patients have no continuing contact with the health care system; there are varying definitions and classifications of mild and moderate TBI; accessible data sets do not exist; and TBI often coexists with other medical problems.

Although practitioners may intuitively distinguish among gradations of TBI, definitions of mild and moderate TBI are imprecise. Moreover, there are no good instruments to discriminate reliably among injury types. Additionally, victims are often seen at a doctor's office or ED, or not seen at all; consequently, they are often excluded from epidemiological databases. The TBI may be concurrent with other injuries that are more prominent and serious and thereby receive primary attention. The GCS is one widely used classification method. However, it may not be sensitive enough to capture the deficits common to these injuries. It is unclear what influence a managed care environment has on the diagnostic and treatment options available to persons with mild TBI.

Mild TBI (GCS = 13 to 15) is a transient event in which there may be a dazed appearance, unsteady gait, and short-term confusion after a blow to the head. The patient feels well after a few minutes; most patients have full recovery without problems. Some will have post-traumatic amnesia and post-concussion syndrome. A subgroup of patients, who seem perfectly fine when seen, develop secondary brain injury and die. The subject of secondary brain injury was previously addressed in this chapter.

No clear criteria exist for diagnosis or management of these patients. Whether all or only certain patients receive CT scans continues to be a clinical judgment of the caregiver. That all patients with a mild TBI need to be observed and monitored for evidence of deterioration is clear. Admission is warranted for patients in the following situations: loss of consciousness; neurological deficits; CSF leak or drainage from the nose or ear; alcohol consumption or other medical condition that makes assessment difficult; and absence of a support person. People exhibiting no significant signs and symptoms may be sent home with a responsible person. Written instructions should outline what signs and symptoms may develop and what should be done if they appear.

The term **moderate TBI** (GS = 9 to 12) indicates that more significant brain damage has occurred than with mild TBI. As this degree of brain injury is often concurrent with other organ system problems, the patient is initially managed as a multisystem trauma patient with all the precautions (e.g., cervical neck injury immobilization) outlined for severe TBI. After the patient has been stabilized, a CT scan should be done as soon as possible. Because the moderate TBI patient is often admitted to an other-than-neurological ICU, the neurological injuries may be underestimated and thus not treated appropriately. An appropriate level of care for patients with moderate TBI requires frequent neurological monitoring and involves the same complement of management considerations outlined for severe TBI. Serious post-injury deficits may develop that can affect the person's ability to work and function effectively in changing roles, such as parent, spouse, or community member. Personality dis-

orders are common. The moderate TBI patient needs to be monitored after discharge and provided with appropriate rehabilitation services and counseling.

Complaints of irritability, fatigue, headache, difficulty concentrating, dizziness, and memory problems, called **post-concussion syndrome,** often arise after moderate TBI. Anxiety and depression are also frequently noted, especially later in the course of the disorder. These symptoms were previously believed to be psychological in origin. However, current evidence supports the existence of a physiological basis for these complaints. Targeted education is helpful in assisting the patient and family cope with post-concussion syndrome. Supportive counseling may be necessary in dealing with emerging problems at work or at home. Symptoms usually subside with time but may last for months before resolution is complete.

Rehabilitation

Traumatic brain injury can bring with it a wide range of physical, behavioral, cognitive, and psychosocial problems. Based on an individual patient's needs, a plan of rehabilitative care is developed. The location for rehabilitation depends, among other factors, on the patient's functional deficits, the managed care options offered, and the available resources. Most discharge and transition planning is coordinated by a case manager. It is the nurse's responsibility to contribute to the database and work with the case manager as an advocate for the needs of the patient and family. Information on available community and national sources of support and information for TBI patients and their families should be provided.

The evidence base for rehabilitation of TBI was addressed in a 1998 report published by the Agency for Health Care Policy and Research (AHCPR).[91] This report makes clear that there are limited scientific data to support evidence-based practice and that there is a need to conduct studies to determine rehabilitation guidelines and standards. See also Chapter 13 for a discussion of rehabilitation of neuroscience patients.

The consequences of TBI are multifaceted and can be devastating, especially with severe TBI. Many of these problems are confronted initially in the rehabilitation setting and then in the community. For further in-depth discussion of this phase of recovery, consult the extensive rehabilitation literature.

▓ PREDICTING OUTCOME FROM TRAUMATIC BRAIN INJURY

Clinical prediction of outcome following TBI is a widely discussed issue in neuroscience practice. Although prognostic indicators are many, no individual variable or cluster of variables is sufficiently reliable to predict outcomes accurately. Because of the interest in enhancing accuracy, many early clinical factors have been identified as possible predictors. A report about traumatic coma indicates that the clinical examination is unreliable, that electrophysiological testing is much more useful, and that brainstem and sensory evoked potentials are helpful within the first week.[92]

In an evidence-based methodological approach to prognostic indicators for severe TBI,[93] a positive predictive value of at least 70% in key criteria was chosen as necessary for an indicator to be included.[94–103] The following indicators met these criteria and are deemed reliable indicators for predicting poor outcome:

- Low score on GCS (≤8)
- Increased age
- Bilaterally absent pupillary light reflex
- Systolic blood pressure less than 90 mm Hg, further strengthened when combined with hypoxia
- Abnormalities on CT scan

The well-known **Glasgow Outcome Scale** places survivors of central nervous system trauma (Chart 18-5) in one of five categories, depending on the degree of their residual function and independence. The scale, which does not evaluate cognitive impairment, conveys only the examiner's general opinion of the patient's status.

Quality of life has become an important framework for describing outcome. However, this concept still has not been properly defined, and a means of measuring it has not been established. The most frequently mentioned indicators for quality of life are independence in performing activities of daily living, ability to maintain social relationships, successful role implementation, gainful employment, and general ability to maintain control of one's life.

PERSONALITY AND BEHAVIORAL DEFICITS

The presence and persistence of behavioral problems in TBI patients are associated with the site and severity of injury, the nature of the premorbid personality, and environmental factors. Personality changes may include silly, childish behavior, as characterized by self-centeredness, an inability to show empathy, impatience, and impulsiveness. Injuries predominantly involving the frontal lobe are characterized by decreased drive and initiative, flat affect, disinhibition, dis-

---

CHART 18–5 • Glasgow Outcome Scale

- *Good outcome*—may have minimal disabling sequelae but returns to independent functioning and a full-time job comparable to preinjury level
- *Moderate disability*—capable of independent functioning but not returned to full-time employment
- *Severe disability*—dependent on others for some aspect of daily living
- *Persistent vegetative state*—no obvious cortical function
- Dead

Jennett, B., & Bond, M. (1975). Assessment of outcome after severe brain damage: A practical scale. *Journal of Neurosurgery, 4,* 673.

---

regard for social protocols, apathy, lethargy, lack of goal-directed behavior, difficulty with impulse control, and an impaired sense of self-identity. Lesions of the temporal lobe are characterized by episodes of violent behavior and possibly seizure disorders. Early intervention is helpful in modifying behavioral patterns and in assisting the patient and family in managing such behaviors before they become established.

FAMILY RELATIONSHIP DEFICITS

The patient's psychosocial and personality deficits, alterations in the patient's roles and responsibilities, and the tremendous burden placed on the family resulting from injury disrupt family function. If the family was dysfunctional before the injury, the added stress of a severely TBI family member compounds that stress. The stress on a marriage is significant when one partner is the victim. The uninjured spouse must become the caregiver for someone quite different from the person he or she married. The enormous stresses on the caregiver, especially those related to fatigue, are well documented in the literature.

SUMMARY

This chapter provides an overview of craniocerebral trauma, including diagnosis, treatment, and collaborative management across the continuum of acute care. The evidence base for practice is discussed, particularly for the management of severe TBI. Research at both the physiological and clinical levels will continue to develop the evidence base for management of TBI to achieve optimal patient outcomes.

REFERENCES

1. Kraus, H. F., & McArthur, D. L. (2000). Epidemiology of brain injury. In P. R. Cooper & J. G. Golfinos (Eds.). *Head injury* (4th ed., pp. 1–26). New York: McGraw-Hill.
2. Saul, T. G., & Kelker, D. (1996). The think first program. In R. K. Narayan, J. E. Wilberger, & J. T. Povlishock (Eds.). *Neurotrauma* (pp. 1031–1037). New York: McGraw-Hill.
3. Adams, J. H., Mitchell, D. E., Scott, G., et al. (1980). Brain damage in non-missile TBI. *Journal of Clinical Pathology, 33,* 1132–1145.
4. Graham, D. I., Adams, J. H., Nicoll, J. A. R., et al. (1995). The nature, distribution, and causes of traumatic brain injury. *Brain Pathology, 5,* 397–406.
5. Gennarelli, T. A. (1994). Animate models of TBI. *Journal of Neurotrauma, 11,* 357–368.
6. Cruz, J., Minoja, G., Mattioli, C., et al. (1998). Severe acute brain trauma. In J. Cruz (Ed.). *Neurological and neurosurgical emergencies* (pp. 405–436). Philadelphia: W. B. Saunders.
7. Dietrich, W. D. (2000). Trauma of the nervous system A. Basic neuroscience of neurotrauma. In W. G. Bradley, R. B. Daroff, G. M. Fenichel, & C. D. Marsden. (Eds.). *Neurology in clinical practice* (3rd ed., pp. 1045–1054). Boston: Butterworth & Heinemann.
8. Gennarelli, T. A., & Thibault, L. E. (1985). Biological modes of TBI. In D. P. Becker & J. T. Povlishock (Eds.). *Central nervous system trauma status report: National Institute of Neurological and*

Communicative Disorders and Stroke (pp. 391–404). Bethesda, MD: National Institute of Health.

9. Graham, D. I., & Gennarelli, T. A. (2000). Pathology of brain damage after TBI. In P. R. Cooper & J. G. Golfinos (Eds.). *Head injury* (4th ed., pp. 133–153). New York: McGraw-Hill.

10. Valsamis, M. P. (1994). Pathology of trauma. *Neurosurgery Clinics of North America, 5*(1), 175–183.

11. Gennarelli, T. A., Thibault, L. E., Tipperman, R., et al. (1989). Axonal injury in the optic nerve: A model simulating diffuse axonal injury in the brain. *Journal of Neurosurgery, 71*, 244.

12. Povlishock, J. T., Becker, D. P., Cheng, C., et al. (1983). Axonal change in minor head injury. *Journal of Neuropathological Experimental Neurology, 42*, 225.

13. Le Roux, P. D., Choudhri, H., & Andrews, B. T. (2000). Cerebral concussion and diffuse brain injury. In P. R. Cooper & J. G. Golfinos (Eds.). *Head injury* (4th ed., pp. 175–199). New York: McGraw-Hill.

14. Maxwell, W. L, Povlishock, J. T., Graham, D. I., et al. (1997). A mechanistic analysis of non-disruptive axonal injury. *Journal of Neurotrauma, 14*, 419–440.

15. Pilz, P. Axonal injury in head injury. (1983). *Acta Neurochirurgica (Suppl) 32*, 119–123.

16. Yaghmai, A., & Povlishock, J. T. (1992). Traumatically induced reactive change as visualized through the use of monoclonal antibodies targeted to neurofilament subunits. *Journal of Neuropathological Experimental Neurology, 23*, 63–78.

17. Bullock, R., & Fujisawa, H. (1992). The role of glutamate antagonists for the treatment of CNS injury. *Journal of Neurotrauma, 9* (Suppl. 2), S443-S462.

18. Siejo, B. (1991). The role of calcium in cell death. In D. Price, A. Aguayo, & H. Thoenen (Eds.). *Neurodegenerative disorders: Mechanisms and prospects for therapy* (pp. 35–69). London: J Wiley & Sons.

19. Mcintosh, T. K., Saatman, K. E., & Raghupathi. (1997). Calcium and the pathogenesis of traumatic CMS: Cellular and molecular mechanisms. *Neuroscientist, 3*, 169–175.

20. Mcintosh, T. K., Saatman, K. E., & Raghupathi. (1998). The molecular and cellular sequence of experimental traumatic brain injury: Pathogenic mechanisms. *Neuropathology Applied Neurobiology, 24*, 251–267.

21. Mcintosh, T. K., Saatman, K. E., & Raghupathi. (1996). Neuropathological sequelae of traumatic brain injury: Relationship to neurochemical and biomechanical mechanisms. *Laboratory Investigation, 74*, 315–342.

22. Young, B. F., Runge, J. M., & Waxman, K. S. (1996). Effects of pegorgotein on neurologic outcome of patients with severe TBI. *Journal of the American Medical Association, 276*, 538–543.

23. Reilly, P. L., Graham, D. I., Adams, J. H., et al. (1975). Patients with TBI who talk and die. *Lancet, 2*, 375–377.

24. Jennett, B., & Carlin, J. (1978). Preventable mortality and morbidity after TBI. *Injury, 10*, 31–39.

25. Povlishock, J. T., Marmarou, A., Mcintosh, T. K., et al. (1997). Impact acceleration injury in the rat: Evidence for focal axolemmal change and related sidearm alteration. *Journal of Neuropathology Experimental Neurology, 56*, 347–359.

26. LeRoux, P., Haglund, M., Newell, D., et al. (1992). Intraventricular hemorrhage in blunt TBI: An analysis of 43 cases. *Neurosurgery, 31*, 678–685.

27. Greenberg, M. S. (1997). *Handbook of neurosurgery* (4th ed., pp. 690–753). Lakeland, FL: Greenberg Graphics.

28. Jennett, B., & Teasdale, G. (1981). *Management of traumatic brain injury*. Philadelphia: F. A. Davis.

29. Adams, J. H., Doyle, D., Ford, I., Gennarelli, T. A., Graham, D. I., & McLellan D. R. (1989). Diffuse axonal injury in TBI: Definition, diagnosis, and grading. *Histopathology, 15*, 49–59.

30. Chedid, M. K., & Flannery, A. M. (1995). Head trauma. In J. E. Parrillo & R. C. Bone (Eds.). *Critical care medicine: Principles of diagnosis and management* (pp. 123–1259). St. Louis: C.V. Mosby.

31. Evans, R. W., & Wilberger, J. E. (1999). Traumatic disorders. In C. G. Goetz & E. J. Pappert (Eds.). *Textbook of clinical neurology* (pp. 1035–1958). Philadelphia: W. B. Saunders.

32. Jallo, J. I., & Narayan, R. K. (2000). Trauma of the nervous system: Craniocerebral trauma. In W. G. Bradley, R. B. Daroff, G. M. Fenichel, & C. D. Marsden (Eds.). *Neurology in clinical practice: The neurological disorders* (3rd ed., pp. 1055–1087). Boston: Butterworth-Heinemann.

33. Graham, D. I., Lawrence, A. E., Adams, J. H., et al. (1994). βAPP is a marker of axonal injury. *Brain Pathology, 4*, P23-24.

34. Crooks, D. A. (1991). The pathological concept of diffuse axonal injury; Its pathogenesis and the assessment of severity. *Journal of Pathology, 165*, 5–10.

35. Slazinski, T., & Johnson, M. C. (1994). Severe diffuse axonal injury in adults and children. *Journal of Neuroscience Nursing, 26*(3), 151–154.

36. Gennarelli, T., Spielman, G., Langfitt, T., et al. (1982). The influence of the type of intracranial lesion on outcome from severe TBI: A multicenter study using a new classification system. *Journal of Neurosurgery, 56*, 26–32.

37. Gennarelli, T. A. (1993). Cerebral concussion and diffuse brain injuries. In P. R. Cooper (Ed.). *Head injury* (3rd ed., pp. 137–158). Baltimore: Williams & Wilkins.

38. Kaufman, H. H. (1993). Civilian gunshot wounds to the head. *Neurosurgery, 32*, 962–964.

39. Rosenberg, W. S., & Harsh IV, G. R. (1999). Penetrating cerebral trauma. In R. G. Grossman & C. M. Loftus (Eds.). *Principles of neurosurgery* (2nd ed., pp. 173–182). Philadelphia: Lippincott-Raven Publishers.

40. Chesnut, R. M., & Marshall, L. F. (1993). Management of severe TBI. In A. H. Ropper (Ed.). *Neurological and neurosurgical intensive care* (3rd ed., pp. 203-246). New York: Raven Press.

41. Brandt, K. E., Burruss, G. L., Hickerson, W. I., White, C. E., & McLellan, D. R. (1991). The management of mid-face fractures with intracranial injury. *The Journal of Trauma, 31*(1), 15-19.

42. Bullock, R., Chesnut, R. M., Clifton, G., et al. (1996). Guidelines for the management of severe head injury. *Journal of Neurotrauma, 13*(11), 639-734.

43. Bullock, R., Chesnut, R. M., Clifton, G., et al. (2000). Guidelines for the management of severe traumatic brain injury. *Journal of Neurotrauma, 17*(6/7), 451–553.

44. ACS-COT. (1998). *American College of Surgeons Committee on Trauma Resources for Optimal Care of the Injured Patient: 1999*. Chicago: American College of Surgeons.

45. Vassar, M. J., Fisher, R. P, O'Brien, P. E., et al. (1993). A multicenter trial for resuscitation of injured patients with 7.5% sodium chloride. The effect of added dextran 70. The Multicenter Group for the Study of Hypertonic Saline in Trauma Patients. *Archives of Surgery, 128*, 1003–1011.

46. Chesnut, R. M., Marshall, L. F., Klauber, M. R., et al. (1993). The role of secondary brain injury in determining outcome from severe TBI. *Journal of Trauma, 34*, 216–222.

47. Fearnside, M. R., Cook, R. J., McDougall, P., et al. (1993). The Westmead TBI Project outcome in severe TBI: A comparative analysis of pre-hospital, clinical, and CT variables. *British Journal of Neurosurgery, 7*, 267–279.

48. Pigula, F. A., Wald, S. L., Shackford, S. R., et al. (1993). The effect of hypotension and hypoxia on children with severe TBI. *Journal of Pediatric Surgery, 28*, 310–316.

49. Rosomoff, H. L., Kochanek, P. M., Clark, R. et al. (1996). Resuscitation from severe brain trauma. *Critical Care Medicine, 24*(Suppl.), S48–S56.

50. Saul, T. G., & Ducker, T. B. (1982). Effects of intracranial pressure monitoring and aggressive treatment on mortality in severe TBI. *Journal of Neurosurgery, 56*, 498–503.

51. Chesnut, R. M. (1995). Medical management of severe TBI: Present and future. *New Horizons, 3*(3), 581–593.

52. Prielipp, R. C., & Coursin, D. B. (1995). Sedative and neuromuscular blocking drug use in critically ill patients with TBI. *New Horizons, 3*(3), 456–468.

53. Murray, M. J., Strickland, R. A., & Weiler, C. (1993). The use of neuromuscular blocking drugs in the intensive care unit: A US perspective. *Intensive Care Medicine, 19*, S40–S44.

54. Ford, E. V. (1995). Monitoring neuromuscular blockade in the adult ICU. *American Journal of Critical Care, 4*(2), 122–130.

55. Kennedy, P. A., & Schalleri, G. (2001). Practical issues and concepts in vagus nerve stimulation: A nursing review. *Journal of Neuroscience Nursing, 33*(2), 105–112.

56. Giannotta, S. L., Weiss, M. H. Apuzzo, M. L. J., et al. (1984). High-dose glucocorticoids in the management in the management of severe head injury. *Neurosurgery, 15*, 497–501.

57. Marshall, L. F., Maas, A. L., Marshall, S. B., et al. (1998). A multicenter trial on the efficacy of using tirilazad mesylate in cases of head injury. *Journal of Neurosurgery, 89*, 519–525.

58. Temkin, N. R., Dikmen, S. S., & Winn, H. R. (1991). Posttraumatic seizures. In H. M. Eisenberg & E. F. Aldrich (Eds.). *Management of head injury* (pp. 425–435). Philadelphia: W. B. Saunders.

59. Yablon, S. A. (1993). Posttraumatic seizures. *Archives of Physical Medicine & Rehabilitation, 74*, 983–1001.

60. Temkin, N. R., Dikmen, S. S., Wilensky A. J., et al. (1990). A randomized, double-blind study of phenytoin for the prevention of post-traumatic seizures. *New England Journal of Medicine, 323*(8), 497–502.

61. Manaka, S. (1992). Cooperative prospective study on posttraumatic epilepsy: Risk factors and the effect of prophylactic anticonvulsant. *Japanese Journal of Psychiatry and Neurology, 46*, 311–315.

62. McQueen, J. K., Blackwood, D. H. R., Harris, P., et al. (1983). Low risk of late post-traumatic seizures following severe head injury: Implications for clinical trails of prophylaxis. *Journal of Neurology, Neurosurgery, and Psychiatry, 46*, 899–904.

63. Vandam, L. D., & Burnap, T. K. (1959). Hypothermia. *New England Journal of Medicine, 261*, 595–603.

64. Bouma, G. J., Muizelaar, J. P., Choi, S. C., Newlon, P. G., & Young, H. F. (1991). Cerebral circulation and metabolism after severe traumatic brain injury: The elusive role of ischemia. *Journal of Neurosurgery, 75*, 685–693.

65. Jaggi, J. L., Obrist, W. D., Gennerelli, T. A., & Langfitt, T. W. (1990). Relationship of early cerebral blood flow and metabolism to outcome in acute head injury. *Journal of Neurosurgery, 72*, 176–182.

66. Marion, D. W., Darby, J., & Yonas, H. (1991). Acute regional cerebral blood flow changes caused by severe head injuries I. *Journal of Neurosurgery, 74*, 407–414.

67. Robertson, C. S., Clifton, G. L., Grossman, R. G., et al. (1988). Alterations in cerebral availability of metabolic substrates after severe head injury. *Journal of Trauma, 28*, 1523–1532.

68. Salvant, J. B., & Muizelaar, J. P. Changes in cerebral blood flow and metabolism related to the presence of subdural hematoma. *Neurosurgery 33*, 387–393.

69. Bouma, G. J., Muizelaar, J. P., Stinger, W. A., et al. (1992). Ultra early evaluation of regional cerebral blood flow in severely head injured patients using xenon enhanced coupled tomography. *Journal of Neurosurgery, 77*, 360–368.

70. Obrist, W. D., Langfitt, T. W., Jaggi, J. L., Cruz, J., & Gennarelli, T. A. (1984). Cerebral blood flow and metabolism in comatose patients with acute head injury. *Journal of Neurosurgery, 61*, 241–253.

71. Obrist, W. D., Gennarelli, T. A, Segawa, H., & Dolinskas, C. A. (1979). Relation of cerebral blood flow to neurological status and outcome in head-injured patients. *Journal of Neurosurgery, 51*, 292–300.

72. Schroder, M. L., Muizellar, J. P., & Kuta, A. J. (1994). Documented reversal of global ischemia immediately after removal of an acute subdural hematoma. *Neurosurgery, 80*, 324–327.

73. Muizelaar, J. P., Marmarou, A., Ward, J. D., et al. (1991). Adverse effects of prolonged hyperventilation in patients with severe TBI: A randomized clinical trial. *Journal of Neurosurgery, 75*, 731–739.

74. Zornow, M. H., & Prough, D. S. (1995). Fluid management in patients with traumatic brain injury. *New Horizons, 3*(3), 488–498.

75. Pulsinelli, W. A., Waldman, S., Rawlinson, D. et al. (1982). Moderate hyperglycemia agents and ischemia brain damage: A neuropathologic study in the rat. *Neurology, 32*, 1239–1246.

76. Lanier, W. L., Stangland, K. J., Scheithauer, B. W. et al. (1987). The effects of dextrose infusion and head position on neurologic outcome after complete cerebral ischemia in primates: Examination of a model. *Anesthesiology, 66*, 39–48.

77. Zornow, M. H., & Prough, D. S. (1995). Fluid management in patients with traumatic brain. *New Horizons, 3*(3), 492.

78. Demopoulous, H. B., Flamm, E. S., Pietronigro, D. D., et al. (1980). The free radical pathology and the microcirculation in the major central nervous system. *Acta Physiologica Scandinavia Supplement, 492*, 91–119.

79. Kassell, N. F., Hitchon, P. W., Gerk, M. K., et al. (1980). Alterations in cerebral blood flow, oxygen metabolism, and electrical activity produced by high-dose thiopental. *Neurosurgery, 7*, 598–603.

80. Clifton, G. L., Miller, E., R., Choi, S., et al. (2001). Lack of effect of induction of hypothermia after acute brain injury. *New England Journal of Medicine, 344*(8), 556–563.

81. Rosner, M. J., Rosner, S. D., & Johnson, A. H. (1995). Cerebral perfusion pressure: Management protocol and clinical results. *Journal of Neurosurgery, 83*, 949–962.

82. Mcilvoy, L., Spain, D. A., Raque, G., Vitaz, T., Baoz, P., & Meyer, K. (2001). Successful incorporation of the severe head injury guidelines into a phased-outcome clinical pathway. *Journal of Neuroscience Nursing, 33*(2), 72–78.

83. Sullivan, J. (2000). Positioning of patients with severe traumatic brain injury: Research-based practice. *Journal of Neuroscience Nursing, 32*(4), 204–209.

84. Tietjen, C. S., Hurn, P. D., Ulatowski, J. A., & Kirsch, J. R. (1996). Treatment modalities for hypertensive patients with intracranial pathology: Options and risks. *Critical Care Medicine, 24*(2), 311–322.

85. Chesnut, R. M. (1993). Medical complications of the TBI patient. In P. R. Cooper (Ed.). *Head injury* (pp. 476–478). Baltimore: Williams & Wilkins.

86. Nih, C. R. (1986). Prevention of venous thrombosis and pulmonary embolism. *Journal of the American Medical Association, 256*, 744–749.

87. Kaufman, H. H., Timberlake, G., Voelker J., & Pait, T. G. (1993). Medical complications of TBI. *Medical Clinics of North America, 77*(1), 43–60.

88. Lam, A. M., Winn, H. R., Cullen, B. F., & Sundling, N. (1991). Hyperglycemia and neurological outcome in patients with TBI. *Journal of Neurosurgery, 75*, 5445–5551.

89. Stechmiller, J., Treloar, D. M., Derrico, D., Yarandi, H., & Guin, P. (1994). Interruption of enteral feedings in head injured patients. *Journal of Neuroscience Nursing, 26*(4), 224–229.

90. Davis, A. E., & White, J. J. (1995). Innovative sensory input for the comatose brain-injured patient. *Critical Care Nursing Clinics of North America, 7*(2), 351–361.

91. Agency for Health Care Policy and Research. (1998). *Rehabilitation for traumatic brain injury. Summary, evidence report/technology assessment, No 2*. Rockville, MD: Agency for Health Care Policy and Research. (http://ww.ahcpr.gov/clinic/thisumm.htm)

92. Attia, J., & Cook, D. J. (1998). Prognosis in anoxic and traumatic coma. *Critical Care Clinics, 14*(3), 497–511.

93. Chesnut, R. M., Ghajar, J., Maas, A. I. R., et al. (2000). Early indicators of prognosis in severe traumatic brain injury. *Journal of Neurotrauma, 17*(6/7), 557–627.

94. Braakman, R., Gelpke, G. J., Habbema, J. D. F., et al. (1980). Systematic selection of prognostic features in patients with severe head injury. *Neurosurgery, 6*, 262–370.

95. Chang, R. W. S., Lee, B., & Jacobs, S. (1989). Accuracy of decisions to withdraw therapy in critically ill patients: Clinical judgment versus a computer model. *Critical Care Medicine, 17,* 1091–1097.

96. Foulkes, M. A., Eisenberg, H. M., Jane, J. A. et al. (1991). The Traumatic Coma Data Bank–Design, methods, and baseline characteristics. *Journal of Neurosurgery, 75,* S8-S13.

97. Jennett, B., & Bono, M. (1975). Assessment of outcome after severe brain damage. A practical scale. *Lancet, 1,* 480-485.

98. Jennett, B., Teasdale, G., Braakman, R., et al. (1979). Prognosis of patients with severe head injury. *Neurosurgery, 4,* 283–289.

99. Kaufmann, M. S., Buchmann, B., Scheidegger, D., Gratzl, O., & Radu, E. W. (1992). Severe head injury: Should expected outcome influence resuscitation and first day decisions? *Resuscitation, 23,* 199–206.

100. Langfitt, T. W. (1978). Measuring the outcome from head injuries. *Journal of Neurosurgery, 48,* 673–678.

101. Marshall, L. F., Becker, D. P., Bowers, S. A., et al. (1983). The national Traumatic Coma Data Bank. Part I. Design, purpose, goals and results. *Journal of Neurosurgery, 59,* 276–284.

102. Marshall, L. F., Gautille, T., Klauber, M., et al. (1991). The outcome of severe closed head injury. *Journal of Neurosurgery, 75,* S28–S36.

103. Teasdale, G., & Jennett, B. (1974). Assessment of coma and impaired consciousness. *Lancet, 2,* 81–84.

Kerr, M. E., & Brucia, J. (1993). Hyperventilation in the TBI patient: An effective treatment modality? *Heart & Lung, 22,* 516–521.

Marmarou, A. (1994). Traumatic brain edema: An overview. *Acta Neurochirurgica, 60*(Suppl.), 421–424.

McIntosh, T. K. (1994). Neurochemical sequelae of traumatic brain injury: Therapeutic implications. *Cerebrovascular and Brain Metabolism Reviews, 6,* 109–162.

Qureshi, A. I., & Suarez, J. I. (2000). Use of hypertonic saline solutions in treatment of cerebral edema and intracranial hypertension. *Critical Care Medicine, 28*(9), 3301–3313.

Richmond, T. S. (1997). Cerebral resuscitation after global brain ischemia: Linking research to practice. *AACN Clinical Issues, 8*(2), 171–181.

Richardson, J. T. (2000). *Clinical and neuropsychological aspects of closed head injury.* Philadelphia: Taylor & Francis.

Rimel, R. W., Giordani, B., Barth, J. T., Boll, T. J., & Jane, J. A. (1981). Disability caused by minor TBI. *Neurosurgery, 9,* 221–228.

Rosenthal, M. (1993). Mild traumatic brain injury syndrome. *Annals of Emergency Medicine, 22*(6), 1048–1051.

Sundrani, S. (1995). Neurologic intensive care unit management and economic issues. *Neurologic Critical Care, 13*(3), 679–693.

Vollmer, D. G., & Dacey, R. G. (1991). The management of mild and moderate TBI. *Neurosurgery Clinics of North America, 2*(2), 437–455.

Wrightson, P., & Gronwall, D. (1999). *Mild TBI: A guide to management.* New York: Oxford University Press.

Young, G. B. (1995). Neurologic complications of systemic critical illness. *Neurologic Clinics, 13*(3), 645–658.

RESOURCES

Professional

Printed Materials

Cruz, J. (1998). *Neurologic and neurosurgical emergencies.* Philadelphia: W. B. Saunders Co.

Cooper, P. R., & Golfinos, J. G. (Eds.). (2000). *Head injury* (4th ed.). New York: McGraw-Hill.

Hilton, G. (2000). Cerebral oxygenation in the traumatically brain-injured patient: Are ICP and CPP enough? *Journal of Neuroscience Nursing, 32*(5), 278–282.

Patient and Family

Gronwall, D., Wrighton, P., & Waddel, P. (1999). *TBI: The facts: A guide for families and caregivers.* New York: Oxford University Press.

Websites for Providers, Patient, and Family

There are hundreds on the Internet; below are a few to begin a search for specific information.

Brain Injury Association USA: http://www.biausa.org/

Intro to Neuroscience Center: http://www.netdirect.net/nsp/

Brain Injury Resource Center: http://www.headinjury.com/

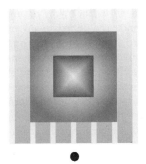

Vertebral and Spinal Cord Injuries

JOANNE V. HICKEY

A PERSPECTIVE

Statistics and Facts

The following information on spinal cord injury (SCI) is taken from a 1999 report of the National Spinal Cord Injury Statistical Center Institute:[1]

- **Incidence:** Annual incidence of SCI, not including those who die at the scene of the accident, is approximately 10,000 new cases each year. Because no overall incidence studies of SCI in the United States have been reported since the 1970s, it is not known whether the pattern of incidence has changed in recent years.
- **Prevalence:** The number of people living with SCIs in the United States is estimated to be 183,000 to 203,000.
- **Age:** 56% occurs in people 16 to 30 years old.
- **Gender:** 82% male.
- **Major categories of causes:** Motor vehicle accidents (44%), acts of violence (17%) (primarily gunshot wounds), falls (22%), recreational sports (7%), and other (10%).
- **Level of injury:** 51.9% had cervical injuries resulting in quadriplegia; 46.7% had lesions in the thoracic, lumbar, or sacral regions of the spinal cord resulting in paraplegia; 0.7% recovered before discharge; and for 0.7%, the level of injury was unknown.
- **Length-of-stay (LOS):** LOS in the hospital has decreased from 26 days in 1974 to 14 days in 1997. Rehabilitation LOS for the same years declined from 115 days to 46 days.
- **Lifetime cost:** The average yearly health care and living expenses related to SCI varies greatly depending on severity and level of injury. The estimated lifetime costs for age 25-years is $1.7 million for a high quadriplegic (C1-C4) and $545,000 for a paraplegic based on 1999 data.[2]
- **Causes of death:** Pneumonia, pulmonary emboli, and septicemia.

Comprehensive Evidence-Based Practice

The model regional SCI care system program was established in 1970 by the Rehabilitation Services Administration. The lessons learned from this program have led to a com-prehensive, cost-effective model for managing SCI patients across the continuum of care, from accident scene through rehabilitation. Currently, 18 model SCI systems across the country provide a continuing source of research and evidence-based practice. Of the resulting changes in care of acute SCI patients, the most important is use of the high-dose steroid protocol established in 1991. This is discussed in the Treatment section.

UNDERSTANDING SPINAL CORD INJURIES

Anatomical Considerations

To appreciate the potential for injury to the spinal axis and its surrounding structures, one must understand the interrelated function of anatomical structures involved, namely, the vertebral column, the spinal cord, the supporting soft tissue, and the intervertebral disks. The vertebrae are irregularly shaped bones that support the muscles and protect the spinal cord. There are 33 vertebrae in the vertebral column: seven cervical, twelve thoracic or dorsal, five lumbar, five sacral (fused as one), and four coccygeal (fused as one). The vertebrae of each area have a distinctive shape. Stacked one on another to form the vertebral column, the vertebrae are laced into position by a series of supporting structures called *ligaments*. The ligaments, muscles, and other supporting structures are considered to be soft-tissue components (Figs. 19-1 and 19-2; see also Chap. 5).

There are two main parts to a vertebra: the body and the arch. The vertebral bodies are separated by intervertebral discs that serve as shock absorbers for the vertebral column during movement. The arch of the vertebra is created by a series of irregularly shaped projections. The fusion of the two pedicles and two laminae along with seven articular processes create a bony ring. The various projections of the vertebral arch allow for alignment, flexion, and movement of the vertebral column. The soft, vulnerable spinal cord passes through the bony arch of the vertebrae, which offer it protection.

The close anatomical relationship of the vertebrae, ligaments, and other soft tissue structures, intervertebral discs,

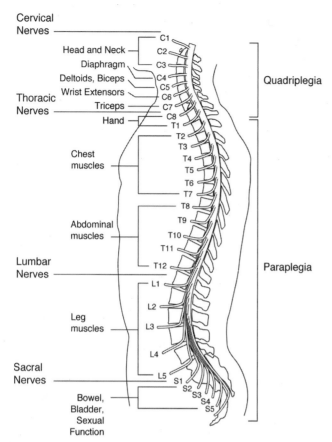

Figure 19–1 • The level of spinal cord injury and functional loss; the higher the spinal cord injury, the more motor, sensory, and autonomic functional losses are incurred.

and spinal cord increases the probability that injury to any one of these structures can cause concurrent injury to any or all of the other structures. In other instances, injury to one structure, such as a vertebral fracture, can create the potential of injury to another structure, such as the spinal cord, if the primary injury is not treated promptly and effectively. Therefore, when discussing injury to the vertebral column and spinal cord, one must consider the interrelatedness of not only these two structures, but also the supporting soft-tissue structures and the intervertebral discs.

Vertebral, spinal cord, and soft-tissue injuries are discussed in this chapter. Intervertebral disc disease is the focus of Chapter 20.

Kinetics of Movement

The seven cervical vertebrae support the head, which weighs 8 to 10 lb. These vertebrae provide substantial movement of the neck and head in various directions, including flexion, extension, and rotation. The total amount of flexion and extension possible at the cervical spine is an 80-degree arc, 75% of which is extension. Rotation is made possible by the uniquely shaped atlas (C-1) and axis (C-2). Beneath the cervical vertebrae are the 12 thoracic vertebrae, which move very little owing to the anchoring of the ribs. Because the cervical spine is not fixed like the thoracic spine, it is extremely vulnerable to injury as a result of acceleration-deceleration forces.

Mechanics of Injury

Vertebral injuries and SCIs result when excessive forces are exerted on the vertebral column. These forces are most often the result of acceleration-deceleration events that result in hyperflexion, hyperextension, deformation, axial loading, and excessive rotation.

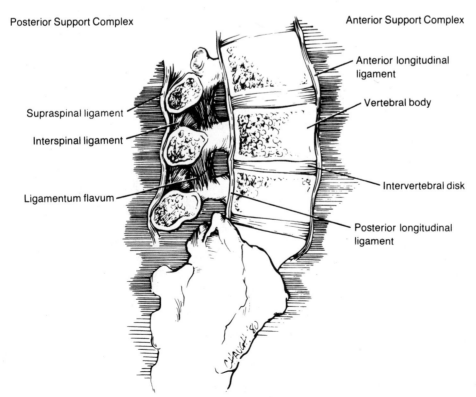

Figure 19–2 • Soft-tissue supporting structures of the spine. Two basic soft-tissue units constitute each spinal segment: the *anterior support complex,* formed by the anterior and posterior longitudinal ligaments, the disc, and the annulus, and the *posterior support complex,* formed by the supra-spinal ligament and interspinal ligament, the ligamentum flavum, and the facet capsules. When the posterior complex is disrupted, the spine is unstable, and surgical fusion is necessary. When the anterior complex is disrupted, the spine is usually more stable and can heal with use of a rigid brace. (From Weiner, W. J., & Goetz, C. G. [Eds.] [1989]. *Neurology for the non-neurologist* [2nd ed.] [p. 261]. Philadelphia: J. B. Lippincott.)

Acceleration-Deceleration Events

Acceleration and deceleration are discussed together because they often occur in split-second sequence. At the moment of impact in a rear-end motor vehicle collision (i.e., external force applied from the rear), there is sudden **acceleration** of the portion of the body in contact with the seat. The head and upper back, which were not in contact with the seat or headrest, are violently thrust backward (hyperextension). After the head strikes the back of the seat or has hyperextended to its limit, it is then thrust forward. The head may strike the steering wheel or dashboard as it slows down (decelerates).

Deceleration is often the major mechanism of injury involved in a head-on motor vehicle collision. While the outside force, exerted from the front, abruptly arrests the vehicle's motion, the head and body continue moving forward until contact is made, usually with the dashboard. The person is forcibly hyperflexed while moving forward, hits the dashboard, and then snaps back into a forced hyperextension position.

Responses to Extreme Acceleration-Deceleration Events

Acceleration-deceleration can produce simultaneous and/or successive actions as detailed in the following descriptions:

- **Hyperflexion** tends to produce compression of the vertebral bodies with disruption of the posterior longitudinal ligaments and the intervertebral discs.
- **Hyperextension** usually causes fractures of the posterior elements of the spinal column and disruption of the anterior longitudinal ligaments.
- **Deformation** refers to the various alterations in the spinal column and supporting soft-tissue structures necessary to accommodate abnormal movements, such as hyperflexion, hyperextension, and excessive rotation. For example, in hyperextension of the cervical neck, the spinal canal shortens, the anterior longitudinal ligaments elongate, and the ligamenta flava are compressed and may bulge into the spinal canal, resulting in injury.
- **Axial loading**, also known as **vertical compression**, occurs when a vertical force is exerted on the spinal column. Axial loading is seen in injuries resulting from diving accidents, landing on the feet when jumping from a height, or landing on the buttocks when falling from a height.
- **Excessive rotation** refers to turning of the head beyond the normal range on the horizontal axis. This can result in compression fractures, tearing or rupture of the posterior ligament, dislocation at the facet joint, and fracture at the articular processes

Classification of Injuries

The velocity and angle of impact, as well as the type of exaggerated mechanical movement produced, influence the type of injury sustained. These factors are considered in the classification of injuries.

Patients who have anatomical abnormalities or disease processes of the spinal column are much more vulnerable to SCI than those who do not. Chronic conditions, such as cervical spondylosis, spinal stenosis, arthritis, and scoliosis, are examples of conditions that increase the probability of injury.

A basic classification of the causes of injury to the vertebral column, spinal cord, and soft tissue includes the following categories and their characteristics.

Hyperflexion Injuries

Hyperflexion injuries (Figs. 19-3 and 19-4) caused by hyperflexion of the head and neck, as in sudden deceleration, are seen in head-on collisions and in diving accidents.

If the posterior ligaments are intact, a **wedge** or **compression fracture** of the vertebral body is common. Because it is a relatively stable fracture type, it does not usually require surgery. A flexion-extension fluoroscopic study may be ordered to rule out a fracture not seen on plain x-rays. If the posterior ligaments are torn, the facets are usually disengaged and dislocated. Because this is an unstable fracture type, surgical stabilization is probably required.

There is a high probability of cord damage with fracture dislocations or bilateral jumped locked facet fractures. These injuries occur most often in the cervical region and involve

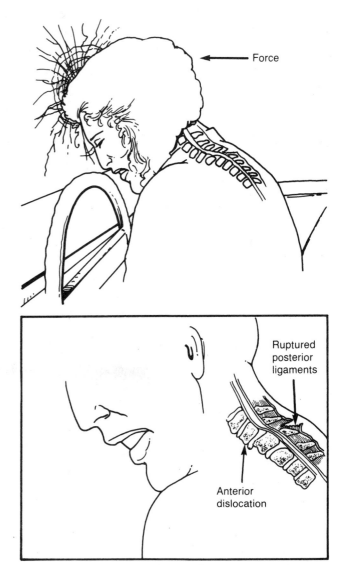

Figure 19–3 • Hyperflexion injury. With hyperflexion to the cervical spine, there may be tearing of the posterior ligamentous complex, resulting in anterior dislocation.

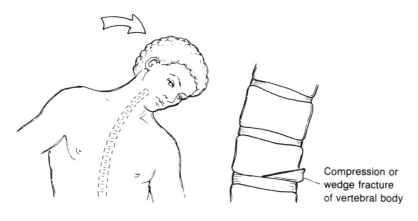

Compression or wedge fracture of vertebral body

Figure 19–4 • Lateral hyperflexion injury. Compression or wedge fracture of the vertebral body.

the greatest areas of stress, levels C-5 and C-6. A lateral hyperflexion injury can result from extreme lateral flexion or rotation of the head and neck.

Hyperextension Injuries

Injuries resulting from hyperextension (Fig. 19-5) of the head and neck, such as from a rear-end vehicular collision, tend to cause greater damage to structures than hyperflexion injuries because backward and downward movement involves a larger arc than flexion. If the head flexes forward, the chin strikes the chest and limits the arc. If the head flexes laterally, the head strikes the shoulder.

In a hyperextension injury, the spinal cord is stretched so that it lies against the ligamenta flava. Despite a negative result on radiographic examination, there may be contusion and ischemia to part of the spinal cord, and neurological deficits may appear. As a rule, ligaments remain intact and no fractures or dislocations occur. The greatest area of stress in a hyperextension injury is at the level of C-4 and C-5. Respiratory compromise, either from direct injury or ascending edema, is a concern.

Hyperextension injuries are commonly seen in an elderly person who has fallen and struck his or her chin. A less severe form of hyperextension injury is called a "whiplash" or acceleration injury, a stress and strain injury to the soft tissue (muscles and ligaments), but with no vertebral injury or SCI.

Compression Injuries

Compression injuries (Figs. 19-6 and 19-7) can result from axial loading; from vertical pressure, for example, falling from a height and landing on the feet or buttocks; or from lateral flexion. Resulting fractures cause wedging, crushing, or bursting of the vertebral body. Compression fractures are sometimes categorized as **burst fracture, simple wedge fracture** (Fig. 19-8), and **teardrop fracture**, depending on the degree of compression or the fracture line noted on x-ray films.

Rotational Injuries

Rotational injuries (Fig. 19-9) are caused by extreme lateral flexion or twisting of the head and neck. Tearing and/or rupturing of the posterior ligaments may occur, allowing dislocation at the facet joint and fracture at the articular processes.

One or two facets may be involved. If one facet is dislocated or locked, usually no neurological deficits or temporary deficits result. In more than half the patients with two facets locked, neurological deficits can be expected. Reduction of the fracture is achieved by traction (cervical traction or halo with or without a jacket) or surgery to disengage the facets and stabilize the

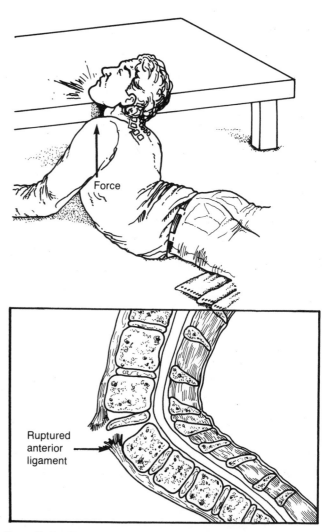

Force

Ruptured anterior ligament

Figure 19–5 • Hyperextension injury in the cervical area. The injury is related to a fall in which the chin is struck, forcing hyperextension of the neck and rupture of the anterior ligament.

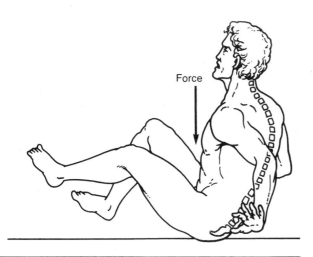

Force

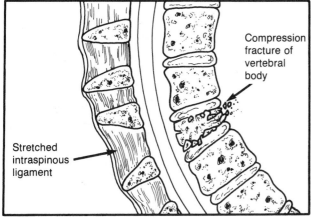

Compression fracture of vertebral body

Stretched intraspinous ligament

Figure 19-6 • Hyperflexion injury in the lumbar area. Injury can be caused by falling onto the buttocks. Note the compression fracture and the stretching of the intraspinous ligament.

vertebral column (Cotrel-Dubousset [CD] rods; see surgical management section later in this chapter).

Penetrating Injuries

Penetrating injuries occur when missiles, such as bullets or shrapnel, or impalement instruments (knives, ice picks) penetrate the spinal column or supporting soft tissue. The object may shatter bone, create bone fragments, or transect a portion or complete plane of the spinal cord or soft tissue.

SPECIFIC CATEGORIES OF INJURIES

Soft-Tissue Injuries

Whiplash

Whiplash is a lay term for an acceleration injury involving hyperextension of the head during a rear-end vehicular collision. The ligaments and muscles of the neck sustain stress and strain injury. The usual signs and symptoms, which include stiff neck, pain in the neck and shoulder, limitation of movement, and muscle spasms, may not begin until 12 to 24 hours after injury. Other signs and symptoms

may include headache, paresthesia, dizziness, vertigo, and tinnitus. The findings on physical examination are normal except for the previously listed signs and symptoms. The radiological examination is negative. The diagnosis is based on the history of injury and the presence of the characteristic signs and symptoms. This is a common injury causing much pain and suffering to the patient, even though no abnormalities are noted on radiographical examination.

The pain caused by whiplash is thought to be attributable to the tearing, stretching, microhemorrhage, and edema incurred by the anterior neck muscles (sternocleidomastoid, scalenus, and longus colli muscles). The muscles, and possibly the ligaments, are strained. Patients with preexisting cervical spondylosis and some with other conditions may have narrowing of the foramina and osteophytes and also increased rigidity of the spinal column. These conditions put them at greater risk of developing neurological problems if a whiplash injury occurs.

Treatment. Treatment of whiplash is directed toward making the patient more comfortable. For less serious injuries treatment involves mild analgesics (e.g., nonsteroidal anti-in-

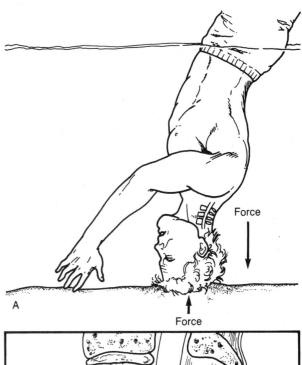

Force

A

Force

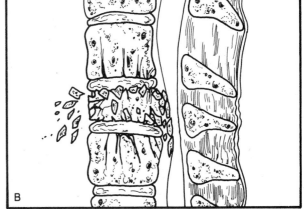

B

Figure 19-7 • Compression fracture secondary to axial loading.

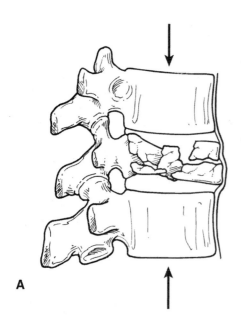
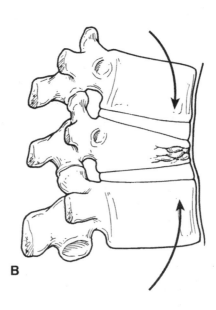

Figure 19–8 • Burst and compression fractures. (*A*) Burst fracture. Axial compressive forces may result in severe vertebral body fractures involving the anterior and middle columns with a collapse of the entire vertebral body, often with retropulsion into the spinal canal. This is a potentially unstable fracture, often with accompanying spinal cord injury. (*B*) Compression fracture. A compression fracture is a wedge-shaped fracture (also called wedge fracture) of the vertebral body involving the anterior column. It occurs in the thoracic and lumbar region, most often in the mid-thoracic and mid-lumbar region. Compression fractures can occur with minor trauma in older patients with osteoporosis and in younger people with significant trauma.

flammatory drugs [NSAIDs], acetaminophen), local ice, and rest. More severe injuries are treated with short-term use of a soft collar, heat and cold application, analgesics, muscle relaxants, and anti-inflammatory agents.

Narcotic analgesics are reserved for severe pain and should be used sparingly to prevent dependency. NSAIDs are commonly ordered both for their anti-inflammatory effect and for their ability to inhibit prostaglandin synthesis, a substance known to be related to pain. Muscle relaxants such as cyclobenzaprine hydrochloride (Flexeril) and methocarbamol (Robaxin) are also used. Extended use of a cervical collar is controversial. Some physicians believe that collars hinder recovery of involved muscles if worn for more than a few days.

Other Soft-Tissue Injuries

The vertebral column depends on soft tissue for its stability. Therefore, any significant soft-tissue trauma (see Fig. 19-2) that occurs with vertebral injury can compromise the vertebral column. The other soft-tissue injuries with significance for vertebral stability are discussed in this chapter in conjunction with vertebral injuries and SCI.

Vertebral Injuries

Classification

Although fractures can occur singularly in any part of the vertebral arch, most injuries occur in combination with vertebral body injuries. The "ends" of the vertebral column, the cervical and lumbar portions, have the greatest built-in mobility, which predisposes them to injury. The thoracic region is less prone to trauma because of the rigidity imparted to it by the rib cage.

Vertebral injuries can be classified based on various perspectives of the injury:

* **Types of fractures**: simple or compression fractures
* **Fracture or dislocation**: pure fracture, pure dislocation, and fracture-dislocation

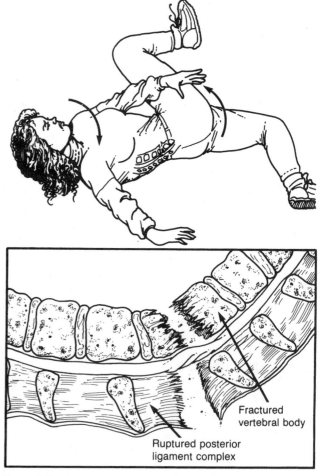

Figure 19–9 • Rotational injury. When rotational force occurs, there is concurrent fracture and tearing of the posterior ligamentous complex.

Fractured vertebral body

Ruptured posterior ligament complex

- **Stability or instability of injury**: according to a three-column framework
- **Segmental involvement**: upper cervical, subaxial cervical, thoracic, or lumbar and sacral

Each category offers a special practical perspective and is discussed in the following section.

Type of Fractures. For the purposes of this discussion, vertebral fractures are subdivided into simple and compression fractures (see Fig. 19-10 for a review of anatomical parts of a vertebra).

- **Simple fractures** appear as a singular break with the alignment of the vertebral parts remaining intact. These types of fractures usually occur to the spinous or transverse process, facets, pedicles, and vertebral body. There is usually no neural compression.
- **Compression fractures** are sometimes further subclassified as *simple wedge fractures, burst fractures,* and *teardrop fractures* (see Fig. 19-8). They are caused by axial loading and hyperflexion.
- **A simple (wedge) compression fracture** is caused by vertical compression when the cervical vertebral column is flexed. A burst fracture is caused by the same mechanical force, but the vertebral column is straight. Because the posterior ligaments are intact, the simple (wedge) compression fracture is stable. No surgery is required. These fractures heal well with hard collar immobilization for about 2 months.[3] A halo jacket may also be used.
- **Burst fractures** are explosive fractures caused by severe axial loading on a straight cervical column. They shatter the vertebral body into several pieces. These fragments then can be driven into the spinal cord, resulting in serious injury. If there is no neurological damage and if the posterior ligaments are stable, wearing a hard collar for 2 months may be adequate therapy (Fig. 19-11). However, burst fractures often require a combined neurosurgical-orthopedic procedure for the removal of bone fragments, cord decompression, and vertebral column stabilization. Stabilization is accomplished by insertion of instrumentation, such as CD rods, a type of segmental rodding that can be accommodated to the individual's

level of injury. See section on surgical management for further discussion.

- **Teardrop fractures** are caused by extreme flexion with axial loading. With this fracture a vertebral body is crushed by the vertebral body superior to it, causing the anterior portion of the compressed body to break away. These fractures, which are usually unstable (i.e., involving disruption of the posterior ligaments, resulting in forward dislocation), are managed with anterior decompression and fusion with halo immobilization.

Fracture or Dislocation. From another perspective, a vertebral injury can be a fracture without a dislocation, a dislocation without a fracture or a fracture combined with a dislocation. **Dislocation** occurs when one vertebra overrides another, and there is unilateral or bilateral facet dislocation. Radiographic studies reveal a disruption in the established alignment of the vertebral column. Usually, the supporting ligaments are also injured, and the spinal cord may or may not be involved.

Subluxation is a partial or incomplete dislocation of one vertebra over another. Damage to the cord and supporting ligaments may or may not be present. With dislocation, reestablishment of alignment is necessary. This may be accomplished by traction followed by immobilization or by surgical stabilization (fusion or sometimes insertion of CD rods if the posterior ligaments are injured).

Fracture-dislocation, as the name implies, denotes a combined injury of a fracture and a dislocation that is usually accompanied by ligament and cord injury. As with simple dislocation, realignment is necessary. The fracture must be allowed to heal, and any bone fragments impinging on the cord must be removed. Therefore, surgery is indicated.

Stability or Instability of Injury. From this perspective, it is critical when considering vertebral fractures to distinguish between stable and unstable fractures and dislocations. This distinction is often based on the posterior ligaments. If the posterior ligaments are intact, the injury is considered stable. If they have been torn, usually by a rotational force, they are considered unstable. Stability of the vertebral-spinal elements is also considered using a three-column theoretical framework. This approach is discussed in Chart 19-1. A stable fracture or dislocation is not apt to displace more than it was at the time of the injury, whereas an unstable fracture or dislocation is highly likely to displace further with extension of injury to the spinal cord. External immobilization or internal fixation may be unnecessary for stable injuries, whereas it is essential for unstable injuries. In addition, when ligaments heal, scar tissue forms. The scarred tissue, being weaker than the preinjury tissue, may result in chronic instability and lead to SCI.

Vertebral Injuries According to Segmental Level

Vertebral injuries can be divided into four groups based on the involved segmental level: upper cervical, subaxial cervical, thoracic and lumbar, and sacral.[4]

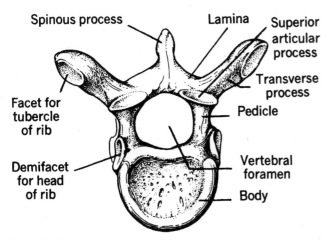

Spinous process
Lamina
Superior articular process
Transverse process
Pedicle
Facet for tubercle of rib
Demifacet for head of rib
Vertebral foramen
Body

Figure 19–10 • The sixth thoracic vertebra with anatomical markings.

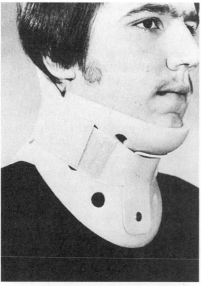
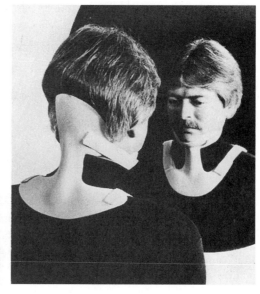
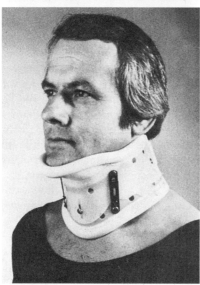

Figure 19–11 • Types of rigid cervical collars.

Upper Cervical Segment

The four most commonly encountered upper cervical segment injuries are atlas fractures, atlantoaxial subluxation, odontoid fractures, and so-called hangman's fractures. Four less common injuries are occipital condyle fractures, atlantooccipital dislocation, atlantoaxial rotary subluxation, and C-2 lateral mass fractures. A summary of upper cervical fractures and lower cervical fractures is presented in Table 19-1.

Subaxial Cervical Segments

Compared with the upper cervical segment, there is an increased risk of cervical cord damage in injuries to the lower cervical vertebrae (subaxial, i.e., below C-2). Two factors account for this: the size of the spinal canal is decreased in the lower spine, and there is an increased prevalence of injuries that narrow rather than expand the canal. Five types of subaxial cervical vertebrae injuries are discussed:

• **Isolated posterior element fractures** of the lamina, articular process, or spinous process occur when there is im-

pact of the posterior elements on one another and compression-extension results.

• **Minor avulsion and compression fractures** of the subaxial cervical vertebrae include anterior compression or avulsion injuries of the vertebral body. Additionally, anterior and posterior concurrent bone injuries with minimal displacement and angulation can occur.

• **Vertebral body-burst fractures**, common in diving accidents, result from axial loading and flexion. The anterior and middle columns are involved, creating instability. Bone may protrude into the spinal canal.

• **With teardrop fractures** flexion and axial loading result in a teardrop fragment on the anteroinferior aspect of the affected body. SCI and three-column instability are usual.

• **Facet injuries causing spinal malalignment** result from a variety of biomechanical forces. Reduction may have to be done in stages to prevent additional injury. If traction is not possible, surgery is necessary. Traumatic disc herniation may also be present and usually requires an anterior discectomy and fusion.

CHART 19 – 1 • The Three-Column Framework: Spinal Stability and Instability*

Spinal stability refers to the ability of the vertebral support column to protect adequately the neural elements from injury during inactivity and activity. This determination is critical in managing patients because an unstable injury can result in extension of or new neurological deficits. Currently, criteria for determining spinal stability or instability are controversial.

Some physicians consider only the condition of the posterior ligaments when determining stability. Another approach is the three-column framework. The three-column approach provides an anatomical framework for considering stability. The cross-section of the spine is organized into three anatomical columns:

- The **anterior column** consists of the anterior longitudinal ligament, anterior half of the vertebral body, annulus fibrosis, and disc.
- The **middle column** consists of the posterior half of the vertebral body, annulus, disc, and posterior longitudinal ligament.
- The **posterior column** consists of the facet joints, ligamentum flavum, posterior elements, and interconnecting ligaments.

Applying this classification system to spinal injuries results in four classification categories, which are determined by the specific column(s) injured.

Type of Injury	Columns Injured		
	Anterior	**Middle**	**Posterior**
Compression fractures	Yes	No	No
Burst fractures	Yes	Yes	No
Flexion-distraction fractures	Yes/no	Yes	Yes
Fracture-dislocations	Yes	Yes	Yes

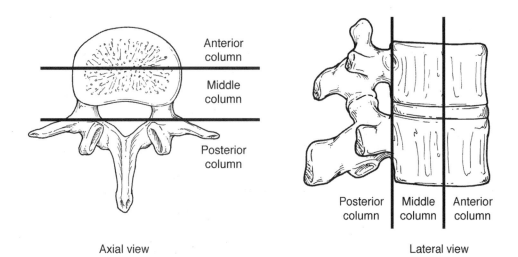

Axial view

Lateral view

*The rule of thumb is that when one column is injured, the spine is usually stable; when two or three columns are injured, the sustained injury is considered unstable.

Lenke, L. G., O'Brien, M. F., & Bridwell, K. H. [1995]. Fractures and dislocations of the spine. In C. R. Perry, J. A. Elstrom, & A. M. Pankovich (Eds.). *The handbook of fractures* [pp. 157–189]. New York: McGraw-Hill

▌▌▌▌ Table 19–1 • CERVICAL VERTEBRAL INJURIES

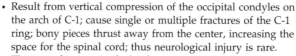

TYPE	DESCRIPTION	TREATMENT

Lower Cervical Vertebral Injuries (Occiput to C-2)

Atlas (C-1) fractures 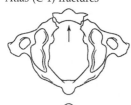	• Result from vertical compression of the occipital condyles on the arch of C-1; cause single or multiple fractures of the C-1 ring; bony pieces thrust away from the center, increasing the space for the spinal cord; thus neurological injury is rare. • There are four types of atlas fractures: 　1. **Isolated anterior arch fractures:** avulsion from anterior part of ring (usually stable) 　2. **Isolated posterior arch fracture (fx):** hyperextension with compression of posterior arch of C-1 between occiput and C-2 (usually stable) 　3. **Lateral mass fx:** fx anterior-posterior to articular surface of C-1 with unilateral displacement; stable fx 　4. **Jefferson's fx:** burst fx into three or four pieces; can result in concurrent rupture of transverse ligament, resulting in instability	• Isolated *anterior or posterior arch fx:* usually no neural injury; about 3 mo in cervical hard collar or halo vest • *Lateral mass fx:* hard collar or halo vest • *Jefferson's fx:* If transverse ligament strong, halo and vest; if weak, cervical traction followed by halo vest for 3–4 mo
Atlantoaxial subluxation	• Caused by a weak or ruptured transverse ligament that stabilizes dens to anterior ring of atlas. • Produces atlantoaxial instability; high risk for spinal injury due to compression of upper cervical cord against the posterior arch of C-1	• Halo vest for 3 mo, only ligament injuries need a C-1 to C-2 posterior fusion • *Type I:* halo vest or hard collar. • *Type II:* difficult to treat; there are 4 options: traction to align then 3 mo in halo vest; halo vest; surgical fixation and fusion; or traction and surgery. • *Type III:* if reduced adequately, halo vest for 3 mo; if not, cervical traction first, then halo vest
Odontoid fractures 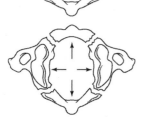  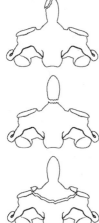	• Need to rule out in all patients with neck pain following a motor vehicle accident (MVA) or in elderly with even minor injury to head or neck • Displacement, anterior or more often, posterior with rare (10%) neurological injury • Odontoid fractures classified into three types: 　1. **Type I:** chip avulsion fx through the tip of the odontoid; stable fracture; heals well 　2. **Type II:** fx through the base of the dens with separation, usually anteriorly, from the body of C-2; most common; poor blood supply to area; nonunion in 40%–50%; treatment depends on severity and response to treatment options 　3. **Type III:** fx line extends into the body of C-2	
Hangman's fractures 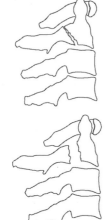	• Bipedicular fx with disruption of the disc and ligaments between C-2 and C-3 resulting from hyperextension and distraction • Named for injury seen in judicial hangings • Further classified according to amount of displacement and angulation of the C-2 body in relation to the posterior elements: 　1. **Type I:** fx of neural arch without angulation and with up to 3 mm of anterior C-2 displacement on C-3; stable fx 　2. **Type II:** <5 mm anterior displacement or angulation of C-2 on C-3 　3. **Type IIA:** severe angulation of C-2 on C-3 with minimal displacement because anterior longitudinal ligament is hinge 　4. **Type III:** bipedicle fx associated with unilateral or bilateral facet dislocations; unstable; often neurological deficits present	• *Type I:* managed with a hard collar • *Type II:* <5 mm, halo vest if reduction maintained; if >5 mm, skeletal traction for 3–6 wk followed by halo vest • *Type IIA:* traction contraindicated; halo vest • *Type III:* open reduction when closed reduction not possible and posterior fusion of C2–3; then halo vest for 3 mo

Table 19 – 1 • CERVICAL VERTEBRAL INJURIES (Continued)

TYPE	DESCRIPTION	TREATMENT
	• Most types unstable; may or may not include neurological deficits depending on amount of displacement or angulation. • Important to know type of fx to determine treatment	
Occipital condyle fractures	• Rare injury caused by concurrent axial loading and lateral flexion • Associated with severe head injury • Two types: avulsion or comminuted compression fx	• Cervical collar, such as Philadelphia type
Atlanto-occipital dislocations	• Rare injury caused by extension or flexion injury • Results in an avulsion of the atlas (C-1) body from the occipital bone and all ligaments • Almost always immediately fatal	• Traction contraindicated; halo vest
Atlantoaxial rotary subluxation	• Rare injury associated with MVAs • Diagnosis often missed	• Cervical traction for alignment, then a halo vest
Lateral mass fractures	• Rare injury associated with a combined axial loading and lateral flexion forces	• Usually hard collar
Lower Cervical Vertebral Injuries (C-3 to T-1)		
Hyperflexion dislocation of C-3 to T-1	Most common cause of paralysis; only neck pain and no neurological deficits may be present	Reduction of the dislocation, then halo immobilization (for 3–6 mo) or a posterior fusion
Flexion-rotational injuries of C-3 to T-1	Usually, anterior subluxation with a unilateral subluxated facet	Reduction of the dislocation with traction; if unstable, posterior fusion
Hyperextension fractures	Usually involves only ligamental and muscle injury; often associated with central cord syndrome	Usually stable fractures; treated with a hard collar for 6–10 wk until the patient is pain-free
Compression fraction of C-3 to T-1	Results from flexion and significant axial loading; may be a simple wedge, burst, or teardrop fracture (see vertebral classification)	Treatment depends on the stability of the fracture; hard collar may be effective for stable fractures, whereas unstable ones may require surgical fusion.

Based on: Lenke, L. G., O'Brien, M. F., & Bridwell, K. H. (1995). Fractures and dislocations of the spine. In C. R. Perry, J. A. Elstrom, & A. M. Pankovich (Eds.). *The handbook of fractures* (pp. 166–189). New York: McGraw-Hill; and on Adams, J. C., & Hamblen, D. L. (1992). *Outline of fractures* (pp. 79–108) [10th ed]. Edinburgh: Churchill Livingstone.

The treatment options for subaxial cervical vertebral injuries include immobilization with sternal-occipital-mandibular orthonic device; halo vest; posterior fusion and stabilization with wires or instrumentation; anterior approaches for decompression; fusion with or without instrumentation; or a combination of these therapies. Treatment choices depend on the specifics of the fracture or malalignment and on the stability of the ligaments.

Thoracic and Lumbar Segments

Vertebral injuries in the thoracic and lumbar regions account for paralysis of the trunk and lower extremities. Compared with the lumbar region, there is normally little movement possible in the vertebrae of the thoracic region because of the inherent structural stability provided by the rib cage. The spinal cord ends at the upper border of the first lumbar vertebra. The cord gradually tapers, beginning at the lower two thoracic vertebrae. As the cord tapers, it forms a cone called the *conus medullaris*, which continues at the filum terminale. The nerve roots coming off the lower segments of the spinal cord, termed the *cauda equina*, hang loosely and are susceptible to injury. However, injury to these nerves is

less likely to be permanent than is injury to the spinal cord. In addition, the emergency procedures of decompression are less likely to be required because the nerve roots tolerate trauma far better than does the spinal cord itself.

There are four general categories of vertebral fractures of the thoracic, thoracolumbar, and lumbar spine:

• **Compression fractures**, caused by axial loading and hyperflexion, are common in the thoracic and upper lumbar regions of the vertebral column. Significant direct force must be applied to produce a fracture in the thoracic area. Injury is usually the result of a direct force applied to one vertebra, which is hyperflexed. The force is then transferred to the underlying cord, putting it at risk of injury. A compression fracture in the thoracic or lumbar region may be compressed anteriorly with or without subluxation of the vertebra. The other possibility is total compression of the vertebral body with anteroposterior protrusion.

• **Burst fractures,** which include injury to the anterior and middle columns and possibly the posterior column, are unstable. Axial loading with flexion creates the biomechanical force responsible for the injury. The vertebral body explodes or "bursts" as a result of the energy associated with injury, and often the vertebral body protrudes into the spinal canal.

- **Flexion-distraction injuries** (also called **Chance fractures**) involve three columns and are thus unstable. The fracture extends through the posterior elements, pedicle, and vertebral body. The mechanism of injury is acute flexion of the torso while restrained with only a lap belt. The flexion-distraction injuries (Chance fractures; Fig. 19-12) are classified according to the involvement of bone and soft tissue components.
- **Fracture-dislocations** of the thoracic and lumbar areas are of three general categories: anterior or posterior dislocation of the whole vertebral body with fracture of the bony parts; comminuted fractures of the vertebral body with anterior or posterior displacement and rotation so that the rotational force usually tears the supporting ligaments; and lateral dislocation of the vertebra with fracture. All three columns are involved so that the fracture is unstable, placing the patient at high risk for neurological injury.

Sacral Segments

Fractures of the sacrum and coccyx usually result from direct trauma, most frequently caused by falls. Any fall in the sitting position, such as falling on ice or being thrown from a horse and landing on the buttocks, can result in such a fracture. Nerve injury in this region can cause bladder, bowel, or sexual dysfunction and saddle anesthesia.

Lesions of the *conus medullaris* can occur with fractures in the lumbar region. These lesions can have confusing clinical presentations. Injury to the conus usually results in lower motor neuron symptoms (muscle flaccidity, muscle atrophy, hyporeflexia) because of the disruption of the anterior gray horn cells. A decompression laminectomy may be necessary if there is pressure on the neural elements. Lesions involving the cauda equina produce selected root syndromes. A decompression laminectomy may also be necessary.

Spinal Cord Injuries

Injury to the spinal cord can be devastating because the resulting loss of body function also involves the loss of independence. The loss of function may be permanent or temporary, depending on the type of injury. The several syndromes related to SCI are summarized in Chart 19-2.

(text continues on page 422)

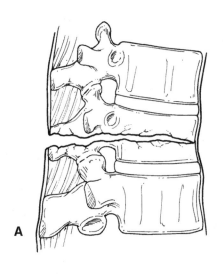

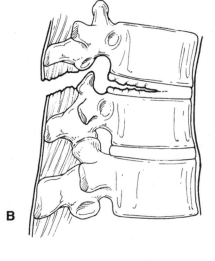

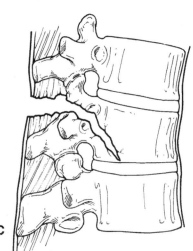

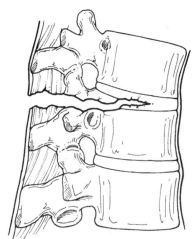

Figure 19–12 • Types of flexion-distraction (Chance) fracture. (*A*) Disruption through the entire bony elements. (*B*) Disruption through the entire ligamentous elements. (*C* and *D*) Disruption through bony and ligamentous elements.

CHART 19–2 • Selected Syndromes Related to Spinal Cord Injury

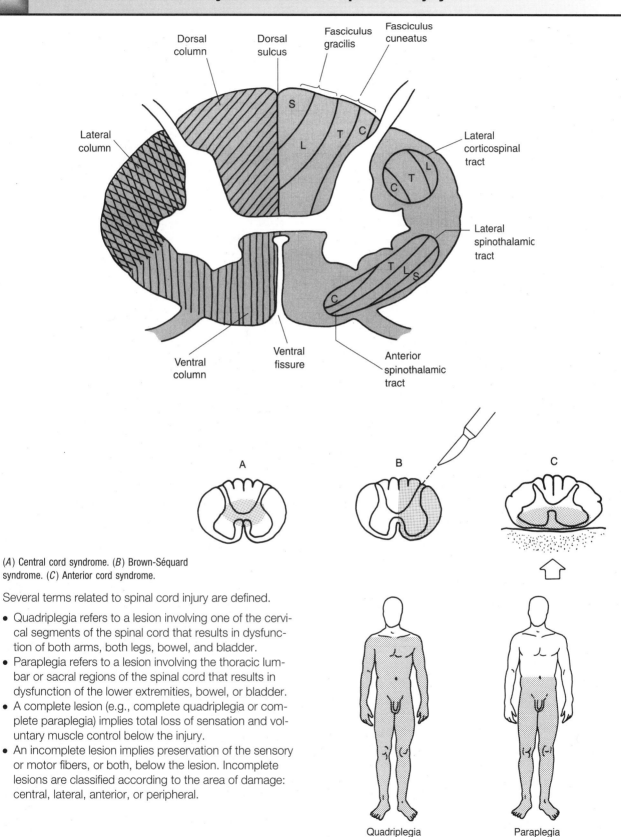

(A) Central cord syndrome. (B) Brown-Séquard syndrome. (C) Anterior cord syndrome.

Several terms related to spinal cord injury are defined.

- Quadriplegia refers to a lesion involving one of the cervical segments of the spinal cord that results in dysfunction of both arms, both legs, bowel, and bladder.
- Paraplegia refers to a lesion involving the thoracic lumbar or sacral regions of the spinal cord that results in dysfunction of the lower extremities, bowel, or bladder.
- A complete lesion (e.g., complete quadriplegia or complete paraplegia) implies total loss of sensation and voluntary muscle control below the injury.
- An incomplete lesion implies preservation of the sensory or motor fibers, or both, below the lesion. Incomplete lesions are classified according to the area of damage: central, lateral, anterior, or peripheral.

The shaded area shows the extent of motor and sensory loss.

(continued)

CHART 19-2 • **Selected Syndromes Related to Spinal Cord Injury (Continued)**

CENTRAL CORD SYNDROME

- Presentation: There are more motor deficits in the upper extremities than the lower extremities; sensory loss varies but is more pronounced in the upper extremities; bowel/bladder dysfunction is variable, or function may be completely preserved.
- Cause: Injury or edema of the central cord, usually of the cervical area, is the underlying cause; hyperextension injuries, particularly if bony spurs are noted, can be causative.
- Result: Edema in the central cord exerts pressure on the anterior horn cells. The cervical fibers of the corticospinal tract are located in a more central position in the cord than the sacral fibers, which are located in the periphery. As a result, motor deficits are less severe in the lower extremities than in the upper extremities.
- Treatment: High-dose steroid (methylprednisolone) protocol for acute cord injury (see pp. 426–427); immobilization or bed rest is the treatment of choice. Flexion-extension radiographs are usually obtained. The prognosis varies.

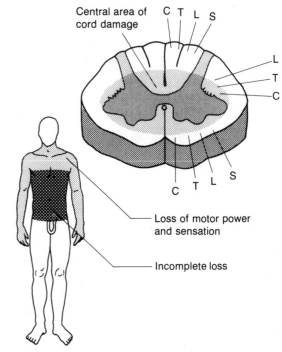

Central cord syndrome
A cross-section of the cord shows central damage and the associated motor and sensory loss (C, cervical; T, thoracic; L, lumbar; S, sacral)

ANTERIOR CORD SYNDROME

- Presentation: Loss of perception pain and temperature, and motor function is noted below the level of the lesion; light touch, position, and vibration sensation remain intact.
- Cause: The syndrome may be caused by acute disc herniation or hyperflexion injuries associated with fracture-dislocation of a vertebra. It also may occur as a result of injury to the anterior spinal artery, which supplies the anterior two thirds of the spinal cord.
- Result: Injury to the anterior part of the spinal cord, which includes the spinothalamic tracts (pain), corticospinal tracts (temperature), and anterior gray horn motor neurons, is noted.
- Treatment: High-dose steroid (methylprednisolone) protocol for acute cord injury (see pp. 426–427); surgical decompression is usually necessary to manage fracture-dislocation. The prognosis varies.

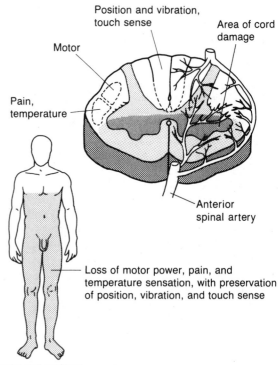

Anterior cord syndrome
Cord damage and associated motor and sensory loss are illustrated.

CHART 19–2 • Selected Syndromes Related to Spinal Cord Injury (Continued)

BROWN-SÉQUARD SYNDROME (LATERAL CORD SYNDROME)

- Presentation: Ipsilateral paralysis or paresis is noted, together with ipsilateral loss of touch, pressure, and vibration and contralateral loss of pain and temperature.
- Cause: Transverse hemisection of the cord (half the cord is transected from north to south), usually as a result of a knife or missile injury, fracture-dislocation of a unilateral articular process, or possibly an acute ruptured disc.
- Result: With right-sided cord transection, for example, the following would occur: paralysis of all voluntary muscles below the level of injury on the right side of the body (lateral corticospinal tract); loss of perception of touch, vibration, and position on the right side of the body below the level of injury (posterior columns, which include the fasciculus gracilis and fasciculus cuneatus); and loss of pain and temperature perception on the left side of the body below the injury (lateral spinothalamic tracts). Fibers that carry pain and temperature cross to the opposite side of the cord immediately after entering the cord and then ascend. The other tracts mentioned do not cross until they reach the brain stem.
- Treatment: High-dose steroid (methylprednisolone) protocol for acute cord injury (see pp. 426–427); no specific treatment is undertaken except fracture-dislocation management.

POSTERIOR CORD SYNDROME

- This is a rare syndrome in which the position and vibration senses of the posterior columns are involved.

ROOT SYNDROMES (PERIPHERAL SYNDROMES)

- Presentation: Root syndromes cause tingling, pain, motor weakness of an isolated muscle or muscle group, and absent or diminished reflexes in the involved area. The spinal cord terminates at T-12 or L-1. The nerve roots that extend from the conus medullaris are collectively called the *cauda equina*. Lesions of L-1 through L-5 denote paraplegia. Patients with this level of involvement can move readily and walk with the assistance of various types of bracing. Lesions of the lumbrosacral region may involve multiple roots of the cauda equina with a varying pattern of motor and sensory loss. Deep tendon reflexes are usually diminished or absent. Isolated nerve root involvement is common in the lumbrosacral region so that saddle hypalgesia—diminished or absence of sensation in the saddle region—is possible. Therefore, careful examination of the patient is necessary to identify the erratic sensory or motor loss. When the sacral roots are involved, the patient may experience bladder or bowel dysfunction. If the cervical region is involved, there is usually tingling in the arm, muscle weakness in the arm or shoulder, and pain radiating down the arm and into the shoulder.
- Cause: Compression secondary to intervertebral disc herniation or vertebral subluxation is the cause of these syndromes. Any area of the cord can be involved.

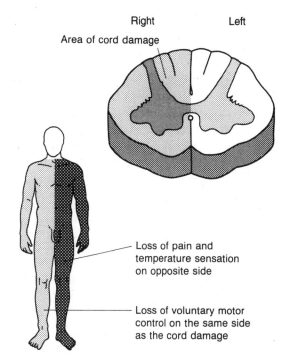

Right   Left

Area of cord damage

Loss of pain and temperature sensation on opposite side

Loss of voluntary motor control on the same side as the cord damage

Brown-Séquard syndrome
Cord damage and associated motor and sensory loss are illustrated

- Result: Compression of one or more nerve roots coming off the spinal cord, rather than compression or injury to the cord itself, occurs. The compression can also cause edema.
- Treatment: Nonsurgical treatment with traction is initiated to release the compressed nerve roots, and drugs may be prescribed to control the associated edema, pain, and muscle spasms. In some cases, surgery for decompression of the nerve roots may be necessary.

HORNER'S SYNDROME

- Presentation: Horner's syndrome, which may be seen with partial spinal cord transection at the level of T-1 or above, includes miosis, ptosis, and loss of sweating on the ipsilateral side.
- Cause: The syndrome is caused by a lesion involving either the preganglionic sympathetic trunk or the cervical postganglionic sympathetic neurons.

Cross-sections of spinal cord in this chart are from Kitt, S. & Kaiser, J. [1990]. *Emergency nursing: A physiological and clinical perspective.* Philadelphia: W. B. Saunders.

Injuries to the spinal cord can be classified by type of injury and by syndrome produced.

Classification by Cause

The spinal cord can be injured by concussion, contusion, compression, laceration, transection, hemorrhage, damage to the blood vessels that supply the cord, or damage to blood vessels within the cord.

- **Concussion:** A jarring, that is, severe shaking, of the spinal cord can result in a temporary loss of function (i.e. spinal shock [see subsequent discussion]) lasting hours to weeks. No identifiable macro-neuropathological changes are noted on examination of the cord.
- **Compression:** As part of the distraction, (i.e., distortion of the normal curvatures), of the spinal cord at the moment of injury, the neural element can be compressed and contused, lacerated, or transected.
- **Contusion:** Contusion is bruising, which can lead to bleeding into the cord, subsequent edema, and possible necrosis from the compression caused by edema or direct damage to the tissue. The extent of the neurological deficits depends on the severity of the contusion and the amount of necrosis, if any. Fractures, dislocations, and direct trauma to the cord can cause a contusion.
- **Laceration:** An actual tear in the cord results in permanent injury to the cord. Contusion, edema, and cord compression accompany a laceration.
- **Transection:** A severing of the cord can be complete or incomplete. Actual complete transection is rare. However, clinical presentations, which mimic complete transections, are frequently seen.
- **Hemorrhage:** Blood in or around the spinal cord is an irritant to the delicate tissue. Changes in the neurochemical environment, edema, and neurological deficits can result.
- **Damage to the blood vessels that supply the cord:** Interference with or damage to the vessels that supply the spinal cord, the anterior spinal artery, or the two posterior spinal arteries results in ischemia and possible necrosis. Episodes of ischemia can cause temporary neurological deficits. Prolonged ischemia and necrosis causes permanent deficits.

Pathophysiology

Spinal cord injury results from both the **primary injury,** which occurs at the time of the impact, and **secondary injury,** which occurs in the first few hours after primary injury. The primary injury is the result of compression, laceration, or disruption of the spinal cord or surrounding vascular components. These disruptions of neural elements and/or injury to the vascular supply within the spinal cord or supplying the spinal cord cause *ischemic injury*. The degree of injury depends on the magnitude of the force applied to the spinal cord and the angle of impact.

Several chemical and vascular changes occur following primary injury, which cause the spinal cord to initiate an intrinsic process of additional injury and self-destruction. These processes are collectively called **secondary injury**. Within minutes of injury, a cascade of concurrent events (including alterations in blood flow, edema, hemorrhage, electrolyte abnormalities, membrane injury, and release of cytotoxic mediators and excitotoxic neurotransmitters) occurs and contributes to cellular membrane injury and post-traumatic ischemia.[5] The secondary injury results from vascular and neuronal pathological changes and the release of vasoactive agents and cellular enzymes. The shift in intracellular calcium activates calcium-dependent proteases and impairs mitochondrial and other intracellular functions. This injury to the blood vessels results in ischemia, increased vascular permeability, and edema. Hypoxia of the gray matter stimulates the release of catecholamines, which contribute to the hemorrhage and necrosis and cause further spinal cord dysfunction. The release of catecholamines and vasoactive substances (norepinephrine, serotonin, dopamine, and histamine) from the injured tissue can cause vasospasm and impede microcirculation. These events further extend necrosis of blood vessels and neurons. The release of proteolytic and lipolytic enzymes from the injured cells causes delayed swelling and necrosis in the spinal cord.[6] The function of highly specialized central nervous system cells is disrupted by ischemia and hypoxia within 30 minutes of injury. Irreversible nerve damage develops as a result of the replacement of normal neural elements with glial and fibrotic scar tissue. As a result, neurological deficits become permanent.

ACUTE SPINAL CORD TRAUMA

Immediate Signs and Symptoms of Spinal Cord Trauma

When the spinal cord is suddenly transected, *spinal shock* (see later discussion) occurs in the portion of the cord that has been severed, and there is complete loss of motor, sensory, reflex, and autonomic function *below* the level of injury. Specific functional losses, based on level of SCI, are listed in Table 19-2.

The following immediate responses occur with sudden, complete **lesions** of the spinal cord and immediate spinal shock:

- Flaccid paralysis of all skeletal muscles below the level of injury
- Loss of all spinal reflexes *below* the level of injury
- Loss of pain perception, light touch, proprioception, temperature, and pressure *below* the level of injury. (Pain may be felt at the site of the injury because of a zone of heightened sensitivity [hyperesthesia] immediately *above* the level of the lesion.)
- Absence of somatic and visceral sensations *below* the level of injury
- Loss of the ability to perspire *below* the level of injury (autonomic function)
- Bowel and bladder dysfunction

Spinal cord lesions can be complete or incomplete. Incomplete spinal cord syndromes are characterized by the presence of some function below the level of injury. If no motor or sensory function is present after spinal shock resolves, the injury is considered complete.

Special Considerations

Spinal Shock

Definition and Description. **Spinal shock** refers to the loss of all neurological function below the level of injury in the acute phase after SCI. In the SCI literature, the term "shock" is used in two ways. **Neurogenic shock** refers to the systemic hypotension caused by loss of sympathetic input. Patients have no motor function, no sensation, and reflexes are absent below the level of SCI.[7] The temperature tends to be lower than normal (96 to 98°F, 35.5 to 36.5°C) because of the break in the connection between the hypothalamus and the sympathetic nervous system. Body heat is lost through two processes: (1) the vascular bed of the skin is passively dilated, and (2) **the ability to sweat** below the level of injury is lost owing to loss of neurological innervation of the sweat glands.

Recovery From Spinal Shock. After a period up to 4 to 6 weeks postinjury, the flaccid, hyporeflexic state is replaced by spastic hyperreflexia and bilateral Babinski responses.[8] Recovery from spinal shock is a gradual process in which the spinal neurons slowly regain their excitability. The earliest indication heralding the end of spinal shock is the return of the perianal reflexes (bulbocavernous and anal-cutaneous reflexes). The bulbocavernous reflex is tested by squeezing the glans penis or pulling the indwelling catheter and observing for slight muscle contraction and retraction of the scrotum. The anal reflex is present if there is a puckering of the anal sphincter ("anal wink") during digital examination of the rectum or scratching of the skin around the anal region. Muscle contraction may also be noted when inserting a rectal thermometer. Perianal reflexes return before deep tendon reflexes.

Neurogenic Shock

Under normal conditions, the sympathetic nervous system, which has its origins in the thoracolumbar region of the spinal cord, receives impulses from the brainstem. The input from the brainstem contributes to basic reflex control of vital signs through the cardiac accelerator and vasoconstriction reflexes. **Neurogenic shock,** which occurs in severe cervical or upper thoracic spinal cord injuries, results from loss of sympathetic input to the systemic vasculature of the heart and subsequent decreased peripheral vascular resistance.[8,9] Clinical manifestations include **hypotension** secondary to the vasodilation of the vascular beds below the level of injury and **bradycardia** resulting from the suppression of the cardiac accelerator reflex. The unopposed vagal tone causes vasodilation and bradycardia. The finding of hypotension with bradycardia is an important clinical clue suggestive of spinal cord injury.[8] Patients with neurogenic shock generally have a heart rate of 50 to 70 beats/minute.

Orthostatic Hypotension

Orthostatic hypotension is defined as a rapid drop in blood pressure when the vertical position is assumed. Because the blood supply to the brain is inadequate, syncope results. Cerebral ischemia or stroke can result if the condition is not rectified. This condition is seen in patients who have been bedridden for a prolonged period, are postoperative from a lumbar sympathectomy, or have new SCI related to neurogenic shock.

Immediately after cord injury, the blood pressure tends to be unstable and lowered. After 1 to 2 weeks, it gradually rises until it is stabilized at a reading that corresponds to the preinjury norm for the patient. Orthostatic hypotension can impede the rehabilitative process if the patient cannot be raised in bed or assume the vertical position. Physiologically, orthostatic hypotension is caused by loss of arteriole vasomotor tone below the level of the lesion, which leads to a drop in arterial blood pressure when the patient assumes an upright position. Pooling of blood in the abdomen and lower extremities hampers adequate blood supply to the brain. Orthostatic hypotension is seen particularly in cord-injured patients with lesions above the T-7 level. Even slightly raising the head of the bed for a new quadriplegic patient can result in a drastic lowering of blood pressure.

Respiratory Insufficiency

The diaphragm is innervated from C-1 to C-4. If such a high cervical injury is sustained, innervation to the diaphragm is affected, and the patient will have a respiratory arrest. Intubation and mechanical ventilation are necessary. If the SCI is below the innervation to the phrenic nerve and above the innervation to the intercostal muscles, diaphragmatic breathing will be noted. This patient may also need varying degrees of respiratory support.[10]

Complications

After recovery from spinal shock, various complications can develop, depending on the type and level of injury. Examples of such problems include autonomic hyperreflexia, sexual dysfunction, bladder dysfunction, and other autonomic dysfunction. These topics and others are discussed later in this chapter.

OVERVIEW OF EARLY MANAGEMENT OF PATIENTS WITH SPINAL CORD INJURY

Prehospital Management

The prehospital management of SCIs is critical to the patient's ultimate neurological outcome.[11] Until proven otherwise, every trauma patient should be treated as if he or she has an SCI. This rule applies to any patient with a head injury and to the inebriated trauma victim whose mental status and cognitive functions are impaired (see Chap. 18).

Table 19–2 • FUNCTIONAL LOSS FROM SPINAL CORD INJURY (BASED ON COMPLETE LESIONS)

LEVEL OF SPINAL INJURY	MOTOR FUNCTION	DEEP TENDON REFLEXES	SENSORY FUNCTION	RESPIRATORY FUNCTION	VOLUNTARY BOWEL AND BLADDER FUNCTION	REHABILITATIVE POTENTIAL
C1-4	• Quadriplegia: loss of all motor function from the neck down	All lost	• Loss of all sensory function in the neck and below (C-4 supplies the clavicles.)	• Loss of involuntary (phrenic) and voluntary (intercostals) respiratory function; ventilatory support and a tracheostomy needed	• No bowel or bladder control	• May be discharged home on a ventilator with home care
C-5	• Quadriplegia: loss of all function below the upper shoulders • **Intact:** sternomastoids, cervical paraspinal muscles, and the trapezius; can control head	C-5, C-6 biceps	• Loss of sensation below the clavicle and most portions of arms, hands, chest, abdomen, and lower extremities • **Intact:** head, shoulders, deltoid, clavicle, portion of forearms (C-5 supplies the lateral aspect of the arm.)	• Phrenic nerve intact, but not intercostal muscles	• No bowel or bladder control	• Use of extremity-powered devices to achieve some upper limb control • Head control facilitates wheelchair (W/C) balance • Adaptive tools, held in mouth, for typing and writing • Some adaptive tools and use of special computer technology
C-6	• Quadriplegia: loss of all function below the shoulders and upper arms; lacks elbow, forearm, and hand control • **Intact:** deltoid, biceps, and external rotator muscles of shoulders	C-5, C-6 brachioradialis	• Loss of everything listed for a C-5 lesion, but greater arm and thumb sensation • **Intact:** head, shoulders, arms, palms of hands, and thumbs (C-6 supplies the forearm and thumb.)	• Phrenic nerve intact, but not intercostal muscles	• No bowel or bladder control	• Needs assistive devices to use arms (may be able to help feed, groom, and dress self) • Needs a motorized wheelchair • Dependent for all transfers
C-7	• Quadriplegia: loss of motor control to portions of the arms and hands • **Intact:** voluntary strength in shoulder depressors, shoulder abductors, internal rotators, and radial wrist extensors	C-7, C-8 triceps	• Loss of sensation below the clavicle and portions of arms and hands • **Intact:** head, shoulders, most of arms and hands (C-7 supplies the middle finger.)	• Phrenic nerve intact, but not intercostal muscles	• No bowel or bladder function	• Can perform some activities of daily living (ADLs) • Can use wrist extensor with a special splint to induce finger flexion • Can push a W/C with special handgrasps • May be able to drive a specially equipped car
C-8	• Quadriplegia: loss of motor control to portions of arms and hands • **Intact:** some voluntary control of elbow extensors, wrist, finger extension, and finger flexors		• Loss of sensation below the chest and in portions of hands • **Intact:** sensation to face, shoulders, arms, hands, and part of chest (C-8 supplies the little finger.)	• Phrenic nerve intact, but not intercostal muscles	• No bowel or bladder function	• Able to push-up in the W/C • Improved sitting tolerance • Can grasp and release hands voluntarily. • Independent in most ADLs from W/C • Independent in use of W/C • Can use hands for catheterization and rectal stimulation for bowel movements

Table 19–2 • FUNCTIONAL LOSS FROM SPINAL CORD INJURY (BASED ON COMPLETE LESIONS) (Continued)

LEVEL OF SPINAL INJURY	MOTOR FUNCTION	DEEP TENDON REFLEXES	SENSORY FUNCTION	RESPIRATORY FUNCTION	VOLUNTARY BOWEL AND BLADDER FUNCTION	REHABILITATIVE POTENTIAL
T1-6	• Paraplegia: loss of everything below the midchest region, including the trunk muscles • **Intact:** control of function to the shoulders, upper chest, arms, and hands		• Loss of sensation below the midchest area • **Intact:** everything to the midchest region, including the arms and hands (T-1 and T-2 supply the inner aspect of the arm; T-4 supplies the nipple area.)	• Phrenic nerve functions independently • Some impairment of intercostal muscles	• No bowel or bladder function	• Full control of upper extremities and completely independent in W/C • Full-time employment possible • Independent in managing urinary drainage and inserting suppositories • Able to live in a dwelling without major architectural changes
T6-12	• Paraplegia: loss of motor control below the waist • **Intact:** shoulders, arms, hands, and long trunk muscles		• Loss of everything below the waist • **Intact:** shoulders, chest, arms, and hands (T-10 supplies the umbilicus; T-12 supplies the groin area.)	• No interference with respiratory function	• No bowel or bladder control	• In addition to the previously described capabilities, there is complete abdominal and upper back control. • Good sitting balance (allows for greater ease of W/C operation and athletics)
L1-3	• Paraplegia: loss of most control of legs and pelvis • **Intact:** shoulders, arms, hands, torso, hip rotation and flexion, and some leg flexion	L2–4 (knee jerk)	• Loss of sensation to the lower abdomen and legs • **Intact:** all of the above plus some sensation to the inner and anterior thigh (L-3 supplies the knee.)	• No interference with respiratory function	• No bowel or bladder control	• Independent for most activities from W/C
L3-4	• Paraplegia: loss of control of portions of lower legs, ankles, and feet • **Intact:** all of the above, plus increased knee extension		• Loss of sensation to portions of the lower legs, feet, and ankles • **Intact:** all of the above, plus sensation to the upper legs	• No interference with respiratory function	• No bowel or bladder control	• Voluntary control of hip extensors; weak abductors • Walking with braces possible
L-4 to S-5	• Paraplegia: incomplete • Segmental motor control L-4 to S-1: abduction and internal rotation of hip, ankle dorsiflexion, and foot inversion L-5 to S-1: foot eversion L-4 to S-2: knee flexion S1-2: plantar flexion S1-2: (ankle jerk) S2-5: bowel/bladder control	S1-2 (ankle jerk)	• Lumbar sensory nerves innervate the upper legs and portions of the lower legs L-5: medial aspect of foot S-1: lateral aspect of foot S-2: posterior aspect of calf/thigh • Sacral sensory nerves innervate the lower legs, feet, and perineum	• No interference with respiratory function	• Bowel and bladder control possibly impaired • S2-4 segments control urinary continence • S3-5 segments control bowel continence (perianal muscles)	• Can walk with braces or may use W/C • Can be relatively independent

Advance Trauma Life Support (ATLS) guidelines are followed.[12] The basic objectives of management at the injury site include (1) rapid assessment to determine the extent of vertebral injury or SCI; (2) immobilization and stabilization of the head and neck to prevent extension of injury; (3) extrication of the patient from the vehicle or injury site; (4) stabilization and control of any other life-threatening injuries; (5) triage to the appropriate facility; and (6) rapid and safe transport. The rescue personnel must be well trained because improper handling at the injury site can turn a minor vertebral injury into a major, irreversible SCI.

Emergency Department Management

On admission to the emergency department (ED), ATLS guidelines are followed. A report of the prehospital management and a history of the injury are collected rapidly. The focus is on rapid stabilization and assessment. After the primary survey and patient stabilization are completed, the secondary survey is conducted.

Transport on a backboard is common; this keeps the patient immobilized in a neutral position to prevent further vertebral spinal injury. The patient is often maintained on the backboard until imaging is completed. However, prolonged immobility on a backboard can lead to development of decubitus ulcers within a few hours, especially if an SCI is present. Therefore, a backboard must be used with great caution and removed quickly. On arrival, the patient may be safely log-rolled off the backboard by well-trained ED personnel. If the patient is admitted to the ICU on a backboard, it should be removed.

History of Accident

The history of the accident can be obtained from various sources, including the patient, a family member, another accident victim, or rescue personnel. Information about the circumstances of the injury, the neurological status of the patient immediately after injury, the treatment at the accident site, and the mode of transport is all vital. At the same time, a baseline assessment (primary survey) is conducted.

Assessment

For victims of trauma, a complete primary and secondary survey must be conducted, as outlined in ATLS. The **ABCs** (i.e., **a**irway, **b**reathing, **c**irculation) of life support are followed. The essential components of assessment include the medical history, physical examination, imaging studies, and other baseline tests. However, emphasis on these components varies depending on the circumstances of injury and patient acuity.[5] After the ABCs (see later discussion) have been stabilized, the clinical examination is conducted to assess the function of the spinal cord and approximate the level of injury.[13] By comparison, the purpose of imaging studies is to identify the extent of bone and ligament injury and to determine the best operative approach for decompression and stabilization, if surgery is indicated.[5]

Treatment

Because hypoxia, hypotension, and hypertension can contribute to secondary injury and other life-threatening complications, a few special considerations related to spinovertebral injury require consideration.[14] In addition, because trauma is involved, it is necessary to rule out the presence of other system injuries that could be life threatening.

Airway and Breathing. The airway is checked for patency, and respirations are evaluated to determine whether the diaphragm and intercostal muscles are functional. Skin color, nail beds, and earlobes are also checked for evidence of proper oxygenation. To prevent hypoxemia and secondary SCI, oxygen saturation should be maintained at 100% by administration of supplemental oxygen to all acute SCI patients. Patients with high cervical injuries may require intubation for ventilatory support with a mechanical ventilator. If a cervical injury is suspected and endotracheal intubation is necessary, a special insertion technique provided by a specially trained physician is necessary to prevent extension of the injury. Any injury compromising ventilation must be treated promptly. Observe those patients not requiring immediate intubation carefully for signs of ascending edema, which may rapidly compromise respirations and require emergent intubation. Continuous respiratory monitoring with pulse oximetry should be provided.

Circulation. Patients with SCIs (particularly in the cervical region) may show signs of hypotension, bradycardia, and lowered body temperature. These are symptoms of neurogenic shock. The lowered blood pressure is attributable to vasodilation, which results from the loss of vasomotor tone below the level of injury. In most instances, treatment will not be necessary unless the hypotension is compounded by hemorrhagic shock. However, if circulation is inadequate because of hemorrhage or cardiac compromise, treatment must be initiated immediately to hemodynamically stabilize the patient. The abdominal and thoracic cavities may be the sites of significant blood loss. A careful physical examination is necessary to rule out hemodynamic instability.

If the patient is cool to touch because of neurogenic shock, adding blankets will usually provide comfort.

Neurological Examination. The goals for the neurological examination include an assessment of the spinal cord function and an approximation of the level of injury. In addition, the possibility of traumatic brain injury must also be assessed and excluded. Two scales for rating functional classification and impairment from SCI have been established by the American Spinal Injury Association (ASIA) and are widely used in practice (Table 19-3 and Fig. 19-13).

Other Organ Systems. As already mentioned, trauma patients frequently have multiple injuries, including cardiac, intrathoracic, or abdominal injuries. The patient should be assessed for possible cardiac complications, especially cardiac contusion, with a 12-lead EKG. The presence of tachycardia with hypotension and cool and clammy skin should raise suspicion of visceral hemorrhage, and a search should commence for signs of intra-abdominal or intrathoracic injury. Because pain perception is diminished or absent, pain will not draw attention to

Table 19–3 • AMERICAN SPINAL INJURY ASSOCIATION (ASIA) IMPAIRMENT SCALE

A **Complete:** No motor or sensory function is preserved in the sacral segments S4–S5

B **Incomplete:** sensory but not motor function is preserved below the neurologic level and includes the sacral segments S4–S5

C **Incomplete:** motor function is preseved below the neurological level, and at least half of key muscles below the neurological level have a muscle grade less than 3

D **Incomplete:** motor function is preseved below the neurological level, and more than half of key muscles below the neurological level have a muscle grade less than 3

E **Normal:** motor and sensory function is normal

Copyright, American Spinal Injury Association, from *International Standards for Neurological and Functional Classification of Spinal Cord Injury,* revised 1996.

a salient, life-threatening ruptured viscera. Neurogenic and hemorrhagic shock can be simultaneously present. Careful assessment and clinical reasoning must be used to recognize the problem and quickly institute appropriate treatment.

Methylprednisolone Protocol. It is critically important to determine whether an SCI patient is a candidate for the **high-dose steroid protocol** (Chart 19-3). Improved motor and sensory outcomes at 6 weeks, 6 months, and 1 year have been reported for both complete and incomplete SCIs when high-dose intravenous [IV] methylprednisolone is administered within 8 hours of the time of injury.[15,16] The most recent studies report that best outcomes occur when the protocol is begun within 3 hours of injury.[17] For those candidates who meet inclusion criteria, the drug is prepared according to the following administration protocol. First, all solutions are mixed as 62.5 mg/mL (e.g., dilute 16 g methylprednisolone with bacteriostatic water to 256 mL). Second, a bolus of 30 mg/kg IV is given over 15 minutes followed by a pause with 45 minutes of saline or other IV fluid. Third, a maintenance infusion of 5.4 mg/kg/hour by continuous infusion is begun. The duration of time to continue the infusion depends on when therapy was initiated in relation to time of injury. If therapy was begun 3 hours or less after injury, the infusion is administered for 23 hours. If therapy was begun between 3 and 8 hours after injury, there is an incremental benefit to providing the infusion for 47 hours.[17] The infusion is maintained even during any necessary surgery, if at all possible.[18] The maintenance rate is calculated by the following: maintenance rate (mL/hr) = patient's weight (kg) × 0.0864 (for 23 or 47 hours, depending on time elapsed since injury). See Chart 19-3 for exclusion criteria and further discussion of administration. Be sure that the patient is receiving supplemental oxygen to prevent hypoxemia and secondary SCI. Pulse oximetry should be used to monitor adequacy of oxygenation. Use of pharmacotherapeutics has significantly improved outcomes for SCI patients.[19,20]

Other Considerations in the Emergency Department. Acute paralytic ileus, characterized by abdominal distention, nausea, vomiting, and the absence of normal peristalsis, occurs with SCIs. A nasogastric tube is inserted and connected to suction to decompress the stomach and prevent vomiting

and aspiration and to facilitate free diaphragmatic movement. Paralytic ileus is not only a sign of neurogenic shock but also can indicate intra-abdominal injury. Normally, the patient with an intra-abdominal injury will experience pain, but with an SCI the sensation of pain may be lost.

The patient with an SCI has an atonic bladder that becomes rapidly overdistended. Urine may be retained and may overflow, and the bladder may feel distended on palpation. An indwelling urinary catheter is inserted to manage urinary output and prevent injury to the bladder from overdistention.

Imaging Examination

Although new imaging techniques have had an important impact on management of SCI patients, conventional radiological examination of the spine continues to play an important role in the initial screening of the entire spinal anatomy (i.e., cervical to sacral) and in the detection of impingement on neural components. Anteroposterior and lateral films are necessary. Careful management to prevent extension of injury is critical. The C-7 to T-1 vertebral level is normally difficult to visualize, especially in obese or heavily muscled patients. To visualize C-7 and T-1, it may be necessary to pull the patient's shoulders downward toward the foot of the bed while the radiographic examination is conducted. If these x-ray films are not satisfactory, positioning in swimmer's position may be helpful. The C1-2 level, especially the odontoid process, is also difficult to visualize. Films are taken with the patient's mouth open to visualize the odontoid process. The physician must decide the specific type of x-ray studies necessary while considering the risk to the patient from assuming the necessary positions.

Computer-assisted imaging greatly enhances the detail with which bony, soft tissue, and SCI can be identified. Both computed tomography (CT) and magnetic resonance imaging (MRI) scans have their particular advantages and provide complementary information for diagnosis and management decisions.[21] CT scan is superior for detail information about bony structures and fractures, whereas MRI provides better detail on soft tissue, including the spinal cord, ligaments, and discs. Metrizamide myelography may be ordered after CT scan to provide more information about soft tissue. However, the patient will need to be turned in the prone position, which may be contraindicated if an unstable cervical or thoracic lumbar fracture is present.[22]

Early Medical Management of Spinal Cord Injury

After initial stabilization and assessment in the ED, the SCI patient will most likely be admitted to the intensive care unit (ICU). In the ICU, a mechanical ventilator and supplemental oxygen, IV fluids, continuous cardiac monitoring, an indwelling urinary catheter, a nasogastric tube, elastic hose (i.e., TEDs), and sequential compression boots are provided. Depending on acuity, invasive monitoring with an arterial

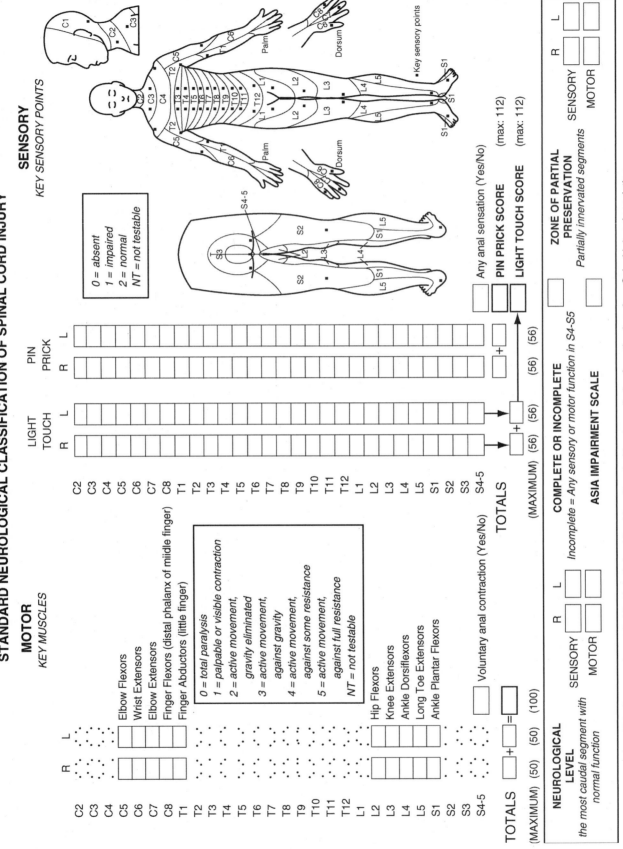

Figure 19–13 • ASIA motor and sensory scales. (Copyright, American Spinal Injury Association, from *International standards for neurological and functional classification of spinal cord injury*, revised 1996.)

CHART 19-3 • High-Dose Methylprednisolone Treatment of Acute Spinal Cord Injury* (Sample)

SUGGESTED PHYSICIAN ORDERS FOR HIGH-DOSE METHYLPREDNISOLONE ADMINISTRATION

1. Record patient weight: _____ kg
2. In the emergency department, begin: methylprednisolone _____ mg (30 mg/kg) IV over 15 minutes
   Record start time _____
   ❏ Check when given
3. Pause 45 minutes. Administer NSS, KVO.

4. Dosage calculation only:
   Methylprednisolone _____ mg
   IV over 23 hours (5.4 mg/kg/h × 23 hours)
5. Start methylprednisolone 3,000 mg IV to run at _____ mg/h (5.4 mg/kg/h)
   Record start time _____
   Record end time _____
   ❏ Check when started

Administer the IV bolus using the chart below. (sample of selected weights)

Initiate maintenance therapy by **first hanging a 3-g methylprednisolone IV bag** as a 62.5 mg/mL solution. Administration rate is found below by weight. Rate calculated for a 5.4 mg/kg/h infusion.

Patient Weight		30 mg/kg IV Bolus over 15 min	For 62.5 mg/mL Solutions		Remaining dose after 3 g given		For 62.5 mg/mL Solutions
lb	kg	Dose (mg)	Dose (mL)	Pause for 45 min	Dose (mg)	Rate (mg/h)	Rate (mL/h)
165.0	75	2,250	36.0		6,315	405.0	6.48
167.2	76	2,280	36.5		6,439	410.4	6.57
169.4	77	2,310	37.0		6,563	415.8	6.65
171.6	78	2,340	37.4		6,688	421.2	6.74
173.8	79	2,370	37.9		6,812	426.6	6.83
176.0	80	2,400	38.4		6,936	432.0	6.91
178.2	81	2,430	38.9		7,060	437.4	7.00
180.4	82	2,460	39.4		7,184	442.8	7.08
182.6	83	2,490	39.8		7,309	448.2	7.17
184.8	84	2,520	40.3		7,433	453.6	7.26
187.0	85	2,550	40.8		7,557	459.0	7.34
189.2	86	2,580	41.3		7,681	464.4	7.43
191.4	87	2,610	41.8		7,805	469.8	7.52
193.6	88	2,640	42.2		7,930	475.2	7.60
195.8	89	2,670	42.7		8,054	480.6	7.69
198.0	90	2,700	43.2		8,178	486.0	7.78
200.2	91	2,730	43.7		8,302	491.4	7.86
202.4	92	2,760	44.2		8,426	496.8	7.95
204.6	93	2,790	44.6		8,551	502.2	8.04
206.8	94	2,820	45.1		8,675	507.6	8.12
209.0	95	2,850	45.6		8,799	513.0	8.21
211.2	96	2,880	46.1		8,923	518.4	8.29
213.4	97	2,910	46.6		9,047	523.8	8.38
215.6	98	2,940	47.0		9,172	529.2	8.47
217.8	99	2,970	47.5		9,296	534.6	8.55
220.0	100	3,000	48.0		9,420	540.0	8.64
222.2	101	3,030	48.5		9,544	545.4	8.73
224.4	102	3,060	49.0		9,668	550.8	8.81
226.6	103	3,090	49.4		9,793	556.2	8.90

Dosage chart based on NASCIS2 guidelines. Bracken, D. et al. [1990]. Randomized controlled trial of methylprednisolone or naloxone in the treatment of acute SCI. *New England Journal of Medicine, 322,* 1405–1411.

*Solu-Medrol (methylprednisolone)—Pharmacia–Upjohn 1 g/16 mL = 62.5 mg/mL.

line and pulmonary artery catheter may be necessary. Other monitoring equipment is ordered as needed. After resuscitation measures are complete, treatment decisions are made. The patient is continuously monitored for potential complications, which are treated promptly as they occur.

SELECTION OF TREATMENT APPROACH: SURGICAL OR NONSURGICAL

The primary goal in treating spinal injury is to optimize outcomes by preserving or improving neurological function.[23] Treatment is directed at neural decompression, spinal realignment, and stabilization through either a nonsurgical or surgical approach. Decompression and stabilization may be done on an emergency basis, especially if neurological deterioration is apparent on serial neurological assessment. Stabilization is important to prevent new or further extension of neurological damage. The management of the patient depends on the type of SCI, the associated injuries, or the patients' other health problems, if any.

- **Neural decompression** of the spinal cord or spinal nerves is the first priority in preserving neurological function. Decompression is necessary to control and/or eliminate ischemia and necrosis in the involved spinal area. For treatment, either skeletal traction or immediate surgery is available. If surgery is chosen, a decompression laminectomy is the usual procedure.
- **Spinal realignment/reduction** of the vertebral column is necessary to reestablish normal spinal alignment and curvatures. Reduction is often associated with decompression management. Skeletal traction, a halo and vest application, and braces have been the mainstays of reduction. If the vertebral facets are locked, surgical intervention may be necessary to unlock the facets and align the vertebrae.
- **Stabilization** of the spinal column is accomplished with surgical instrumentation or by spontaneous fusion during the natural healing process. Skeletal traction and immobilization promote the natural healing process. These treatment options can be used alone or in combination with surgery to achieve the desired outcome. If surgery is indicated, stabilization is achieved either by fusing the spine using an analogous bone graft or by stabilizing the spine with the insertion of instrumentation (see later discussion).

SURGICAL MANAGEMENT OF SPINAL CORD INJURY

Neurological assessment data and imaging studies provide the foundation for determining the best approach to treatment. If surgery is indicated, selecting the best time for surgery is critical. Early surgery (within the first 12 to 24 hours) can preserve or improve spinal cord function. However, other clinicians prefer to have the patient well stabilized before proceeding to surgery. The following are reasons for early surgery:

- Evidence of cord compression

- Progressive neurological deficit
- Compound fracture of the vertebra (potential for bony fragments to dislodge and penetrate the cord)
- Penetrating wounds of the spinal cord or surrounding structures
- A bone fragment evident in the spinal canal

Early surgery is usually postponed in the following circumstances:

- When rapid and significant improvement in neurological function is demonstrated
- When staging is necessary, for instance, the need before surgery to first realign the vertebral column or to reduce dislocations or fracture-dislocations through traction or immobilization
- When a life-threatening injury or disease exists elsewhere in the body. With severe trauma, the patient may have other injuries such as a brain injury, contused kidney, cardiac contusion, intestinal rupture, or other problems in addition to SCI. Emergency surgery for life-threatening injuries, such as a ruptured spleen, may be necessary. The patient's condition may not be stable enough to tolerate prolonged anesthesia and spinal surgery.

Types of Procedures

For neural decompression, a posterior (most common), anterior, or lateral laminectomy is performed. For stabilization, the most common procedure is a posterior laminectomy. An open reduction and internal fixation with instrumentation is performed that utilizes plates, screws, wires, and rods. A fusion, using autologous iliac bone graft, may also be performed. It is beyond the scope of this text to summarize the selection criteria for surgical options or surgical instrumentation. Laminectomy and spinal fusion, along with nursing care, are discussed in Chapter 20.

All instrumentation systems have the same basic components that include a vertical device and a fixation or anchoring device.[5] The *vertical device* is a rod or a plate that is attached lengthwise to the vertebral column to provide stabilization. *Fixation or anchoring devices*, which attach the vertical rod or plate to the vertebra, are wires, screws, or hooks oriented at right angles to the vertical device. All systems pose potential complications because of system failure as well as postoperative wound infection. Available systems include Harrington rods, Luque rods, the Cotrel-Dubousset (CD) system, and the Texas Scottish Rite Hospital (TSRH) screw-rod system.[24]

Harrington rods, developed in the early 1960s, were originally the cornerstone of spinal surgery instrumentation. The Harrington rod system consists of a rod or rods and wires affixed to the base of spinous processes and to the rod. This provides multiple fixation points for stabilization. In some cases, loss of reduction with progressive kyphotic deformity occurred in patients treated with Harrington instrumentation.[25] Current instrumentation systems are much more rigid and allow for segmental spinal fusion. **CD rods,** introduced in the early 1990s, are an example. These rods, used in conjunction with lamina hooks or pedicle screws, are the current approach for thoracic lumbar instrumentation.[26]

This system provides for multiple points of fixation and greater stabilization. CD rod placement, although technically more difficult, does not usually require postoperative immobility. Ideally, use of CD instrumentation facilitates early mobility of the patient.

NONSURGICAL MANAGEMENT OF SPINAL CORD INJURIES

Nonsurgical management of the patient with a SCI commonly involves immobilization with a halo vest or brace and traction for reduction and realignment, singularly or more often in combination. Vertebral subluxation with or without cord involvement is often managed with immobilization with a halo vest and traction.

Approaches to Management Based on the Level of Injury

Cervical Injuries

Cervical Traction. Cervical traction is used much less frequently with the advent of earlier and better surgical stabilization. When cervical traction is used, its purpose is realignment or reduction of cervical vertebral dislocations. Gardner-Wells, Crutchfield, Vinke, and other types of cervical tongs have been almost eliminated in favor of the versatile halo traction system (described below), the most common type of cervical traction. Skeletal traction greatly facilitates care and enhances patient comfort. After traction is in place, pain is greatly decreased or completely relieved. Traction ameliorates pain by separating and aligning the injured vertebrae and by reducing or eliminating spasms in the distracted muscles.

A regular, firm hospital bed is used with cervical traction. Some physicians prefer using a special bed, such as a Roto Rest (Fig. 19-14). Depending on the type of injury and method of immobilization, other special beds may be used to decrease the possibility of pressure areas. When in traction, a special technique is used to safely turn the patient for skin care and to change position to reduce pressure.

The Halo System. The halo is the most frequently ordered method for cervical and high thoracic vertebral injuries. The following are two uses for the halo:

- Direct skeletal traction involving the application of hanging weights; the patient is maintained on complete bed rest and managed with special nursing care techniques (Fig. 19-15).
- With a special body vest to stabilize the spine and allow

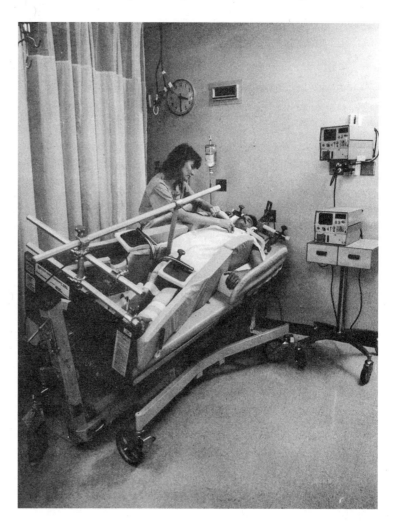

Figure 19–14 • Roto Rest bed. (Courtesy of Kinetic Concepts, San Antonio, TX.)

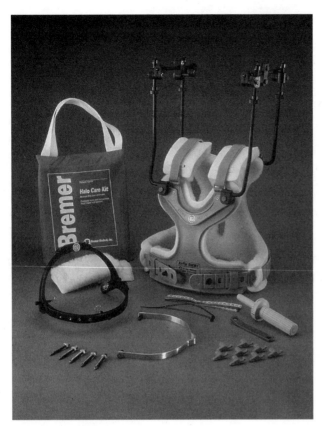

Figure 19–15 • Halo cervical skeletal traction. (Courtesy of Acromed Corp., Cleveland, OH).

Thoracic and Lumbar Injuries

Depending on the specific type of injury, various treatment options are available for a patient with a thoracic or lumbar fracture or fracture-dislocation. If indicated, the surgical procedure most frequently performed is a laminectomy with instrumentation for stabilization, with or without a fusion. The following may be used to maintain thoracic or lumbar alignment either as an adjunct to surgery or as the only management protocol for the injury:

- A fiberglass or plastic vest (the vest, which is fitted to the patient, provides immobilization and support to the injured area)
- A canvas corset
- A Jewett brace, which extends the length of the spinal column (i.e., provides support to the lower thoracic and lumbar region)
- Other specially designed braces or orthotics

Sacral and Coccygeal Injuries

The usual treatment for sacral and coccygeal fractures is bedrest. The affected area is supported by a low support corset or special brace. A rubber ring can provide relief from

healing. Ambulation is possible if the patient is neurologically intact (Fig. 19-16).

Using local anesthesia,[27] the halo (a metal ring) is inserted into the external bony table of the cranium and fixed with four pins, two posterior and two anterior. If direct traction is desired, a rope with hanging weights is applied. If immobilization and stabilization are desired, a vest with external metal rods is attached to the halo ring.[28] Small, dry, sterile dressings are placed around the pin sites.[29] Despite its appearance, the halo is comfortable, although some patients may develop a headache initially. In addition, any sound caused by bumping the halo can result in annoying vibrations. Rubber tips may be added to the pins to reduce this problem.

Using the halo for immobilization and fixation or stabilization allows for a shorter period of hospitalization, an outstanding cost advantage. If no paralysis exists, the patient is able to ambulate, thereby counteracting the multitude of potential problems associated with bed rest and immobility. The halo with vest is beneficial in cervical and very high thoracic fractures.

Another feature of the halo is that surgery can be performed while the patient is in halo traction. This avoids the risk of malalignment of the injured area or extension of cord injury that could occur without the traction device.[30] One should remember that the physician often applies skeletal traction before surgery to reduce the injury. When the best alignment possible is achieved, surgery (usually spinal fusion) is scheduled.

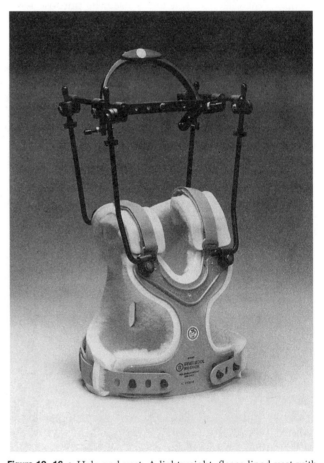

Figure 19–16 • Halo and vest. A lightweight, fleece-lined vest with a halo may be used to stabilize cervical vertebrae. Note that the vest comes in various sizes and does not need to be removed for magnetic resonance imaging studies. (Courtesy of Bremer Medical, Inc., Dawin Road, Jacksonville, FL 32207.)

pain and discomfort in the supine position. Pain is increased by sitting on a hard surface, so this should be avoided. The patient should be evaluated for bowel, bladder, and sexual dysfunction. Surgery is considered if there is evidence of compression.

FOCUS ON COLLABORATIVE MANAGEMENT IN THE ACUTE AND POSTACUTE PHASES

Acute Phase

Managing the patient with an acute SCI requires coordinated and collaborative interdisciplinary care that focuses on the patient. A clinical pathway provides a structure to map and integrate all components of care, in a timely manner, to achieve optimal measurable outcomes. The clinical pathway unites interdisciplinary team members and fosters collaboration around patient needs and outcomes. The pathway facilitates timely communications among the disciplines and assists the case manager in understanding the comprehensive needs of the patient. The core of the professional multidisciplinary team is composed of physicians, nurses, a physical therapist, an occupational therapist, a respiratory therapist, a case manager, a nutritionist, and a social worker. The major areas of focus for the collaborative team are included in Table 19-4.

After the patient has been physiologically stabilized and the vertebral column is also stable, rehabilitation efforts are begun. An increasingly precise picture of the extent of the overall deficits and how they will affect the patient's former lifestyle begins to emerge. Because LOS in acute care hospitalization is short, coordinated care is critical. In the current health care delivery system the continuum of care may also include subacute care, day hospitals, and community based care. Careful coordination is necessary to move the patient along the continuum to provide seamless care. In conceptualizing the rehabilitation process, it must be recognized that rehabilitation is not complete until integration back into the community and into previous functional roles is achieved to the degree possible.

MAJOR PATIENT MANAGEMENT RESPONSIBILITIES OF THE NURSE

Selection of a Bed

Special beds are available that have been designed to provide support to the vertebral column, decrease the risk of multisystem complications associated with immobility, and facilitate administration of nursing care. Because of the additional cost associated with use of these beds, criteria should be established to determine appropriate bed use. The Roto Rest bed (Kinetic Treatment Table; see Fig. 19-14) is one model that may be selected for the patient with SCI. A motor-powered bed, it provides continual turning of the patient through a maximal arc of 124 degrees at a minimal

rate of 3.5 minutes. It also has three hatches on the undersurface at the cervical, thoracic, and lumbosacral (rectal) regions that allow easy access to all parts of the patient's body, including the entire back and rectal area for providing back care and rectal care. With the trend toward early surgery for spinal stabilization, other bed options are available that are designed for the stabilized patient.

Signs and Symptoms of Acute Spinal Cord Trauma

The signs and symptoms of spinal cord trauma have been discussed in the previous section. The higher the level of injury, the greater will be the loss of motor, sensory, and reflex function. See Table 19-3 for a description of the functional loss that relates to specific levels of injury. The following section discusses several concurrent conditions associated with an acute SCI.

Neurogenic Shock

The temporary loss of autonomic function, termed **neurogenic shock,** affects vital signs. Blood pressure is low (especially with cervical injuries), and bradycardia is present. A cardiac monitor may be ordered to monitor the patient for cardiac arrhythmias. The low blood pressure is related, in part, to orthostatic hypotension. Because there is pooling of blood in the lower parts of the body below the level of injury, the rate of return of blood to the heart is slowed. Orthostatic hypotension is a major consideration in cervical injuries.

The ability to perspire is lost below the level of injury, so body temperature is responsive to the ambient room temperature. Most often, the temperature is low (possibly dropping to 95°F). In hot weather, the body temperature may be elevated, if climate control is not available.

Atonic Bladder

An atonic bladder is initially managed with an indwelling catheter. The nurse should follow meticulous aseptic technique in managing the catheter to prevent infections. As soon as possible, the catheter is removed and an intermittent catheterization program is initiated. There is urgency attached to early catheter removal because extended use of an indwelling catheter predisposes the patient to risk of urinary tract infection.

Ascending Spinal Cord Edema

With spinal cord trauma, edema develops soon after injury as a physiological response. The swelling results in cord compression and compounds the functional loss. This is potentially life threatening, especially in association with cervical or high thoracic injury. Because edema can ascend the cord quickly and affect the C-4 level and above (the phrenic nerve innervates the diaphragm), a patient with previously adequate respirations may rapidly develop respiratory difficulty.

(text continues on page 437)

▓▓▓ Table 19-4 • SUMMARY OF THE COLLABORATIVE MANAGEMENT OF MULTISYSTEM PROBLEMS IN THE ACUTE PHASE AFTER SPINAL CORD INJURY

SYSTEM-SPECIFIC CONSIDERATIONS	NURSING DIAGNOSES AND COLLABORATIVE PROBLEMS	ASSESSMENT AND MONITORING DATA	MANAGEMENT AND INTERVENTIONS
Neurological System • The level and pattern of neurological loss depend on the level of injury and need to be assessed and monitored for change; change can result from extension of injury or ascending edema. • As a result of spinal shock, many motor, sensory, and reflex functions are lost. Many specific deficits are listed under the body system that they primarily affect. • Hypothermia and orthostatic hypotension are commonly seen in the acute phase. • The patient who is quadriplegic is completely dependent on the care provider for self-care and mobility. • Often a cerebral concussion was also sustained at the time of injury; often memory is impaired for the circumstance of injury.	**Nursing diagnoses** • Risk for Altered Body Temperature • Hypothermia • Knowledge Deficit • Impaired Memory • Pain, acute • Impaired Physical Mobility • Self Care Deficit, complete • Self Care Deficit, instrumental • Sensory/Perceptual Alterations • Sexual Dysfunction • Sleep Pattern Disturbance • Impaired Swallowing • Risk for Injury **Collaborative problems** • Increased intracranial pressure if also sustained a brain injury	**Clinical data** • Assess baseline and monitor highest sensory level, motor function, and reflexes. • Monitor vital signs. • Assess baseline and monitor routine neurological signs for evidence of a concomitant brain injury. **Laboratory data** • Magnetic resonance imaging (MRI) or computed tomography (CT) scan • Plain x-rays of spine	• Provide for total care needs of patient. • Make sure that the patient is on the right type of bed based on the stability of the fracture and personal characteristics of the patient, such as weight. • Provide information to patient and family as requested; recognize that information will need to be repeated because of inability to comprehend fully the impact of the injury. • Be alert for decreased neurological function as a result of edema.
Respiratory System • Can develop varying degrees of respiratory difficulty depending on the level of injury: Injury at C-4 or above: Paralysis of diaphragm requires ventilator support. C-5 to T-6: Diaphragm is spared, but intercostals (T1-6) are involved; patient is at high risk for respiratory problems and may need oxygen and special respiratory support. Even with lower injuries (T6-12 innervating the abdominal muscles), there may be minor respiratory deficits. Also, immobilization and bed rest will decrease respiratory function (e.g., vital capacity), regardless of the level of injury. • The probability of certain respiratory complications decreases the lower the injury because the diaphragm and intercostals are spared. • Patients who cannot cough or manage their own secretions need a special respiratory management program. • Cervical surgery (both the procedure itself and the associated anesthesia) increases the risk of postoperative respiratory complications; thus, an optimal time for surgery (when the respiratory system is in the best condition possible) is recommended.	**Nursing diagnoses** • Ineffective Airway Clearance • Risk for Aspiration • Ineffective Breathing Pattern • Impaired Gas Exchange • Inability to Sustain Spontaneous Ventilation • Risk for Respiratory Infection • Risk for Altered Respiratory Function **Collaborative problems** • Hypoxemia • Atelectasis, pneumonia • Pneumothorax • Respiratory arrest	**Clinical data** • Determine baseline respiratory status. (Auscultate chest; note breathing pattern; assess the patient's ability to cough and deep breathe effectively.) **Laboratory data** • Chest x-ray studies • Blood gas levels • Complete blood count (CBC) • Sputum cultures • Pulmonary function studies (e.g., vital capacity)	• Intubate and provide ventilator support if the diaphragm is paralyzed or if respiratory function is ineffective. (The mode setting will depend on the needs of the patient.) • Provide supplementary oxygen as necessary. • Perform respiratory regimen (chest percussion; respiratory toilet; suctioning for patency; deep breathing if on a ventilator or sighing on ventilator setting). • Consult with a pulmonary physician as necessary. • Provide tracheostomy care every 4 h to maintain patency. • Provide chest physical therapy (PT) and deep breathing exercises every 2–4 h; if the patient is unable to cough effectively, assist with coughing by firmly depressing the abdomen when the patient coughs (place hands below the rib cage and above the umbilicus.)*

Table 19–4 • SUMMARY OF THE COLLABORATIVE MANAGEMENT OF MULTISYSTEM PROBLEMS IN THE ACUTE PHASE AFTER SPINAL CORD INJURY (Continued)

SYSTEM-SPECIFIC CONSIDERATIONS	NURSING DIAGNOSES AND COLLABORATIVE PROBLEMS	ASSESSMENT AND MONITORING DATA	MANAGEMENT AND INTERVENTIONS
• Other risk factors contributing to altered respiratory function include immobilization; bed rest; smoking; pre-existing pulmonary disease (e.g., chronic obstructive pulmonary disease); concurrent chest trauma (e.g., fractured ribs, contused lungs); anemia; and gastric distention or paralytic ileus. Gastric distention may be associated with vomiting, aspiration, and compromised lung expansion. □ • Alert: Ascending edema can rapidly cause respiratory difficulty that requires immediate intervention; monitor rate and pattern frequently. □	—	—	• Provide for intermittent positive-pressure breathing (IPPB) every 4 h. • Provide for use of incentive spirometer every 4 h.
Cardiovascular System • Loss of sympathetic input from the higher brain centers results in bradycardia and vasomotor paralysis (vasodilation of blood vessels below the level of injury), so blood pressure is lowered. • Orthostatic hypotension results in pooling of blood below the level of injury because of vasodilation; this causes hypotension and decreased blood return to the heart. • Pooling of blood, coupled with immobility, greatly increases the risk of vascular stasis and orthostatic hypotension.	**Nursing diagnoses** • Impaired Gas Exchange • Decreased Cardiac Output • Altered Tissue Perfusion • Risk for Peripheral Neurovascular Dysfunction **Collaborative problems** • Decreased cardiac output • Dysrhythmias • Deep vein thrombosis (DVT) • Hypovolemia	**Clinical data** • Monitor vital signs. • Provide cardiac monitoring. • Monitor response to elevation of head (orthostatic hypotension). • Observe for signs and symptoms of thrombophlebitis, DVT, and pulmonary embolus. **Laboratory data** • Electrocardiogram • Electrolyte, coagulation studies	• Treat any life-threatening arrhythmias. • Apply elastic hose sequential compression boots. • Prophylactic use of heparin (5,000 U every 12 h) helps prevent DVTs; this is *contraindicated* if any internal bleeding is present or if surgery has been performed. • Use vasopressors as necessary. • Cardiology consult may be necessary, especially if a cardiac contusion is suspected. • Assess for arrhythmias by observing the cardiac monitor. • Monitor patient's response to elevation of the head (orthostatic hypotension). • Observe for signs and symptoms of DVT and pulmonary embolus.
Integumentary System (Skin) • Loss of vasomotor tone, paralysis, and bedrest contribute to the development of pressure areas and skin breakdown. • Once developed, broken areas of skin are very difficult to heal; therefore, use of a bed type to relieve continuous pressure while maintaining alignment should be considered.	**Nursing diagnoses** • Risk for Peripheral Neurovascular Dysfunction • Impaired Skin Integrity • Impaired Tissue Integrity • Altered Peripheral Tissue Perfusion **Collaborative problems** • Pressure ulcers	**Clinical data** • Monitor for signs and symptoms of redness or breakdown.	• Provide skin care and turn patient every 2–4 h. • When a special bed (e.g., a Roto Rest bed) is in use, adapt care measures appropriately.

(continued)

Table 19 – 4 • SUMMARY OF THE COLLABORATIVE MANAGEMENT OF MULTISYSTEM PROBLEMS IN THE ACUTE PHASE AFTER SPINAL CORD INJURY (Continued)

SYSTEM-SPECIFIC CONSIDERATIONS	NURSING DIAGNOSES AND COLLABORATIVE PROBLEMS	ASSESSMENT AND MONITORING DATA	MANAGEMENT AND INTERVENTIONS
Musculoskeletal System • Prolonged immobility and paralysis have significant effects on bone, joints, and muscles (see Table 19–5).	**Nursing diagnoses** • Disuse Syndrome • Impaired Physical Mobility • Altered Protection **Collaborative problems** • Contractures • Ankylosis • Muscle atrophy • Osteoporosis	**Clinical data** • Monitor range of motion of joints for development of deformities, spasticity, or ankylosis.	• Consult with physical therapist to develop individualized PT program. • Provide range-of-motion exercises once daily. • Position the patient's extremities in proper body alignment.
Gastrointestinal (GI) System • Peristalsis is lost with spinal shock, resulting in paralytic ileus. • A distended abdomen interferes with adequate respirations. • Stress ulcers and gastric hemorrhage can also occur; because sensation is lost, the patient cannot feel the pain of ulceration. • Monitor for constipation.	**Nursing diagnoses** • Ineffective Breathing Pattern • Risk for Altered Respiratory Function • Risk for Injury • Bowel Incontinence • Constipation **Collaborative problems** • Paralytic ileus • GI bleeding • Constipation	**Clinical data** • Perform abdominal auscultation for bowel sounds. • Monitor stools for occult blood. • Monitor gastric pH. **Laboratory data** • CBC • Decreased hemoglobin	• Immediately insert a nasogastric tube to intermittent suction (low) for GI decompression. • Maintain patient's NPO status until bowel sounds return and the nasogastric tube is removed. • Initiate a bowel program as soon as possible. • Maintain a pH >5.0 by using Maalox, 30 mL every 3 h. • Administer drugs (e.g., cimetidine) for gastric prophylaxis. • Stool softeners/laxatives to facilitate a bowel program.
Genitourinary System • Bladder reflexes and control of micturition from higher brain centers are lost with cord injury; atonic bladder results. • An atonic bladder (loss of bladder tone) is distended and predisposes the patient to urinary tract infections (UTIs).	**Nursing diagnoses** • Reflex Incontinence • Altered Pattern of Urinary Elimination • Urinary Retention • Risk for Infection **Collaborative problems** • Acute urinary retention • Urinary tract infection	**Clinical data** • Palpate suprapubic area for bladder distention. • Review intake and output record. **Laboratory data** • Urine C&S, U/A, BUN, and creatinine	• Insert an indwelling urinary catheter immediately • Remove catheter and initiate intermittent catheterization program every 6–8 h once the patient is stable • Aggressively treat UTI. • Maintain an intake and output record. • Use aseptic technique when managing the indwelling catheter.
Metabolic (Nutritional) System • The method of providing nutrition will depend on the associated injuries, level of consciousness, and the presence or absence of peristalsis. • The body needs sufficient fluid, carbohydrates, and protein for energy and tissue repair.	**Nursing diagnoses** • Altered Nutrition: Less than body requirements • Fluid Volume Deficit • Fluid Volume Excess **Collaborative problems** • Negative nitrogen balance • Electrolyte imbalances • Acidosis • Alkalosis • Hypoglycemia, hyperglycemia	**Clinical data** • Assess skin turgor and mucous membranes for adequacy of hydration. • Monitor weight two times a week. • Monitor muscle mass of extremities. **Laboratory data** • Albumin, electrolytes, and other indications of nutritional levels	• Maintain NPO status until peristalsis returns. • Nutrition consult is necessary as soon as possible. • May need to consider total parenteral nutrition. • Use GI tract, if not contraindicated, as soon as peristalsis returns.

Table 19 – 4 • SUMMARY OF THE COLLABORATIVE MANAGEMENT OF MULTISYSTEM PROBLEMS IN THE ACUTE PHASE AFTER SPINAL CORD INJURY (Continued)

SYSTEM-SPECIFIC CONSIDERATIONS	NURSING DIAGNOSES AND COLLABORATIVE PROBLEMS	ASSESSMENT AND MONITORING DATA	MANAGEMENT AND INTERVENTIONS
Psychological or Emotional Response			
• If the patient is conscious, he or she is usually in a state of shock and denies what has happened and the impact on lifestyle. • Allow the patient to ask questions when ready. • The family may require the most support as they begin to comprehend what has happened and its impact on personal and family function.	**Nursing diagnoses** • Impaired Adjustment • Anxiety • Body Image Disturbance • Confusion • Decisional Conflict • Defensive Coping • Ineffective Denial • Diversional Activity Deficit • Grieving • Ineffective Individual Coping • Personal Identity Disturbance • Powerlessness • Impaired Social Interaction **Collaborative problems** • Depression • Anxiety	**Clinical data** • Assess the patient to determine what he or she is ready to hear. • Assess the family unit and its response to the injury and its impact.	• Be supportive of the patient and family. • Provide comprehensive information. • Make appropriate referrals for support.

The spinal cord tolerates cord compression poorly. Permanent loss of function may result from frank damage to the cord itself, or temporary loss may occur related to exaggerated edema. With resolution of the edema, some functional return is possible, provided that irreversible damage has not been sustained. It is of critical importance for the nurse to observe the patient's status frequently for signs of deterioration from baseline function, especially in the early, acute phase of injury (during the first 72 hours or so).

Respiratory Insufficiency

With C-1 to C-4 injuries, the intercostal muscles and often the diaphragm are paralyzed. The patient depends on a ventilator for respiratory support. Although the diaphragm is spared in injuries at C-5 or below, a ventilator may be necessary in the acute phase owing to ascending cord edema. Related nursing diagnoses are listed in Table 19-4.

Nursing Assessment

The nursing database begins with the nursing history and assessment at the time of admission. Data collected in the history are part of the database for discharge planning, which is initiated during admission. Information about the family unit, work and leisure activities, and previous coping patterns is helpful in individualizing the plan of care.

Assessment includes vital signs, neurological signs, spinal cord assessment, monitoring of laboratory data, and overall body systems assessment. Many physiological assessment data are collected from instrument monitoring and a computer interface.

Vital Signs

Vital signs must be monitored frequently. A lower than expected blood pressure, bradycardia, and abnormal temperature may be noted, especially with cervical cord injuries. The basis for these changes in relationship to spinal cord trauma is discussed in the section of this chapter on neurogenic shock. However, SCI patients who have sustained trauma to other body systems may be exhibiting changes in the vital signs related to these other injuries. Because some injuries may not be noted immediately, a change in vital signs may be the first sign of occult internal hemorrhage or other potentially life-threatening problems. Therefore, frequent monitoring of vital signs for change and trends is important.

Neurological Signs

An abbreviated neurological assessment is conducted periodically, including evaluation of the level of consciousness and pupillary response. Patients with SCIs often have concurrent brain injuries of varying severity. A standard neurological assessment sheet may be used.

Spinal Cord Assessment Sheet

To determine exactly which functional levels remain intact, an extensive motor, sensory, and reflex assessment is necessary. A facility-created form, the ASIA Motor and Sensory Assessment form, or Chart 19-4 may be used for systematic assessment. Information collected in this database helps the nurse monitor the patient for neurological change and facilitates development of an individualized plan of care based on functional loss.

CHART 19–4 • Nursing Assessment of Spinal Cord Function

Part I. Motor Function			Part II. Reflexes		
Left	Muscle Action	Right	Left	Deep Tendon Reflexes	Right
	Abduct upper arm			Ankle Jerk — S-1, S-2	
	Adduct upper arm			Knee Jerk — L-3, L-4	
	Extend upper arm			Biceps — C-5, C-6	
	Flex elbow			Triceps — C-7, C-8	
	Extend elbow			Superficial Reflexes	
	Flex wrist			Perineal — S3-5	
	Extend wrist			Abdominals, upper — T8-10	
	Flex fingers			Abdominals, lower — T10-12	
	Extend fingers			Gag — cranial nerve IX and X	
	Thumb opposition				
	Upper abdominals				
	Lower abdominals				
	Flex upper leg				
	Extend upper leg				
	Flex knee				
	Extend knee				
	Dorsiflex foot				
	Plantarflex foot				
	Extend big toe				

A few selected reflexes are assessed.

The grading of deep tendon reflexes is assessed using the following scale:

- 4+ = very brisk; markedly hyperactive, often with associated clonus
- 3+ = more brisk than average
- 2+ = average or normal
- 1+ = diminished response
- 0 = no response

The grading of superficial reflexes is assessed using the following scale:

- 1 = present
- 0 = absent

Motor function is assessed using the following scale:

- 5 = normal strength
- 4 = slight weakness; can tolerate only a moderate amount of resistance
- 3 = moderate weakness; full range of movement against gravity only (no resistance)
- 2 = severe weakness; can move only when gravity is eliminated
- 1 = very severe weakness; a weak muscle contraction palpated but no visible movement noted
- 0 = complete paralysis

CHART 19 – 4 • Nursing Assessment of Spinal Cord Function (Continued)

Part III. Sensory Function

| Left | | Level | Right | | Left | | Level | Right | |
Pain	POS/VIB	Cervical	Pain	POS/VIB	Pain	POS/VIB	Sacral	Pain	POS/VIB
		1					1		
		2					2		
		3					3		
		4					4		
		5					5		
		6							
		7							
		8							
		Thoracic							
		1							
		2							
		3							
		4							
		5							
		6							
		7							
		8							
		9							
		10							
		11							
		12							
		Lumbar							
		1							
		2							
		3							
		4							
		5							

Two sensory modalities are assessed: pain (pinprick), which is controlled by the lateral spinothalamic tract, and position (or vibration), which is controlled by the posterior columns. Pain perception is tested with pinprick. Position is tested by moving the thumbs and big toes up and down. If vibration is tested, a 256-Hz tuning fork is used. Using a dermatome, dermatomic areas are tested on each side of the body separately.

Sensory function is assessed using the following scale:

- 2 = normal
- 1 = present but abnormal
- 0 = absent

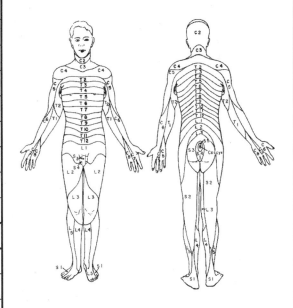

Dermatomes
Cutaneous distribution of the spinal nerves (See Figure 2-33, page 40. From Barr, M.L., and J.A. Kiernan 1988. The human nervous system, 5th ed. Philadelphia: J. B. Lippincott.)

▌▌▌ Table 19-5 • MUSCULOSKELETAL CHANGES CAUSED BY PROLONGED IMMOBILIZATION

	INITIAL	ADVANCED
Bone	Skeletal malalignment; loss of calcium	Skeletal deformities and generalized osteoporosis, which can result in an increased amount of cavities and pathological fractures
Joints	Joint stiffness; shortening or stretching of ligaments	Ankylosis
Muscles	Muscle weakness; shortening or stretching of muscles	Muscle atrophy; fibrotic changes; muscle contractures

Body Systems Review

There are two reasons for conducting a systematic assessment of body systems in the patient with SCI. The first is to determine the location and extent of injuries to body systems other than the neurological system. The second is to determine the impact of the neurological injuries on other body systems (see Table 19-4).

Injuries to Other Body Systems. As discussed previously, patients with SCIs often sustain injury to other body systems as well. It is therefore important to consider the possibility of other injuries when assessing the patient.

This assessment is complicated by the fact that all sensations are lost, including pain (often an indicator of a problem), below the level of injury. Because pain cannot be used as an objective indicator of dysfunction in affected patients, the nurse must rely on other indicators, such as laboratory data, to assess the patient. For example, gastric hemorrhage may be heralded by pain, decreased levels of hematocrit and hemoglobin, and a decline in central venous pressure. The nurse will need to concentrate on indications other than pain to monitor the patient for hemorrhage especially if the SCI is cervical or high thoracic.

Impact of Neurological Injury on Other Body Systems. Assessment data for problems arising in the acute phase of SCI are included in Table 19-4.

Laboratory Data

Laboratory data obtained during the acute phase of SCI include blood chemistry values (e.g., electrolyte studies, glucose and blood gas levels), microbiological tests (e.g., cultures), and hematological studies (e.g., complete blood count, hematocrit, hemoglobin). Also included among the diagnostic data are results from radiology (e.g., chest x-ray films, spinal films), special procedures (e.g., CT scans, MRI), and other data. Review of this database helps to correlate clinical observations of signs and symptoms with laboratory findings, to identify the need for special assessment and monitoring, and to determine specific nursing interventions.

Summary

Sources of data are numerous, and the needs of the patient can change dramatically, especially in the acute phase of SCI. Therefore, ongoing comprehensive assessment is required to provide a basis for analysis and to establish appropriate nursing diagnoses.

Nursing Interventions

General Considerations

Given that patients admitted to the hospital with SCIs have self-care deficits, the nurse must determine to what degree the patient can perform such basic functions as bathing and hygiene, dressing and grooming, feeding, and toileting. The patient may be completely independent, in need of assistance, or completely dependent. An appropriate level of care is provided to meet basic needs. Other nursing interventions are included in Table 19-4. Based on the level of injury, the nurse can make some assumptions about patient needs (see Table 19-3).

Management of Cervical Skeletal Traction

Special protocols are used to manage patients who are being treated with halo cervical skeletal traction alone or combined with a vest used in association with the halo (Charts 19-5 and 19-6). Patients maintained in cervical traction are on complete bedrest and are at high risk for the multiple problems associated with immobility (Table 19-5).

Acute and Subacute Problems With Spinal Cord Injury

In considering the comprehensive needs of patients along the continuum of care, several conditions can develop as the patient moves from the acute to the subacute phase. They include autonomic hyperreflexia, spasticity, bladder dysfunction, bowel dysfunction, sexual dysfunction, and psychosocial maladaption.

Autonomic Hyperreflexia

Autonomic hyperreflexia, also termed *autonomic dysreflexia,* is characterized by strong muscle spasms and autonomic dysfunction precipitated by cutaneous or visceral stimuli.[31] It is seen only *after* recovery from spinal shock when reflex activity has returned and *only in patients with spinal cord lesions at or above T-6.* Noxious stimuli that can precipitate autonomic hyperreflexia include a distended bladder secondary to a plugged catheter, urinary calculus, or cystitis; constipation or fecal impaction; acute abdominal lesions; operative incisions; uterine labor contractions; pressure on the glans penis; and, stimulation from skin lesions, such as inguinal rash, pressure ulcer, or ingrown toenail. It can also be caused by small objects that were left in the bed.

Clinically, the patient suddenly develops severe hypertension associated with a severe pounding headache, nasal obstruction, shortness of breath, nausea, and blurred vision. The patient also exhibits bradycardia, arrhythmias, sweating, goose flesh, and cutaneous vasodilation with flushed face, neck, and upper chest, *above* the injury level. Pallor is noted *below* the level of injury. The blood pressure may rise as high as 240/120 or higher. The significance of the rise in blood pressure should be judged based on the patient's usual baseline. If severe hypertension is left untreated, retinal hemorrhage, hemorrhagic stroke, subarachnoid hemorrhage, seizures (including status epilepticus), pulmonary edema, or myocardial infarction may result.[32–34]

The pathophysiology of autonomic hyperreflexia is complex (Fig. 19-17). Afferent impulses ascend the spinal cord, but because of the spinal injury, upward ascension to higher centers is interrupted. A mass reflex stimulation of the sympathetic chain and nerves *below* the spinal injury occurs. This causes arteriolar spasms of the pelvic and abdominal viscera and of the skin, resulting in vasoconstriction *below* the lesion. The vasoconstriction produces cold skin and goose flesh in the involved area and raises blood pressure. Baroreceptors in the aortic arch and carotid sinus are stimulated, and a message is sent through the vagus nerve to the vasomotor center (in the medulla), causing reflex slowing of the heart (bradycardia) and vasodilation *above* the lesion. The bradycardia represents an attempt by the body to cause vasodilation and lower the blood pressure.

Management. Nursing management is aimed at preventing conditions that are known to trigger autonomic hyperreflexia. If autonomic hyperreflexia occurs, treatment is directed toward removal of the noxious stimuli and lowering of the blood pressure. Management includes elevation of the head of the bed, lowering of the lower legs and feet over the side of the bed, and rapid assessment to determine the underlying cause. This situation represents a *medical emergency* and should be treated accordingly.

- Assess the bladder for distention. If a catheter is in place, check it for evidence of obstructed flow, such as a kink in the tubing. If the catheter is plugged, immediately irrigate it with a small amount (about 30 mL) of solution. If it still does not drain, replace the catheter immediately.
- In patients who are being catheterized intermittently, catheterize the patient immediately, regardless of the time that has elapsed since the last catheterization.
- Autonomic hyperreflexia is often triggered during bowel care or defecation. If symptoms develop, cease all activities until symptoms subside. Assess the lower bowel for the presence of stool. Apply a topical anesthetic ointment (e.g., Nupercaine) to the anus and also insert the ointment 1 inch into the rectum. Wait 5 to 10 minutes, then attempt disimpaction.
- If a pressure ulcer is present, spray the area with a topical anesthetic agent.
- Monitor vital signs frequently.
- Antihypertensive drugs may be ordered to lower severe hypertension.

Skin and Decubitus Ulcers

Patients with SCI are at high risk for development of decubitus ulcers. The high risk associated with use of backboards was discussed earlier in this chapter. Areas insensitive to sensory input are also at high risk for skin breakdown if relief from pressure is not provided. Special beds designed to relieve pressure are useful and cost effective for prevention. After the patient is seated, relieve weight on the ischial tuberosities at frequent intervals, for example, every 15 minutes initially, and gradually increase the time. Gel pads and other devices designed to relieve pressure are useful. A skin management and prevention program is an important responsibility, which is discussed in Chapter 13.

Deep Vein Thrombosis and Pulmonary Embolus

Patients with SCIs are at high risk for development of deep venous thrombosis (DVT) and pulmonary embolus (PE). The contributing factors are immobility, flaccidity, and decreased vasomotor tone in the blood vessels below the level of injury. Prevention strategies include use of thigh-high elastic stockings, sequential compression boots, low-molecular-weight heparin, and early mobilization. Fatal PE is reported in 1% to 2% of all patients with SCI within the first 3 months of injury. Focal pain, a common symptom of DVT, may not be noticed by SCI patients because of sensory deficits. Testing for those patients at higher risk of DVT includes impedance plethysmography, Doppler ultrasound, and duplex study, all of which provide good sensitivity and specificity.[22]

Heterotopic Ossification

Heterotopic ossification (HO) is the development of calcification around a joint, most often the hip. Approximately 20% of patients with traumatic brain injury or SCI exhibit HO within 12 weeks after injury.[35] The signs and symptoms mimic those of acute arthritis with the exception that pain in SCI patients may be absent because of loss of sensation. Limitation in range of motion may be the first sign noted, followed by swelling of the affected limb. Because swelling is also a common finding associated with DVT, a careful evaluation is necessary to differentiate between these problems. The third sign is an elevated alkaline phosphatase level, which confirms the diagnosis of HO. Radiographic changes follow these three signs.

The treatment for HO includes irradiation, NSAIDs, and disodium etidronate (20 mg/kg for the first 2 weeks followed by 10 mg/kg for 2.5 months for a total treatment period of 3 months).[36,37] Because HO that exists at the time of diagnosis is not reversible, treatment is directed at prevention of further progression of the process. For patients with significant limitation of range of motion, surgery may be considered in 12 to 18 months. The time lapse allows for the maturation of the heterotopic bone that minimizes the likelihood of recurrence. Surgery is directed at increasing the range of motion of the hip so that the patient can sit in a wheelchair without undue pressure. Because HO can be the cause of significant pain and limitation of range of motion, its presence can significantly impede the rehabilitation phase and the achievement of an optimal outcome.

(text continues on page 446)

CHART 19 – 5 • Summary of the Nursing Management of a Patient in Cervical Skeletal Halo Traction

Nursing Diagnoses	Nursing Interventions	Expected Outcome(s)
Orthopedic Traction Equipment • Risk for Injury	• Check the orthopedic frame and traction daily to ensure that nuts and bolts are secure. • Check tongs daily to be sure that they are secure. • Be sure that traction weights are hanging freely and not resting on the floor or frame. (Releasing the traction is dangerous because cord injury could be extended.)	• The orthopedic frame will remain intact. • Tongs will not slip. • Traction weights will hang freely. • There will not be any extension of cord injury secondary to slippage of the traction apparatus.
Skin Integrity • Risk for Infection • Impaired Skin Integrity	• Inspect tong sites, and clean and dress daily as ordered (may be referred to as "pin care"). • Turn the patient every 2 h from side to back to other side using a triple log roll technique as described below if a patient is on a regular hospital bed. • Nurse # 1 stands behind the head of the bed and places hands firmly on the patient's head and neck, maintaining it in a neutral position; the head and neck are turned as a unit. • Nurse #2 stands at the patient's side and moves the patient's shoulders. • Nurse #3 stands at the patient's side and moves the patient's hips and legs. • Plan ahead, identifying desired position and pillow placement *before* moving the patient. When all three nurses are ready, turn the patient as a log on the count of three. Leave the patient positioned in the middle of the bed (if not, he or she will be uncomfortable); use pillows to support the patient's body in alignment. • Nurse #1 should hold the head and neck until the patient is supported adequately (if traction slips, manual traction can be supplied by Nurse #1).	• The pin site will remain free of infection. • Skin integrity will be maintained. • The vertebral column will be maintained in a neutral position and in proper alignment.
Basic Care • Self-Care Deficits	• Provide for basic care needs that the patient cannot do for self.	• Basic care needs will be met.
Respiratory System • Risk for Aspiration • Ineffective Airway Clearance • Risk for Infection • Impaired Gas Exchange • *Note:* The patient on a ventilator will need special care.	• Have suction available to maintain a patent airway. • Provide respiratory care. • Provide for deep-breathing, assistive coughing, and incentive spirometer exercises every 1 to 2 h.	• Airway patency will be maintained. • The patient will not aspirate. • The patient will not develop a respiratory infection.

CHART 19-5 • Summary of the Nursing Management of a Patient in Cervical Skeletal Halo Traction (Continued)

Nursing Diagnoses	Nursing Interventions	Expected Outcome(s)
Cardiovascular System		
• Impaired Tissue Integrity (venous stasis) • Altered Peripheral Tissue Perfusion • Decreased Cardiac Output	• Maintain thigh-high elastic (TED) stockings and sequential compression boots. • If the patient is receiving heparin, observe for signs and symptoms of bleeding. • Monitor for deep vein thrombosis (DVTs) and pulmonary emboli. (May be receiving minidoses of subcutaneous heparin q 12 h, if not contraindicated.)	• Air boots and TEDs will be worn at all times. • Vital signs will be maintained within normal limits. • The patient will be observed for DVTs and pulmonary emboli.
Musculoskeletal System		
• Risk for Disuse Syndrome • Pain (related to muscle spasm) • Sensory Perceptual Alterations: visual and tactile	• Provide comfort measures. • Provide range-of-motion exercises q.i.d. • Position the patient in proper body alignment. • Reposition the patient frequently. • Stretch the patient's heel cord with exercises.	• The patient will be free from pain. • Contractures will not develop. • Strategies will be used to manage spasticity if it occurs.
Gastrointestinal System		
• Colonic Constipation	• Institute a bowel-retraining program. • Auscultate the abdomen for bowel sounds. • Record the frequency and consistency of stool.	• Pattern of bowel evacuation every 1 to 2 d will be established.
Genitourinary System		
• Altered Urinary Elimination • Risk for Infection • Sexual Dysfunction	• Monitor intake and output • Force fluids. • If an intermittent catheterization protocol is initiated, use aseptic technique. • If the patient is voiding on his or her own, monitor postvoid residuals. • Provide information about sexual function.	• Intake will be 3,000 mL unless contraindicated. • Postvoid residuals will be less than 100 mL. • Strict aseptic technique will be used for catheter protocols. • Sexual function and spinal cord injury are discussed with the patient when he or she is ready.
Nutrition		
• Altered Nutrition: Less than body requirements • Fluid Volume Deficit	• Encourage an adequate diet. • Ask the dietician to see the patient. • Provide for adequate fluid intake up to 3,000 mL daily. • Encourage the patient to take small portions of food into the mouth and chew well to prevent aspiration. • Keep suction equipment handy.	• A diet high in protein and carbohydrates, which includes a fluid intake of up to 3,000 mL, will be provided. • Aspiration will be prevented.
Emotional and Psychological Support		
• Powerlessness • Social Isolation • Ineffective Individual Coping • Diversional Activity Deficit • Body Image Disturbance • Knowledge Deficit	• Provide for social interaction and diversion based on the patient's functional level. • Reinforce a positive self-image. • Allow the patient to participate in decision making as much as possible. • Provide for patient teaching.	• The patient's mental health will be supported. • Social interaction and diversion will be provided based on the patient's ability to participate. • A positive body image will be supported. • Necessary information will be provided.

CHART 19 – 6 • Summary of Nursing Management of the Patient in a Halo With Vest

Nursing Responsibilities	Rationale
Management of the Halo Device and the Body Vest	
• Check the pins on the halo ring to be sure they are secure and tight.	• Ensures safety and integrity of the treatment
• Check the edges of the fiberglass vest for comfort and fit by inserting the small finger or index finger between the vest and the patient's skin. If the vest is too tight, skin breakdown, edema, and possible nerve injury can occur.	• Provides for comfort and prevents skin irritation
• The vest should be supported while the patient is in bed.	• Maintains proper body alignment
• Place a rubber cork over the tips of the halo device to diminish magnification of sound if the pin is bumped.	• Provides for comfort
Meticulous Skin Care	
• Inspect and cleanse the pin site once or twice daily, as prescribed, to prevent infection.	• Maintains skin integrity and monitors the patient for infections.
• Turn the patient in bed every 2 h by means of the triple log-roll technique to prevent the development of hypostatic pneumonia, atelectasis, and skin breakdown.	• Maintains proper body alignment and prevents injury
• Provide sponge pads to prevent pressure on prominent body areas, such as the forehead and shoulder, while the patient is in bed.	• Prevents injury and irritation to the skin
• Inspect under the vest, and keep all areas of skin dry.	• Provides early identification of skin irritation or breakdown
Altered Body Image	
• Help the patient adjust to the distorted body image that the halo device can create.	• Supports the patient's emotional well-being
Control of Pain: Comfort	
• Administer mild analgesics to control headache and discomfort, which are common, around the pin site.	• Provides for comfort
• Provide a soft diet, because many patients have jaw pain if they attempt to chew.	• Provides for comfort
Basic Hygienic Care	
• Encourage self-care as much as possible.	• Maintains the patient's independence and supports self-esteem
Support of Body Systems	
• Maintain an intake and output record.	• Provides information on urinary tract function and adequacy of fluid intake
• Provide for a bowel program.	• Prevents constipation and maintains a normal pattern of bowel evacuation
• Provide for range-of-motion exercises for all extremities.	• Maintains muscle tone
• Provide for deep-breathing exercises at least four times daily.	• Encourages hyperinflation of the lungs and prevents infections and atelectasis
• Apply thigh-high elastic hose (TED) to the legs to improve blood return to the heart.	• Decreases the possibility of thrombus or embolus formation
• Observe the legs for development of thrombophlebitis or deep vein thrombosis.	• Allows early identification of potential problems so that treatment can be initiated
Assessment Data	
• Monitor neurological signs, vital signs, and vital capacity.	• Establishes a baseline and indicates change

---

CHART 19 – 6 • Summary of Nursing Management of the Patient in a Halo With Vest (Continued)

Nursing Responsibilities	Rationale
Ambulation	
If the patient's neurological function is intact, he or she will be able to ambulate in the halo ring and vest.	
• Start to assess the patient's tolerance of the upright position by having him or her sit on the edge of the bed ("dangle"). Check vital signs. (Orthostatic hypotension may be a problem to overcome in the early stages.)	• Prevents development of untoward side effects
• Teach the patient to compensate for lost head and neck movement by making increased use of eye movement to scan the area.	• Provides for safety needs
• Accompany patients when ambulating because they are more accident prone owing to a displaced center of gravity, a tendency for loss of balance, and decreased peripheral vision.	• Same as above
• Consider the patient's use of a walker for ambulation as a means of support and greater safety.	• Same as above
Patient Teaching	
• If the patient is to go home with the halo and vest, begin a patient and family teaching plan using a booklet or other printed material. Review any written material prepared by the manufacturer for accuracy before giving it to the patient or family.	• Provides for safety and independence • Meets the patient's and family's knowledge needs

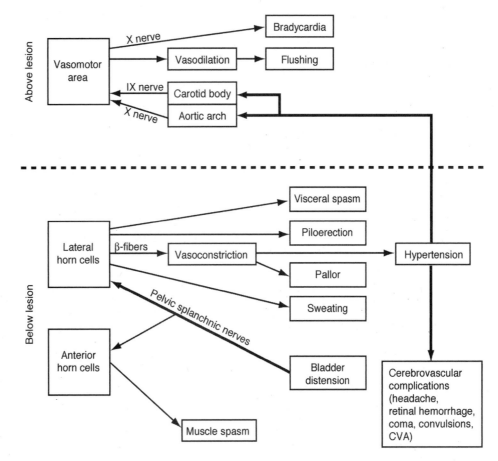

Figure 19–17 • Mechanism of autonomic hyperreflexia.

Spasticity

Spasticity, a condition with excessive tonus of selected muscles and with exaggerated deep tendon reflexes, gradually develops in both complete and incomplete SCI patients after they recover from spinal shock. A common problem, it can occur any time from a few weeks (4 to 6) to several months (7 to 8) after SCI. Typically, the magnitude of spasticity gradually increases, reaching its limit in 1.5 to 2 years, after which its intensity gradually diminishes. The flexors of the arms and the extensors of the legs are predominantly affected, and the predominant pattern is flexion or extension.

The pathophysiology of spasticity involves interruption of the descending inhibitory pathways, causing increased tonic activity of gamma motor neurons through spindle afferent impulses, and centrally through reticulospinal and vestibulospinal pathways that act mainly on alpha motor neurons. Clinically, there may be little or no change in the tonus when the limb is moved slowly. However, when the muscle is stretched rapidly, the "clasp-knife" phenomenon is seen. **Clonus,** a series of involuntary muscle contractions, describes a hyper-reflexic response to abrupt stimuli, seen in spasticity. The clasp-knife analogy used to explain spasticity compares the action of the muscles with the "catch" and "give" of a spring-loaded jack-knife blade. Through the initial phase of passive movement on a spastic limb, there is resistance to stretching, as with the opening of a knife blade. With continued pull, abrupt loss of muscle resistance occurs, with the muscle completely submitting to the movement, similar to the final phase of blade action.

The major day-to-day nursing problems encountered with spasticity are the difficulty of positioning the patient and the impact of spasticity on rehabilitation of the patient's mobility. Flexor spasticity develops first, with the patient's extremities assuming a flexed position. Development of contractures further complicates the problems of positioning.

The initial appearance of spasticity may be a false ray of hope for the patient. The "movement" noted is often misinterpreted by the patient or family as a return of normal voluntary function, rather than a heightened reflex response. Spasticity must be explained clearly and concisely to prevent any misinterpretation of its significance.

Management. Spasticity is a difficult problem best managed in collaboration with a physical therapist. Treatment depends on the severity of the spasticity and requires a combined regimen of proper positioning, exercises (e.g., passive range-of-motion exercises and stretching exercises), and specific therapies (e.g., application of cold and heat, electrical stimulation, and drug therapy). Baclofen (Lioresal), dantrolene sodium (Dantrium), and diazepam (Valium) are frequently administered.[38] Newer forms of adjunctive therapy include oral and transdermal forms of clonidine (Catapres) and tizanidine (Zanaflex). Botulism toxin A (Botox) and intrathecal baclofen are also useful for spasticity management.[22] Surgical options include tendon lengthening, capsular release, rhizotomy, and dorsal root zone ablation.

The following are nursing interventions directed at preventing, controlling, or reducing spasticity:

- Provide passive range-of-motion exercises at least four times a day. Stiffness increases spasticity.
- Avoid circumstances that precipitate noxious stimuli known to increase spasticity (e.g., extremes in temperature, remaining in one position for an extended period, anxiety, pain, bladder or bowel distention, tight clothing or equipment, and decubitus ulcers).
- Turn and reposition the patient at least every 2 hours. Avoid rubbing or irritating the skin.
- Prevent the development of contractures. Flexor spasticity and contractures gravely limit the patient's ability to participate in activities of daily living (ADLs). Use proper positioning and consult with the physical therapist on the use of splints and for positioning options.
- Regard a sudden increase in spasticity as evidence of underlying noxious stimuli (e.g., a kink in the urinary drainage; fecal impaction; a skin abrasion or pressure ulcer; cold; and stiffness). The underlying cause should be treated or eliminated promptly.

Neurogenic Bladder and Retraining

The ability to control urination may be lost in SCI patients because of loss of control of the external urethral sphincter.[39] Because prolonged use of a urinary catheter poses a major risk of urinary tract infections, earliest possible removal is indicated,[40] and intermittent catheterization protocol should be begun as soon as possible.[41] Aseptic technique, as well as careful handling of the catheter, drainage bag, and tubing, helps prevent urinary tract infections while the catheter is in place. As spinal shock resolves, a bladder retraining program can be instituted. Cystometric studies to evaluate bladder function may be scheduled.[42] Various neurogenic bladder disorders are discussed in Chapter 13.

Drug therapy to acidify the urine may be ordered. A urinary antiseptic, such as methenamine mandelate (Mandelamine), is often administered. A urinary pH of 5.5 must be maintained for the drug to be effective; therefore, a urinary acidifier, such as vitamin C, is often prescribed. The average adult dose is 1 to 2 g four times daily. The patient is instructed about the necessity for consuming large amounts of liquid (3,000 to 5,000 mL every 24 hours). Because cranberry juice and apple juice are urinary acidifiers, they should be included as part of the fluid intake. Vitamin C is incorporated into the pharmacological plan for patients, because one would have to drink 2.5 quarts of cranberry or apple juice daily to acidify the urine. See Chapter 13 for a further discussion of bladder retraining.

Bowel Dysfunction and Bowel Retraining

Most patients with SCIs are able to regain bowel control with an appropriate bowel training program.[43] An individualized bowel program is instituted and managed by the nurse (see Chap. 13). Prevention of constipation and fecal impaction is important for many reasons, including the risk of triggering autonomic hyperreflexia and of aggravating spasticity. The large bowel has its own neural center within the intestinal wall that responds to distention caused by feces. Dietary intake and digestive activities from the upper intestinal tract also influence bowel evacuation. The SCI affects bowel evacuation in the following way:

- Loss of the sensation of fullness in the lower abdomen or bowel

- Loss of awareness of bowel evacuation
- Loss of the ability to control the rectal sphincter
- Loss of the ability to contract the abdominal muscles and to expel the stool

In SCI patients, the abdominal muscles and diaphragm are used to facilitate bowel evacuation. If possible, position the patient comfortably with feet flat on the floor. If the abdominal muscles are impaired, he or she may be taught to exert pressure on the abdomen with the hands, or an abdominal belt may be recommended for someone who cannot strain at stool.

A well-balanced diet that is high in roughage, combined with an adequate fluid intake, produces softer stools and stimulates peristalsis. Medications, such as stool softeners, bulk producers, and lubricants, are also helpful. Mild cathartics and suppositories may be ordered. Digital dilation may be recommended. If these methods are not successful, a mild enema of limited fluid content can be administered.

A final important consideration is that selected body rhythms can be effectively used to help achieve bowel evacuation at predictable times. For example, the stimulus for defecation commonly occurs after meals because food is a stimulus for peristalsis, and peristalsis aids in moving the contents of the GI tract. The gastrocolic reflex responsible for strong contractions and peristalsis in the GI tract can be initiated by feeding the patient warm fluids and food at any time of the day. Therefore, planning for bowel evacuation and retraining should capitalize on normal body rhythms.

Bowel training must be a planned activity and must be individualized. Collaboration among the patient, nurse, and physician is necessary for successful outcomes. Patience and an optimistic attitude are necessary to provide a climate for success.

Sexual Dysfunction

Sexuality and sexual adjustment should be an integral part of the overall rehabilitation for SCI patients. Sexual function is controlled by spinal levels S-2, S-3, and S-4. Therefore, several complete and incomplete SCI syndromes can affect sexual function. The initial step is referral to a physician who focuses on sexual dysfunction, such as a urologist, for diagnosis of specific problems and to provide information and options to a patient. Further counseling and education by a health care professional skilled in SCI and sexual function, both alone or with the patient's partner, are useful for successful adaptation.

Sexually active patients need counseling in birth control methods. Because the use of certain types of oral contraceptives may increase the risk of thrombophlebitis for women, careful determination of the best choice is important for the SCI patient.

Psychological Maladaption

The impact of catastrophic illness, coupled with devastating functional loss, is overwhelming to the patient and family. Comprehensive patient and family education and support are required, as are sensitivity and compassion. The nurse should acknowledge the losses while being optimistic for the future. The patient and family will need comprehensive information to make appropriate decisions. The proper timing of information, that is, what information needs to be provided at what point in the illness, is critical to prevent overwhelming the patient and family. In addition to the support provided by the individual practitioner, patient-centered conferences or family meetings incorporating an interdisciplinary team approach may be helpful in supporting the patient and family. A psychiatric consultation may be helpful for some patients.

Psychological Response to Injury

The rapidity with which patients move from acute care settings to rehabilitation has been accelerated by managed care policies. Patients often do not have sufficient time to begin to process what has happened to them and what it means to their personhood. Wide ranges of emotional responses are experienced by the patient with an SCI as he or she progresses from the acute phase to the rehabilitation phase. The sensory losses associated with SCI and the subsequent immobilization create sensory and perceptual alterations. Immobilization and confinement to bed by traction or paralysis limit and distort visual and auditory stimuli. For instance, vision may become distorted for the patient on bed rest, so that although fully aware of the ceiling, the upper half of the walls, and people from the waist up, he or she may not visualize most objects in their totality.

Immobility is an extreme hardship for a paralyzed patient who may not even be able to scratch his or her nose. Confinement represents limited territoriality, with lack of control over access to one's surroundings. For those accustomed to using physical activity to relieve stress, immobility negates this stress-reduction strategy. As a result, physical immobility can lead to psychological distress.

As the nurse assesses the patient and family, several of the following nursing diagnoses may be applicable:

- Anxiety
- Fear
- Body Image Disturbance
- Ineffective Individual Coping
- Loneliness
- Dysfunctional Grieving
- Personal Identity Disturbance
- Powerlessness
- Self Esteem Disturbance
- Hopelessness
- Social Isolation
- Spiritual Distress

In addition, the emotional and psychological responses of the family may require intervention. Family-focused nursing diagnoses include ineffective family coping and altered family processes.

Psychological Response: A Model for Intervention. Sudden catastrophic injury precipitates a crisis. Crisis theory and adjustment to long-term disability provide the nurse with a framework for viewing SCI and an approach to intervention.

Spinal trauma, a catastrophic event, is met with shock, disbelief, and denial. Initially, much of the activity in the hospital is directed toward life-saving measures and stabilization of the patient. The focus is on survival. If the patient is conscious, he or she is usually in a state of emotional shock. Shock and disbelief then evolve into denial. Patients who are experiencing denial do not believe that what they are being told has any bearing on their lives. They may acknowledge some of their injuries but may deny or downplay the seriousness of others. For example, a patient may recognize and acknowledge that his or her legs are dysfunctional but may believe that this is just a temporary state. Such patients may be convinced that next week or the week after, they will be back to normal. The nurse should listen but give no false hope. Focusing on the present helps to keep the patient firmly grounded in reality.[44]

The next stage is one of reaction, and it often lasts for a long time. There may be an acknowledgment that significant losses of body function have occurred that affect the patient's degree of independence and lifestyle. Reactions, which are varied, may include anger, rage, depression,[45] bargaining, verbal abuse of caregivers and family, ideation of suicide, and inappropriate sexual behavior. Listening, gentle reminders of intact functions, and support are helpful during this stage. Any suggestions of suicide should be taken seriously and the patient protected from self-harm.

Next, the person begins to seek information about the injury, what can be expected in terms of outcome, and how care will be managed. At this stage, he or she becomes an active participant in care and rehabilitation. The nurse should allow the patient as much independence as possible and encourage the patient's efforts to maintain control of decision-making.

Finally, the person begins to cope effectively, provided adaptation has progressed. During this phase the patient develops a plan for a productive life, considering the limitations imposed by the injury. At this time, the patient can be integrated into the community.

The entire adjustment process just described can take many years to achieve. The nurse should be aware that because many patients are transferred almost immediately to specialized care centers from other hospitals, they may be only at the stage of denial or early reaction at the time of transfer.

The Nurse's Role. Caring for a patient who has sustained a SCI requires an awareness of the impact that the illness has had on the patient's emotional and psychological equilibrium. The following general suggestions are offered as an approach to providing patient care:

- Establish a therapeutic nurse—patient relationship.
- Cultivate a climate of trust.
- Allow the verbalization of feelings.
- Accept behavior without being judgmental.
- Let the patient know that it will take time to adjust to the disability.
- Encourage questions, referring those that you are unable to answer to the appropriate resource.
- Include written documentation of emotional and psychological reaction.
- Incorporate steps for meeting emotional and psychological needs into the care plan.
- Promote a good self-concept and body image by encouraging good grooming.

- Use team conferences to discuss the patient's emotional and psychological status.
- Encourage participation in the decision-making process related to care to foster a feeling of self-control.

Discharge Planning

In a managed-care environment, major decisions related to discharge planning are made almost immediately, that is, during initial evaluation of the patient.[46] The case manager who assumes the leadership role in facilitating and coordinating discharge planning and placement relies on assessments by the interdisciplinary team to provide a comprehensive database for matching patient needs with available resources. The assessments of health care team members should include specific recommendations for comprehensive patient management and long-term needs. Patient and family input and preferences must also be considered in planning. In addition to providing comprehensive assessment and recommendations, the nurse assumes an advocacy role for the patient and family.

Rehabilitation is a complex relearning process that addresses the holistic needs of the person. The continuum of care from critical care to rehabilitation is designed to help the patient achieve the highest level of independence and quality of life possible. The ultimate goal of the rehabilitation is the highest possible level of reintegration into the community and roles. The recovery of a patient with a SCI can be viewed in the context of Maslow's hierarchy of needs (Fig. 19-18).

If the patient is not already at a SCI center, transfer to a rehabilitation facility offers an opportunity for implementing a comprehensive and individualized program. The pro-

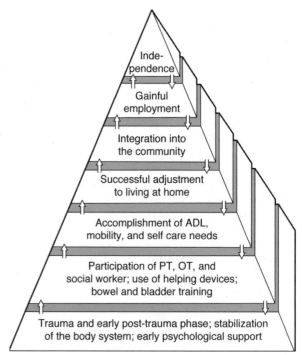

Figure 19–18 • The rehabilitation process following spinal cord injury. (PT = physical therapy; OT = occupational therapy; ADL = activities of daily living.)

gram may last from several weeks to several months. A multidisciplinary staff, including physicians, nurses, physical therapists, occupational therapists, social workers, psychologists, vocational counselors, and other specialists, collaboratively provides a comprehensive rehabilitation program. Individual, group, and family counseling helps the patient and family accept and adjust to disabilities and changes in lifestyle resulting from the injury. Advice is also offered on necessary environmental modifications that allow the patient to live at home. The social worker can help identify available resources to help meet the needs of the person with an SCI. For example, some states and private agencies provide funds to build ramps and purchase special equipment for the home.

The care within a rehabilitation facility is beyond the scope of this text. The reader is directed to other sources in the rehabilitation literature for this information.

Summary

This chapter has provided an overview of SCI with an emphasis on stabilization and acute care management. Patients who sustain an SCI require a collaborative interdisciplinary approach to achieve optimal patient outcomes. Patients with paraplegia and quadriplegia require comprehensive rehabilitation and life-long management and care to reduce the risk of complications and to optimize independence. New options for delivering health care in the home and in subacute and long-term care facilities promise independence and improved quality of life. The most promising news for SCI victims, however, is new research, which is now under way. One day, new treatment protocols, including the actual regeneration of spinal cord tissue, may eliminate the devastating functional losses associated with SCI and restore mobility to those who, under current circumstances, have lost their ability to walk.[47]

REFERENCES

1. The National SCI Statistical Center. (1999). SCI: Facts and figures at a glance. Birmingham, AL: Author (http://www.spinalcord.uab.edu/docs/factsfig.htm).
2. DeVivo, M. J. (1997). Causes and costs of spinal cord injury in the United States. *Spinal Cord, 35*, 809–813.
3. Lenke, L. G., O'Brien, M. F., & Bridwell, K. H. (1995). Fractures and dislocations of the spine. In C. R. Perry, J. A. Elstrom, & A. M. Pankovich (Eds.). *The handbook of fractures* (pp. 166–189). New York: McGraw-Hill.
4. Adams, J. C., & Hamblen, D. L. (1992). *Outline of fractures* (10th ed., pp. 81–85). Edinburgh: Churchill Livingstone.
5. Marcotte, P. J., Shaver, E. G., & Weil, R. J. (1998). Acute spinal injury. In J. Cruz. *Neurological and neurosurgical emergencies* (pp. 363–403). Philadelphia: W. B. Saunders.
6. Porth, C. M. (1994). *Pathophysiology: Concepts of altered health states* (4th ed., pp. 1052–1053). Philadelphia: J. B. Lippincott.
7. Chesnut, R. M., & Marshall, L. F. (1990). Early assessment, transport and management of patients with posttraumatic spinal instability. In P. E. Cooper (Ed.). *Management of posttraumatic spinal instability* (pp. 1–17). Park Ridge, IL: AANS.
8. Peterson, P. L., O'Neil, B. J., Alcantra, A. L., & Michael, D. B. (1998). Initial evaluation and management of neuroemergencies. In J. Cruz (Ed.) *Neurological and neurosurgical emergencies* (pp. 1–20). Philadelphia: W. B. Saunders.
9. Pararin, G., & Green, B. (1993). Emergency room assessment and stabilization of spinal injury. In J. Greenberg (Ed.), *Handbook of head and spinal trauma* (p. 413.). New York: Marcel Dekker.
10. Lemons, V. R., & Wagner, F. C., Jr. (1994). Respiratory complications after cervical SCI. *Spine, 19*(20), 2315–2320.
11. Yarkony, G. M., Formal, C. S. & Cawley, M. F. (1997). SCI rehabilitation. 1. Assessment and management during acute care. *Archives of Physical Medicine Rehabilitation, 78*, S-48–S-52.
12. Committee on Trauma. (1993). *Advanced trauma life support manual* (5th ed.) Chicago: American College of Surgeons.
13. Bondurant, F. J., Cotler, H. B., Kulkarni, M. V., et al. (1990). Acute SCI: A study using physical examination and magnetic resonance imaging. *Spine, 15*, 161–168.
14. Tator, C. H., & Fehlings, M. G. (1991). Review of the secondary injury theory of acute spinal cord trauma with emphasis on vascular mechanisms. *Journal of Neurosurgery, 75*, 15–26.
15. Bracken, D., Shepard, M., Collins, W., et al. (1990). Randomized controlled trial of methylprednisolone or naloxone in the treatment of acute SCI. *New England Journal of Medicine, 322*, 1405–1411.
16. Bracken, M. B. (1992). Pharmacological treatment of acute SCI: Current status and future prospects. *Paraplegia, 30*, 102–107.
17. Bracken, M. B., Shepard, M. J., Holford, T. R., et al. (1997). Administration of methylprednisolone for 24 or 48 hours or tirilazad mesylate for 48 hours in the treatment of acute spinal cord injury. *JAMA, 227*, 1597–1604.
18. Greenberg, M. S. (2001). *Handbook of neurosurgery* (5th ed., p. 691). Lakeland, FL: Greenberg Graphics.
19. Segatore, M., & Miller, M. (1995). The pharmacotherapy of spinal spasticity, A decade of progress. I. Theoretical aspects. *SCI Nursing, 11*(3), 66–69.
20. Segatore, M., & Miller, M. (1995). The pharmacotherapy of spinal spasticity, A decade of progress. II. Therapeutics. *SCI Nursing, 12*(1), 2–7.
21. Tracy, P. T., Wright, R. M., & Hanigan, W. C. (1989). Magnetic resonance imaging of spinal injury. *Spine, 14*, 292–301.
22. Apple, D. F. (2000). Medical management and rehabilitation of the spinal cord injured patient. In J. M. Cotler, J. M. Simpson, H. S. Au, & C. P. Sliveri (Eds.). *Surgery of spinal trauma* (pp. 157–178). Philadelphia: Lippincott Williams & Wilkins.
23. Wolf, A., Levi, L., Mirvis, S., et al. (1991). Operative management of bilateral facet dislocation. *Journal of Neurosurgery, 75*, 883–890.
24. Greenberg, M. S. (2001). *Handbook of neurosurgery* (5th ed., pp. 686–735.) Lakeland, FL: Greenberg Graphics.
25. Gertzbein, S. D., Macmicheal, D., & Title, M. (1982). Harrington instrumentation as a method of fixation in fractures of the spine. *Journal of Bone & Joint Surgery, 64B*, 526–529.
26. Cotrel, Y., Dubousset, J., & Guillaumat, M. (1988). New universal instrumentation in spinal surgery. *Clinical Orthopaedics and Related Research, 277*, 10–23.
27. Hickey, J. V. (2001). External fixation device insertion (assist). In D. J. Lynn-McHale & K. K. Carlson (Eds.). *AACN procedure manual for critical care* (4th ed., pp. 620–624). Philadelphia: W. B. Saunders.
28. Hickey, J. V. (2001). Halo traction care. In D. J. Lynn-McHale & K. K. Carlson (Eds.). *AACN procedure manual for critical care* (4th ed., pp. 625–630). Philadelphia: W. B. Saunders.
29. Hickey, J. V. (2001). Tong and pin care. In D. J. Lynn-McHale & K. K. Carlson (Eds.). *AACN procedure manual for critical care* (4th ed., pp. 631–633). Philadelphia: W. B. Saunders.
30. Hickey, J. V. (2001). Traction maintenance. In D. J. Lynn-McHale & K. K. Carlson (Eds.). *AACN procedure manual for critical care* (4th ed., pp. 634–638). Philadelphia: W. B. Saunders.
31. Barker, I., Alderson, J., Lydon, M., & Franks, C. I. (1985). Cardiovascular effects of spinal subarachnoid anesthesia: A study in patients with chronic spinal cord injuries. *Anaesthesia, 40*, 533–536.

32. Jane, M. J., Freehafer, A. A., Hazel, C. et al. (1982). Autonomic dysreflexia: A cause of morbidity and mortality in orthopedic patients with spinal cord injury. *Clinical Orthopedics, 169,* 151–154.

33. Kiker, J. D., Woodside, J. R., & Jelinek, G. E. (1982). Neurogenic pulmonary edema associated with autonomic dysreflexia. *Journal of Urology, 128,* 1038–1039.

34. Yarkomy, G. M., Katz, R. T., & Wu, Y. C. (1986). Seizures secondary to autonomic dysreflexia. *Archives of Physical Medicine Rehabilitation, 67,* 834–835.

35. Sandel, M. E., Robinson, K. M., Goldberg, G., Graziani, V., & Michaud, L. J. (1998). Neurorehabilitation. In J. Cruz (Ed.). *Neurological and neurosurgical emergencies* (pp. 503–546). Philadelphia: W. B. Saunders.

36. Spielman, G., Gennarelli, T., & Rogers, R. (1983). Disodium etidronate: Its role in preventing heterotopic ossification in traumatic brain injury. *Archives Physical Medicine Rehabilitation 64,* 539–542.

37. Garland, D. E. (1991). A clinical perspective of common forms of acquired heterotopic ossification. *Clinical Orthopedics Research, 263,* 13–29.

38. Campbell, S. K., Almeida, G. L., Penn, R. D., & Corcos, D. M. (1995). The effects of intrathecally administered baclofen on function in patients with spasticity. *Physical Therapy, 75*(5), 352–362.

39. Green, B. G., Foote, J. E., & Gray, M. (1993). Urologic management during acute care and rehabilitation of the spinal cord-injured patient. *Physical Medicine and Rehabilitation Clinics of North America, 4*(2), 249–272.

40. Cardenas, D. D. & Hooten, T. M. (1999). Urinary tract infections in persons with SCI. *Archives of Physical Medicine Rehabilitation, 76,* 272–280.

41. Giannantoni, A., Scivoletto, G., Di Stasi, S. M., Silecchia, A., Finazzi-Agri, E., Macli, I. & Castellano, V. (1998). Clean intermittent catheterization and prevention of renal disease in spinal cord patients. *Spinal Cord, 36,* 29–32.

42. Chancellor, M. B. (1993). Urodynamic evaluation after SCI. *Physical Medicine and Rehabilitation Clinics of North America, 4*(2), 272–298.

43. Kirshblum, S. C., Gulati, M., O'Connor, K. & Voorman, S. J. (1998). Bowel care practices in chronic SCI patients. *Archives of Physical Medicine Rehabilitation, 79,* 20–23.

44. Dijkers, M. (1997). Quality of life after SCIs: A metaanalysis of the effects of disablement components. *Spinal Cord, 35,* 829–840.

45. Elliott, T.R. & Frank, R. G. (1996). Depression following SCI. *Archives of Physical Medicine Rehabilitation, 77,* 816–823.

46. DeVivo, M. J. (1999). Discharge disposition form model SCI care system rehabilitation programs. *Archives of Physical Medicine Rehabilitation, 80,* 785–790.

47. Barbeau, H., Ladouceur, M., Norman, K. E., Pepin, A. & Leroux, A. (1999). Walking after SCI: evaluation, treatment and functional recovery. *Archives of Physical Medicine Rehabilitation, 80,* 225–235.

RESOURCES

Professional

BOOKS

Cotler, J. M., Simpson, J. M., Au, H. S., & Sliveri, C. P. (Eds.). *Surgery of spinal trauma.* Philadelphia: Lippincott Williams & Wilkins.

Cruz, J. (Ed.) (1998). *Neurological and neurosurgical emergencies.* Philadelphia: W. B. Saunders.

Greenberg, M. S. (2001). *Handbook of neurosurgery* (5th ed., p. 691). Lakeland FL: Greenberg Graphics.

Grossman, R. G., & Loftus, C. M. (1999). *Principles of neurosurgery* (2nd ed.). Philadelphia: Lippincott-Raven.

PERIODICALS

Bergman, S. B., Yarkony, G. M. & Stiens, S. A. (1997). SCI rehabilitation. 2. Medical complications. *Archives of Physical Medicine Rehabilitation, 78,* S-53–S-58.

Brady, W. J., Moghtader, J., Cutcher, D., Exline, C., & Young, J. (1999). ED use of flexion-extension cervical spine radiography in the evaluation of blunt trauma. *American Journal of Emergency Medicine, 17*(6), 1456–1466.

Cantu, R. C. (2000). Cervical spine injuries in the athlete. *Seminars in Neurology, 20*(2), 173–178.

Chiles, B. W. & Cooper, P. R. (1996). Acute spinal cord injury. *New England Journal of Medicine, 334*(8), 514–520.

Formal, C. S., Cawley, M., & Stiens, S. A. (1997). SCI rehabilitation. 3. Functional outcomes. *Archives of Physical Medicine Rehabilitation, 78,* S-59–S-64.

Kirshblum, S. C. & O'Connor, K. C. (1998). Predicting neurologic recovery in traumatic cervical SCI. *Archives of Physical Medicine Rehabilitation, 79,*1456–1466.

McKinley, W. O., Seel, R. T. & Hardman, J. T. (1999). Nontraumatic SCI: Incidence, epidemiology, and functional outcome. *Archives of Physical Medicine Rehabilitation, 80,* 619–623.

Marino, R. J., Ditunno, J. F., Donovan, W. H. & Maynard, F. (1999). Neurologic recovery after traumatic SCI: Data from the model SCI system. *Archives of Physical Medicine Rehabilitation, 80,* 1391–1396.

Marion, D. W. (1998). Head and spinal cord injury. *Neurologic Clinics of North America, 16*(2), 485–502.

Lu, J. & Waite, P. W. (1999). Advances in spinal cord regeneration. *Spine, 24*(9), 926–930.

Lyles, K. W. (1999). Management of patients with vertebral compression fractures. *Pharmacotherapy, 19*(1), 21S–24S.

Petri, R. & Gimbel, R. (1999). Evaluation of the patient with spinal trauma and back pain: An evidence based approach. *Emergency Medicine Clinics of North America, 17*(1), 25–39.

Stiens, S. A., Bergman, S. B. & Formal, C. S. (1997). SCI rehabilitation. 4. Individual experience, personal adaptation, and social perspectives. *Archives of Physical Medicine Rehabilitation, 78,* S-65–S-72.

WEBSITES

American Spinal Cord Injury Association: http://www.asia.com
University of Alabama: http://www.spinalcord.uab.edu

Patient and Family

Published Material

See www.asia.com for recommended readings.

WEBSITES

See above.

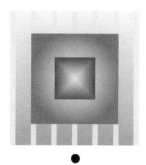

CHAPTER **20**

Back Pain and Intervertebral Disc Injury

JOANNE V. HICKEY

Back pain is a common and challenging health problem. Low back pain affects almost 90% of us at some time during our lifetimes. It is second only to upper respiratory tract disease as a cause of temporary disability in all age groups. Because it ranks so high among the reasons for seeking health care, back pain has an enormous economic impact on providing health care. The economic toll to society is further increased by the lost productivity of sufferers and the income-associated disability costs. Most patients with low back pain suffer from lumbosacral strain and will recover in 4 weeks. Others with more serious underlying causes require more aggressive treatment. Acute back problems often become chronic conditions characterized by periods of exacerbation and temporary relief. Even after surgical intervention, some patients continue to experience symptoms of varying severity or have "failed back surgery." Management of acute back pain is a controversial issue especially in a managed care environment.

CONDITIONS RELATED TO BACK PAIN

Several conditions such as normal degenerative changes of aging increase the risk of back pain and disc disease. Other conditions are "red flags" for serious underlying problems and must be addressed rapidly (Table 20-1). Degenerative changes of aging are discussed later in this chapter. Other conditions mentioned elsewhere are summarized in Table 20-2 (see also Figs. 20-1 and 20-2).

Degenerative Changes Associated With Aging

The normal aging process affects the vertebrae and supporting soft tissue (ligaments, intervertebral discs) in three ways. First, the fluid content of the nucleus pulposus gradually decreases from 88% in people in their early 30s to 66% in later years, causing the discs to become less efficient shock absorbers. As the discs become somewhat smaller, they can more easily slip from their normal anatomical position. Second, the aging process causes degeneration of the annulus fibrosus and the pos-

terior longitudinal ligaments that secure the vertebral bodies together. As these ligaments degenerate, they are less able to respond to the various alterations required in movement so that stresses, strains, and injuries are much more easily precipitated.

Third, **osteoporosis,** which is demineralization of the bone matrix related to hormonal changes, occurs in women during the postmenopausal period. It is also seen in patients with Cushing's syndrome and those receiving long-term steroidal therapy. The vertebrae are particularly vulnerable. The patient may be completely asymptomatic or may complain of back pain. Slight trauma can cause collapse, dislocation, or fracture of the fragile, demineralized vertebrae. Compression of the spinal cord or nerve roots by the collapsed vertebrae can result, and surgical decompression may be necessary.

These normal anatomical degenerative processes of aging, plus the cumulative effects of everyday activity, predispose the back to injury.

Low Back Pain

The *Quick Reference Guide for Clinicians: Acute Low Back Problems in Adults: Assessment and Treatment* (1994)[1] published by the Agency for Health Care Policy and Research, an excellent evidence-based resource, sets a national standard for patient management. The *Guide's* recommendations, based on scientific evidence, are the consensus of expert practitioners. The *Guide* defines acute low back problems as activity intolerance resulting from lower back or back-related leg symptoms of shorter than 3 months' duration. The *Guide's* recommendations form the basis for the guidelines outlined in this chapter.

About 90% of patients recover spontaneously from low back pain within 1 month. A subsequent episode of low back pain is managed as a new acute episode. The focus of guidance has shifted from managing pain to helping patients improve activity tolerance.

Diagnosis of Back Problems

Because back pain is a symptom in many conditions and disease processes, proper diagnosis is critical for treatment and a satisfactory outcome. During the initial encounter, usually at

Table 20–1 • "RED FLAGS" TO RECOGNIZE IN THE HISTORY AND PHYSICAL EXAMINATION OF PATIENTS WITH BACK PAIN

- Possible fracture
- Major trauma (e.g., motor vehicle accident, fall from height)
- Minor trauma or even strenuous lifting in older patients or those who potentially have osteoporosis
- Possible tumor or infection
- Tumor: pain in people under 20 or age 50 or over; history of cancer
- Infection: fever, chills, unexplained weight loss (note risk factors for spinal infection that includes recent bacterial infection, e.g. urinary tract infection, IV drug abuse, immunosuppression)
- Either tumor or infection: pain that worsens when lying down or the severity of which increases at nighttime
- Possible cauda equina syndrome
- Lost or diminished sensation in the saddle area (e.g., perianal, perineal)
- Recent onset of bladder dysfunction (e.g., retention, increased frequency, overflow)
- Severe or progressive neurological deficit in the lower extremity
- Poor rectal tone
- Major motor weakness (quadriceps—weakness for knee extension; ankle plantar flexors, evertors, and dorsiflexors [foot drop])

a clinic or primary care physician's office, the history and physical examination are directed at the following:

- Rule out signs or symptoms of potentially dangerous underlying conditions, that is, "red flags"; see Table 20-1.
- Collect a detail-focused history emphasizing limits to normal lifestyle, functional loss, and degree of pain.
- Perform a regional back examination (e.g., deformity, vertebral point tenderness, muscle spasm).
- Perform a neurological screening examination with particular attention to muscle strength, sensory dermatomes (pinprick and light touch), reflexes, evidence of muscle atrophy, and, if low back pain is present, observation of the patient walking (e.g., posture, walking tandem, on toes, on heels, squat).
- Perform the straight leg raising (SLR) test for low back pain (sometimes called Lasegue's sign); Figure 20-3 shows a way of testing for sciatic nerve root tension.

The *Guide* states that, in the absence of signs of serious problems, there is no need for special diagnostic studies because 90% of patients recover spontaneously within 4 weeks. These are patients who have a lumbosacral sprain. However, if a *serious underlying condition* is found or if there is *rapid progression of neurological deficits*, immediate urgent diagnostic studies and definitive care should be sought.

Initial Management

Patients with back problems are almost always treated on an outpatient basis. The cornerstones of early management are education and reassurance, patient comfort, and activity alterations.

Education and Reassurance

In the absence of "red flags," patients need to be reassured that most people recover from back problems within 4 weeks. Education is a key element to recovery and prevention of future problems. The nurse often assumes the role of educator.

Patient Comfort

Pain and discomfort are the usual reasons for seeking health care. The safest effective medication for acute low back problems is acetaminophen. Nonsteroidal anti-inflammatory drugs (NSAIDs), such as ibuprofen, are also recommended, but caution must be exercised because they may cause gastric irritation and renal and allergic side effects. Narcotics are avoided if at all possible because of possible dependency. Muscle relaxants may also be ordered. About 30% of patients experience drowsiness, which interferes with daytime activities. Application of heat or cold to the concentrated area of pain may provide some relief. No evidence supports the use of skin traction or massage as treatment modalities.

Activity Alteration

Activity is altered to avoid undue back irritation and debilitation from inactivity. Most patients do not require bed rest. Prolonged bed rest (i.e., more than 4 days) has potentially debilitating effects, and its efficacy in the treatment of acute back problems is unproved. For people with severe limitations resulting from leg pain, 2 to 4 days of bed rest may be helpful.

To avoid undue stress to the back, patients need education on body mechanics (how to lift, sit, walk, bend). Sitting, although a safe activity, may aggravate symptoms for some patients. Avoiding debilitation is accomplished by low-stress aerobic conditioning, such as walking, stationary biking, and swimming, with the time of exercise gradually increasing. Temporary activity restrictions for the workplace may be necessary, depending on the type of work an individual performs. Depending on gender and severity of symptoms, restrictions may need to be placed on the number of pounds that should be lifted without assistance. These recommendations range from 20 lb for patients with severe symptoms regardless of gender, to 60 lb and 35 lb, respectively, for men and women with mild symptoms.

After 1 Month

If after 1 month the patient has not recovered, and there is a question of an underlying problem or physiological evidence of tissue insult or nerve impairment, imaging and possibly conduction studies are ordered.

- Magnetic resonance imaging (MRI) is now the gold standard for diagnosis of neural and soft tissue problems (Fig. 20-4); a myelogram is rarely ordered.
- Computed tomography (CT) scans are the standard for imaging bone.

- Nerve conduction studies are ordered for nerve root compromise.
- Other laboratory tests (e.g., erythrocyte sedimentation rate, complete blood count, and urinalysis) are helpful to screen for nonspecific medical problems; a bone scan is helpful if a spinal cord tumor, infection, or occult fracture is suspected.

More specific information is found in the *Clinical Practice Guidelines* already cited in this section.

▥ HERNIATED INTERVERTEBRAL DISCS

Herniation of intervertebral discs is the major cause of severe acute and chronic back pain. The cervical and lumbar regions, as the most flexible areas of the spine, are most susceptible to injury and stress. The lumbar area is most frequently affected by herniated disc disease. Thoracic herniation is uncommon. Patients may complain of arm or leg pain and be diagnosed with **radiculopathy,** a disease of the spinal nerve roots.

▥ Table 20–2 • CONDITIONS RELATED TO BACK PAIN

CONDITIONS	DESCRIPTION, SIGNS AND SYMPTOMS	MANAGEMENT OR TREATMENT
Developmental Problems		
• Scoliosis; kyphosis —Predispose the patient to disc and vertebral disease	Cause anatomical alterations; may result in • Malalignment of one vertebra with the next • Disproportionate stress to selected areas of the vertebral column • A narrowed space within the spinal canal	Possible management approaches depend on the degree of dysfunction: • Physical therapy • Braces • Harrington rods • Fusion
Neoplasms		
• Metastatic lesions involving the vertebrae or spinal cord • Primary tumors of the dura or spinal cord	• Metastases are most often from prostate, lungs, breast, or gastrointestinal tract; deficits depend on the level of the lesion. —They cause pain, neurological deficits (e.g., bowel or bladder dysfunction, paresis, paresthesia). • With primary tumors, deficits depend on the spinal level involved; signs and symptoms are the same as for metastatic lesions.	Surgical decompression may be necessary; alternatively, irradiation with or without surgery (see Chap. 23) may be advised
Infections		
• Abscess secondary to infections elsewhere in the body, especially the lungs • Infections related to surgical procedures • Possible organisms include *Staphylococcus,* tubercle bacillus, *Aspergillus,* and *Streptococcus*	• Pain is the chief complaint; other deficits relate to the dermatomal level.	Management may include: • Bed rest • Immobilization • IV antibiotics for 4–6 wk • Surgical drainage • Spinal fusion, if necessary
Degenerative Diseases of the Vertebral Column		

• *Spondylosis:* degeneration of the vertebral bodies or of the intervertebral discs with abnormal fusion of two or more vertebrae and narrowing of the intervertebral space
  —An *osteophyte* (bone spur) can develop as a result of the irritation.
  —The cervical region is commonly involved.
	• Pain results from fatigue and additional stress on the vertebral column.
	• This is most common in cervical region.
	• Disc protrusion can cause collapse of the disk space, resulting in narrowing of the intervertebral foramen and compression of the nerve roots.
		Conservative management (effective in more than 50% of patients):
		• Bed rest and immobility
		• Cervical traction
		• Drug therapy (nonnarcotic analgesics; nonsteroidal anti-inflammatory agents [ibuprofen]; other types of anti-inflammatory drugs)
		Surgical approach:
		• If conservative treatment is ineffective, a laminectomy is performed to remove osteophytes and decompress any neural elements

• *Osteoarthritis:* degeneration of the articular cartilages
  —Most frequently the cervical region is involved; the next most common site is the lumbar region
  —It is related to long-term stress on the back and is seen in older people.
	• Clinical symptoms relate poorly to x-ray findings.
	• Signs and symptoms include stiffness, limitation of movement, and pain aggravated by movement.
	• Marked osteophytic overgrowth with osteophyte development occurs.
	• Nerve root spinal cord compression, or both, occur, resulting in myelopathy.
		• Treatment is the same as for spondylosis

(continued)

Table 20-2 • CONDITIONS RELATED TO BACK PAIN (Continued)

CONDITIONS	DESCRIPTION, SIGNS AND SYMPTOMS	MANAGEMENT OR TREATMENT
Inflammatory Diseases		
• *Marie-Strümpell spondylitis:* also known as ankylosing spondylitis —Predominantly affects young men —Sacroiliac joints primary sites —Involves destruction of the joints and ankylosis —Slowly progressive disease; can result in complete calcification of the anterior longitudinal ligament with resulting immobilization of the spine	• The chief symptom is pain in the center lower back. Morning stiffness is common, and decreased hip mobility may also occur. • Slow, progressive course lasts several years. • In early disease, symptoms precede roentgenographical changes; as the disease advances, the spine looks like a "bamboo spine" on x-ray studies. • Back pain, stiffness, and limitation of movement are the most common symptoms.	Management is symptomatic: • Pain control • Physical therapy • Other approaches, depending on the age of the patient and the degree of disability
• *Rheumatoid arthritis:* a generalized disease process affecting the connective tissue of the spine, hips, and hands —Cervical atlantoaxial area commonly affected —Women aged 25 to 45 years affected three times more often than men	• As the disease progresses, pain occurs in the lower back owing to disc displacement or possible cord compression.	Treatment is the same as for Marie-Strümpell spondylitis.
Trauma		
• *Sprains and strains,* including whiplash (see Chap. 19) • *Spondylolysis:* breakdown of the structure of the vertebra; usually involves a fracture of the isthmus • *Spondylolisthesis:* a defect on both sides of the vertebra through the isthmus, with the anterior section displacing forward and the posterior elements (spinous process and laminae) remaining in place • *Intervertebral disc disease:* discussed in the next section of this chapter	• Spondylolysis precedes spondylolisthesis. • The most frequently affected area is L-5, followed by L-4. • Symptoms are mild early in the course of the disease, then progress (lower back pain radiating to the thighs and legs; tenderness over L-4 and L-5; sensory and motor weakness). • Narrowing of the spinal canal and cord compression are possible as a result of disc displacement.	• Management includes conservative pain control and physical therapy • In slippage of a vertebra or disc, surgery for cord decompression or laminectomy for disc displacement may be necessary
Referred Pain from Viscera		
• A patient may have back pain secondary to referral from viscera, such as the gallbladder and kidneys.	• A thorough physical examination will reveal underlying cause.	Treatment depends on underlying cause

Men suffer from intervertebral herniation much more frequently than women. Most patients with disc disease are between 30 and 50 years old. About 90% to 95% of lumbar herniations occur at the L4-5 to S-1 levels. When the cervical region is involved, the most common levels are C6—7 and then C5–6. Multiple herniations occur in 10% of patients.

Etiology

Trauma accounts for approximately 50% of disc herniations. Examples of traumatic incidents include lifting heavy objects while in a flexed position (most common), slipping, falling on the buttocks or back, and suppressing a sneeze. In some patients, no history of trauma can be identified. The cumulative result of repeated minor injuries is a chronic condition that places the patient at high risk for herniation. The herniation syndrome also occurs in association with other degenerative processes, such as osteoarthritis or ankylosing spondylitis (Marie-Strümpell spondylitis). Patients with congenital anomalies, such as scoliosis, appear to be predisposed to disc injury because of malalignment of the vertebral column.

Pathophysiology

As previously mentioned, degenerative changes weaken the posterior longitudinal ligaments and the annulus fibrosis in middle and later life. Simultaneous degenerative changes

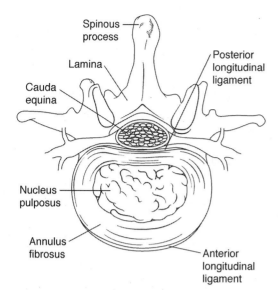

Figure 20–1 • Axial view of the lumbar spine, showing an intervertebral disc, the contents of the spinal canal, and the elements of the posterior bony arch.

occur in the intervertebral discs, beginning after a peak level of development is reached in the early 30s. Fraying and tearing of the annulus fibrosis make the disc vulnerable to posterior displacement in response to a prolapse of the nucleus pulposus. This can occur with slight provocation, such as making an awkward movement, sneezing, or lurching forward. The nucleus pulposus can also protrude through the annulus fibrosus. A fragment may be laterally or centrally thrust into the spinal canal, where it encroaches on nerve roots (see Fig. 20-2). The herniation may be spontaneously reduced or reabsorbed, but most often it persists as a source of chronic root irritation. The presence of symptoms, particularly pain, depends on the quantity of disc material that has herniated into the spinal canal, the degree of narrowing of the spinal canal from herniation and edema, the number of discs involved, and the degree of encroachment on nerve roots.

Signs and Symptoms by Location

Lumbar Area

Herniation of a lumbar disc is usually lateral and only occasionally central. More than 90% of all clinically significant lower extremity radiculopathy is due to disc herniation at the L4–5 or L5 to S1 level. The signs and symptoms of herniated lumbar discs are grouped in the following general categories: pain, postural deformity, motor changes, sensory changes, alterations of reflexes, and specific diagnostic signs.

Pain. After injury, the severity of pain, the first and most characteristic symptom of a herniated disc, varies in terms of aching and sharpness. The alleged etiology of the pain is stimulation of the pain fibers of the posterior annulus and the posterior longitudinal ligament. Low back pain persists for varying periods, with radiation across the buttock, thigh, and one entire leg. In some patients, buttock and leg pain

develops without back pain. The term **sciatica** is sometimes used to describe a syndrome of lumbar back pain that spreads down one leg to the ankle and is intensified by coughing and sneezing. The nerve roots L-4, L-5, S-1, S-2, and S-3 give rise to the sciatic nerve. The pain in the buttocks is described as deep, aching, or gnawing. The intensity of pain is influenced by leg position.

Pain from a herniated disc is aggravated and intensified by coughing, sneezing, straining, stooping, standing, sitting, blowing the nose, spasms of the paravertebral muscles, and any jarring movement while walking or riding. The character of pain ranges from mild discomfort to excruciating agony. Prolonged sitting is particularly painful. In the acute phase, the patient is most comfortable lying on the back with knees flexed and a small pillow at the head. Other patients prefer the lateral recumbent position, lying on the unaffected side with the knee flexed on the affected side.

Postural Deformity. The normal lumbar lordosis is absent in about 60% of patients with herniated discs. This sign is also accompanied by lumbar scoliosis and spasms of the paravertebral muscles. Movement of the lumbar spine is limited, and lateral flexion is restricted.

In the standing position, the patient exhibits a typically flattened lumbar spine (Fig. 20-5), slight tilting forward of the trunk, and slight flexion on the affected side of the hip and knee. These alterations of normal posture are assumed to compensate for the pathophysiological changes. The paravertebral muscles contract to prevent traction on the affected nerve roots, which would intensify the pain if the spine were extended. The patient walks cautiously, bearing as little weight as possible on the affected side. The gait may be described as stiff, and movement is deliberate to prevent jarring. Climbing stairs is particularly painful.

Motor Deficits. Hypotonia is common with motor root compression. Slight motor weakness may be experienced, although major weakness is rare. Motor weakness is difficult

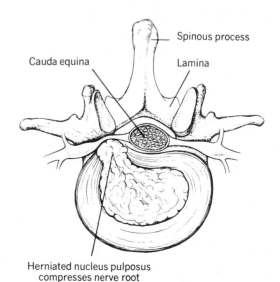

Figure 20–2 • Ruptured vertebral disc. (From Chaffee, E. E., & Lytle, I. M. [1980]. *Basic physiology and anatomy.* Philadelphia: J. B. Lippincott.)

Clinical test for sciatic tension

The straight leg raising (SLR) test (A) can detect tension on the L5 and/or S1 nerve root. SLR may reproduce leg pain by stretching nerve roots irritated by a disc herniation.

A. Instructions for the Straight Leg Raising (SLR) Test

(1) Ask the patient to lie as straight as possible on a table in the supine position.

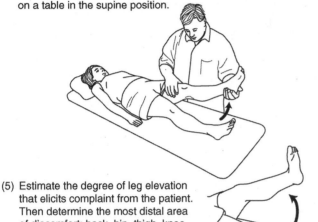

(5) Estimate the degree of leg elevation that elicits complaint from the patient. Then determine the most distal area of discomfort: back, hip, thigh, knee, or below the knee.

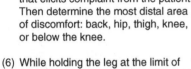

(6) While holding the leg at the limit of straight leg raising, dorsiflex the ankle. Note whether this aggravates the pain. Internal rotation of the limb can also increase the tension on the sciatic nerve roots.

Pain below the knee at less than 70 degrees of straight leg raising, aggravated by dorsiflexion of the ankle and relieved by ankle plantar flexion or external limb rotation, is most suggestive of tension on the L5 or S1 nerve root related to disc herniation. Reproducing back pain alone with SLR testing does not indicate significant nerve root tension.

(2) With one hand placed above the knee of the leg being examined, exert enough firm pressure to keep the knee fully extended. Ask the patient to relax.

(3) With the other hand cupped under the heel, slowly raise the straight limb. Tell the patient, "If this bothers you, let me know, and I will stop."

(4) Monitor for any movement of the pelvis before complaints are elicited. True sciatic tension should elicit complaints before the hamstrings are stretched enough to move the pelvis.

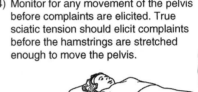

Crossover pain occurs when straight raising of the patient's well limb elicits pain in the leg with sciatica. Crossover pain is a stronger indication of nerve root compression than pain elicited from raising the straight painful limb.

Sitting knee extension (B) can also test sciatic tension. The patient with significant nerve root irritation tends to complain or lean backward to reduce tension on the nerve.

B. Instructions for sitting knee extension test

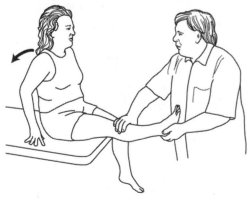

With the patient sitting on a table, both hip and knees flexed at 90 degrees, slowly extend the knee as if evaluating the patella or bottom of the foot. This maneuver stretches nerve roots as much as a moderate degree of supine SLR.

Figure 20–3 • Straight leg raising (SLR) test. (*A*) Instructions for SLR when the patient is lying down. (*B*) Instructions for SLR when the patient is sitting. (Bigos, S., Bowyer, O., Braen, G., et al. [1994]. *Acute low back problems in adults.* Clinical Practice Guideline, Quick Reference Guide Number. 14. Rockville, MD: U.S. Department of Health and Human Services, Public Health Service, Agency for Health Care Policy and Research, AHCPR Pub. No. 95-0643.)

Figure 20–4 • MRI views of herniated discs. *A* (cervical). Midsaggital T1-weighted MRI shows herniated disc (*arrow*) at C5–6 producing compression of the spinal cord. *B* (thoracic). Midsagittal T2-weighted MRI shows hypointense herniated disc (*arrow*) in mid-thoracic region resulting in compression of the spinal cord. *C* (lumbar). Midsagittal post-contrast T1-weighted MRI of the same patient shows that herniated disc (*arrow*) is not attached to any parent disc. There is peripheral disc enhancement. (Castillo, M. [1999]. *Neuroradiology companion* [2nd ed.]. Philadelphia: Lippincott-Raven.)

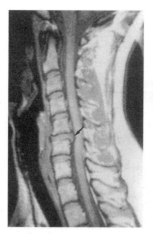 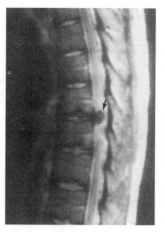 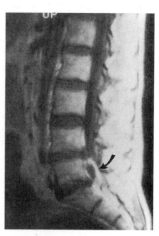

A (cervical) **B (thoracic)** **C (lumbar)**

to evaluate because of the defensive reaction precipitated by pain. Weakness may be evident on plantar flexion or dorsiflexion of the foot and occasionally of the hamstring and quadriceps muscles. Atrophy of the affected muscles may develop, although it is not a common finding and can be minimal. Foot drop has been evident in some patients. Motor weakness is sometimes accompanied by difficulty with micturition and sexual activity.

Sensory Deficits

The most common sensory impairments from root compression are paresthesias and numbness, particularly of the leg and foot. Note the specific areas of decreased sensation in the foot and leg using the pinprick method of sensory testing. Tenderness is noted over the L-5 and S-1 vertebral spines and along the tracking of the sciatic nerve (Fig. 20-6).

Alterations of Reflexes. Depending on the level of the disc herniation, knee or ankle reflexes are absent or diminished.

Other Diagnostic Signs. Other diagnostic methods commonly associated with evaluating patients with possible lumbar

herniated disc disease include straight leg raising test, Neri's sign, Naffziger's test, and Kernig's sign (Figs. 20-7 and 20-8).

The **straight leg raising test** (also called **Lasègue's sign**) is helpful in determining limitations of lower limb range of motion and pain location (see Fig. 20-3). Normally, it is possible when lying on the back to move the straightened leg about 90 degrees with only some slight discomfort in the hamstring muscles. The sciatic nerve becomes stretched with movement and creates traction on the proximal nerve roots. Traction and stretching of the nerve roots begin when the leg is at a 30- to 40-degree angle. In the patient with a herniated low back disc,

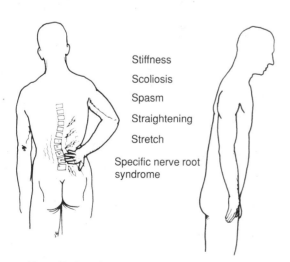

Stiffness
Scoliosis
Spasm
Straightening
Stretch
Specific nerve root syndrome

Figure 20–5 • The signs of lumbar disc herniation.

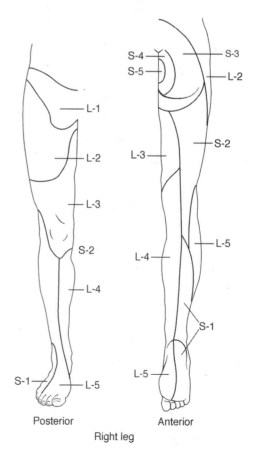

Figure 20–6 • Dermatomes of the leg.

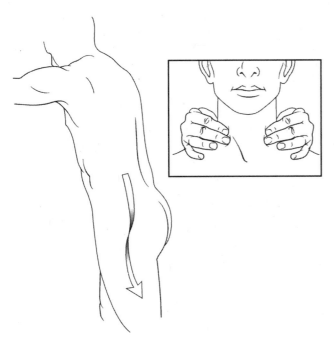

Figure 20–7 • Naffziger's test is conducted by compressing the jugular veins simultaneously while the patient is standing erect. Radiating components of the pain are usually accentuated by this maneuver. The examiner must avoid bilateral compression of the carotid arteries when performing Naffziger's test.

the stretching of the sciatic nerve during passive, straight leg raising creates traction on the irritated nerve roots, thereby producing severe pain. Patients with severe sciatica will not be able to raise their legs beyond 20 to 30 degrees. Less severe involvement allows straight leg raising to 50 or 60 degrees. Repeating the Lasègue's maneuver on the unaffected leg produces pain of decreased severity on the contralateral side.

Neri's sign is elicited when the patient bends forward, resulting in knee flexion on the affected side. This is a protective mechanism to prevent stretching the sciatic nerve.

Naffziger's test requires simultaneous compression of both jugular veins while the patient is standing (see Fig. 20-7). This maneuver will produce pain in the patient with a herniated disc. Physiologically, compression of the jugular veins obliterates venous drainage from the brain, thereby increasing intraventricular pressure of the cerebrospinal fluid (CSF). The result is an increase in intraspinal pressure, which will produce pain if a herniated disc is present.

Kernig's sign is elicited by attempting to flex the patient's hip and knee while he is in the dorsal recumbent position (see Fig. 20-8). With the hip flexed at a 90-degree angle, the knee is slowly extended. Normally, the knee can be extended about 90 degrees. In a patient with a low-back herniated disc, knee extension will precipitate severe pain because of stretching of the irritated nerve roots. Therefore, it will not be possible to extend the knee to the normal range in the patient with a herniated disc. Any manipulation of the leg is painful.

Specific Lumbar Levels

The most common sites for lumbar disc herniation are the L4–5 and the L-5 to S-1 levels, in that order. Lesions at the L3–4 level are rare. Each level presents a characteristic syndrome of symptoms that is distinct from that of other levels.

L4–5 Level. Pain is perceived in the hip, groin, posterolateral thigh, lateral calf, dorsal surface of the foot, and the first or second and third toes. Paresthesias may be experienced over the lateral leg and web of the great toe. There is tenderness at the femoral head and lateral gluteal region. There is some weakness with dorsiflexion of the great toe and foot. Foot drop can occur. The patient has difficulty walking on the heels. Atrophy, if present, is minor. Reflexes are usually not diminished.

L-5 to S-1 Level. Pain is perceived in the midgluteal, posterior thigh, and calf regions down to the heel and the outer surface of the foot on the side of the fourth and fifth toes. Paresthesias are found in the posterior calf and in the lateral heel, foot, and toe. Tenderness is especially apparent in the area about the sacroiliac joint. Weakness in plantar flexion of the foot and the great toe is noted. The patient has difficulty walking on the toes. The hamstring muscles may also show signs of weakness. If atrophy is present, the gastrocnemius and the soleus muscles are affected. The ankle jerk reflex is diminished or absent.

L3–4 Level. Pain is located in the lower back, hip, posterolateral thigh, and anterior leg. Paresthesias are experienced in the middle section of the anterior thigh. Weakness is noted in the quadriceps muscles, which may also demonstrate atrophic changes. The knee-jerk reflex is diminished.

Remission of Pain. Pain associated with herniated disc disease is recurrent. Patients typically present with a history of one or several episodes of low back pain radiating across the buttocks and into one leg to the ankle. Between acute episodes, pain may be completely absent or at least substantially diminished so that the patient is able to cope with the discomfort. Remissions of acute episodes are probably attributable to recovery of the protruding disc, decreased local

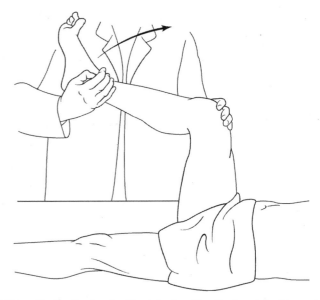

Figure 20–8 • Testing for Kernig's sign. Flex the leg at the hip and the knee, then straighten the knee. Note resistance or pain. Repeat with the other leg.

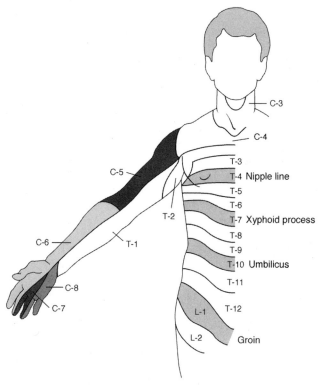

Figure 20–9 • Dermatomes of the cervical, thoracic, and upper lumbar regions.

edema, relief of root compression, and reabsorption of disc exudate.

Cervical Area

The cervical region of the spine is also prone to trauma, degeneration, and spondylitic changes, which predispose the affected person to a wider range of pathological conditions. A serious potential consequence of nerve root or spinal cord compression is interference with vital respiratory functions.

One of the most common causes of neck, shoulder, and arm pain in middle-aged and older people is disc herniation of the lower cervical region. Symptoms can develop without any apparent injury, or they may follow trauma, such as whiplash or hyperextension injuries. On radiological investigation, salient disc degeneration, arthritis, and spondylitis are frequently identified. The most common sites of cervical herniation are at the C5-6 and C6-7 levels, with pain along the affected sensory dermatomes (Fig. 20-9). Herniation may be lateral or central.

Anatomically, there is little free room within the spinal canal to accommodate any extraneous material. The cervical spinal cord is firmly positioned by the ligamenta denticulata. Disc protrusion in the cervical area can result not only in root compression but also in cord compression because of the lack of free space. The particular presenting symptoms depend on the anatomical point of disc protrusion. The possible locations of disc protrusion include lateral, paracentral, or central herniation.

Lateral Herniation. Symptoms of lateral cervical disc herniation include root pain in the shoulders, neck, and arms (Fig.

20-10) and paresthesias along the dermatome of the compressed nerve root. Paravertebral muscle spasms, which cause a stiff neck, accompany the pain. Reflex loss and possible motor weakness follow. Neck movement is often restricted to some degree in all directions. Tenderness may be experienced when pressure is exerted over the involved cervical spine. Weakness of the hand muscles and forearm may be noted. Atrophy may also be detected on physical examination. Arm reflexes are absent or diminished.

Paracentral or Central Herniations. Herniation of the paracentral or central regions have somewhat different symptoms than lateral herniations. Pain, if present, is usually mild, insidious, and intermittent (Fig. 20-11). Onset of spinal cord compression can be acute or gradual. Weakness of the lower extremities and an unsteady gait become apparent. As the compression increases, spasticity is noted. There may be difficulty with voiding and sexual function. Reflexes of the lower extremities become hyperactive, whereas those in the upper extremities vary.

Specific Cervical Levels

The most common cervical herniations are at C5–6 and C6–7. Each level presents a characteristic syndrome of symptoms that is distinct from that of other levels.

C5–6 Level (Lateral Herniation). Pain is experienced in the neck, shoulder, anterior portion of the upper part of the arm, radial forearm, and possibly the thumb and forefinger. Less frequently, pain extends to the scapular and clavicular regions. Paresthesias and sensory loss are found in the thumb, forefinger, radial and lateral forearm, and lateral aspects of the upper arm. Weakness is noted with flexion of the forearm (biceps). Tenderness is found in the supraspinal area of the scapula and the biceps region. The biceps and supinator reflexes are diminished or absent. The triceps reflex is either exaggerated or left intact.

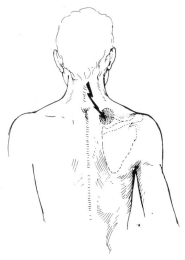

Figure 20–10 • Pattern of pain radiation accompanying lateral protrusion of a cervical disc. (From Hoppenfeld, S. [1977]. *Orthopaedic neurology.* Philadelphia: J. B. Lippincott.)

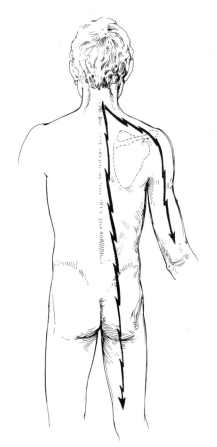

Figure 20–11 • Pattern of pain radiation with a midline herniated cervical disc. (From Hoppenfeld, S. [1977]. *Orthopaedic neurology*. Philadelphia: J. B. Lippincott.)

C6–7 Level (Lateral Herniation). Pain is experienced in the neck, shoulder blade, and lateral surfaces of the upper arm and forearm. The index finger, the little finger, and sometimes the ring finger are plagued by pain, although all fingers may be involved. Paresthesias and sensory loss are most prominent in the second and third fingers and lateral forearm. Weakness is found in the triceps and extensor carpi radialis (extensors for forearm and hand grips). Occasionally, wrist drop may result. Tenderness is most apparent in the area over the medial shoulder blade. The biceps and supinator reflexes are preserved, whereas the triceps reflex is diminished or absent.

Diagnosis

Intervertebral disc herniation must be differentiated from other diseases causing back pain, such as primary metastatic neoplasms. Diagnosis based on clinical examination alone is difficult, if not impossible. Additional information needed includes location, quality and severity of pain, history of trauma, and an abnormal MRI or CT scan. MRI is preferred because it provides better visualization of the soft tissue. X-ray films, although not specific, can indicate a narrowing of the intervertebral disc space, osteophytes (spurs), or hypertrophic osteoarthritis. In special cases, an electromyogram may be performed to differentiate between neural and

muscle injury. Myelograms, previously the mainstay of diagnosis, have been replaced by the MRI scan.

Treatment

There are two possible paths for treatments of herniated disc disease: *conservative treatment* or *surgery*. The belief that disc disease is caused by repeated trauma with degenerative changes is generally accepted. Most physicians, therefore, propose a course of treatment that will protect the involved area from added trauma and provide an environment that will allow for healing of the injured degenerative discs by fibrosis. This two-pronged approach, together with pain control, constitutes conservative treatment.

Conservative Treatment

Conservative treatment may be tried for 4 weeks. The three cornerstones of management are education and reassurance, patient comfort, and readjusting activity level to prevent further injury. The need for bed rest and restriction of activity depends on the severity of symptoms. A patient with mild or moderate symptoms is generally advised to do the following:

- Decrease general activity for a short time.
- Avoid any flexion of the spine, such as lifting, bending, or twisting.
- Use a firm mattress.
- Take non-narcotic analgesics, anti-inflammatory drugs, and possibly muscle relaxants.
- Self-application of heat or cold therapy for temporary symptoms may provide temporary comfort.

The patient with *severe* symptoms is treated with bed rest for a short time. Resumption of light activity is advised to avoid undue back irritation and debilitation. Use of traction or of physical modalities such as massage, diathermy, ultrasound, cutaneous laser treatment, biofeedback, and transcutaneous electrical nerve stimulation (TENS) have no proven efficacy in the treatment of low back pain.

Nursing Management During Conservative Treatment

With the advent of diagnosis-related groupings and managed care, conservative management of the patient with disc disease often takes place in the home with the assistance of the family and possibly the home care nurse. Hospitalization is reserved for the patient with extreme symptoms who will likely be taken to surgery in the near future. The focus of care for this population, as with all patients, is education and reassurance, patient comfort, and activity alterations. Goals of care are maintaining altered activity restrictions, administering medications, and preventing complications. Chart 20-1 provides a summary of nursing management during conservative treatment.

Bed Rest. Bed rest for patients with severe pain in the lumbar region is limited to a short course (less than 4 days), followed by resumption of light activity. When on bed rest,

CHART 20-1 • Summary of Nursing Management During Conservative Treatment of the Patient With a Herniated Intervertebral Disc*

Nursing Diagnosis	Nursing Interventions

Acute or Chronic Pain related to (R/T) inflammation or rupture of an intervertebral disc	• Maintain a regimen of bed rest (patient usually retains bathroom privileges).
	• Instruct family to apply heat or hydroculator packs as ordered.
	   —Protect skin from burns.
	   —Often sensation is decreased to involved area, and burns can easily occur.
	• Use pain-relieving strategies, such as imagery, relaxation technique. Administer analgesics and muscle relaxants as necessary; assess the patient's severity of pain to decide which pain medication to give if more than one is prescribed.
	• Monitor the patient's response to pain-reducing treatments; use the visual analogue scale (scale of 1–10) for the patient to rate pain before and after interventions.

Risk for Trauma: extension of back injury R/T environmental factors and improper body mechanics	• Provide firm mattress. • Use a log-rolling technique when turning the patient. • Teach proper body mechanics; caution the patient against twisting, stretching, pulling, or bending. • Maintain the patient in proper body alignment to decrease stress and strain. • For those with a herniated *cervical* disc, provide a small pillow in the nape of the neck. • For those with a herniated *lumbar* disc, provide a small pillow under the knees to relieve pressure; a small pillow can also be placed under the head (avoid pressure on the popliteal areas).
Risk for Constipation related to decreased activity, bed rest, and drugs that decrease peristalsis	• Provide high-bulk diet. • Increase fluid intake. • Monitor the frequency of bowel movements and their consistency. • Institute a bowel program according to the physician's preference (e.g., stool softeners, laxatives.)
Impaired Physical Mobility R/T pain, numbness/tingling, fatigue, and muscle weakness	• Monitor degree of intact motor function. • Teach the patient to perform range-of-motion exercises at least four times daily. • Provide for progressive mobilization. • Assist patient with ambulation as necessary. • Monitor the patient for use of proper body mechanics. • Provide assistive devices (e.g., brace, walker) as necessary.
Sensory/Perceptual Alterations: tactile, R/T diminished interpretation of tactile sensation secondary to inflammation or injury of the spinal nerves.	• Monitor degree of intact tactile perception in the affected areas. In patients with *cervical* disk, monitor sensation to arms, upper back, shoulders, and neck; in those with *lumbar* disk, monitor sensation to the lower back, buttocks, and legs. • Protect involved area from injury. • Teach the patient to compensate for diminished function, such as by visually checking the position of an extremity.
Knowledge Deficit R/T body mechanics, modification of lifestyle, treatment plan, or use of braces, traction, or drugs	• Develop a teaching program tailored to the patient's needs; include proper body mechanics, a discussion of lifestyle adjustments, use of equipment, the prescribed treatment plan, use of drugs, and exercises, such as semisitups, pelvic tilt, knee-chest bends, and gluteal setting (Fig. 20–12) when patient is ready.
Risk for Disuse Syndrome R/T bed rest and immobility	• Provide for basic maintenance interventions. • Monitor vital signs and neurological signs periodically. • Apply elastic stockings to prevent deep vein thrombosis. • Encourage deep breathing exercises at least four times a day. • Monitor urinary output for urinary retention or urinary stasis. • Monitor for musculoskeletal changes, such as atrophy, contracture, foot drop.

(continued)

CHART 20 – 1 • Summary of Nursing Management During Conservative Treatment of the Patient With a Herniated Intervertebral Disc* (Continued)

Nursing Diagnosis	Nursing Interventions
Anxiety R/T pain, immobility, hospitalization, uncertainty of outcome, and interference with previous lifestyle	• Explore areas of concern with the patient. • Help patient develop strategies to reduce stress and anxiety. • Teach relaxation techniques and imagery techniques to control anxiety. • Help the patient set realistic goals. • Contact appropriate resources, such as a social worker, to assist in special problem solving.

* Differences in the management of a patient with a cervical or lumbar disc are noted when there is a variation.

proper positioning on the back with knees flexed is recommended. A pillow may be placed under the knees to prevent excess tension on the nerve roots. In addition, pressure must not be allowed to build up on the popliteal nerve. A small pillow may be placed under the head for comfort. For a patient with cervical pain, a small pillow may be placed in the nape of the neck. Because the purpose of bed rest is to reduce strain and pulling on the nerves, any items the patient may need should be within easy reach to avoid any undue stretching or moving. The nurse should discuss the overall purpose and goals of the bed rest regimen, as well as the duration, with the patient. Most physicians want the patient to resume walking as soon as possible; proper body mechanics should be reviewed and stressed during ambulation.

Activity Restrictions. Following a period of bed rest, the length of which is determined by the patient's progress, mobilization is indicated. The patient may begin by walking short distances within the home, being careful to use good body mechanics. Bending, stooping, pushing, and pulling should be avoided. If symptoms and pain subside, activity restriction can be decreased.

Drug Therapy. Analgesics, anti-inflammatory drugs, muscle relaxants, and sedative-tranquilizers are the major categories of drugs ordered to control the symptoms associated with back pain and intervertebral disc disease. All these drugs have side effects for which the patient should be monitored.

Analgesics. Analgesics are often necessary to manage mild to severe pain. Analgesics are classified as non-narcotics or narcotics. For mild to moderate pain, non-narcotic drugs are usually ordered. The following drugs are commonly used:

• NSAIDs
• Propoxyphene hydrochloride (Darvon)
• Narcotic analgesics are reserved for severe pain (e.g., acetaminophen with codeine 30 mg is a common choice)

Pain is best controlled with a multifaceted treatment approach. Pain-relieving protocols include positioning, anxiety reduction, relaxation therapy, imagery, heat or cold local application, and analgesics. Analgesics are most effective when given before the pain becomes severe. Pain should be treated appropriately according to the guidelines for acute pain management. When chronic pain cannot be controlled adequately and interferes with a person's quality of life, referral to a multidisciplinary pain clinic may be helpful.

Anti-inflammatory Drugs. Inflammation is triggered as part of a normal response to tissue injury. In the last decade or so, complex chemical substances, known as prostaglandins, have been identified as important mediators in the inflammatory process. Prostaglandins are synthesized and released in the presence of cellular injury. Drugs that treat inflammation are subclassified as steroidal or nonsteroidal.

Steroidal agents are chemically related to cortisone (a hormone excreted by the adrenal cortex). Nonsteroidal agents are synthetic compounds that are *not* chemically re-

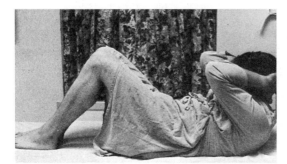
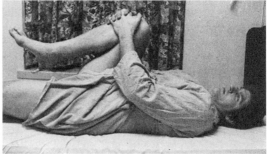

Figure 20–12 • An exercise program for patients with a herniated disc may include semi-sit-ups (*left*) and knee–chest exercises (*right*).

lated to substances produced by the body. NSAIDs are now the most important class of drugs used to treat inflammatory processes. These drugs have varying degrees of analgesic and antipyretic effects. They act by inhibiting the synthesis of prostaglandins.

NSAIDs are classified into salicylates and nonsalicylates. Aspirin is the most common and most prescribed of the salicylate group. In the nonsalicylate group, the following drugs are commonly used:

- Ibuprofen (Motrin, Advil)
- Naproxen (Anaprox, Naprosyn)

Muscle Relaxants. Several muscle relaxants are used. A few of the more frequently ordered drugs include:

- Cyclobenzaprine (Flexeril)
- Methocarbamol (Robaxin)
- Carisoprodol (Soma)
- Chlorzoxazone (Paraflex)
- Metaxalone (Skelaxin)

Most drugs are given orally, although in the hospitalized patient, rapid intravenous (IV) administration of certain muscle relaxants, such as diazepam (Valium) and methocarbamol, is possible. For example, IV methocarbamol 500 mg in 5% dextrose in water may be given because its dilution in solution decreases the highly irritative quality of the drug. The nurse who administers any drugs should be familiar with the many side effects and precautions for each.

Sedative-Tranquilizers. Sedative-tranquilizers are administered to decrease anxiety, which in turn decreases muscle tension and pain. One of the drugs frequently used is diazepam.

Summary of Nursing Management

The expected outcomes for the patient who is being managed conservatively for intervertebral disc disease include the following:

- Control of pain
- Improved mobility
- Tolerance of a progressive exercise program to strengthen muscles and improve posture
- Patient teaching and education to reduce the risk factors for additional disc trauma (e.g., going to a "back school" program)
- Resumption of previous lifestyle, within reason or with some modifications

Most patients treated conservatively will have a good recovery (see Chart 20-1). Unfortunately, some continue to have unresolved pain and may be considered as candidates for surgery.

Surgical Intervention

Within the first 3 months of acute low back symptoms, surgery is considered only when serious spinal pathology or nerve root dysfunction due to herniated disc is determined. These are patients who do not respond to conservative

treatment or who, by the nature of the herniation or symptoms, require immediate surgical intervention to preserve neurological function. This latter group includes patients with:

- Massive central herniations that compress the cauda equina and results in sensory loss, paresis, and loss of sphincter control
- Compression, resulting in quadriceps weakness or foot drop
- Severe and unrelenting pain
- Slow-to-resolve or recurrent sciatica that interferes with normal lifestyle and employment

The surgical procedure selected depends on the location of the herniation (cervical, thoracic, or lumbar), the stability of the spine, and the findings on diagnostic workup. If surgery is being considered, the surgical options and the reasonably expected outcome of each option must be discussed with the patient.

Possible surgical procedures for a ruptured intervertebral disc include:

- **Discectomy**: Removal of the nuclear disc material of an intervertebral disc; it is done with or without a laminectomy. In the lumbar region, a **posterior approach** is always used; the entire disc and cartilaginous plate are usually removed (to prevent recurrent disc protrusion). In the cervical region, there are options. If a **posterior discectomy** is performed, only the extruded disc fragments are removed (the annulus is not entered). If an **anterior discectomy** is done, the total disc is usually removed.
- **Hemilaminectomy**: Part of the lamina and part of the posterior arch of the vertebra are excised.
- **Laminectomy**: The lamina, a part of the posterior arch of the vertebra, is removed. Both the posterior approach (traditional method) and the anterior approach are used for hemilaminectomy and laminectomy.
- **Spinal fusion**: Specific vertebrae are immobilized by insertion of a wedge-shaped piece of bone or bone chips between the vertebrae. The bone graft is usually obtained from the iliac crest (donor site) or the bone bank. The purpose of the fusion is to immobilize and thus stabilize the vertebral column that is weakened because of degenerative disease or multilevel laminectomy. With a spinal fusion the patient must become accustomed to a permanent area of stiffness.
  - **Lumbar fusion**: When the *lumbar* spine is fused, the patient is often unaware of stiffness after a short time because motion increases above the fusion.
  - **Cervical fusion**: When the *cervical* spine is fused, increased limitation of movement is noted. **Anterior cervical fusion** through an incision in the anterior neck is performed when the cervical spine is unstable. An **anterior cervical discectomy with fusion** is performed when the total disc is removed *and* a fusion is done.
- **Foraminotomy**: The intervertebral foramen is surgically enlarged to increase the space for exit of a spinal nerve. By enlarging the foramen, pressure on the spinal nerve that may be entrapped will be reduced, resulting in decreased pain, compression, and edema. This procedure is performed

most often in the cervical region, because anatomically the cervical foramina are smaller than the lumbar foramina.

Microsurgical Approaches to Disc Surgery. Microsurgical techniques offer improved magnification and illumination for surgery, easier identification of anatomical structures, and improved precision in removal of small fragments or exudate. Microdiscectomy can be performed through a small incision and reduces the risk of:

- Dural laceration (resulting in CSF leak)
- Traction on nerve roots (which can cause muscle spasm and possible nerve root injury)
- Stripping of muscle from the spinal fasciae
- Trauma to blood vessels (hematoma) by improving homeostasis
- Infection

With the smaller incision and increased precision of microdiscectomy, tissue trauma and pain are lessened. The patient is able to ambulate sooner, and the length of hospitalization is shorter than with conventional disc surgery.

Percutaneous Discectomy

Percutaneous discectomy is a technique sometimes used for removing "contained" lumbar disc herniations in which the outer border of the annulus fibrosis is intact. The procedure is done through a posterolateral approach with the aid of a high-power system comprising a suction shaver and cutter. It is monitored using an endoscope and performed with the patient under local anesthesia and with an anesthesiologist available. Percutaneous discectomy is indicated only in cases of disc-related root compression accompanied by minor neurological deficits. Results are positive and indicate that percutaneous discectomy is a viable alternative to microdiscectomy for patients who fit the stringent criteria of a contained and small lumbar disc herniation.

Nursing Management of the Patient Undergoing Laminectomy

Laminectomy and hemilaminectomy are similar procedures except for the amount of bone removed. Because these are the most frequently performed surgical procedures, our nursing management discussion is limited to them (Chart 20-2).

General Considerations

By the time a patient with a herniated disc is admitted for surgery, severe and debilitating pain has usually been present for some time. The decision to undergo surgery is often made because conservative treatment has failed, pain control is inadequate, and the quality of life is unacceptable. Other patients may have already undergone a surgical procedure but have experienced continued or renewed pain. For others, rapid onset of neurological deterioration has precipitated the need for urgent surgical decompression.

The length of hospitalization for a laminectomy or hemilaminectomy is very short. Clinical pathways move a patient through surgery and recovery in 23 hours or in a timeframe that includes one overnight stay. For a more complicated procedure or for surgery related to other primary problems such as spinal cord injury, hospitalization is longer.

Preoperative Teaching

Preoperative teaching may be provided in the physician's office before admission to the hospital or within the hospital setting if the surgery is related to other primary problems. Generally, patients must understand that they are likely to experience some pain because of nerve root irritation and edema, which will gradually subside. The possibility of muscle spasms should also be discussed. Tactful handling by the nurse creates a feeling of trust. Many patients experience uncomfortable muscle spasms in the low back, thighs, and abdomen (following lumbar laminectomy) during the early postoperative period. The nurse might say, "You may experience muscle spasms after surgery. It is a temporary occurrence that passes in a few days. It does not indicate that your surgery was not successful. You will be receiving your pain medication after surgery to keep you comfortable." Included in patient teaching is the need to turn the patient as a unit (log roll) and remove any undue stress on the back with the use of good body mechanics.

The preoperative patient teaching plan should include a discussion of the following:

- Basic preoperative routines, such as nothing by mouth (NPO) status before surgery and where the patient will go after the surgery (often provided by the primary care nurse)
- Basic postoperative routines (e.g., vital sign monitoring, frequent checking of dressing, deep breathing exercises)
- Logrolling technique for turning the patient in bed
- Rationale for maintaining proper body alignment at all times and ways in which alignment can be maintained
- The risks of twisting, pulling, stretching, or straining after surgery
- The correct technique for getting out of bed after surgery

Preoperative Nursing Management

In addition to the routine preoperative preparation of the patient, thigh-high elastic stockings (TEDs) will be applied. This is done to facilitate blood return to the heart and to decrease venous stasis, which would place the patient at high risk for deep vein thrombosis. Vasomotor changes in the lower extremities secondary to autonomic stimulation can also contribute to stasis of blood.

Postoperative Nursing Management

General Care. The patient should be returned to a bed with a firm, supportive mattress. A bedboard may be added if necessary. Basic postoperative nursing management, such as frequent monitoring of vital signs, care of dressings, administration of IV fluids, and monitoring of intake and output,

CHART 20-2 • Summary of the Nursing Management of Patients Following a Posterior Laminectomy*

Nursing Diagnosis	Nursing Interventions

Pain related to (R/T) tissue trauma, muscle spasms, and nerve root compression associated with surgical trauma and inflammation
• *Lumbar laminectomy:* pain and spasms in lower back, abdomen, or thighs
• *Cervical laminectomy:* pain and spasms in upper back, shoulder, neck, or arms; may have sore throat after surgery as a result of intubation (medicated throat lozenges may be ordered for comfort)
• *Anterior cervical discectomy:* pain and spasms in upper back, shoulder, neck, or arms; may have sore throat and difficulty swallowing postoperatively as a result of manipulation of the esophagus during the procedure.
	• Maintain the patient's bed-rest regimen using a firm mattress initially.
	• Position bed to reduce stress to the operative site.
	  —*Cervical laminectomy:* The head of bed is usually elevated to a comfortable position.
	  —*Lumbar laminectomy:* Keep the bed flat or slightly elevated (5 to 10 degrees, as ordered).
	  —*Anterior cervical discectomy:* Head of bed is usually elevated to a comfortable position.
	• Provide pillow for comfort
	  —*Cervical laminectomy:* A small pillow may be positioned under the head; a soft cervical collar is worn for comfort (Fig. 20-13).
	  —*Lumbar laminectomy:* A small pillow may be placed under the head and one may be placed under the knees periodically (Fig. 20-14) to reduce strain.
	  —*Anterior cervical discectomy:* A small pillow may be positioned under the head; a hard collar (i.e., Philadelphia) is worn to prevent flexion, extension, or rotation of the neck.
	• Use a log rolling technique for turning the patient during the first 12 h postoperatively.
	• Maintain the patient in proper body alignment at all times so that spine remains in neutral position.
	• Reposition patient every 2 h.
	• Reinforce patient preoperative teaching to refrain from twisting, flexing, hyperextending, or pulling on the side rails.
	• Use pain-relieving strategies, such as imagery, relaxation techniques.
	• Administer analgesics as necessary; assess severity of the patient's pain to decide which pain medication to give if more than one is prescribed.
	• Monitor the patient's response to pain-reducing treatments; use the visual analogue scale (scale of 1–10) to allow the patient to rate pain before and after interventions.

Urinary Retention R/T difficulty voiding in a horizontal position, the depressant effects of perioperative drugs, or sympathetic fiber stimulation during lumbar laminectomy	• Provide for privacy and comfort. Assist patient to the bathroom, if possible. • Provide male patients with an opportunity to stand for urination if the physician permits. • Palpate the bladder for distention. • Monitor the intake and output (I&O) record for adequate intake. • Intermittent catheterization may be ordered if the patient is unable to void during the early postoperative period.
Constipation R/T decreased activity, bed rest, and drugs that decrease peristalsis	• Provide a diet high in bulk. • Increase fluid intake. • Monitor the frequency of bowel movements and their consistency. • Auscultate the abdomen in all four quadrants for bowel sounds. • Institute a bowel program according to physician's preference (e.g., stool softeners, laxatives, etc.).

Sensory/Perceptual Alterations: tactile R/T nerve root compression associated with surgical trauma and inflammation	• Monitor patient's perception of light touch and pain.
	  —*Cervical laminectomy/discectomy:* monitor sensation to the arms, upper back, shoulders, and neck
	  —*Lumbar laminectomy:* monitor sensation to the lower back, buttocks, and legs
	• Protect the involved area from injury.
	• Teach the patient to compensate for diminished function, such as by visually checking the position of the extremity.

(continued)

CHART 20–2 • Summary of the Nursing Management of Patients Following a Posterior Laminectomy* (Continued)

Nursing Diagnosis	Nursing Interventions
Impaired Physical Mobility R/T pain, numbness, tingling, and muscle weakness	• Monitor the patient's ability to move legs and arms freely in bed; compare with pre-operative baseline data. • Perform range-of-motion exercises at least four times daily; the patient may be taught to do this independently. • Provide assistive devices (e.g., brace, walker, etc.) as necessary. • Provide for progressive mobilization as ordered.† —*Lumbar laminectomy:* the physician may write an order for the evening of surgery or the first postoperative day; follow the physician's protocol for getting the patient out of bed.‡ —*Cervical laminectomy/discectomy:* roll the head of the bed up, align the patient at the edge of the bed, and gently assist the patient to a standing position by placing your arms across the patient's upper back and under the knees. The patient should *not* place his or her arm on the nurse's shoulder.
Risk for Infection R/T surgical incision	• Observe the dressing for evidence of drainage (blood or cerebrospinal fluid). • Monitor the incision for swelling, redness, drainage, irritation, or pain. • Maintain strict aseptic technique when changing the dressing. • With a lumbar laminectomy, check the dry, sterile dressing to ensure that it has not become wet; if this occurs, change the dressing immediately.
Risk for Disuse Syndrome R/T surgery, perioperative drugs, bed rest, and immobility	• Provide for basic maintenance interventions. • Monitor vital signs and neurological signs periodically. • Apply sequential compression boots to prevent deep vein thrombosis. • Encourage deep breathing exercises at least every 2 h; patients with a *cervical laminectomy* tend to have shallow respirations because of pain; such patients are at high risk for development of atelectasis and pneumonia. • Auscultate the chest for breath sounds every 4 h. • Monitor the patient for musculoskeletal changes, such as atrophy, contracture, foot drop.
Knowledge Deficit R/T body mechanics, modification of lifestyle, treatment plan, or use of braces, traction, or drugs	• Develop a discharge teaching program to decrease the risk of recurrent disc herniation by reducing stress on the back or neck; include the following information: —Proper body mechanics —Use of adequate support when on a mattress and in a chair —Maintenance of optimal weight (A weight reduction program may be necessary.) —Proper technique for any exercises prescribed by the physician, or reinforcement of exercises taught by the physical therapist, such as semisitups, pelvic tilt, knee-chest bends, and gluteal setting (see Fig. 20-12). —Any modifications in activity (e.g., for climbing stairs, lifting) • Explore areas of concern with the patient. • Help the patient develop strategies to reduce stress and anxiety. • Teach relaxation techniques and imagery techniques to control anxiety. • Help the patient set realistic goals. • If possible, provide written discharge instructions.

* Differences in the management of a patient with a cervical or lumbar laminectomy are noted where there is variation.

† *Variations in postoperative management protocols after a laminectomy:* The procedure for ambulation of patients varies from physician to physician. Some surgeons may ask that their patients dangle their feet from the edge of the bed on the evening of the day of surgery or the first postoperative day. Other surgeons do *not* allow their patients to dangle their feet at all, believing that excessive stress would be placed on the suture line. The individual protocols of the surgeon must be followed.

‡ *Technique for getting the laminectomy patient out of bed:* If possible, the head of the bed is raised with the patient comfortably positioned on the bed close to the edge of the side where he or she will be getting out of the bed. If the bed must remain flat, the patient is positioned on his or her side with knees and hips slightly flexed near the side of the bed from which he or she will rise. In either case, two nurses are necessary. One nurse grasps the patient under the arm and around the upper back and neck. The patient is instructed to place his or her arm around the nurse's shoulders. The other nurse grasps the patient's hips and legs. At the count of three, the nurses assist the patient to the upright position. If the patient is to walk, the support of two nurses is advisable, because weakness, dizziness, and light-headedness are common. A few steps to the door and back are sufficient for the first venture out of bed. Gradually, the patient will be able to tolerate ambulation for greater distances.

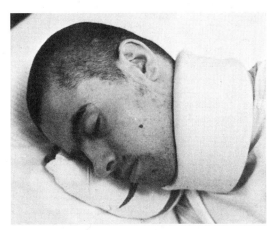

Figure 20–13 • A Thomas collar is applied following cervical laminectomy.

should be instituted. Follow the clinical pathway for a laminectomy.

Special Assessment. In the postoperative period, the nurse should frequently assess sensory and motor function in the extremities. If the operative site is proximal to the cervical region, assessment should concentrate on arm strength. With lumbar surgery, the legs should be the focus of attention. When assessing motor and sensory function, the nurse compares present motor and sensory function with preoperative function. The patient is asked to move the extremities, wiggle the fingers or toes, and identify the part of the extremity that has been touched or squeezed. If there is apparent motor weakness, paralysis, or lack of awareness of touch or temperature in the postoperative period, nerve root compression should be suspected. Such deficits should be reported to the physician immediately.

Several problems may arise following a laminectomy, including urinary retention, paralytic ileus, and muscle spasms. The common nursing diagnoses associated with the postoperative laminectomy patient are discussed in Chart 20-2. In addition, many patients have an elevated temperature (up to 102.2° F, 39° C) for a day or two after surgery. Use acetaminophen (Tylenol) 650 mg orally to lower the temperature. Fluid intake should also be increased.

Table 20-3 presents special nursing considerations for the patient who has undergone spinal fusion or an anterior cervical fusion or discectomy.

Complications of Laminectomy: Collaborative Nursing Problems

Several complications can develop following a laminectomy or spinal fusion. Some are more apt to occur in the immediate postoperative period, whereas others usually arise later. Discharge teaching should include a discussion of signs and symptoms that should be reported to the physician immediately.

Complications after a laminectomy or spinal fusion, when they arise, require medical assessment and intervention and are therefore collaborative problems. Hematoma at the operative site is usually an early complication. Later complications include CSF fistula; arachnoiditis; and nerve root

injury resulting in foot drop, hand or arm weakness (depending if the laminectomy was cervical or lumbar), and/or postural deformity.

Hematoma at the Operative Site. In rare instances, a hematoma can develop postoperatively as a result of bleeding at the incision site. The most prominent symptom is severe, localized incisional pain that may or may not be described as throbbing. The nurse will note that the postoperative administration of analgesics does not keep the patient comfortable. On assessment, there is a decrease in motor function of the legs or arms (depending on the location of the laminectomy) and a decrease in sensation to the involved area. This combination of severe incisional pain and decreased motor and sensory function suggests a hematoma; the physician should be notified immediately. If a hematoma is present and is causing neurological deficits (decreased or lost motor and sensory function), the physician will probably reoperate immediately to evacuate the hematoma. A hematoma, if left untreated, can result in irreversible motor and sensory deficits, including paraplegia and bowel or bladder dysfunction.

CSF Fistula. A **CSF fistula** is an abnormal connection between the subarachnoid space and the incision, which causes CSF drainage; this will be evident on the dressing, either alone or in combination with serosanguinous drainage. The dressing is usually wet, and increased drainage occurs when the patient is lying on the back or standing. Of major concern is infection at the fistula site and meningitis, because microorganisms can ascend the fistula and flourish in the ideal environment of the cerebrospinal space.

Formation of a fistula is not an early postoperative complication. It often takes 1 week for evidence of a fistula to appear. Because CSF drainage on the dressing is the major sign of a fistula, it is important to monitor the dressing. The drainage may be tested for sodium content (see Chap. 14) to verify the presence of CSF. Continuous drainage on the dressing should be reported to the physician. If the fistula does not spontaneously seal itself, surgical closure will be necessary. Prophylactic antibiotics may be ordered to prevent infection. If leakage of CSF is suspected, maintaining the patient on flat bed rest, thereby decreasing pressure on the meningeal defect, may help the leak to seal spontaneously.

Arachnoiditis. **Arachnoiditis**, an inflammation of the arachnoid layer of the spinal meninges, can result from infection

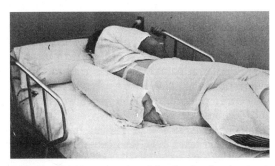

Figure 20–14 • Position of patient following lumbar laminectomy.

Table 20–3 • SPECIAL NURSING CONSIDERATIONS IN SPINAL FUSION AND ANTERIOR CERVICAL FUSION OR DISCECTOMY*

PROBLEM OR PROCEDURE	SPECIAL CONSIDERATIONS	POSTOPERATIVE NURSING CONSIDERATIONS
Spinal fusion (in general) • Bone graft	A bone graft will be obtained from the patient or from a bone bank. • If from the patient, the donor site is the iliac crest. • If from a bone bank, there will not be a donor site.	If a donor site is present: • Monitor the incision for bleeding or drainage. • Assess the incision daily; change the dry sterile dressing as ordered. • Position the patient so that no undue pressure is placed on the donor site.
• Immobilization of the operative site	Some form of immobilization will be ordered. • *Cervical:* soft or rigid collar will be ordered; alternatively, a halo apparatus with jacket may be applied. • *Thoracic or lumbar:* a brace or body jacket may be ordered.	• Maintain the collar or brace as ordered. • Monitor the patient's skin for irritation. • Teach proper body mechanics. • Teach the patient the proper application of collar or brace. • If a halo apparatus has been applied, provide for patient teaching.
Anterior cervical fusion	Postoperatively, management is similar to that of posterior cervical laminectomy except that the patient may be • Out of bed on the first postoperative day wearing a cervical collar • Relatively pain free • Bothered by a sore throat or experiencing difficulty swallowing as a result of irritation from endotracheal anesthesia	• Assess the patient for the presence of gag and swallowing reflexes before beginning oral intake. • Provide comfort measures (viscous lidocaine [Xylocaine] may be ordered by the physician).
Anterior cervical discectomy with fusion	Postoperatively, the patient is managed in a manner similar to patients undergoing anterior cervical fusion. Additional complications are related to soft-tissue injuries. The esophagus and trachea are retracted during surgery, and irritation of the laryngeal nerve and tracheal edema can result in hoarseness and difficulty coughing.	• The approach to management is the same as for anterior cervical fusion. • In addition, assess the quality of the patient's voice and the ability to cough; do not initiate oral intake if the patient cannot protect the airway adequately.

* See Chart 20–2 for general principles of postoperative care.

caused by contamination of the surgical site at surgery or contamination of the dressing. If there is clinical evidence of infection (an increase in temperature and white blood cell count, malaise, headache, redness at the incision, or drainage on the dressing), antibiotic therapy is initiated. Arachnoiditis is a particularly worrisome complication because the scar tissue and adhesions that can form cause severe and chronic pain within weeks of surgery. The pain can be so severe that surgical intervention to remove the adhesions may be necessary.

Nerve Root Injury. Foot drop or hand or arm weakness can occur as a result of sustained pressure on a nerve root (spinal nerve). If the patient has sustained nerve root injury, an aggressive program of physiotherapy is needed, along with slings, braces, or splints, depending on the involved extremity and the extent of injury. A short course of steroids (e.g., dexamethasone [Decadron]) may decrease the surrounding edema and improve function. Range-of-motion exercises should be incorporated into the nursing care plan, and careful attention must be directed toward preventing contractures, musculoskeletal deformities, and injury to the involved limb. The patient may sustain permanent disability even with an aggressive treatment program.

Postural Deformity. A laminectomy at more than one level of the vertebral column can cause spinal column instability and postural deformity. Such abnormalities may be noted by observing the patient while ambulating or by assessing the patient's posture in bed. When the surgeon performs a laminectomy on two or more vertebral levels, a spinal fusion may be necessary to ensure stability of the spinal column and prevent disability. If postural deformity develops after a simple laminectomy at a few levels, a spinal fusion may be necessary.

Recurrent Symptoms After Surgery

Surgery is not always synonymous with relief of pain and other symptoms. For example, a patient who has experienced long-term pain radiating down the leg before surgery will probably continue to have some pain after surgery. It may persist for several weeks postoperatively. If there has been considerable sensory loss because of nerve root compression preoperatively, pain perception may actually increase because of improvement of the sensory deficit. Such patients may experience paresthesias for several months after surgery.

Surgery for a herniated disc does not negate the possibility of recurrence of a disc herniation at the same level on the same or opposite side or at other levels. Repeated laminectomies in the same patient are not unusual. This possibility does underscore the need for patient teaching related to body mechanics, posture, and protection from injury. However, degenerative changes may already be present that predispose the patient to future problems, even if a teaching program is judiciously followed.

SUMMARY

Although this chapter has focused primarily on low back pain and the recommendations of the *Clinical Practice Guidelines for Low Back Pain*, a similar approach can be used with neck pain and cervical disc disease with modification for regional differences. Back pain is an affliction that affects most people at some time in their lives. The evidenced-based and comprehensive *Clinical Practice Guideline* helps enormously in determining the most clinically effective and cost-effective approach to management.

REFERENCES

1. Bigos, S., Bowyer, O., Braen, G., et al. (1994). *Acute low back problems in adults.* Clinical Practice Guideline, Quick Reference Guide Number 14. AHCPR Pub. No. 95-0643. Rockville, MD: U. S. Department of Health and Human Services, Public Health Service, Agency for Health Care Policy and Research.

RESOURCES
Professional

Published Material

BOOKS

Bigos, S., Bowyer, O., Braen, G. et al. (1994). *Acute low back problems in adults.* Clinical Practice Guideline, Quick Reference Guide Number 14. AHCPR Pub. No. 95-0643. Rockville, MD: U.S. Department of Health and Human Services, Public Health Service, Agency for Health Care Policy and Research.

Braddom, R. L. (1997). Approach to the patient with failed back syndrome. In J. Biller (Ed.). *Practical neurology* (pp. 269–281). Philadelphia: Lippincott-Raven.

Hoppenfeld, S. (1976). Physical examination of the lumbar spine. In S. Hoppenfeld. *Physical examination of the spine and extremities* (pp. 237–262). New York: Appleton-Century-Crofts.

Martinex-Arizalo, A. (2000). Low back and lower limb pain. In W. G. Bradley, R. B. Daroff, G. M. Fenichel, & C. D. Marsden (Eds.). *Neurology in clinical practice: Principles of diagnosis and management* (3rd ed., pp. 451–464). Boston: Butterworth Heinemann.

Nelson, P. B. (1997). Approach to the patient with low back pain and lumbosacral radiculopathy. In J. Biller (Ed.). *Practical neurology* (pp. 238–244). Philadelphia: Lippincott-Raven.

Nussbaum, E. S., & Rengachary, S. S. (1994). Cervical disc disease and spondylosis. In S. S. Rengachary & R. W. Wilkins (Eds.). *Principles of neurosurgery* (pp. 44-1–44-16). St. Louis: Mosby Wolfe.

Rodts, M. F. (1994). Disorders of the spine. In A. B. Maher, S. W. Salmond, & T. A. Pellino (Eds.). *Orthopedic nursing* (pp. 581–616). Philadelphia: W. B. Saunders.

Rothman, R., & Simone, F. (Eds.). (1992). *The spine* (Vols. 1 and 2). Philadelphia: W. B. Saunders.

Shapiro, S. A. (1997). Approach to the patient with neck pain, with and without associated arm pain. In J. Biller (Ed.). *Practical neurology* (pp. 229–237). Philadelphia: Lippincott-Raven.

Wilkins, R. W. (1994). Lumbar intervertebral disc herniation. In S. S. Rengachary & R. W. Wilkins (Eds.). *Principles of neurosurgery* (pp. 451–459). St. Louis: Mosby Wolfe.

PERIODICALS

Bazzoli, A. S. (1992). Chronic back pain: A common sense approach. *American Journal of Physical Medicine & Rehabilitation, 7*(1), 53.

Chase, J. A. (1992). Outpatient management of low back pain. *Orthopaedic Nursing, 11*(1), 11–21.

Della-Giustina, D. (1998). Acute low back pain: Part 1: Recognizing the "red flags" in the work-up. *Consultant, 38*(4), 995–1002.

Della-Giustina, D. (1998). Acute low back pain: Part 2: Guidelines for treating common–and uncommon–back pain syndromes. *Consultant, 38*(6), 1528–1544.

Gates, S. J. (1987). Conservative management of lumbar disc herniation. *Orthopedic Nursing, 6,* 37–41.

Herzog, R. J. (1991). Selection and utilization of imaging studies for disorders of the lumbar spine. *Physical Medicine and Rehabilitation Clinics of North America, 2*(1), 7–59.

Lukert, B. P. (1994). Vertebral compression fractures: How to manage pain, avoid disability. *Geriatrics, 49*(2), 22–26.

Malmivaara, A., Hakkinen, U., Aro, T., Heinrichs, M., Kokenniemi, L., Kuosma, E., Lappi, S., Paloheimo, R., Servo, C., Vaaranen, V., & Hernerg, S. (1995). The treatment of acute low back pain–bedrest, exercises, or ordinary activity? *New England Journal of Medicine, 332*(6), 332–351.

Mayer, H., & Brock, M. (1993). Percutaneous endoscopic discectomy: Surgical technique and preliminary results compared to microsurgical discectomy. *Journal of Neurosurgery, 78*(2), 216–225.

Michelsen, C., Jackson, R., Lowe, T., Farcy, J., & Deinlein, D. (1998). A multi-center prospective study of the CD spinal system in patients with Degenerative disc disease. *Journal of Spinal Disorders, 11*(6), 465–470.

Patel, P. R., & Lauerman, W. C. (1997). The use of magnetic resonance imaging in the diagnosis of lumbar disc disease. *Orthopedic Nursing, 16*(1), 59–65.

Patel, A. T. & Ogle, A. A. (2000). Diagnosis and management of acute low back pain. *American Family Physician, 61*(6), 1779–1786.

Rodriquez, A. A., Bilkey, W. J., & Agre, J. C. (1992). Therapeutic exercise in chronic neck and back pain. *Archives of Physical Medicine & Rehabilitation, 73*(9), 870–875.

Vanichkachorn, J. S., & Vaccaro, A. R. (2000). Thoracic disk disease: Diagnosis and treatment. *Journal of American Academy of Orthopedic Surgery, 8,* 159–169.

WEBSITES

Back Pain Resource Center: http://www.backpainreliefonline.com
Comprehensive information on neck/back problems: http://www.sofamordanek.com
Information on neck and back pain: http://www.neckreference.com

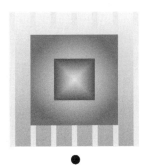

C H A P T E R **21**

Peripheral Nerve Injuries

JOANNE V. HICKEY

Injury to peripheral nerves can occur in the following three ways: *acute trauma* associated with vehicular accidents, mechanized industry, falls, and sports; *chronic entrapment syndromes* such as carpal tunnel syndrome; and exposure to toxins (e.g., alcohol), as well as some kinds of drug therapy; and through chronic disease (e.g., diabetes mellitus). In this chapter, peripheral injuries resulting from acute trauma are discussed. Chronic entrapment syndromes and other neuropathies are discussed in Chapter 32.

MECHANISMS OF INJURY

The possible acute traumatic events by which peripheral nerves can be injured include partial or complete nerve transection, contusion, stretching, and electrical or thermal injury.

- A **partial or complete transection** of a nerve is a structural loss of integrity of some or all of the fascicles of a nerve, usually the result of severe traumatic injury of a type that lacerates the nerve, such as a chainsaw injury or impact from a sharp instrument.
- With a **contusion**, the nerve remains intact structurally, but with undetermined axonal injury. The injury can occur from a direct blow to a nerve located close to the body surface, such as may occur when an elbow is bumped, causing injury to the superficial ulnar nerve. It may also occur from a missile, such as a bullet or shrapnel, careening close to the nerve.
- **Stretch injuries** may result from traction exerted on the nerve related to trauma such as vehicular accidents or possibly from improper use of orthopedic traction. In traumatic conditions, an unrestrained driver or passenger may be thrown into abnormal positions that stretch a peripheral nerve. A shoulder injury is common and may result in a brachial injury. Excessive application of weight in orthopedic traction can also cause traction on a nerve. For example, the peroneal nerve may be injured by excessive traction.
- **Avulsion** is a tearing away from a structure or part of a structure by traction. This is a particular consideration in brachial plexus injuries. Root avulsions may be complete or incomplete, but all avulsions are generally irreparable.

- **Electrical or thermal injuries** of peripheral nerves are often related to acute trauma. Electrical nerve injury results from a current passing through the peripheral nerve when contact is made with electrical wires. The resulting injuries produce severe muscle and nerve coagulation, in addition to burns of the skin and destruction of bone. Prognosis for muscle reinnervation in these instances is generally poor. Thermal nerve injury causes similar types of local responses, with major damage resulting from burning and necrosis of tissue.

PATHOPHYSIOLOGY

Peripheral nerves are composed of nerves and connective tissue. The anatomy of a peripheral nerve includes the **endoneurium,** which is the connective tissue that surrounds both myelinated and unmyelinated axons. Each unit is grouped with many other axons into bundles of *fascicles* by the **perineurium.** Groups of fascicles are bound together by an outer covering of connective tissue called the **epineurium** (Fig. 21-1). Nerves are composed of afferent and efferent fibers. These axons can be differentiated on the basis of their size and presence or absence of myelin (i.e., myelinated or unmyelinated fibers). Each nerve fiber is composed of an axon encased in a series of *Schwann cells* that cover the length of the axon. The junctional points between Schwann cells are called the *nodes of Ranvier.* As nerves develop, one of two events can occur. Many unmyelinated axons become embedded in the Schwann cell, or the Schwann cell wraps around one axon in concentric circles to fuse together to form the myelin of the myelinated nerve fiber. The electrical activity of each nerve fiber is independent of the activity in all the other fibers in the nerve even though the fibers are close to each other. The endoneurium and the myelin isolate the action potentials of each fiber from other adjacent fibers.[1]

Axonal transport is the continuous and regulated flow of material from the cell body to the axons and synaptic terminals as well as in the reverse direction (antegrade and retrograde transport). This action is critical for neuronal function through the transport of material synthesized in the cell body and dendrites to reach the axon terminals, and for

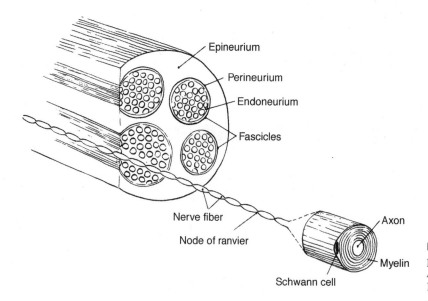

Figure 21–1 • Anatomical components of the peripheral nerve. (Benanoch, C. et al. [1998]. *Medical neurosciences* [4th ed.]. Philadelphia: Lippincott-Raven.)

the material in the axon terminals to reach the cell body of the nerve. Without an operational axonal transport system, the nerve dies.[1] The resting and action potentials of axons are discussed in Chapter 5.

Axons may be affected by acute disorders of the axoplasm (i.e., cytoplasm of an axon). This may occur with a complete or partial laceration of the nerve or with severe local crushing, traction, or ischemia. In laceration the connective tissue framework is destroyed, whereas in the other lesions cited it remains intact. Common to all injuries mentioned are the loss of axonal continuity and the loss of the axonal transport system. Three degenerative reactions occur in response to this: changes in the cell body (chromatolysis), changes in the nerve fiber segment between the cell and body and the point of transection (primary degeneration), and changes in the distal nerve fiber or amputated stump distal to the injury (secondary or wallerian degeneration; Fig. 21-2). Chromatolysis appears within 24 hours after the axon is cut and progresses until a maximum is reached between the second and third weeks.[3] Concurrently, most degenerated debris at the distal stump undergoes wallerian degeneration and is removed. Peripheral muscle atrophy accompanies wallerian degeneration. In lesions with a partial transection, not all axons are destroyed and some function may remain intact. If a nerve is completely severed, reinnervation is poor because the axonal buds or sprouts have no pathway to follow. They may grow haphazardly, form large abnormal tips, or form a painful neuroma.[1]

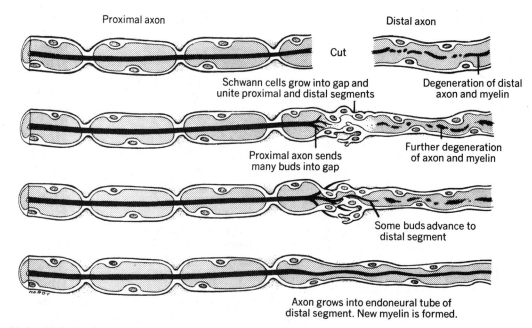

Figure 21–2 • Wallerian degeneration: Diagram of changes that occur in a nerve fiber that has been cut and then regenerates.

CLASSIFICATION OF PERIPHERAL NERVE INJURIES

Nerve injuries can be classified using the Seddon[3] or Sunderland[4] classification systems. For the purposes of this chapter, peripheral nerve injury is based on the simpler Seddon system, which classifies injury according to whether nerve or connective tissue is disrupted. Classification of injury is important to facilitate interpretation of clinical findings, provide guidance for treatment decisions, and suggest prognosis of any nerve injury. If neither the nerve nor its connective tissue covering is disrupted, the injury is called a **neuropraxia**. It is a physiological rather than an actual transection, but the axonal transport is impaired. Additionally, no wallerian degeneration occurs. Recovery may occur in hours to months, with an average of 6 to 8 weeks. If the neuronal components are disrupted but the connective tissue through which the nerve travels remain intact, the injury is called an **axonotmesis**. This type of injury is associated with wallerian degeneration of the involved neurons (see Fig. 21-2). Because the connective tissue components remain intact, the neurons are able to regenerate, albeit at a very slow rate. If the neuronal and connective tissue elements are disrupted, the injury is called a **neurotmesis**, and recovery depends on prompt and effective surgical intervention.

If a peripheral nerve has been completely severed, however, there is still a possibility for regeneration after surgical reapproximation of the severed nerve ends (see Fig. 21-1). Changes occur in the cell body of the injured peripheral nerve, for instance, swelling, chromatolysis, and side displacement of the nucleus. Chromatolysis usually indicates increased RNA and protein synthesis, an example of metabolic activity necessary for the regeneration of severed axonal fibers. In the isolated axonal segment, secondary degeneration occurs (wallerian degeneration). The axis cylinder and myelin sheath degenerate and are removed by the phagocytic cells. The only remaining evidence of the severed axonal segment is the Schwann (neurolemma) cells.

After surgical repair, the regeneration process begins with the proliferation of Schwann cells in the proximal stump near the transection and in the distal stump. These cells divide by mitosis to form continuous cords of Schwann cells, covering an area that encompasses the proximal stump, the gap across the transected area, the distal stump, and the area up to the sites of the sensory receptors and motor endings. The neurolemma cords act as guidelines for the regenerating axon.

Meanwhile, the cell body is directing synthesized protein and metabolites distally to provide the nutritional machinery for axonal regeneration. The axis cylinder of the proximal axon at the transection begins to generate tiny, unmyelinated sprouts that grow longitudinally. There may be as many as 50 sprouts. The random growth of buds or sprouts, which is accompanied by connective tissue proliferation, forms an enlargement called a *neuroma*; this can often be a source of intractable pain. Some sprouts will be misdirected and stray, but some will be successful in crossing the transected gap through the guidance of the neurolemma, finding their way to the distal stump. The rate of growth of a regenerating sprout is 1 to 4 mm per day. If the union is well aligned so that the axon will grow back into its former channel, functional return will be good.[1]

Successfully realigned nerves will remyelinate, grow to their former size, and eventually claim a conduction velocity equivalent to 80% of their former capacity. If the nerve realignments are mismatched, functional weakness, unintentional movements of muscles, and poor sensory discrimination and localization of stimuli may result. Sprouts that are unsuccessful in making connections degenerate. Nerves proximal to the injured neurons are stimulated to produce collateral innervation to denervated areas. This process provides innervation long before the axon has regenerated to provide innervation. Therefore, some sensory return may occur before regeneration can realistically occur. This process is possible in the central and peripheral nervous systems.

DIAGNOSIS OF PERIPHERAL NERVE INJURIES

Diagnosis of plexus and peripheral nerve injury is based on a history of injury or presence of an irritative or injurious lesion and a complete neurological examination. The clinical examination is a very important step in establishing the type, degree, and site of injury. A motor and sensory examination must be conducted, and pain characteristics must be evaluated. For upper-extremity nerve injuries, Tinel's sign and evidence of Horner's sign are important. Plain x-rays of the chest (for upper-extremity problems), computed tomography (CT) or magnetic resonance imaging (MRI), electromyography (EMG), and nerve conduction velocity (NCV) studies are conducted. The EMG and NCV studies are two diagnostic tests most useful to assess function nerve and muscle function.

General Signs and Symptoms of Peripheral Nerve Trauma

Motor, sensory, autonomic, and trophic signs and symptoms are the usual functional changes occurring in association with peripheral nerve injuries. The degree of deficit in any area depends on the type and extent of injury. The general signs and symptoms include:

- Flaccid paralysis of the muscle or muscle groups supplied by the nerve. A paresis results if some, but not all, of the lower motor neurons innervating the muscle are functional.
- Absence of deep tendon reflexes in the affected area if all neurons are affected. If some neurons are functional, deep tendon reflexes are weak.
- Atonic or hypotonic muscles.
- Progressive muscle atrophy that begins early (reaches peak in several weeks).
- Fibrillations and fasciculations that peak 2 to 3 weeks after the muscle is denervated. (**Fibrillations** are transitory muscle contractions caused by spontaneous stimulation of a single muscle fiber and can only be detected during

EMG studies. **Fasciculations** are spontaneous contractions of several muscle fibers innervated by a single motor nerve filament and can be observed during the physical examination.)

- Diminished or complete sensory loss.
- Warm or dry skin (anhidrosis; does not perspire) caused by transection of the postganglionic sympathetic fibers.
- Trophic skin changes, which can be separated into a warm phase followed by a cold phase. The *warm phase* lasts about 3 weeks, during which time the skin in the affected areas is dry, warm, and flushed. The *cold phase* is characterized by cold, cyanotic skin; brittle fingernails; loss of hair; dryness and ulceration of skin; and lysis of bones and joints. The digits are affected most. In some incomplete lesions of the median, ulnar, or sciatic nerve with causalgia (see below), the warm phase may persist and may be accompanied by sweating.

Types of Peripheral Nerve Trauma

Common Traumatic Syndromes

The **peripheral nerves** are the major nerve trunks in the extremities and are derived from the plexuses. Each nerve has a well-defined anatomical course in an extremity and innervates specific areas of the skin and muscles. A **plexus** is a complex network of axons that come together to form new combinations. The three major plexuses are the brachial, lumbar, and sacral plexuses. Specific traumatic syndromes

commonly seen include brachial plexus injuries, upper-extremity injuries (medial, ulnar, and radial nerves), and lower-extremity injuries (femoral, sciatic, and common peroneal nerves).[5]

Brachial Plexus Injuries

Anatomical Considerations. The brachial plexus (Fig. 21-3) is created from spinal nerves C-5, C-6, C-7, C-8, and T-1. (To make the difficult task of learning the anatomy of the brachial plexus easier, see Peck's study.[6]) By a series of division and recombination, three major trunks result: the upper trunk (C-5 and C-6), the middle trunk (C-7), and the lower trunk (C-8 and T-1). Again, these trunks divide and recombine to create three cords that give rise to the following nerves:

- Lateral cord (chiefly derived from C-5 and C-6): musculocutaneous and the lateral half of the median nerve
- Median cord (chiefly derived from C-8 and T-1): ulnar nerve and the medial half of the median nerve
- Posterior cord (C-5, C-6, and C-7): axillary and radial nerves

Patterns of Injury. There are two common patterns of brachial plexus injury: an *upper plexus injury* that usually results from direct downward pressure on the shoulder; and a *lower plexus injury* from hyperabduction on the arm with traction and stretching. The upper brachial injury produces a weak

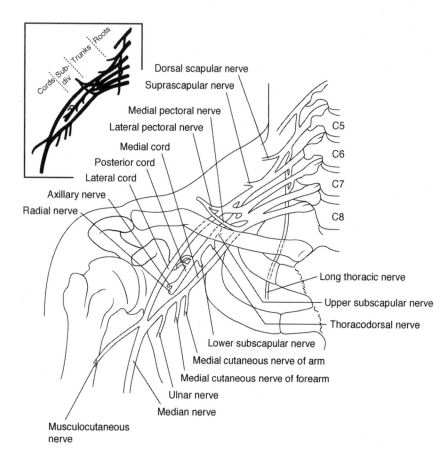

Figure 21-3 • Brachial plexus showing its various constituents and their relationship to structures in the region of the upper chest, axilla, and shoulder.

arm and shoulder with a functioning hand, whereas a lower brachial injury results in a strong arm, but a hand held in flexion.

A severe traction injury usually involves avulsion of two or more spinal roots from the spinal cord. Simultaneously, other roots have probably experienced severe stretching. The result is total and permanent functional loss to both the avulsed and stretched nerves. The presence of Horner's syndrome strongly suggests C-8 and T-1 avulsion. (**Horner's syndrome** includes the sinking of the eyeball, ptosis of the upper eyelid, slight elevation of the lower eyelid, constriction of the pupil, and anhidrosis caused by paralysis of the cervical sympathetic nerve supply.) Table 21-1 lists specific injuries.

Upper Extremity Injuries

The radial, median, and ulnar nerves are the major peripheral nerves of the arm (Fig. 21-4). The radial nerve is most frequently injured at the point where the nerve winds around the humerus. A fracture of the humerus is the usual cause of injury, although a radius fracture may be the underlying cause. The median nerve may be injured in the upper arm by a shoulder dislocation or in the forearm or wrist by a laceration or a gunshot wound (Fig. 21-5). The ulnar nerve is most often injured at the elbow because of a fracture or dislocation of the elbow joint. Injury may also occur from a blow to the elbow that results in a contusion to the ulnar nerve. **Volkmann's contracture** refers to a muscle contraction of the arm and hand resulting from ischemic injuries at the elbow (Fig. 21-6). Table 21-2 shows specific motor and sensory deficits associated with each injury.

Lower Extremity Injuries

The lumbar plexus gives rise to the femoral, sciatic, and common peroneal nerves (Fig. 21-7). The femoral nerve may be injured from compression of a pelvic tumor or a laceration during pelvic surgery. The sciatic nerve may be injured

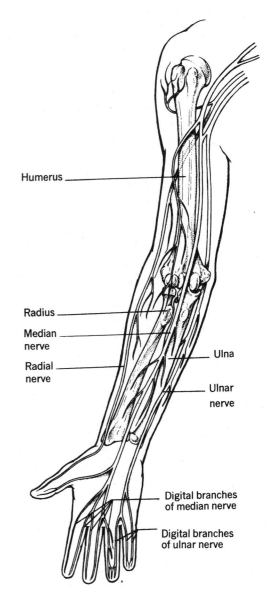

Figure 21–4 • Distribution of peripheral nerves of the arm.

Labels: Humerus, Radius, Median nerve, Radial nerve, Ulna, Ulnar nerve, Digital branches of median nerve, Digital branches of ulnar nerve

Table 21–1 • BRACHIAL PLEXUS INJURIES: NERVE ROOTS, TRUNKS, MOTOR LOSS, AND SENSORY LOSS

NERVE ROOTS	TRUNK	MOTOR LOSS	SENSORY LOSS
C-5 and C-6 Also called Duchenne-Erb palsy	Upper	Most shoulder muscles are involved, except the pectoralis major Loss or difficulty in abduction and external rotation of the arm and weak supination and flexion of the forearm	Deficit in the deltoid region and radial surface of the forearm
C-7	Middle	Incomplete triceps loss and some involvement of the forearm flexors and extensors Difficulty in extending the forearm	Deficits in the middle fingers
C-8 and T-1 Also called Klumpke's palsy or Duchenne-Aran palsy	Lower	Forearm muscle flexors and the hand muscles are chiefly involved Paralysis and atrophy of the small hand muscles and wrist flexors, giving the appearance of a "claw hand"	Deficit is in the medial side of the arm, forearm, and small finger

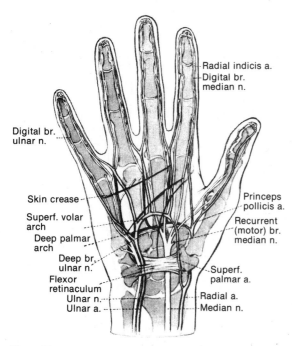

Figure 21–5 • Distribution of peripheral nerves of the hand.

by pelvic or femoral fractures or gunshot wounds. Pelvic tumors and herniated intervertebral discs are other possible causes of sciatic compression. The common peroneal nerve can be injured from prolonged traction, prolonged application of a tourniquet, or compression at the lateral aspect of the knee during surgery. Table 21-3 provides specific motor and sensory losses with major peripheral nerve injuries of the leg.

Causalgia

In 1865, S. Weir Mitchell coined the term **causalgia** to describe a rarely seen (except in wartime) type of peripheral neuralgia caused by partial injury to the median or ulnar nerve and occasionally the sciatic nerve. True causalgia is associated with penetrating injuries in which some sensory fibers, and usually some muscle fibers, are left intact. The pain, beginning shortly after injury, is described as a constant and intense burning. Symptoms are most pronounced in the digits, palm of the hand, or sole of the foot. Any minor stimulus, such as a draft of air, contact with clothes, or loud noise, can aggravate the pain. The patient is most comfortable when left alone with a cool moist cloth wrapped around the limb.

Abnormalities of the sweat glands and vasomotor tone in the affected area are caused by alteration of autonomic function. The involved hand (or foot) is moist, warmer or colder, and either pinker or bluer than the other hand. Trophic changes soon occur in the skin (shiny and smooth and then scaly and discolored). The underlying pathophysiology is thought to be a short-circuiting of the efferent sympathetic impulses to the sensory somatic fibers at the point of injury. True causalgia may respond to procaine blocks and sympathectomy but often progresses to an intractable pain syndrome.

PERIPHERAL NERVE INJURIES: TREATMENT

Treatment options must be individualized to the particular problem. If nerve injury is secondary to a primary problem, such as a tumor, attention is first directed to treatment of the primary problem. Fresh lacerations or transactions should be explored and repaired with tension-free end-to-end anastomosis within 72 hours of injury.[7] Ideally, any associated injuries should be clean and healed. Selecting the optimal time for surgery, however, is most important.[8] To determine the extent of nerve injury, surgical exploration may be planned immediately after injury. Primary nerve repair is usually scheduled for 3 weeks to 2 months after injury. Severed nerves may require resection and suturing to reapproximate the ends. Nerve grafts and transplantation are other options for treating injury.

During surgical anastomosis of the severed nerve, the two nerve segments will have contracted, with each having formed scar tissue at the stump. Dissection of the stumps further decreases the lengths of the ends to be joined. To compensate for this, the extremity is positioned in exaggerated flexion with a cast or splint applied to maintain the position after surgery. However, healing at the suture site takes 3 or 4 weeks. After healing has been ensured, the cast or splint is revised several times, with the degree of extension gradually increased by approximately 10 degrees each time. Cable grafting with autologous nerve tissue is a newer surgical technique that allows for anastomosis of nerves over large gaps, without the need for the exaggerated flexion position.

Because denervated muscle begins to atrophy almost immediately after injury, it is important to use all available means to retard the process. As previously noted, axonal growth occurs at the rate of 1 to 4 mm per day. Some muscle atrophy will be evident before the slow process of nerve regeneration is completed.

As soon as satisfactory healing has occurred, a physiotherapy program should be implemented to deal with the problems of immobility (stiffness, atrophy, and joint ankylosis). Special spring braces may be used to prevent foot drop or wrist drop. Daily regimens of galvanic stimulation to minimize the atrophic change of muscle to fibrotic tissue may be

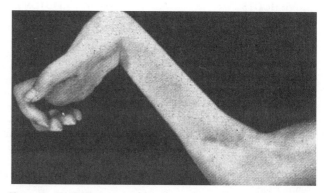

Figure 21–6 • Volkmann's contracture. (From Boyes, J. H. [1970]. *Bunnell's surgery of the hand* [5th ed]. Philadelphia: J.B. Lippincott.)

Table 21-2 • INJURIES TO THE RADIAL, MEDIAN, AND ULNAR NERVES

	RADIAL NERVE (FROM C-5 TO C-8 NERVE ROOTS)	MEDIAN NERVE (FROM C-6 TO T-1 NERVE ROOTS)	ULNAR NERVE (FROM C-7 AND T-1 NERVE ROOTS)
Motor paresis or paralysis	Loss of extension and abduction of the wrist, fingers, and thumb Wrist drop Inability to grasp an object or make a fist Forearm is pronated and flexed	Weakness of pronation of the forearm Weakness of wrist flexion Difficulty in abducting and opposing the thumb Inability to flex the distal phalanges of the index finger and thumb	Weakness of flexion of the wrist Flexion of the fourth and fifth fingers Inability to abduct and adduct the thumb See Volkmann's contracture (Fig. 21-6)
Sensory impairment or loss	Loss over the posterior aspect of the forearm and the radial aspect of the dorsum of the thumb or dorsum of hand	Loss of radial half of the palm, the palmar surface of the thumb, index and middle fingers, and the radial half of ring finger	Loss of the fifth finger, the ulnar aspect of the fourth finger, and the ulnar border of palm With a nerve contusion, the chief symptom may be pain with little, if any, motor deficit
Atrophy	Extensor carpi ulnaris, extensor digitorum, extensor digiti minimi, abductor pollicis longus and brevis, and extensor indicis	Thenar muscles of hand and the flexor-pronator group of the forearm	"Claw hand" deformity (from wasting of the small hand muscles with hyperextension of the fingers at the metacarpophalangeal joints)
Other	Trophic changes at minimum	Loss of ability to sweat in affected areas	

instituted until the affected muscle demonstrates, on electromyography, that it has been reinnervated. Massage, whirlpool treatments, and an exercise program to reeducate the muscles are important components of an aggressive physiotherapy program.

The rehabilitation program is long and arduous. The prognosis varies depending on the type and location of the injury. It may be necessary to offer a total rehabilitation program at a center that provides vocational rehabilitation if permanent disability will prevent the patient from assuming his or her former place in society and returning to previous employment. The patient should be kept comfortable with appropriate analgesics, as necessary. The pain that sometimes accompanies peripheral nerve injury may seriously limit the functional rehabilitation of these patients and should be dealt with aggressively.

COLLABORATIVE AND NURSING MANAGEMENT OF THE PATIENT WITH PERIPHERAL NERVE TRAUMA

The major collaborative problems associated with peripheral nerve injuries are **peripheral nerve impairment**, **paresis/paralysis**, **paresthesia**, and **pain management**. The medical or surgical plan will address the primary peripheral nerve problem. The loss of motor and sensory function in the involved area requires a multidisciplinary approach to care. In addition, pain management through a variety of strategies may be necessary.

Specific nursing care depends on the particular problem, type, and degree of injury. The patient with a peripheral injury may be hospitalized for surgery and discharged to recuperate at home. In other instances, a peripheral injury may be only one of several injuries seen as a result of multiple trauma. Management of the peripheral injury is incorporated into the total nursing management of the patient. However, general principles can be identified and followed when caring for patients with a peripheral nerve injury. These principles can be categorized into the following areas: assessment of function, maintenance of function, and rehabilitation.

Assessment of Function

A neurological assessment of the limb is made to determine which neurological functions remain intact. The assessment is initially conducted by the nurse to establish a baseline with which subsequent assessments can be compared. After the baseline has been established, subsequent assessments are conducted every 4 hours or at less frequent intervals, depending on the patient's condition.

Motor Function. Motor function is assessed by asking the patient to engage the limb through the normal range of motion, provided there is no contraindication to movement. In an acute traumatic injury, the injury is evaluated by the physician initially to determine whether movement is contraindicated, as would be the case if there were danger of a broken bone severing a nerve. If movement of the involved extremity is not contraindicated, range of motion is assessed. Any

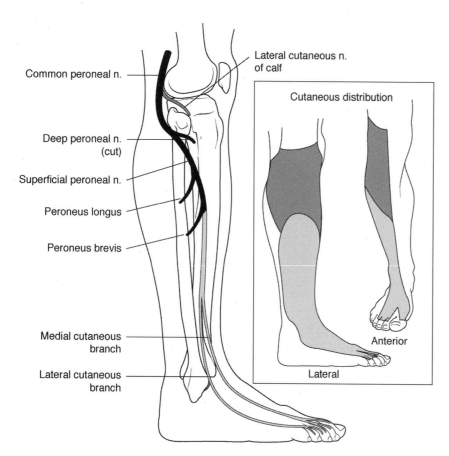

Figure 21–7 • Distribution of peripheral nerves of the leg.

evidence of abnormal movements, such as tremors, fibrillation, or fasciculations, should be documented. Atrophy, contractions, paresis, and paralysis are abnormal findings. Deep tendon reflexes should also be assessed.

Sensory Function. Light touch, pain, position, and temperature are assessed. The patient should be questioned about whether he or she has experienced any abnormal sensations,

such as tingling, a crawling sensation, or pain. All are examples of reportable findings.

Other Assessment Parameters. The involved limb should also be assessed for color, warmth, and texture. If the skin is cool to the touch or appears cyanotic, circulatory impairment or vasomotor tone may be indicated. Warm, dry, reddish skin indicates possible early trophic changes associated with au-

Table 21–3 • INJURIES TO THE FEMORAL, SCIATIC, AND COMMON PERONEAL NERVES

	FEMORAL NERVE (FROM THE L-2, L-3, AND L-4 NERVE ROOTS)	SCIATIC NERVE (FROM L-4 TO S-3 NERVE ROOTS)	COMMON PERONEAL NERVE (FROM L-4 TO S-1 NERVE ROOTS)
Motor paresis or paralysis	Weakness of extension of the knee Weakness of hip flexion (if injury is near the psoas muscle)	Inability to flex the knee Weakened gluteal muscles Foot drop	Paralysis of dorsiflexion of foot and toes (foot drop) Difficulty with eversion of the foot (with involvement of the superficial peroneal nerve)
Sensory impairment or loss	Anterolateral thigh	Outer aspect of the leg and dorsum of the foot and sole and inner aspect of foot	Medial part of the dorsum of the foot and outer side of the leg
Atrophy	Wasting of the quadriceps muscles	Hamstrings and all muscles below the knee	Extensor digitorum brevis, peronei (foot eversion)
Other	Absence of the knee-jerk reflex	Loss of hair, changes in toenails, and changes in skin texture in distal leg below knee	—

tonomic alterations. Any evidence of scaling, brittle nails, or loss of body hair should be recorded.

Planning and Implementation

Following an assessment of the involved area, the nurse plans and implements the nursing care plan with consideration of the goals of medical management. If the physician has ordered immobilization of the involved area, the immobilization may be accomplished by a splint, cast, or traction. The purpose of immobilization is to allow for the healing of a surgical incision in which there has been a reanastomosis or other surgical intervention for a severed nerve.

The following outlines major points of nursing management.

Splint and Cast Care. The splint is usually held secure with an Ace-bandage wrap or Velcro. The splint and wrap can become tight because of edema. The skin around the splint or cast should be checked for tightness, warmth, and color. If the splint or cast is too tight, as evidenced by tingling, blanched color, or coolness, steps can be taken to provide a better fit. In the case of a tight cast, the physician will need to decide which adjustments need to be made to ensure a better fit. It is best to refer the need for adjustments to the department that made the splint or brace originally, because all braces and most splints are custom-made to fit the contour of the wearer. A blanched appearance of the skin and coolness to the touch indicate interference with autonomic function and adequate blood supply. Any indications of drainage under the cast or splint should be addressed immediately.

Positioning of Extremity. If a cast or splint has been applied to the arm, a sling may be used to prevent dependence. In the case of a leg cast, the physician usually wants the leg to be supported and elevated on pillows to reduce the likelihood of edema.

Skin Care. Trophic changes of the skin are common signs and symptoms associated with peripheral nerve injury that make the skin susceptible to breakdown and injury. The skin should be examined for evidence of irritation or injury. Washing and careful drying are important, especially between the toes or fingers. If the skin is dry and scaly, lubricate with a lanolin preparation or other prescribed treatment. The nails should be filed and cut straight across to prevent skin injury.

Temperature. The involved extremity should be carefully protected from extremes in temperature. Because of lost or compromised sensory function, the area can be easily injured by extreme heat or cold without the patient being alerted to this through pain or discomfort.

Ambulation. Depending on the extent of injury of the involved extremity, the physician may limit ambulation and other activities of daily living (ADLs). The nurse should

adjust the plan of care based on the limitations imposed by the injury and the medical treatment.

Rehabilitation

The length and complexity of the rehabilitative process can vary greatly. Patient education and support are important components of care. Patient education is directed at regaining the greatest possible level of independence. Help may be needed in developing alternative methods of performing ADLs. For example, if the dominant arm and hand are encircled by a splint, the patient will need to be helped to learn to eat with the other hand. If food is adequately prepared for the patient (beverage poured, food cut, and so forth), he or she will be able to manage with practice. In addition, anxiety is decreased, and the patient is better able to cope with the limitations imposed by the injury.

When an exercise program is initiated for the involved extremity, the patient will have to learn the active and passive (prescribed) exercises. Protect the involved limb from injury. The process of regaining motor and sensory function can be slow and thus lead to discouragement. Encourage the patient to commit to the outlined physiotherapy program to prevent skeletal deformities and slowly regain as much function as possible.

A decreased level of independence precipitates various emotional and psychological reactions. The patient experiences changes in body image, self-esteem, and lifestyle. Sensory deprivation, social isolation, and powerlessness result from the limitations imposed by the disability. Common behavioral manifestations from the various physical, emotional, and social disabilities include frustration, hostility, anger, and depression. Many patients go through a process of loss, grief, and bereavement over the lost function. The process of recovery is very slow (approximately 1 year with nerve transections). Physiotherapy is the major approach after surgical intervention has been completed. It is a slow process characterized by ups and downs, so it is easy for patients to become discouraged with the lack of apparent improvement. If the disability is permanent, the emotional impact imposes increased demands on the person's coping skills and adjustment patterns; therefore, it is extremely important that the nurse provide appropriate psychological and emotional support.

REFERENCES

1. Benarroch, E. E., Westmoreland, B. F., Daube, J. R., Reagan, T. J., & Sandok, B. A. (1999). *Medical neurosciences: An approach to anatomy, pathology, and physiology by systems and levels* (4th ed., pp. 382–384). Philadelphia: Lippincott Williams & Wilkins.
2. Chuang, D. C. (1999). Management of traumatic brachial plexus injuries in adults. *Hand Clinics, 15*(4), 737-755.
3. Seddon, H. J. (1942). A classification of nerve injuries. *British Medical Journal, 1,* 237–288.
4. Sunderland, S. (1968). *Nerves and nerve injuries.* Baltimore: Williams & Wilkins.
5. Black, P., & Rossitch, E., Jr. (1995). *Neurosurgery: An introduction text.* New York: Oxford University Press.

6. Peck, D. (1978). A "five-fingered" mnemonic for the brachial plexus. *Journal of Kentucky Medical Association, 76,* 70–72.
7. Greenberg, M. S. (2001). *Handbook of neurosurgery* (5th ed., pp. 520-548). Lakeland, FL: Greenberg Graphics.
8. Cruz, J. (Ed.). (1998). *Neurologic and neurosurgical emergencies* (pp. 348–362). Philadelphia: W. B. Saunders.

RESOURCES

Books

Greenberg, M. S. (2001). *Handbook of neurosurgery* (5th ed., pp. 520–548). Lakeland, FL: Greenberg Graphics.
Samii, M., & Penkert, G. (1998). Traumatic disorders of the peripheral nervous system. In J. Cruz (Ed.). *Neurological and neurosurgical emergencies* (pp. 349–362). Philadelphia: W. B. Saunders.

Sunderland, S. (1991). *Nerve injuries and their repair: A critical approach.* New York: Churchill Livingstone.
Victor, M., & Ropper, A. H. (2001). *Principles of neurology* (7th ed., pp. 1370–1445). New York: McGraw-Hill.

Periodicals

Bartels, R. H., Menovsky, T., Van Overbeeke, J. J., & Verhagen, W. I. (1998). Surgical management of ulnar nerve compression at the elbow: An analysis of the literature. *Journal of Neurosurgery, 89,* 722–727.
Chuang, D. C. (1999). Management of traumatic brachial plexus injuries in adults. *Hand Clinics, 15*(4), 737–755.
Krivickas, L. S., & Wilbourn, A. J. (2000). Peripheral nerve injuries in athletes: A case series of over 200 injuries. *Seminars in Neurology, 20*(2), 225–232.

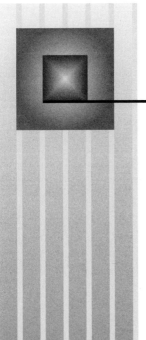

Nursing Management of Patients With Neoplasms of the Neurological System

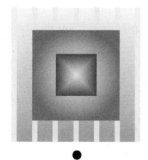

C H A P T E R **22**

Brain Tumors

JOANNE V. HICKEY

▥ OVERVIEW OF BRAIN TUMORS

The diagnosis of a brain tumor begins a journey of uncertainty, fear, and hope for the patient and family. The human saga is laden with confounding issues, including loss of neurological function ranging from subtle to significant, often including cognitive function; treatment options; quality of life; and often, end-of-life decisions. To care for the patient and family in a sensitive, compassionate, hopeful, and humanistic manner, the health care professional needs a broad knowledge base and particular skills. Within this framework of fundamental principles, concepts related to brain tumors and related management are explored in this chapter.

The Surveillance, Epidemiology, and End Results (SEER) program projected 16,500 new brain and other nervous system cancers for the year 2000 in the United States (9,500 males and 7,000 females).[1] In 1998, there were approximately 13,300 deaths from "brain and other nervous system tumors." Incidence of brain and other nervous system tumors is second after leukemia in children under the age of 15 years, third for those between 15 to 34 years, and fourth for men between ages 35 and 54.[2] About two thirds of all childhood tumors are found in the posterior fossa (infratentorial region). In contrast, most adult brain tumors are located in the anterior and middle fossae (supratentorial region). Among children, the most common primary brain tumors are astrocytomas (31%), medulloblastomas (21% to 25%), and ependymomas (9% to 19%).[3] Gliomas, particularly those of astrocytic origin, are the most common type of primary brain tumors and account for more than 40% of all neoplasms of the central nervous system (CNS).[4] The number of gliomas has been reported to be rising in the elderly whereas other types of cancers are in decline; the reason is unclear. Metastasis to the brain is found in 10% to 15% of cancer patients, which totals 80,000 annually.

The cause of most nervous sytem tumors remains unknown. Some inherited genetic syndromes predispose patients to brain tumor development (e.g., neurofibromatosis types 1 and 2, tuberous sclerosis, von Hippel-Lindau disease). Specific chromosomal locations are related to specific types of tumors. For example, neurofibromatosis type 1 is located on chromosome 17q11 and is associated with astro-

cytomas or peripheral neurofibromas. In contrast, neurofibromatosis type 2, located on chromosome(s) 22q12, is associated with acoustic and other neuromas, meningiomas, astrocytomas, ependymomas, and central neurofibromas.[5] Other tumors have a congenital basis (e.g., epidermoid, dermoid, and teratoid tumors and craniopharyngiomas). Some environmental agents, ionizing radiation in particular, clearly are implicated as causes of brain tumors, but they also appear to account for few cases.[5]

Classification of Brain Tumors

Classification of brain tumors is based primarily on histopathological characteristics, which are important considerations for determining treatment options. For clinical purposes, other conventional classifications are also helpful in understanding the nature of brain tumors.

Histopathological Basis of Classification

In recent years, tumors of the nervous system as a focus of basic research have led to interest in improving classification systems. Although gliomas are assumed to be derived from only three cell types (i.e., astrocytes, oligodendrocytes, and ependymal cells), subsequent tumors display a broad spectrum of different histopathological features. These features represent marked differences in incidence, location, preferential age of affected patients, clinical course, and outcome. Variations in the phenotype (the outward, visible expression of the hereditary constitution of an organism) and biologic behavior of gliomas reflect the type of transformation-associated genes function in neoplastic development.[4]

The World Health Organization (WHO) classifies CNS tumors into nine categories (Chart 22-1).[6] Tumors originating from neuroepithelial tissue account for the most prevalent glial tumors. The neuroepithelial category is further subclassified in Chart 22-2. Astrocytic tumors, which have been the focus of much classification discussion, are included.[7]

Historically, histological grading according to Kernohan and colleagues' four-tiered (1949)[8] and Ringertz's three-tiered (1950)[9] grading systems for astrocytic tumors have been used for many years. The variations in approach have

CHART 22-1 • World Health Organization Classification of Central Nervous System Tumors

1. Tumors of neuroepithelial tissue
2. Tumors of cranial and spinal nerves
3. Tumors of the meninges
4. Hematopoietic neoplasms
5. Germ cell tumors
6. Cysts and tumor-like lesions
7. Tumors of the anterior pituitary
8. Local extensions from regional tumors
9. Metastatic tumors

led to confusion. Currently, the WHO classification is more widely accepted.[6,10] For diffusely infiltrating astrocytomas, the St. Anne/Mayo[11] grading system has proved to be both highly reproducible and predictive of patient survival.[4] Table 22-1 compares the WHO and St. Anne/Mayo classifications and describes histopathologic changes.

The WHO's definition of astrocytic tumors is based on the degree of growth potential (i.e., nuclear and cellular

CHART 22-2 • Classification of Major Brain Tumors

Gliomas
  Astrocytic tumors
    Pilocytic astrocytomas (grade 1)
    Astrocytoma (grade 2)
    Anaplastic astrocytoma (grade 3)
    Glioblastoma multiforme (grade 4)
  Ependymomal tumors
    Ependymoma (variants)
    Anaplastic (malignant) ependymoma
    Myxopapillary ependymoma
    Subependymoma
  Oligodendroglial tumors
    Oligodendroglioma
    Anaplastic (malignant) oligodendroglioma
  Medulloblastoma
  Unclassified (mostly gliomas)
Meningiomas
  Menigiomas (multiple histologic types)
  Atypical types
  Anaplastic (malignant) meningioma
Pituitary adenoma
Neurinoma (schwannoma, acoustic neuroma)
Craniopharyngioma, dermoid, epidermoid, teratoma
Angiomas
Sarcomas
Miscellaneous (pinealoma, chordoma, granuloma, lymphoma)

Adapted from the WHO classification.

atypia, mitotic activity, endothelial proliferation, vascular changes, and necrosis). The term **pleomorphism**, used to describe nuclear and cellular atypia, is defined as the occurrence of widely different forms of the same species. In brain tumors, it is applied to bacteria and malignant cells. For example, a glioblastoma is a highly cellular tumor with nuclear and cellular variations, endothelial proliferation, mitotic changes, and often, necrosis. Necrosis is a hallmark of this lesion and often occurs, but its presence is not required for classification as a glioblastoma according to the WHO classification system.[12] By comparison, anaplastic astrocytomas are less cellular, pleomorphic, mitotically altered, and lack necrosis whereas astrocytomas have few cells and minimal pleomorphic changes. Note that the grade I (pilocytic astrocytoma) is a tumor seen frequently in children. It is circumscribed, slow growing, and rarely undergoes progression to anaplasia.

The St. Anne/Mayo system, often used by pathologists, is a different grading method based on the presence or absence of four criteria: atypia, mitosis, endothelial proliferation, and necrosis.[11] Grade 1 neoplasms have none of these features, grade II have one feature, grade III have two features, and grade IV have at least three features present.

Conventional Classifications

Other conventional classifications are based on several distinguishing clinical considerations. These include primary versus secondary, neuroembryonic origins, anatomical location, and malignant versus benign.

• Primary versus metastatic brain tumors: *Primary brain tumors* originate from the various cells and structures that constitute the brain. *Metastatic brain tumors* originate from sites outside the brain, most often from primary tumors of

Table 22-1 • COMPARISON OF THE WORLD HEALTH ORGANIZATION (WHO) AND ST. ANNE/MAYO GRADING SYSTEM FOR ASTROCYTOMAS

WHO GRADE	WHO CLASSIFICATION	ST. ANNE/ MAYO	HISTOPATHOLOGY
I	Pilocytic astrocytoma	Pilocytic astrocytoma	Bipolar, "piloid" cells, Rosenthal fibers, eosinophilic granular bodies
II	Low grade astrocytoma	Astrocytoma grades 1 and 2	Neoplastic fibrillary, or gemistocystic astrocytes; nuclear atypia
III	Anaplastic astrocytoma	Astrocytoma grade 3	Neoplastic fibrillary, or gemistocystic astrocyte; nuclear atypia, mitotic activity
IV	Glioblastoma multiforme	Astrocytoma grade 4	Cellular anaplasia, nuclear atypia, mitoses, vascular proliferation, necrosis

the lung (84%), breast, and melanomas. Brain tumors rarely metastasize outside the brain. Medulloblastomas, common in children, can seed into the spinal cord. *Carcinomatosis* is a condition in which carcinoma is widespread throughout the body. The term is sometimes used to describe multiple metastatic lesions to the brain or meninges.

• *Neuroembryonic origins:* The nervous system originates from the ectodermal (outer) layer of the embryo. Chapter 5 briefly describes early embryonic development. At 16 days the *neural plate* appears, changing to the *neural groove* and *neural tube* by the third week. Those neuroectodermal cells not incorporated into the neural tube form *neural crests*. The neural tube and neural crests contain two types of undifferentiated cells called neuroblasts and glioblasts (spongioblasts). The *neuroblasts* become the basic unit of structure in the nervous system and are then called *neurons*. The *glioblasts* form a variety of cells that support, insulate, and metabolically assist the neurons. They are collectively called *glial cells.*[13] Glial cells are subclassified into *astrocytes* (star-shaped cells), *oligodendrocytes* (glial cells with few processes), and *ependymal cells* (line the ventricles). This is the basis for the broad category of brain tumors called *gliomas.* Gliomas are further subdivided into *astrocytomas, oligodendrogliomas,* and *ependymomas.*

• Anatomical location: The anatomical location of the lesion affects signs and symptoms as well as presentation. The location of the tumor can be described by the specific site of the lesion such as the frontal or temporal lobe, pons, or cerebellum (Fig. 22-1). Location may be noted by using the tentorium as a reference point to differentiate between *supratentorial,* located above the tentorium (i.e., cerebral hemispheres), and *infratentorial,* located below the tentorium (i.e., brain stem or cerebellum). Knowing the location of the lesion helps to predict probable deficits based on an understanding of the normal function of that anatomical area. In addition, location is an important variable in selecting treatment options and prognosis.

• Malignant versus benign: Using the word "benign" in the classification of brain tumors can be somewhat misleading. When a neoplasm is designated as benign, one suggests that a complete cure is possible; conversely, a ma-

lignant tumor would suggest a poor prognosis. The benign-versus-malignant distinction is made on the basis of histological properties. Cells that are well differentiated are related to a better prognosis than poorly differentiated cells. However, when a tumor is located within the brain, other factors are equally important. A tumor that is considered to be histologically benign may be surgically inaccessible, as with a deep tumor requiring extensive dissection of tissue or one located in a vital area, such as the pons or medulla. A benign tumor that is partially or completely surgically inaccessible may continue to grow, and cause neurological deficits, if the tumor does not respond to other treatment options such as chemotherapy or radiation. These deficits can result in loss of significant neurological function and life.

Pathophysiology of Brain Tumors

The pathophysiology of brain tumors can be viewed from the perspective of molecular considerations and the effects of the tumor, both directly on cerebral tissue and indirectly through the development of increased ICP.

Molecular Considerations

Transformation of glial or neuronal cells into brain tumors is a complex process that is still incompletely understood. Brain tumors arise in association with multiple, specific structural molecular genetic alternations (i.e., mutations) within cells. These mutations can cause the cell to proliferate inappropriately as well as result in other malignancy attributes, such as the loss of differentiated characteristics of the tissue of origin, acquisition of the ability to invade surrounding normal tissues and metastasize, and the ability to resist antineoplastic therapies.[14] Two types of genetic molecular alterations trigger these changes in cellular behavior. The first change results in the complete cessation or partial decrease in cellular activities that physiologically restrain growth. These genes are known as *tumor suppressor genes.* The second change inappropriately activates genes that typically enhance cellular proliferation. Known as *proto-oncogenes,* these genes encode proteins that act as growth factors or growth factor receptors, mediators of signaling pathways, or regulators of gene expression. Mutations convert proto-oncogenes to oncogenes, which function in various ways to promote neoplastic changes, such as alterations in cell cycle progression, abnormalities in signal transduction pathways, glial cell invasion, and angiogenesis.[12,14]

The Effects of a Space-Occupying Lesion Within the Brain

Tumors directly affect the brain through *compression of cerebral tissue, through invasion or infiltration of cerebral tissue,* and sometimes through *erosion of bone.* A brain tumor usually grows as a spherical mass until it encounters a more rigid structure, such as bone or the falx cerebri. The encounter with an aplastic substance necessitates a change in the contour of the neoplasm. Neoplastic cells can also grow diffusely, with multiple cells infiltrating tissue spaces without

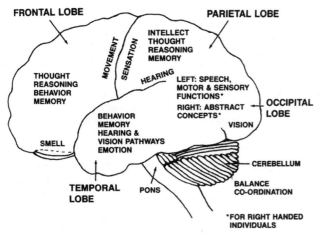

Figure 22–1 • Cerebral function and associated anatomical areas. (Reproduced with permission from the American Brain Tumor Association.)

forming a definite mass. The tumor enlarges because of cell proliferation, necrosis, fluid accumulation, hemorrhage, or the accumulation of degenerative by-products within the mass.

The clinical effects of a tumor within the brain and cranial vault depend on the location of the tumor, rate of growth, and consequences of increased intracranial pressure (ICP). A slow-growing tumor may become large before clinical signs and symptoms of increased ICP are noted. This happens because the tumor's volume is accommodated in the intracranial space over a long period of time, often years. A meningioma is a slow-growing tumor that can become large before signs and symptoms of increased ICP are noted. Conversely, depending on its location, evidence of a meningioma may be noted early because of focal deficits. With a fast-growing tumor, such as a glioblastoma multiforme, there is little time for the intracranial compartment to accommodate the lesion, and signs of increased ICP may be noted in a shorter time frame. In summary, an understanding of the pathophysiological effects of brain tumors requires an understanding of the Monro-Kellie hypothesis and increased ICP along with the specific tumor type, location, and related focal deficits. See Chapter 14 for a discussion of increased ICP and its management.

In most patients with brain tumors, vasogenic edema develops in the surrounding tissue as a result of compression. At the cellular level, an increase in permeability of capillary endothelial cells of the cerebral white matter results in seepage of plasma into the extracellular space and between the layers of the myelin sheath. This alters the electrical potential of cells, impairing cellular activity. Cerebral edema may also develop rapidly from alterations in the blood-brain barrier caused by substances released from tumor cells.[4] As cerebral edema increases, a mass effect develops, and signs and symptoms of increased ICP become apparent. These signs and symptoms continue to develop as a tumor grows. The resulting increase in cerebral edema can result in cerebral herniation syndromes and death (see Chap. 14).

SIGNS AND SYMPTOMS OF BRAIN TUMOR

Given that brain tumors present in widely variable clinical patterns, there are no classic signs and symptoms. The particular clinical presentation depends on the size, location, compression or infiltration of specific cerebral tissue, related cerebral edema, and the development of increased ICP. Brain tumors are sometimes discovered as asymptomatic masses. Initially, neurological symptoms are subtle. Some symptoms found in association with brain tumors are also those found in less serious conditions, so patients need to be carefully evaluated. Patients often present with two categories of signs and symptoms, general or focal:

- General: headaches, nausea and vomiting, changes in the level of consciousness, and seizures
- Focal: specific *focal deficits,* such as monoparesis or *syndromes related to specific cerebral areas,* such as acromegaly

General Signs and Symptoms

The most common initial signs and symptoms of brain tumors are headache, nausea and vomiting, changes in the level of consciousness, and seizures.

Headache. Headache is an early symptom in approximately one third of patients with brain tumors. The location and characteristics of the headache cover a wide range of possibilities. Headache is often described as intermittent and moderately severe; is usually worse in the morning because of irritation, compression, or traction of the blood vessels; and may be aggravated by acts known to increase ICP such as coughing or straining at stool. Onset of a new headache pattern, especially if it is worse in the morning or awakens the patient at night, deserves investigation. The area affected by the headache may be generalized or localized to the site of the tumor. As ICP rises, headache is generally bifrontal or bioccipital, regardless of the tumor location.

Nausea and Vomiting. Vomiting may indicate increased ICP or a posterior fossa tumor, and it may or may not be accompanied by headache. Nausea or abdominal discomfort may accompany vomiting, although in most instances vomiting occurs without these symptoms. Vomiting associated with brain tumor is usually unrelated to meals, occurs most commonly in the morning, and can be projectile. The cause may be direct stimulation of the vomiting center (located in the medulla), especially with a posterior fossa lesion.

Change in the Level of Consciousness. Initially, alterations in consciousness may be very subtle, progressing from slight confusion, irritability, and somnolence to stupor and finally to coma. Blatant changes in consciousness, such as stupor and coma, are related to increased ICP.

Seizures. A new onset of seizures in an adult should prompt an immediate search for the underlying cause. Many patients experience seizures in the course of their illness. Seizures are either the initial symptom or occur during the illness in about 30% of patients. About 70% of patients with slower-growing tumors are likely to have seizure activity, whereas those with more rapidly growing tumors have a seizure rate of 30% to 40%.[12]

With brain tumors, hyperactive cells caused by cerebral edema and alterations in normal electrical potential produce abnormal paroxysmal discharges or seizure activity that may be generalized or focal. Focal seizures can aid in the localization of the tumor. Seizure activity is seen primarily with supratentorial tumors. Please refer to Chapter 29 for a more detailed review of seizure management and nursing implications.

The recommended workup for a patient who presents with new onset of seizures is included in Figure 22-2. The workup is divided into toxic/metabolic and structural factors. Possible metabolic factors include electrolyte imbalance, liver or renal failure, or side effects from radiation or chemotherapeutic agents. Structural causes include parenchymal metastases, dural metastases, or leptomeningeal disease. Additionally, hemorrhage, thrombosis, or meningitis can cause seizures in the patient with known brain tumor.

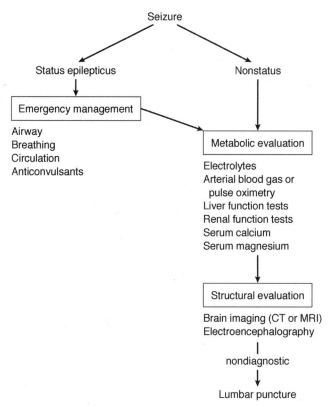

Figure 22–2 • Algorithm for initial evaluation of patients with suspected brain tumor based on type of seizure in presenting symptoms.

Focal Signs and Symptoms

Regardless of the histological structure, location of a tumor will often give rise to focal signs and symptoms. Focal findings are often present and assist the health care provider in localizing the tumor. The possible manifestations of a brain tumor are many and include a new onset of seizures; gradual neurological deficits such as weakness or numbness on one side of the body; headache; new onset of vomiting; visual loss or field cuts; papilledema; loss of the gag reflex; ataxia; confusion; listlessness, somnolence or irritability; change in behavior or personality; memory deficits; and speech deficits. In addition, deficits may be noted in specific cranial nerves, including unilateral hearing loss or tinnitus; loss of smell; numbness on one side of the face; swallowing difficulty; and diplopia or blurred vision.[16] The next section reviews focal signs and symptoms as they relate to specific anatomical cerebral locations.

Frontal Lobe

Multiple higher cognitive, executive, behavioral, speech, and motor functions are controlled by the frontal lobe. Focal deficits can be traced to either anterior frontal and posterior frontal findings.

Anterior Frontal Lobe. Patients with tumors in the *anterior frontal lobe* present with a wide range of higher-level function and personality changes such as short- and long-term memory deficits, difficulty in concentration and vigilance, slowing of mental processes and reaction time, abulia, and difficulty with calculations, problem solving, insight, abstraction, and synthesis of ideas. Collectively, anterior frontal lobe symptoms are called the *frontal lobe syndrome.* Personality and behavioral changes may include emotional lability, flat affect, lack of initiative and spontaneity, loss of self-restraint, and loss of social behavior.

Posterior Frontal Lobe. Broca's area is located in the posterior-inferior frontal lobe. If a tumor is located in or around Broca's area in the dominant hemisphere, fluent speech deficits such as word finding may be noted. The primary motor strip is located in the posterior frontal lobe. Tumors in this area can cause focal findings of motor weakness such as monoparesis or focal seizure activity.

Parietal Lobe

The parietal lobe contains the sensory discrimination and association areas for body orientation, vision, and language. Parietal lobe tumors cause deficits in sensation, inability to recognize common objects, and neglect syndromes such as the lack of awareness of the opposite side of the body. If the lesion is in the dominant hemisphere and is located in the left angular gyrus of the parietal lobe, Gerstmann's syndrome may be present (finger agnosia, loss of right-left discrimination, acalculia, and agraphia). Seizure activity and homonymous hemianopsia are also possible with a parietal lobe tumor. A collection of symptoms associated with parietal lobe dysfunction is called the *parietal lobe syndrome.* Common symptoms include the following:

SENSORY CHANGES
- Hypo- or hyperesthesia (impaired sensation with increased or decreased tactile sensitivity)
- Paresthesia (abnormal sensation involving tingling, crawling, or burning feeling on the skin)
- Loss of two-point discrimination (unable to determine by feeling if the skin is touched by one or two points simultaneously)

RECOGNITION DEFICITS
- Inability to recognize letters or numbers
- Astereognosis (inability to recognize an object by feeling its size and shape)
- Autotopagnosia (inability to locate or recognize parts of the body)
- Anosognosia (loss of awareness or denial of specific motor or sensory deficits)
- Finger agnosia (inability to identify or select specific fingers of the hand such as thumb)

ORIENTATION DEFICITS AND NEGLECT SYNDROMES
- Loss of right-left discrimination
- Difficulty in going through doorways without knocking self on one side
- Neglect syndrome (a tendency to ignore the part of the environment or body opposite to the tumor)
- Construction apraxia (if asked to draw a face of a clock, ignoring the side of the clock opposite to the tumor)

Temporal Lobe

Neoplasms of the temporal lobe may cause psychomotor seizures, weakness, visual field deficits (often loss in the upper quadrant opposite the lesion), and memory deficits, most often for recent events. When the dominant side is involved, speech and language deficits are frequent because Wernicke's area is located in the dominant temporal lobe. Psychomotor seizures with visual, auditory, or olfactory hallucinations; automatism; and amnesia for events of the attack can occur. They may begin with an aura of peculiar sensations of the abdomen, epigastrium, or thorax.

Occipital Lobe

Tumors of the occipital lobe are infrequent compared with lesions involving the other cerebral lobes. When neoplasms do occur, the symptoms tend to be associated with vision. Symptoms include homonymous quadrantanopia (loss of vision in one fourth of the visual field), visual hallucinations, and failure to recognize familiar objects.

Pituitary and Hypothalamus Region

The pituitary gland and hypothalamus are closely related by location and endocrine production. Common symptoms resulting from tumors in these areas are visual deficit caused by optic atrophy and paralysis of one or more of the extraocular muscles; headache; and endocrine dysfunction of the pituitary gland with the subsequent precipitation of various syndromes, such as Cushing's syndrome, giantism, acromegaly, and hypopituitarism. In addition, tumors of the hypothalamus can affect fat and carbohydrate metabolism, water balance, sleep patterns, appetite, and sexual drive.

Lateral and Third Ventricles

If the tumor remains small, the patient may be asymptomatic. If the tumor grows into the cerebral hemispheres, deficits will depend on the particular function of the area involved. Tumors that grow within the ventricle may become of sufficient size to obstruct the flow of cerebrospinal fluid (CSF). If this occurs, headache, vomiting, and other symptoms of rapidly increased ICP will be noted. The patient may experience relief of symptoms by changing the position of the head. In this case, the position of the obstructing tumor is altered, thereby allowing the normal CSF flow pattern to be reestablished.

Brain Stem

Tumors of the brain stem may produce multiple symptoms such as lower cranial nerve deficits (swallowing, articulation, gag reflex), motor and sensory deficits, vertigo, hiccups, ataxia, incoordination, nystagmus, dysphagia, nausea, and vomiting throughout the illness. Sudden death can occur from encroachment on vital centers (respiratory or car-

diac arrest). Obstructive hydrocephalus may develop from encroachment on the ventricular system.

Midbrain

Neoplasms of the midbrain are rare. If present, they may result in occlusion of the cerebral aqueducts, cerebellar symptoms if the red nucleus is involved, Parinaud's syndrome (conjugate paralysis of upward gaze) if the quadrigeminal plate is involved, abnormal posturing, and ptosis and diminished light reflex as the tumor enlarges.

Fourth Ventricle

Tumors of the fourth ventricle obstruct the flow of CSF (obstructive hydrocephalus) and infiltrate and compress the brain stem or cerebellum. Headache, vomiting, and nuchal rigidity are common symptoms. Sudden death caused by compression of the cardiorespiratory center is possible. The lower cranial nerves, which control the gag and swallowing reflexes, become impaired, making aspiration a constant concern.

Cerebellum

Growth of a tumor in the cerebellar area is accompanied by cerebellar signs (ataxia, incoordination, nystagmus, vertigo, nausea), obstruction of flow of CSF, and potential for brain stem compression. The usual signs of increased ICP (headache, vomiting, and classical changes in vital signs) are common, particularly with CSF obstruction.

ASSOCIATED INCREASED ICP SIGNS

Many tumors are associated with increased ICP and present with or without localizing signs. They include medulloblastoma, ependymoma of the fourth ventricle, hemangioblastoma of the cerebellum, pinealoma, colloid cyst of the third ventricle, and craniopharyngioma. These tumors are listed in Table 22-2.

The signs and symptoms associated with increased ICP are discussed in Chapter 14. Only papilledema and obstruction of CSF flow, as it relates to brain tumors, are discussed in this section.

Papilledema

Papilledema, seen in about 70% of patients with brain tumors, is associated with visual changes, such as decreased visual acuity, diplopia, and deficits in the visual fields. The visual pathways extend through the four lobes of the cerebral hemispheres. Therefore, it is reasonable to expect a high incidence of visual disturbances with supratentorial lesions. Dysfunction of the abducens nerve (cranial nerve VI), a symptom commonly seen in brain tumor lesions, results in an inability to move the eye outward on the horizontal

(text continues on page 494)

Table 22–2 • BRAIN TUMORS

TYPE OF TUMOR	DESCRIPTION	LOCATION OR DEMOGRAPHIC DATA	SIGNS AND SYMPTOMS	TREATMENT	PROGNOSIS
Common Brain Tumors					
Astrocytoma (grades I and II) Constitutes 25%–30% of all cerebral gliomas	Grade I: well-defined cells Grade II: cell differentiation less defined ↑ Cellularity	Usually found in cerebrum, cerebellum, hypothalamus, optic nerve and chiasma, and pons Cerebral hemisphere tumors most often found in adults 20–40 years	Neurological deficits depend on specific location of tumor and if it is supra- or infratentorial Onset of a focal or generalized seizure in previously seizure-free person is most common first sign	*Surgery:* gross total removal is treatment of choice, but complete removal rarely possible; partial removal may prolong life; tumor recurrence often associated with malignant progression. *Radiation:* controversial; not done for Grade 1	5–6 yr survival on average Range, 2–20 yrs
Anaplastic astrocytoma (grade III)	Cellularity anaplastic: cellular atypia, ↑ mitosis				15–28 mo average survival
Glioblastoma multiforme (GBM) (also known as astrocytoma, grades IV) Constitutes 20% of all intracranial tumors and 55% of all gliomas	Malignant, rapidly growing Composed of heterogeneous cells Necrotic and hemorrhagic areas within tumor common	Usually found in a frontal lobe 40–60 yr most common and with increasing age Male predilection	Memory loss, neurobehavioral changes, seizures, speech deficits, hearing/auditory (H/A), visual deficits Diffuse cerebral symptoms	*Surgery:* resection and debulking to relieve compression and ICP *Radiation* and sometimes *chemotherapy* (BCNU or PCV)	12 mo avg. survival
Astrocytoma of optic nerves and chiasma (spongioblastoma) Most common in children; sometimes seen in young adults	As the tumor grows, it enlarges the optic foramen with little distortion of surrounding structures Slow-growing tumor	Found along the optic nerves Girls > boys, with 2:1 predilection	Early symptoms include Dim vision Hemianopsia Optic atrophy Blindness Proptosis Hypothalamic imbalance	*Surgery:* removal possible but tumor often inaccessible *Radiation:* usually poor response	10 years or more
Ependymoma (low grade and anaplastic) Tumor of childhood and young adults	Arises from lining of ventricles Slow-growing	In ventricles, particularly fourth; can attach itself to roof or floor of ventricle, or grow directly into cerebral hemisphere Seen in children and adults up to 30 y, most often in men Supratentorial more common in adults; infratentorial in children	Rapid elevation in ICP secondary to CSF obstruction S&S vary by location If 4th ventricle, ↓ level of consciousness, severe H/A, VS changes with ↑ ICP, N/V, pupillary changes, hemiplegia, hemiparesthesia, seizures If in cerebellar area, ataxia	*Surgery:* removal if surgically accessible; depends on location *Radiation:* for most *Chemotherapy:* usually not helpful *Shunting procedure:* prn to reduce ↑ ICP from obstructive hydrocephalus	About 5–10 yr, depending on location
Oligodendroglioma (low grade and anaplastic)	Calcification noted on radiological examination in about 50% of patients	Cerebral hemispheres, particularly frontal and temporal lobes Found in patients 20–40 yrs	Depends on location Seizures are first symptoms in 50% of patients	*Surgery, radiation, and chemotherapy*	5–10 yrs, depending on grade

(continued)

▌▌▌ **Table 22–2** • BRAIN TUMORS (Continued)

TYPE OF TUMOR	DESCRIPTION	LOCATION OR DEMOGRAPHIC DATA	SIGNS AND SYMPTOMS	TREATMENT	PROGNOSIS
Mixed gliomas Named for predominant tumor cell present	Composed histologically of two or more cell types of astrocytoma/glioblastoma, oligodendroglioma, or ependymoma in any combination	Any place where various glioma types can be found	Depend on location of tumor	Depends on type of tumor *Surgery, radiation, chemotherapy*	≥5 years or more
Meningioma	Extra-axial tumor arising from dural elements Firm, encapsulated; can erode into bone Have estrogen and progesterone receptors; grow rapidly during pregnancy Slow-growing; can become large before symptoms appear Recur if not completely removed; can become malignant with reoccurrence Compresses brain	Predilection for areas proximal to venous sinuses Most common in women; average age, 50 yrs Parasagittal sinus Lateral convexities Sphenoid ridge Suprasellar Olfactory groove	Neurological deficits caused by compression and depending on area involved Progressive H/A, memory loss, or cognitive changes; paraparesis; seizures; urinary incontinence Gradual development of hemiparesis, speech abnormalities; other related to area of compression Extraocular nerve palsy, proptosis, seizures Bitemporal hemianopsia, optic atrophy, pituitary related hormonal imbalance Anosmia, visual deficits, dementia, pupillary abnormalities	*Surgery:* complete removal, if possible, or partial dissection *Radiation:* after subtotal resection and at tumor recurrence Immunotherapy for atypical meningiomas	"Cure" with total removal Many years with partial excision with radiation
Metastatic brain tumors	20%–40% of cancer patients have metastasis to brain from other parts of the body (lungs, breast, lower GI most common) Spread to brain by blood Usually well differentiated from other brain tissue; lesion may be single or multiple	Can occur anywhere Seen as individual tumor or multiple tumors	Depend on location H/A, paresis, and cognitive deficits most common	*Surgery:* resection if possible, for singular lesion *Radiation:* with multiple lesions Gamma knife radiosurgery (for >3 lesions) Chemotherapy: similar as for primary tumor; methotrexate with oral leucovorin rescue common	Prognosis usually based on primary cancer 1–3+ year avg
Malignant melanomas	Rare	Cerebral hemispheres from a primary lesion in skin	Depend on location	Surgery, radiation, chemotherapy	Few months to few years
Primary cerebral lymphoma	Cellular tumor Behaves much like a glioblastoma Occurs in adults 40–50 y; more common in immunocompromised patients (immunosuppressive therapy for organ transplant or people with AIDS)	May arise in any part of brain May be either monofocal or multifocal	Neurocognitive and personality changes Focal signs or ↑ ICP signs	Radiation followed by Decadron *or* Chemotherapy Both radiation and chemotherapy are effective	After initial response, relapse common; Average survival, 1–4 yrs

▚▚ **Table 22-2** • BRAIN TUMORS (Continued)

TYPE OF TUMOR	DESCRIPTION	LOCATION OR DEMOGRAPHIC DATA	SIGNS AND SYMPTOMS	TREATMENT	PROGNOSIS
Cerebellopontine Angle Tumors (includes several categories of tumors located in this anatomical area)					
Miscellaneous astrocytomas and meningiomas	Can be confused with an acoustic neuroma without visualization Definitive diagnosis made by surgical exposure, biopsy, and histological examination	Cerebellopontine angle	Variation of those seen with acoustic neuroma (see below)	*Surgery:* if possible; difficult surgical access (near vital centers) *Radiation:* may be selected over surgery	Depends on the type of tumor
Acoustic neuroma (schwannoma)	Arises from sheath of Schwann cells Usual size: pea to walnut Considered a benign tumor but located in an often inaccessible area Slow-growing Bilateral tumors are possible; when they occur, they result from a hereditary problem of chromosome 22; the tumors are part of central neurofibromatosis	Seen most often in patients 30–49 yrs Involves vestibular branch of CN VIII *Small tumors* are confined to internal auditory canal and involve CN VIII *Large tumors* extend outside internal auditory meatus *Large tumors* displace CN VII and compress CN V along with CN VIII; they may also encroach on CN IX and CN X, and possibly cerebellum	Depend on size; deficits noted on affected side *Small tumor (confined to internal auditory canal and involving CN VIII) and include:* Tinnitus/vertigo Hearing loss; most notable when using telephone or when source of sound is close to affected ear Dizziness *Large tumor (outside auditory meatus):* S&S listed above and *Facial:* loss of taste on anterior tongue, difficulty closing lower eyelid, facial weakness *Trigeminal:* facial paresthesia/anesthesia, difficulty chewing *Glossopharyngeal and vagus* (difficulty swallowing, hoarseness) *Cerebellar involvement* (ataxia/incoordination, possibly hydrocephalus, ↑ ICP from obstruction of CSF flow secondary to displacement of pons and medulla)	*Surgery:* microsurgical complete removal or debulking of larger tumors (debulking to preserve CNs involved in the tumors) Suboccipital retrosigmoid approach for smaller tumors Translabyrinthine approach for larger tumors With large tumors, the tumor may entwine other cranial nerves that would cause *severe* deficits if tumor were completely excised *Radiation:* focused radiation (proton beam, gamma knife) alternative in older patients; scar tissue a possible problem if later surgery needed. Also used in younger patients	Cure with small tumor and total resection; generally good outcome Tumor regrowth possible if subtotal resection Possible permanent hearing loss, loss of facial sensation on affected side, or facial droop Decreased or absent corneal reflex
Chordoma	Arises from embryonic remnants May appear as a cerebellopontine angle tumor	Predilection M > F Occurs in patients 30–49 yrs Found in clivus (35%) dorsum of sellae to foramen magnum and (50% in sacrococcygeal area)	Loss of vision Extraocular muscle paralysis Paralyzed muscles of swallowing Noted on MRI or CT scan	*Surgery:* excision (approach varies depending on tumor location) *Radiation:* conventional or proton beam	Tumors tend to recur Poor prognosis with aggressive and metastatic tumors

(continued)

Table 22-2 • BRAIN TUMORS (Continued)

TYPE OF TUMOR	DESCRIPTION	LOCATION OR DEMOGRAPHIC DATA	SIGNS AND SYMPTOMS	TREATMENT	PROGNOSIS
Pituitary Tumors					

Pituitary adenomas*
Classified by type of:
  Hormones secreted
  Effects (functioning
    or nonfunctioning)
  Grade of sella tur-
    cica enlargement
    or erosion
  Suprasellar extension
	Hormone(s) secreted
	  Prolactin (most
	    common)
	  Growth hormone
	  ACTH
	  Nonfunctioning:
	    produce S&S from
	    compression of
	    adjacent structures
	    (e.g., optic nerves,
	    bitemporal
	    hemianopsia)
	    Functioning (hor-
	    mone-secreting):
	    cause endocrine
	    syndromes (e.g.,
	    acromegaly)
	Enclosed adenomas:
	  I—sella normal;
	    floor may be
	    indented
	  II—sella enlarged,
	    floor intact
	  III—invasive adeno-
	    mas; localized ero-
	    sion of the floor
	  IV—entire floor dif-
	    fusely eroded
	Classified A–D by su-
	  prasellar extension
	  A: No suprasellar
	    extension
	  B: Suprasellar bulge
	    does not reach
	    floor of 3rd
	    ventricle
	  C: Tumor reaches
	    3rd ventricle, dis-
	    torting chiasmatic
	    recess
	  D: Tumor fills 3rd
	    ventricle almost to
	    foramen of Munro
		Most pituitary tu-
		  mors in anterior
		  lobe
		Both lobes can be
		  damaged from
		  compression of
		  parasellar tumors
			In general:
			  Visual disorders (di-
			    minished vision
			    with a scotoma;
			    bitemporal
			    hemianopsia)
			  Paresis of extraocu-
			    lar muscles
			  H/A
			  Various endocrine
			    disorders (see
			    below)
			  Abnormal sella tur-
			    cica region on CT
			    scan
			Endocrine disorders:
			Prolactin-secreting
			  adenoma
			  Galactorrhea
			  Amenorrhea
			  Infertility
			  Loss of pubic hair
			  Impotence
			  ↑ Serum prolactin
			ACTH-secreting
			  adenoma
			  Adrenal hyperplasia
			  Cushing's
			    syndrome*
			Growth hormone–
			  secreting adenoma
			  Giantism before pu-
			    berty or closure of
			    epiphyses
			  Acromegaly after
			    puberty or closure
			    of epiphyses (en-
			    larged jaw, nose,
			    tongue, hands,
			    feet)
			  Thickening of soft
			    tissue of face
			  Enlarged heart and
			    pulmonary disease
			  Diabetes mellitus
			  Serum growth hor-
			    mone levels >10
			    ng/mL
			Serious complications:
			Pituitary apoplexy
			  syndrome: acute on-
			  set of ophthalmople-
			  gia, blindness,
			  drowsiness, and
			  coma; death possible
				Depends on the size
				  and type of the
				  tumor, patient's
				  age, and endocrine
				  and visual deficits;
				  surgery, radiation,
				  or drug therapy
				  separately or in
				  combination
				Surgery:
				  For smaller tu-
				    mors, transsphe-
				    noidal microsur-
				    gery to remove
				    total tumor and
				    preseve or nor-
				    malize pituitary
				Radiation: Conven-
				  tional radiation
				  therapy or proton
				  beam, if available
				Hormonal replacement:
				  Postsurgery, hor-
				  monal replacement
				  possible
				Other drug treatment:
				  Bromocriptine
				  may be used to
				  inhibit prolactin;
				  for some patients,
				  this is only treat-
				  ment necessary for
				  prolactin-secreting
				  tumors
					Curable with
					  complete
					  resection
					In others, very
					  good out-
					  come

▌▌▌ **T a b l e   2 2 – 2** • BRAIN TUMORS (Continued)

TYPE OF TUMOR	DESCRIPTION	LOCATION OR DEMOGRAPHIC DATA	SIGNS AND SYMPTOMS	TREATMENT	PROGNOSIS
Developmental Tumors (seen sometimes in adults)					
Craniopharyngioma	Thought to arise from Rathke's pouch Solid or cystic tumors Can compress the pituitary and may even amputate the pituitary stalk About 75% with calcified areas Tumor growth is directed upward, resulting in invagination of the 3rd ventricle and possible blockage of CSF flow Optic chiasm elevated by tumor, resulting in traction on optic nerves	In or about the sella pituitary area Usually affects children	Signs and symptoms of grossly ↑ ICP because of CSF flow blockage Pituitary or hypothalamic dysfunction Visual disturbance	*Surgery:* resection by intracranial or transsphenoidal approach *Radiation:* after surgery; tumor radiosensitive	Excellent if tumor is excised with microsurgery, cure rate, 80% Recurrence if only subtotal resection performed, even with radiation
Epidermoid and dermoid cysts	Cysts of congenital origin arising from the ectodermal layer; cysts lined with stratified squamous epithelium Epidermoid cysts contain keratin, cellular debris, and cholesterol; dermoid cysts contain hair and sebaceous glands	On bones of skull or within brain	Depends on location	*Surgery:* complete removal is usually possible	Very good
Genetically Related Autosomal Dominant Diseases					
Von Recklinghausen's disease (neurofibromatosis)	Genetic origin because of autosomal dominant mendelian trait Skin, nervous system, bones, endocrine glands, and other organs are sites of congenital anomalies, in addition to the multiple tumors of skin Firm, encapsulated lesions attach to the nerve	Benign, multiple, circumscribed dermal and neural tumors with increased skin pigmentation (cosmetically offensive) Tumors late in childhood or in early adolescence	Spots of hyperpigmentation (café au lait) and cutaneous and subcutaneous tumors	*Surgery:* possible, depending on the location of the tumor *Radiation:* tumor is radioresistant	Depends on involved area
Hemangioblastoma (with von Hippel-Lindau disease)	Vascular tumor Slow-growing	Cerebellum (as a single or multiple lesion); less common in the medulla and cerebral hemispheres; tumor in adults	Dizziness Unilateral ataxia Signs and symptoms of ↑ ICP Possible spinal cord involvement	*Surgery:* complete removal, if possible *Radiation:* with recurrence	Usually curable

(ICP, intracranial pressure; CN, cranial nerve; CSF, cerebrospinal fluid; GI, gastrointestinal; CT, computed tomography; AIDS, acquired immunodeficiency syndrome; MRI, magnetic resonance imaging; ACTH, adrenocorticotropic hormone; H/A, headache; VS, vital signs; S&S, signs and symptoms; N&V, nausea and vomiting.)

* Cushing's syndrome comprises moon facies, "buffalo hump," abdominal striae, pendulous abdomen; ecchymosis, hypertension, muscle weakness, osteoporosis, and high cortisol levels.

plane. It is common that deterioration in vision is the main reason for referral to a neurologist by an optometrist or ophthalmologist, provided that the first examiner recognized the visual deficits as possibly being related to an intracranial lesion.

Obstruction to Flow of Cerebrospinal Fluid

Tumor encroachment from within or outside the ventricles or subarachnoid space interferes with the normal flow of CSF. This obstruction of CSF results in obstructive hydrocephalus. If the tumor encroachment occurs slowly, the development of hydrocephalus will be gradual. However, rapid tumor growth produces acute precipitation of signs and symptoms, such as a massive spike in ICP with rapid deterioration in neurological status.

▥ APPROACH TO THE PATIENT WITH A BRAIN TUMOR

Patients and families going through the process of diagnosis and treatment of a brain tumor have multiple needs that can only be met by a collaborative interdisciplinary team of health care professionals who are knowledgeable about the disease. A partnership must be formed among the patient, family, and team to work together to create the best plan for the individual patient. There is an ongoing need for patient and family education as the patient's trajectory progresses through the various stages of illness. Education provided in a supportive, honest environment empowers the patient and family to take control of the illness by making informed decisions. Through this process, good communication among the interdisciplinary team provides the support structure to assist the patient with the holistic impact of the illness.

Several potential collaborative problems should be addressed by the interdisciplinary team. Among potential neurological complications related to a brain tumor are increased ICP, seizures, hydrocephalus, cranial nerve impairment, paresis/paralysis, and peripheral nerve impairment. Other body systems are at risk for complications related to treatment options such as sepsis, myelosuppression, gastric ulcer, and electrolyte imbalance. These more common problems seen in patients along the continuum of illness, as well as less common problems, require interdisciplinary effort for successful management.

Diagnosis

The clinical manifestations of brain tumors span a wide range of signs and symptoms, depending on the type, size, and location of the tumor. After a neurological examination, magnetic resonance imaging (MRI) or computed tomography (CT) with and without gadolinium contrast is the procedure of choice for imaging all types of brain tumors. There are many reasons to recommend MRI: it has high sensitivity; it can identify small tumors located near bone, especially in the posterior fossa, pituitary fossa, internal auditory canal, and floor of the middle cranial fossa; it can identify cerebral edema accurately; and it can differentiate low-grade and high-grade tumors, in most instances.[17] It is relatively easy to acquire multiplanar images that provide accurate localization and identification of the tumor without loss of detail (Fig. 22-3 to 22-10).[18] A CT scan provides satisfactory imaging in patients who have contraindications for an MRI, such as those with a pacemaker, who are claustrophobic, or who need rapid screening. The CT should be done with and without gadolinium contrast. In most instances, MRI, or sometimes CT, is the only necessary test to diagnose a brain tumor.

For tumors around the optic chiasm such as pituitary tumors or gliomas, careful mapping of the visual fields by an ophthalmologist is necessary to determine the degree of visual deficits. With cerebellopontine angle tumors, such as

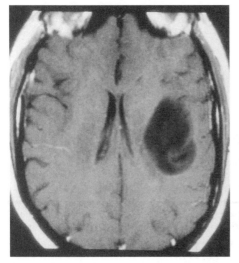

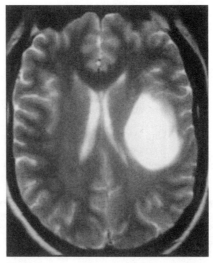

A   B

Figure 22–3 • Low-grade astrocytoma. (*A*) Axial post-contrast T1-weighted MR image shows low-grade nonenhancing astrocytoma in the left temporal region. (*B*) Corresponding T2-weighted image shows well-defined margins and absence of surrounding edema. There is little mass effect.

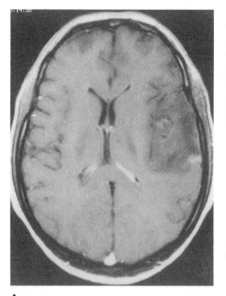 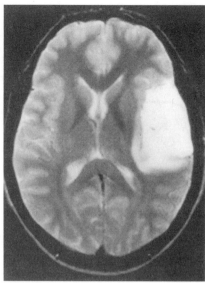

Figure 22–4 • Anaplastic astrocytoma. (*A*) Axial post-contrast T1-weighted MR image shows left insular anaplastic astrocytoma with ill-defined margins and patchy enhancement. There is no obvious necrosis. (*B*) Corresponding T2-weighted image shows the tumor to have ill-defined margins.

A   **B**

acoustic neuromas, audiometric studies are helpful in determining the degree of hearing loss.

Endocrine studies (blood and urine levels of hormones controlled by the pituitary gland) are helpful when a pituitary adenoma or a craniopharyngioma is suspected. Common tests and their normal values are found in Table 22-3.

After a brain lesion has been identified, surgery is required to make an accurate diagnosis. In almost all patients, a biopsy is attempted using CT-guided and/or MRI-guided techniques. The biopsy identifies the specific tumor type and grade, information necessary in making appropriate treatment decisions. Biopsy is not recommended for vascular tumors or tumors in the brain stem for fear of precipitating hemorrhage or respiratory distress. In the case of brain-stem

tumors, they tend to be grade II or III astrocytomas and are not resectable because of location.[12]

Medical Treatment

After the diagnosis of a brain tumor is established, the next major consideration is medical management. The three general methods for treatment of brain tumors are surgery, radiation, and chemotherapy alone or in combination. The variables that are considered when selecting appropriate treatment include the type and grade of tumor, its location and size, surgical accessibility, presenting signs and symptoms, and the general condition of the patient. Informed consent for treatment must include the patient in the decision-making process.

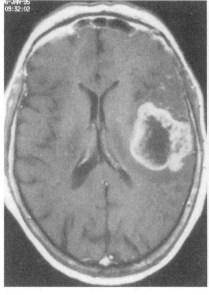 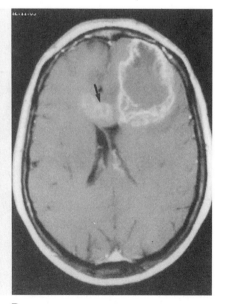

Figure 22–5 • Glioblastoma multiforme. (*A*) Axial post-contrast T1-weighted MR image shows glioblastoma multiforme (GBM) in the left temporal lobe. Note irregular and thick ring enhancement. There is central necrosis. (*B*) Axial post-contrast T1-weighted MR image shows large and irregular enhancing GBM in the left frontal lobe with extension across the genu of the corpus callosum (*arrow*).

A   **B**

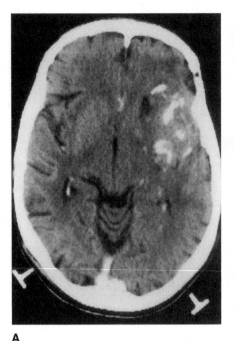

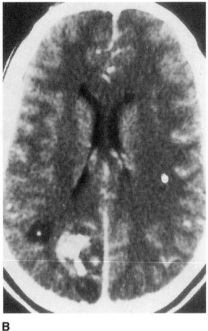

Figure 22–6 • Oligodendroglioma. (*A*) Axial post-contrast CT scan shows an oligodendroglioma with multiple calcifications in the left frontotemporal region. (*B*) Post-contrast CT scan shows heavily calcified oligodendroglioma in the medial left occipital lobe. There is a tumor cyst lateral to the calcification.

General Drug Therapy

Most patients benefit from administration of corticosteroids (dexamethasone, prednisone, or methylprednisolone) to decrease cerebral edema. The reversal of symptoms can be remarkable. In the case of a CNS lymphoma, complete resolution of the enhancing tumor on scan can occur within weeks of initiating corticosteroids (although this is often a transient effect). A corticosteroid is usually begun when the tumor is diagnosed and the presence of cerebral edema and increased ICP is confirmed. If surgery is recommended, dexamethasone is administered preoperatively, continued postoperatively, and during radiation therapy to control radiation-induced edema. Known side effects of steroid therapy include gastritis, peptic ulcer disease, alterations in healing, increased blood glucose levels, fluid retention, Cushing's

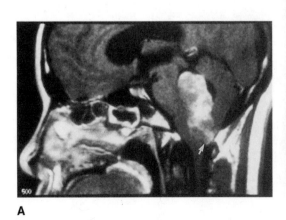

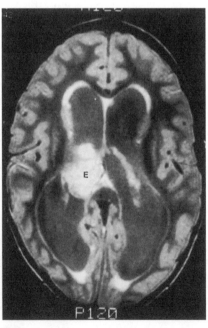

Figure 22–7 • Ependymoma. (*A*) Midsagittal post-contrast T1-weighted MR image shows enhancing ependymoma in the fourth ventricle. The tumor extrudes (*arrow*) through the foramen of Magendie. (*B*) Proton density image shows ependymoma (*E*) inside the right lateral ventricle.

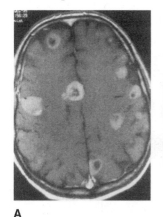
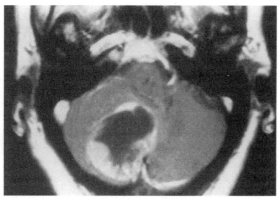

Figure 22–8 • Metastatic tumors. (*A*) Axial post-contrast T1-weighted MR image shows multiple enhancing metastases (breast primary) at the gray-white junctions. (*B*) Axial post-contrast T1-weighted MR image of a different patient shows single necrotic metastasis from squamous cell carcinoma of the lung.

A

B

syndrome (most commonly called "moon face" and "buffalo hump"), and corticosteroid-induced proximal myopathy. An H2 blocker (e.g., famotidine [Pepcid] or ranitidine [Zantac]) must be administered concurrently with corticosteroids to prevent gastric irritation.

Most patients with supratentorial lesions will be placed on an anticonvulsant drug to prevent seizures, and phenytoin and carbamazepine are often the drugs of choice. If the patient is to be treated with chemotherapy, phenytoin should be used, because carbamazepine can potentiate thrombocytopenia associated with chemotherapeutic therapy. In some instances, a combination of two or three anticonvulsants is necessary to achieve seizure control. Phenobarbital and gabapentin (Neurontin) can both be added to the primary anticonvulsant for this purpose. Proper dosing and knowledge of signs of toxicity are important, because a toxic phenytoin level can mimic signs of increased tumor growth.

Surgery

In most instances, surgical biopsy is the first step in an accurate diagnosis of a brain tumor. Examination of the tissue by the pathologist will identify the tumor histological type and grade, thus assisting in selecting treatment options and determining prognosis. In addition, location and surgical accessibility must be considered. A surgically accessible tumor is one that can be removed without causing severe neurological damage to adjacent tissue. In most cases, surgical removal or "debulking" of as much tumor as possible is the first step in treating a brain tumor. There are several reasons for this approach. First, because all of the cells of the tumor are not of the same grade (i.e., heterogeneous), the biopsy sample may have underestimated the aggressiveness and malignancy of the tumor. Second, the debulking of the tumor can rapidly relieve symptoms related to mass effect and increased ICP. Third, when the remaining postsurgical tumor is as small as possible, further treatment is more

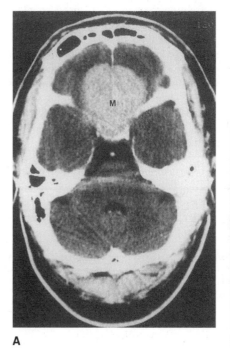
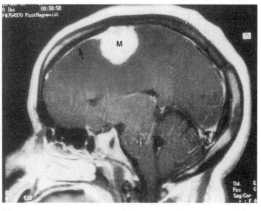

A

B

Figure 22–9 • Meningioma. (*A*) Contrast-enhanced CT scan shows large frontobasal meningioma (*M*). (*B*) Parasagittal post-contrast T1-weighted MR image shows parafalcine meningioma (*M*) with dural tail (*arrow*) of enhancement. There is surrounding edema.

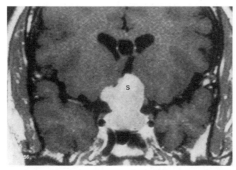

Figure 22–10 • Pituitary adenoma. Coronal post-contrast T1-weighted MR image shows macroadenoma with typical figure-of-eight shape and suprasellar (*s*) extension.

effective. Fourth, more extensive debulking or resection in symptomatic lesions usually results in rapid clinical improvement.

Several surgical options are available.[12] In some cases, complete tumor removal is possible, achieving a surgical "cure." This is true for many benign tumors such as juvenile pilocytic astrocytomas and meningiomas (as long as they have not encroached around the optic nerves or tracts). A complete surgical resection may be the only therapy necessary, thus avoiding the need for radiotherapy, which can have long-term negative effects, particularly on children and the elderly. Some tumors, although histologically benign, cannot be completely removed; nonetheless, even a partial resection will relieve symptoms temporarily. If the tumor is a slow-growing neoplasm, such as a meningioma, the patient may be asymptomatic for years. In other situations, nonsurgical treatment may be very effective and further surgery beyond a biopsy to establish the specific tumor type and grade will not be necessary to relieve symptoms or extend survival. For example, primary CNS lymphomas have responded well to chemotherapy and radiotherapy without surgery. Finally, in more malignant tumor forms, there appears to be a relationship between the extent of tumor resection and length of survival, although many unanswered questions still exist. Currently, neurosurgical and imaging techniques provide a safe means of partial or complete resection with a complication rate of less than 5% for most tumors.

A craniotomy, either above or below the tentorium, is the surgical procedure most patients undergo. A bone flap is created by removing a portion of bone from the skull, allowing access to the dura, which can be opened. The tumor is either partially or completely resected and the bone flap replaced. Current technologies, such as stereotaxis and other image-guided systems, allow neurosurgeons to localize a tumor and other anatomical sites precisely. By identifying the margins of the tumor, surgery is minimally invasive and normal tissue preserved. Stereotaxis uses a computer to create a three-dimensional map of the tumor from CT or MRI information. Intraoperative MRI also enables increased accuracy in resection. Stereotaxis is combined with microsurgical technology. Microsurgery enhances the neurosurgeon's visualization of the operative field through high-powered magnification. Ultrasonic aspirators combine two actions: high-frequency sound waves to break up the tumor and an aspirator to suction away the tumor fragments. La-

sers, alone or in combination with conventional surgery, provide a beam of concentrated light energy capable of destroying tissue. A laser is useful for complete resection of a tumor, or it may be used in combination with partial surgical resection.[19]

Other technologies allow treatment of tumors previously inaccessible to neurosurgeons such as those deep in the brain, those located on the motor strip or speech areas, or those at the base of the skull. Evoked potential electrophysiological mapping of the brain's cortical surface is useful to measure electrical potential of nerves in response to stimulation with small electrodes. Surgery can also be conducted under local anesthesia with brain-mapping techniques to allow for removal of tumors from the speech and motor areas. Finally, tumors at the base of the skull can now be successfully removed through the collaborative efforts of ear, nose, and throat (ENT) specialists, plastic surgeons, and neurosurgeons optimizing their skill and knowledge with available technology. See Chapter 15 for management of neurosurgical patients.

Radiation Therapy

Radiation therapy is the second major option in the treatment of most brain tumors, whether they are benign or malignant. The objective of radiation therapy is to destroy tumor cells without injuring normal cells. Tumor cells are more radiosensitive than normal cells. Damage to DNA is the mechanism by which radiation destroys tumor cells. Large numbers of hypoxic tumor cells are present in the core of malignant tumors. These cells are more resistant to the DNA-damaging effects of radiation, which may explain why radiation has a time-limited beneficial effect for malignant tumors.

Planning is essential in controlling both the short-term and long-term complications of radiation. Three-dimensional treatment planning is used to maximize radiation dose to the tumor and limit radiation damage to the adjacent area to spare healthy tissue. (See Chap. 15 for discussion of stereotactic procedures.) Whole-brain radiation is not recommended for most patients with primary astrocytic tumors, although it is used for medulloblastoma and primary CNS lymphoma. Data from the CT scan are used for dose calculation, but an MRI is necessary to identify tumor margins.[12]

In most cases, surgery is used for initial diagnosis and resection of as much tumor as possible. Radiation therapy is

Table 22–3 • COMMON TESTS FOR PATIENTS WITH SUSPECTED PITUITARY TUMORS

HORMONE	NORMS FOR WOMEN	NORMS FOR MEN
Prolactin	Premenopausal women: 2.2–19.2 mEq/L Postmenopausal women: 1.0–12.8 mEq/L	Men: 1.9–11.7 mEq/L
Growth hormone	Women: 0–30 ng/mL	Men: 0–8 ng/mL
Cortisol	6:00 to 8:00 AM: 10–25 g/L	Same

then employed to target the residual tumor with the goal of reducing or stabilizing its size. For malignant lesions, resection is never complete. Even if all visible tumor has been resected, there is usually microscopic seeding into normal adjacent tissue. Therefore, a course of postoperative radiation therapy is recommended to prevent or delay recurrent growth. Radiotherapy is usually recommended postoperatively for some benign tumors that have undergone subtotal resection and may be life threatening if growth continues. Other benign brain tumors may be treated with radiation to prevent recurrence.

Patients usually receive dexamethasone when radiation therapy is provided. The steroid helps to control the cerebral edema that often occurs with radiation. In addition, H2 blockers are given to protect the stomach from irritation and prevent gastric bleeding related to steroid use.

Various options may be used to deliver radiation therapy. Standard radiation therapy and, more recently, hyperfractionation are the cornerstones of radiation therapy. Several newer forms of radiation used are stereotactic radiosurgery, interstitial brachytherapy, and stereotactic radiotherapy. Each is briefly discussed.

Standard Radiation Therapy. Standard fractionated external beam radiation therapy uses x-rays or gamma rays to destroy tumor cells. With a conventional radiation protocol, the amount of radiation is based on individual differences previously cited. The total radiation dose varies depending on the tumor's histological type, location, radioresponsiveness, and tolerance of the patient. The total radiation dose ranges from 4 to 6 Gy in daily fractions of 150 to 200cGy to the tumor plus a 2-cm margin for malignant lesions and is administered over 4 to 8 weeks.[20] Radiation for lower-grade gliomas prolongs survival. Use of radiation therapy after surgical resection is unquestionably the standard of care and doubles the survival rate for patients with anaplastic astrocytomas and glioblastoma multiforme. Radiation therapy is useful to prevent recurrence of benign tumors (i.e., meningiomas, acoustic neuroma). Corticosteroids are given during radiation therapy to control cerebral edema associated with treatment.

Hyperfractionation. The biological effect of radiation depends not only on the total dose, but also on the time course in which it is given. Therefore, the fractionation plan and the dosage are important to the biological effect. Hyperfractionation is a modified version of traditional radiation therapy.[20] This protocol provides smaller, more frequent daily doses (fractions) of radiation for a specified length of time for tumors resistant to standard radiation therapy plans. This means that radiation is given two to three times a day for the prescribed length of time. The advantage of hyperfractionation is that it allows for a higher overall dose to be given without necessarily increasing the risk to normal brain tissue.[12]

Stereotactic Radiosurgery. Stereotactic radiosurgery is a system that uses focused radiation with a sophisticated planning system in a *single dose*. The term **radiosurgery** is misleading because it does not involve surgery. The initial technique, developed by Lars Leksell, allows multiple source beams (more than 200) to converge on a small, targeted focus to deliver a calculated radiation dose.[21] Various instrumentations have been designed to accomplish this goal.

The first system uses a *linear accelerator (LINAC)*. Using the linear accelerator, non-coplanar arcs are produced to deliver the radiation focused on the tumor target. The second system is the *gamma knife* (not a knife as suggested by the name). The gamma knife uses multiple point sources of gamma radiation from cobalt 60 to converge on one focused area.[22] The third system, proton beam radiation, uses a cyclotron to deliver high-energy proton beams (positively charged atomic particles) to a focused area. The linear accelerator and gamma knife technologies are available at many centers, but the cyclotron is available in only two locations (Massachusetts and California).

Stereotactic radiosurgery is useful to treat small tumors (i.e., those smaller than 4 cm) located deep in the brain that were previously considered inoperable. It is being used increasingly to treat small metastatic brain tumors in people who are otherwise doing well. Stereotactic radiosurgery is also useful to radiate small residual tumor areas after surgery or as a boost for conventional radiotherapy.[19] The risk of radiation injury must be considered. The larger the tumor treated, the greater will be the chance of symptomatic cell necrosis. That is why small tumors are best treated with this technique.

Interstitial Brachytherapy. For brachytherapy, radioactive "seeds" are implanted in the tumor bed using stereotactic techniques. The radiation source can be implanted on a temporary or permanent basis. For temporary therapy, *high-activity* iodine 125 sources are implanted at surgery or in a separate procedure under local anesthesia. The required dose is carefully calculated, and the radiation sources are removed in 4 to 5 days. The procedure is generally low risk and well tolerated. However, there is a late effect in which the patient becomes symptomatic as a result of tissue necrosis. Brain tissue has a low capacity to remove dead tissue, cell debris, fluid, and drugs because there is no lymphatic drainage in the brain. About 40% of patients require surgical removal of the necrotic cerebral tissue in 6 months to 2 years.[23]

Stereotactic Radiotherapy. Stereotactic radiotherapy combines stereotactic focused radiation with multiple fraction (small, daily) doses.[20] It is used with radiosensitive tumors such as meningiomas and craniopharyngiomas.

Responses to Radiation Therapy. Unfortunately, not all patients respond well to radiation therapy. Failure to completely annihilate malignant cells is the problem. This failure is attributed, in part, to the presence of hypoxic cells. Hypoxic cells are approximately three times more resistant to radiation than are well-oxygenated cells[24] and can remain viable after radiation therapy. The use of radiosensitizer drugs—drugs that make tumor tissue more sensitive to radiation—is currently being explored. Etanidazole and tirapazamine are two drugs designed to make poorly oxygenated cells in the center of a tumor more sensitive to radiation therapy. The limiting factor in the use of radiation therapy is cerebral cell intolerance with resulting necrosis.

Side effects from radiation depend on location, total dose administered, and the technique used to provide radiation. The most common side effects of radiation in the acute phase are somnolence, hair loss, and skin disorders. Chronic side effects include loss of pituitary function, diminished intellectual function, hydrocephalus, and, less commonly, cerebral necrosis. In addition to follow-up for recurrence of the tumor, neuropsychological testing and endocrine evaluation may be helpful.

Chemotherapy

Chemotherapy is most often used as part of a multimodal approach together with surgery and radiation. It may be given before, during, or after radiation therapy or at the time of tumor recurrence. Chemotherapeutic drugs work by interfering with the transmission of genetic information necessary for cellular replication. Rapidly dividing cells, such as malignant cells, are targeted. One method used to classify chemotherapeutic drugs has been by cell cycle, that is, cell cycle–specific agents (only active during certain phases of the cell's life cycle) and cell cycle–nonspecific agents (effective during all phases of the cell cycle). Some treatment protocols combine both categories of drugs to be effective against the maximum number of malignant cells. Although chemotherapy has been the mainstay of treatment for various malignancies in other body systems, its use in brain tumor treatment has had limited success because of the blood-brain barrier, which is a network of blood vessels and cells that protect the brain and prevent certain molecules from passing through the cellular barrier. If chemotherapeutic drugs cannot be delivered to the focus of need, they will not be effective in killing the targeted tumor cells. A major challenge in brain tumor chemotherapy research has been to find drugs that will cross the blood-brain barrier without causing neurological injury to normal cells.

Chemotherapeutic Drugs

The most commonly used chemotherapeutic drugs are alkylating agents, particularly the nitrosoureas. Carmustine (BCNU), lomustine (CCNU), Gliadel wafers (i.e., carmustine), procarbazine, or a combination of procarbazine, CCNU, and vincristine (PCV) are frequently used. Given that many malignant tumors have heterogeneous cells with varied vulnerability to the same drug, a combination of drugs is sometimes used. The mainstay of drugs for brain tumor chemotherapy has been the same for many years. However, in 1999, the U. S. Food and Drug Administration (FDA) approved temozolomide (Temodar), the first new chemotherapeutic drug for recurrent brain cancer in 20 years.

Most chemotherapeutic drugs are administered by the intravenous or oral route. More recently the interstitial, intra-arterial, and intrathecal routes have become options, depending on the particular drug. These newer routes allow increased drug dosage, increasing the attack on malignant cells while limiting side effects. By focusing the delivery of the drug to a specific site, less of the drug spreads to other organs of the body, thus reducing toxicity. With *interstitial*

administration, disc-shaped wafers impregnated with a biodegradable chemotherapeutic drug are placed directly into the surgical cavity after a tumor is removed to provide slow, direct drug to the tumor site without the drug spreading elsewhere in the body. The *intra-arterial* route helps to focus the chemotherapeutic agent as compared with an intravenous infusion in which the drug is mixed into the general circulation. *Intrathecal infusion* delivers a chemotherapeutic agent directly into the spinal fluid. This method has been used to treat some brain, spinal cord, and metastatic tumors.

The acute side effects of chemotherapy include anemia, leukopenia, thrombocytopenia, nausea, vomiting, and fatigue. The long-term effects are neurotoxic, hepatic, and pulmonary. The dosage of a drug is limited by potential toxicity to normal cells, called *dose-limiting toxicity*. Special concerns when treating a malignant lesion of the brain using chemotherapeutic agents include the following: cerebral edema affects drug entry into the tumor; drug resistance can occur; and the heterogeneity of tumor cells results in different chemosensitivity among cells within the same tumor.[25]

The major chemotherapeutic drugs are briefly discussed in the next section and also summarized in Table 22-4. Patients receive routine drugs along with the chemotherapeutic agent. Expect that the patient will receive intravenous hydrating agents and anticonvulsants, dexamethasone, and an H2 blocker. A diuretic, such as furosemide, is often given after the chemotherapeutic protocol is completed. See the discussion of drugs earlier in this chapter in the treatment section.

BCNU (carmustine) is a synthetic alkylating agent and nitrosourea approved by the FDA in 1977 for primary brain tumors that cross the blood-brain barrier. It has been the standard, first-line treatment for glioblastoma multiforme for many years. The action of BCNU is that of alkylating DNA and RNA and inhibiting several enzymatic processes of amino acids and proteins. BCNU is available as an intravenous preparation and, more recently, as a drug-impregnated biodegradable wafer (Gliadel; see discussion of Gliadel Wafers below). The dosage varies depending on whether BCNU is being administered alone or in combination with other chemotherapeutic agents. As a single agent in previously untreated patients, the recommended dosage is 150 to 200 mg as a single intravenous dose every 6 weeks. The most common and severe toxic side effects are bone marrow suppression, anemia, diarrhea, thrombocytopenia, leukopenia, kidney damage, pulmonary toxicity, stomatitis, and swallowing difficulty.[26] Therefore, complete blood count (CBC), blood urea nitrogen (BUN), creatinine, and close monitoring for adverse signs and symptoms are necessary. Possible adverse reactions are numerous and varied. Pulmonary toxicity in the form of fibrosis is a dose-related possible long-term effect. Patients complain about extreme fatigue.

BCNU and CCNU are closely related. The drug actions, side effects, and adverse reactions are similar except that pulmonary fibrosis is less common in CCNU. To counteract the unacceptable effects on bone marrow, some centers use a combination of high-dose chemotherapy with autologous bone marrow transplantation to protect the bone marrow.

CCNU (lomustine) is a synthetic alkylating agent and nitrosourea approved by the FDA in 1977 for therapy of brain tumors and Hodgkin's disease.[27] The action of CCNU is that of alkylating DNA and RNA and inhibiting several

Table 22-4 • CHEMOTHERAPEUTIC DRUGS COMMONLY USED TO TREAT BRAIN TUMORS

DRUG AND CLASSIFICATION	EARLY OR DELAYED TOXICITY	LABORATORY MONITORING	NURSING RESPONSIBILITIES

Carmustine (BCNU)
Major drug used in treatment of malignant brain tumors
Cell-cycle nonspecific
Nitrosoureas: causes breaks and cross-linking in DNA strands
Crosses BBB
	Early
	  Nausea and vomiting
	  Local phlebitis
	Delayed
	  Bone marrow depression in 3–6 wk
	  Pulmonary fibrosis (may be irreversible) with doses >200 mg/m² IV
	  Renal and liver damage
	  Veno-occlusive disease (hepatic or pulmonary) with high doses
		Baseline data
		  Weekly monitoring of CBC and BUN, creatinine, uric acid, SGOT, SGPT, and alkaline phosphatase levels
		  Periodic chest x-ray studies
			Administer antiemetics before and during drug administration.
			Apply ice to puncture site.
			Protect the patient from and monitor for infections.
			Monitor for respiratory, liver, and kidney dysfunction.

Lomustine (CCNU)
Cell cycle nonspecific
Nitrosourea
Similar to BCNU
	Early
	  Nausea and vomiting
	Delayed
	  Bone marrow depression (may be prolonged)
	  Elevated AST level
	  Pulmonary fibrosis
	  Renal damage
		Baseline data
		Same as for BCNU
			Same as for BCNU

Cisplatin (Platinol)
Heavy metal compound
Exact mechanism of action unknown; appears to bind DNA
Cell cycle nonspecific
	Early
	  Nausea and vomiting
	  Anaphylactic reactions
	  Fever
	  Electrolyte imbalances
	Delayed
	  Renal damage
	  Ototoxicity
	  Peripheral neuropathy
	  Bone marrow depression
	  Electrolyte imbalance
	  Hypocalcemia
		Baseline data
		Weekly monitoring of CBC and BUN, creatinine, electrolyte, and calcium levels
			Administer antiemetics as necessary.
			Hydrate well
			Monitor intake and output
			Assess for hearing loss
			Assess for numbness or tingling of fingers and toes
			Monitor hearing
			Monitor the patient for electrolyte imbalance

Procarbazine hydrochloride
Exact mechanism of action is unclear; probably inhibits protein, RNA, and DNA synthesis
Given orally
Rapidly absorbed
Crosses BBB
	Early
	  Nausea and vomiting
	  CNS depression
	Delayed
	  Bone marrow depression
	  Stomatitis
	  Peripheral neuropathy
	  Pneumonia
	  Interaction with tyramine in food: hypertensive crisis
		Baseline data
		CBC monitored weekly
		Chest x-ray studies
			This is usually given as 28-d course (usually for first 72 h)
			Administer antiemetics as necessary
			Monitor for signs of neurotoxicity
			Monitor the patient for and protection from infection
			Teach avoidance of foods high in tyramine (e.g., beer, ripe and aged cheeses).
			Teach avoidance of alcohol consumption (can cause severe GI toxicity because of Antabuse-like drug activity).
			Provide for special mouth care.
			Monitor peripheral nerve function.
			Monitor patient for respiratory problems.

Etoposide (VePesid)
Also called VP16
Cell-cycle nonspecific
Appears to interfere with synthesis of DNA or RNA
	Early
	  Nausea and vomiting
	  Red urine (not hematuria)
	  Diarrhea
	  Fever
	  Hypotension
	Delayed
	  Bone marrow depression
	  Alopecia
	  Peripheral neuropathy
	  Mucositis
	  Hepatic damage
		Urinalysis
		CBC, AST and ALT levels monitored weekly
			Administer antiemetics as necessary.
			Monitor vital signs
			Monitor the color of the urine
			Monitor patient for, and protect from, infection.
			Prepare patient mentally for hair loss; support positive body image.
			Monitor peripheral nerve function.

(continued)

Table 22-4 • CHEMOTHERAPEUTIC DRUGS COMMONLY USED TO TREAT BRAIN TUMORS (Continued)

DRUG AND CLASSIFICATION	EARLY OR DELAYED TOXICITY	LABORATORY MONITORING	NURSING RESPONSIBILITIES
Vincristine Plant alkaloid Inhibits mitosis Does not cross BBB Given IV Excreted by liver in bile	*Early* Leukopenia Neuritic pain Constipation *Late* Hair loss	CBC	Interacts with many drugs; consult pharmacists or other resources to determine possible interactions. Monitor blood levels of anticonvulsants (drug interaction with vincristine, which lowers blood level).
Temozolomide (Temodar/Temodal) First oral chemotherapeutic drug that crosses BBB Interferes with tumor growth	*Early* Nausea Vomiting Headache *Late* ↓ WBC Fatigue	CBC —	Provide antiemetic as needed. Monitor and treat headache. Monitor WBC. Protect from infection. Assist patient in developing strategies for fatigue.

CBC, complete blood count; BBB, blood-brain barrier; IV, intravenous; BUN, blood urea nitrogen; AST, aspartate aminotransferase; WBC, white blood cells; GI, gastrointestinal; CNS, central nervous system; ALT, alanine aminotransferase.

enzymatic processes of amino acids and proteins. The drug is administered orally and is excreted in 24 hours. It crosses the blood-brain barrier. The dosage varies depending on whether CCNU is being administered alone or in combination with other chemotherapeutic agents. As a single agent in previously untreated patients, the recommended dosage is 130 mg as a single oral dose every 6 weeks. The side effects are similar to those associated with BCNU except that pulmonary fibrosis is less common.

Gliadel Wafers are dime-sized, discoid, biodegradable polymers impregnated with BCNU as a means of providing interstitial chemotherapy directly to the tumor bed area, bypassing the blood-brain barrier. Up to eight Gliadel Wafers are implanted directly into the surgical cavity created by resection of the tumor.[28] The wafers slowly dissolve over 3 weeks (70% gone in the first 3 weeks), delivering a high concentration of BCNU to the tumor bed, and do not need to be removed.[29] This approach delivers a higher dose of BCNU to the tumor bed with fewer and less severe side effects in other parts of the body. Gliadel Wafers have been approved only for recurrent glioblastoma multiforme. Studies have shown increased survival in patients treated with Gliadel Wafers as compared to placebo. The most commonly reported side effect of Gliadel Wafers is delayed wound healing, which occurs in 14% of patients treated with Gliadel versus 5% without Gliadel. Usually, there is no nausea, vomiting, hair loss, or drop in blood counts.[30]

Procarbazine (Matulane) is a synthetic antineoplastic agent approved by the FDA in 1969 for Hodgkin's disease. The exact action of the drug is unclear, but it appears to inhibit protein RNA and DNA synthesis. After oral administration, it crosses the blood-brain barrier and equilibrates between plasma and CSF. Procarbazine is rapidly and completely absorbed following oral administration, with a maximum peak plasma concentration reached in 60 minutes. Approximately 70% of the drug is excreted in the urine within 24 hours. Because procarbazine exhibits monamine oxidase inhibitory activity, a diet that restricts foods high in tyramine should be followed; this includes avoiding all cheeses, smoked or pickled fish, nonfresh meats, liver, wines, broad beans, meat extracts, yeast extracts/brewer's yeast, dry sausage, sauerkraut, and beer and ale including nonalcoholic variations. Foods that may be used with caution include avocados, raspberries, soy sauce, red and white port wines, distilled spirits, and yogurt and cream cheese made from unpasteurized milk.

Undue toxicity can occur if there is impairment of renal or hepatic function. The most frequently occurring reactions are leukopenia, anemia, thrombocytopenia, nausea, and vomiting. There are many possible drug interactions with procarbazine. In addition to foods high in tyramine, over-the-counter drugs such as antihistamines or sympathomimetics, barbiturates, narcotics, hypotensive agents and phenothiazines, and ethyl alcohol are listed. Onset of CNS signs or symptoms such as paresthesias, neuropathies, or confusion, low counts of white blood cells (WBCs) or platelets, stomatitis, diarrhea, and hemorrhage or bleeding require evaluation and possible discontinuation of the drug. The list of possible adverse reactions is lengthy and cuts across most physiological systems. Pharmacological texts should be consulted for a thorough review.

Vincristine (Oncovin) is a plant alkaloid approved by the FDA in 1963 for various non-CNS tumors and for neuroblastoma. The clinical action of vincristine is not completely understood, but its action has been attributed to the inhibition of microtubule formation in the mitotic spindle, resulting in an arrest of dividing cells at the metaphase state. Vincristine is excreted by the liver into bile. It does not appear to cross the blood-brain barrier. Vincristine is given intravenously and *should not be given intrathecally*. Several drug interactions have been reported. They include reduction of blood levels of anticonvulsant drugs, so adjustment of anticonvulsants will be necessary based on blood levels. The most common adverse reaction is hair loss. Leukopenia, neuritis pain, and constipation occur initially, but subside after a week. There are other possible adverse reactions that can occur. Other pharmacological resources should be consulted for the complete listing.

A **combined PCV (procarbazine, CCNU, and vincristine) protocol** has reported advantages over single drugs, including BCNU. It has been used as first-line treatment for malignant gliomas (oligodendrogliomas, anaplastic astrocytomas, glioblastoma multiforme) and can be used in combination with radiation therapy and/or surgery. This protocol is not a cure for malignancy but does appear to slow tumor progression and thus prolong survival.

Temodar or Temodal (temozolomide) is the first oral chemotherapeutic agent found to cross the blood-brain barrier. Unlike many traditional chemotherapeutic agents that require metabolic activation to exert their effects, Temodar can convert spontaneously to a reactive agent that directly interferes with tumor growth. Temodar does not interact with other drugs commonly taken by patients, such as anticonvulsants, corticosteroids, and antiemetics. It can be administered for up to 24 months, with drug administration and necessary lab work conducted on an outpatient basis. No dietary restrictions are necessary; although fasting for 1 hour before taking the drug is required. Most side effects are mild to moderate in severity and include a decreased WBC count (a dose-limiting factor), nausea, vomiting, headache, and fatigue.[31]

Clinical Uses of Chemotherapeutic Drugs

Chemotherapy for brain tumors in children must address special developmental concerns that are not discussed in this adult-focused text. Anaplastic astrocytomas and anaplastic oligodendrogliomas respond well to a combination of procarbazine, CCNU, and vincristine. Given in 6-week intervals, the combination doubles survival. Some glioblastomas respond to BCNU or procarbazine and increase survival by 2 to 6 months.[32] In adults, oligodendrogliomas and CNS lymphomas often respond to chemotherapy and radiation.

Chemotherapy has its most effective application in treating primary, malignant brain tumors. Metastatic lesions to the brain generally do not respond well to chemotherapy because they are isolated by the blood-brain barrier. With metastatic tumors, most centers use the treatment that has been found to be most effective against the primary tumor. Chemotherapy is rarely used with benign brain tumors with the exception of some recurrent meningiomas, which respond well to anti-progesterone agents.[19]

Investigational Treatments and Future Directions

Various novel treatments are being investigated in an effort to increase the response rates to drugs and control tumor growth. There are currently no perfect chemotherapeutic drugs for brain tumors, so research continues. The development of new drugs and new methods of delivery begins with laboratory investigations and proceeds to clinical trials. Drug trials progress in four phases:

- Phase I establishes an optimal safe dose and defines toxicity.
- Phase II determines the action of the drug against specific tumors.
- Phase III compares the new drug with standard therapy for a specific tumor.

- Phase IV adopts the new treatment as part of standard treatment.

Current therapies under investigation are summarized in Table 22-5.[12,19,33–35] Some of these novel drugs may eventually be used in combination with current standard drug protocols or in combination with other novel drugs currently under investigation.

Medical Management Along the Illness Continuum

For a patient with a brain tumor, great variability in outcome can occur depending on the type of tumor, the location, the treatment plan, and the multiple patient characteristics already discussed. The patient is at risk for developing complications from advancement of the disease process and treatment side effects. For example, a patient who has been seizure free may have a seizure. This suggests advancement of the disease process or failure to maintain a therapeutic blood level of an anticonvulsant drug.

Patients may also develop complications from treatment protocols such as myelosuppression or gastric bleeding. Both disease progression and treatment complications are opportunities for collaboration among the physician, the nurse, and other health care professionals to manage problems effectively across the continuum of the illness.

NURSING MANAGEMENT OF THE PATIENT WITH A BRAIN TUMOR

An Overview

The nurse is a member of a collaborative interdisciplinary team caring for the patient. The nurse's role comprises both independent and interdependent aspects. Many collaborative problems confront the team caring for the patient. The specifics of nursing management for patients with brain tumors depend on the nursing history and neurological assessment, with physical care focusing on the functional deficits incurred. The patient is monitored for neurological changes that suggest deterioration in neurological function, and as the patient's needs change, modifications are made in the plan of care.

The patient's and the family's responses to a brain tumor are influenced by the type, grade, location, and presenting symptoms of the tumor. They are also influenced by the age, disabilities, family dynamics, and coping skills of the patient and family. Patients and families have an ongoing need for information and emotional support, which should be addressed by the nurse as part of the management plan.

The appropriate nursing diagnosis for addressing informational needs of the patient and family is *Knowledge Deficit*, and the nursing intervention for Knowledge Deficit is an individualized teaching plan for the patient and family. It includes information about the medical plan of care, management of current deficits and disabilities, and future needs. Helpful information concerning brain tumors in gen-

▐▐▐▐ T a b l e 2 2 – 5 • NOVEL TREATMENTS IN CLINICAL TRIALS FOR MALIGNANT BRAIN TUMORS

CATEGORY	DESCRIPTION/ACTION OF DRUGS THAT:	DRUGS/COMMENT
BBB modifiers	Increases permeability of BBB to allow chemotherapeutic and radiation sensitizing agents access to the brain tumor	RMP-7 *selectively* ↑ BBB permeability in the region of tumor; mannitol is an osmotic diuretic that ↑ permeability of the brain *globally*
Angiogenesis inhibitors	Interfere with growth of tumor-associated blood vessels, thus cutting off tumors from critical nutrients and oxygen	Thalidomide; TNP-470 (given IV after surgery or radiation); interferon; angiostatin
Imidazotetrazines	Prevent the replication of cells that divide rapidly in tumors; an oral cytotoxic alkylating agent	Temozolomide
Metalloproteinase inhibitors	Interfere with cellular growth factors necessary for tumor growth thus reducing the invasiveness of tumors	Phenylbuteric and phenylacetic acids both deprive tumor cells of glutamine, an amino acid that is a building block for protein
Protein kinase C inhibitors	Block signal transduction in multiple pathways of enzymes necessary for tumor proliferation	Tamoxifen, UCN-01, bryostatin, transretinoic acid, SU101
Cyclin-dependent kinase inhibitors	Inhibit cell cycle progression by inhibiting cyclin-dependent kinase family of genes	Flavopiridol; PDGF; fibroblast growth factor
Other drugs to destroy tumor cells	Destroy tumor cells; these newer drugs related to other drugs that have severe side effects (i.e., MX2 related to doxorubicin, which injures cardiac muscle); MX2 not harmful to cardiac muscle	Paclitaxel (Taxol); MX2
Immunotherapy	Boost immune system to fight tumors; tumor cells removed from patient are modified using a gene transfer technique, irradiated, and then injected back to patient subcutaneously. Various cytokines used for this purpose.	Poly ICIC; interferons; granulocyte-macrophage colony-stimulating factor (GM-CSF)
Gene therapy	Inject modified viruses carrying toxic genes directly into tumor making tumor vulnerable to drug therapy; Herpes simplex thymidine kinase gene (HSVtk) encodes for the viral enzyme thymidine kinase that phosphorylates ganciclovir. The phosphorylated metabolite is toxic to the tumor cells.	HSVtk first gene to be used in humans with recurrent malignant tumors; P53 gene (transfer P53 gene into tumor cells using adenoviral vector)

BBB, blood-brain barrier.

eral, treatment of brain tumors, coping with brain tumors, and other related topics is available in publications from the Association for Brain Tumor Research, the National Brain Tumor Foundation, and the American Brain Tumor Association.

The emotional needs of the patient and family members are also within the province of nursing. Common nursing diagnoses related to emotional needs include:

• Fear
• Anxiety
• Personal Identity Disturbance
• Anticipatory Grieving
• Dysfunctional Grieving
• Altered Role Performance
• Social Isolation
• Impaired Social Interaction
• Altered Family Processes
• Impaired Adjustment
• Ineffective Individual and Family Coping
• Ineffective Denial

Nursing interventions are based on individual needs. In addition, referrals are made to appropriate and available resources. Patients and family members should be made aware of brain tumor support groups and counseling options.

In medical and nursing management of the patient with a brain tumor, quality of life for the patient is an ongoing concern. The *Karnofsky Performance Status Scale* (KPS) is widely used to quantify the functional status of cancer patients.[36] Functional status is an indicator of quality of life. The KPS is an 11-point rating scale ranging from normal functioning (100) to dead (0). The increment from one category to another is 10 points (*e.g.*, 10, 20, 30). Loss of function is viewed as being related to the cumulative physical, physiological, and psychological effects of the illness. The KPS is helpful for monitoring the patient's quality of life over time.

Along with quality-of-life issues come decisions related to end-of-life care and intensity of care. (Chapter 4 discusses end-of-life decisions and palliative care.)

Nursing Management During Diagnosis

One of the nurse's main responsibilities during the diagnostic period is to provide information about the tests to be conducted. Since the possibility of a brain tumor can subject the patient to extreme emotional stress, the nurse must take the patient's deficits into account. The impact of such a diagnosis depends on the patient's ability to comprehend what the diagnosis means and how it will affect his or her life. Many patients have lost short-term memory. A patient who has an altered level of consciousness or impaired mental functions, such as memory loss, may not grasp the total impact of the situation but may react merely to the strangeness of the health care environment and interventions or loneliness. Memory loss has a major impact on patient teaching. The nurse must recognize if memory loss is present as well as the severity of loss. Depending on the severity of loss, teaching strategies may be modified to help the patient understand and remember. In severe memory loss, patient teaching is not possible and the focus of teaching is the family.

The patient who understands what is happening may initially deny the diagnosis. If this is the case, the patient will refuse to consider treatment, so informed consent is impossible. If the patient does accept the diagnosis, he or she may react with anger and hostility. Fear of death, mutilation, and loss of independence and mental functions are terrifying concerns. Mental images of other people with similar diagnoses may loom in the patient's mind and threaten body image and self-concept. A sense of powerlessness can overwhelm the patient.

A positive, supportive approach by the nurse can help the patient cope with the reality of the condition. Encourage questions and expression of feelings. The nurse should provide realistic reassurance about expected outcomes. At the same time, the patient should be included in the decision-making process as often as possible. Memory deficits have an impact on the process of providing support, because the patient may not recall previous information provided. Repetition of information is often necessary, and even repetition may not be sufficient to keep the patient informed.

Some organizations (and their telephone numbers) that provide information related to treatment options and support are listed below.

- National Brain Tumor Foundation, 800-934-CURE
- American Brain Tumor Association, 800-886-2282
- American Cancer Society, 800-ACS-2345
- Cancer Information Service, 800-4-CANCER

Nursing Management Before and After Surgery

Nursing management for brain tumor surgery is the same as that outlined for other intracranial surgical procedures in Chapter 15.

Nursing Management During Radiation Therapy

As the patient's advocate, the nurse facilitates collecting satisfactory answers to the patient's questions. If the patient's level of consciousness or mental functions have been impaired, the family will be afforded help so that informed consent can be ensured. The nurse's role during radiation therapy is to provide emotional support to the patient and family, assess patient needs, manage side effects of treatment, and provide general comfort and hygienic needs.

The specific nursing responsibilities during radiation therapy include:

1. Before the start of treatment, inform the patient and family of the various activities that will occur in the radiation therapy department. As with most patient preparation of this kind, informing the patient of what to expect will help allay any fears caused by unfamiliarity with the procedure.
2. Provide proper skin care of the radiation site. Radiation dermatitis can be anticipated (the epidural layer is denuded in a 4- to 6-week period). The skin becomes reddened, tanned, and desquamated. Because the skin is sensitive, do not rub, apply tape, expose to sunlight, or apply alcohol, powder, cream, or cosmetics. The skin markings used to localize radiation exposure should not be washed off.
3. If the patient suffers from nausea, vomiting, or diarrhea, administer antiemetics and antidiarrheal agents as necessary.
4. To manage anorexia, offer small portions of foods that are easy to digest and liked by the patient.
5. For fatigue and general malaise, schedule activities to allow for rest periods. (Fatigue is a very common problem and needs to be vigorously addressed to customize treatment plans.)
6. Note the results of CBCs, with special attention to WBC and platelet counts. Bone marrow depression decreases platelets, which in turn increases the possibility of hemorrhage (petechiae, purpura, nosebleeds, or, most critical, intratumoral hemorrhage).
7. Monitor neurological signs for indications of increased ICP.
8. Provide emotional support by reassuring the patient that side effects will resolve after the treatment has been completed.

See Chart 22-3 for a summary of common nursing diagnoses.

Nursing Management During Chemotherapy

As previously discussed, the role of systemic therapy is increasingly at the forefront of treatment for patients with CNS tumors, especially malignant gliomas. The nurse should know which drugs the patient is receiving and the common side effects related to specific drugs. The patient and family should also be aware of this information. The most common side effects of intravenous chemotherapy include nausea, vomiting, diarrhea, stomatitis, anorexia, alopecia, and bone marrow depression (see Table 22-4).

Collaborative activities involving the nurse and physician include monitoring of vital signs and specific laboratory data and monitoring of the patient's response to the chemotherapy. The specific laboratory data to be collected depend on the toxicity of the drug, which may involve the kidney, liver, blood, or lungs. Clinical pathways, at the forefront of today's care, streamline care delivery and are helpful for drug protocols. With a clinical pathway, care and use of resources are standardized and streamlined, and expected outcomes are carefully monitored.

CHART 22–3 • Summary of Nursing Diagnoses During Radiation Therapy

Nursing Diagnosis	Nursing Interventions	Expected Outcome(s)
Knowledge Deficit related to (R/T) purpose, method, and goals of treatment protocol	• Ask the patient to tell you his or her understanding of the treatment protocol. • Clarify misconceptions. • Expand on areas of partial understanding. • Introduce new information as necessary. • Encourage the patient to ask questions. • Refer questions to another person, if necessary. • Develop a written teaching plan.	The patient will be able to verbalize and describe the purpose, goals, and method of administering the prescribed protocol.
Anxiety R/T approaching or current treatment	• Observe the patient for verbal and nonverbal cues indicating anxiety. • Provide emotional support. • Anticipate the needs of the patient.	The patient's anxiety will be reduced or controlled.
Altered comfort: acute nausea/vomiting R/T chemotherapy	• Assess the patient for nausea. • Provide small, frequent feedings that are easy to digest. • Administer antiemetic as ordered (give as prophylactic and as necessary). • Give nothing by mouth if vomiting occurs. • Offer mouth care frequently.	Nausea will be controlled or minimized; vomiting will be absent or controlled.
Altered Nutrition: Less than body requirements, R/T nausea and vomiting	• Assess the patient's nutritional intake on a 24-hour basis. • Assess the patient's dietary preferences. • Offer small meals frequently (choose easy-to-digest foods).	The patient will maintain adequate nutritional intake.
Altered Oral Mucous Membrane, R/T stomatitis	• Provide frequent mouth care. • Administer a soothing oral rinse or topical solution for oral comfort, such as glycerin swabs or viscous lidocaine suspension, as directed. • Avoid potentially irritating foods, such as citrus fruits. • Provide a soft, bland diet.	Discomfort from stomatitis will be eliminated or controlled.
Body Image Disturbance R/T hair loss	• Discuss the cause of alopecia, as well as the regrowth process. • Provide for meticulous personal hygiene. • Encourage female patients to use makeup and wear attractive head coverings. • Suggest the use of wigs when the patient is able to wear one. • Correct any misconceptions. • Allow the patient to verbalize feelings.	The patient will accept altered body image.
Fatigue R/T chemotherapy or radiation	• Allow the patient to express his or her feelings about general malaise. • Encourage and plan a schedule that allows for frequent rest periods. • Assess the patient's ability to perform activities of daily living (ADLs). • Provide for frequent rest periods. • Adjust the patient's schedule as necessary to conserve energy.	The feeling of fatigue will be minimized by frequent rest periods.

CHART 22-3 • Summary of Nursing Diagnoses During Radiation Therapy (Continued)

Nursing Diagnosis	Nursing Interventions	Expected Outcome(s)
Altered Cerebral Perfusion R/T cerebral edema	• Assess the patient's neurological signs periodically. • Identify any signs of neurological deterioration; report any such changes to the physician and record findings. • Elevate the head of the bed 30 degrees. • Administer drugs and other protocols as ordered. • Continue to monitor the patient.	Neurological changes will be identified early and definitive action taken to control deterioration.
Risk for Infection R/T bone marrow depression	• Protect the patient from exposure to infections. • Monitor the patient for signs and symptoms of infection. • Teach the patient and family the meaning of a decreased white blood cell (WBC) count and nadir (i.e., lowest point of WBC).	The patient and family will verbalize an understanding of preventive measures.
Risk for Injury R/T thrombocytopenia	• Monitor the complete blood count (WBC and platelet) and coagulation study results. • Be aware of and discuss with the patient delayed onset of bone marrow suppression (after 3 weeks). • Assess the patient for occult bleeding (stools, urine, gastric). • Assess the patient for easy bruising, petechial bleeding, nosebleeds, and bleeding from the gums.	The patient and family will verbalize an understanding of the precautions against and the risk factors for injury.
Risk for Impaired Skin Integrity R/T radiation-induced dermatitis (with radiation dermatitis, the skin becomes reddened, tanned, desquamatized, and sensitive)	• Institute special precautions for skin care at the site of radiation. • Protect the skin from rubbing, application of tape, and exposure to sunlight. • Do not use alcohol, powder, cream, or cosmetics on this area. • Do not wash off the skin markings used to localize the radiation exposure site.	Skin integrity will be maintained.
Knowledge Deficit R/T discharge and follow-up care	• Develop a written teaching plan for discharge. • Stress the importance of follow-up care. • Provide a written list of signs and symptoms that should be reported to the physician. • Caution against use of any drugs (e.g., aspirin) without prior approval of the physician. • Help the patient understand that some side effects of the treatment have a delayed onset. • Arrange for a follow-up appointment.	The patient will verbalize an understanding of the discharge plans and care.

Note: Some of the nursing diagnoses listed may not apply to all patients; however, those identified do include major nursing concerns.

▚▚ SUMMARY

Nursing management for the patient with a brain tumor spans a wide variety of circumstances, situations, and treatment modalities. Perhaps no role is more important than that of providing sensitive, supportive care of the patient and family.

REFERENCES

1. Greenlee, R. T., Murphy, T., Bolden, S., & Wingo, P. A. (2000). Cancer statistics, 2000. *CA: Cancer Journal for Clinicians, 50,* 7–33.
2. Sugar, S. M., & Israel, M. A. (1998). Tumors of the nervous system. In A. S. Fauci, et al. (Eds.). *Harrison's principles of internal medicine* (14th ed, p. 2398). New York: McGraw-Hill.
3. Feigenbaum, F., Manz, H., Platenberg, C., & Martuza, R. L. (1999). Primary intrinsic tumors of the brain. In R. G. Grossman

& C. M. Loftus (Eds.) *Principles of neurosurgery* (2nd ed., pp. 469–520). Philadelphia: Lippincott-Raven Publishers.

4. Kleihues, P., Soylemezoglu, F., Schauble, B., Scheithauer, B. W., & Burger, P. C. (1995). Histopathology, classification, and grading of gliomas. *Glia, 15,* 211–221.

5. Preston-Martin, S. (1996). Epidemiology of primary CNS neoplasms. *Neurologic Clinics, 14*(2), 273–290.

6. Kleihues, P., Burger, P. C., & Scheithauer, B. W. (1993). The new WHO classification of brain tumors. *Brain Pathology 3,* 255–268.

7. Adams, R. D., Victor, M., & Ropper, A. H. (1997). *Principles of neurology* (6th ed., pp. 642–694). New York: McGraw-Hill.

8. Kernohan, J. W., Mahon, R. F., Svien, H. J., & Adson, A. W. (1949). A simplified classification of gliomas. *Proceedings of Staff Meetings of the Mayo Clinic, 24,* 71–75.

9. Ringertz, J. (1950). Grading of gliomas. *Acta Pathologica Microbiologica Scandinavia, 27,* 51–64.

10. Kleihues, P., Burger, P. C., & Scheithauer, B. W. (1993). *Histological typing of tumours of the central nervous system: World Health Organization international histological classification of tumours.* Berlin: Springer.

11. Daumas-Duport, C., Scheithauer, B., O'Fallon, J., & Kelly, P. (1988). Grading of astrocytomas: A simple and reproducible method. *Cancer, 62,* 2152–2165.

12. Prados, M. D., Berger, M. S., & Wilson, C. B. (1998). Primary central nervous system tumors: Advances in knowledge and treatment. *CA: Cancer Journal for Clinicians, 48,* 331–360.

13. Barr, M. L., & Kiernan, J. A. (1988). *The human nervous system: An anatomical viewpoint* (5th ed., p. 4). Philadelphia: J. B. Lippincott.

14. Barker, F. G., & Israel, M. A. (1995). The molecular biology of brain tumors. *Neurologic Clinics, 13*(4), 701–717.

15. Gilbert, M., & Armstrong, T. (1995). Management of seizures in the adult patient with cancer. *Cancer Practice, 3*(3), 143–49.

16. The Brain Tumor Society. (2000). Clinical presentation of patients with brain tumor. http:www.thts.org/mono/chap2.htm

17. Gilman, S. (1998). Imaging the brain. *New England Journal of Medicine, 338*(13), 889–896.

18. Castillo, M. (1999). *Neuroradiology companion: Methods, guidelines, and imaging fundamentals* (2nd ed., pp. 106–134). Philadelphia: Lippincott-Raven.

19. The Brain Tumor Society. (2000). Available treatment. http://www.tbts.org.treatment.htm.

20. The Brain Tumor Society. (2000). Radiation therapy for brain tumors. http://www.tbts.org/mono/chap7.htm.

21. Leksell, L. (1951). The stereotactic method and radiosurgery of the brain. *Acta Chirurgica Scandinavia, 102,* 316–319.

22. Larson, D. A., Flickinger, J. C., & Loeffler, J. S. (1993). Stereotactic radiosurgery: Technique and results. In V. T. De Vita, S. Hellman, & S. A. Rosenberg (Eds.). *Cancer: Principles and practice of oncology updates* (pp. 1–19). Philadelphia: J. B. Lippincott.

23. McDermott, M. W., Gutin, P. H., Larson, D. A., et al. (1990). Interstitial brachytherapy. *Neurosurgical Clinics of North America, 1,* 801–824.

24. Nelson, D. F., Urtasum, R. C., Saunders, W. M., Gutin, P. H., & Sheline, G. (1986). Recent and current investigations of radiation therapy of malignant gliomas. *Seminars in Oncology, 13*(1), 46–55.

25. Shapiro, W. R., & Shapiro, J. R. (1986). Principles of brain tumor chemotherapy. *Seminars in Oncology, 13*(1), 56–69.

26. DiPiro, J. T., Talbert, R. L., Yee, G. C., Matzke, G. R., Wells, B. G., & Posey, L. M. (Eds.) (1999). *Pharmacotherapy: A pathophysiologic approach* (4th ed., p. 1990). Stamford, CT: Appleton & Lange.

27. Acquafredda, D., & Hunter, G. (1999). Clinical trials and noteworthy treatments for brain tumors: PCV for brain tumors. http://www.virtualtrials.com/pcv.cfm.

28. Brem, H., Mahaley, M., Vick, N., Black, K., Schold, S., Burger, P., Friedman, A., Ciric, I., Eller, T., Cozzens, J., et al. (1991). Interstitial chemotherapy with drug polymer implants for the treatment of recurrent gliomas. *Journal of Neurosurgery, 74,* 441–446.

29. Guilford Pharmaceuticals. (2000). *Gliadel.* Http://www.virtual trials.com/gliadel.

30. Guilford Pharmaceuticals. (2000). *Gliadel Wafers Patient Information: Frequently asked questions.* http://www.virtualtrials.com/gliadel/faq.cfm.

31. The Brain Tumor Society. (2000). New brain tumor treatment approved by FDA. http://www.tbts.org.temodar.htm.

32. The Brain Tumor Society. (2000). Chemotherapy for brain tumors. http://www.tbts.org/mono/chap8.htm.

33. Merchant, R., McVicar, D., Merchant, L., & Young, H. (1992). Treatment of recurrent malignant glioma by repeated intracerebral injections of human recombinant interleukin-2 alone or in combination with systemic interferon-alpha. Results of a phase I clinical trial. *Journal of Neuro-oncology, 12,* 75–83.

34. Jaeckle, K. (1994). Immunotherapy of malignant gliomas. *Seminars in Oncology, 21,* 249–259.

35. Malkin, M. G. (2000). New medical therapies for malignant brain tumors. http://www.tbts.org.newmed.htm.

36. Mor, V., Laliberte, L., Morris, J. N., & Wiesmann, M. (1984). The Karnofsky performance status scale. *Cancer, 53,* 2002–2007.

RESOURCES

Professional

Published Material

Abramowicz, M. (Ed.). (2001). Drugs of choice for cancer chemotherapy. *The Medical Letter, 42*(1087–1088), 83–92.

DeAngelis, L. M. (2001). Brain tumors. *New England Journal of Medicine, 344*(2), 114–123.

Gilman, S. (1998). Imaging the brain. *New England Journal of Medicine, 338*(13), 889–896.

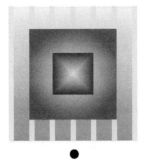

C H A P T E R **23**

Spinal Cord Tumors

JOANNE V. HICKEY

EPIDEMIOLOGY

Primary tumors of the spinal cord constitute approximately 0.5% of newly diagnosed tumors and 7% of primary central nervous system neoplasms.[1] Their causes are unknown. From a histological perspective, most primary spinal cord tumors are benign. The incidence and types of spinal cord tumors vary greatly between children and adults. Only tumors affecting adults are discussed in this chapter.

Spinal cord tumors are classified as either primary or metastatic tumors. **Primary spinal cord tumors** include neurofibromas and meningiomas usually found in the extramedullary area, and ependymomas and other gliomas usually found in the intramedullary area. Other types of primary spinal cord tumors include sarcomas, vascular tumors, chordomas, and epidermoids (Table 23-1). **Metastatic spinal cord tumors** are mostly extradural tumors. Although malignancies from almost any site can metastasize to the vertebral column, lesions from the lungs, breast, prostate, colon, kidney, and uterus, as well as lymphomas and multiple myelomas, are the most common.

Classification of Spinal Cord Tumors

Spinal cord tumors are classified according to their anatomical location with reference to the dural meningeal covering and the spinal cord, or to the vertebral column.

Location in Relation to Dura and Spinal Cord. Primary spinal cord tumors may be classified as extramedullary or intramedullary with respect to the dura and spinal cord.

Extramedullary tumors are located outside the spinal cord and account for about 80% to 90% of primary tumors. Extramedullary tumors are subdivided into:
Extradural: outside the spinal dura; within the epidural space (mostly chordomas and sarcomas–20% of all spinal cord tumors)
Intradural: within the spinal dura, but not within the spinal cord (mostly meningiomas and neurofibromas–60% of all spinal cord tumors)
Intramedullary tumors are located within the substance of the spinal cord (mostly ependymomas and gliomas–about

10% to 20% of all primary spinal cord tumors). The locations of primary spinal cord tumors are shown on cross section in Figure 23-1.

Location in Relationship to the Vertebral Column. Spinal cord tumors are roughly distributed as follows: cervical, 30%; thoracic, 50%; and lumbosacral, 20%. Locating a tumor more precisely helps to correlate the dermatome with specific functional assessment for that level (see Chaps. 5 and 20). Conversely, identifying sensory deficits on examination can help to diagnose a spinal cord tumor and identify its location according to the involved dermatome.

Pathophysiology

Regardless of the type or location of a spinal cord tumor, the associated pathophysiological changes can lead to cord dysfunction and neurological deficits. These changes result from direct cord compression, ischemia secondary to arterial or venous obstruction, or, in the case of intramedullary tumors, direct invasion (Figs. 23-2 and 23-3). Cord compression can cause traction on or irritation of the spinal nerve roots, displacement of the spinal cord, interference with the spinal blood supply, or obstruction of cerebrospinal fluid (CSF) circulation. Cord compression alters the normal physiology involved in providing an adequate blood supply, maintaining stable cellular membranes, and facilitating afferent and efferent impulses for specific sensory, motor, and reflex functions of the spinal cord and related spinal nerves. Invasive infiltration of the spinal cord is seen in association with intramedullary tumors. Edema associated with cord compression is seen in both extramedullary and intramedullary tumors. Edema can ascend the spinal cord, causing additional deficits to the sensitive cord. Control of edema is a major focus in management. Focal (localizing) signs depend on the spinal level, the cross-section location, and the rate of growth and density of the spinal tumor.

Spinal Level

Spinal level refers to the specific location of the tumor in the cervical, thoracic, or lumbosacral area. Sensory distribution from the spinal nerves at each level is mapped at dermatome

▌▌▌ Table 23-1 • COMMON SPINAL CORD TUMORS

TUMOR TYPE	HIGHEST INCIDENCE	GENDER	DESCRIPTION
Neurofibroma	30–50 yrs	Equally affected	60% above L-1, causing spastic paraparesis; 30% below L-1, causing a lateral cauda equina syndrome
Meningioma		M/F ratio 1:9	Most in mid-thoracic (T3–6); a few in foramen magnum
Ependymomas	Average age 30 yrs	M/F ratio 2:1	Either intrinsic within the spinal cord at C-6–T-2 or on the filum terminate (central cauda equina syndrome). Very high incidence of associated syringomyelic cavitation, making the lesion seem much more extensive than its actual size.
Gliomas	35–45 yrs	Equally affected	Almost all in cervical cord
Dermoids	15–20 yrs	No data	Located in sacrococcygeal area, usually associated with spina bifida
Chordoma	No data	Mostly males	Most in sacrococcygeal area; bone destruction and pain are major feature
Hemangioblastoma	Before the age of 40	No data	Well-circumscribed, encapsulated vascular tumor that can usually be completely removed; accounts for 3%–8% of intramedullary tumors

levels (see Chaps. 5 and 20). Loss of sensation depends on the level of the tumor and correlates with the dermatome level. Motor deficits are also related to the tumor level, because motor components of various spinal nerves come together to innervate specific areas.

Location on Cross Section

A neoplasm affecting the vertebral elements can cause cord compression. The compression is often anterior because metastatic tumors frequently involve the vertebral body. In the anterior location, a pathological fracture of the vertebral body with bone fragments driven back into the cord or tumor growth can encroach on the anterior aspect of the spinal cord. Isolated posterior element involvement is much less common.[2]

The major sensations conveyed by the spinal cord are light touch, pain and temperature, and position and vibration. A specific tract located in a designated anatomical area, noted on cross section (see Chap. 5), carries each sensation. The **posterior columns** (fasciculus gracilis and fasciculus cuneatus) convey *position and vibration sensations*. The **lateral spinothalamic tracts** convey *pain and temperature*. The **anterior** **spinothalamic tract** conveys *light touch*. On cross section, the spinothalamic tracts are located in the anterolateral area of the spinal cord (see Fig. 23-2). Therefore, the location of the tumor on cross section will help determine functional loss.

Rate of Growth and Density

The development of neurological deficits is directly related to the tumor's rate of growth and its density (i.e., soft or hard). A slow-growing tumor can accommodate itself to the limited space of the vertebral-spinal cord space within compensatory limits. Many primary spinal cord tumors grow very slowly over years, compressing the cord into a thin, ribbon-like structure with minimal neurological deficits. However, with a rapidly growing tumor, such as a primary malignant spinal cord tumor or a metastatic lesion, the cord fares poorly. Physiologically, the tumor produces major compression of the cord, resulting in substantial edema and, possibly, rapid paralysis (within hours).

A soft tumor can be of a consistency similar to that of the spinal cord. If it grows slowly, it causes gradual compression of the spinal cord. However, the cord's blood supply is able to

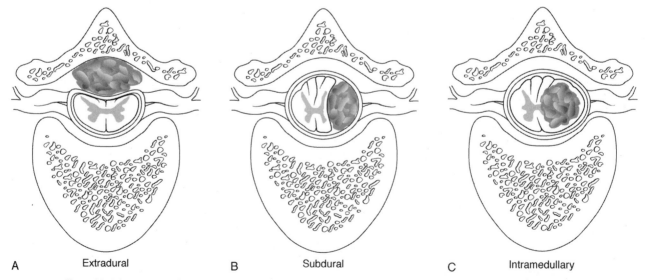

| A   Extradural | B   Subdural | C   Intramedullary |

Figure 23–1 • Location of intramedullary and extramedullary (subdural and extradural) tumors on cross-section.

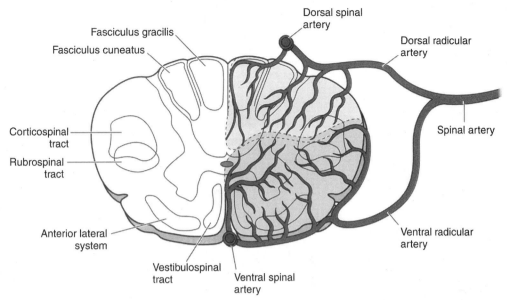

Figure 23–2 • Perfusion patterns of the spinal cord. (Kingley, R. E. [2000] *Concise text of neuroscience.* Philadelphia: Lippincott Williams & Wilkins.)

respond to this alteration and adequately supply the vascular needs without interruption. The tumor adjusts to the available space for growth, becoming elongated, as necessary. Neither movement of the spinal column nor normal alterations in blood flow to the cord will produce injury by contusion or ischemia. By contrast, a hard tumor will respond to movement or vascular changes with spinal contusion, ischemia, and irreversible cord damage. Encroachment on neurological function is apparent earlier with hard tumors than with soft tumors because hard tumors do not conform to the available space.

Morphologically, spinal cord tumors are described as encapsulated or sharply outlined. Soft tumors are irregularly elongated and can extend for two or more segments whereas hard tumors are more circumscribed. Some tumors have a fluid-filled cystic cavity called a *syrinx* that requires drainage.

Metastatic Spinal Cord Tumors

Compression of the spinal cord occurs in about 5% to 10% of patients with cancer. An epidural spinal tumor is the first sign of a malignancy in about 10% of patients.[3] The vertebral column is the most common site in the bony skeletal system for metastases. As mentioned previously, the most common primary sites of metastatic spinal cord tumors are the lungs, breast, prostate, colon, kidneys, and uterus. The malignant lesion tends to spread proximally from the primary organ affected to the adjacent vertebral body, spinous or transverse process, or pedicle. Vertebral metastases are essentially bone-marrow metastases. Retroperitoneal neoplasms (especially lymphomas or sarcomas) may enter the spinal canal through the intervertebral foramina; typically they produce radicular pain and signs of root involvement prior to cord compression. The thoracic area (70%) is most commonly involved, followed by the lumbosacral area (20%), and the cervical area (10%). Prostate cancer tends to spread to the lumbar region (T-8 to T-10) and lumbosacral region whereas ovarian cancer almost always involves the lumbosacral region. In both prostatic and

breast metastases, multiple sites are often involved. Metastatic lesions most commonly exert their effects on the spinal cord by direct compression, enlargement of a vertebral body or pedicle, collapse of an eroded vertebra, or direct extension of a paravertebral lesion through the intervertebral foramen. Edema, a consequence of compression, increases the degree of the deficit.

Signs and Symptoms Associated With Spinal Cord Tumors

Symptoms may develop insidiously and progress gradually, or they may progress rapidly as is common with metastatic lesions. The specific signs and symptoms depend on the anatomical location of the tumor (location on cross section), its location in relation to the level of the vertebral column (thoracic, lumbosacral), and the specific spinal nerves involved. Focal signs and symptoms aid in determining the level of the lesion; however, they can also be indistinct, misleading, and intermittently variable. Table 23-2 summarizes signs and symptoms according to the anatomical level of the tumor on or within the spinal cord.

Pain is the initial symptom in almost all patients. About 95% of patients with vertebral or spinal cord tumors have pain without neurological deficits as the *initial* symptoms, and 75% have pain and weakness, sensory disturbance, or sphincter dysfunction at time of diagnosis.[4]

Pain

The pain may be aching and localized or sharp and radiating (radicular pain). *Localized pain and point tenderness* are common over the involved vertebral area when pressure is applied to the spinous process. *Radicular pain* is defined as pain within the sensory distribution of a spinal nerve root. Pain, which can localize to the back or to an extremity, is caused by irritation, tension/traction, or compression of the nerve root. The quality

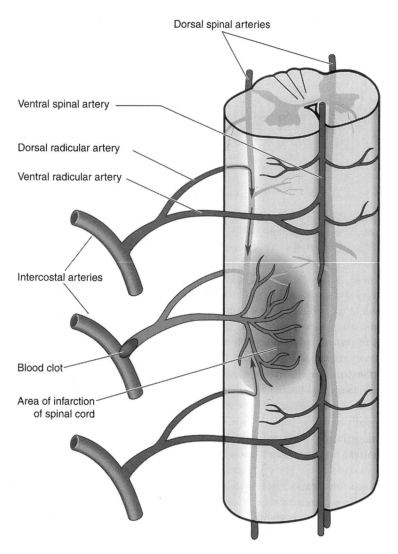

Dorsal spinal arteries

Ventral spinal artery

Dorsal radicular artery

Ventral radicular artery

Intercostal arteries

Blood clot

Area of infarction
of spinal cord

Figure 23–3 • Radicular arteries of the spinal cord. Not all of the 31 potential pairs of spinal arteries develop completely. Therefore, some parts of the spinal cord are perfused by only one or two radicular spinal arteries. Loss of a single artery at these sites can result in ischemic infarction of the spinal cord. The upper lumbar and thoracic spinal cord are particularly vulnerable. (Kingley, R. E. [2000]. *Concise text of neuroscience.* Philadelphia: Lippincott Williams & Wilkins.)

of pain can vary from mild to severe and from dull to piercing, but it is almost always present. Any activity that increases intraspinal pressure, such as the Valsalva maneuver (as occurs with coughing, sneezing, or straining) and movement, can cause pain to intensify and radiate. Pain can also be exaggerated by reclining, because this position stretches the spinal nerves. As a result, pain may awaken the patient at night.

Pain typically precedes signs of cord compression by weeks or even months, but after cord compression occurs, it is always progressive and may advance rapidly.[3] Because the dermatomes supplying a particular area of the body overlap, pain can be diffuse, mimicking such conditions as angina, an acute abdominal lesion, or intercostal neuralgia.

Motor Deficits

The presenting signs and symptoms depend on the degree of involvement of the spinal nerve root and the spinal cord (Fig. 23-4). For example, involvement of the *anterior spinal nerve root* leads to a *lower motor neuron syndrome*. This is characterized by motor weakness; wasting and fasciculations of involved muscles; hypotonia (flaccidity); loss of tendon reflexes when neurons responsible for those reflexes are affected; and normal abdominal and plantar reflexes

unless the neurons responsible for those reflexes are directly involved, in which case the reflex response is lost.

When the spinal cord becomes compressed, other motor deficits develop. Involvement of motor tracts results in an upper motor neuron deficit below the level of the lesion. An *upper motor neuron syndrome* includes weakness or paralysis, spasticity, increased tendon reflexes, a positive Babinski sign, loss of abdominal reflexes, and little or no muscle atrophy.[4] The patient can have a *mixed presentation* of lower motor neuron disease and upper motor neuron disease, depending on the degree of compression present and the anatomical structures affected. Additionally, a combination of sensory and motor deficits may be noted as a Brown-Sequard syndrome (loss of motor function, light touch, vibration, and position sense on the side of the lesion, and contralateral loss of pain and temperature sense).

Sensory Deficits

Which specific sensory deficits develop depends on the presentation of the tumor on cross section. A lateral presentation affects pain and temperature sensation. Numbness or paresthesias, especially of the legs, appear as early symptoms. Light touch sensation is preserved in the presence of a unilateral

Table 23-2 • SIGNS AND SYMPTOMS OF SPINAL CORD TUMORS BY VERTEBRAL LEVEL

LOCATION	SIGNS AND SYMPTOMS	COMMENTS
Cervical Levels		
C-4 and above • Especially dangerous because of innervation to the diaphragm (C1–4) and the potential effect on respirations. • High cervical tumors can affect the lower cranial nerves (VIII to XII).	• Possible respiratory difficulty • Quadriparesis or quadriplegia • Paresthesia • Occipital headache • Stiff neck • CN VIII: downbeat nystagmus • CNs IX to X: dysphagia; dysarthria • CN XI: difficulty shrugging shoulders; atrophy of shoulder and neck muscles • CN XII: deviation of tongue; difficulty speaking; unilateral tongue atrophy	Difficult surgical access; may consider proton beam therapy or another nonsurgical modality Downward gaze is controlled by pathways that extend from the brain stem to the upper cervical cord.
Below C-4	• Pain in shoulders and arms • Paresthesia • If the C5 to C6 root is involved, there will be pain along the medial aspect of the arm. • If C7 to C8 is involved, there will be pain along the outer side of the forearm and hand. • Weakness follows pain. • Atrophy of the shoulder, arm, and intrinsic hand muscles is often associated with fasciculation. • Horner's syndrome (ptosis, miosis, and anhidrosis on the affected side) • Hyperactive reflexes	Attributable to interference with sympathetic innervation
Thoracic Levels		
T1–12 • Most metastatic lesions involve the thoracic region.	• Pain in chest/back • Use of motor deficits to localize the lesion is difficult; spastic paresis may be evident • Sensory deficits are more accurate in identifying the lesion's level: —Know landmark areas, such as T-4 (nipple line) and T-10 (umbilicus). —A band of hyperesthesia is often found above the level of the lesion. • A positive Babinski sign is noted. • Bowel and/or bladder dysfunction • Sexual dysfunction	See Chapter 19 for an explanation and illustration of dermatomes.
Lumbosacral		
S-1 to S-5	• Pain in lower back, which often radiates to legs; may also be felt in the perineal area • Paresis/spasticity of lower extremities, usually in one leg and later in the other • Sensory loss in legs and/or saddle area • Bowel and/or bladder dysfunction • Sexual dysfunction • Reflexes—ankle and knee jerk reflexes are diminished or absent	• Footdrop is common. • Atrophy may affect certain muscle groups.

tumor resulting from the crossed and uncrossed components to the tract. Awareness of vibration and proprioception of body parts are affected if the posterior columns are involved. Compression from a tumor affects function below the lesion. Therefore, the highest intact sensory level should be determined.

Bowel, Bladder, and Sexual Dysfunction

Bowel, bladder, or sexual dysfunction is common. Constipation and, later, paralytic ileus are common bowel deficits. Early bladder deficits may present as urgency or difficulty in initiating urination gradually progressing to urinary retention. De-

creased motor function and paresthesias of the perineum occur with some tumors, and impotence or other sexual dysfunction is possible. With a cervical intramedullary tumor (uncommon tumor location), *sacral sparing* may occur. Because perineal sensation is controlled by the spinothalamic tract located on the periphery of the spinal cord, sensation to the perineum may be spared.

Other Findings

As a tumor grows, it consumes all the space around the spinal cord, thus isolating the CSF below the tumor from normal CSF circulation. Examination of the CSF reveals

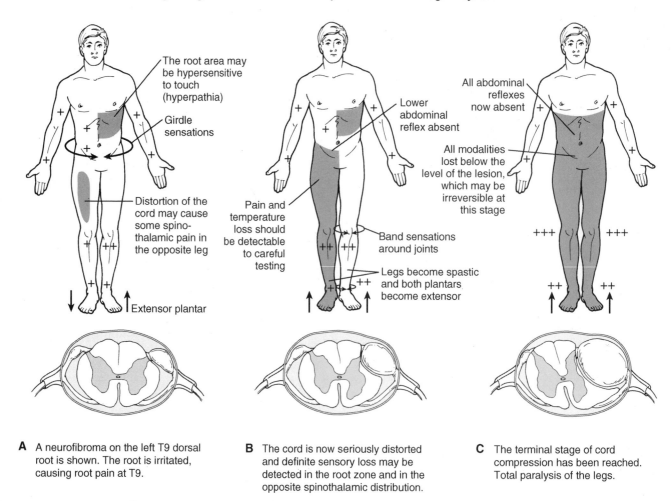

A A neurofibroma on the left T9 dorsal root is shown. The root is irritated, causing root pain at T9.

B The cord is now seriously distorted and definite sensory loss may be detected in the root zone and in the opposite spinothalamic distribution.

C The terminal stage of cord compression has been reached. Total paralysis of the legs.

Figure 23–4 • Progression of deficits as the size of the mass and cord distention increases.

xanthochromia, an increased protein count, few or no cells, and immediate clotting. Collectively, these findings are called **Froin's syndrome**. Some types of spinal cord tumor cause a syringomyelic syndrome from a syrinx found in the central intramedullary gray matter. This syndrome causes a chronic degenerative disorder of the spinal cord accompanied by motor weakness, spasticity, and pain.

DIAGNOSIS

Diagnosis begins with a complete medical history and physical examination, including a focused neurological examination. Diagnostic testing follows, with the urgency of some tests based on clinical findings.

Clinical Findings

In the early stages, subtle symptoms may not be evident. Collect a history of pain, including onset, location, and aggravating symptoms. Palpate the back and spine for localized point tenderness or spasms. Assess muscle strength and abnormal tone (flaccidity or spasticity) and look for signs of muscle wasting. Test deep tendon reflexes, superficial abdominal reflexes, and the Babinski sign.

Sensory assessment (i.e., pain, vibration, position, light touch) begins at the toes and moves upward to determine the highest intact functional level. The lesion level is often accompanied by a narrow band of hyperesthesia (abnormally increased sensitivity to stimuli) directly above its location. Assess for bladder dysfunction (urinary retention, urinary dribbling), bowel dysfunction (constipation), and sexual dysfunction (impotence).

Diagnostic Methods

The diagnostic test of choice for a patient with a suspected spinal cord lesion is magnetic resonance imaging (MRI) with contrast enhancement (gadolinium). This procedure exhibits superior sensitivity in detecting lesions in bony areas such as in the vertebral bodies. A noninvasive procedure, MRI allows multiple axial and midsagittal views demonstrating intramedullary pathology without radiological exposure. Figure 23-5 shows an intradural-extramedullary meningioma. Optimal MRI imaging requires that the patient remain motionless for a period of time during the procedure. This can be difficult if the patient is in pain. There are contraindications for MRI, such as previous surgery for placement of metal plates or rods. In these cases, alternative, less sensitive tests such as computed tomography (CT) may be used. However, in most circumstances, MRI has replaced myelography and CT as the standard of care.

With spinal cord tumor, the MRI demonstrates an enlarged or thickened cord. Often, the spinal cord is enlarged around the area of the slowly expanding tumor. The entire spinal axis should be examined to determine presence of areas of involvement. Although a specific type of tumor may be suggested by its location and pattern, the definitive histological tumor type must be known before beginning treatment. Neurosurgical evaluation for possible biopsy or evacuation should be considered. Evoked potentials are useful to determine cord involvement and also to follow the patient preoperatively and postoperatively.[5] Patients are at risk for sustaining significant neurological deficits both from the impact of the tumor on the spinal cord and from treatment modalities that may cause secondary cord injury.

PRINCIPLES OF TREATMENT

For patients with suspected or diagnosed spinal cord tumors, the primary goals of treatment are preservation of neurological function, control of pain, and initiation of a treatment plan directed at tumor removal or control. A combination of surgical, medical, and radiological approaches is often required. The degree of neurological dysfunction and the location of the lesion determine the urgency of treatment. For example, in a patient with mild right upper extremity weakness who has a cervical spine lesion, immobilization of the neck is mandatory until stability has been obtained.

Preservation of Neurological Function

Spinal cord tumors are often associated with localized edema. The spinal canal is narrow and provides little space for swelling without accompanying neurological dysfunc-

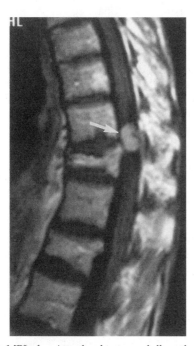

Figure 23–5 • MRI of an intradural-extramedullary thoracic meningioma. Note the incidental old compression fracture in the midthoracic region. (Castillo, M. [1999]. *Neuroradiology companion: Methods, guidelines, and imaging fundamentals* [2nd ed.]. Philadelphia: Lippincott-Raven.)

tion. Extensive pressure can compromise venous and arterial blood flow, resulting in ischemia and irreversible infarction of the spinal cord. The immediate administration of corticosteroids, most commonly dexamethasone (Decadron), can rapidly reverse this edema. The dosage and schedule of administration are controversial. Some recommend a bolus dose followed by a slow tapering dose over several days or until symptoms increase. Corticosteroids are often given with chemotherapy and radiation protocols to control edema and preserve function.

Various supportive care measures may be necessary. If stability of the spinal cord is in question or a cervical spine lesion is involved, the patient should be immobilized with a cervical collar until the stability of the vertebral column can be assessed and surgical stabilization, if needed, can be undertaken. With a high cervical tumor, respiratory support may be necessary. Close monitoring of respiratory function is imperative. Difficulty with swallowing suggests the need for a feeding tube to prevent aspiration and support nutritional needs. For the patient with urinary retention, an indwelling catheter is useful. As soon as possible, an intermittent catheterization program is started. Improvement in function may occur after corticosteroid therapy is established and has become therapeutic. Physical therapy may also be necessary to assist with impaired ambulation related to paresis, muscle wasting, fatigue, and the concurrent high risk for falls.

With metastatic tumors, prompt diagnosis and treatment are the keys to preserving function. Most patients diagnosed with metastatic tumors have pain for an average of 3 months before the appearance of neurological deficits, which prompt a search for a cause.

Treatment Options

The treatment plan for a specific spinal cord tumor depends on the type of tumor, its location, and the rapidity with which signs and symptoms are developing. The overall medical condition of the patient is also an important consideration. Intradural-extramedullary tumors, such as neurofibromas, meningiomas, vascular tumors, chordomas, and epidermoid tumors, are usually treated with surgical excision alone. The management of intramedullary tumors, such as astrocytomas, ependymomas, and metastatic lesions, is much more difficult. These tumors often require a combination of surgery, radiotherapy, and possibly chemotherapy.

Surgery

Surgical intervention is the primary treatment for most types of spinal cord tumors. Surgery is undertaken to establish a diagnosis through biopsy and to partially or completely resect the tumor. Rapid loss of motor, sensory, and bowel/bladder function indicates the need for *immediate surgery* to preserve or restore neurological function. Advances in surgical technique, such as intraoperative spinal cord evoked potential monitoring, intraoperative ultrasound localization, microneurosurgical approaches, and newer instrumentation (e.g., ultrasonic aspirators, lasers), are improving surgical outcomes. If a laminectomy is performed involving two or more levels, spinal fusion may be necessary.

For rapidly growing metastatic lesions, surgical decompression may be advised to maintain bowel, bladder, or motor function, thus preserving a reasonable quality of life even if the prognosis for the primary tumor is poor. The outcome of surgery is good if extradural metastatic lesions are diagnosed early (when only back pain is present and no neurological deficits have occurred). A poor outcome is likely if neurological deficits are already present. Paralysis, once present, usually is irreversible. Extramedullary tumors, such as meningiomas or neurofibromas, can often be completely excised surgically. After complete resection, recurrence is rare for both tumor types. For neurofibromatosis patients with multiple spinal cord tumors, tumor removal is limited to symptomatic lesions. For intramedullary tumors, which are frequently malignant and often have microscopic infiltration of spinal cord parenchyma, attempts at complete surgical excision pose substantial risk of loss of neurological function. Therefore, the goals of surgery are limited to establishing a diagnosis and decompressing the spinal cord before embarking on additional treatment.

Radiation

Most patients with primary spinal cord tumors do not require radiation therapy. However, radiation therapy is the mainstay of treatment for patients with spinal cord compression due to metastatic cancer. Some primary malignant spinal cord tumors (i.e., malignant gliomas, malignant ependymomas, and metastatic lesions) are treated with radiation. Radiation therapy is rarely used for benign or low-grade spinal cord tumors that cannot be completely removed surgically.

The spinal cord is less tolerant of radiation therapy than the brain and other organs. The thoracic spinal cord, where half of all spinal tumors occur, is the most sensitive spinal tissue and least tolerant of the effects of radiation. Radiation oncologists work to minimize the risk of radiation-induced damage to normal spinal tissue by limiting the amount of radiation exposure. Studies suggest that the spinal cord can tolerate a maximum of 4,500 cGy. Higher doses are associated with an increased risk of *radiation myelopathy*. This irreversible complication of radiation exposure begins insidiously at least 6 months after completion of radiation therapy and, more frequently, 12 to 15 months after therapy. Radiation myelopathy is a chronic, progressive condition initially seen as sensory impairment to the areas supplied by the affected cord. Pain is absent initially. Motor deficits and changes in pain and temperature sensation develop, so that a Brown-Sequard syndrome is observed. This eventually converts to a transverse myelopathy with spastic paraplegia, loss of sensation in the affected areas, and loss of bowel and bladder control.

Chemotherapy

The role of chemotherapy for spinal cord tumors is limited. Chemotherapy, similar to that used for brain tumors, may be recommended in adults for spinal gliomas that progress after surgery and radiation. Chemotherapy may also be useful in a few chemosensitive cancers such as lymphomas and small-cell lung cancer, as well as for some metastatic lesions from breast cancers, or when surgery and additional radiation are not recommended.[6]

Adjunctive therapy such as hormonal manipulation may be useful for specific tumors. For example, tamoxifen (Megace) may be helpful for breast cancer, and androgen

inhibition, either through chemical means (i.e., diethylstilbestrol) or orchiectomy, may be beneficial in prostate cancer. Intrathecal chemotherapy for patients with known leptomeningeal involvement may be instituted. This involves direct administration of chemotherapy into the CSF either by lumbar puncture or an Ommaya reservoir. Unfortunately, there is a very limited selection of suitable drugs, and the results are often disappointing.

Prognosis and Discharge Planning

Prognosis will vary greatly, depending on the type of tumor and the neurological deficits present. With primary tumors, some resolution of neurological deficits may occur gradually over a period of approximately 2 years, especially with physiotherapy. Each patient should be evaluated to identify individual rehabilitation needs. Most patients with neurological deficits will benefit from a short-term, aggressive rehabilitation program. Patients with metastatic lesions do not fare as well because of the advanced stage of the primary tumor. For these patients, further treatment of the primary cancer may be planned. For others, palliative care with hospice care or placement in a chronic care facility may be chosen.

NURSING MANAGEMENT OF THE PATIENT WITH A SPINAL CORD TUMOR

Some commonalties in nursing management exist in the care of patients with spinal cord injuries and those with spinal cord tumors (see Chap. 19). Specifics of care depend on the segmental level of the tumor and the presenting signs and symptoms. If the patient is treated surgically, nursing management follows that outlined for a laminectomy patient (see Chap. 20). Some patients develop metastatic lesions to the spinal cord as a complication of a primary cancer. The nurse will need to consult a text on oncological nursing for specific management and treatment that should be integrated into the plan of care.

The objectives of care for the hospitalized patient with a spinal cord tumor include early recognition of neurological change through ongoing monitoring; control of pain; management of sensory and motor deficits and their impact on activities of daily living (ADLs); and management of bowel and bladder dysfunction. See Chart 23-1 for a summary of assessment parameters.

Assessment

The nurse should conduct a baseline assessment of vital and neurological signs. Neither the level of consciousness nor pupillary signs are apt to be affected unless the sympathetic innervation of the cervical spinal nerves is involved. In this instance, Horner's syndrome will be seen. The key areas of assessment include pain, motor, sensory, bowel, and bladder function.

Pain. Assess the quality (on a scale of 1 to 10), location, and type (e.g., dull, piercing) of pain present, using the Visual Analog Scale. Note any circumstances that exacerbate the pain.

Motor Function. Assess motor strength and grade on a 0 to 5 scale as outlined in Chapter 7. Palpate the muscles for signs of atrophy. Note presence of abnormal motor tone, involuntary movement, and limited range of motion. If the patient is able to walk, assess the gait. Note any functional deficits that impact on ADLs.

Sensory Function. All sensory modalities must be evaluated, including light touch, pain and temperature, vibration, and position sensations (see Chap. 7). With the patient's eyes closed, begin at the toes and work your way up the body, assessing each side of the body and comparing findings. Determine which modalities are absent or diminished. A band of hyperesthesia often exists over the level of sensory loss. Note any abnormal sensations (paresthesias), such as burning.

Bowel Function. Auscultate the abdomen for bowel sounds in all four quadrants. Determine the normal pattern of bowel function, and ascertain whether there has been a change in bowel patterns such as constipation, diarrhea, or incontinence of stool. A bowel program may need to be instituted.

Bladder Function. Note the urinary voiding pattern. Determine whether there is evidence of urinary retention (a common problem with spinal cord tumors) or incontinence.

Urinary retention will place the patient at high risk for urinary tract infection. Monitor intake and output. A bladder retraining program may be necessary.

Collaborative Problems and Nursing Diagnoses

After assessment data have been collected, a list of collaborative problems and nursing diagnoses with interventions is developed (Chart 23-2). The major collaborative problems are:

- Spinal cord compression
- Paresis/paresthesia/paralysis
- Fecal impaction
- Urinary retention
- Infection
- Intractable pain

Management

In preparation for discharge, the nurse will make a complete assessment of the patient to determine the level of independence in performing ADLs, home activities, and activities

---

CHART 23–1 • Assessment Parameters for a Patient With a Spinal Cord Tumor

SENSORY ASSESSMENT

- With patient's eyes closed, assess the following sensory modalities:
  - Light touch
  - Pain (pinprick)
  - Position
- Beginning at the feet and working upward systematically, assess each side of the body and compare findings; often, sensory loss is asymmetrical. (See Chap. 7 for technique.)
- Note the highest level of sensation recorded in relation to an anatomical marking (e.g., umbilicus) or dermatome level. (See Chaps. 5, 7, and 19.)
- If pain is present, describe the characteristics of pain using standard pain assessment criteria.
- Assess progression/change in pain over time.
- Assess for cervical vertebral, thoracic vertebral, and lumbar vertebral pain for *tenderness* while palpating vertebrae.
- Identify highest level of intact sensory function on each side of body.
- Document highest level of function for pain so pain level can be monitored over time.

MOTOR ASSESSMENT

- Systematically assess each side of the body for muscle strength and muscle tone; compare findings. (See Chap. 7 for technique.)
- Observe the patient's gait pattern, if ambulatory.

- Note the presence of spasticity or other abnormal movement.
- Assess deep tendon reflexes and coordination.

BOWEL ASSESSMENT

- Assess the normal bowel evacuation pattern for the patient (frequency, consistency, time of day, etc.).
- Assess for any changes in bowel habits.
- Assess use of any home remedies for regularity (food, drugs).
- Auscultate the abdomen for bowel sounds and distention.

BLADDER ASSESSMENT

- Assess the patient's normal voiding pattern.
- Assess the patient for any changes or discomfort in voiding pattern.
- Palpate the suprapubic area for distention or pain.

RESPIRATORY ASSESSMENT (FOR CERVICAL TUMORS)

- Assess rate, depth, and rhythm of respirations.
- Observe chest movement for asymmetry, abdominal breathing, or abnormal chest movement.
- Auscultate the chest bilaterally for breath sounds.

OTHER NOTATIONS

- Assess the patient for orthostatic hypotension.
- Note any absence of perspiration (e.g., Horner's syndrome).

CHART 23-2 • Summary of Nursing Management of the Patient With a Spinal Cord Tumor

Nursing Diagnoses	Nursing Interventions	Expected Outcome(s)

Pain Related to (R/T) Spinal Cord and/or Spinal Nerve Compression and Muscle Spasms	• Monitor pain at least every 4 hours.
	  —Monitor quality (dull, piercing), location, and other characteristics.
	  —Monitor the severity of pain by asking the patient to use the Visual Analogue Scale (VAS) to report pain severity on a scale of 1 to 10.
	  —Monitor nonverbal signs of pain (e.g., facial expression, emotional control).
	  —Monitor the effect of pain on activities of daily living (ADLs).
	• Identify activities/factors that aggravate pain.
	
	• Administer analgesics and steroids as ordered, and before the pain intensity has escalated.
	• Provide physical comfort measures.
	  —Reposition the patient every 1 to 2 hours.
	  —Maintain proper body alignment.
	  —Administer massage (e.g., a back rub).
	• Apply a special mattress based on any limitations (e.g., a water mattress, an alternating pressure mattress).
	• Teach stress-reducing techniques for pain control (e.g., relaxation, imagery, distraction activities).
	• Assist the patient to plan individual pain control strategies that are most effective.
		The patient will
		• Accurately describe pain phenomena.
		• Identify changes in pain intensity using the VAS.
		
		• Participate in controlling activities/factors that aggravate pain.
		• Report the patient's response to analgesics using the VAS.
		• Identify measures that facilitate comfort.
		
		• Learn and use stress-reducing techniques to control pain.
		• Participate in developing an overall pain control plan.

Impaired Physical Mobility R/T muscle weakness, paralysis, spasticity, and pain	• Monitor motor function every 8 hours (muscle strength, muscle tone, gait, ability to move in bed). • Teach the proper use of assistive devices. • Provide assistance, as necessary, in transfer and ambulation once spinal cord is stabilized. • Administer range-of-motion exercises every 4 hours. • Position the patient in proper body alignment every 2 hours; use supportive devices as necessary.	• The comparison of data to baseline data will identify any changes.
Related Nursing Diagnosis: • Self-Care Deficits • Risk for Impaired Skin Integrity • Risk for Disuse Syndrome	• Monitor the effect of impaired mobility on ADLs. • Develop specific interventions to compensate for deficits. • If spasticity is present, keep the involved extremity warm; reposition periodically; seek suggestions from the physical therapist. • Provide analgesics at least 30 minutes before a planned activity. • If bedrest is ordered, consider protocols to counter the effects of immobility (deep breathing exercises, skin care, turning schedule, etc.) • Request physical therapy (PT) and occupational therapy (OT) consults once patient's spinal cord is stabilized.	• Any ADLs that the patient cannot do independently will be provided by the nurse, or an alternative way of doing the activity with an adaptive device will be developed. • The patient will report a decrease in pain and an increase in activity tolerance. • Interventions will be in place to prevent the development of disuse syndrome.
Sensory/Perceptual Alterations: Tactile and Kinesthetic, R/T neurological sensory deficits (spinal cord compression, edema) Related Nursing Diagnosis: • High Risk for Injury	• Monitor sensory function; identify the highest level of intact sensory function. • Teach the patient to compensate for any deficits by checking the position of the involved area visually. • Protect the involved area from injury (e.g., burns, bruising). • Monitor ability to ambulate secondary to sensory deficits.	• Comparison of data to baseline data will identify any changes. • The patient will find ways to compensate for the lost sensory modality so that the effect on performance of ADLs will be minimized.

CHART 23–2 • Summary of Nursing Management of the Patient With a Spinal Cord Tumor (Continued)

Nursing Diagnoses	Nursing Interventions	Expected Outcome(s)
Urinary Retention R/T spinal cord compression and edema	• Monitor the patient's voiding pattern and amount per voiding. • Maintain an accurate intake and output record. • Monitor the patient for suprapubic distention or pain. • Explain the rationale for treatment and management. • Insert indwelling catheter or establish intermittent catheterization schedule.	• Accurately report his or her former voiding pattern. • Verbalize an understanding of the treatment regimen and the underlying rationale.

Related Nursing Diagnosis:
• Risk for Urinary Tract Infection
	• Remove the indwelling catheter as soon as possible.
	• Develop a bladder retraining program:
	  —Teach the Credé and stretch maneuvers.
	  —Measure postvoid residuals after attempts to empty the bladder.
	  —Teach intermittent catheterization.
	  —Set a catheterization time schedule to obtain about 500 mL of urine each time.
		• The patient will establish a regular pattern of urinary elimination.
		
		• The patient will learn self-catheterization technique.

Constipation R/T decreased peristalsis secondary to spinal cord compression/edema	• Establish the patient's previous bowel elimination pattern. • Auscultate the abdomen for bowel sounds. • Palpate the abdomen for distention. • Increase bulk in diet. • Encourage an adequate fluid intake. • Begin a bowel protocol that will provide for satisfactory bowel elimination.	• The patient will accurately report the previous bowel elimination pattern. • Presence of peristalsis will be monitored. • A diet high in bulk and fluids will be encouraged unless contraindicated by the medical plan. • A bowel protocol will be established that ensures bowel movements (with stools of soft consistency) every 1 to 2 days.

Risk for Injury R/T sensory/perceptual alterations and impaired physical mobility	• Teach the patient to:
	  —Check the position of the affected limbs visually.
	  —Check the integrity of the skin daily, especially affected parts, for evidence of injury.
	  —Check the temperature of the unaffected limb before applying heat to affected areas.
	  —Use heating devices very cautiously.
	• Assist the patient with ambulation.
		• The patient and family will recognize the patient's high-risk status secondary to neurological deficits.
		• Strategies will be developed to prevent injury.
		
		• The patient will seek assistance in ambulation.

Anxiety R/T pain, uncertainty about the disease process, and outcome	• Allow the patient to express his or her feelings. • Correct misinformation and clarify information as necessary. • Refer the patient to appropriate resource people, as necessary. • Help the patient set realistic goals. • Be supportive. • Help the patient find ways to reduce anxiety (e.g., relaxation techniques; diversion).	• Anxiety will be reduced to a manageable level.

Other possible nursing diagnoses—general:
• Knowledge Deficit R/T
  —Disease process
  —Treatment modalities (surgery, irradiation, chemotherapy)		

(continued)

CHART 23-2 • Summary of Nursing Management of the Patient With a Spinal Cord Tumor (Continued)

Nursing Diagnoses	Nursing Interventions	Expected Outcome(s)
• Sexual Dysfunction • Functional Incontinence • Fatigue • Fear • Ineffective Individual Coping • Ineffective Family Coping • Powerlessness For patients with cervical tumors: • Ineffective Breathing Pattern • Ineffective Airway Clearance • Impaired Swallowing		

within the community. Working collaboratively with other health team members, a discharge plan is developed. These patients need a case manager to assist with the planning of care that is often complex and long-term. As mentioned previously, some patients will benefit from a short-term rehabilitation program through an in-house rehabilitation facility or through outpatient services. For the patient with a metastatic lesion, contacting the primary physician managing the cancer and any community resources previously involved in the patient's care will help ensure continuity of care. Hospice care in the home or nursing home is an option for patients in the terminal stages of illness.

Follow-Up in the Community

Patients with either primary or secondary spinal cord tumor need long-term follow-up and management. From the nursing perspective, functional ability in ADLs, nutrition, comfort (pain control), and quality of life provide a framework for assessment and care. In addition to monitoring motor, sensory, bowel, and bladder function, other functional deficits may become apparent, such as impotence. Persistent problems may require further evaluation and possible referral for resolution.

REFERENCES

1. Goetz, C. G., & Pappert, E. J. (1999). *Textbook of clinical neurology* (p. 947). Philadelphia: W. B. Saunders.
2. Cruz, J. (1998). *Neurologic and neurosurgical emergencies* (pp. 379–380). Philadelphia: W. B. Saunders.
3. Gucalp, R., & Dutcher, J. (1999). Oncologic emergencies. In Fauci, A. D., et al. (Eds.). *Harrison's principles of internal medicine* (14th ed., pp. 628–630). New York: McGraw-Hill.
4. Aminoff, M. J., Greenberg, D. A., & Simon, R. P. (1996). *Clinical neurology* (3rd ed., pp. 153–154, 163–164). Stanford, CT: Appleton & Lange.
5. Yung, W. K. A., & Janus, T. (1999). Primary neurological tumors. In C. G. Goetz & E. J. Pappert (Eds.). *Textbook of clinical neurology* (pp. 933–956). Philadelphia: W. B. Saunders.
6. The Brain Tumor Society. (2000). Spinal cord tumors. http://www.tbts.org/sctumors.htm.

RESOURCES
Professional

Published Material

Bell, G. R. (1997). Surgical treatment of spinal tumors. *Clinical Orthopedics, 335,* 54–63.
Hamilton, A. J., Lulu, B. A., Fosmire, H., & Gossett, L. (1996). LINAC-based spinal stereotactic radiosurgery. *Stereotactic Functional Neurosurgery, 66*(1–3), 1–9.
Janjan, N. A. (1996). Radiotherapeutic management of spinal metastases. *Journal of Pain and Symptom Management, 11*(1), 47–56.
Newton, H. B., Newton, C. L., Gatens, C., Herbert, R., & Pack, R. (1995). Spinal cord tumors: Review of etiology, diagnosis, and multidisciplinary approach to treatment. *Cancer Practice, 3*(4), 207–218.

Patient and Family

Published Material

General information about the effects of spinal cord disease can be assessed from the National Spinal Cord Injury Association at (800) 962-9629.
American Brain Tumor Association. *About metastatic tumors to the brain and spine.* Available by phone at (800) 886-2282.
Brain and Spinal Cord Tumors: *Hope through research* (NIH Publication No. 93-504). Available by phone at (800) 352-9424.
Murphy, R. F. (1990). *The body silent.* New York: W. W. Norton (written by an anthropologist coping with an inoperable ependymoma).
Price, R. (1994). *A whole new life: An illness and a healing.* New York: Atheneum Press (a prize-winning author who has survived more than 15 years with a malignant spinal cord astrocytoma).

Websites

Brain and Spinal Cord Tumors: *Hope through research* (NIH Publication No. 93-504); available at http://www.ninds.nih.gov/healinfo/disorder/brtumors/braintum.htm.

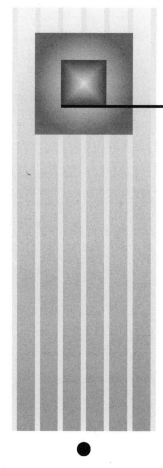

SECTION 7

Nursing Management of Patients With Cerebrovascular Problems

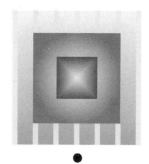

JOANNE V. HICKEY
DEIDRE M. BUCKLEY

C H A P T E R **24**

Cerebral Aneurysms

OVERVIEW

A **cerebral aneurysm** is a saccular outpouching of a cerebral artery. Intracranial saccular aneurysms or berry aneurysms account for approximately 80% to 90% of all intracranial aneurysms and are the most common cause of nontraumatic subarachnoid hemorrhage. These small, berry-like projections occur at arterial bifurcations in the circle of Willis, with other shapes such as pedunculated, sessile, and multilobulated aneurysms occasionally seen.[1] Rupture of a cerebral aneurysm usually results in a **subarachnoid hemorrhage (SAH)**, which is defined as bleeding into the subarachnoid space. Autopsy studies have shown that the overall frequency of unruptured intracranial aneurysms in the general population ranges from 0.2% to 9.9% (mean about 5%).[2] It is estimated that approximately 10 to 15 million Americans have a cerebral aneurysm, most of which are small, innocuous and do not bleed throughout life.[3] Most studies have found an increased occurrence of aneurysms in women compared with men, although in childhood and adolescence the ratio appears to be opposite, with male:female ratio of 2:1.[1]

Eighty-five percent of aneurysms in adults occur in the anterior circle of Willis in the proximal arterial bifurcations. The most common sites in the anterior circulation include the anterior communicating artery to anterior cerebral junction, internal carotid artery bifurcation in the posterior communicating artery origin, and the proximal middle cerebral artery. In the posterior circulation, the most common locations include the basilar tip, the superior cerebellar artery, and the anterior inferior cerebellar arteries. In children and adolescents, approximately 40% arise from the posterior circulation. Multiple aneurysms occur in 10% to 20% of the people affected.[1]

Each year in the United States there are approximately 30,000 new cases of SAH secondary to rupture of intracranial aneurysm.[4] Despite considerable advances in diagnostic, surgical, anesthetic, and perioperative techniques, the outcome for patients with ruptured aneurysms remains poor; in fact, only one third of people who experience aneurysmal SAH recover without major disability.[5] Cerebral aneurysm rupture is most prevalent in the 35- to 60-year-old age group, with 50 being the mean age of occurrence. Aneurysmal SAH occurs more often in women than men by a ratio of 3:2.[6]

FAMILIAL ANEURYSMS

There have been many families with documented intracranial aneurysms. *Familial intracranial aneurysms* are generally defined as the presence of two or more family members among first- and second-degree relatives with proven aneurysmal SAH or incidental aneurysms.[7-10] Incidence of familial aneurysms among SAH patients is 6% to 20%.[11-13] It has been estimated that the prevalence of familial intracranial aneurysms among patients with SAH is somewhere in the order of 7% to 10%. Ogilvy states that in his experience with patients with ruptured and unruptured aneurysms, approximately 22% will have family members with aneurysms. Familial intracranial aneurysm is defined as two or more blood relatives who harbor intracranial aneurysms.[14] Le Blanc and colleagues reviewed 13 families with intracranial aneurysms and found the occurrence in the same decade in two affected siblings in 10 of 12 cases (83%). Although the usual incidence of morbidity and mortality from initial rupture of hemorrhage is about 40%, when familial patients are reviewed, the incidence of patients who suffered death or disability in the initial hemorrhage is 70%.[15]

The familial occurrence does suggest the possibility of a genetically determined defect of the arterial wall. Several studies suggest that individuals with familial intracranial aneurysms are more likely to have multiple aneurysms and that these aneurysms are more likely to rupture at a smaller size than those patients with an isolated aneurysm.[16] Thus, treatment considerations are different than for patients with an unruptured isolated aneurysm. The mode of transmission of familial intracranial aneurysms remains unknown. No genetic locus has yet been identified. To date, there is no biological marker that can identify patients with familial intracranial aneurysms. The likelihood of finding such a genetic locus is highest in patients with multiple lesions and familial tendency, so blood samples can be obtained from many members of the same family possibly harboring the gene.

Various genetically determined conditions have been associated with intracranial aneurysm; a definite link has only been associated with autosomal dominant polycystic kidney disease. The percentage of these patients that have cerebral aneurysms varies from 10% to 40%. There is no identified definitive pattern of inheritance. Other disease frequently mentioned such as Marfan's syndrome, Ehlers-Danlos syndrome type 4, neurofibromatosis, and pseudoxanthoma elasticum are more often associated with carotid cavernous fistulas than with aneurysms.[14] The current recommendation for screening is that each family member should undergo magnetic resonance imaging (MRI), magnetic resonance angiography (MRA), or computed tomography angiography (CTA). It is recommended that family members be screened in their twenties and every 8 to 10 years thereafter. It is thought that patients who have a family history of aneurysm may develop them at a younger age than those with spurious aneurysms, although there is no conclusive study.[14]

After an aneurysm is identified in a patient with a family history of aneurysms, treatment is often recommended. Endovascular, surgical or combined options are considered, and the treatment with the lowest risk and highest efficacy of obliterating the aneurysm is recommended to the individual.[14]

ETIOLOGY

Although the precise etiology of cerebral aneurysms remains unclear, many extrinsic, congenital, and genetic factors have been implicated in the formation and rupture of intracerebral aneurysms. One theory suggests that a congenital/developmental defect exists in the medial and adventitial layers of the artery in the circle of Willis. There is little scientific basis for this theory, because these defects are commonly found postmortem in persons without aneurysms.[17] The degenerative theory is strongly supported by current research and ascribes causation to hemodynamically induced degenerative vascular disease.[18] According to this theory, the intima, covered only by the adventitia, bulges from a local weakness. By late midlife, stress causes vessel ballooning and rupture. There may be a predisposition to aneurysm formation in individuals with hypertension and in those in whom connective tissue disease promotes fragility of the arterial wall.[18] More recently, research has demonstrated an association between the presence of specific human leukocyte antigen alleles and the genetic role they may play in aneurysm formation.[19] There are some families in which several members are found to have aneurysms. When this occurs, other close family members should be monitored for vascular lesions.

Although the etiology of most aneurysms is as yet unknown, there are types of intracerebral aneurysms in which the etiology has been well demonstrated. Head trauma can result in traumatic intracranial aneurysms resulting from localized arterial tear. Bacterial and fungal infections have also been known to cause infectious (mycotic) aneurysms. Infectious aneurysms form when bacteria, usually from sep-

tic emboli, break off and actually invade and destroy the vessel wall. Atherosclerotic aneurysms can form in vessel walls that have been damaged by deposits of atheromatous material, resulting in fusiform aneurysms. Fusiform aneurysms are rarely associated with SAH.

ANEURYSM HEMODYNAMICS

The occurrence, growth, thrombosis, and rupture of intracranial saccular aneurysms can be directly related to the effect of hemodynamic forces. Strong evidence favors the idea that aneurysms of this nature occur because of hemodynamically induced degenerative vascular injury.[18] Despite in vitro studies over the last decade, the exact mechanisms of action of these stresses remain to be completely understood, and guidelines for determining the likelihood that a particular aneurysm will grow, rupture, regress, or thrombose do not exist.

Because of the capacity of evolving and available imaging techniques to depict vascular morphology accurately as well as to assess and in some instances quantify particular aspects of cerebral hemodynamics, there is an opportunity to add to the natural history of saccular aneurysms.[20]

An assessment of the chance of rupture of an asymptomatic saccular aneurysm is almost entirely based on a statistical analysis of the natural history of "similar lesions." Several factors combine to influence the magnitude of this risk (history of smoking, age, gender, number of aneurysms), and they all play a role in formulating techniques that would allow a more objective and individual estimation of risk. Research directed at the use of several evolving techniques in angiography, MR, and ultrasound aimed at the improved imaging of hemodynamic stresses that affect aneurysms may better define the relationship between the stresses and the vascular remodeling seen in aneurysm wall degeneration and healing.[20]

Aneurysm growth is a dynamic process that results from complex and incompletely understood interactions between hemodynamic forces and production of structural components that compose an aneurysm's wall. Because of physical limitations in the collagen present at the site where an aneurysm forms, it would be expected that a growth much larger than 8 mm in diameter would result in rupture. However, in most instances this does not occur. Changes in various hemodynamic factors (shear stress, pressure, and impingement force) as well as the presence of several humoral factors (inflammatory mediators and adhesion molecules) are potential signs of arterial injury. Sensing these signs, endothelium has the capacity to regulate the activity of substances that either act to promote or inhibit the repair of an aneurysm wall.[20]

Combinations of CT, MRI, MRA, and ultrasound can in some instances measure both geometric relationships and physiological parameters such as shear stress, pulse pressure, and compliance before and after a given intervention. As these techniques evolve, improve, and become more widely used, they will provide data that will be valuable in both the laboratory and in a clinical setting.[20]

CLASSIFICATION

Cerebral aneurysms present in a variety of sizes, shapes, and etiologies. When classified by size, the following categories are used:

- Small: to 10 mm
- Medium: 10 to 15 mm
- Large: 15 to 25 mm
- Giant: 25 to 50 mm
- Super-giant: larger than 50 mm

Classification by shape and etiology yields the following categories:

- **Berry aneurysm:** most common type; berry- or saccular-shaped with a neck or stem (Fig. 24-1)
- **Fusiform aneurysm:** an outpouching of an arterial wall, without a stem (see Fig. 24-1)
- **Traumatic aneurysm:** any aneurysm resulting from a traumatic head injury (accounts for a small number)
- **Mycotic (infectious) aneurysm:** rare; caused by septic emboli from infections, such as bacterial endocarditis; may lead to aneurysmal formation
- **Charcot-Bouchard aneurysm:** microscopic aneurysmal formation associated with hypertension; involves the basal ganglia and brain stem
- **Dissecting aneurysm:** related to atherosclerosis, inflammation, or trauma; an aneurysm in which the intimal layer is pulled away from the medial layer and blood is forced between the layers

LOCATION

Cerebral aneurysms usually occur at the bifurcations and branches of the large arteries at the base of the brain (circle of Willis). Eighty-five percent of aneurysms develop in the anterior part of the circle of Willis. The remaining 15% are found in the posterior circulation, known as the vertebro-basilar system.

The most common sites of saccular aneurysms are:

- 85% to 95% in the carotid system, with the following three most common locations:

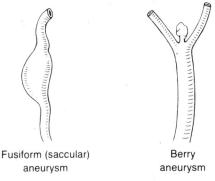

Fusiform (saccular)   Berry
aneurysm   aneurysm

Figure 24–1 • Berry and fusiform aneurysms.

- Anterior communicating artery is the single most common: 30%
- Anterior communicating artery and anterior cerebral artery are more common in males
- Posterior communicating artery: 25%
- Middle cerebral artery (MCA): 20%
- 5% to 15% in the posterior circulation (vertebrobasilar arteries)
  - About 10% on basilar artery: basilar bifurcation, known as basilar tip, most common followed by basilar artery–superior cerebellar artery (BA-SCA), basilar artery–vertebral artery (BA-VA) junction, and anterior inferior cerebellar artery (AICA)
  - About 5% on vertebral artery (VA) and posterior inferior cerebellar artery (PICA) junction is the most common
- Fusiform aneurysms are more common in the vertebrobasilar system
- 20% to 30 % of patients who suffer an aneurysm will have multiple aneurysms[21]

RUPTURED ANEURYSM

Subarachnoid hemorrhage is a type of intracranial hemorrhage in which bleeding occurs into the subarachnoid space. It accounts for 6% to 8% of all strokes and continues to be a significant cause of morbidity and mortality. Approximately 30% of people die within the first 2 weeks following the acute event,[22] and many survivors have persistent long-term deficits. Although advanced imaging techniques have allowed the noninvasive detection of an aneurysm or atriovenous malformation (AVM) as the potential source of a bleed, most aneurysms are detected following rupture. After SAH has occurred, medical complications are aggressively treated, but morbidity from factors other than rebleeding is still common.

Natural History and Incidence of Subarachnoid Hemorrhage

Many questions regarding natural history of SAH can be answered from available data. SAH of any cause represents from 4.5% to 13% of all strokes. Age-adjusted incidence rates of SAH are available from numerous studies, with reported rates from 7.9 per 100,000 persons per year in Oxfordshire, England to 15.1 per 100,000 in Helsinki, Finland. In Japan, there have been higher incident rates reported—21 to 25 per 100,000. Long-term trends are only available from Rochester, Minnesota in population-based studies, which demonstrate that there is no change in the incidence rate of SAH through 1989. There are some gender-related differences, with female incidence higher than male in some population-based studies.[23]

There is a possible reduced occurrence of SAH in some premenopausal women, especially those without a smoking history. In the same study, hormone replacement reduced the risk in postmenopausal women who had never smoked.[24] Racial differences have been infrequently studied, although there are data that indicate that the incidence rate in the African-American population is twice that of whites.[25] Age-related differences are detected, with increasing incidence of SAH with age.

Pathophysiology

At the time of aneurysmal rupture, blood under high pressure is forced into the subarachnoid space at the base of the brain (circle of Willis), spreading by way of the sylvian fissures into the basal cisterns. Less often the aneurysm ruptures into one of the following areas of the brain, resulting in formation of a hematoma: the brain parenchymal tissue (intracerebral hematoma); the ventricles (intraventricular hematoma); the subarachnoid space (subarachnoid hematoma); or the subdural space (subdural hematoma). When rupture occurs, it usually occurs at the thin-walled dome of the aneurysm, causing blood to enter into the subarachnoid space. Tissue pressure surrounding the aneurysm stops the bleeding, and fibrin, platelets, and fluid form a plug that seals off the site of bleeding. The resulting clot can occlude the area or interfere with cerebrospinal fluid (CSF) absorption. The blood released irritates the brain tissue, setting up an inflammatory response that enhances cerebral edema.

Concurrent with the time of rupture, significant SAH occurs, raising intracranial pressure (ICP) toward the mean arterial pressure and lowering cerebral perfusion pressure. These hemodynamic changes probably account for the transient loss of or altered level of consciousness. Clinically, a stroke syndrome with associated increased ICP develops. The specific signs and symptoms associated with the event depend on the location of the hemorrhage and the degree of ICP.

▌▌▌▌ SIGNS AND SYMPTOMS

Signs and symptoms arising from an aneurysm can be divided into two categories: those presenting before rupture or bleeding (**unruptured**), and those appearing after rupture or bleeding (**ruptured**).

Unruptured Aneurysms

Most patients are completely asymptomatic until the time of bleeding. A recent publication of the American Heart Association outlines the recommendations for management of patients with unruptured intracranial aneurysms.[26] In approximately 40% of cases, there are warning signs, often called *prodromal signs*, that are either ignored or attributed to other causes. Prodromal signs may suggest the location of the aneurysm or enlargement of the lesion. Localizing signs and symptoms include:

- Dilated pupil (loss of light reflex; oculomotor nerve [cranial nerve (CN) III] deficit)
- Extraocular movement deficits of the oculomotor (CN III), trochlear (CN IV) or abducens (CN VI) cranial nerves

- Possible ptosis (oculomotor nerve [CN III] deficit)
- Pain above and behind eye
- Localized headache
- Nuchal rigidity (neck pain on flexion)
- Possible photophobia

Small intermittent aneurysmal leakage of blood may result in generalized headache, neck pain, upper back pain, nausea, and vomiting. Management of unruptured intracranial aneurysms is controversial because of the lack of knowledge of the natural history of these lesions and the risks of repairing them.[27] A large multicenter study was conducted to determine the risk of rupture and the risks associated with the repair of unruptured intracranial aneurysms.

Whether all unruptured aneurysms should be treated has been debated for years. Clinical outcomes depend on various factors and require balancing early and delayed risks. There are relatively few data regarding the natural history of unruptured aneurysms.[28] A published study of the natural history of aneurysm studies observed 130 patients for a follow-up that lasted 8.3 years. None of the aneurysms smaller than 1 cm in maximal diameter at discovery ruptured during follow-up, whereas 15 of 51 aneurysms 1 cm or larger ruptured during follow-up. In a review of 142 patients harboring 181 unruptured aneurysms (some had multiple aneurysms), 27 hemorrhages occurred during 1,944 patient years of follow-up (mean 13.9 years) with annual rupture rate of 1.4%. The size of the aneurysm was a predictor of hemorrhage. Other studies have suggested that there was not an insignificant risk of hemorrhage in small aneurysms and in others, selected locations, such as anterior communicating artery aneurysms, had been associated with increased rupture rate.[1]

International Study of Unruptured Intracranial Aneurysms (ISUIA)

In 1998, the investigators of the ISUIA reported results from the initial aspects of the international collaborative study of unruptured intracranial aneurysms. The retrospective cohort study included patients with unruptured intracranial aneurysms diagnosed among 53 participating centers from 1970 to 1991. Patients with and without SAH were included, but analysis was performed based on the following categories:

- Group 1: patients without an SAH
- Group 2: patients with an earlier SAH from an aneurysm, but with that ruptured aneurysm definitively treated, and having had another unruptured aneurysm

Patients with traumatic, mycotic, or fusiform aneurysms were not eligible. A prospective component including those with and without surgical or endovascular treatment was also conducted, and the surgical results were reported in 1998. Hard copies of cerebral angiograms from all patients were reviewed at the Mayo Clinic. Long-term follow-up was conducted in both prospective and retrospective groups. In the retrospective cohort, 1449 patients with 1937 unruptured intracranial aneurysms (727 Group 1 and 722 Group 2) were observed during follow-up. There were 1,085 (75%) who had a single unruptured intracranial aneurysm, and 364 had multiple unruptured intracranial aneurysms. Signs and symptoms leading to diagnosis of unruptured intracranial aneurysms included ischemic cerebrovascular disease, headaches, cranial nerve deficits, aneurysmal mass effect, ill-defined spells, and convulsive disorders.[1]

Several aneurysm characteristics were analyzed, including site, size, presence of daughter sac, and presence of multiple lobes. During the follow-up period, 32 of the 1,449 patients had an aneurysm rupture, with 28 of 32 ruptures within the first 7.5 years of follow-up. Among Group 1 patients with SAH, 1 of 12 was smaller than 10 mm in diameter whereas 17 of 20 patients in Group 2 with ruptures had aneurysms smaller than 10 mm in diameter.[1]

In Group 1 patients, the only significant predictors of rupture were size and location of aneurysm. Aneurysms smaller than 10 mm were less likely to rupture than those 10 to 24 mm. There were other selected sites—basilar tip, vertebrobasilar and posterior communicating—that were at increased risk of rupture. In Group 2, the relative risk of rupture was 5.1 for aneurysms at the basilar tip and 1.31 for older age. Size of aneurysm did not predict rupture in group 2 patients.

The cumulative rates of rupture for patients were:

- Group 1 patients (no previous SAH) with aneurysms smaller than 10 mm in diameter were .05% per year.
- Group 1 patients with aneurysm larger than 10 mm in diameter were 20 times higher—approaching 1% per year.
- Group 2 patients—smaller aneurysms (i.e., smaller than 10 mm) were 11 times more likely to rupture as aneurysms of the same size in Group 1, at about 0.5% per year.
- The rupture rate of larger aneurysms (i.e., larger than 10 mm) was similar in Group 2 patients compared with those in Group 1, at about 1% per year.

Mortality for SAH was 66%. The paper also reported surgical intervention-related morbidity and mortality of the prospective cohort. At 1 month, Group 1 patients' surgical mortality was 2.3%. Overall morbidity and mortality for all patients in Group 1 were 17.5% at 1 month and 15.7% at 1 year.[1] A meta-analysis was performed in 1997 that reviewed 23 studies of prevalence and risk of rupture of intracranial saccular aneurysms. For adults without specific risk factors, the prevalence of intracranial saccular aneurysm was 2.3%, which increased with age. Nine studies were used to analyze risk of rupture, totaling 3,907 patient years. The highest risk per year was 1.9%. For aneurysms equal to 10 mm, the annual risk was 0.7% per year. The risk was slightly higher in women. The risk was also higher for those aneurysms larger than 10 mm in diameter, those that were symptomatic, and those in the posterior circulation.[29]

Ruptured Aneurysm

The most frequent presentation of aneurysms is rupture, which most often produces SAH. Intracerebral hemorrhage occurs in 20% to 40% of cases (more common in those with aneurysms distal to the circle of Willis, e.g., middle cerebral artery [MCA]). Intraventricular bleeding occurs in 13% to 28% (most common in anterior communicating artery aneurysm; prognosis appears worse with about 64 % mortality),

whereas subdural blood is present in 2% to 5% of cases.[21] At the time of rupture or bleeding, blood is forced into the subarachnoid space. The patient experiences a violent headache, often described as "explosive" or "the worst headache of my life." Immediate loss of consciousness may occur, or the level of consciousness may decrease. Vomiting is common. Other signs and symptoms include:

- Cranial nerve deficits (especially cranial nerves [CNs] III, IV, and VI); non-pupil sparing CN III palsy produced by expanding posterior communicating artery aneurysm
- Those related to meningeal irritation, including nausea, vomiting, stiff neck, pain in the neck and back, and possible blurred vision or photophobia. Signs of meningeal irritation usually appear 4 to 8 hours after the SAH. Mild temperature elevation may accompany SAH.
- Those related to a stroke syndrome, including signs and symptoms related to the vascular territory involved and intracerebral hemorrhage (e.g., hemiparesis, hemiplegia, aphasia, cognitive deficits)
- Those related to cerebral edema and increased ICP (mass effect), including seizures, hypertension, bradycardia, and widening pulse pressure
- Those related to pituitary dysfunction secondary to irritation or edema resulting from the proximity of the gland to common locations of aneurysms and possibly causing diabetes insipidus and hyponatremia[21]

Hunt-Hess Classification

Many different SAH grading systems have been proposed; the most widely used is the Hunt-Hess Classification.[30] This system was initially designed for patients with SAH. It is a helpful tool to guide the physician in diagnosing the severity of SAH secondary to aneurysmal bleeding, as well as in timing surgical intervention if surgery is an option. The patient is assigned to a category on admission to the hospital (Table 24-1). Changes in the patient's condition are then

Table 24–1 • HUNT-HESS CLASSIFICATION OF SUBARACHNOID HEMORRHAGES

GRADE	DESCRIPTION
I	Asymptomatic, or mild headache and slight nuchal rigidity
II	Cranial nerve (CN) palsy (e.g., oculomotor [CN III], abducens [CN VI]), moderate-to-severe headache, nuchal rigidity
III	Mild focal deficit, lethargy, or confusion
IV	Stupor, moderate to severe hemiparesis, early decerebrate rigidity
V	Deep coma, decerebrate rigidity, moribund appearance
	Add one grade for serious systemic disease (e.g. hypertension, chronic obstructive pulmonary disease) or severe vasospasm on angiography
	Modified classification adds the following:
0	Unruptured aneurysm
1a	No acute meningeal/brain reaction, but with fixed neurological deficit

monitored according to baseline. The original paper did not consider the patient's age, site of aneurysm, or time since hemorrhage; patients were graded on admission and preoperatively.

IIIII DIAGNOSIS

Diagnosis of a cerebral aneurysm is based on:

- History and results of neurological examination.
- CT scan, without contrast media; a good-quality fourth-generation CT will detect SAH in 95% or more of cases if scans are done within 48 hours of SAH. Blood appears as high density (i.e., appears white) within subarachnoid spaces.
- If the CT findings are negative, lumbar puncture is used in selective cases. Red blood cell (RBC) counts usually exceed 100,000 per mm³.
- CTA is now being used in many institutions as the first radiographic tool. It is a more recent development than MRA, and its role is being refined, with a reported sensitivity of 95% and specificity of 83%. Unlike conventional angiography, CTA provides a three-dimensional image and demonstrates the relationship to nearby bony structures.
- MRI is not sensitive within the first 24 to 48 hours, especially with thin layers of blood; it is more satisfactory after 4 to 7 days. MRA is also used.
- Cerebral angiography remains the *gold standard* for evaluation of cerebral aneurysms. It demonstrates a source of the aneurysm in about 80% to 85% of cases and radiologic vasospasm (i.e., a narrowing of the cerebral blood vessels as seen on radiographic films).[21]

Imaging

Computed Tomography

CT remains the mainstay of initial detection of SAH, with 90% or better sensitivity in detecting a clinically significant SAH in the first 2 days after the event. It is important to realize that a negative CT scan never excludes SAH and that a clinical suggestion of an SAH, even in the face of a negative CT scan, still requires a lumbar puncture.[31]

A plain CT scan obtained within 48 hours of aneurysmal rupture is usually the initial diagnostic procedure ordered. If the scan is performed within 24 hours of the initial SAH , a high-density clot in the subarachnoid space can be demonstrated in 92% to 95% of cases; if done within 48 hours, the clot can be demonstrated in 75% to 85% of cases.[4,32,33] A CT scan also aids in establishing the extent and location of subarachnoid bleeding and is useful for identifying patients at high risk for the development of vasospasm and for pinpointing the potential vascular territory of the vasospasm.[31]

The Fisher Grading Scale[97] (Table 24-2) is used to assist in prediction of outcome. The amount of blood on CT scan correlates with the severity of cerebral vasospasm.

If an angiogram is ordered and multiple aneurysms are seen, the CT scan is helpful in identifying which aneurysm bled, based on the presence of a clot.

T a b l e 2 4 – 2 • FISHER GRADING SCALE (AMOUNT OF BLOOD ON CT SCAN IS A PREDICTOR OF VASOSPASM)

FISHER GROUP	BLOOD ON CT
1	No subarachnoid blood detected
2	Diffuse or vertical layers <1 mm thick
3	Localized and/or vertical layers ≥1 mm
4	Intracerebral or intraventricular clot with diffuse or no subarachnoid hemorrhage

Spiral Computed Tomography Angiography

Spiral CTA using the slip ring technology allows visualization of arterial anatomy after IV administration of a timed bolus of contrast material and can acquire images in a very short time. This new technique is often used as a first step in evaluation of patients with a diagnosis of SAH who are being transferred into a tertiary care facility. The images can provide an immediate diagnosis for the physician managing the patient. Patients have been brought to the operating room or endovascular suite based on these images to reduce any further time from treatment of the lesion. Imaging time is generally 30 to 40 seconds. This is an extremely helpful technology in the primary evaluation of patients with diagnosis of SAH. One disadvantage of the technique is the load of contrast material that is administered, although the benefits often outweigh the risks.[31]

The examination is begun in the location of interest, either the circle of Willis or the carotid bifurcation, using contiguous unenhanced 5-mm thick axial sections. After the area of interest is determined, the time to peak arterial enhancement is calculated by using preliminary IV bolus infusion of 20 mL of contrast material, which is usually nonionic. This is administered using a power injector at 3 mL/sec and a 20-gauge catheter needle in the antecubital vein. For the actual CTA acquisition, contrast material is administered at 3 mL/ sec for 30 seconds, a total of 90 mL. Images are transferred to an off-line workstation and projections are obtained. Source images must always be consulted when interpreting CTA.

CTA is a reliable alternative to MRA in evaluating the circle of Willis and carotid bifurcation. At some institutions, specific applications include triaging patients for possible superselective thrombolysis, following patients with carotid stents, and evaluating multiperspective approaches to intracranial aneurysms. Additionally, CTA may ultimately demonstrate advantages in the screening of aneurysms in the appropriate patient population.[31]

Angiography

Cerebral angiography (Fig. 24-2) is still the mainstay of diagnosis for cerebral aneurysms, but with the advent of CTA this may change. Angiography provides visualization of all four major cerebral vessels and their branches. Angiography is commonly scheduled immediately following diagnosis of SAH by CT scan or CTA in patients who are deemed clinically stable. If not clinically stable, the CTA may provide

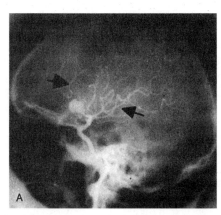

Figure 24–2 • Carotid angiography indicates a large aneurysm of the anterior communicating artery. The anterior cerebral artery (*larger arrow* on left) and the middle cerebral artery (*smaller arrow*) are also illustrated.

enough information to offer reasonable treatment of the aneurysm. Early angiography allows for definitive diagnosis and enables the cerebrovascular team of physicians (neurosurgeon, interventional neuroradiologist, and neurologist) to advocate a treatment plan for the patient. In addition to the specific location of the aneurysm, the following points can be identified using angiography:

- The particular characteristics of the aneurysm (shape, size, presence of daughter sac)
- Any anomalies of cerebral vasculature (e.g., involving the circle of Willis) that will affect treatment decision
- The presence of vasospasm, which may influence the urgency to obliterate the aneurysm either surgically or endovascularly, so that so-called triple H (hypervolemic, hemodilution and hypertensive) therapy can be initiated.

Repeat Angiography. Repeat angiography may be performed for the following reasons:

- Confirmation of diagnosis when no aneurysm is found on early angiography (small aneurysms can be missed, particularly in the posterior circulation). Angiogram is usually repeated 10 days to 2 weeks after the initial study.
- Identification of reversal of previously observed vasospasm
- Detection and treatment of vasospasm when there is deterioration of neurological function (change in level of consciousness is the most common situation.)

Negative Angiogram and Subarachnoid Hemorrhage. It is generally believed that if an aneurysm is not found with a thorough cerebral angiogram in a patient with a documented SAH, in approximately 5% of the cases, this represents a false-negative result. Explanations range from transient thrombosis of the aneurysm, to vasospasm, technical error, or ruptured pial vascular malformation. Repeat angiography is generally recommended in such patients 1 to 2 weeks after the initial angiogram. A third angiogram is often recommended by many neurosurgeons and neuroradiologists, usually at 3 months after the initial angiogram, often including spinal angiography.

Perimesencephalic nonaneurysmal SAH is a distinct entity and considered a benign condition with a good outcome. This group has less risk of rebleeding and vasospasm than other patients with SAH of unknown etiology. The actual etiology is yet to be determined, but it may be secondary to rupture of a small perimesencephalic vein or artery.[21].

Small aneurysms may obliterate themselves after rupture, leaving no aneurysm to be found on angiography. This type of aneurysm may be referred to as a *cryptic aneurysm.*

Magnetic Resonance Imaging

Magnetic resonance imaging (MRI) plays only a minor role in the diagnosis of acute SAH because of the unstable condition of many of these patients and the relatively high insensitivity of MRI to acute subarachnoid blood. The inherent contrast of MRI depends on clot retraction and deoxygenation of the hemoglobin. In the acute stages of a bleed, this clot retraction does not occur readily when blood is mixed with CSF. The hemoglobin molecule remains better oxygenated after an SAH than after bleeding into the parenchyma. Thus, CT scan remains the examination modality of choice in the evaluation of an acute SAH.[31]

Magnetic Resonance Angiography

Magnetic resonance angiography (MRA) evaluation of aneurysms yields the best results with aneurysms 0.5 to 1.5 cm. MRA can assist in the evaluation of aneurysms, particularly when they are larger than 3 mm in diameter. MRI and MRA should be reserved as tools to assist in the evaluation of patients with possible symptoms of aneurysm and not used in those who have had an acute hemorrhage. This procedure will also screen for possible causes that may elicit symptoms relative to headache or mass effect, such as an arteriovenous malformation or arterial fistula. Given these limitations, high-resolution angiography may still be necessary to exclude aneurysms smaller than 3 mm.[31,34]

Lumbar Puncture (LP)

An LP is used only if a CT scan is unavailable, if there is no evidence of increased ICP (e.g., papilledema) and the CT scan results are negative, and there is also the need to establish evidence of SAH. A LP is contraindicated in the presence of increased ICP because of the risk of brain-stem herniation; it also increases the risk of rebleeding. CSF analysis reveals blood; xanthochromia (discoloration of CSF) is noted when the CSF is centrifuged.

Transcranial Doppler (TCD)

Transcranial Doppler (TCD) series is newer technology that is used on a daily basis in neurological intensive care units (NICU) in patients who have suffered SAH to monitor flow velocities in major cerebral arteries so that early vasospasm can be detected and treated.

INITIAL APPROACH TO MEDICAL MANAGEMENT

The patient who survives the initial rupture of a cerebral aneurysm is beset by various potential problems and complications that can lead to additional morbidity and mortality. Consideration of whether to treat or how to treat a ruptured cerebral aneurysm depends on various factors: age of the patient, the neurological condition of the patient (Hunt-Hess grade), Fisher grade, or size of the aneurysm. The patient's current or previous medical condition may also factor into the decision-making process.

Initial Management Concerns

- Rebleeding—the major concern during the initial work-up. Maximal frequency of rebleeding is in the 1st day (4% on day 1, then 1.5% daily for 13 days). Between 15% and 20% rebleed within 14 days, and 50% will rebleed within 6 months; thereafter, the risk is 3%/year with a mortality of 2%/year.
- Acute hydrocephalus—usually obstructive because of obstruction of CSF by a blood clot.
- Delayed ischemic neurological deficit most likely related to vasospasm
- Hyponatremia with hypovolemia
- Deep venous thrombosis (DVT) and pulmonary embolism
- Seizure
- Determining source of bleeding; four-vessel cerebral angiography is required.

The **goals of initial medical management** include:

- Augmenting cerebral blood flow (CBF) by:
  - Increasing cerebral perfusion pressure (CPP)
  - Improving blood rheology
  - Maintaining euvolemia (the majority of patients become hypovolemic in the first 24 hours after SAH)
  - Maintaining normal ICP
- Neuroprotection

Patients are admitted to the NICU where the following can be provided:

- An arterial line is placed (for those patients who are hemodynamically unstable, stuporous or comatose).
- Patient is intubated (comatose or unable to protect airway).
- Pulmonary artery catheter (PAC) line is placed for those with a Hunt-Hess grade of 3 or higher, syndrome of inappropriate antidiuretic hormone (SIADH), or who are hemodynamically unstable.
- Cardiac monitor attached—SAH may be associated with cardiac arrhythmias and there are changes measurable on electrocardiogram in more than 50% of cases.
- Intraventricular catheter is placed in patients developing hydrocephalus and with a Hunt-Hess grade of 3 or higher.[21]

Nursing orders include:

- Vital signs with neurological checks every hour
- Bedrest with head of bed (HOB) elevated by 30 degrees
- Low level of external stimulation, restricted visitation
- Strict intake-and-output (I&O) record
- Daily weights
- Thigh-high antiembolism (TED) hose and pneumatic compression boots
- Indwelling urinary catheter if patient is lethargic, incontinent, or unable to void

Fluid Volume Control

One of the goals of medical management is to maintain fluid volume within a normal range (euvolia). The underlying reason for this is that dehydration increases hemoconcentration, which is thought to increase the incidence of cerebral vasospasm. If cerebral edema is present, a regimen of moderate fluid restriction and steroids may be ordered. Mannitol may be ordered to decrease cerebral edema. Early aggressive fluid therapy may prevent cerebral salt wasting.

- Normal saline IV solution with 20 mEq KCl /L at 2 ml/kg per hour
- 5% albumin, 500 mL over 4 hours, started immediately at admission

Blood Pressure Control

In the early hours after rupture, blood pressure is commonly elevated, probably reflecting a physiological response to increased ICP. As ICP is decreased, the blood pressure also decreases. If the blood pressure continues to be elevated owing to increased ICP from mass effect of cerebral edema or a hematoma, mannitol may be administered. The drug is beneficial for two reasons: (1) it decreases cerebral edema and neurological deficits, and (2) it improves CBF. Decreased cerebral edema lowers the ICP and blood pressure.

Hypertension is controlled to prevent rebleeding. The goal of therapy is to maintain the systolic blood pressure between 120 and 150 mm Hg. Systolic pressures above this level are treated with drugs such as labetalol or nitroprusside. Nitroprusside is used in conjunction with an arterial line. It is a vasodilator and may increase the risk of rupture with an unsecured aneurysm. These drugs effectively lower the pressure without sudden drops in the systolic pressure and are easily titrated.

Electrocardiographic Changes

The association between SAH and electrocardiography (EKG) has been known since 1954 when Burch and colleagues noted an EKG pattern of Q-T prolongation and T-wave inversion in patients with SAH.[35] Subsequent investigations have determined that EKG abnormalities occur in 25% to 75% of patients with SAH.[36]

The pathophysiology of cardiac injury in patients with SAH appears to result from an excess of catecholamines in the myocardium. The "catecholamine hypothesis" remains controversial, and other proposed mechanisms include coronary arterial spasm, coronary artery disease, and injury caused by elevated myocardial wall stress in the setting of tachycardia and hypertension.[37]

The prognostic importance of EKG changes in association with SAH has been examined in small studies with varying results. It is unclear whether these EKG changes are predictive of cardiac mortality or are simply a reflection of the underlying central nervous system process.

Zaroff and associates[38] conducted a retrospective study of 439 patients with SAH with abnormal EKG changes and determined the incidence of cardiac and all-cause mortality. They found that 27% of the study population had EKG readings that met the criteria for myocardial ischemia or infarction. This study indicates that patients with SAH and ischemic EKG readings are at low risk for cardiac mortality, with or without aneurysm surgery. One may conclude that surgery should not be withheld from patients with SAH on the basis of ischemic EKG changes alone. The patients with a higher Hunt-Hess grade may be at greater risk for poor neurological outcomes without aggressive therapy such as surgery or endovascular treatment.[38]

Drug Therapy

The following drugs are usually ordered for the patient with an aneurysmal rupture:

- The calcium channel blocker nimodipine (Nimotop) 60 mg q 4 hours orally or through nasogastric tube, initiated within 96 hours of SAH, is given for 21 consecutive days. Nimodipine has been shown to enhance collateral blood flow and improve long-term outcomes in patients with SAH from aneurysm rupture.
- Anticonvulsants may be given as prophylaxis against seizures. Phenytoin is the usual agent used—load with 17 mg/kg, maintenance with 100 mg three times daily.
- Stool softeners prevent constipation and straining at stool, which results in initiation of Valsalva's maneuver, increased ICP, and increased blood pressure, which in turn can cause rebleeding of the aneurysm.
- Use of steroids is controversial; however, some believe it is beneficial for treatment of cerebral edema and the inflammatory effect of the meningeal irritation.
- Analgesics (acetaminophen or codeine) are administered as necessary to control headache.
- Sedatives may be prescribed, because an agitated patient is at risk for elevated blood pressure.

Monitoring for Complications

In the acute phase, most patients are managed in the NICU where they can be observed frequently and monitored with invasive hemodynamic monitoring equipment by a well-trained and knowledgeable nursing staff. The rationale for monitoring of neurological signs and other parameters is early detection of complications. The major complications of aneurysmal rupture are *rebleeding, cerebral vasospasm* and *hydrocephalus*, which are discussed in a later section of this chapter. Other problems associated with aneurysmal rupture/bleed are reflected in laboratory studies and the results of an electrocardiogram. The following are pertinent data.

Blood Studies

- White blood cell (WBC) count: often elevated (15,000 to 18,0000) as a result of meningeal irritation
- Hematocrit, fibrinogen, and platelets; bleeding time and osmolality: indicators of development of cerebral vasospasm
- Electrolytes: hyponatremia often develops as a result of SIADH or salt wasting
- Blood gases: monitor adequacy of oxygenation

Electrocardiogram

Changes related to hypothalamic dysfunction result in elevated serum catecholamine levels. Catecholamines stimulate alpha-adrenergic receptors in the myocardium, possibly causing ST changes, prolonged QRS, prolonged Q-T interval, and tall T waves. EKG changes may be consistent with endocardial damage and sometimes myocardial ischemia. Consultation with a cardiologist experienced in the care of patients with SAH is beneficial and can avoid delay in treatment with early intervention.

SURGICAL/INTERVENTIONAL TREATMENT

Surgery historically has been the treatment of choice for a ruptured or bleeding cerebral aneurysm. With the advent of interventional procedures using such devices as the Guglielmi detachable coil (GDC), balloons, and stents, there are now options in the modality of treatment. Placement of GDCs into cerebral aneurysms is rapidly gaining acceptance as an alternative to surgical clipping and in many centers is the treatment of choice. Consideration of various factors, including age of the patient, size of the aneurysm, location of the aneurysm, the neurological condition of the patient (Hunt-Hess grade), and previous medical conditions, is necessary when deciding the best treatment option. The goal of treatment, either surgical or interventional, is to prevent rebleeding by sealing off the aneurysm so that the aneurysm is totally obliterated with either a clip or coil. In situations in which the patient is gravely ill, the decision may be to coil the dome of the aneurysm (where rupture occurred) and after the patient's condition stabilizes, operate and clip the entire aneurysm.

Timing of Treatment

Timing of treatment is critical to patient outcome. As a result of studies demonstrating improved outcomes from earlier treatment, there has been a definite trend toward early (within 24 to 48 hours after hemorrhage) treatment for those patients who present with aneurysmal SAH. Even patients whose condition is assessed as poor (Hunt-Hess Grades 4 and 5) are considered for early treatment, depending on the stability of their overall medical condition. The following are the benefits of early treatment:

- Results in superior management in overall care
- Eliminates the problem of rebleeding

- Allows for removal of basal cistern clots associated with vasospasm
- Permits institution of previously mentioned triple H (hypervolemic, hemodilution and hypertensive) therapy for postoperative vasospasm without the risk of rebleeding

Surgical Approaches and Considerations

Microsurgical techniques and improved anesthesia allow for a precise surgical approach and clipping of aneurysms. The surgical approach and method of aneurysmal obliteration depends on the location and characteristics of the aneurysm. An aneurysm with a stem or neck is usually managed with a surgical clip on the neck (Figs. 24-3, 24-4, and 24-5; see also Chapter 15). Depending on the location and size of the aneurysm, more than one clip may be necessary to obliterate it. The surgeon may choose from a wide selection of commercial clips of different sizes, shapes, and angulations. For aneurysms that are difficult to reach, the surgeon may have to modify a clip to accommodate the vessels and structures at the aneurysmal site. Before permanent clips are positioned, temporary clips are often applied medial or distal to the aneurysm to minimize blood flow to the aneurysm so as to improve the exposure to the aneurysm and to ensure proper placement of the permanent clip. The temporary clips, which are softer and gold tipped, are removed after the aneurysmal neck has been securely clipped. The adequacy of vascular territory circulation is verified before the permanent clips are applied. Figure 24-6 is the arteriogram of a 54-year-old woman with an incidental finding of an unruptured anterior cerebral artery (ACA) aneurysm. Figure 24-7 is an intraoperative photo of the aneurysm, and Figure 24-8 shows a clipping of an ACA aneurysm.

Intraoperative angiography, CBF studies, or intraoperative Doppler studies may be conducted during surgery to verify the adequacy of circulation and the security of the clip. Some aneurysms, such as fusiform aneurysms, are not amenable to clipping because of their shape or location. In such situations, the aneurysm may be surgically wrapped in muslin, which provides support to the weakened arterial

wall and also induces scarring. Newer techniques for obliterating fusiform aneurysms include a bypass and an end-to-end anastomosis of arteries once the fusiform section is dissected and removed.

If multiple aneurysms are present, it may not be possible to obliterate all lesions at one surgery. The priority site is the aneurysm that has bled, after it has been identified by CT scan and angiography. A second surgical procedure may be planned for a later date, if indicated. Alternatives to surgical treatment of an aneurysm include:

- Wrapping—although this is usually not the goal of surgery, situations may arise in which little else can be done (e.g., fusiform aneurysms).
- Trapping—effective treatment requires distal and proximal arterial interruption by direct surgical means (ligation or occlusion with clip), by placement of a detachable balloon, or combination. It may also necessitate extracranial-intracranial (EC-IC) bypass to maintain flow distal to the trapped segment proximal ligation.[21]

Certain situations require special considerations by the neurosurgeon. For example, with a large aneurysm involving the basilar tip, special precautions must be taken to prevent injury to the small perforating branches emitted from this area. If these vessels are compromised, the patient may not awaken and may develop thalamic infarcts, depending on the extent of the injury. Some neurosurgeons consider using cardiac arrest bypass surgery to clip these large posterior circulation lesions. Prolonged cardiac arrest can be tolerated under deep hypothermia and artificial extracorporeal circulation. The techniques involved are very complicated, and a skilled surgeon who is confident in the use of this technique is necessary.[39]

Special considerations are also warranted with a mycotic aneurysm. Mycotic aneurysms account for approximately 4% of intracranial aneurysms and occur in 3% to 15% of patients with subacute bacterial endocarditis. Usually located at the distal end of a vessel, the most common location is the distal MCA branches (75% to 80%). Treatment with antibiotics for 4 to 6 weeks may result in disappearance of

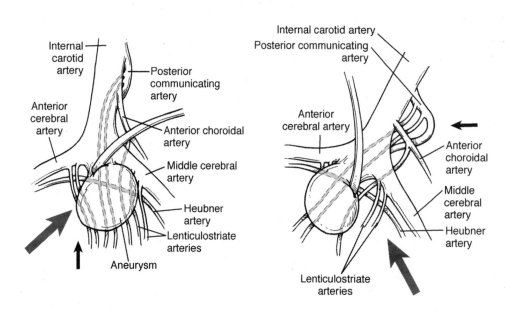

Figure 24–3 • Microexposure and visualization of the perforating vessels near the aneurysm. *Striped arrows* indicate frontal and temporal surgical access. *Open arrow* indicates lateral carotid accesses. *Small black arrow* points to Sylvian accesses. (Courtesy of Chris Ogilvy, MD, Massachusetts General Hospital, Boston, MA.)

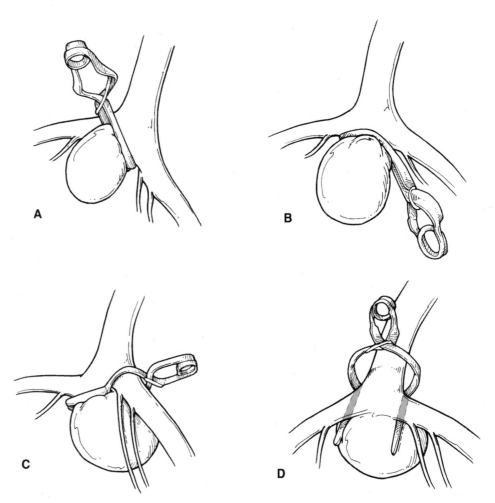

Figure 24-4 • Clipping techniques. (A) Straight clip for small aneurysms. (B) Curved clip to reconstruct the vessel. (C) Fenestrated clip encircles the middle cerebral artery to keep it open while clipping the aneurysm. (D) Fenestrated clip encircles the internal carotid artery to occlude the neck of an inferiorly directed aneurysm. (Courtesy of Chris Ogilvy, MD, Massachusetts General Hospital, Boston, MA.)

the lesion. However, if the aneurysm remains and enlarges, surgical or endovascular treatment may be necessary.[21]

Asymptomatic Aneurysms

During the last two decades, detection of unruptured intracranial aneurysms has increased because of new and improved diagnostic tests (MRA, digital subtraction angiography, and three-dimensional CTA) and a more active treatment approach for patients with ruptured intracranial aneurysms. In addition, older patients are more likely to be treated than in the past.[40]

The natural history of unruptured intracranial aneurysms is poorly understood, as are the risk factors. This is due to the lack of studies with sufficient patient numbers and follow-up years. The current knowledge of the natural history of unruptured aneurysm is based on only a few studies, with the risk factors being even more controversial because of the differing results published from these studies. Therefore, treatment decisions for unruptured aneurysms vary.[41–49]

In a long-term cohort study of 142 patients with unruptured aneurysms, Juvela and colleagues conducted follow-up of 2,575 person-years. They found an approximate rupture rate of 1.3% per year for an unruptured aneurysm. This overall rupture rate is similar to earlier observations of 1% to 2% per year[42,44–46,49] but somewhat lower than those re-

ported in another study (2.3% per year),[48] and it is higher than that in the ISUIA study (0.3% per year).[43]

Aneurysms may be acquired degenerative lesions that develop as a result of hemodynamic stress, or they may be familial or associated with connective tissue diseases.[50] There may be unknown factors that increase the risk of aneurysm formation or SAH. Some of these factors include hypertension, cigarette smoking, use of oral contraceptives, female gender, atherosclerosis, aging, alcohol consumption, arterial deficiency in collagen type III, viral infections, arteriovenous malformations, asymmetry of the circle of Willis, pituitary tumors, and certain human leukocyte antigen–associated factors.[41,51,52]

The results of studies conducted by Juvela and colleagues suggest that unruptured aneurysms should be treated regardless of size, at least in patients younger than 50 years.[41,51,52] In older patients with small aneurysms, smoking cessation alone may be treatment enough. In North America and Europe, the prevalence of smoking in patients who suffer SAH ranges from 45% to 75%, whereas in the general adult population the range is 20% to 35%.[52,53] These studies concluded that unruptured intracranial aneurysms should be surgically treated, regardless of size, if technically possible, and that patient age and concurrent diseases do not increase surgical risk. Although cigarette smoking seems to increase the risk of aneurysm rupture, surgery should not be withheld in these cases because of the devastation that

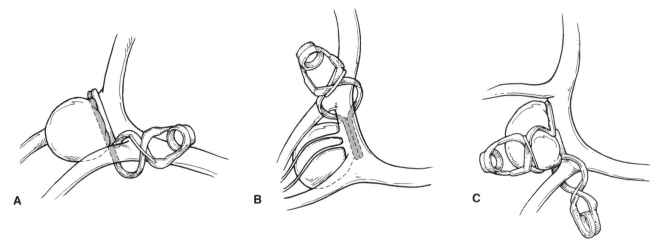

A   B   C

Figure 24–5 • Clipping strategies with fenestrated clips. (*A*) Here, a side-deflected fenestrated clip is used to occlude the aneurysm neck while reconstructing the neck of the A2 vessel. (*B*) An angled fenestrated clip reconstructs the anterior communicating artery, saving perforating branches. (*C*) Two fenestrated clips are used to clip a wide neck aneurysm. (Courtesy of Chris Ogilvy, MD, Massachusetts General Hospital, Boston, MA.)

can result from aneurysmal rupture compared with the success rates attained in surgical treatment of unruptured aneurysms.[41]

Endovascular Treatment of Aneurysms

Despite recent advances in neurological surgery and intensive care management, the morbidity and mortality rates of patients who survive an initial SAH remain high. A high percentage of patients may not be surgical candidates for various reasons. The management of intracranial aneurysms continues to evolve, particularly the endovascular management component. The use of electrically detachable platinum coils for the endovascular treatment of intracranial aneurysms was first described by Guglielmi and col-

leagues.[54,55] Guglielmi detachable coils (GDCs) were prospectively evaluated in selected North American medical centers to determine their use in treating intracranial aneurysms that were not amenable to direct surgical treatment. Electrothrombosis occurs when a positively charged electrode that has been placed in the bloodstream attracts negatively charged blood elements—RBCs and WBCs, platelets, and fibrinogen. Electrolysis occurs when two electrodes positioned in a solution are connected to a direct current. When direct current is applied to the coil system, the positively charged platinum coils promote electrothrombosis while at the same time electrolysis of the junctional stainless steel wire occurs, detaching the coil in the aneurysm without traction.[56]

The platinum coils are soft and have their own preformed helix of 2 to 14 mm. Once released from the catheter tip, the coil forms loops to prevent unnecessary stress to the aneu-

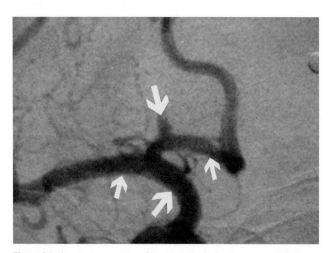

Figure 24–6 • Arteriogram of an unruptured anterior cerebral artery (ACA) aneurysm. The *left arrow* is the middle cerebral artery (MCA), the *bottom arrow* is the internal carotid artery (ICA), the *right arrow* is the ACA, and the *top arrow* points to the dome of the ACA aneurysm. (Courtesy of Chris Ogilvy, MD, Massachusetts General Hospital, Boston, MA.)

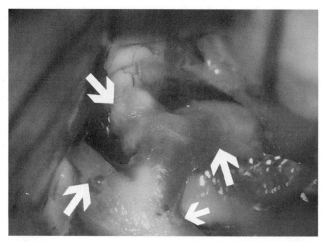

Figure 24–7 • Intraoperative photo of the ACA aneurysm. The *bottom left arrow* is the MCA, the *bottom right arrow* the ICA, the *top right arrow* the ACA, and the *top left arrow* the dome of the ACA aneurysm. (Courtesy of Chris Ogilvy, MD, Massachusetts General Hospital, Boston, MA.)

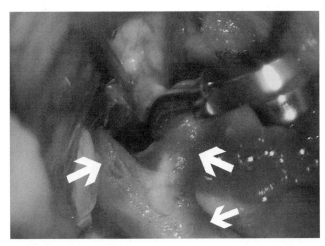

Figure 24–8 • Intraoperative photo of the clipping of the ACA aneurysm. The *left arrow* is the MCA, the *bottom right arrow* the ICA, and the *top right arrow* with lines the ACA. The clip on the neck of the ACA aneurysm is at right. (Courtesy of Chris Ogilvy, MD, Massachusetts General Hospital, Boston, MA.)

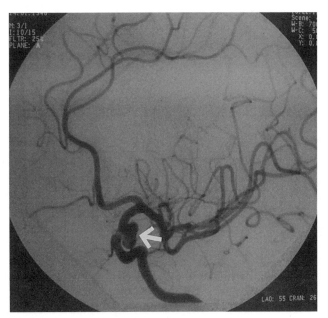

Figure 24–9 • Arteriogram of a 52-year-old female with a left internal carotid artery (ICA) back wall supraclinoid aneurysm presented for elective GDC embolization of the aneurysm. The *arrow* shows the left ICA aneurysm on her pre-embolization arteriogram. (Courtesy of Chris Ogilvy, MD, Massachusetts General Hospital, Boston, MA.)

rysm wall. When the correct size coil is introduced into the aneurysm, it adopts the shape of the lumen, not deforming the aneurysm.

GDC Technique

Using proper angiographic technique, a 5-Fr to 7-Fr guiding catheter, is introduced into the carotid artery or VA under systemic heparinization. The microcatheter, either Tracker 10 or 18, depending on the size of the aneurysm, is coaxially advanced into the aneurysm. It is necessary to use a soft tip guidewire when entering the aneurysm, not only to direct the catheter into the lumen but also to minimize risk of rupture to the aneurysm wall.

Once the microcatheter is in the proper position, a detachable coil is introduced into the lumen. If the coil migrates, it can be repositioned. When the coil is in the proper position, the positive end of a direct current source is connected to the proximal end of the detachable wire and the negative end is connected to a needle inserted in the groin. Current of 0.5 or 1 mA is provided by a battery-operated generator. The detaching end must be beyond the catheter tip to promote electrolysis. This can be ensured by markers on the catheter (3 cm from the tip) and the wire (28 mm from the uninsulated segment).[56]

The direct current induces thrombus formation around the platinum coil. More than one coil and often multiple coils (depending on aneurysm size) are used to sufficiently pack the aneurysm. These patients have follow-up angiograms 6 months to 1 year after the procedure to ensure complete obliteration of the aneurysm and to assess whether recanalization has occurred. If recanalization does happen, the patient will most likely require repeated GDC procedures to obliterate the remaining open portion.[56] Endovascular treatment of intracranial aneurysms by using GDCs is proving to be a safe method of preventing aneurysm rupture. The treatment of aneurysms by using electrically detachable electrothrombolytic coils was developed by Guglielmi in 1989, and the first patient was treated in

1990.[54,55,57] Since 1990 many centers have published their experience with the GDC modality, and these data show this procedure to be both safe and effective in preventing most intracranial aneurysms from rupture.[58–61] Figures 24-9, 24-10, and 24-11 show details related to coiling of an aneurysm.

The exception to this usually favorable outcome is seen in patients with giant intracranial aneurysms measuring 2.5 cm or larger. In the early GDC series, it was demonstrated that although post-GDC aneurysm rupture was exceedingly un-

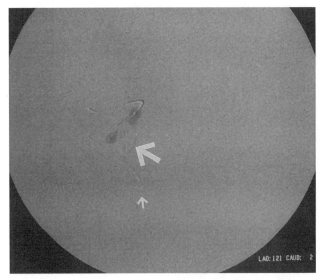

Figure 24–10 • The arteriogram during coil insertion. The *smaller arrow* points to the catheter, and the *larger arrow* points to the aneurysm with some coils in place. (Courtesy of Chris Ogilvy, MD, Massachusetts General Hospital, Boston, MA.)

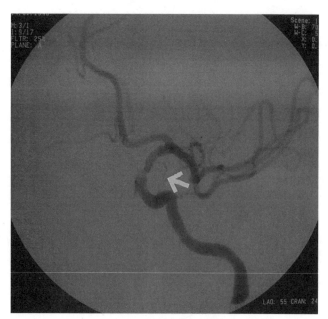

Figure 24-11 • Arteriogram demonstrating completion of coil embolization. The *arrow* points to the coil mass. (Courtesy of Chris Ogilvy, MD, Massachusetts General Hospital, Boston, MA.)

common in all aneurysms smaller than 2.5 cm in diameter, a significant number of giant aneurysms bled after GDC treatment.[54] It is important to stress that protection of the aneurysm from hemorrhage is the primary goal of any treatment. In September of 1995, the United States Food and Drug Administration approved the GDC, which is now widely used.[62]

In an attempt to improve outcome, endovascular embolization of aneurysms performed using GDCs has been evaluated as a viable treatment option and as an adjunct to the proven definitive treatment of surgical clipping in selected cases in which clipping is not desirable or feasible. Patients in poor medical condition and those who have aneurysms that are inaccessible may benefit from endovascular treatment because it may at least provide protection from early rebleeding during the acute period.[58]

GDC embolization of ruptured basilar tip aneurysms not amenable to surgical clipping appears to decrease morbidity and mortality rates compared with available natural history data on ruptured aneurysms treated conservatively. Some patients with ruptured basilar tip aneurysms who are not surgical candidates should be offered GDC embolization as a treatment option. The role of endovascular treatment in patients with unruptured basilar tip aneurysms remains unclear.[63]

In those patients in whom giant aneurysms can be surgically clipped with acceptable risks of morbidity and mortality, that approach remains the treatment of choice because the GDC option does not appear to offer the same durability of protection from rupture. GDC does offer an alternative in those cases in which patients presenting with mass effect symptoms on CNs cannot be surgically treated with acceptable risks of morbidity and mortality.[57]

Parent Vessel Occlusion

Another treatment approach involves occluding the parent vessel that supplies blood to the aneurysm. Before occlusion of the vessel is considered, it is important to establish whether the vessel can be sacrificed without neurological impairment. Various methods have been documented as effective, but not as absolute predictors of tolerance. A basic method is to constantly monitor motor, sensory, and cognitive functions in an awake patient during temporary occlusion (15 to 20 minutes).[56] A patient's electroencephalogram (EEG) can be monitored to detect any ischemic focus that may lead to clinical symptoms.

Preparation for temporary occlusion testing is similar to routine angiography. The occlusion balloon is inflated with contrast material until internal carotid artery flow is completely stopped. An experienced neurologist monitors neurological functions continuously for 20 minutes. Some centers may be monitoring EEG changes or stump pressure measurements during this interim. A challenge test may be applied by reducing systolic blood pressure to approximately 80 mm Hg. If the patient tolerates this occlusion and has sufficient collateral circulation on high volume angiogram, the patient is ready for permanent occlusion.

Indications for Permanent Occlusion

Most aneurysms treated by parent vessel occlusion are those of the cavernous or petrous extracranial internal carotid artery or extracranial VA. Giant subarachnoid aneurysms inoperable because of their size or undefined neck have also been treated. Aneurysms that are unclippable and located below the level of the circle of Willis or carotid bifurcation have been effectively managed with proximal occlusion. Additionally, dissecting aneurysms of the internal carotid or vertebral arteries and fusiform aneurysms without a well-defined neck can be eliminated by trapping or proximal occlusion.[56]

Post-occlusion Care

Hemodynamic changes following carotid occlusion can persist for at least a week. Low-level heparinization (partial thromboplastin time [PTT] level 40 to 60) should be maintained for 4 to 5 days postoperatively and the patient's activity regulated. For the first 48 hours, the patient is on complete bed rest; on the third day, the head of the bed is gradually elevated. By the fourth or fifth day, the patient is ambulating. If symptoms of cerebral ischemia are detected, the blood pressure is further elevated and blood volume expanded by increasing fluid intake. Gradual increase in activity helps the proper adjustment of cerebral circulation to post-occlusion hemodynamic changes, thus minimizing the risk of cerebral ischemia.

Patients are usually discharged home on some type of anticoagulation therapy, often one aspirin daily. If proximal occlusion of the parent artery is achieved, aneurysms of the internal carotid artery below the ophthalmic artery or VA undergo complete obliteration. For those internal carotid artery aneurysms above or at the level of the ophthalmic artery and for basilar aneurysms, the rate of complete obliteration drops to the 50% range. This is as a result of persistent flow in the aneurysm lumen through collateral circulation.[56]

Balloon Remodeling Technique

Aneurysms selected for GDC treatment are usually spherical and have a dome:neck ratio greater than or equal to 2. The absolute diameter of the aneurysm neck should be less than 4 mm and less than one half the diameter of the parent vessel.[64,65] Many aneurysms do not fall within these guidelines and are not considered for coil placement. Recent reports in the literature discuss the feasibility, efficacy, and safety of the balloon-assisted technique first described by Jacques Moret as the "remodeling technique."[64,66–71] The technique involves temporary occlusion of the aneurysm neck with a detachable balloon while a GDC is in place. The balloon prevents coil migration out of the aneurysm or protrusion into the parent vessel, allowing for an increased percentage of successful aneurysm treatment. There are several types of balloons that can be used, including over-the-wire occluded balloons and ones without end holes. Each type has distinct advantages and disadvantages.

Many aneurysms are amenable to coil treatment using the Moret balloon-assisted technique.[69,72] The balloon is placed across the neck of the aneurysm, which prevents coil protrusion and migration. The remodeling technique is a practical extension of endovascular coil embolization of cerebral aneurysms and increases the number of aneurysms that can be treated. It may offer a second treatment approach in aneurysms in which surgical clipping has failed and may provide an alternative treatment in aneurysms that are surgically inaccessible or require a different surgical approach. It provides an alternative to second or third craniotomies in patients with multiple aneurysms and a less invasive treatment in patients with severe concomitant medical problems.[70]

Findings to date show that aneurysms completely occluded postprocedure remain occluded on follow-up examination. Aneurysms that are subtotally occluded (i.e., more than 95%) immediately after coil placement tend to remain stable (30%), have progressive thrombosis (14%), or progress to occlusion (22%). Neck remnant growth in aneurysm subtotally occluded is not unique to aneurysms treated with GDCs and can be found in the surgical literature. Some believe that growth of a neck remnant in aneurysms treated with GDCs is directly related to the density of the coil packing within the treated aneurysm and the relationship of the neck remnant to the parent artery.

Future of Interventional Endovascular Treatment

Interventional endovascular technology has great potential for the future. The current combined morbidity and mortality rate related to the neurosurgical clipping of an incidental cerebral aneurysm is between 5% and 10%. The indication for surgical treatment of incidental surgical aneurysms is influenced by the location and size of the aneurysm and the patient's age and medical condition. The overall morbidity and mortality in patients treated in a series by Murayma and coworkers are comparable to the best neurosurgical series for the treatment of incidental aneurysms. The combined clinical and procedural morbidity and mortality rate of the GDC technology has dramatically decreased over the last couple of years because of the development of better delivery systems and softer GDCs and the increased experience of the neurointerventional teams. The long-term anatomical results have also been improved by the combined use of three-dimensional coils, soft coils, and GDC balloon-assisted technology.[73]

Stents

Stent refers to a device used to hold a skin graft in position that was originally composed of a substance invented by British dentist Charles Thomas Stent (1807 to 1901), called Stent's mass, which he used to make impressions of teeth. The origin of the term stent is controversial. Another belief is that the word may have derived from the word "stint," which means to restrain within certain limits.[74]

According to Palmaz, a stent is a coil or mesh tube that is introduced into the body through a catheter in a constrained form. The device is deployed by various mechanisms. The device's original role was thought to be to:

1. Prevent elastic recoil of a vessel after balloon angioplasty by holding a vessel open to a predetermined diameter
2. Prevent dissection after balloon angioplasty by pushing the dissected layers against one another and against the arterial wall
3. Provide a cylindrical vessel lumen wall by forcing asymmetrical plaques eccentrically[75]

The application of stenting to internal carotid artery (ICA) disease grew out of the success that such procedures had in both the coronary and peripheral arenas. In the mid-1990s , interest grew in the use of stents in the management of pseudoaneurysms and arterial dissections.[76] One of the limitations of coil embolization of wide neck aneurysms or fusiform aneurysms is permanent obliteration. Stents may provide a means of covering an aneurysmal neck to allow for coil deposition within the fundus without the fear of parent vessel occlusion or stenosis. In 1997 Higashida and associates successfully placed a Palmaz-Schatz PS 1540 articulated stent (Johnson & Johnson Interventional Systems) across the neck of a ruptured fusiform basilar aneurysm and used the stent to hold coils in the aneurysmal fundus and out of the basilar artery lumen.[77] In 1998, Lanzino and associates used an AVE (Arterial Vascular Engineering [Santa Rosa, CA]) coronary stent in the management of a paraclinoid aneurysm.[78]

Others have used stents to assist with coil embolization of wide neck vertebral artery (VA) aneurysms. Stenting is an exciting new neurointerventional procedure that assists the practitioner with the management of some challenging and otherwise unmanageable neurovascular disease processes. As new devices are developed and as controlled trials are undertaken to assess their effectiveness, older surgical procedures may be replaced in favor of less costly and less debilitating endovascular procedures.[76]

COMPLICATIONS OF ANEURYSMAL RUPTURE/BLEEDING

The major complications of aneurysmal rupture/bleeding, which can lead to significant mortality and morbidity, include rebleeding, vasospasm, and hydrocephalus.

Aneurysmal Rebleeding

Of the 18,000 persons who survive the initial rupture of an aneurysm annually, 3,000 either die or are disabled from rebleeding. Some believe the incidence of rebleeding is as high as 30%. The highest incidence occurs in the first 2 weeks after initial hemorrhage. Peaks in the incidence of rebleeding occur in the first 24 to 28 hours and at 7 to 10 days. Rebleeding within the first 24 to 48 hours is the leading cause of death in persons surviving the initial bleed. Peaking of rebleeding episodes at about 7 to 10 days appears to correlate with normal clot dissolution by natural fibrinolysis or from hypertension. Approximately 70% of patients who rebleed will die.[4]

Signs and Symptoms/Treatment

The onset of rebleeding is usually accompanied by sudden severe headache, often associated with severe nausea and vomiting; a decrease in or loss of consciousness; and new neurological deficits. Death may occur. Rebleeding can be confirmed by a CT scan or a sudden spike in ICP with new blood seen in the bag if a ventricular drain is in place. Early treatment, with either surgical or endovascular methods, of the aneurysm is the most effective means of preventing rebleeding.

Cerebral Vasospasm

Of the 18,000 persons annually who survive initial aneurysmal rupture, 3,000 either die or are disabled from cerebral vasospasm. Vasospasm occurs in approximately 30% of patients. By definition, *cerebral vasospasm* is narrowing of a cerebral blood vessel and causes reduced blood flow distally, which may lead to delayed ischemic deficit and cerebral infarction if left untreated. Besides the damage done by the initial SAH, brain damage produced by vasospasm is an important cause of morbidity and mortality after hemorrhage, with 14% to 36% of patients suffering disability and death.[79] Clinical signs of vasospasm are evident in about one third of patients after SAH, whereas angiographic and transcranial Doppler studies reveal spasm in 70% of cases.

When the patient's condition deteriorates 3 to 14 days after SAH, vasospasm should be considered as the possible cause. A CT scan should be performed immediately to rule out hydrocephalus, infarction, or rebleeding. Vasospasm can decrease cerebral perfusion to an area, causing ischemia and perhaps infarction, and can lead to further deterioration of neurological function. The etiology of vasospasm is unknown, although many hypotheses have been proposed. Current hypotheses range from the suggestion that spasmogenic agents are re-

leased as the clot breaks down, to the more recent hypothesis that an endothelium relaxing factor, such as nitric oxide, is somehow inhibited from exerting its relaxing effect because of changes in the endothelial cells that produce nitric oxide. These cellular changes may be induced by the release of blood into the extravascular compartment.

Vasospasm may be differentiated as either angiographic or symptomatic. **Angiographic vasospasm** refers to narrowing of a cerebral arterial territory, as noted on angiography, without clinical symptoms. **Symptomatic vasospasm** is the clinical syndrome of delayed cerebral ischemia associated with angiographically documented narrowing of a major cerebral arterial territory and TCD elevation of a specific arterial territory. Vasospasm develops 3 to 14 days after SAH (peaking at 7 to 10 days), although the onset may be delayed up to 21 days.[1]

Signs and Symptoms

Vasospasm is characterized by a gradual neurological deterioration related to a vascular territory. The clinical manifestations of vasospasm are variable. At least 50% of patients remain asymptomatic, whereas some 20% to 30% will have some delayed neurological ischemia. These deficits may be focal, but a clinician may also see confusion, decreased level of consciousness, and coma. The neurological deficits may be specific to a particular vascular territory, such as ACA or MCA, or they may be multifocal and diffuse, as when the cortical areas and boundary zones are involved. Most patients will have impaired level of consciousness. Deficits may include paresis/paralysis of a limb or side of the body, cranial nerve deficits, and aphasia. As a consequence of the severity and location of the ischemia caused by the vasospasm, cerebral infarction may develop, thus contributing to increased permanent neurological deficits or death.

Prediction of Vasospasm and Vascular Territory

An initial CT scan taken at the time of the bleed has gained credibility as a predictor of the incidence, location, and severity of vasospasm (see Fisher Grading Scale, Table 24-2). The extent and location of clots in the basal cisterns of the subarachnoid space and cerebral fissures are the specific determinants considered. Patients who have subarachnoid clots larger than 5×3 mm in the basal cisterns or who have layers of blood 1 mm thick or more in the cerebral fissures have a high incidence of vasospasm. Fisher has demonstrated that the amount of blood in the basal cisterns, as shown by the initial CT scan, can reliably predict which patients will develop symptomatic vasospasm, with the amount of blood directly related to the incidence and severity of vasospasm.[97] Bleeding into the brain or ventricles does not result in vasospasm.

Information concerning the probability and location of vasospasm can be helpful to the physician and nurse. Correlation of the vascular territory supplied by the artery at risk with the specific neurological functions of that territory helps to focus attention on those specific functions during neurological assessments. A decreased level of consciousness, the presence of focal signs, or both, together with a CT scan correlated to the cerebral territory, along with elevated TCDs, are indicative of vasospasm *when no other changes can explain the neurological deterioration*. When subtle or significant deficits occur, the nurse can quickly alert the physician to these findings so that prompt interventions can prevent extension of the neurological deficits or even death.

High-Risk Factors: Hyponatremia and Fluid Restriction

Hyponatremia is the most common electrolyte abnormality following SAH, detected in 10% to 25% of the cases, whereas mild hyperkalemia occurs less frequently. This is an important clinical finding because hyponatremia and decreased fluid volume are recognized high-risk factors for development of vasospasm. In aneurysmal hemorrhage, hyponatremia can be caused by SIADH or salt wasting (see Chap. 10). If hyponatremia is caused by true SIADH, an expanded blood volume is present that requires fluid restriction. If hyponatremia is attributed to salt wasting (in which case there is also hypernatriuria), blood volume is decreased. The treatment for salt wasting is fluid replacement.

Widjicks and colleagues measured plasma volume, fluid and sodium balance, and serum vasopressin (i.e., ADH) levels in patients with ruptured saccular aneurysms.[80] They found that vasopressin values were elevated at the time of the patient's admission but declined in the first week, regardless of the presence of hyponatremia. By definition, SIADH is associated with an increased serum ADH level. The conclusion drawn was that the natriuresis and hyponatremia were the result of primary salt wasting rather than SIADH. Further, they suggested that the natriuresis and hyponatremia should be corrected by fluid replacement rather than by fluid restriction, which is the treatment of SIADH.

The degree of hyponatremia is usually mild, occurring within 2 to 4 days of SAH, reaching a peak occurrence at about 7 days, and then becoming less frequent. Management should be with salt repletion, either orally or parenterally as needed to maintain sodium balance. Volume restriction is rarely necessary and often dangerous in the setting of vasospasm. Clinical manifestations may include a decreased level of consciousness or seizures, with delayed ischemic deficit and vasospasm reported as outcomes of previously used treatment with fluid restriction. The overall clinical outcome is worse for patients with hyponatremia.[81]

Seizures

The frequency of seizures following SAH is not known with certainty. In the early period, seizures occur between 16% and 90%.[98] Risk factors for seizures in the early period after SAH include previous history of hypertension, CT-documented presence of focal intraparenchymal blood, occurrence of a cerebral infarction, middle cerebral aneurysm location, and duration of coma after SAH.[1] Seizures generally occur within 18 months (if they do occur) and may be generalized, focal, or complex. On the basis of available data, many treat all aneurysmal SAH patients with anticonvulsants. If the hemorrhage is mild, anticonvulsants are tapered after 1 month. If the hemorrhage is more severe and if intraparenchymal brain injury has occurred, extended therapy and EEG monitoring are employed. Phenytoin 100 mg every 8 hours is given after an initial loading dose with 1 g (or 15 mg/kg) given slowly.[79]

Treatment

The result of vasospasm is decreased cerebral perfusion (blood flow) to the clinically affected arterial territory. Currently, treatment for symptomatic vasospasm is directed at the primary goal of increasing cerebral perfusion pressure, using hypervolemic, hypertensive, and hemodilution (triple H) therapy. With a craniotomy, there is usually a 300 to 400 mL blood loss that produces hemodilution with a hematocrit of 30% to 32%.[79] Hemodilution improves CBF. The balance of oxygen-carrying capacity and viscosity is optimized at a hematocrit level of 32% to 35%. To maintain the hematocrit in the desired range, albumin and packed RBCs may be used as volume expanders, or blood may be removed and mannitol may be administered (to decrease volume).

Central venous pressure is maintained at approximately 8 to 10 mm Hg, and the pulmonary capillary wedge pressure is 14 to 18 mm Hg. This is achieved by administration of colloid (5% albumin) on a regular basis (every 6 or 8 hours) to expand the intravascular volumes. Therapy is also aimed at maintaining a heart rate of greater than 70 beats per minute and a 30% rise in mean arterial blood pressure (160 to 170 mm Hg) for the duration of the vasospasm. If necessary, hypertension can be induced with vasopressors—dopamine (Intropin), phenylephrine (Neo-Synephrine), or dobutamine. The level of hypertension may be carefully controlled in the case of an unclipped aneurysm because of the concern for rebleeding. If vasospasm occurs after surgical clipping of the aneurysm, systolic blood pressure is often maintained between 180 and 200 mm Hg. Special care is warranted in patients with cardiac, pulmonary, or renal dysfunction. Central venous pressure monitoring is indicated in these cases, and some patients will need pulmonary artery catheters to guide therapy. One must watch for pulmonary edema, electrolyte imbalances, and cerebral edema in such complex patients.

Mannitol has been shown to increase CBF in the setting of vasospasm, with improvement in neurological function. A calcium channel blocker, nimodipine, has been standard treatment for nearly a decade and has been shown to have a beneficial effect on stroke after SAH, and a beneficial effect on blood flow as well. Nimodipine is begun at 60 mg PO or through nasogastric tube every 4 hours. Multiple studies demonstrate a modest effect in neurological outcome, although no clear angiographic demonstration of improved spasm was noted. It is believed that the site of effect is at the cellular level where it acts as a neuronal protector. Nimodipine therapy seems reasonable as long as the ability to treat with hypertension is not compromised. If it does lead to unmanageable drops in blood pressure, the dose is split or reduced or use of the drug is eliminated.[82]

TCD is an invaluable tool in the management of vasospasm. It is noninvasive, rapidly interpretable, and can be done on a daily basis to guide therapy. TCD gives flow velocities in the basal segments of the cerebral vessels, and increases in velocities may be seen in increased perfusion states or with narrowing of the basal segments. It is difficult to precisely correlate ischemic symptoms with TCD velocities because of variability of collateral supply. Vasospasm of the anterior cerebral artery (ACA) and middle cerebral artery (MCA) will be symptomatic at lower velocities than isolated MCA spasm. As TCD velocities increase, the intensity of medical management is also increased.

Medical therapy may be nearly exhausted by the time ischemic symptoms appear, and emergency and invasive alternatives are immediately begun. Angiography with the intention of angioplasty or intra-arterial papaverine can be extremely useful. The major goal is to proceed with invasive therapy before prolonged clinical deficits to maximize neurologic function.

Endovascular Therapy

Not all patients who develop anatomical spasm will develop clinical vasospasm. If a patient develops a new deficit that is suggestive of clinical vasospasm despite maximal medical prophylaxis, cross-sectional imaging is required (CT is preferable and easier than MRI). This will allow exclusion of other conditions that can produce such a deficit (such as rehemorrhage, hydrocephalus, or postoperative extra-axial hematoma) and permit identification of infarction or hemorrhagic transformation if already present in ischemic territory. If infarction has already occurred in the zone of the vasospastic arteries, endovascular therapy is precluded.

Two forms of endovascular therapy are available: balloon angioplasty and intra-arterial transcatheter infusion of a potent vasodilator drug, papaverine. Balloon angioplasty uses a low-pressure nondetachable microballoon to dilate the spastic segment mechanically. This is done under systemic anticoagulation. Once dilated, arteries generally do not experience spasm again unless a second hemorrhage occurs. The use of intra-arterial papaverine, although technically easier, is less effective because the duration of the drug's effect is often limited (24 to 48 hours). Papaverine infusion can be efficacious in situations in which spasm is quite distal in the arterial bed or inaccessible by balloon.

Outcomes are clearly best when such intervention is early. The risks of either angioplasty or papaverine include reperfusion hemorrhage in an already infarcted territory, mechanical arterial rupture, arterial dissection, and thromboembolism. The risks are warranted in the hands of an experienced endovascular therapist at $2,000 to $10,000 per procedure, which is a small price compared with the potential life-long cost of stroke in a patient in whom it could have been prevented.[83]

Communicating Hydrocephalus

Hydrocephalus is a condition in which there is either an obstruction to the flow of CSF within the ventricular system or subarachnoid space (noncommunicating hydrocephalus) or a problem with reabsorption of CSF (communicating hydrocephalus). The type of hydrocephalus that occurs with SAH is communicating hydrocephalus. Hydrocephalus can be classified as acute, subacute, or delayed. The profiles for each are different and are briefly discussed here. With SAH, hydrocephalus develops as a result of blood in the CSF, which plugs the arachnoid villi, thus interfering with the reabsorption of CSF. Diagnosis is established on the basis of

CT findings, which will reveal dilated ventricles with blood within the ventricles.

Signs and Symptoms/Treatment

The following summarizes the signs and symptoms of the three types of hydrocephalus, as well as the appropriate treatment for each.

ACUTE
- Occurs within the first 24 hours after hemorrhage
- Occurs in up to 20% to 67% of affected patients within 3 days following SAH
- Associated with intraventricular hemorrhage or excessive blood in the basal cisterns of posterior fossa
- Characterized by the abrupt onset of stupor or persistence of coma
- Management: immediate ventriculostomy to drain the CSF periodically, especially when ICP is elevated above a predetermined level such as 20 mm Hg

SUBACUTE
- Occurs within the first few days to 7 days after hemorrhage
- Associated with blood in the CSF secondary to SAH
- Characterized by drowsiness, the onset of which is gradual, although an abrupt onset is possible
- Management: ventriculostomy, or serial lumbar puncture or lumbar drainage of CSF

DELAYED
- Occurs 10 or more days after hemorrhage
- Associated with blood in the CSF secondary to SAH
- Characterized by a gradual onset of symptoms when the patient is recovering from surgery; symptoms include gait difficulty, behavioral changes (dull, quiet, and blunted animation)
- Management: surgical placement of a ventriculoperitoneal shunt

Because signs and symptoms of hydrocephalus are nonspecific, changes in responsiveness may be attributed to other problems, thus delaying appropriate treatment.

▌▌▌▌ NURSING MANAGEMENT OF THE PATIENT WITH AN ANEURYSM

Nursing management of the patient with a cerebral aneurysm can be divided into three areas: management before treatment, management during complications, and management after treatment.

Nursing Management Before Treatment

The patient who has sustained aneurysmal rupture/bleeding requires ongoing neurological and systems assessment, supportive care, preventive strategies, implementation of specific protocols (e.g., drug therapy), and management of increased ICP.

Assessment/Monitoring

The initial and ongoing neurological and systems assessment and monitoring require not only a focus on neurological function but also include other body systems such as the cardiovascular, respiratory, renal, and endocrine systems. These symptoms can be directly affected by cerebral aneurysm pathophysiology as well as by multiorgan dysfunction associated with severe illness. Cardiac monitoring for arrhythmias and ischemic events has already been discussed, along with respiratory and other system concerns. The initial assessment and ongoing monitoring of the neurological system includes:

- Level of consciousness*
- Pupillary size, shape, and reaction to light*
- Motor function (e.g., hand grasps, pronator drift, motor strength of extremities)*
- Other CN deficits (blurred vision or diplopia, extraocular movement deficits, ptosis, facial weakness)
- Aphasia
- Headache and facial pain (e.g., pain behind the eyeball)
- Nuchal rigidity (stiff neck, pain in neck and back pain with flexion of neck), photophobia

Neurological assessments are conducted periodically. The frequency of assessments depends on the acuity and stability of the patient. Those assessment components marked with an asterisk (*) are the most sensitive to change in neurological function. The neurological assessment may be conducted every 15 minutes to 4 hours, depending on the stability of the patient and care setting. New assessment data are compared with previous findings to determine change and trends. Accurate documentation and intershift sharing and reporting of information are essential in identifying trends in neurological function.

On confirmation of diagnosis of cerebral aneurysm, the patient is assigned a grade category according to Hunt-Hess classification and the Fisher Grading Scale. Both classification systems alert the nurse to the acuity of the patient and give an indication of the probable treatment. Usually, patients who present with a SAH are admitted to an intensive care setting where the technology and proper monitoring devices are available to assist in neurological and other body systems monitoring. See Chapter 17 for a discussion on neurological critical care.

Altered consciousness diminishes the patient's ability to comprehend the significance and implications of the events happening around him or her. Because there may not be one clear cause to which altered consciousness can be attributed, determining the etiology of deterioration in the level of consciousness, restlessness, or agitation may be difficult. Such alterations may result from rebleeding, hydrocephalus, ischemia, vasospasm, hypoxia, increased ICP, or electrolyte imbalance. Alterations may also be caused by the psychological effects of immobility, sensory deprivation, powerlessness, or other responses to hospitalization.

Common Nursing Diagnoses and Collaborative Problems

The most common nursing diagnoses are found in Chart 24-1. The following are the major collaborative problems associated with aneurysmal SAH:

- Aneurysmal rebleeding
- Hydrocephalus
- Cerebral vasospasm
- Increased ICP (i.e., secondary brain injury)
- Seizures
- Stroke
- Cardiac ischemic injury, dysrhythmias
- DVT
- Electrolyte-endocrine imbalance (hyponatremia, SIADH, diabetes insipidus, cerebral salt wasting, hyperglycemia)
- Neurogenic pulmonary edema
- Infections, especially aspiration or bacterial pneumonias

Most of these have been discussed briefly. Rebleeding, hydrocephalus, and vasospasm are the most critical complications in which astute nursing care and assessment can lead to early treatment and ultimate prevention of permanent neurological disability or death. The affected patient is also prone to DVT and related pulmonary emboli, for unknown reasons. The nurse needs to keep these potential problems in mind when caring for the patient.

Nursing Care: Additional Points of Care

Nurses are responsible for preventing complications. These responsibilities are singled out as being extremely important because they are within the realm of the nurse to monitor and control. First, a bowel program is initiated to prevent straining at stool. Most patients receive a narcotic for headache control. A side effect is decreased peristalsis, which can result in constipation if action is not taken to counteract this trend. In addition, bedrest and immobility also contribute to constipation. A bowel management program must be instituted immediately on hospitalization. By the time constipation becomes a problem, the peak time for high incidence of rebleeding is reached. Straining at stool (initiating Valsalva's maneuver) is dangerous because it can cause rebleeding and increase ICP.

The second concern is that the patient who is maintained on bedrest is at high risk for DVT and pulmonary emboli. This risk factor can be controlled by the use of elastic hose (TEDs) and sequential compression boots. It is the nurse's responsibility to make sure TEDs and boots are worn at all times. The patient's legs should be monitored periodically for the development of DVT.

Third, *seizure precautions* are instituted. As a precaution in the event of seizure activity, aspiration, or deterioration, a standby suction setup is kept in readiness at the bedside along with an oral airway. Padded side rails are also in place to protect the patient from injury.

Drug Therapy. In addition to care, the nurse is responsible for administering prescribed medications and for being aware of the action, toxicity, and interactions of the various drugs used. In this way, pertinent observations can be made in assessing the patient's response to the drug therapy. Nimodipine is given

CHART 24–1 • Summary of Nursing Diagnoses Associated With Cerebral Aneurysms

Nursing Diagnosis	Nursing Interventions	Expected Outcomes
Pain (headache, neck/back pain) related to (R/T) meningeal irritation	• Assess the type, location, and specific characteristics of the headache. • Assess the patient for pain and other signs and symptoms of meningeal irritation. • Reposition the patient gently, avoiding any unnecessary movement of the neck or head. • Administer analgesics as ordered. • Darken the patient's room. • Apply a cold, wet cloth or ice pack to the patient's head for comfort.	• The characteristics of the headache will be noted and recorded. • Analgesics and comfort measures will be administered. • The patient will provide objective evidence that the pain has been relieved.
Sensory/Perceptual Alterations, Visual, R/T photophobia secondary to meningeal irritation	• Note any evidence of discomfort when assessing direct light response of the pupils. • Maintain a darkened room by drawing the blinds or shades and avoiding direct light.	• Photophobia will be controlled by maintaining a darkened room.
High Risk for Injury R/T seizure activity secondary to cerebral irritation	• Maintain seizure precautions. • Monitor the patient for any signs of seizure activity and document in the patient's chart. • Administer anticonvulsant drugs prophylactically, as ordered.	• Seizure activity will be prevented. • If a seizure does occur, the patient will not be injured.
Anxiety (mild, moderate, or severe) R/T illness and/or restrictions of aneurysm precautions	• Assess the patient for objective and subjective evidence of anxiety. • If anxiety is present, try to identify the specific causes. • Attempt to clarify, control, or change the circumstances surrounding the anxiety. • Make appropriate referrals, as necessary. • Reassure the patient. • Depending on the patient's level of consciousness, use imagery, relaxation techniques, and other methods to control anxiety. • Administer sedatives, if ordered.	• Depending on the patient's level of consciousness, he or she will demonstrate an understanding of the purpose of the aneurysm precautions. • The patient will be informed of the plan of care and reassured. • The specific causes of anxiety will be identified. • Anxiety will be minimized or controlled.
High Risk for Secondary Brain Injury R/T rebleeding or cerebral vasospasms	• Assess neurological signs frequently for evidence of neurological deterioration. • Report immediately any significant changes in the patient's condition. • Recognize the peak times of occurrence of rebleeding and vasospasm. • If deterioration occurs, implement nursing protocols and standing orders so that ischemic response is treated.	• The patient will be carefully monitored so that any signs or symptoms of neurological deterioration will be identified quickly. • If there is evidence of deterioration, the physician will be notified immediately. • Nursing interventions and standing orders will be implemented quickly.

for 21 days to all patients who have suffered a SAH. With discharge from the hospital occurring earlier, it is important to ensure that the patient's pharmacy has the medication available before the patient is sent home. It is also necessary that the patient and family comprehend the importance of completing the drug.

Psychological Support

Considering the sudden diagnosis, it is important to monitor the patient's and family members' psychological and emotional responses. If the patient presents with an unruptured aneurysm, they may want to talk to another patient who has already experienced treatment—either surgical or endovascular. This may alleviate fears and anxieties that only "survivors" can share. Providing written material is also helpful to explain treatment and recovery. Patients may want to contact organizations such as the Brain Aneurysm Foundation (see Resources section at end of chapter) for additional support and educational material.

When a patient has suffered a SAH, he or she will need reassurance and frequent orientation to the hospital environment. If the Hunt-Hess grade is high (associated with unconsciousness), it is often the family that will need education and guidance through a tenuous and often uncertain hospitalization course. A calm and reassuring approach to the patient and family is most therapeutic.

The following are general suggestions to prevent adverse behavioral or psychological responses in the patient who has suffered a SAH secondary to immobility, sensory deprivation, and powerlessness:

- Orient the patient frequently to time, place, and person.
- Familiarize the patient/family with the environment.
- Be alert for cues from the patient/family indicating areas of concern.
- Provide information in a clear and simple manner to clarify any concerns.
- Clarify any misconceptions and quickly reorient the patient.
- Report any severe responses to the patient's restrictions that may indicate the need for modification by the physician.
- Be supportive and available to the family throughout the hospitalization and follow-up.

Nursing Management After Surgery/Endovascular Therapy

Nursing management after a craniotomy for aneurysm clipping follows that outlined in Chapter 15. Because there is some incidence of vasospasm even after surgery, the nurse must monitor the patient for any neurological deterioration that may herald the onset of vasospasm. (Note that such onset may be gradual, as evidenced by a slight pronator drift or confusion.) Cerebral angiography is often ordered after surgery to assure adequacy of clip placement. A CT scan is often done when new neurological change occurs.

For the patient who has undergone endovascular therapy with either coils or balloon occlusion, nursing management focuses on monitoring vital signs and neurological signs for evidence of vasospasm or ischemia. In addition, the femoral puncture site where the sheath is placed is monitored for evidence of bleeding, and the pedal pulses are assessed for evidence of occlusion. The patient is maintained on bed rest with the involved leg extended for a period of time until the sheath is removed. If the patient is receiving intra-arterial treatment for vasospasm, the sheath may be left in for a longer time. It is important to assess for potential signs and symptoms of a retroperitoneal bleed, such as decreased hematocrit, low systolic blood pressure, and abdominal pain and discomfort. Such symptoms need to be reported to the physician immediately.

Discharge Planning

Even with the technological advances that have been made in the management of patients with aneurysms, the outcome for patients includes significant neurological deficits. Throughout hospitalization, there needs to be interdisciplinary patient management to address the patient holistically and ensure early diagnosis and treatment of deficits. Many patients will need further rehabilitation after discharge from the acute care setting. Discharge planning should begin at admission or shortly thereafter and should address the individual needs of the patient. Much patient and family teaching is necessary to assist them in making decisions and coping with the multiple problems that may arise.

Cost Analysis and Predictors of Outcomes

There is a growing concern in our health care environment to minimize cost while maintaining quality care. It is a major challenge to all health care personnel and requires a collaborative effort of the managers of the health care delivery system and the providers of health care. Patient outcomes are such indicators and should be the focus in evaluating the achievement of quality, effectiveness, and appropriateness of patient care. Nurses should be active in collaborative decision making to optimize patient outcomes.

Although there are 28,000 reported cases of aneurysmal SAH in the United States annually, most aneurysms remain asymptomatic and undetected. In the past, unruptured aneurysms came to the attention of a neurosurgeon only after an SAH in a patient with multiple aneurysms. Since the development of microneurosurgical techniques, most neurosurgeons advocate elective surgical repair of an unruptured, asymptomatic, intracranial aneurysm. The superiority of elective aneurysm surgery has not been tested in any prospective clinical trials, although decision analysis models show more favorable outcomes with surgery.[84] Economic implications of treatment decisions are in the forefront of the minds of physicians and society. Cost-effectiveness analysis is a technique designed to evaluate treatment options by using both economic and clinical outcome data. In this era of economic health care constraints, treatments that are not cost effective will be increasingly denied public and private insurance reimbursement.[84]

Advances in treatment of patients who present with an unruptured intracranial aneurysm have changed the outlook for those who receive surgical or endovascular treatment. Substantial improvements in surgical morbidity and mortality do not seem to have had much of an impact on the clinical course of SAH when the total patient population is studied.[85] The mortality rate from SAH is as high as 50%, and the many patients who do survive incur significant morbidity.[86]

The search for more accurate outcome predictors and the continued development of ever more precise outcome-based measures and their relationship to the management of cerebral aneurysms and SAH are critical.[87] The neurological deficits that occur after aneurysmal SAH may vary according to location of the lesion. Saccular intracranial aneurysms are the most common cause of SAH. The Hunt-Hess classification (previously described) is based on a patient's clinical condition and correlates with surgical risk. A newer grading system, the Massachusetts General Hospital (MGH) Scale, has been proposed to better predict outcome of aneurysm patients. It recognizes several predictive variables such as age, Fisher Grading Scale (amount of blood on CT scan), clinical presentation, and location of the aneurysm that the traditional Hunt-Hess classification ignores. The Hunt-Hess classification only looks at the clinical condition of the patient. The MGH Scale is designed to better predict cost and length of stay for aneurysm patients.[88]

Much of the literature states that clinical grade on admission is strongly associated with outcome and encompasses many of the reported outcome predictors, such as extent of the initial hemorrhage and age. Economic concerns require a concomitant improvement in methods for assessing and predicting management costs. Length of stay (LOS) provides a reasonable estimate of medical resource use.[87] Health care professionals realize that the risk of disability and death and the cost of medical care is particularly high, especially in those patients who have suffered a SAH and are 65 years or older. Increasing knowledge about predictors that can help determine patient outcome can only serve to enhance our care for these patients and families. Treatment options must be evaluated in terms of quality of life, functional outcome, and financial details.

Nurses do not ignore health care cost containment. The current and anticipated health care environment demands that nurses and other health care providers shift focus from planned care to a managed care system. The emphasis on "care planning" is moving toward ensuring the achievement of acceptable patient outcomes within an efficient time frame with the appropriate use of resources. The changing health environment requires health care professionals to explore alternative ways to deliver quality patient care, reduce length of stay, and manage resources.[89]

Stachniak and colleagues looked at age as an influence on cost and effectiveness of treatment in patients with SAH.[90] The results from their study suggest that elderly patients, certainly those over 65 years, can benefit from aggressive treatment. Stachniak determined that cost was indeed higher in every area of care for those aged 65 years or older compared with younger patients. Interestingly, when evaluated by decade, there were no significant cost differences. The data analyzed indicates that aggressive treatment is appropriate unless and until the patient or family determines that for nonmedical reasons, nonsurgical treatment is preferred. Even though hospital costs may be higher for treating elderly patients with SAH, the decision of whether access to care should be based on the cost of care provision is a moral and ethical question that cannot be answered based on financial data.

To better understand the effect of severity of hemorrhage and the clinical course on resource use, researchers compared demographic and clinical information as well as hospital costs for the following four groups of patients: patients with unruptured aneurysms, those with acute aneurysmal SAH, those with SAH and vasospasm, and those with SAH and a negative angiographic result. The results of the study revealed three high-cost areas that accounted for almost 50% of the total costs in the care and treatment of patients with SAH: ICU stay, arteriography, and medical/surgical supplies. Strategies for cost containment include minimizing the ICU stay, limiting stays to those patients who need aggressive management—for example, patients in vasospasm.[91] A step-down unit may be a viable alternative for some of these patients. This is an area in which nurses could collaborate in critical decision making to determine which patients could be safely managed in a less acute setting. A major cost savings in this population could be reduced consumption of disposable supplies. Development of new treatment modes

to manage vasospasm may also reduce the need for angiograms and papaverine infusions, thus reducing costs.

After reviewing 543 SAH patients over a 10-year period, Elliot and colleagues correlated clinical grade on admission (Hunt-Hess grade) with hospital LOS and cost.[87] As the Hunt-Hess grade increased, so did LOS. The patients with the worst clinical grade (i.e, grade 5) showed a reduction in both LOS and cost because of devastating bleeding followed by death soon after admission. More than 50% of the costs of patients with cerebral aneurysms, both ruptured and unruptured, are associated with LOS and surgery.[87,91] Surgical repair of aneurysms before rupture could represent tremendous savings in expense and use of neurosurgical and other hospital resources. This conclusion is supported by other reports of direct costs for patients with SAH to be 1.5 times greater than costs for the care of patients with unruptured aneurysms.[92] These studies emphasize a need for a more detailed evaluation of how preoperative and postoperative factors influence LOS, particularly in regard to nursing and medical interventions. Further research needs to be done to stratify radiographic, clinical, and treatment factors that will better predict cost and LOS for each grade of aneurysm patient. Such information could be useful in nursing research allocation.[93] Therefore, there are several factors to consider when deciding to treat a patient with a ruptured intracranial aneurysm. Age, size of the lesion, neurological condition of the patient, and aneurysm location are important factors.

Advances in aneurysmal SAH management have been documented by decrease in mortality after surgical management. Ropper and Zervas highlighted that significant neurological morbidity and decreased rates of patients returning to work are common, even in patients presenting in the best neurological condition.[94] Recently, outcome analysis has assumed a prominent role for caregivers, patients, and payers who are interested in standardized assessments of the clinical sequelae of different treatment practices. With the advent of multiple-modality treatment of SAH, as well as advanced intensive care units and endovascular options for vasospasm treatment, there is little doubt that regional variations in the practice of SAH management will continue to evolve. To document the effect of these practice variations accurately, specific standardized assessment of outcomes are essential.[95]

Most data about outcomes after SAH have relied on physician-oriented global assessments, such as the Glasgow Outcome Scale (GOS). This reliable tool is used to assess outcomes in various illnesses and has five categories: dead, persistent vegetative state, severe disability, moderate disability or fair recovery, and good recovery. Good recovery describes the patient's neurological and physical status and the assessor's perception of the patient's capacity to return to work and return to "normal" or "near normal" functioning. The nature of this scale has made it difficult to analyze specific factors that may contribute to global outcome. The assessment of "good recovery" is not usually based on a full evaluation of both the patient's cognitive and behavioral changes. Standardized neuropsychological tests provide objective measures of cognitive function, but if they are used alone, disabling behavioral changes and problems in everyday life may be underestimated.[96]

Buchanan and coworkers[96] assessed behavioral and personality changes, psychosocial function, and family burden in a mixed sample of 28 patients who underwent surgery for SAH and were viewed by their neurosurgeon as having a "good recovery" or "moderate disability." Despite good physical recovery 19 months after SAH, more than half the patients had not returned to their previous level of employment. Their daily lives were affected by mental and physical fatigability. Intolerance to being rushed, to groups of people, to small children, to lack of order or routine, and to normal sound levels were common complaints. It is difficult to measure these problems objectively, and they can compromise personal relationships and employment. Family relationships suffered, and intimate relationships were affected by lack of libido. Carter and colleagues[95] examined the prevalence of physical disability and depression in a cohort of patients who had sustained aneurysmal SAH who presented initially in good neurological condition (Hunt-Hess grades I to III). Other factors analyzed included patient age and initial neurological status; a standard global outcome assessment, Reintegration to Normal Living Status Index; and the patient's self-report of work status.[95]

Measures such as the GOS or Rankin Scale provide for a ready assessment of outcome, and the use of a standardized self-reported outcome assessment has the ability to further our understanding of deficits after SAH from a patient's perspective. By identifying and analyzing factors associated with quality of life, it may be possible to identify specific interventions (i.e., antidepressive therapy or cognitive rehabilitation programs) that may help quality-of-life perceptions.

REFERENCES

1. Brown, R. (1999). Natural history of intracranial aneurysms. Syllabus for course: Neurovascular Update: Present Practices and Future Directions, June 2 to 4,1999, Swissotel, Boston, MA.
2. Jakubowski, J., & Kendall, B. (1978). Coincidental aneurysms with tumours of pituitary origin. *Journal of Neurology Neurosurgery Psychiatry, 41,* 972–979.
3. McCormick, W. F. & Acousta-Rua, G. J. (1980). The size of intracranial saccular aneurysms: An autopsy study. *Journal of Neurosurgery, 33,* 422–427.
4. Mayberg, M. R., Batjer, H. H., Dacey, R., Diringer, M., et al. (1994). Guidelines for the management of aneurysmal subarachnoid hemorrhage. *Stroke, 25*(11), 2315–2328.
5. Herrick, I. A., & Gelb, A. W. (1992). Anesthesia for intracranial aneurysm. *Journal of Clinical Anesthesia, 4,* 73–82.
6. Heiserman, J. E. & Bird, C. R. (1994). Cerebral aneurysms. *Neuroimaging Clinics of North America, 4*(4), 799–821.
7. Kasuya, H., Onda, H., Takeshita, M., Hori, T., & Takakura, K. (2000). Clinical features of intracranial aneurysms in siblings. *Neurosurgery, 46*(6), 1301–1306.
8. LeBlanc, R. (1997). Familial cerebral aneurysms. *Canadian Journal of Neurologic Science, 24,* 191–199.
9. Ronkaien, A., Miettinen, H., Karkola, K., Papinaho, S., Vanninen, R., Puranen, M., & Hernesniemi, J. (1998). Risk of harboring an unruptured intracranial aneurysm. *Stroke, 29,* 359–362.
10. Schievink, W. I., Schaid, D. J., Rongers, H. M., Piepgras, D. G., & Michels, V. V. (1994). On the inheritance of intracranial aneurysms. *Stroke, 23,* 1024–1030.
11. LeBlanc, R. (1996). Familial cerebral aneurysms: A bias for women. *Stroke, 27,* 1050–1054.
12. Raymakers, T. W. M., Rinkel, G. J. E., & Ramos, L. M. P. (1998). Initial follow-up screening for aneurysms in families with familial subarachnoid hemorrhage. *Neurology, 51,* 1125–1130.
13. Ronakainen, A., Hernesniemi, J., & Ryynanen, M. (1993). Familial subarachnoid hemorrhage in East Finland, 1977–1990. *Neurosurgery, 33,* 787–797.
14. Ogilvy, C. S. (2000). Familial intracranial aneurysms. *Circle of Friends—The Brain Aneurysm Foundation Newsletter, 4*(2), 1–2.
15. LeBlanc, R., Melanson, D., Tampieri, D., & Guttmann, R. D. (1995). Familial cerebral aneurysms: A study of 13 families. *Neurosurgery, 37,* 633–639.
16. Schievink, W. I., Schaid, D. J., Michels, V. V., & Piepgras, D. G. (1995). Familial aneurysmal subarachnoid hemorrhage: A community based study. *Journal of Neurosurgery, 83,* 426–429.
17. Camarata, P. J., Latchaw, R. E., Rufenacht, D. A., & Heros, R. C. (1992). Intracranial aneurysms. *Investigative Radiology, 28*(4), 373–382.
18. Stebhens, W.E. (1989). Etiology of intracranial berry aneurysms. *Journal of Neurosurgery, 70,* 823–831.
19. Ryba, M. Grieb, P., Iwanska, K., et al. (1992). HLA antigens and intracranial aneurysms. *Acta Neurochirurgica, 116,* 1–5.
20. Strother, C. (2000). Aneurysm hemodynamics. Syllabus from course: Neurovascular Update: The New Millennium, The Fairmont Hotel, San Francisco, CA.
21. Greenberg, M. (2001). Cerebral aneurysms. In M. Greenberg (Ed.). *Handbook of neurosurgery* (5th ed.). Lakeland, FL: Greenberg Graphics.
22. Ingall, T. J. & Wiebers, D. O. (1993). Natural history of subarachnoid hemorrhage. In Whisnant, J. P. (Ed.). *Stroke: Populations, cohorts, and clinical trials.* Boston: Butterworth-Heinemann.
23. Brown, R. (2000). Ruptured intracranial aneurysms: Morbidity and mortality. Syllabus from course: Neurovascular Update: The New Millennium. The Fairmont Hotel, San Francisco, CA.
24. Longstreth, W. T., Jr, Nelson, L. M., Koepsell, T. P., & van Belle, G., (1994). Subarachnoid hemorrhage and hormonal factors in women: A population based case control study. *Annals of Internal Medicine, 121,* 163–173.
25. Broderick, J. P., Brott, T., Tomsick, T., Huster, G., & Miller, R. (1992). The risk of subarachnoid and intracerebral hemorrhages in blacks as compared to with whites. *New England Journal of Medicine, 326,* 733–736.
26. Bederson, J. B., Awad, I. A., Wiebers, D. O., et al. (2000). Recommendations for the management of patients with unruptured intracranial aneurysms: A statement for healthcare professionals from the Stroke Council of the American Heart Association. *Circulation, 102,* 2300–2308.
27. Wiebers, D. O., & The International Study of Unruptured Intracranial Aneurysm Study Investigators. (1998). Unruptured intracranial aneurysms–Risk of rupture and risk of surgical intervention. *The New England Journal of Medicine, 339* (24), 1725–1733
28. Ojemann, R. G., (1981). Management of the unruptured intracranial aneurysm. Editorial. *New England Journal of Medicine, 304,* 725-726.
29. Raaymakers, T. W., Rinkel, G. J., Limburg, M., & Algra, A. (1998). Mortality and morbidity for surgery of unruptured intracranial aneurysms: A meta-analysis. *Stroke, 29,* 1531.
30. Hunt, W. E. & Hess, R. M. (1968). Surgical risk as related to time of intervention in the repair of intracranial aneurysms. *Journal of Neurosurgery, 28,* 14–20.
31. Norbash, A. (2000). Traditional and contemporary imaging of intracranial aneurysms: The changing face of diagnosis. Syllabus from course: Neurovascular Update: The New Millennium. The Fairmont Hotel, San Francisco, CA.
32. Davis, K. R., Kistler, J. P., Heros, R. C., & Davis, J.M. (1982). Neuroradiologic approach to the patient with a diagnosis of subarachnoid hemorrhage. *Radiology Clinics of North America, 20,* 87–94.

33. Fleisher, A. S., Patton, J. M., & Tindall, G. T. (1975). Cerebral aneurysms of traumatic origin. *Surgical Neurology, 4,* 233–239.

34. Sevick, R. J., Tsuruda, J. S., Schmalbrock, P. (1990). Three-dimensional time of flight MR angiography in the evaluation of cerebral aneurysms. *Journal of Computed Assisted Tomography, 14*(6), 874–881.

35. Burch, G. E., Meyers, R., & Abildskov, J. A. (1954). A new electrocardiographic pattern observed in cerebrovascular accidents. *Circulation, 9,* 719–723.

36. Davis , T. P., Alexander, J., & Lesch, M. (1993). Electrocardiographic changes associated with acute cerebrovascular disease: A clinical review. *Progressive Cardiovascular Disease, 36,* 245–260

37. Marion, D. W., Segal, R., & Thompson, M. E. (1986). Subarachnoid hemorrhage and the heart. *Neurosurgery, 18,* 101–106.

38. Zaroff, J. G., Rordorf, G. A., Newell, J. B., Ogilvy, C. S., & Levinson, J. R. (1999). Cardiac outcome in patients with subarachnoid hemorrhage and electrocardiographic abnormalities. *Neurosurgery, 44*(1), 34–40.

39. Heros, R. C. (1995). Giant aneurysms. In: R. G. Ojemann, C. S. Ogilvy, R. C. Heros, & R. M. Crowell (Eds.). *Surgical management of neurovascular disease* (3rd ed.). Baltimore: Williams & Wilkins.

40. Fogelholm, R., Hernesniemi, J., & Vapalahti, M. (1993). Impact on early surgery on outcome after aneurysmal subarachnoid hemorrhage: A population based study. *Stroke, 24,* 1649–1654

41. Juvela, S., Porras, M., and Poussa, K. (2000). Natural history of unruptured intracranial aneurysms: Probability of and risk factors for aneurysm rupture. *Journal of Neurosurgery, 93,* 379–387

42. Heiskanen, O. & Marttila, I. (1970). Risk of rupture of second aneurysm in patients with multiple aneurysms. *Journal of Neurosurgery, 32,* 295–299.

43. International Study of Unruptured Intracranial Aneurysm Investigators (1998). Unruptured intracranial aneurysms—risks of rupture and risks of surgical intervention. *New England Journal of Medicine, 339,* 1725–1733.

44. Jane, J. A., Kassell, N. F., Torner, J. C., et al. (1985). The natural history of aneurysms and arteriovenous malformations. *Journal of Neurosurgery, 82,* 945–952.

45. Juvela, S., Porras, M., & Heiskanen, O. (1993). The natural history of unruptured aneurysms: A long term follow-up study. *Journal of Neurosurgery, 79,* 174–182.

46. Taylor, C. L., Yuan, Z., Selman, W., et al. (1995). Cerebral arterial aneurysm formation and rupture in 20,767 elderly patients: hypertension and other risk factors. *Journal of Neurosurgery, 83,* 812–819.

47. Wiebers, D. O., Whisnant, J. P., Sundt, T. M, Jr., et al. (1987). The significance of unruptured intracranial saccular aneurysms. *Journal of Neurosurgery, 66,* 23–29.

48. Yasui, N., Suzuki, A., Nishimura, H., et al. (1997). Long-term follow-up study of unruptured intracranial aneurysms. *Neurosurgery, 40,* 1155–1160.

49. Winn, H. R., Almaani, W. S., Berga, S. L., et al. (1983). The long-term outcome of patients with multiple aneurysms. Incidence of late hemorrhage and implications for treatment of incidental aneurysms. *Journal of Neurosurgery, 59,* 642–651.

50. Ronkaninen, A, Miettinen, H., Karkola, K., et al (1998). Risk of harboring an unruptured intracranial aneurysm. *Stroke, 29,* 359–362.

51. Juvela, S. (1996). Prevalence of risk factors in spontaneous intracerebral hemorrhage and aneurysmal subarachnoid hemorrhage of unknown etiology. *Archives of Neurology, 53*(8), 734–740.

52. Juvela, S., Hillbom, M., Numminen, H., et al. (1993). Cigarette smoking and alcohol consumption risk factors for aneurysmal subarachnoid hemorrhage. *Stroke, 24,* 639–646.

53. Weir, B. K. A., Kongable, G. L., Kassell, N. F., et al. (1998). Cigarette smoking as a cause of aneurysmal subarachnoid hemorrhage and risk for vasospasm: A report of the Cooperative Aneurysm Study. *Journal of Neurosurgery, 89,* 405–411.

54. Guglielmi, G., Vinuela, F., Duckwiler, G., et al. (1991). Electrothrombosis of saccular aneurysms via endovascular approach. Part 2. Preliminary Clinical Experience. *Journal of Neurosurgery, 75,* 8–14.

55. Guglielmi, G., Vinuela, F., Sepetka, I., et al. (1991). Electrothrombosis of saccular aneurysms via endovascular approach. Part 1: Electrochemical basis, technique, and experimental results. *Journal of Neurosurgery, 75,* 1–7.

56. Choi, I. S. (1995). Endovascular treatment of aneurysms. In: R. G. Ojemann, C. S. Ogilvy, R. C. Heros, & R. M. Crowell (Eds.). *Surgical management of neurovascular disease* (3rd ed.). Baltimore, MD: Williams & Wilkins.

57. Malisch, T., Guglielmi, G., Vinuela, F., Duckwiler, G., Gobin, Y. P., Martin, N. A., Frazee, J.G.,& Chiml, J. S. (1998). Unruptured aneurysms presenting with mass effect symptoms: Response to endovascular treatment with Gugliemi detachable coils. Part I. Symptoms of cranial nerve dysfunction. *Journal of Neurosurgery, 89,* 956–961.

58. Graves, V. B., Strother, C. M., Duff, T. A., et al. (1995). Early treatment of ruptured aneurysms with Guglielmi detachable coils: Effect on subsequent bleeding. *Neurosurgery, 37,* 640–648.

59. Malisch, T., Guglielmi, G., Vinuela, F., et al. (1997). Intracranial aneurysms treated with the Guglielmi detachable coil: Midterm clinical results in a consecutive series of 100 patients. *Journal of Neurosurgery, 87,* 176-183.

60. Martin, D., Rodesch, M. D., Alavarez, H., et al. (1996). Preliminary results of nonsurgical intracranial aneurysms with GD coils: The 1st year of their use. *Neuroradiology, 38* (Suppl 1,: S142–S150.

61. Guglielmi, G., Vinuela, F., & Duckwiler, G. (1995). Coil induced thrombosis of intracranial aneurysms. In R. J. Marcunias (Ed.). *Endovascular neurological intervention* (pp. 179–188). Park Ridge, IL: American Association of Neurological Surgeons.

62. McDougall, C. G., Halbach, V.V., Dowd, C.F., Higashida, R. T., Larsen, D. W., & Hieshima, G. B. (1998). Causes and management of aneurysmal hemorrhage occurring during embolization with Guglielmi detachable coils. *Journal of Neurosurgery, 89,* 87–92.

63. Eskridge, J. M., Song, J. K., and the Participants (1998). Endovascular embolization of 150 basilar tip aneurysms with Guglielmi detachable coils: Results of the Food and Drug Administration multicenter clinical trial. *Journal of Neurosurgery, 89,* 81–86.

64. Debrun, GM., Aletich, V. A., Kehrli, P., et al. (1998). Selection of cerebral aneurysms for treatment using Guglielmi detachable coils. *Neurosurgery, 43,* 1281–1297.

65. Fernandez Zubillaga, A., Gugliemi, G, Vinuela, F., et al. (1994). Endovascular occlusion of intracranial aneurysms with electrically detachable coils: Correlation of aneurysm neck size and treatment results. *American Journal of Neuroradiology, 15,* 815–820.

66. Levy, D. I. (1997). Embolization of wide neck anterior communicating artery aneurysm: Technical note. *Neurosurgery, 41,* 979–982.

67. Levy, D. I. & Ku, A. (1997). Balloon assisted coil placement in wide neck aneurysms: Technical note. *Journal of Neurosurgery, 70,* 556–560.

68. Mericle, R. A., Wakhloo, A. K., Rodriguez, R., et al. (1997). Temporary balloon protection as an adjunct to endovascular coiling of wide necked cerebral aneurysms: Technical note. *Neurosurgery, 41,* 975–978.

69. Moret, J., Cognard, C., Weill, A., et al. (1997). The "remodeling technique" in the treatment of wide necked intracranial aneurysms: Angiographic results and clinical follow-up in 56 cases. *Interventional Neuroradiology, 3,* 21–35.

70. Moret, J., Pierot, L., Boulin, A., et al. (1994). "Remodeling" of the arterial wall of the parent vessels in the endovascular treatment

of intracranial aneurysms [abstract]. *Proceedings of the Society for Neuroradiology, 36* (Suppl. 1), S83.

71. Takahashi, A., Ezura, M., Yoshimoto, T. (1997). Broad neck basilar tip aneurysm treated by neck plastic intra aneurysmal GDC embolization with protective balloon. *Interventional Neuroradiology, 3,* 167–170

72. Aletich, V. A., Debrun, G. M., Misra, M., Charbal, F., & Ausman, J.I. (2000). The remodeling technique of balloon assisted Guglielmi detachable coil placement in wide neck aneurysms: Experience at the University of Illinois at Chicago. *Journal of Neurosurgery, 93,* 388–396.

73. Murayma, Y., Vinuela, F, Duckwiler, G. R., Gobin, Y. P., and Guglielmi, G. (1999). Embolization of incidental cerebral aneurysms by using the Guglielmi detachable coil system. *Journal of Neurosurgery, 90,* 207–214.

74. Kutryk, M. J. B., & Serruys, P. W. (1998). Stenting. In E. J. Topol (Ed.). *Comprehensive cardiovascular medicine* (pp. 2307–2338). Philadelphia: Lippincott-Raven.

75. Palmaz, J. C. (1992). Intravascular stenting: From basic research to clinical application. *Cardiovascular Interventional Radiology, 15,* 279–284.

76. Horowitz, M. B. & Purdy, P. D. (2000). The use of stents in the management of neurovascular disease: A review of historical and present status. *Neurosurgery, 46*(6), 1335–1343.

77. Higashida, R. T., Smith, W, Gress, D., Urwin, R., Dowd, C., Balousek, P. A., & Halbach, V. V. (1997). Intravascular stent and endovascular coil placement for a ruptured fusiform aneurysm of the basilar artery. *Journal of Neurosurgery, 87,* 944–949.

78. Lanzino, G., Wakhloo, A. K., Fessler, R. D., Mericle, R. A., Guterman, L. R., & Hopkins, L. N. (1999). Efficacy and current limitations of intravascular stents for intracranial internal carotid, vertebral and basilar artery aneurysms. *Journal of Neurosurgery, 91,* 538–546.

79. Crowell, R. M., Ogilvy, C. S., Gress, D. R., & Kistler, J. P. (1995). General management of aneurysmal subarachnoid hemorrhage. In R. G. Ojemann, C. S. Ogilvy, R. C. Heros, & R. M. Crowell (Eds.). *Surgical management of neurovascular disease* (3rd ed.). Baltimore: Williams & Wilkins.

80. Widjicks, E. F. M., Vermeulen, M., Hijdra, A., et al. (1985). Hyponatremia and cerebral infarction in patients with ruptured intracranial aneurysms: Is fluid restriction harmful? *Annals of Neurology, 17,* 137–140.

81. Hasan, D., Wijdicks, E. F., Vermeulen, M. (1990). Hyponatremia associated with cerebral ischemia in patients with aneurysmal subarachnoid hemorrhage. *Annals of Neurology, 27,* 106–108.

82. Gress, D. R. (2000). Medical management of vasospasm in subarachnoid hemorrhage. Syllabus from course: Neurovascular update: The new millennium. The Fairmont Hotel, San Francisco, CA.

83. Dowd, C. 1999. Endovascular treatment of vasospasm. Neurovascular update: Present practices and future direction—Syllabus, June 2–4, 1999. Boston, MA.

84. King, Jr., J. T., Glick, H. A., Mason, T. J., & Flamm, E. S. (1995). Elective surgery for asymptomatic, unruptured, intracranial aneurysms: A cost effectiveness analysis. *Journal of Neurosurgery, 83,* 403–412.

85. Hijdra, A., Braakman, R., van Gijn, J., Vermeulen, M., & van Crevel, H. (1987). Aneurysmal subarachnoid hemorrhage–complications and outcome in a hospital population. *Stroke, 18*(6), 1061–1067.

86. Taylor, C. L., Yuan, Z., Selman, W. R., Ratcheson, R. A., & Rimm, A. A. (1997) Mortality rates, hospital length of stay, and the cost of treating subarachnoid hemorrhage in older patients: Institutional and geographical differences. *Journal of Neurosurgery, 86,* 583–588.

87. Elliott, J. P., Le Roux, P. D., Ransom, G., Newell, D. W., Grady, M. S., & Winn, H.R. (1996). Predicting length of hospital stay and cost by aneurysm grade on admission. *Journal of Neurosurgery, 85,* 388–391.

88. Ogilvy, C. S. & Carter, B. S. (1998). A proposed comprehensive grading system to predict outcome for surgical management of intracranial aneurysms. *Neurosurgery, 42*(5), 959–970.

89. Kowal, N. S., & Delaney, M. (1996). The economics of a nurse-developed critical pathway. *Nursing Economics, 14*(3), 156–161.

90. Stachniak, J. B., Layon, A. J., Day, A. L., & Gallagher, J. (1996). Craniotomy for intracranial aneurysm and subarachnoid hemorrhage: Is course, cost, or outcome affected by age? *Stroke, 27*(2), 276–281

91. Yundt, K. D., Dacey, R. G., & Diringer, M. N. (1996). Hospital resource utilization in the treatment of cerebral aneurysms. *Journal of Neurosurgery, 85,* 403–409.

92. Wiebers, D. O., Torner, J. C., & Meisser, I. (1992). Impact of unruptured intracranial aneurysms on public health in the United States. *Stroke, 23*(2), 1416–1419.

93. Stewart-Amidei, C. (1997). Resource use in aneurysmal subarachnoid hemorrhage. *Journal of Neuroscience Nursing, 29*(1), 60.

94. Ropper, A., & Zervas, N. (1984). Outcome 1 year after SAH from cerebral aneurysm: Management morbidity, mortality, and functional status in 112 good risk patients. *Journal of Neurosurgery, 60,* 909–915.

95. Carter, B. S., Buckley, D. A., Ferraro, R., Rordorf, G. & Ogilvy, C. S. (2000). Factors associated with reintegration to normal living after subarachnoid hemorrhage. *Neurosurgery, 46*(6), 1326–1334.

96. Buchanan, K. M., Elias, L. J., & Goplen, G. B. (2000). Differing perspectives on outcome after subarachnoid hemorrhage: The patient, the relative, the neurosurgeon. *Neurosurgery, 46*(4), 831–840.

97. Fisher, C. M., Kestler, J. P., & Davis, J. M. (1980). Relation of cerebral vasospasm to subarachnoid hemorrhage visualized by CT scanning. *Neurosurgery, 6,* 1–9.

98. Giroud, M., Gras, P., Fayolle, H., Andre, N., Soichot, P., & Dumas, R. (1994). Early seizure after stroke: A study of 1,640 cases. *Epilepsia, 35*(5), 959–964.

RESOURCES

Professional

Published Material

Arford, P. H., & Allred, C. A. (1995). Value = quality + cost. *Journal of Nursing Administration, 25*(9), 64–69.

Caroselli, C. (1996). Economic awareness of nurses: relationship to budgetary control. *Nursing Economics, 14*(5), 292–298.

Dieter, D. C. (1996). Cost effectiveness and quality nursing care. *Clinical Nurse Specialist, 10*(3), 153.

Elliott, J. P., Le Roux, P. D., Ransom, G., Newell, D. W., Grady, M. S., & Winn, H.R. (1996). Predicting length of hospital stay and cost by aneurysm grade on admission. *Journal of Neurosurgery, 85,* 388–391.

Fridriksson, S. M., Hillman, J., Saveland, H., & Brandt, L. (1995). Intracranial aneurysm surgery in the 8th and 9th decades of life: Impact on population-based management outcome. *Neurosurgery, 37*(4), 627–632.

Gerber, C. J., Lang, D. A., Neil-Dwyer, G., & Smith, W.F. (1993). A simple scoring system for accurate prediction of outcome within four days of a subarachnoid haemorrhage. *Acta Neurochirurgica, 122,* 11–22.

Hicks, L. L. (1985). Using benefit-cost and cost-effectiveness analyses in health-care resource allocation. *Nursing Economics, 3,* 78–84.

Hijdra, A., Braakman, R., van Gijn, J., Vermeulen, M., & van Crevel, H. (1987). Aneurysmal subarachnoid hemorrhage–complications and outcome in a hospital population. *Stroke, 18*(6), 1061–1067.

Inagawa, T. (1994). Timing of admission and management outcome in patients with subarachnoid hemorrhage. *Surgical Neurology, 41,* 268–276.

Kowal, N. S., & Delaney, M. (1996). The economics of a nurse-developed critical pathway. *Nursing Economics, 14*(3), 156–161.

Lanzino, G., Kassell, N. F., Germanson, T. P., Kongable, G. L., Truskowski, L. L., Torner, J. C., Jane, J. J., & the Participants (1996). Age and outcome after aneurysmal subarachnoid hemorrhage: Why do older patients fare worse? *Journal of Neurosurgery, 85,* 410–418.

Micek, W. T., Berry, L., Gilski, D., Kallenbach, A., Link, D., & Scharer, K. (1996). Patient outcomes–the link between nursing diagnoses and interventions. *Journal of Nursing Administration, 26*(11), 29–35.

Niskanen, M. M., Hernesniemi, J. A., Vapalahti, M. P., & Kari, A. (1993). One year outcome in early aneurysm surgery: Prediction of outcome. *Acta Neurochirurgica, 123,* 25–32.

Stachniak, J. B., Layon, A. J., Day, A. L., & Gallagher, J. (1996). Craniotomy for intracranial aneurysm and subarachnoid hemorrhage: Is course, cost, or outcome affected by age? *Stroke, 27*(2), 276–281.

Taylor, C. L., Yuan, Z., Selman, W. R., Ratcheson, R. A., & Rimm, A. A. (1997). Mortality rates, hospital length of stay, and the cost of treating subarachnoid hemorrhage in older patients: Institutional and geographical differences. *Journal of Neurosurgery, 86,* 583–588.

West, D. A., Hicks, L. L., Balas, E. A., & West, T. D. (1996). Profitable capitation requires accurate costing. *Nursing Economics, 14*(3), 162–170.

Websites

American Heart Association: www.americanheart.org
Aneurysm Information Project: www.colombia.edu/~mdtl
See also Chapter 26 for other recommendations.

Patient and Family

Published Material/Organizations

Brain Aneurysm Foundation, 295 Cambridge St., Boston, MA 02114, Tel: 617 -723-3870.

Websites

American Heart Association: www.americanheart.org.

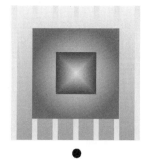

C H A P T E R **25**

Arteriovenous Malformations and Other Cerebrovascular Anomalies

JOANNE V. HICKEY
DEIDRE A. BUCKLEY

Cerebrovascular malformations are believed to be developmental vascular anomalies that result from failure of the embryonic vascular network to develop properly.[1] The incidence of cerebrovascular malformations is unclear because many lesions are asymptomatic and are found only incidentally at autopsy.

CLASSIFICATIONS OF VASCULAR MALFORMATIONS

Cerebrovascular malformations are classified into four major categories: capillary telangiectases, cavernous malformations, venous malformations, and arteriovenous malformations.[1] The term *malformation* is preferable to the previously used *angioma*. Angioma has a connotation of neoplasia that does not occur in these lesions. The incidence of vascular malformations varies from 0.1% to 4% in various autopsy studies. Because some of these lesions do not have direct arterial vessel input, they may not be visible on angiography.[1–3]

Telangiectases

Telangiectases are small (0.3 to 1.0 cm) capillary lesions that are composed of clusters of vessels that look something like dilated capillaries separated by normal-appearing parenchyma. These lesions have little clinical significance because they rarely cause hemorrhage; they are not apparent on radiological examination. Telangiectases are an incidental finding at autopsy and are most commonly located in the brain stem.

Cavernous Malformations

Cavernous malformations, also called cavernous hemangiomas, are nodular lesions composed of sinusoidal-type vessels that are not separated by normal-appearing parenchyma (neural tissue). These low-flow lesions are not apparent on angiography but may be visualized on computed tomography (CT) scan and magnetic resonance imaging (MRI). Cavernous malformations are well-defined, purple lesions that may grow to an appreciable size and may be mistaken for a brain tumor on CT scan. Other cavernous malformations are found incidentally at autopsy. Microscopic examination often reveals small hemorrhages with numerous, hemosiderin-laden macrophages and gliotic tissue in the adjacent parenchyma. Calcification within the lesion is common. Some cavernous malformations may cause seizures and intracerebral hemorrhage. With larger, clinically significant lesions, surgical removal is indicated.

Venous Malformations

Venous malformations, also referred to as venous anomalies, are composed of anomalous veins, separated by normal parenchyma, which drain into a dilated venous trunk. They are the most common vascular anomaly of the brain. These lesions have no recognizable direct arterial input. Calcification within the lesion is rare. The predominant location of venous malformations is in the cerebrum, although some are found in the cerebellum (3:1 ratio). Clinically, the patient may present with seizures. Venous malformations may be evident on CT scan, MRI, or angiography. Those found in the cerebrum rarely cause hemorrhage and are treated conservatively. However, cerebellar venous malformations are associated with an increased incidence of intracerebral hemorrhage; affected patients are, therefore, considered for surgery.

Arteriovenous Malformations

An arteriovenous malformation (AVM) is composed of a tightly tangled collection of abnormal-appearing, dilated blood vessels that directly shunt arterial blood into the venous system without the usual connecting capillary network (Fig. 25-1). Blood vessels of the AVM are thin-walled and tortuous and lack the normal characteristics of veins or arteries. The three morphologic components of an AVM are the nidus, the feeding arteries, and the draining veins. (The literature often refers to the nidus when discussing AVMs; a nidus is defined as the focus of the AVM, that is, the tangle of abnormal vessels.) The vessels of the AVM vary greatly in diameter, but the veins are generally larger than the arteries. The arterial vessels, also called feeder arteries, supply the AVM. The lesion is drained by dilated veins without the usual intervening capillary network. As a result of the absence of the capillary network, blood flow is accelerated and the pressure is elevated within the fragile vessels of the AVM. These conditions predispose the lesion to hemorrhage.

AVMs may be small and focal, or they may be large, involving an entire hemisphere. Some are conical, with the apex pointing inward and the base positioned on the surface of the cerebral cortex. In rare instances, the lesion is so deep that the ventricles and choroid plexus are involved, thus predisposing the person to intraventricular hemorrhage. The parenchyma between the vessels of the AVM is usually abnormal, with nonfunctional gliotic tissue (proliferation of neuroglia [i.e., supporting tissue] in the brain). Frequently, there is evidence of old hemorrhage and hemosiderin deposits (iron-containing glycoprotein pigment found in tissue, excessive amounts of which occur in pathological conditions). Patients may have a radiographic hemorrhage without clinical signs or symptoms of hemorrhage.

The AVM is the most common cerebrovascular lesion that causes symptoms and is, therefore, clinically significant. Over the last decade, there have been significant developments in the treatment of intracranial AVMs. There has been an evolution in microsurgical, endovascular, and radiosurgical techniques to treat these lesions. As the management options have evolved, combined modality treatment protocols have developed in various institutions. AVMs are found in both children and adults. AVMs in adults constitute the focus of most of this chapter.

ARTERIOVENOUS MALFORMATIONS IN THE ADULT: AN OVERVIEW

Several important points can be made to describe AVMs: they account for 8.6% of subarachnoid hemorrhages; this means that 1% of strokes are attributable to ruptured AVMs. The Harvard Cooperative Stroke Registry did a 3-year study documenting 9 AVM cases among 494 cases of stroke from all causes of stroke in a population of 100,000. This yields an incidence of about 3 per 100,000 annually.[2,5] The ratio of AVMs to intracranial aneurysms is 1:10.[2,5] Approximately 90% of AVMs are located in the supratentorial area and involve the cerebral hemispheres; only 10% of this group are located in the deep subcortical areas (e.g., basal ganglia, thalamus, corpus callosum). The location of 10% of AVMs is within the cerebellum and brain stem. Of those patients with AVMs, 80% develop symptoms between the ages of 20 and 40 years of age; the remaining 20% develop symptoms before the age of 20 years.

Pathophysiology and Pathological Characteristics

There are two pathophysiological characteristics related to AVMs. The first is the effect of shunting of blood from the arterial to the venous system without the intervening capillary network. Normally, the capillary network provides capillary resistance to blood flow, thus decreasing the intravascular pressure. However, when an AVM is present, blood is shunted from the high-resistance normal vascular bed to the low-resistance vessels within the AVM, thus exposing the draining venous channels to elevated intravascular pressure. These dynamics predispose the vessels to rupture and hemorrhage.

The second is the effect of impaired perfusion of the cerebral tissue adjacent to the AVM. Elevated intravascular and venous pressure impairs cerebral perfusion pressure. When the AVM is large and has a high flow, the diversion of blood to the AVM may cause ischemia to the adjacent normal tissue. Clinically, this is evidenced by slowly progressive neurological deficits. The diversion of blood to the AVM is called the *vascular steal phenomenon.*

AVMs are circumscribed vascular lesions that displace, rather than encompass, normally functioning brain tissue. They are separated from normal tissue by abnormal and nonfunctional gliotic parenchyma. Evidence of microscopic or gross hemorrhage is very common. This is true even in patients who have no clinical manifested hemorrhage. Partial thrombosis of an AVM is not uncommon and can occur spontaneously. This may explain why some AVMs appear smaller on repeat angiography than on a previous study. This may also explain why some AVMs that are classified as "occult" are not seen on angiography.

Clinical Manifestations

The major clinical manifestations of AVMs are hemorrhage, seizures, headache, and progressive neurological deficits. The following section provides a brief discussion of each.

Hemorrhage

Hemorrhage is the most common initial manifestation of AVMs. Approximately 50% of clinically evident AVMs present with intracranial hemorrhage. When an AVM ruptures, it usually causes intraparenchymal hemorrhage.[6,7] If the AVM is superficial, a subarachnoid hemorrhage can occur. In the rare instance of an AVM that involves the choroid plexus, rupture can result in intraventricular hemorrhage. Mortality associated with initial AVM rupture is reported to be between 6% and 30% with an average of about 15%. Serious morbidity is between 15% and 80% with an average of about 30%. The combined morbidity and mortality rates from an AVM bleed may be as high as 15% to 80%.[8–11] The chance of rebleeding during the first year is approximately 6%.[12] After the first year, the incidence of recurrent hemorrhages decreases to 4% per year. This is the same as the rate of hemorrhage from AVMs that have never bled. The hemorrhage associated with rupture of an AVM is not so devastating as that associated with a ruptured cerebral aneurysm. In addition, the vasospasm and acute rebleeding (20% to 40% rebleed within 14 days) associated with aneurysms are not characteristic of AVMs.[3] Vasospasm does not occur within the AVM because there is no blood in the basilar subarachnoid cistern around the major intracranial arteries as is commonly found with aneurysmal rupture.

Seizures

Seizures are the second most common manifestation of AVMs.[6,12] Seizures occur in approximately 20% to 25% of patients.[13,14] It has been suggested that approximately 70% of patients with AVMs have seizures at some time.[7] Of those patients who have seizures, about 50% experience the focal type. The natural history of a patient with an AVM presenting with seizures is still not certain.

The etiology of seizures in patients with AVMs is also not clear, but two explanations have been suggested. First, cortical injury from hemorrhage into areas adjacent to the AVM may cause foci for seizure activity. Second, chronic ischemia from the vascular steal phenomenon may also cause abnormal cells that may become the foci for seizure activity.[5]

In patients who present with seizure, there is a 25% chance of hemorrhage within 15 years, or 4% per year.[15] It is thought that medical therapy is generally successful in the control of seizure activity. The prognosis for patients who have surgery or embolization in combination with surgery to resect the AVM is favorable in that the frequency of seizures lessens in most patients.[16] It is also thought that seizures improve after radiosurgery.[17]

Headache

Other presentations of AVMs include headaches in 15% of affected patients.[18] Recurrent headache that does not respond to usual drug therapy may be the only symptom of an AVM. Some patients experience migraine-like headaches. A headache workup with an MRI scan may suggest the presence of an AVM. It is important to remember that some types of headaches are related to AVMs. Some AVMs in the occipital lobe cause migraine-like headaches. Often after the removal of the AVM, the patient's headaches resolve.[19] Because of the high frequency of headaches in the population, the relationship of AVM to headache is difficult to define. As technology improves and becomes more readily available, MRI scans are being ordered by physicians for headaches or other complaints, and an AVM or other lesion may be found incidentally. In certain circumstances headaches are clearly related to an underlying AVM, but in other situations there is a much less well-defined relationship. In cases in which differentiation of symptoms from lesions is less clear, it would be dangerous to assume the headaches are caused by the malformation and will be relieved by treatment, either partial or complete. The patient must understand that symptoms may be incidental to the lesion.

Progressive Neurological Deficits

The development of progressive neurological deficits is primarily attributed to cerebral ischemia resulting from vascular steal. The signs and symptoms will depend on the specific area of cerebral tissue deprived of adequate blood supply. Progressive deficits may also be related to repeated small hemorrhages that have not been clinically apparent.

Venous hypertension from arterialization of the venous system may account for neurological deterioration. Hydrocephalus is another mechanism that plays a role in progressive neurological deficits caused by ventricular compression from dilated veins.

Neuropsychiatric Manifestations

AVMs may cause neuropsychiatric manifestations. Approximately 10% of patients with an AVM manifest some sort of neuropsychiatric behavior. The vascular steal syndrome is thought to be responsible for such symptoms.[5]

Diagnosis

Diagnostic Procedures

CT Scan. The CT scan is one of the initial screening tools for AVMs. It is a diagnostic test in which cross-sections of the brain are examined through the use of x-rays and a computer. The picture of the various layers produced by the scan accurately reflects anatomical structures inside the brain, such as the ventricles, basal ganglia, and thalamus. A CT scan without contrast is often ordered to rule out the presence of an acute hematoma. If the AVM has hemorrhaged, serial CT scans are helpful in monitoring blood clot and observing for resolution of blood over time.

MRI/Magnetic Resonance Angiography (MRA). MRI is an initial diagnostic tool and is ordered more commonly than a CT scan for complaints such as headaches. The MRI is critical in defining the treatment plan of the AVM to determine the site of its nidus (the central part of the AVM), as well as its relationship to other critical anatomical structures in the brain. It is also better than CT scanning in demonstrating subtle changes in tissue composition (e.g., edema and old hemorrhage).

MRA is the same procedure as MRI, but with the difference that blood vessels are examined instead of body tissue. MRI and MRA are both noninvasive types of studies.

Angiography. Cerebral angiography is the definitive diagnostic procedure for AVMs. It demonstrates the feeding arteries, the nidus, and the draining veins. This information is important for making decisions about the advisability of surgery, endovascular therapy, or radiosurgery. Cerebral angiography is also useful for following the progress and development of the AVM over time.

As mentioned earlier, some AVMs are angiographically occult lesions. These lesions are discovered in the diagnostic workup of patients presenting with intracranial hemorrhage or in patients with seizures.

Treatment

Decisions regarding the best approach to management of AVMs are complex. Among the factors that influence patient outcomes, the two that are critical are the reputation of the hospital and, in particular, the experience and skill of the neurosurgeon and interventional neuroradiologist with AVMs. The natural history of the lesion for hemorrhaging, along with the specific characteristics of the particular lesion for an individual patient, must be carefully weighed. The physician must compare the long-term risk presented by an untreated AVM with the more immediate risk of surgery or other treatment options. See Case Studies 25-1 and 25-2.

Case Study 25-1

Ms. L. E. is a 30-year-old white female who spent the day snowmobiling. Toward the end of the day, she developed a headache and ultimately had a seizure that involved the right leg and right arm. She presented to the emergency room, where a CT scan showed a high left parietal hemorrhage. An MRI/MRA was subsequently done, which demonstrated a left parietal arteriovenous malformation. The patient underwent a left parietal craniotomy for microsurgical resection of the AVM. The following intraoperative photos were taken. Under the microscope, one can visualize the AVM with the arteries and a large dark draining vein extending posteriorly (Fig. 25-1). The arteriogram is a lateral view, with injection of the left internal carotid artery demonstrating a left paramedian parietal AVM. There is direct arterial supply directly through an anterior parietal branch of the anterior cerebral artery. The venous drainage is through the superior sagittal sinus, medullary veins, and vein of Galen (Fig. 25-2). The final photo is the

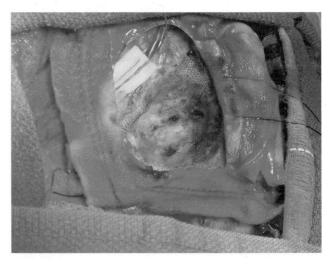

Figure 25–3 • Final photo of the resected cavity after removal of the AVM.

resected cavity after removal of the AVM (Fig. 25-3). A follow-up angiogram showed complete resection of the AVM.

Case Study 25-2

This is a 45-year-old woman who presented with a generalized seizure. Figure 25-4 shows the arteriovenous malformation (AVM) on magnetic resonance imaging; the arrow points to the lesion, which is approximately 3 × 4 × 2 cm. Figure 25-5 is an angiogram showing the size and location of the AVM as well as pertinent feeding vessels which come from the posterior cerebral artery, as well as feeders from the middle cerebral artery and anterior cerebral artery. The patient was treated with two sessions of embolization followed by surgery. Figure 25-6 is the angiogram pre-embolization, Figure 25-7 is an angiogram taken post-embolization, and Figure 25-8 is an angiogram taken after surgery. Patient discharged on anticonvulsant drugs.

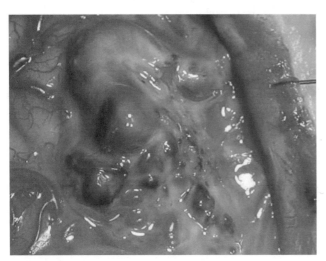

Figure 25–1 • Arteriovenous malformation as seen under the microscope at surgery.

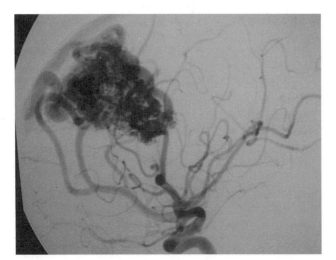

Figure 25–2 • Intraoperative arteriogram (lateral view). Injection of the left internal carotid artery demonstrates a left paramedian parietal AVM.

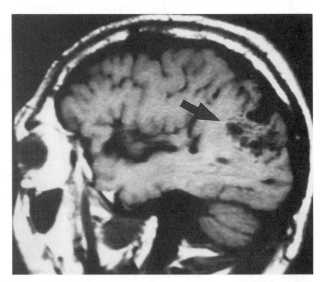

Figure 25–4 • AVM on MRI; the *arrow* points to the lesion, which is approximately 3 × 4 × 2 cm.

Case Study 25-2 (Continued)

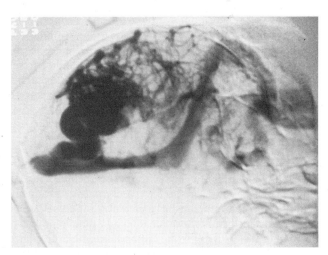

Figure 25–5 • Angiogram showing the AVM with feeder vessels from the anterior, middle, and posterior arteries.

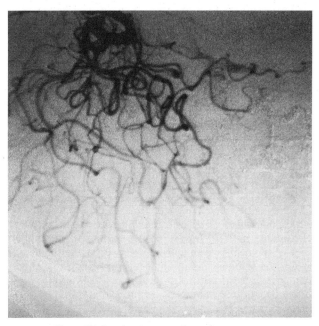

Figure 25–8 • Angiogram taken after surgery.

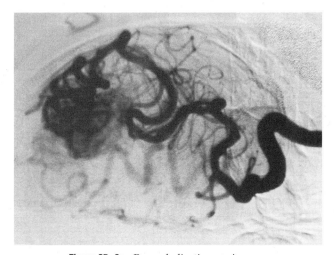

Figure 25–6 • Pre-embolization angiogram.

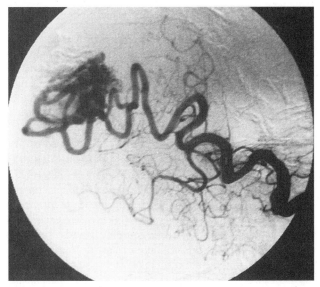

Figure 25–7 • Post-embolization angiogram.

Seen in follow-up, 2 1/2 years later, she has had one seizure since treatment. She has remained on anticonvulsants and has been seizure free. Neurologically, she is intact and enjoys a very good quality of life.

Natural History of Arteriovenous Malformations

The biological behavior or natural history of AVMs is helpful in weighing treatment approaches. The following provides statistics about the natural history of AVMs.

Unruptured AVM. There is approximately a 3% risk of bleeding per year, with about a 1% risk of death per year.

Ruptured AVMs. *Peak age for hemorrhage is between 15 to 20 years.* The mortality rate for the first hemorrhage is about 10%; morbidity exists in the 30% to 50% range (neurological deficit from each bleed). Small AVMs tend to present more often as hemorrhages than larger ones.[20] It was postulated that larger AVMs presented as seizure simply because their size made them more likely to involve the cortex. The smaller AVMs are now thought to have a much higher pressure in the feeding arteries. Thus, smaller AVMs are assumed to be more lethal than larger ones.

The average risk from hemorrhage from an AVM is approximately 2% to 4% per year.[21] The risk of rebleeding is approximately 6% during the first year; it then declines to approximately 3% per year after that, up to about 15 years.

The mortality associated with a second hemorrhage is approximately 13%; subsequent hemorrhages carry a mortality rate of about 20%.

With wider use of MRI for screening of patients for various neurological signs and symptoms, asymptomatic AVMs are being detected more frequently. The risk of hemorrhage is about 4%.[21] Of all patients with AVMs who have no previous clinical history of hemorrhage, 25% to 33% demonstrate evidence of previous hemorrhage.[19]

The natural history of AVMs suggests a high probability for hemorrhage at some time. Statistics also suggest that the incidence of rebleeding is the same regardless of whether the AVM is unruptured or ruptured. Although the physician makes the decisions about medical management, it is important for the nurse to understand the basis for the decision. This information is helpful in teaching both the patient and family and in reinforcing the information provided to the patient and family by the physician.

Aneurysms and Arteriovenous Malformations. Seven percent of patients with AVMs have aneurysms. Approximately 75% of such aneurysms are located on a major feeding artery, most likely resulting from increased flow. Aneurysms may form within the nidus or on draining veins. When treating tandem lesions, the symptomatic aneurysm or AVM is usually the one treated first. When feasible, they both may be treated at the same time with either surgery or embolization. If it is not clear which had produced the bleeding, the odds are usually with the aneurysm.[22]

Grading of Arteriovenous Malformations

The most commonly used grading system for AVMs is that described by Spetzler and Martin, who developed their system according to their degrees of surgical difficulty.[23] The Spetzler-Martin AVM Grading Scale provides a simplified scheme based on size, location, and venous drainage:

SIZE

0–3 cm	1
3.1–6.0 cm	2
>6 cm	3

LOCATION

Non-eloquent	0
Eloquent	1

DEEP VENOUS DRAINAGE

Not present	0
Present	1

Eloquence refers to areas of the brain that have readily identifiable neurological function; if injury to any of these areas occurs, a disabling neurological deficit will be noted. According to this grading system, the eloquent areas are the sensorimotor, language, and visual cortex; the hypothalamus and thalamus; the internal capsule; the brain stem; the cerebellar peduncles; and the deep cerebellar nuclei.

Each of these three variables becomes a subscale that is assigned a numerical value. The scores of each subscale are added together, and the total score indicates an AVM grade from I to V. Angiographic findings are used to collect data for each subscale.

Within this system, grades I and II lesions have a low morbidity, whereas higher-grade lesions are associated with gradually increasing morbidity. Spetzler and Martin recommend surgery for all grades I and II lesions. Grade III lesions should be treated case by case; however, they usually recommend surgery for both symptomatic and asymptomatic lesions. Grades IV and V lesions necessitate a multidisciplinary approach. There are other grading systems that focus on anatomical, hemodynamic, and physiological properties associated with AVMs; however, it was found that the three factors identified in the Spetzler-Martin systems were most accurate in predicting surgical outcomes.[18]

Treatment Options

The treatment options available for AVMs include surgery, embolization, radiosurgery, and conservative treatment. Comprehensive evaluation of a patient with an AVM includes a detailed clinical examination and radiological clarification of the anatomy with MRI and arteriography. After the comprehensive evaluation, decisions can be made regarding the best management approach by comparing the natural history of the lesion with the intervention-related morbidity and mortality.

There is evidence suggesting that the radiological parameters may be predictive of hemorrhage risk. There is a complex combination of variables that may predict the risk of hemorrhage from AVM. Some have noted that patients with seizures may be at slightly higher risk, but this has not been noted consistently.[8,12] There are also data to suggest that prior hemorrhage is a strong predictor of hemorrhage.[24] Small AVM size in maximal diameter[12] or volume may also be a predictor for higher hemorrhage risk.[25] AVMs in the intraventricular or periventricular location may also be at an increased risk to bleed,[26] although this is not found consistently.[27]

The angiographic characteristics of an AVM are complex. There are both arterial and venous factors that are predictive of an increased risk of hemorrhage, although studies are not *definitive*. Characteristics of the venous drainage system, including the presence of deep venous drainage, have been reported to be a predictor of presentation with hemorrhage.[28,29]

Surgery. With rare exceptions, surgery for an AVM is always elective. Only if there is an intracerebral hematoma or subdural hematoma is early surgery considered. Even when surgery is anticipated after hemorrhage, it is usually delayed for about 3 weeks. This timetable allows for the patient to be stabilized and for the brain to recover from the effects of hemorrhage.

Applying the grading system for AVMs discussed earlier, the experienced neurosurgeon is able to assess the degree of surgical difficulty. The physician considers the age of the patient along with the anatomical location of the lesion and other characteristics that influence the technical approach to the lesion. The goals of surgery are (1) complete excision of the AVM to prevent hemorrhage completely and (2) excision of the lesion without causing hemorrhage or injury to adjacent tissue during the surgery. Ligation of the feeder vessels does not provide protection from hemorrhage.[30] Lesions are typically excised using standard microsurgical techniques with the microscope. The arterial feeders are generally attacked first, followed by excision of the nidus of the lesion and then resection of the draining vein. To ensure complete obliteration of the lesion, intraoperative or postoperative angiogram is recommended. If there is residual lesion, immediate resection should be considered to avoid potential hemorrhage from the remaining vessels. If it is thought not to be safe to resect remaining vessels, alternative treatment should be considered, which may include stereotactic radiosurgery. There is a risk of hemorrhage during the interval period until the lesion has been obliterated.[18] The lesion may have to be treated in stages with a combination of embolization and surgery. (See Case Study 25-1.)

A special concern related to surgery for large AVMs (i.e., larger than 4 to 5 cm) is normal perfusion pressure breakthrough.[31] Normal perfusion pressure breakthrough is a rare occurrence and is described as severe, protracted, and unexplained brain edema accompanied by diffuse hemorrhage or focal deep hemorrhage in the parenchyma immediately adjacent to the area of resection. To prevent this occurrence, the interventional neuroradiologist plans one, two, or more stages of endovascular treatment to reduce the blood supply to the AVM.

Embolization. Embolization of brain AVMs is a subspecialty of interventional neuroradiology that has made tremendous strides over the past few years. Improvement in catheters—that is, flow-directed and flow-assisted microcatheters—have made navigation of intracranial vessels safer and have allowed more accurate delivery of embolic material. Improvement in imaging equipment has led to safer, more effective treatment. Depending on size, location, symptoms, hemodynamics, and anatomical vasculature of AVMs, embolization may be curative, palliative, or adjunctive to surgery or radiosurgery.[32]

As with surgery, the interventional neuroradiologist's experience with embolization procedures greatly influences outcomes for the patient. Improvements in microcatheter technology have allowed for superselective catheterization of distal vessels as well as intranidal aneurysms. Digital subtraction angiography and the development of "road mapping" technique are essential to endovascular treatment. The use of heparin during the procedure has been proved to minimize thromboembolic complications and is a necessary adjunct to embolization.

Current embolic materials are divided into solid and liquid agents. Solid agents consist of polyvinyl alcohol particles, microcoils, fibers, and microballoons.[33,34] Liquid agents consist of cryanacrylate monomers, such as I-butyl cyanoacrylate (IBCA) and n-butyl-cyanoacrylate (NBCA), which is a short-acting liquid polymerizing agent. In its solidified form, it is relatively soft, making it easy for the surgeon to resect.[30] NBCA has recently been officially approved by the Food and Drug Administration for use in cerebral AVMs. Another agent that is a polymer solution is ethylene vinyl alcohol (i.e., EVAL copolymer).[35] Other liquid agents include absolute ethanol, with and without the use of contrast agents for visualization under fluoroscopy.

Polyvinyl alcohol (PVA) and Gelfoam particles are easier to use but are non-permanent embolic agents. Microcoils and silk thread are highly thrombogenic, although not per-manent. The goal of embolization for definitive or palliative treatment is permanent occlusion of the nidus and feeding vessels and to attempt to occlude deep surgically inaccessible or deep arterial feeding vessels to facilitate surgical excision. Other goals of preoperative embolization are to occlude intranidal aneurysms and high-flow fistulas to promote thrombosis of the AVM's nidus (see Case Study 25-2).

Radiosurgery. The underlying goal of radiation therapy for AVMs is to induce an inflammatory response in the vessel walls of the lesion that will result in permanent thickening of pathological vascular channels, with ultimate thrombosis and obliteration of the lesion.[5] The success in achieving this goal is determined, in part, by the ability to provide partial or total radiation to the lesion. If obliteration is incomplete, the patient is at risk for hemorrhage.

Pre-radiosurgical embolization for AVM's is also a consideration. Three potential goals when endovascular therapy is to be undertaken before radiosurgery are (1) to decrease target size to less than 3 cm in diameter, because it is known from the radiosurgical data that smaller volumes have a higher cure rate; (2) to eradicate angiographic predictors of hemorrhage, such as intranidal aneurysms or venous aneurysms; and (3) to attempt to reduce symptoms related to venous hypertension.[18] There has been no ideal embolic agent identified for pre-radiosurgical use.[36,37]

Various types of ionizing radiation have been used in the treatment of AVMs, including x-rays (produced by x-ray tubes or megavoltage linear accelerators); gamma rays (produced by cobalt); and Bragg peak therapy (proton beam and helium beam).[38] A delayed complication common to all types of radiation therapy is radionecrosis of healthy neural tissue. This can occur in a matter of months (3 to 11 months) or years (1 to 8 years) after radiation therapy. It is evidenced by development of new neurological deficits or worsening of previous deficits.

Conventional Radiation Therapy. Conventional radiation therapy is defined as orthovoltage or megavoltage external beam radiation or cobalt-60 gamma rays without stereotactic technique. Its use has generally not been considered effective in treating AVMs. However, recent publications recommend a reexamination of the use and patient selection criteria for conventional radiation therapy. The literature suggests that desirable changes within the wall of lesions are induced by this type of radiosurgery.

Gamma Knife Radiosurgery. Stereotactically directed gamma radiation has been pioneered by Leksell.[39] This so-called bloodless surgery is used to treat surgically inaccessible lesions that are 2 to 3 cm in diameter (see Chap. 15). For larger lesions, only partial radiosurgery can be offered.

Bragg Peak Proton Beam Therapy. For surgically inaccessible AVMs, proton beam radiosurgery has been useful as an ablative approach to shrink the lesion.[10] This is a noninvasive procedure that uses the radiation emitted by protons that have been accelerated in a cyclotron. Stereotactic technique controls the focus of the beam to the target area.

The major advantage of proton beam radiosurgery is that, after the diagnostic workup has been completed, radiation therapy is administered on an outpatient basis or during a brief hospitalization. There is no immediate risk to the patient from such irradiation. The major drawback is the possibility of hemorrhage before the effect of the therapy is realized. Radiosurgery effects develop gradually, requiring 12 to 24 months to reach a therapeutic level that provides protection against hemorrhage. As a result of radiosurgery, the walls of the lesion thicken, and there may be some obliteration of the lesion and reduction in its size. Complications related to proton beam therapy are uncommon, although radiation-induced necrosis has been reported. The physician attempts to keep the risk below 3% to 5%. The possibility of complications in a patient reflects the location of the AVM relative to brain structures.

Conservative Management. In some instances, the treatment of choice may be conservative management. A discussion of any restrictions on activities, such as contact sports, is necessary. For patients who present with seizures, seizure activity can be well controlled with anticonvulsant therapy.

Summary of Treatment

Regardless of the treatment approach recommended to a particular patient, it is necessary to monitor him or her over time. In addition to follow-up appointments, periodic cerebral angiography, MRI, or both are ordered to check the progress of the lesion.

Arteriovenous Malformations and Pregnancy

The incidence of hemorrhage from brain AVMs during pregnancy has been a controversial topic over the years. Earlier studies suggested a high incidence of hemorrhage during pregnancy when a patient had a true high-flow AVM.[31,39] The implication is that when the AVM did present in a pregnant woman, it did so in the form of a hemorrhage.

A retrospective study by Horton and associates found the incidence of hemorrhage in pregnant women with unruptured AVMs during the interval of time during and immediately after gestation to be 3.5% annually.[40] These women had no previous history consistent with hemorrhage. In women with a previous clinical history of hemorrhage, the risk was increased to a 5.8% chance of hemorrhage during pregnancy. In non-pregnant patients, the incidence of hemorrhage is 4% per year. It was concluded by the investigators that pregnancy was not a significant risk factor for hemorrhage in women with unruptured AVMs.

Studies have shown that there is no increase in the rate of hemorrhage during labor or the immediate postpartum period. Therefore, when a woman presents during pregnancy with an AVM, the recommendation is that the pregnancy be carried to term. The patient can also be reassured that the risk of hemorrhage during delivery is very small, as is the case throughout the entire pregnancy. Data suggest in most cases that vaginal delivery is safe, but caesarean section may decrease the already low incidence of hemorrhage during delivery. There are no data to support or deny this statement.[39] The patient, neurosurgeon, and obstetrician need to discuss the safety and efficacy of the mode of delivery carefully on a case-by-case basis. All must be comfortable with the decision. According to the

statistics, the actual incidence of problems encountered during pregnancy is low.

If the woman presents with a hemorrhage during pregnancy, care should proceed as in the non-pregnant patient. The nurse plays an important role in reassuring the patient while anticipating potential neurological problems. If a hematoma is currently causing significant mass effect, it should be evacuated. Ogilvy and Tattler recommend removal of the clot only and operating on the AVM on an elective basis.[39] Early angiography is often done. This is preferable and is used to define the anatomy of the lesion. If possible, the angiogram should be done during the second or third trimester to avoid added risk to the fetus. As with non-pregnant patients, the treatment modality, either surgery, embolization, radiosurgery, or a combination, is decided on based on size, location, and surgical accessibility of the lesion. Women with known AVMs should be carefully counseled before conception. If possible, the lesion should be treated before pregnancy. As previously stated, although the risk of hemorrhage in a pregnant woman with an unruptured AVM is very low, it is not zero. Safe management of pregnant patients with neurological diseases, such as an AVM, requires close collaboration of the health care team, including the neurosurgeon, neurologist, obstetrician, anesthesiologist, and nurses.[39] Reassuring the patient and reinforcing the information given to her by her physicians is an important role of the nurse during this critical time. Providing written information is most helpful.

Nursing Management

The patient who is suspected of having a cerebral AVM is at risk for hemorrhage. If hemorrhage has not occurred, management is directed toward preventing hemorrhage by controlling hypertension, preventing seizures, and modifying the patient's lifestyle (e.g., avoiding contact sports and lifting) to prevent surges in blood pressure. In the hospital, the nurse can expect to perform the following:

- Conduct a baseline neurological assessment as well as ongoing monitoring of neurological signs
- Monitor vital signs for evidence of hypertension
- Assess and monitor characteristics of headache, if present
- Monitor the patient for evidence of seizure activity
- Administer drug therapy as necessary

If the AVM has ruptured, the patient will be managed in a similar manner to that of other patients who have had a cerebral hemorrhage (see Chap. 24). The severity of the hemorrhage and the patient's clinical presentation will determine the medical treatment selected and the related nursing management. Hemorrhage is usually intracerebral. However, less frequently, subarachnoid hemorrhage, a subdural hematoma, or an intraventricular hematoma may occur. Unlike patients with ruptured aneurysms, vasospasm is not a concern after hemorrhage. There is some risk of rebleeding, and the patient should be monitored for evidence of rapid neurological deterioration. If surgery, embolization, or both are intended, they are usually delayed for about 3 weeks to allow for planning and for recovery of the brain from hemorrhage.

In addition to carrying out baseline and ongoing monitoring of neurological and vital signs, a major role of the nurse is in providing emotional support and teaching to the patient and family. Most patients with AVMs are young, and the thought of having a serious lesion within the brain is very frightening to them. These patients undergo various diagnostic procedures to collect data about the lesion, and they are given much information, including the advantages and disadvantages of each treatment option. Finally, a decision is made regarding the appropriate course of treatment. The nurse is very much involved in the related patient teaching, as well as in reinforcing the information provided by the physician. Anxiety and fear are common responses of the patient and family. Nursing interventions are directed at alleviating these responses and supporting effective coping strategies. A support group specifically for patients with brain AVMs may help both the patient and family members.

Perioperative Nursing Management

If surgery is planned, the nurse will be responsible for providing basic preoperative teaching (see Chap. 15). Postoperative nursing management for patients with AVMs is similar to that outlined for a craniotomy patient (see Chap. 15). If a large lesion has been resected, there is the concern that normal perfusion pressure breakthrough can occur, as discussed previously. Clinically, there would be evidence of significant neurological deterioration.

The management of the patient after endovascular therapy includes continuous use of intravenous heparin, which will decrease the possibility of a thromboembolic complication while being carefully monitored in the neurological intensive care unit. The arterial sheath remains in place for 12 to 24 hours. The patient is kept well hydrated, with tight blood pressure control. Mild systemic hypotension may be helpful in allowing flow changes to occur gradually in the brain tissue surrounding the AVM during the first 24 hours after the procedure. Sometimes, affected patients will complain of headache. This can be attributed to changes in flow dynamics in the brain. The nature of the headache should be documented, and the physician should be notified. If the indication of embolization is adjuvant to surgery, the patient is prepared for surgery 24 to 48 hours after endovascular treatment.[32]

After recovery from surgery, the patient is discharged with orders for anticonvulsant therapy. Depending on the presence of neurological deficits, there may be need for rehabilitation. For some patients, a neuropsychological evaluation may be ordered after a few months to evaluate the presence of cognitive deficits. The patient's progress is followed by the physician. If the lesion has not been obliterated completely, the patient remains at risk for hemorrhage.

Future Trends

Advances in functional imaging, microsurgical technique, neuroanesthesiology, endovascular therapy, and stereotactic radiosurgery have contributed to the ongoing therapeutic care and management of vascular malformations. Also important have been advances in biological knowledge, which form the foundation for modern success in treatment.[41]

Research continues on various interventional materials, including glue (i.e., NBCA), PVA, and other liquid agents that are injected into the feeders of these complex lesions. Fractionated radiation is currently being researched as a mode to treat larger AVMs that were once deemed untreatable. Although technology and knowledge of vascular malformations have increased tremendously over the years, and will continue to do so, one cannot dismiss the importance of characteristics of individual patients, such as age, medical condition, vocation, and psychological factors in the process of evaluating management options and coming to treatment decisions.

REFERENCES

1. Tatter, S. B., & Ogilvy, C. S. (1995). Vascular malformations: General considerations. In C. W. Mitchell (Ed.). *Surgical management of neurovascular disease* (pp. 387–403). Baltimore: Williams & Wilkins.
2. Mohr, K., Caplan, L., Melski, J. W., et al. (1978). The Harvard Cooperative Stroke Registry: A prospective registry. *Neurology, 28,* 754.
3. Guidetti, B. & Delitala, A. (1980). Intracranial arteriovenous malformations: Conservative and surgical treatment. *Journal of Neurosurgery, 53,* 149–152.
4. McCormick, W. F. (1978). Classification, pathology, and natural history of angiomas of the central nervous system. *Neurology and Neurosurgery Weekly Update, 1,* 3–7.
5. Ondra, S. L., Troupp, H., George, E. D., & Schwab, K. (1990). The natural history of symptomatic arteriovenous malformations of the brain: A 24-year follow-up assessment. *Journal of Neurosurgery, 73,* 387–391.
6. Parkinson, D. & Bachers, G. (1980). Arteriovenous malformations: Summary of 100 consecutive supratentorial cases. *Journal of Neurosurgery, 53,* 285–299.
7. Pertuiset, B., Sichez, J. P., Philippon, J., Fohanno, D., & Horn, Y. (1979). Mortality and morbidity after complete surgical removal of 162 intracranial arteriovenous malformations. *Review of Neurology, 135,* 319–327.
8. Brown, R. D., Jr., Weibers, D. D., & Forbes, G. S. (1990). Unruptured intracranial aneurysms and arteriovenous malformations: Frequency of intracranial hemorrhage in relation to lesions. *Journal of Neurosurgery, 73,* 859–863.
9. Fults, D. & Kelly, D. L., Jr. (1984). Natural history of arteriovenous malformations of the brain: A clinical study. *Neurosurgery, 15,* 658–662.
10. Kjellberg, R. N., Hanamura, J., Davis, K. R., Lyons, S. L., & Adams, R. D. (1983). Bragg Peak proton-beam therapy for arteriovenous malformations of the brain. *New England Journal of Medicine, 308,* 269–274.
11. Luessenhop, A. J. & Rosa, L. (1984). Cerebral arteriovenous malformations: Indications for and results of surgery, the role of intravascular techniques. *Journal of Neurosurgery, 60,* 14–22.
12. Graf, C. J., Perret, G. E. & Torner, J. C. (1983). Bleeding from cerebral arteriovenous malformations as part of their natural history. *Journal of Neurosurgery, 58,* 331–337.
13. Brown, R. D. Jr, Wiebers, D. O., Forbes, G., O'Fallon, W. M., Piepgras, D. G., Marsh, W. R., & Maciunas, R. J. (1988). The natural history of unruptured intracranial arteriovenous malformations. *Journal of Neurosurgery, 16,* 421–430.
14. Wilkins, R. H. (1985). The natural history of intracranial vascular malformations: A review. *Neurosurgery, 16,* 421-430.
15. Forster, D. M., Steiner, L., & Harkanson, S. (1972). Arteriovenous malformations of the brain: A long-term clinical study. *Journal of Neurosurgery, 37,* 562–570.

16. Piepgras, D. G., Sundt, T. M., Jr., Ragoowanse, A. T., & Stevens, L. (1993). Seizure outcome in patients with surgically treated cerebral arteriovenous malformations. *Journal of Neurosurgery, 78*, 5–11.

17. Pollock, B. E., Lunsford, L. D., Kandziolka, D., Maitz, A., & Flickinger, J. C. (1994). Patient outcomes after sterotactic radiosurgery for "operable" arteriovenous malformations. *Neurosurgery, 35*, 1–8.

18. Ogilvy, C. S., Stieg, P. E., Awad, I., Brown, R. D. Jr, Kondziolka, D., Rosenwasser, R., Young, W. L., & Hademenos, G. (2001). American Heart Association scientific statement: Recommendations for the management of intracranial arteriovenous malformations: A statement from health care professionals from a special writing group of the Stroke Council, American Stroke Association. *Stroke, 32*, 1458–1471.

19. Heros, R. C. & Tu, Y. K. (1986). Unruptured arteriovenous malformations: A dilemma in surgical decision making. *Clinical Neurosurgery, 33*, 187–236.

20. Spetzler, R. F., Hargraves, R. W., McCormick, P. W., et al. (1992). Relationship of perfusion pressure and size to risk of hemorrhage from arteriovenous malformations. *Journal of Neurosurgery, 36*, 918–923.

21. Kondziolka, D. McLaughlin, M. R., & Kestle, J. R. W. (1995). Simple risk predictions for arteriovenous malformation hemorrhage. *Neurosurgery, 37*, 851–855.

22. Greenberg, M. S. (2001). Vascular malformations. In M. S. Greenberg (Ed.). *Handbook of neurosurgery* (5th ed., pp. 804–813). Lakeland, FL: Greenberg Graphics.

23. Spetzler, R. F., & Martin, R. A. (1986). A proposed grading system for arteriovenous malformations. *Journal of Neurosurgery, 65*, 476–483.

24. Harmann, A., Mast, H., Mohr, J. P., et. al. (1998). Morbidity of intracranial hemorrhage in patients with cerebral arteriovenous malformation. *Stroke, 29*, 931–934.

25. Duong, D. H., Young, W. L., Vang, M. C., et al. (1998). Feeding artery pressure and venous drainage pattern are primary determinants of hemorrhage from cerebral arteriovenous malformations. *Stroke, 29*, 1167–1176.

26. Nagata, S., Matsushima, T., Takeshita, Il, Fukui, M., & Yasumoori, K. (1991). Lateral ventricular arteriovenous malformations: Natural history and surgical indications. *Acta Neurochirugica (Wien), 112*, 37–46.

27. Turjman, F., Massoud, T. F., Vinuela, F., Sayre, J. W., Guglielmi, G., & Duckwiler, G. (1995). Correlation of the angioarchitectural features of cerebral arteriovenous malformations with clinical presentation of hemorrhage. *Neurosurgery, 37*, 856–860.

28. Miyasaka, Y., Yada, K., Ohwada, T., Kurata, A. & Irijura, K. (1992). An analysis of the venous drainage system as a factor in hemorrhage from arteriovenous malformation. *Journal of Neurosurgery, 76*, 239–243.

29. Kader, A., Young, W. L., Pile-Spellman, J., Mast, H., Sciacca, R. R., Mohr, J. P. & Stein, B. (1994). The influence of hemodynamic factors on hemorrhage from cerebral arteriovenous malformations. *Neurosurgery, 34*, 801–807.

30. Purdy, P. D., Batjer, H. H., Risser, R. G., & Samson, D. (1992). Arteriovenous malformation of the brain: Choosing embolic materials to enhance safety and ease of excision. *Journal of Neurosurgery, 77*, 217–222.

31. Robinson, J. L., Hall, C. S., & Sidzimir, C. B. (1972). Subarachnoid hemorrhage in pregnancy. *Journal of Neurosurgery, 36*, 27–33.

32. Hacien-Bey, L., Pile-Spellman, J., & Ogilvy, C. S. (1995). Embolization of brain arteriovenous malformations. In C. W. Mitchell (Ed.). *Surgical management of neurovascular disease* (pp. 404–418). Baltimore: Williams & Wilkins.

33. Fournier, D., TerBrugge, K. G., Willinsky, R., Lasjunias, P., & Montanera, W. (1991). Endovascular treatment of intracerebral arteriovenous malformations: Experience in 49 cases. *Journal of Neurosurgery, 75*, 228–233.

34. Scweitzer, J. S., Chang, B. S., Madsen, P., Vinuela, F., Martin, M. A., Marroquin, C. E., & Vinters, H. V. (1993). Pathology of arteriovenous malformations treated by embolotherapy, part 2: Results of embolization with multiple agents. *Neuroradiology, 35*, 468–474.

35. Wallace, R. C., Flom, R. A., Khayata, M. H., et al. (1995). The safety and effectiveness of brain arteriovenous malformation embolization using acrylic and particles: The experience of a single institution. *Neurosurgery, 37*, 606–618.

36. Gobin, U. P., Laurent, A., Merriene, L., Schlienger, M., Aymard, A., Houdart, E., Casasco, A., Lefkopoulos, D., George, B., & Merland, J.J (1996). Treatment of brain arteriovenous malformations by embolization and radiosurgery. *Journal of Neurosurgery, 85*, 19–28.

37. Dion, J. E., & Mathis, J. M. (1994). Cranial arteriovenous malformations: The role of embolization and stereotactic surgery. *Neurosurgery Clinics of North America, 5*, 459–474.

38. Ondra, J. L., Doty, J. R., Mahla, M. E., & George, E. D. (1988). Surgical excision of a cavernous hemangioma of the rostral brainstem: Case report. *Neurosurgery, 23*, 490–493.

39. Ogilvy, C. S., & Tatter, S. B. (1995). Surgical management of vascular lesions and tumors associated with pregnancy. In H. H. Schmidek & W. H. Sweet (Eds.). *Operative neurosurgical techniques, indications, methods and results* (pp. 1163–1173). Philadelphia: W. B. Saunders.

40. Horton, J. C., Chambers, W. A., Lyons, S. L., et al. (1990). Pregnancy and the risk of hemorrhage from cerebral arteriovenous malformations. *Neurosurgery, 27*, 867–871.

41. Martin, N. A. & Vinters, H. V. (1995). Arteriovenous malformations. In L. P. Carter & R.F. Spetzler (Eds.). *Neurovascular surgery* (pp. 875–903). New York: McGraw-Hill.

RESOURCES

Professional

Published Material

Martin, N. A., & Vinters, H. V. (1995). Arteriovenous malformations. In L. P. Carter, & R. F. Spetzler (Eds.). *Neurovascular surgery* (pp. 875–903). New York: McGraw-Hill.

Edwards, M. S. B., & Hoffman, H. J. H. (Eds.). (1989). *Cerebral vascular disease in children and adolescents.* Baltimore: Williams & Wilkins.

Lunsford, E. D. (Ed.). (1988). *Modern stereotactic neurosurgery.* Boston: Martinus Nijhoff.

Malik, G.M., Pasqualin, A., & Ausman, J. I. (1992). A new grading system for cerebral arteriovenous malformations. In A. Pasqualin, & R. Dapin (Eds.). *New trends in management of cerebral vascular malformations.* New York: Springer-Verlag.

Ojemann, R. G., Ogilvy, C. S., Crowell, R. M., & Heros, R. C. (1995). *Surgical management of cerebrovascular disease* (3rd ed). Baltimore: Williams & Wilkins.

Websites

See Chapter 24 and stroke websites.

Patient and Family

Websites

See Chapter 24 and stroke websites.

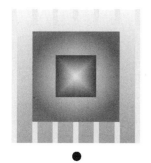

C H A P T E R 26

Stroke and Other Cerebrovascular Diseases

JOANNE V. HICKEY
NANETTE H. HOCK

Stroke represents an enormous public health burden. In the United States, it is the third leading cause of death, with 160,000 deaths resulting from stroke reported annually. In 1993 the U.S. stroke mortality rate increased for the first time in four decades, from 26.2 deaths per 100,000 to 26.5 deaths per 100,000. The mortality rate inched up again in 1995 to 26.7, with a slight decline in 1996 to 26.4.[1] The dramatic decrease in stroke mortality from the 1960s to 1992 paralleled the decrease in high blood pressure attributed to antihypertensive medication and may now be paralleling increasing patient noncompliance with antihypertensive drugs. Every year approximately 730,000 Americans have a new or recurrent stroke. Of the 580,000 Americans who survive a stroke each year, approximately 10% to 18% will have another stroke within 1 year.[1] Stroke risk increases with age. For each decade after age 55, the risk of stroke doubles. Two thirds of all strokes occur in people over age 65. Stroke is a major and increasing factor in the late-life dementia that affects more than 40% of Americans over age 80. Women account for approximately 43% of the strokes that occur each year, yet they account for 62% of stroke deaths (97,467 of the 159,942 annual deaths).[1] The explanation may be that stroke risk increases with age, and women generally live longer than men. Women over age 30 who smoke and take high-estrogen oral contraceptives have a stroke risk 22 times higher than average. Incidence rate for first stroke among African Americans is significantly greater than that of white Americans: 288 per 100,000 African-Americans, compared with 179 per 100,000 whites.[2] Stroke mortality in the African-American population is nearly double that for whites. Stroke represents a major public health expenditure, approaching $41 billion per year.

In the past decade, management of stroke has undergone a fundamental transformation as a result of research and technological advances, including improved pathophysiological models of stroke to understand changes on the biochemical and cellular levels; superior neuroimaging using magnetic resonance (MR) imaging, MR angiography, MR with diffusion-weighted (DW) and perfusion-weighted (PW) imaging, and improved computed tomography (CT) scanning techniques; the introduction of new pharmacological neuroprotective agents and techniques such as hypothermia; the definitive role of thrombolytic agents in early treatment; advances in radiological interventional procedures, such as angioplasty, cerebrovascular stenting, and embolic protection; the preventive benefit of carotid endarterectomy in patients with symptomatic high-grade stenosis; neurotransplantation; and other studies and investigative tools that continue to shape and refine patient management.

The term *brain attack* has become more popular in describing stroke, as appreciation has grown of the timeline associated with the development of neurological deficits and the window of opportunity that exists for reversal of neurological deficits with new interventions. Cardiac resuscitation training programs in basic life support (BLS) and advanced cardiac life support (ACLS) have been revamped with a focus on saving brain tissue as well as saving cardiac muscle. Improved emergency medical systems triage and the creation of dedicated stroke programs at institutions have significantly enhanced rapid stroke interventions.

Research is the foundation of both primary and secondary prevention of stroke and the management of stroke victims along a continuum of care with emphasis on early rehabilitation. Several research-based guidelines and consensus reports, such as the guidelines for the management of transient ischemic attacks, acute ischemic stroke, and carotid endarterectomy, are now available to guide health care providers in making informed decisions about treatment options.[3–6] In addition, in 1995 the Agency for Health Care and Policy Research (AHCPR) published clinical guidelines for post-stroke rehabilitation that set a national standard for management of stroke patients.

With more and more care being provided in managed-care environments, many institutions have developed interdisciplinary clinical pathways for stroke. The emphasis is on providing cost-effective care with measurable outcomes. This has resulted in frequent outcomes assessment, which has contributed to further refinement of care along the continuum. Nurses and other health care providers will continue to be challenged to demonstrate efficacy and cost effectiveness of interventions and care.

DEFINITION AND CLASSIFICATION OF STROKE

Stroke is a heterogeneous, neurological syndrome characterized by gradual or rapid, nonconvulsive onset of neurological deficits that fit a known vascular territory and that last for 24 hours or more. Stroke occurs when oxygen supply to a localized area in the brain is interrupted, resulting in a series of intricate processes that lead to the destruction of neural tissue and consequent brain damage. Stroke includes cerebral infarction (ischemic stroke) and intracerebral hemorrhage (ICH) and subarachnoid hemorrhage (hemorrhagic stroke). The two categories are further subdivided, as discussed later (Fig. 26-1). The type and severity of neurological deficits encompass a wide range and gradation of signs and symptoms. The severity and permanence of symptoms are the factors that differentiate between so-called minor stroke and major stroke.

Classification of stroke is based on the underlying problem created within the cerebral artery and the blood supply to the brain. An analogy to home plumbing pipes can be made. Only two events create problems with household plumbing: plugging of the pipe so that effluence cannot proceed to its destination; and bursting or rupturing of the pipe so that fluid within the pipe flows into the surrounding areas. In the brain, plugging by atherosclerosis or a clot creates a narrow lumen, preventing adequate flow of blood to cerebral tissue. Alternatively, rupture resulting from a weakened vessel causes leakage of blood into the brain or subarachnoid space.

Thus, stroke is divided into the two major categories of *ischemic stroke* and *hemorrhagic stroke*. The ischemic stroke category has been refined from the previous classification of thrombotic and embolic stroke to include additional categories.

Ischemic Stroke

Ischemic stroke accounts for 85% of all strokes and is subdivided into atherosclerotic cerebrovascular disease (20%); penetrating artery disease, or "lacunae" (25%); cardiogenic embolic (20%); cryptogenic (30%); and other (5%). Atherosclerosis of large and small cerebral arteries that results in thrombosis is the most common cause of ischemic stroke in North America and Europe and accounts for 45% of strokes in United States.

Terms Related to Ischemic Stroke

Transient ischemic attacks (TIAs) are temporary focal brain or retinal deficits, caused by vascular disease, that fit a known vascular territory and clear completely in less than 24 hours. Most TIAs are much shorter; most reverse completely within 1 hour. TIAs are classified into TIAs associated with the carotid and TIAs associated with vertebrobasilar vascular territories. One of the most important warning signs of a stroke is a TIA.

TIAs of the carotid (anterior circulation) cause lateralizing signs. When the carotid territory is involved, the symptoms reflect ischemia to the ipsilateral eye or cerebral hemisphere. A common eye symptom is temporary monocular blindness (TMB). Hemispherical ischemia usually causes weakness or numbness of the contralateral face or limb; language deficits and cognitive and behavioral changes may also occur.

TIAs of the vertebrobasilar (posterior) circulation cause diffuse signs. When the vertebrobasilar territory is involved, the symptoms often include dysarthria, vertigo, dizziness, ataxia, abnormalities of eye movement resulting in diplopia, and unilateral or bilateral motor and sensory deficits (Table 26-1).

A **penumbra** is a zone of compromised neuronal cells that are unable to function but remain viable and are located around an area of lethal injured cells; such a zone is amenable to reversal from ischemia (Fig. 26-2).

A **watershed** or **border zone infarction** is an infarcted area that occurs between the terminal distributions of two adjacent arteries, such as the anterior cerebral and middle cerebral arteries. Because the terminal distributions are at the end of the pipeline, they are subject to low, marginally adequate arterial pressure under normal circumstances (Fig. 26-3). They are also the first to fail when systemic blood pressure drops further. If systemic hypotension occurs, there is failure to maintain adequate cerebral perfusion.

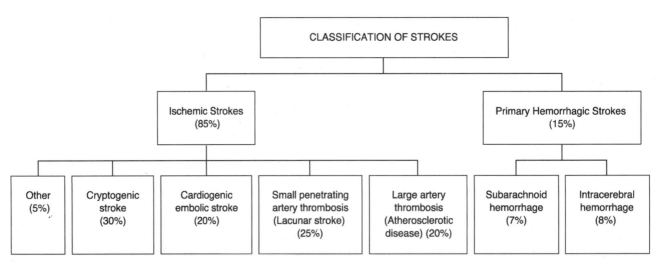

Figure 26-1 • Classification of stroke types.

Table 26–1 • COMPARISON OF SIGNS AND SYMPTOMS OF CAROTID AND VERTEBROBASILAR TRANSIENT ISCHEMIC ATTACKS

CAROTID TERRITORY	VERTEBROBASILAR TERRITORY
Related to Ophthalmic Artery	*Related to Posterior Cerebral Artery*
Amaurosis fugax (temporary monocular blindness)	Dysarthria
Transient graying, fogging, or blurred vision	Dysphagia
	Diplopia
A "shade" descending over line of vision	Bilateral blindness
	Unilateral or bilateral motor and sensory weakness
Related to Middle Cerebral Artery	Quadriparesis
Hemiparesis (more arm than leg weakness)	*Related to Cerebellar Arteries*
Hemianesthesia	Ataxia
Contralateral motor or sensory deficits to face or limbs	Vertigo
	Dizziness
Related to Anterior Cerebral Artery	
Hemiparesis (more leg than arm weakness)	

Atherosclerotic Cerebrovascular Disease Stroke

The large extracranial and intracranial arteries are subject to atherosclerosis with an associated atheroma that narrows the lumen of the vessel. The atheroma can also be the site for thrombus formation. Both conditions can lead to hypoperfusion, ischemia, and ischemic stroke. About 40% of patients have TIAs before a large-vessel ischemic stroke.

The patient typically awakens with neurological deficits or is sedentary when the symptoms occur. During sleep or at rest, blood pressure tends to be lowered, and there is less pressure to push the blood through the narrowed arterial lumen. Systemic hypoperfusion, decreased cerebral perfusion, ischemia, and ischemic stroke can develop. The area of cerebral ischemia depends on the vascular territory involved and the location within the vascular territory (proximal or distal) of the thrombus.

If a major artery is involved, large areas of both gray and white matter become ischemic, infarcted, and necrotic. Neuronal ischemia causes changes in the cell membrane, resulting in intracellular edema and compression of the capillaries, further compromising adequate blood supply. Cerebral edema peaks approximately 2 to 4 days after the stroke. Symptoms of ischemic stroke often develop in a step-wise progression relating to cerebral edema and infarction, reaching a peak in 1 to 3 days before stabilizing.

Small Penetrating Artery Stroke (Lacunar Stroke)

The term **lacuna** describes the small cavity remaining in the brain tissue that develops after the necrotic tissue of a small, deep infarct has been removed. A **lacunar stroke** is a type of ischemic stroke caused by microatheroma and thrombosis of a small penetrating artery, resulting in a small, softened area in the deep white matter structures of the brain. As the softened tissue sloughs away, a small cavity or lake remains, the lacuna (diameter of 0.5 mm or less). Occlusion occurs in the presence of lipohyalinosis, a condition characterized by pathological thickening of these small vessels, and leads to a specific clinical stroke syndrome. Hypertension is the principal risk factor for lacunar strokes. Lacunar strokes are seen predominately in the basal ganglia, especially the putamen, the thalamus, and the white matter of the internal capsule and pons; they occur occasionally in the white matter of the cerebral gyri. They are rare in the gray matter of the cerebral surface, in the corpus callosum, visual radiations, or medulla (Fig. 26-4). Most lacunae occur in the lenticulostriate branches of the anterior cerebral artery and middle cerebral artery, the thalamoperforant branches of the posterior cerebral arteries, and the paramedian branches of the basilar artery.[7]

There are distinct signs and symptoms associated with several recognized lacunar syndromes, including pure motor hemiplegia, pure sensory stroke, homolateral ataxia and leg paresis, dysarthria, clumsy hand syndrome, sensorimotor stroke, and basilar branch syndromes. Even though a lacunar stroke is small, it can cause considerable deficits if a critical area, such as the internal capsule, is involved. Patients may have several lacunae, as evidenced on CT or MR imaging, and have diffuse white matter changes associated with dementia.

Cardiogenic Embolic Stroke

About 20% of ischemic strokes result from cardiogenic embolism from atrial fibrillation (the most common), valvular disease, ventricular thrombi, myocardial infarction, congestive heart failure, patent foramen ovale (PFO), atrial septal aneurysm, and other cardiac problems. Atherosclerosis and atherogenic plaques of the proximal aorta are another source of cardiac emboli detectable with the use of transesophageal echocardiography. The atherogenic plaques commonly found in coronary vessels, in the heart, and at the bifurcation of the aorta are precursors for hypertension and atrial fibrillation. Unstable plaques can break off and become microemboli to the brain, causing stroke. Microemboli from the heart are mobilized and enter the cerebral system most often through the carotid arteries, flowing until the vessel is too narrow to allow further passage of the embolus and the vessel becomes occluded. The left middle cerebral artery is affected most often because it is a relatively straight vessel and provides the path of least resistance for the embolus. Cardiogenic strokes associated with PFO occur in approximately 20% to 25% of persons older than 30 years of age and usually occur when the patient is awake and active. The development of the ischemia is very rapid with maximal deficit present within minutes.

Cryptogenic Stroke

About 30% of ischemic strokes are cryptogenic in origin, which means that no cause of the stroke could be found after diagnostic evaluation.

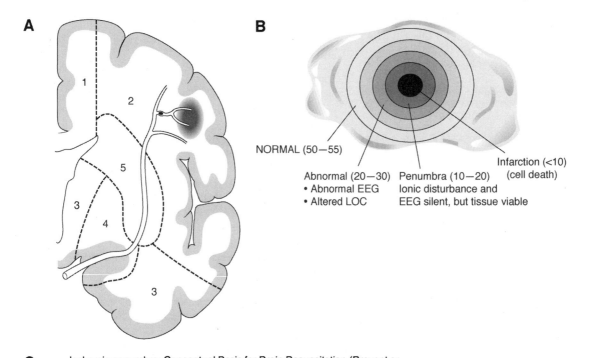

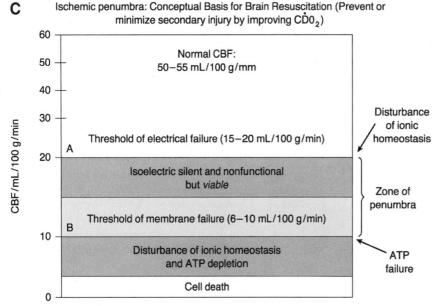

Figure 26–2 • (*A*) See distribution of middle cerebral artery and occlusion of a branch. Note area of infarction and surrounding penumbra with viable but nonfunctional cells. These cells will either become infarcted or recover, depending on treatment. (*B*) Ischemic penumbra: normal CBF = 50–55 mL/100 g/min. Variations in CBF are noted. Penumbra is the critical area that may be salvageable with appropriate treatment, or cell death will occur if adequate CBF is not restored. (EEG, electroencephalogram; LOC, level of consciousness; CBF, cerebral blood flow.) (*C*) Ischemic penumbra: conceptual basis for brain resuscitation.

Stroke From Other Causes

About 5% of ischemic stroke results from coagulopathies, arteritis, migraine/vasospasm, infection, and drug abuse, such as that of cocaine.

Hemorrhagic Stroke

Intracerebral hemorrhage (ICH), or ICH stroke, represents 15% of all strokes and involves primary rupture of a blood vessel. Although ICH represents a relatively small fraction of total strokes, it is a formidable disease, with a 30-day mortality rate twofold to sixfold higher than that for ischemic stroke. The mortality rate in the first 30 days after ICH is 35% to 50%, with more than half of these deaths occurring in the first 2 days and

6% of patients dying before they reach the hospital. The high mortality and morbidity associated with ICH are caused primarily by the blood mass itself and by the mechanical effects it creates.

Hemorrhagic stroke is divided into two categories based on the underlying mechanism. **Intracerebral stroke**, also called **intraparenchymal stroke**, is caused by bleeding into the brain tissue as a result of rupture of a small artery, most often a deep, penetrating vessel. **Subarachnoid hemorrhagic stroke** or simply **subarachnoid hemorrhage** (SAH) is the result of bleeding into the subarachnoid space, most often in relation to a ruptured aneurysm or arteriovenous malformation–in both cases, the result of hemorrhage. In this chapter, only intracerebral hemorrhagic stroke is discussed. Cerebral aneurysms and arteriovenous malformations were addressed in Chapters 24 and 25.

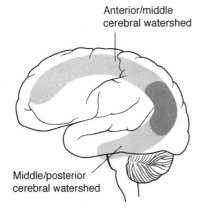

Anterior/middle
cerebral watershed

Middle/posterior
cerebral watershed

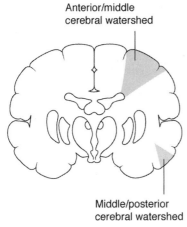

Anterior/middle
cerebral watershed

Middle/posterior
cerebral watershed

Figure 26–3 • Location of watershed.

Intracerebral Hemorrhagic Stroke

The cause of intracerebral hemorrhagic stroke is a spontaneous hemorrhage related to hypertension and cerebral amyloid angiopathy. The typical profile is that of an older person with a long history of poorly controlled hypertension. At the moment of hemorrhage, the person is active and usually has not experienced any warning signs. A typical situation is one of a patient straining at stool, and then developing a severe headache, decreased consciousness, hemiplegia, and possible focal seizures and vomiting. Subarachnoid hemorrhage is commonly seen in younger people. Hemorrhagic stroke occurs rapidly, with steady development of symptoms over a period of minutes to hours (1 to 24 hours). The most common sites of intracerebral hemorrhage, each of which has distinguishing signs and symptoms, are the following:

• Putamen (part of the basal ganglia) and adjacent internal capsule (50%)
• Thalamus (30%)
• Cerebellum (10%)
• Pons (10%)

Arterial Dissection

Arterial dissection is an unusual cause of stroke and accounts for 1% to 5% of all strokes, occurring commonly in younger persons (aged between 25 and 45 years), usually in the absence of atherosclerosis. Arterial dissection is typically caused by trauma to a vessel wall (as in the case of iatrogenic trauma associated with catheter passage during an angiographic procedure), vessel abnormality, migraine, and fibromuscular dysplasia. After injury to the vessel wall, hematoma forms in the medial layer and breaks through the intimal wall. Injury to the intimal wall allows blood to dissect through the medial layer, resulting in luminal narrowing; a pseudoaneurysm may result in some cases. The patient with an arterial dissection is at risk for ischemic stroke due to resulting thrombosis, embolization, or subarachnoid hemorrhage due to vessel rupture. The most common locations for dissection are the cervical carotid, intracranial carotid (usually in the middle cerebral or supraclinoid internal carotid artery), and the vertebral artery. Vertebral dissections are often associated with trauma.

The signs and symptoms of an arterial dissection may evolve over hours to days. The patient commonly experiences a severe unilateral headache, scalp throbbing, and/or neck pain. Other presenting signs and symptoms include transient monocular blindness, oculosympathetic paralysis, pulsatile tinnitus, TIAs, or stroke in evolution.

Emergency MRA or cerebral angiography is indicated if an arterial dissection is suspected. After the diagnosis has been established, cautious heparinization is initiated; other measures such as stenting, angioplasty, grafting, and bypass may be undertaken as appropriate. Chronic oral anticoagulation may be necessary in unresolved cases.

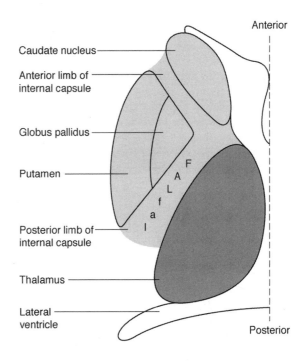

Caudate nucleus

Anterior limb of
internal capsule

Globus pallidus

Putamen

Posterior limb of
internal capsule

Thalamus

Lateral
ventricle

Anterior

Posterior

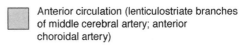
Anterior circulation (lenticulostriate branches
of middle cerebral artery; anterior
choroidal artery)

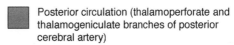
Posterior circulation (thalamoperforate and
thalamogeniculate branches of posterior
cerebral artery)

Figure 26–4 • Primary location of lacunar strokes.

ANATOMY, ATHEROGENESIS, AND PATHOPHYSIOLOGY RELATED TO STROKES

Anatomical Basis for and Correlations Related to Stroke

There are four major cerebral arteries that supply the brain: two internal carotid arteries (ICAs) that constitute the anterior circulation, and two vertebral arteries (VAs) that constitute the posterior circulation. The ICAs ascend from the common carotid bifurcation, enter the cranium at the petrous portion of the temporal bone between the layers of dura, and then begin to branch. The first major small branch is the ophthalmic artery, which supplies the eye. Temporary ischemia to this vessel results in transitory monocular blindness in one eye (also called *amaurosis fugax*). The major cerebral arteries arising from the ICAs are the middle cerebral artery (MCA), the anterior cerebral artery (ACA), the anterior communicating artery, and the posterior communicating arteries. The MCA supplies the lateral portion of the cerebral hemisphere (Fig. 26-5). The ACA supplies the frontal pole and medial surface of the frontal and parietal lobes (Fig. 26-6).

The two VAs enter the cranial vault through the foramen magnum. They then unite to form the basilar artery (Fig. 26-7). The basilar artery then divides to form the posterior cerebral artery (PCA), which supplies the medial and inferior surfaces and lateral portions of the temporal and occipital lobes (see Figs. 26-5 and 26-6). The basilar artery also gives off a number of cerebellar and brain-stem arteries. The circle of Willis, at the base of the skull, joins the anterior and posterior circulation. Collateral circulation for an occluded vessel is possible owing to anastomosis between the vessels. However, anomalies of cerebral vessels are common, so it is difficult to predict if a patient will receive collateral circulation to an occluded area. Chapter 5 provides further details regarding cerebral circulation.

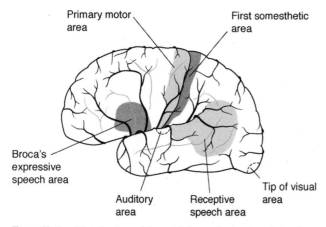

Figure 26–5 • Distribution of the middle cerebral artery (lateral surface of the brain).

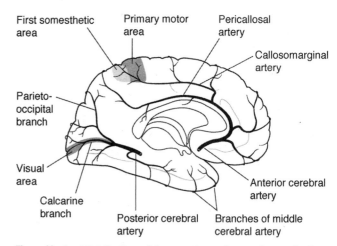

Figure 26–6 • Distribution of the anterior and posterior cerebral arteries on the medial surface of the cerebral hemisphere.

Atherogenesis and Ischemic Stroke

Atherogenesis is the pathological process of the development of atherosclerosis. Stroke due to atherosclerosis remains the most common neurological disorder among adults in the U.S. There are two dominant theories of atherogenesis: reaction to injury and the lipid hypotheses. Regardless of the specific mechanism of injury, the arterial wall undergoes a series of morphological changes that result in structural alteration and pathogenesis.

Pathogenesis in Larger Arteries

The earliest lesions of atherosclerosis are seen as yellowish, fatty streaks of the intimal surface of large to medium arteries, which are widely distributed throughout the arterial vasculature and may be seen as early as late childhood or early adolescence. On microscopic examination, the fatty streaks consist of lipid-laden macrophages known as foam cells (some foam cells are smooth muscle cells and some come from circulating monocytes) and extracellular lipid.

Over the course of years the fatty streaks progress, and by middle to old age, fibrosis plaques (atheromas) begin to develop in more localized sites than fatty streaks, typically occurring at arterial branches or opposite arterial bifurcation of extracranial vessels. The maturated fibrous plaque consists of an intact endothelial lining overlaying a fibrous cap (containing foam cells, transformed smooth muscle cells, lymphocytes, a connective tissue matrix, and a central necrotic core of cellular debris, free extracellular lipid, and cholesterol crystals) extruding from the intima and producing varying degrees of alterations in blood flow. As plaques advance, there may be central necrosis and associated changes such as fibrosis, intraplaque hemorrhage, ulceration, and mineralization. Platelet adhesion and aggregation may occur at this later stage, increasing the plaque size. Fibrin and fibrinogen may also be incorporated into the plaque. Small arterioles, commonly observed at the plaque periphery, may be the genesis of possible hemorrhagic transformation in some fibrous plaques that contain hemosiderin, areas of intraplaque calcification, and disruption of the endothelial lining. The plaque destabilization and

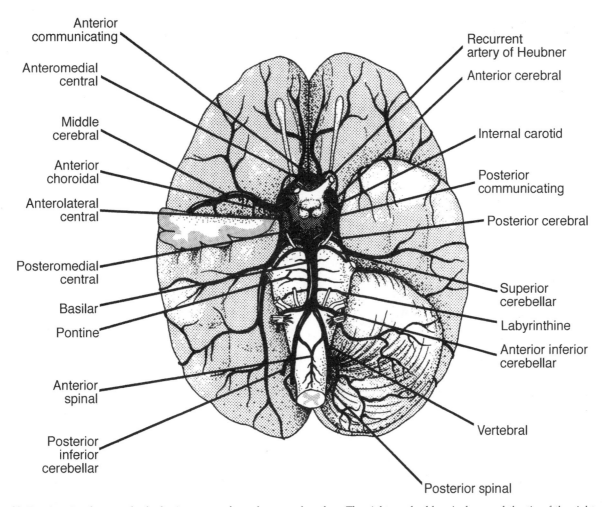

Figure 26-7 • Arteries that supply the brain, as seen from the ventral surface. The right cerebral hemisphere and the tip of the right temporal lobe have been removed.

luminal thrombi result in endothelial injury and clinical symptoms.[3,4]

Plaque enlargement occurs slowly over decades, and the person is asymptomatic until the plaque intrudes on a substantial percentage of the arterial lumen diameter. Typically, luminal thrombi are associated with luminal surface disruption or ulceration of the endothelial lining, leading to arterial obstruction. Blood within the plaque or intraplaque hemorrhage appears to be secondary to the luminal disruption, with dissection of luminal blood into the plaque.

Pathogenesis in Smaller Arteries

The underlying pathological process for smaller penetrating arteries, such as the lenticulostriate arteries, basilar penetrating arteries, and medullary arteries that supply deep cerebral white matter, is probably different than for atherosclerosis found in the larger arteries. The underlying pathological changes in the small penetrating arteries are attributable to a process called **lipohyalinosis**, in which a hyaline-lipid material coats the small penetrating arteries, which causes thickening of the walls. Eventually, the vessel thromboses create a lacunar stroke.

Pathophysiology of Ischemic Stroke

The pathophysiology of ischemic stroke due to atheromas, thrombi, or emboli is the same. The lumen of the blood vessel becomes narrowed or occluded, resulting in ischemia in that vascular territory (Fig. 26-8). As shown mainly in animal models, occlusion seldom completely abolishes the delivery of oxygen and glucose to the affected vascular territory because blood flow to the affected vascular territory is usually partly maintained by dense vascular collaterals.

Cerebral Blood Flow and Metabolism

Normally, the rate of blood flow to the entire brain is relatively constant, and it does not change in response to alterations in mean systemic blood pressure over a range of 50 to 150 mm Hg. This phenomenon, known as *autoregulation*, protects the brain from the effects of hypotension and from cerebrovascular hemorrhage caused by excessive intravascular pressure. The severity of neuronal injury in ischemic brain tissue is proportional to the reduction of cerebral blood flow (Table 26-2). In the center of an infarct, blood flow is greatly reduced or absent, whereas at its margin, maximum

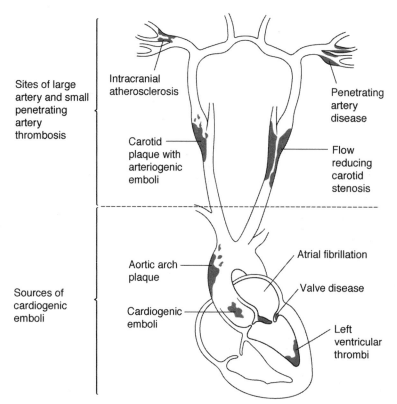

Figure 26-8 • Major sites and sources related to ischemic stroke.

vasodilation results from the lactic acid formed during anaerobic glycolysis. When CO_2 is inhaled or a cerebral vasodilator is administered to patients with focal infarction, only the vessels in normal areas of the brain dilate, resulting in an intracerebral steal of blood away from the infracted zone. This same phenomenon can result if hypertension is treated too aggressively during an acute infarct. Judicious use of antihypertensive agents is critical during an acute infarct.

Time Course of Cerebral Infarction

Animal data so far provide the information for the current understanding of the pathogenesis of brain damage. After 5 minutes to 1 hour of severe focal ischemia—that is, ischemia that causes persistent loss of membrane potentials in the gerbil—persistent loss of neuronal membrane potentials results in the death of some or all of the selectively vul-

 Table 26-2 • THRESHOLDS OF CEREBRAL ISCHEMIA

Normal range	40–50 mL/100 g/min
Oligemia	30–40 mL/100 g/min
Mild ischemia	30–30 mL/100 g/min
	Electrical function is affected
Moderate ischemia (penumbra)	10–120 mL/100 g/min
	Reversible cellular damage
Severe ischemia (lesion core)	0–10 mL/100 g/min
	Irreversible cellular damage

Hock, N.H. (1999). Brain attack. The stroke continuum. *Nursing Clinics of North America, 34*(3), 697.

nerable cells in the affected vascular bed. After approximately 1 hour, infarction begins and its volume enlarges progressively.[10]

The time required for progression toward the maximum volume of infarction differs in different species. In nonhuman primates with reversible cerebral artery occlusion, clinical improvement and limited infarct size are observed when occlusion lasts 3 hours or less. When occlusions persist between 2 to 3 and 6 to 7 hours, neurological deficits are more pronounced and produced in a higher percentage of animals. If complete cerebral artery occlusion persists for longer than 4 to 6 hours, animal studies suggest that rescue of neuronal tissue may not be possible. The time to maximum volume of infarction in nonhuman primates may be 6 to 8 hours. Such a time has not been determined in humans. Cerebral blood flow and metabolic studies and autopsy in humans supplant data from animal studies and have provided the basis for determining the treatment window in acute stroke clinical trials and the current thinking on emergent stroke interventions.

Ischemia can cause primary cellular injuries resulting from no blood flow and from secondary cellular injury due to the effects of biochemical and molecular cascades precipitated by ischemia. Ischemia severe enough to kill cerebral cells is called **cerebral infarction**. Consider the injured cerebral area that occurs with ischemic stroke. A core of necrotic tissue often exists from a lack of oxygen and nutrients. In the core zone, which is an area of severe ischemia (blood flow below 10% to 25%), the loss in adequate supply of oxygen and glucose results in rapid depletion of energy stores. However, around the necrotic core is another circumscribed area called the *ischemic penumbra* (see Fig. 26-2). Although the neuronal cells of the penumbra are unable to function, they remain viable. This is because the penumbral zone is supplied with blood by collateral arteries anastomosing with branches of the occluded vessel. However, even cells in this region die if reperfusion is not established during the early hours because collateral circulation is inadequate to maintain neuronal demand for oxygen and glucose indefinitely.[11] The penumbra is where pharmacological interventions are likely to be most valuable. Neuroprotective agents, including the use of mild-to-moderate brain cooling, are being tested in clinical trials to assess their safety and efficacy in protecting the cells from the secondary injury associated with ischemia.

The blood supply to the brain can be compromised due to the so-called no-flow phenomenon (e.g., following cardiac arrest resulting in global ischemia) or a low-flow phenomenon (e.g., following stroke resulting in focal ischemia). Low-perfusion states can result in more tissue damage than no-perfusion states because the presence of glucose in an inadequately oxygenated area enhances lactate production.[12] Brain tissue lactate causes severe tissue necrosis and extracellular acidosis that results in infarction. In addition, low-flow states also provide a continued supply of both water, which exacerbates edema, and activated white blood cells, platelets, and coagulation factors, which contribute to tissue damage by further impeding the microcirculation.

Secondary cellular injury associated with ischemia occurs in response to deprivation of oxygen and cessation of oxidative metabolism. Complex biochemical and molecular cascades result in ischemic damage to neurons. From 2 and 5 minutes of complete oxygen deprivation is the general benchmark for irreversible neuronal damage. However, extreme hypothermia can significantly increase the viability time, and hypothermia has been used therapeutically to save neurons. Without oxygen, adenosine triphosphate (ATP) energy-dependent cell functions (e.g., the cellular respiratory chain, lipid metabolism, and maintenance of the transmembrane ion channels) rapidly cease. Impairment of the respiratory chain results in anaerobic glycolysis of remaining available glucose. Anaerobic glycolysis proceeds only to pyruvate, which reduces to lactate. Lactic acid and free fatty acid accumulation causes intracellular acidosis, further inhibiting mitochondrial function.

Concurrently, other cell destruction processes occur that include *excitotoxicity, increased intracellular calcium,* and *generation of free radicals.* Hypoxia impairs the reuptake of the excitatory neurotransmitter glutamate at the presynaptic membrane. The excessive extracellular glutamate opens sodium, chloride, and calcium channels, resulting in an influx of sodium and chloride ions with water into the cell, causing acute cellular swelling; the voltage-dependent calcium channels allow influx of calcium into the cytosol and efflux of potassium. (Intracellular calcium is normally maintained at a low level by active transport mechanisms.) The high intracellular calcium activates calcium-dependent degradative enzymes (proteases, phospholipases, and endonucleases) that attack the cell membranes and DNA and further inhibit mitochondrial function. Oxygen free radicals with resultant lipid peroxidation occur in inadequately perfused areas and during reperfusion of previously ischemic areas. Oxygen free radicals, superoxide peroxide, and hydroxyl ions destroy fatty acids and disrupt calcium homeostasis, further contributing to cellular demise. Approximately 8 to 12 hours

after the insult, the neuron becomes smaller and more angular. The cytoplasm and nucleus shrink, followed by complete dissolution of the cell and cell death.[13]

The ischemic cascade and cellular changes that follow oxygen deprivation are outlined earlier in this chapter.

Reperfusion Injury in Stroke

During ischemia, hypoxic cell injury and death occur distal to the occluded vessel. The injured and dying cells produce pro-inflammatory mediators that cause inflammation in the area around the infarction. As inflammation subsides, scar tissue develops in the infarcted region. Neurons that have died are replaced by fibrogliotic scar tissue, and neurological function is lost.

Another type of injury to neurons results from reperfusion to previously ischemic areas. The cellular injury due to activated oxygen free radicals that occurs after the blood supply to the ischemic area has been restored is called **reperfusion injury**. Although reperfusion has been shown to be beneficial in experimental systems, evidence suggests that the process of reperfusion may also injure the ischemic brain.[14] This injury involves acute inflammation in the ischemic tissue. During periods of ischemia, endothelial cells secrete many pro-inflammatory cytokines that attract and activate leukocytes. When reperfusion occurs, neutrophils migrate through the vessel wall into the ischemic brain tissue, potentially releasing various toxic substances, such as oxygen free radicals and proteinases, that may further injure the compromised but viable tissue. Oxygen free radicals, which are partially reduced oxygen molecules that are highly reactive with other molecules, are implicated in post-ischemic membrane injury. The buildup of adenosine diphosphate (ADP) and pyruvate during ischemia results in rapid production of electrons when the oxygen supply is reestablished. The oxygen free radicals are formed when the electrons are transferred to oxygen. They allegedly injure the cell membrane by stealing hydrogen molecules and by forming abnormal molecular bonds.[15] As a result of reperfusion injury, additional injury to neuronal cells is incurred.

Although reperfusion is best exemplified by the use of thrombolytic therapy, it is also likely to be relevant even without pharmacological thrombolysis. Advanced imaging studies have demonstrated increased uptake in the brain following a stroke and correlate with neurological outcome.[16] Presumably, circulating leukocytes reach the infarcted area as a result of either spontaneous reperfusion or collateral circulation. It is important to note that when pharmacological thrombolytic therapy is used, the patient may manifest new or identical stroke symptoms after a successful recanalization. It is therefore critical to observe the patient for reperfusion injury following thrombolytic therapy. Another example of perfusion injury is the natural break-up of an embolic thrombus and the onset of expanded deficits.

Pathophysiology of Hemorrhagic Stroke

The pathophysiology of hemorrhagic stroke is associated with an immediate rise in intracranial pressure (ICP), ischemic cellular responses, cerebral edema, compromised cerebral perfusion pressure, and possible herniation. With ICH, the usual hemorrhage sites are small, deep cortical arteries or subarachnoid hemorrhage due to aneurysmal rupture (see Chap. 24). At the time of ICH, blood is forced into the surrounding cerebral parenchyma, creating a hematoma. The pathology is a dynamic one that continues to evolve over the first few days after onset. In 20% to 30% of cases, clot volume increases over the first 24 hours. The hematoma displaces and compresses the adjacent cerebral tissue and ischemic cellular responses and cerebral edema occur, resulting in increased ICP. The final outcome of ICH could also include potential neurotoxicity from the blood degradation products and associated neuronal ischemia. A major ICH can cause midline displacement and herniation syndromes and has a high mortality rate of about 50%.

Hemorrhagic Conversion of an Ischemic Stroke

An embolus that represents all or part of a thrombus has a spontaneous tendency to lysis and dispersion; thrombotic occlusions may also lyse spontaneously. In hemorrhagic infarction, or *hemorrhagic conversion* or *transformation*, varying amounts of red blood cells are found among the necrotic tissues, with hemorrhagic foci ranging from a few scattered petechiae to petechial hemorrhages that merge to form a significant hemorrhagic mass.[17] The timing of hemorrhagic infarction varies from a few hours to as late as 2 weeks or longer after an arterial occlusion. Surges of arterial hypertension or rapid rise of blood pressure might explain hemorrhagic infarction in many cases. Marked hyperglycemia has also been implicated in some cases.[18] Examination of biochemical changes that correlate with hemorrhage into infarcts suggested that marked tissue energy depletion accompanied by acidosis damages brain vessels and renders them penetrable by edema fluid and, ultimately, red blood cell extravasation.

▌▌▌ SIGNS AND SYMPTOMS OF STROKE SYNDROMES ACCORDING TO THE INVOLVED VESSEL

The presenting signs and symptoms of stroke depend on the extent and location of the insult. When a cerebral artery is occluded by a thrombus or embolus, classical syndromes are said to develop. The clinical features of stroke are commonly classified as carotid artery (anterior circulation) syndromes and vertebrobasilar (posterior circulation) syndromes. In reality, syndromes frequently overlap one another rather than appearing in their pure form.

Carotid Region

ICA Syndrome

Symptoms of the typical ICA syndrome include the following:

- Paralysis of the contralateral face, arm, and leg
- Sensory deficits of the contralateral face, arm, and leg

- Aphasia, if the dominant hemisphere is involved
- Apraxia, agnosia, and unilateral neglect, if the nondominant hemisphere is involved
- Homonymous hemianopsia

MCA Syndrome

Middle cerebral syndrome is by far the most common of all cerebral occlusions. If the main stem of the MCA is occluded, a massive infarction of most of the hemisphere results. Initially, there may be vomiting and a rapid onset of coma, which may last a few weeks. Cerebral edema is extensive.

Symptoms of MCA syndrome include:

- Hemiplegia (involving the face and arm on the contralateral side; the leg is spared or has less deficits than the arm)
- Sensory deficits (same area as hemiplegia)
- Aphasia (global aphasia if the dominant hemisphere is involved)
- Homonymous hemianopsia

ACA Syndrome

The ACA is least often occluded. If the occlusion occurs proximal to a patent anterior communicating artery, the blood supply may be compromised. If the occlusion is distal or if the communicating artery is inadequate, there will be infarction of the medial aspect of one frontal lobe. Bilateral medial frontal lobe infarction occurs if one ACA is occluded and the other artery is small and dependent on blood flow.

Symptoms of ACA syndrome (note that aphasia and hemianopsia are not part of the syndrome) include:

- Paralysis of the contralateral foot and leg (foot drop is a consistent finding)
- Impaired gait
- Sensory loss over the toes, foot, and leg
- Abulia (slowness and prolonged delays to perform acts voluntarily or to respond)
- Flat affect, lack of spontaneity, slowness, distractibility, and lack of interest in surroundings
- Cognitive impairment, such as perseveration and amnesia
- Urinary incontinence

Vertebrobasilar Region

Occlusion of the vessels within the vertebrobasilar system produces unique syndromes. The vertebral and basilar arteries and their branches supply the brain stem and cerebellum. The posterior cerebral arteries are the terminal branches of the basilar artery and supply the medial temporal and occipital lobes, as well as part of the corpus callosum.

VA Syndrome

The following signs and symptoms are characteristic of VA occlusion:

- Wallenberg's syndrome (lateral medullary syndrome)
- Dizziness
- Nystagmus

- Dysphagia and dysarthria
- Pain in face, nose, or eye
- Ipsilateral numbness and weakness of face
- Staggering gait and ataxia
- Clumsiness

Basilar Artery Syndrome

The following signs and symptoms are characteristic of basilar artery occlusion:

- Quadriplegia
- Possibly the "locked-in" syndrome
- Weakness of facial, lingual, and pharyngeal muscles

Anterior Inferior Cerebellar Artery Syndrome

Occlusion of the anterior inferior cerebellar artery is also known as the lateral inferior pontine syndrome. Symptoms of the anterior inferior cerebellar artery syndrome include vertigo, nausea, vomiting, tinnitus, and nystagmus.

IPSILATERAL SIDE
- Paresis of lateral conjugate gaze
- Horner's syndrome
- Cerebellar signs (ataxia, nystagmus)

CONTRALATERAL SIDE
- Impaired pain and temperature sensation in trunk and limbs (may also involve face)

Posterior Inferior Cerebellar Artery Syndrome (Wallenberg's Syndrome)

Posterior inferior cerebellar artery syndrome involves the lateral portion of the medulla as a result of the occlusion of the posterior inferior cerebellar artery.
  Symptoms include:

- Nausea and vomiting
- Dysphagia and dysarthria
- Horizontal nystagmus
- Ipsilateral Horner's syndrome
- Cerebellar signs (ataxia and vertigo)
- Loss of pain and temperature sensation on contralateral side of trunk and limbs

PCA Syndrome

Few strokes involve the PCA. The usual consequence of the superficial occlusion (peripheral areas) of a PCA is contralateral homonymous hemianopsia. If the penetrating branches (central areas) are occluded, the cerebral peduncle, thalamus, and upper brain stem are involved. There is wide variation in the manifestations of the syndrome.
  Symptoms of PCA syndrome include:

PERIPHERAL AREA
- Homonymous hemianopsia
- Memory deficits
- Perseveration

- Several visual deficits (cortical blindness, lack of depth perception, failure to see objects not centrally located, visual hallucinations)

CENTRAL AREA
- If the thalamus is involved, sensory loss of all modalities, spontaneous pain, intentional tremors, and mild hemiparesis
- If the cerebral peduncle is involved, Weber's syndrome (oculomotor nerve palsy with contralateral hemiplegia)
- If the brain stem is involved, deficits involving conjugate gaze, nystagmus, and pupillary abnormalities, with other possible symptoms of ataxia and postural tremors

Deep Cortical Syndromes

Four syndromes are associated with intracerebral hemorrhagic stroke. In addition to an altered level of consciousness (confusion to coma), headache, nausea, vomiting, nuchal rigidity, hypertension, and bradycardia related to increased ICP, each syndrome has its own distinguishing characteristics.

Putamen Hemorrhage (Often Involves the Internal Capsule)

- Contralateral hemiplegia
- Contralateral hemisensory deficits
- Hemianopsia
- Slurred speech

Thalamic Hemorrhage

- Contralateral hemiplegia
- Contralateral hemisensory deficits
- Deficits of vertical and lateral gaze

Pontine Hemorrhage

- "Locked-in" syndrome
- Deficits in lateral eye movement

Cerebellar Hemorrhage

- Occipital headache
- Dizziness
- Ataxia
- Vertigo

General Comparison of Left-Sided and Right-Sided Stroke

Some generalizations can be made about the deficits incurred with left-sided and right-sided stroke (Table 26-3).

Table 26–3 • COMPARISON OF SIGNS AND SYMPTOMS ASSOCIATED WITH RIGHT-SIDED AND LEFT-SIDED HEMIPLEGIA

STROKE SYNDROME ON LEFT SIDE OF BRAIN (RIGHT-SIDED HEMIPLEGIA)	STROKE SYNDROME ON RIGHT SIDE OF BRAIN (LEFT-SIDED HEMIPLEGIA)
• Expressive aphasia or • Receptive aphasia or • Global aphasia • Intellectual impairment • Slow and cautious behavior • Defects in right visual fields	• Spatial-perceptual deficits • Denial and the deficits of the affected side require special safety considerations • Tendency for distractibility • Impulsive behavior; apparently unaware of deficits • Poor judgment • Defects in left visual fields

Summary of Deficits Incurred With Stroke Syndrome

A stroke syndrome is a form of cerebral injury. The injury to the brain results from a ruptured blood vessel, in the case of hemorrhagic stroke, or from ischemia that develops over time or suddenly, as may be the case in thrombotic or embolic strokes. In all cases of stroke syndrome, areas of the brain are deprived of an adequate oxygen supply. If the blood supply is cut off for an extended period, the involved cerebral tissue may become necrotic, resulting in permanent neurological deficits. In instances of ischemia, temporary neurological impairment may result. Similar hemodynamic changes occur with other forms of cerebral injury, such as brain injuries, cerebral aneurysms, or cerebral edema.

The particular type and degree of neurological deficits depend on the particular area of the brain involved. Because the brain is composed of the most highly specialized tissue in the body, the deficits incurred depend on the area compromised. The rehabilitation and management of these deficits are discussed in Chapter 13.

Diagnosis of Stroke

Hyperacute Diagnosis of Stroke

To determine and provide the most judicious therapy for stroke, an accurate hyperacute diagnosis must be made. Only recently has it become possible to save brain tissue by acting quickly in treating stroke. Prompt action is also necessary to prevent recurrence, because most recurrences take place within hours to days of a first stroke. Evidence-based practice supports the fact that patients admitted to stroke units have been shown to have better outcomes than those patients admitted to general units.[19]

A patient seen with a possible TIA or stroke must be carefully evaluated. A complete medical history and comprehensive physical and neurological examination begin the compiling of the database. In addition to the neurological examination, a neurovascular examination that includes the following components is necessary:[20]

• Blood pressure measurement in both arms and in the reclining and standing positions; especially important when vertebrobasilar ischemia is suspected. Care must be taken when checking standing blood pressures to prevent sudden postural hypotension.
• Cardiac auscultation and rhythm check
• Auscultation of the head and neck for bruit
• Palpation of the neck and facial pulses; palpation of superficial temporal arteries for tenderness and edema
• Funduscopic examination for platelet or fibrin, cholesterol, or calcific emboli

A thorough cardiac examination, including a search for a carotid bruit (a marker of generalized atherosclerosis and a source of atherogenic microemboli), is important because of the possibility of cardiogenic emboli. Many patients who have significant extracranial occlusive ideas will not have a bruit. In patients with cervical bruits, about 50% have significant carotid stenosis. About 70% of people who have bruits located near the jaw angle, especially when these bruits extend into diastole, have carotid stenosis. Ocular bruit may signify high-grade carotid stenosis or a vascular anomaly.[20]

The onset of neurological deficits is not necessarily a sign or symptom of TIAs or stroke, so a detailed history about the onset, signs, and symptoms, frequency, progression, and other characteristics is important. Although the clinical presentation of TIA/stroke is heterogeneous, the symptoms are dictated by three key variables: affected vascular territory, duration and severity of ischemia, and underlying mechanism of cerebral hypoperfusion.[21] A review of the history and physical examination is helpful in identifying risk factors for stroke (Table 26-4). A comparison of signs and symptoms related to carotid and vertebrobasilar TIAs is found in Table 26-1. An understanding of the vascular territories and related functional levels is critical in helping the care provider relate presenting symptoms to vascular territories.

In the diagnosis of acute stroke, risk factor analysis and clinical assessment are useful but cannot substitute with certainty for diagnostic brain imaging techniques. Numerous imaging tools are now available for the assessment of stroke patients, and each has unique advantages and disadvantages in the clinical setting. Table 26-5 describes the commonly required diagnostic procedures and laboratory tests used to diagnose a stroke.

Table 26–4 • MAJOR RISK FACTORS FOR STROKE

• Hypertension • Atrial fibrillation • Hyperlipidemia • Diabetes mellitus • Stress • Excessive alcohol consumption	• Clinical symptoms of coronary heart disease (CHD) • EKG or radiographic evidence of CHD • Sedentary lifestyle • Smoking • Obesity • Valvular disease (e.g., mitral valve)

▌▌▌ **Table 26–5** • STROKE AND TIAs: DIAGNOSTICS*

CT scan without contrast	Important immediate diagnostic to differentiate between ischemic and hemorrhagic stroke; if hemorrhagic, antiplatelets or anticoagulants are not given because of the increased risk of more bleeding; important for treatment decisions
CT scan with contrast	Useful to rule out lesions that many mimic a TIA, especially when symptoms are related to hemispheric deficits; hypodense areas on CT scan suggest infarction
Magnetic resonance imaging (MRI)	Offers excellent soft tissue contrast discrimination with superior demarcation of mass lesion from surrounding structures including areas of ischemia and infarction; good visualization of vascular structures when questioning a vascular lesion; useful for diagnosis of stroke in first 72 hours; a diffusion-weighted MRI can show ischemia in first few hours
Magnetic resonance angiography (MRA)	Less available and higher cost; noninvasive imaging of the carotid, vertebral, basilar, and major intracranial and extracranial arteries to determine occlusion; useful for clot visualization
Carotid ultrasonography	Noninvasive imaging; widely used initial diagnostic in patients with carotid territory symptoms for whom CEA is considered; cervical carotid artery imaging often required to exclude high-grade stenosis, which is an exclusion for CEA; less sensitive in assessing mild-to-moderate stenosis
Transcranial Doppler (TCD)	TCDs are now part of standard work-up for stroke, especially when CEA is considered; useful to detect severe intracranial stenosis, evaluate the carotid and vertebrobasilar vessels, assess patterns and extent of collateral circulation in patients with known arterial stenosis or occlusion, and detection of microemboli[†]
Blood flow studies	PET, SPECT, and Xenox CT are used to determine global and focal blood flow; used mostly for clinical research
Cerebral angiography	Ordered for patients considered candidates for CEA to define precisely the percentage of occlusion and in patients with unusual presentation with aneurysm, vasculitis, high-grade stenosis
Transthoracic echocardiography (TTE)	Helpful in search for cardioemboli sources; TTE is particularly helpful for diagnosing of left ventricular thrombi, left atrial myxomas, and thrombi that protrude into the atrial cavity; they are less reliable for small tumors, laminated thrombi, and thrombi limited to the left or right atrium[‡]
Transesophageal echocardiography (TEE)	Benefit of TEE is in greater sensitivity for source of cardioemboli (except ventricular disease); TEE provides better visualization of cardiac structures, especially those at greater depth from chest wall and lesions of the atria (atrial appendage thrombi associated with atrial fibrillation), interarterial septum defects (patent foramen ovale, atrial septal defects), mitral valvular vegetation, and atherosclerotic disease of ascending aortic arch[‡]
Electrocardiogram (EKG)	Useful when cardiogenic embolic stroke or concurrent coronary artery disease is suspected
Ambulatory EKG monitoring	Reserved for patients who have suspicious palpitations, arrhythmias, or enlarged left atrium
Prothrombotic states	Protein C, protein S, antithrombin III, thrombin time, hemoglobin, electrophoresis, anticardiolipin antibody, lupus anticoagulant, and syphilis serology

CT, computed tomography; CEA, carotidendarterectomy; PET, positron emission tomography; SPECT, single photon emission computed tomography.

* Feinberg, W. M., Albers, G. W., Barnett, H. J. M., Biller, J., Caplan, L. R., Carter, L. P., Hart, R. G., Hobson, R. W., Kronmal, R. A., Moore, W. S., & Robertson, J. T. (1994). Guidelines for the management of transient ischemic attacks. *Stroke, 25*(6), 1320–1335.

† Tong, D. C., Bolger, A., & Albers, G. W. (1994). *Stroke, 25*, 2138–2141.

‡ Reeder, G. S., Khandheria, B. K., Seward, J. B., & Tajik, A. J. (1991). Transesophageal echocardiography and cardiac masses. *Mayo Clinic Proceedings, 66*:(11) 1101–1109.

Transient Ischemic Attacks

If a person is having TIAs, by definition, the signs and symptoms clear completely in less than 24 hours. The TIAs should be understood to be forewarnings of possible stroke. The focus of care includes diagnosis of TIAs versus other problems; prevention of stroke by modification of risk factors; treatment with antiplatelet drugs or surgical intervention if indicated; ongoing monitoring for change in risk factors or condition; and patient education.

The person needs to be aggressively worked up and treated *before* a stroke occurs. Diagnostic evaluation proceeds in a stepwise progression. Initially, the following tests are generally ordered: complete blood cell count, platelets, electrolytes, blood urea nitrogen, creatinine, glucose, fasting lipid panel (total cholesterol, low-density lipoproteins, high-density lipoproteins), prothrombin time, activated partial thromboplastin time, and sedimentation rate. Other studies include an electrocardiogram (EKG), a CT scan (particularly in hemispheric TIAs), noninvasive computed imaging, and transcranial Doppler (TCD). Further investigation to resolve persistent diagnostic uncertainty may include transthoracic echocardiography (TTE), transesophageal echocardiography (TEE), TCDs if not already completed, MRI, MR angiography (MRA), cerebral arteriography, and antiphospholipids. Recent studies show that the use of MR with DWI and PWI allows rapid definition of areas of perfusion defects and localizes regions of ischemic injury within minutes after onset of ischemia. Information obtained from DWI and PWI will be instrumental in further identifying and predicting stroke onset more objectively, and help guide the treatment window for acute stroke interventions. When continuing to pursue cardiogenic source (for silent myocardial ischemia), an ambulatory EKG, an exercise EKG, or a thallium perfusion may be ordered. Other tests for prothrombotic states are listed in Table 26-5, which also includes a description of all diagnostic procedures.

Stroke

In the patient who has neurological deficits consistent with a stroke, several diagnostics are helpful in determining the type of stroke, which then determines treatment options (see Table 26-5). The most important initial diagnostic is an emergency CT scan without contrast medium to differentiate ischemic and hemorrhagic stroke. Early treatment for ischemic stroke includes thrombolytic therapy and anticoagulation, both of which are contraindicated if hemorrhagic stroke is present. Therefore, differentiating ischemic and hemorrhagic stroke is critical to treatment decisions.

After a patient has been stabilized from acute stroke, further diagnostic investigation may follow to determine primary problems related to the stroke (e.g., cardiac disease, carotid or vertebrobasilar occlusion), which will need to be addressed to prevent future strokes.

TREATMENT OF TRANSIENT ISCHEMIC ATTACKS AND ISCHEMIC STROKE

In the next section, management of stroke is discussed according to stroke preventive therapy, including medical management and treatment, cerebral revascularization, and endovascular treatment; hypervolemic hemodilution therapy; reperfusion therapy; neuroprotective agents; and rehabilitation.

Paradigm Shift to Prevention

The overall approach to patients with risk factors for stroke–TIAs, stroke, and poststroke–is toward prevention of a first stroke or, in the person who has already had a stroke, prevention of another stroke. Prevention is geared toward identification of all risk factors; modification of modifiable risk factors; drug therapy; surgical interventions, when appropriate; and education of the patient and family. Education is directed at helping the person understand his or her risk factors and the need to make a commitment to lifestyle changes and adherence to treatment plans to prevent stroke. Mass general education directed at educating all people to understand a "brain attack" as a medical emergency that warrants immediate emergency department care must be undertaken. The general public understands that a heart attack is a medical emergency that requires a call to 911 for emergency help to save lives and heart muscle. People need to apply the same sense of urgency to a brain attack. Educating the public about the signs and symptoms of a brain attack and the definitive action to be taken is very cost effective and can save human potential and quality of life.

Medical Management and Treatment

Risk factor management and antiplatelet and antithrombotic therapy are the mainstays of medical management. Guidelines for antithrombotic therapy, which have been outlined by expert consensus based on clinical research, include the recommendations included in Table 26-6.[4] Risk factor management guidelines, taken from the same expert consensus, are also outlined in Table 26-7.

The mainstay of drug therapy is the use of either an antiplatelet or anticoagulant agent. Antiplatelet agents deter the adherence of platelets to the wall of an injured blood vessel or to other platelets. Current antiplatelet drugs include aspirin, ticlopidine, clopidogrel, and extended-release dipyridamole and aspirin combined in a single formulation. Combination of one or two drugs is not uncommon, but this increases the risk of adverse drug responses such as bleeding.

Intravenous anticoagulation therapy with intravenous heparin is used to decrease further development of thrombi

Table 26–6 • USE OF ANTITHROMBOTIC AGENTS IN PATIENTS WITH TIAs

EVENT	RECOMMENDED THERAPY	THERAPEUTIC OPTIONS	COMMENT
TIAs or minor ischemic stroke	ASA 50–325 mg/d	ER-DP 200 mg + 25 mg, bid (single formulation) Clopidogrel 75 mg/d Ticlopidine 250 mg, bid ASA 50–1300 mg/d	Monitor for diarrhea, rash; CBC q/2/wk for 3 months for neutropenia if on ticlopidine; GI upset and headaches are common with ER-DP
TIA (atherothrombotic) and aspirin intolerant or if TIA occurs during ASA therapy	ER-DP 200 mg + ASA 25 mg bid (single formulation) Clopidogrel 75 mg/d	Ticlopidine 250 mg bid Warfarin (INR 2–3) ASA 50–1300 mg/d	If on warfarin schedule, regular INR levels to monitor and adjust dose. Watch for excessive bleeding if INR exceeds therapeutic range; patient at risk for thromboembolic event if INR falls below therapeutic range. Long-term oral anticoagulation with warfarin recommended for patients with atrial fibrillation who have a TIA (INR 2–3)
TIA (cardioembolic)	Warfarin target INR 2.5 (range, 2–3)	ASA 50–325 mg/d (if contraindications to warfarin)	

ASA, (acetylsalicylic acid, aspirin); ER-DP, extended release-dipyridamole; CBC, complete blood count; INR, international normalized ratio.

▌▌▌▌ **T a b l e 2 6 – 7** • RECOMMENDATIONS FOR RISK FACTOR MANAGEMENT

RISK FACTOR	RECOMMENDATION
Hypertension	Maintain blood pressure <104 mm Hg and diastolic blood pressure <90 mm Hg
	For people with diabetes, blood pressure levels <13/85 mm Hg
Cigarette smoking	Discontinue smoking
	Counseling, nicotine replacement therapies, bupropion, and formal smoking cessation programs may all be helpful
Coronary artery disease, cardiac dysrhythmias, congestive heart failure, and valvular disease	Treat disease and underlying cause as appropriate
Excessive alcohol intake	Eliminate excessive alcohol intake; formal alcohol cessation programs are recommended; mild-to-moderate use of alcohol (1–2 drinks/d) has been associated with a reduction in stroke rates
Hyperlipidemia	AHA Step II diet (≤30% of calories derived from fat, <7% from saturated fat, and <200 mg/d cholesterol consumed)
	Maintain ideal body weight
	Regular exercise
	If lipids remain elevated (LDL >130 mg/dL), use of a lipid-lowering agent, preferably a statin drug, to keep LDL <100 mg/dL
Diabetes mellitus	Diet and oral hypoglycemics or insulin to keep fasting blood glucose levels <126 mg/dL, maintain hemoglobin A1c level between 3%–6%

LDL, low density lipoprotein.

and occlusion. An intravenous heparin infusion for 3 to 5 days during acute care management of progressive ischemic stroke is common. Use of warfarin for anticoagulation is now generally reserved for high-grade artery stenosis, large vessel disease, and cardioembolic sources, especially atrial fibrillation and patent foramen ovale. Anticoagulation is also a reasonable choice for patients with TIA or a stroke while receiving antiplatelet agents, crescendo TIAs, cervical artery dissection, severe carotid artery stenosis before endarterectomy, antiphospholipid antibody syndrome, or coagulation factor deficiencies. High-dose low-molecular-weight heparin, given subcutaneously, is now being used in some centers rather than IV heparin; this has the added advantage of a reduced length of stay.[22] It is also given at the beginning of warfarin therapy to aid in reaching therapeutic international normalized ratio (INR) levels faster.[23]

There has been much written in the literature to support the use of the INR to monitor anticoagulation therapy rather than prothrombin time (PT). Because of laboratory variability in reagents used to perform PT, the use of INR is recommended nationally.[23]

Surgical Interventions

Selected patients with extracranial or intracranial atherosclerotic disease that is located in accessible sites (areas previously mentioned) may be good candidates for surgery. The goal of the surgical procedures is to prevent TIAs or stroke. Carotid endarterectomy or extracranial graft may benefit the patient with narrowing of the extracranial artery. A bypass grafting procedure may be of value for the patient with an intracranial occlusion, such as of the internal carotid or MCA. The procedure often used for intracranial involvement is superior temporal artery/middle cerebral artery (STA-MCA) anastomosis. For patients who have an identified thrombus, a thrombectomy may be done to restore

circulation. Chart 26-1 provides key points in the acute management of stroke patients after special interventions.

Endovascular Therapy

Endovascular therapies encompass interventional radiological procedures to treat intracranial vascular lesions with high morbidity and mortality. These procedures use vascular superselective catheterization and navigation with microcatheters. A form of endovascular therapy is *percutaneous angioplasty* of a large cerebral vessel (typically the carotids, vertebral, basilar, and middle cerebral arteries). The procedure involves stretching the media of the stenosed vessel and breaking the atherosclerotic plaque by inflating a balloon at the site of the stenosis. Another form of therapy, *intravascular stenting*, is used in conjunction with the angioplasty to maintain vessel patency. Stenting has been proposed as an alternative therapeutic modality for patients with significant carotid, MCA, and vertebrobasilar artery stenoses.[24] It may be particularly suited for patients who are at too high a risk for carotid endarterectomy. Studies are currently under way to evaluate the efficacy of cerebral protection device to entrap emboli during percutaneous angioplasty and stenting of the carotid arteries.

Cerebral Revascularization

Carotid Endarterectomy

The North American Symptomatic Carotid Endarterectomy Trial (NASCET) clearly demonstrated that carotid endarterectomy (CEA) is superior to medical therapy alone for stroke prevention in patients with 70% or greater symptomatic internal carotid artery stenosis. Patients with 70% or greater carotid stenosis, without major operative risk factors, have a relative reduction of about 60% and absolute risk reduction

CHART 26 – 1 • Key Points in Acute Care Nursing Management of Stroke Patients After Treatment With Special Interventions

NURSING MANAGEMENT OF PATIENTS WHO HAVE UNDERGONE THROMBOLYTIC THERAPY

- Monitor vital signs for evidence of extracranial bleeding (e.g., gastric hemorrhage).
- Monitor neurological signs for evidence of deterioration and increased intracranial pressure (ICP) that may be caused by intracerebral hemorrhage or increasing cerebral edema.
- Monitor for reperfusion injury.*
- Monitor for bleeding at catheter site; bleeding may also be noted in urine or stool, or from mouth.
- Monitor coagulation studies and maintain in therapeutic parameters.
- Protect femoral catheter, which is left in place for as long as 24 hours.

NURSING MANAGEMENT OF PATIENTS WHO HAVE UNDERGONE CEREBRAL ANGIOGRAPHY/STENT PLACEMENT

- Monitor vital signs for hemodynamic instability.
- Monitor for bleeding at catheter site; bleeding may also be noted in urine, stool, GI tract, or mouth.
- Monitor neurological signs for evidence of intracerebral hemorrhage and reperfusion injury.*
- Monitor coagulation studies and maintain in therapeutic range using international normalizing ratio (INR) parameters.

NURSING MANAGEMENT OF PATIENTS WHO HAVE UNDERGONE A CAROTID ENDARTERECTOMY

- Monitor blood pressure and rigorously maintain within set parameters, usually about 150 mm Hg systolic (hypertension predisposes to intracerebral hemorrhage,

and hypotension to ischemic stroke); instability of blood pressure is common particularly in the first 12 to 24 hours postoperatively so expect to monitor and manage blood pressure frequently.
- Monitor for cardiac arrhythmias and evidence of myocardial ischemia (myocardial infarction is not uncommon).
- Monitor neurological signs frequently and observe for early signs of deterioration.
  - Monitor for cranial nerve deficits (especially facial and vagal) as a result of surgery.
  - Monitor for signs of intracerebral hemorrhage (increased ICP, new onset of neurological deficits).
  - Monitor for vascular headache and seizures (hyperperfusion syndrome).
- Monitor for reperfusion injury.*
- Maintain head of bed according to physician orders; because of vascular instability, the head of the bed may be flat for the first 24 hours.
- Observe operative site for hemorrhage, hematoma, or tearing of suture site.

NURSING MANAGEMENT OF PATIENTS WHO ARE RECEIVING INTRAVENOUS HEPARIN ADMINISTRATION

- Monitor neurological signs for evidence of deterioration and increased ICP that may be caused by intracerebral hemorrhage or increasing cerebral edema.
- Monitor coagulation studies and maintain in therapeutic range using INR parameters.
- Adjust intravenous heparin infusion according to coagulation parameters.
- Monitor for bleeding at catheter site and from urine, stool, GI tract, or mouth; note evidence of bruising easily.
- Monitor for reperfusion injury.*

* Reperfusion injury: observe for signs and symptoms of cerebral edema, increased ICP, and recurrence stroke symptomology or expansion of neurological deficits after successful recanalization.

---

of 5% to 10% per year within the subsequent 2 years.[25] In one study, patients with 50% to 69% stenosis with a recent TIA or minor stroke have a reduced stroke rate with endarterectomy versus medical treatment.[26] However, the absolute benefit of surgery is less than that for patients with higher degrees of stenosis and among women and patients with retinal TIAs. Patients with less than 50% stenosis with recent symptoms do not benefit from CEA. Antiplatelet therapy is recommended for these patients.

The "hot spots" for atheroma build-up are noted in Figure 26-8. A CEA consists of careful removal of the atherosclerotic plaque and intraluminal clot, if present, from the artery after a temporary bypass shunt has been created to provide adequate cerebral perfusion. The plaque is removed after the artery is temporarily occluded both above and below the atheroma. In some instances, a bypass graft is used to improve circulation. The major danger during surgery is em-

bolization of atherogenic plaque and thrombi from excessive manipulation of the carotid bifurcation. On completion, a Jackson-Pratt drain may be inserted at the operative site to prevent development of a hematoma.

The major postoperative concerns are blood pressure instability, stroke or transient neurological deficits, cranial nerve injury (facial, vagal), wound hematoma, suture line rupture, TIAs, and hyperperfusion syndromes.[27] After surgery, patients experience a period of postoperative blood pressure instability that lasts for approximately 12 to 24 hours, probably as a result of a carotid sinus malfunction and loss of effective baroreceptor action. After blood flow has been restored, maintenance of the systolic pressure at a constant level of approximately 150 mm Hg is critical. The sudden restoration of high flow, especially after removal of a tight stenosis and in the presence of heparin (used during surgery) or antiplatelets, can lead to intracerebral hemorrhage. Hypotensive episodes are just as disastrous and can result in ischemic stroke or TIAs. The potential for cranial nerve injury results from the proximity of these nerves to the operative site.

Hyperperfusion syndromes are related to the marked increase in cerebral blood flow after CEA. Patients often have paralysis of autoregulation ipsilateral to the surgical site so that the profound increase in blood flow is not blunted. When this occurs, blood pressure must be meticulously maintained in the 120 to 130 mm Hg range. Patients may experience vascular headaches or catastrophic intracerebral hemorrhage. Seizures may occur about 7 to 10 days postoperatively. Finally, a leading cause of death after CEA is myocardial infarction, either immediate or delayed. The patient should be monitored carefully for evidence of myocardial ischemia or infarction.

STA-MCA Anastomosis

Extracranial/intracranial anastomosis, most often of the superficial temporal artery to the MCA, is a microsurgical bypass procedure used to provide collateral circulation to the areas of the brain supplied by the MCA. Currently, it is used infrequently because of the negative results reported in the EC/IC Bypass Trial.[28]

Thrombectomy

An emergency thrombectomy may have some dramatic results. Major concerns are the development of severe cerebral edema owing to reperfusion of necrotic tissue. Thrombectomy has been replaced by thrombolytic therapy.

Hypervolemic-Hemodilution Therapy

To support cerebral hemodynamics, hypervolemic hemodilution therapy is used (see Chap. 24). This therapy helps to maintain a stable, slightly higher blood pressure, which increases and maintains cerebral perfusion pressure by lowering blood viscosity. The hematocrit is reduced to 33 to 35 mg/dL, and hypervolemia is achieved with saline and albumin.

Reperfusion

Both intravenous recombinant tissue plasminogen activator (t-PA) and intraarterial thrombolytic agents (e.g., t-PA and prourokinase) have been used in acute ischemic stroke to restore cerebral blood flow, reduce ischemia, and limit neurological disability. The recanalization of an occluded cerebral artery may assist the recovery of ischemic tissue within a brief time span after onset of stroke. The major concerns with these therapies are hemorrhage and reperfusion injury. Risk for hemorrhage is further increased by systemic fibrinolytic drug effects.

The use of intravenous defibrinogenating agents is also being studied as an alternative to thrombolytic therapy. A defibrinogenating agent lowers the fibrinogen level, a prothrombotic factor. A reduction in fibrinogen level is associated with a risk of hemorrhagic complications.

Emergency Intervention With Intravenous Tissue Plasminogen Activator

Intravenous t-PA should be considered for all patients with acute ischemic stroke who meet the inclusion and exclusion criteria used in the National Institute of Neurological Disorders and Stroke (NINDS) trial and who can be treated within 3 hours of stroke onset.[29] (Chart 26-2 shows these selection criteria.) The recommended dose is 0.9 mg/kg (maximum 90 mg). The initial 10% is given as an intravenous bolus over 1 minute and the remaining t-PA infused over 60 minutes. Anticoagulants or aspirin should not be given in the first 24 hours after t-PA treatment.

Thrombolytic therapy with t-PA is not without risk. Symptomatic intracranial hemorrhage occurred in 6.4% of patients treated with t-PA in the NINDS-sponsored study. Following initiation of therapy, patients must be assessed in an intensive care setting. Frequent assessment of blood pressure during the first 24 hours, with treatment of blood pressure elevations of more than 185 mm Hg systolic or 110 mm Hg diastolic, may help prevent thrombolysis-related ICH. Frequent neurological assessment can allow early detection of decreased levels of consciousness, headache, nausea and vomiting, or an increase in focal neurological deficits (signs and symptoms that could indicate onset of ICH).

Patients with acute stroke who are ineligible to receive t-PA should be carefully evaluated by repeated neurological examinations over the next few hours to be sure the stroke is not progressing. Use of t-Pa is not recommended in patients presenting with rapidly improving neurological deficit or minor deficits with a National Institutes of Health (NIH) Stroke Scale score of less than 3 or 4 (see Chart 26-3 for the NIH Stroke Scale) because they usually have excellent recovery without therapy.

Administration of t-PA should only be used in hospitals fulfilling the following requirements:

- Neurological or emergency department expertise should be available for prompt clinical investigation of the patient and interpretation of the initial CT brain scan, and expert radiographic opinion should be available if needed for CT interpretation.
- Facilities such as a stroke unit or an intensive care unit (ICU) should be available for close monitoring of the patient's vital signs and neurologic status for at least 24 hours after treatment.
- A management plan should be available for possible intracranial hemorrhage, including access to neurosurgical care and expertise.

Emergency Intervention With Intra-arterial Thrombolysis

Intra-arterial thrombolysis with t-PA, prourokinase, and streptokinase has been used in both controlled and uncontrolled cases in patients with a demonstrable occlusion of the MCA and the vertebrobasilar arteries. This treatment is not yet FDA approved and is used primarily for compassionate care in patients who have had severe strokes and where the futility of continuing with available approved measures has been established. Clinical research continues evaluating the definitive role of intraarterial t-PA in acute ischemic stroke.

CHART 26–2 • Eligibility Criteria for Thrombolytic Therapy

INCLUSION CRITERIA

1. Symptom onset of <3 hours
2. Clinical diagnosis of ischemic stroke with measurable deficit on National Institutes of Health Stroke Scale
3. Age >18 years
4. Criteria for computed tomography: absence of high-density lesion consistent with intracerebral hemorrhage; absence of significant mass effect or midline shift; absence of parenchymal hypodensity, and/or effacement of cerebral sulci >33% of the middle cerebral artery territory

EXCLUSION CRITERIA

1. Stroke or serious head trauma within past 3 mo
2. Systolic blood pressure (BP) >185 mm Hg or diastolic BP >110 mm Hg, or BP readings that require aggressive treatment
3. Conditions that could precipitate or suggest parenchymal bleeding (subarachnoid and intracranial hemorrhage, recent myocardial infarction, seizures at stroke onset, major surgery within past 14 d, gastrointestinal or urinary tract hemorrhage within previous 21 d, and arterial puncture of a noncompressible site or lumbar puncture within previous 7 d)
4. Glucose <50 mg/dL or >400 mg/dL; INR >1.7, platelet count <100,000/mm^3
5. Rapidly improving or deteriorating neurological signs or minor symptoms
6. Recent myocardial infarction
7. Recent treatment with intravenous or subcutaneous heparin within past 48 hours and with elevated partial thromboplastin time
8. Woman of child-bearing age who has a positive pregnancy test result

From Hock, N. H. (1999). Brain attack: The stroke continuum. *Nursing Clinics of North America, 34*(3), 718–719.

Neuroprotective Agents

Neuroprotective or cytoprotective agents are designed to protect the brain from delayed injury by interfering in the steps of the ischemic cascade and reperfusion injury. Several of these investigational agents are undergoing clinical trials. The disturbance in calcium flux and calcium-activated enzyme systems, production of free radicals, membrane destruction, and disturbance in protein synthesis are targets of investigation. Neuroprotective agents that have been considered represent a broad spectrum of compounds with disparate mechanisms of action: sodium-channel blockers, calcium-channel antagonists, free radical scavengers, membrane stabilizers, glutamate receptor antagonists, gamma-aminobutyric acid (GABA) agonists, and monoclonal antibodies that curtail inflammatory cascades. A number of compounds have undergone clinical trials in the past decade without proven success in improving clinical outcome in the human population of patients with stroke. Newer drugs, changes in clinical trial design, and combination therapy with thrombolytics, as well as the use of neuroimaging markers of drug effectiveness (i.e., DWI), promise to improve the chance of finding an effective neuroprotective treatment.

Mild Hypothermia as a Neuroprotectant

In recent years there has been increasing interest in the use of hypothermia, as well as aggressive control of hyperthermia (elevated temperature), in acute stroke patients. Deep hypothermia has been used in the setting of neurosurgical and cardiothoracic surgery for its neuroprotective benefits, but it also carries tremendous risks.[30] Secondary effects include fatal cardiac dysrhythmias and coagulopathies that predispose patients to hemorrhagic, cardiac, and systemic complications. Mild hypothermia (i.e., 32° to 34°C) is evolving as a safer alternative to deep hypothermia. It has been shown to improve neurological outcome in experimental models of ischemia and head injury as well as in head injury clinical trials.[31–33] In patients with large hemispheric strokes, hypothermia seems to control cerebral edema. The neuroprotective effects include reduced oxygen consumption in the brain, reduced release of excitatory amino acids, and decreased free-radical production.

Hypothermia is achieved using various methods. Lowering the room temperature, placing cooling blankets under the patients while convective air blankets cover them, gastric lavage with iced saline, and placement of ice packs at selected skin folds are employed. Endovascular and intravenous catheters to achieve rapid systemic hypothermia are now in clinical trials in stroke, cardiothoracic, shock-trauma, and neurosurgical settings. In stroke, the patient selected typically has a large hemispheric and severe stroke and will require intensive care stay and astute nursing observation throughout the cooling and rewarming phases. In this patient group, hypothermia is usually induced within 12 hours of stroke onset, and gradually achieved over a 2- to 3-hour period. The patient will require intubation and ventilatory support, continuous sedation, hemodynamic and ICP monitoring, continuous EEG monitoring, and frequent blood draws to determine electrolytes and coagulation status. Body temperature is continuously monitored using core temperature. If the temperature falls below the desired level, cooling procedures are stopped and gradual rewarming procedures (over a period of 2 to 3 hours) are undertaken. Measures must be taken to prevent shivering. Rewarming

CHART 26-3 • National Institutes of Health Stroke Scale

1a. Level of consciousness (LOC)
   alert — 0
   drowsy — 1
   stuporous — 2
   coma — 3
1b. LOC questions
   answers both correctly — 0
   answers one correctly — 1
   answers neither correctly — 2
1c. LOC commands
   performs both correctly — 0
   performs one correctly — 1
   performs neither correctly — 2
2. Best gaze
   normal — 0
   partial gaze palsy — 1
   forced deviation — 2
3. Visual
   no visual loss — 0
   partial hemianopsia — 1
   complete hemianopsia — 2
   bilateral hemianopsia — 3
4. Facial palsy
   normal — 0
   minor paralysis — 1
   partial paralysis — 2
   complete paralysis — 3
5. Motor arm
   no drift — 0
   drift — 1
   some effort against gravity — 2
   no effort against gravity — 3
   no movement — 4
   amputation, joint fusion (explain) — 9
6. Motor leg
   no drift — 0
   drift — 1
   some effort against gravity — 2
   no effort against gravity — 3
   no movement — 4
   amputation, joint fusion (explain) — 9
7. Limb ataxia
   absent — 0
   present in one limb — 1
   present in two limbs — 2
8. Sensory
   normal — 0
   mild to moderate loss — 1
   severe to total loss — 2
9. Best language
   no aphasia — 0
   mild-to-moderate — 1
   severe — 2
   mute — 3

From Hock, N. H. (1999). Brain attack: The stroke continuum. *Nursing Clinics of North America, 34*(3), 709.

can be achieved by turning off the cooling blankets, room temperature elevation, warm bladder irrigations, and placement of warm blankets over the patient.

Hyperthermia (more than 37.5°C) has been associated with poorer outcome and poorer prognosis following acute stroke. This finding is consistent with experimental studies, which consistently indicate that increased temperature is associated with more severe neuronal injury. Vigilant nursing observation of the patient's temperature and taking active and immediate measures to prevent and control fever are key functions in the care of the stroke patient.

Neurotransplantation

Fundamental advances in stem cell research, gene therapy, and neurotrophic factors have contributed to the success of neurotransplantation in animal stroke models.[34] Various studies using different experimental stroke paradigms have demonstrated neurological function following neuronal grafts. In some cases the transplanted grafts have been shown to survive, differentiate into neuronal cells appropriate for the infarct size, make functional connections, and induce angiogenesis. Various types of neuronal grafts have been tried experimentally, including cortical grafts, fetal tissue, neuronal stem cells, postmitotic tumor cells, and bone marrow cells. The goal of cell transplant therapy is to facilitate cell regeneration to improve the patient's neurologic status and functional outcome.

Rehabilitation

Early rehabilitation is important to making optimal recovery; rehabilitation needs to be addressed immediately. Figure 26-9 provides a flow diagram for stroke rehabilitation from the clinical practice guidelines, *Post-Stroke Rehabilitation*.[35] This is an outstanding resource that sets the national standard for stroke rehabilitation and should be familiar to all care providers of stroke patients (see Chap. 13 for rehabilitation content).

Acute Management of ICH Stroke

For persons who sustain an intracerebral hemorrhagic stroke, acute management is directed toward management of increased ICP as outlined in Chapter 14. Care is often provided in an intensive care environment. To control increased ICP, a ventriculostomy may be necessary. Surgical decompression and stereotactically guided removal of the hematoma may be necessary in certain cases. Care of the postoperative neurosurgical patient is discussed in Chapter 15. Vasospasms are not considered a problem with an intracerebral hemorrhage. Chapter 24 also provides guidance for patient management.

For patients who survive, rehabilitation is necessary. In addition, identification and modification of risk factors need to be undertaken. Nursing management is outlined in Chapters 14 and 24.

GENERAL NURSING MANAGEMENT OF THE STROKE PATIENT

Nursing management of patients with stroke varies according to the specific stroke syndrome and neurological and functional deficits. However, there are several areas to consider,

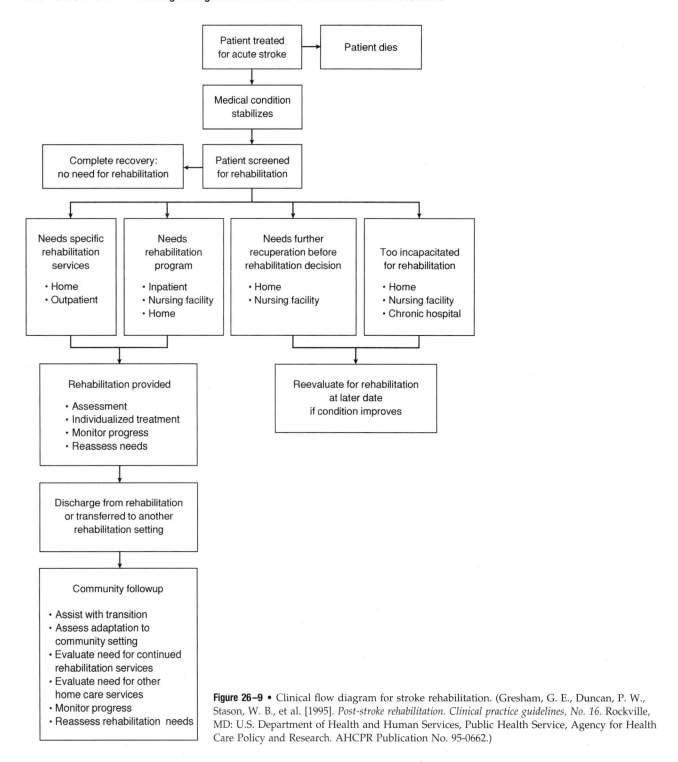

Figure 26–9 • Clinical flow diagram for stroke rehabilitation. (Gresham, G. E., Duncan, P. W., Stason, W. B., et al. [1995]. *Post-stroke rehabilitation. Clinical practice guidelines, No. 16.* Rockville, MD: U.S. Department of Health and Human Services, Public Health Service, Agency for Health Care Policy and Research. AHCPR Publication No. 95-0662.)

including primary and secondary prevention of stroke, initial management during the acute phase, early focus on rehabilitation, discharge planning and continuity of care, and patient education. Assessment and nursing diagnosis guide nursing management.

Primary and Secondary Prevention of Stroke

The paradigm shift from treatment to prevention has redefined the nurse's role in identification of risk factors and working with the patient not only to modify risk factors but also to promote a healthier lifestyle. The major risk factors for stroke are listed in Table 26-4. These major risk factors are the same for stroke and heart disease, the number one and number three causes of death in the U.S. Nurses are particularly effective in helping patients think through how they can modify risk factors within the context of their lifestyles. Secondary prevention becomes the focus after a stroke to prevent another stroke, regardless of whether the patient is followed in a stroke prevention clinic or by the primary care provider. Along with education and motivation, the patient must be monitored collaboratively by the nurse and physician. Prevention is cost effective and results in savings.

Possible nursing diagnoses related to stroke prevention include:

- Knowledge Deficit
- Noncompliance
- Ineffective Management of Therapeutic Regimen

Initial Management During the Acute Phase

Early treatment of stroke is recognized as a key factor in optimizing outcomes. Care may be rendered in a neurological ICU or special acute care unit. Having been stabilized, the patient may receive therapies to protect the brain from secondary injury related to the ischemic cascade. The current approved window of opportunity to use t-PA is 0 to 3 hours after onset of ischemic stroke. The acute care management goals for intracranial occlusive disease include maintaining the following:

- An adequate airway and oxygenation to avoid hypoxia
- Stable, slightly higher blood pressure to maximize cerebral perfusion pressure
- Serum glucose in a range below 150 mg/dL with insulin as necessary to avoid the increased risk of cerebral edema and hemorrhage
- Aseptic technique, following procedures to prevent infections (e.g., aspiration pneumonia, urinary tract infection)

The treatment options include thrombolytic therapy, antiplatelet agents, anticoagulation with heparin, hypervolemic hemodilution, and measures to control ICP.[36]

Many patients will be managed in ICUs to monitor closely for effects from therapies such as thrombolytics. The nurse works collaboratively with the physician to achieve the goals already listed.

The following nursing diagnoses and collaborative problems may be made in the acute phase of illness:

POSSIBLE NURSING DIAGNOSES
- Ineffective Airway Clearance
- Risk of Aspiration
- Impaired Swallowing
- Altered Cerebral Tissue Perfusion
- Risk of Infection
- Ineffective Breathing Pattern
- Sensory Perceptual Alterations
- Impaired Physical Mobility
- Impaired Verbal Communication

POSSIBLE COLLABORATIVE PROBLEMS
- Hypoxemia
- Hypoglycemia and hyperglycemia
- Increased intracranial pressure
- Stroke
- Paresis/paresthesia/paralysis
- Gastrointestinal bleeding
- Hypertension

- Reperfusion injury
- Electrolyte imbalances
- Dysrhythmias
- Anticoagulant therapy adverse effects
- Thrombolytic therapy adverse effect

Frequent neurological, hemodynamic, and respiratory monitoring is necessary to determine early changes and the need to adjust management. Cerebral edema develops with all ischemic strokes, but it is a major concern with a large stroke. Severe hypertension increases the risk of hemorrhage. Both cerebral edema and hemorrhage are associated with increased ICP. Increased ICP may result from the original hemorrhage, but hemorrhage can also occur 2 to 4 days after massive infarction of the cerebral hemisphere. The development of edema is heralded by a gradual deterioration in neurological signs, such as drowsiness and sluggish pupillary response. Increased ICP is treated with osmotic diuretics and hyperventilation. Supportive therapy depends on the extent of the deficits and complications present. In the conscious patient, assess for fluent and nonfluent aphasia.

Careful cardiac monitoring is necessary to determine the need to adjust therapy to maximize hemodynamic parameters. It is also necessary to observe for secondary insult such as myocardial infarction. The level of the head of the bed will depend on hemodynamics and ICP, but it is generally elevated to 30 degrees. Respiratory parameters are also monitored closely for evidence of secondary problems, such as neurogenic pulmonary edema, atelectasis, and pneumonia. For patients on ventilatory support, weaning should begin as soon as possible. The awake patient should be maintained on "nothing by mouth" status until a swallowing study has been conducted and problems of aspiration have been ruled out.

Both hypoglycemia and hyperglycemia are detrimental to the injured brain. Hyperglycemia above 150 mg/dL increases infarct size in experimental stroke models and contributes to poorer outcomes. Serum glucose levels should be monitored and kept in the normal range with regular insulin. In addition, intravenous solutions should be *saline and not glucose.* For patients receiving anticoagulants such as heparin, monitor the activated partial thromboplastin time and observe for bleeding. Electrolytes, creatinine, and blood urea nitrogen are monitored. Electrolyte imbalance, particularly sodium, is common and should be managed.

For details about the key points in acute care nursing management of stroke patients after treatment with special interventions, see Chart 26-1. Chart 26-4 summarizes the common nursing diagnoses associated with stroke. Chart 26-5 summarizes the common deficits and emotional reactions related to stroke. See also Chapter 16 for management of the unconscious patient and Chapter 14 for ICP management. After the patient's condition has stabilized, nursing management is refocused on rehabilitation and prevention of another stroke (Chart 26-6).

Early Focus on Rehabilitation

Rehabilitation begins as soon as the patient is stabilized. Figure 26-9 provides an overview of stroke rehabilitation. The nurse collaborates with other health care professionals to develop a

(text continues on page 583)

CHART 26 – 4 • Summary of Common Nursing Diagnoses for Stroke Patients in Acute Phase

Nursing Diagnoses (Potential or Actual)	Nursing Interventions	Expected Outcomes
Ineffective Airway Clearance related to (R/T) unconsciousness or ineffective cough reflex	• Position the patient to facilitate drainage of oropharyngeal secretions; turn the patient from side to side every 2 hours. • Elevate the head of the bed to 30 degrees. • Clear secretions from the airway using suction, as necessary; provide for pulmonary hygiene. • Provide for chest physical therapy. • Provide for coughing and deep breathing exercises. • If the patient is receiving oxygen therapy, be sure that it is adequately humidified.	• The airway will be patent, allowing for increased air exchange. • The risk of aspiration will be decreased. • The risk of elevated CO_2, which contributes to cerebral hypoxia and cerebral edema, will be decreased.
Risk of Aspiration R/T inability to protect airway or unconsciousness	• Maintain nothing-by-mouth status. • Swallowing studies needed to evaluate swallowing function before oral intake is tried. • When oral intake is resumed, take precautions to prevent aspiration (elevate head of bed, hold head up, etc.).	• Aspiration and aspiration pneumonia will not develop.
Altered Tissue Perfusion, cerebral, R/T ischemia, cerebral edema, or increased intracranial pressure (ICP)	• Monitor vital and neurological signs. • Maintain venous outflow from the brain by elevating the head of the bed 30 degrees. • Maintain the patient's head in a neutral position. • Avoid positions that increase intra-abdominal/intrathoracic pressure (hip flexion, prone position, etc.; see Chap. 14). • Maintain normothermia. • Avoid activities known to increase ICP (clustering activities, etc.; see Chap. 14). • Maintain the patient's blood pressure within the range set for sufficient cerebral perfusion pressure.	• Vital signs will be maintained within normal limits. • Cerebral perfusion pressure will be maintained.
Risk of Infection	• Aseptic technique will be followed. • Urinary catheter will be removed as soon as possible. • Measures will be taken to prevent respiratory infections.	• Infections will not develop in lungs, urinary tract, catheter sites.
Sensory/Perceptual Alterations: • Kinesthetic • Tactile • Visual R/T altered consciousness, impaired sensation, or impaired vision	• Provide appropriate stimulation to involved areas of sense. • Monitor the level of sensation. • Patch one eye and alter the patch to control diplopia. • Place materials on and approach the patient from the unaffected side if homonymous hemianopia is present. • Provide tactile stimulation to hands and limbs affected by decreased sensation. • Protect the patient from injury. • Develop compensatory strategies to meet particular patient needs.	• Optimal sensory input will be received and interpreted accurately. • Safety will be maintained.
Impaired Verbal Communication R/T cerebral injury/altered level of consciousness	• Assess type of communication deficit present. • Develop appropriate methods for communications.	• An alternative method of communication will be established. • The patient's attempts to communicate will be supported.
Impaired Physical Mobility R/T neurological deficits	• Assess the type and degree of impairment. • Provide slings, braces, support shoes, and so forth, as necessary. • Teach the patient alternative methods of mobility. • Provide for range-of-motion exercises four times/d.	• Alternative methods of mobility will be used. • Passive movement will be provided to prevent the negative effects on the nervous system that are associated with immobility.

CHART 26 – 5 • Common Deficits and Emotional Reactions to Stroke and Related General Nursing Interventions

Common Motor Deficits

1. Hemiparesis or hemiplegia (side of the body opposite the cerebral episode)
2. Dysarthria (muscles of speech impaired)
3. Dysphagia (muscles of swallowing impaired)

Nursing Interventions

1. Position the patient in proper body alignment; use a hand roll or splint to keep the hand in a functional position.
   - Provide frequent passive range-of-motion exercises.
   - Reposition the patient every 2 hours.
2. Provide for an alternative method of communication.
3. Test the patient's palatal and pharyngeal reflexes before offering nourishment.
   - Keep NPO with swallowing screen completed and oral intake approved by physician.
   - Elevate and turn the head to the unaffected side.
   - If the patient is able to manage oral intake, place food on the unaffected side of the patient's mouth.

Common Sensory Deficits

1. Visual deficits (common because the visual pathways cut through much of the cerebral hemispheres)
   a. Homonymous hemianopia (loss of vision in half of the visual field on the same side)

Left   Right

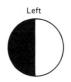

   b. Double vision (diplopia)
   c. Decreased visual acuity
2. Absent or diminished response to superficial sensation (touch, pain, pressure, heat, cold)

3. Absent or diminished response to proprioception (knowledge of position of body parts)
4. Perceptual deficits (disturbance in correctly perceiving and interpreting self and/or environment)
   a. Body scheme disturbance (amnesia or denial for paralyzed extremities; **unilateral neglect syndrome**)
   b. Disorientation (to time, place, and person)

   c. Apraxia (loss of ability to use objects correctly)

Nursing Interventions

1. Be aware that variations of visual deficits may exist and compensate for them.
   a. Approach the patient from the unaffected side; remind the patient to turn the head to compensate for visual deficits.

   b. Apply an eye patch to the affected eye
   c. Provide assistance as necessary.
2. Increase the amount of touch in administering patient care.
   - Protect the involved areas from injury.
   - Protect the involved areas from burns.
   - Examine the involved areas for signs of skin irritation and injury.
   - Provide the patient with an opportunity to handle various objects of different weight, texture, and size.
   - If pain is present, assess its location and type, as well as the duration of the pain.
3. Teach the patient to check the position of body parts visually.
4. Compensate for the patient's perceptual-sensory deficits.

   a. Protect the involved area.
   - Accept the patient's self-perception.
   - Position the patient to face the involved area.
   b. Control the amount of changes in the patient's schedule.
   - Reorient the patient as necessary.
   - Talk to the patient; tell him or her about the immediate environment.
   - Provide a calendar, clock, pictures of family, and so forth.
   c. Correct misuse of objects and demonstrate proper use.

(continued)

CHART 26-5 • Common Deficits and Emotional Reactions to Stroke and Related General Nursing Interventions (Continued)

Common Sensory Deficits

d. Agnosia (inability to identify the environment by means of the senses)
e. Defects in localizing objects in space, estimating their size, and judging distance
f. Impaired memory for recall of spatial location of objects or places

g. Right-left disorientation

Nursing Interventions

d. Correct misinformation.

e. Reduce any stimuli that distract the patient.

f. Place necessary equipment where the patient will see it, rather than telling the patient "It is in the closet" for example.
g. Phrase requests carefully, like "Lift this leg." (Point to the leg.)

Language Deficits

1. Nonfluent aphasia (difficulty in transforming sound into patterns of understandable speech)—can speak using single-word responses
2. Fluent aphasia (impairment of comprehension of the spoken word)—able to speak, but uses words incorrectly and is unaware of these errors
3. Global aphasia (combination of expressive and receptive aphasia)—unable to communicate at any level

4. Alexia (inability to understand the written word)

5. Agraphia (inability to express ideas in writing)

Nursing Interventions

1. Ask the patient to repeat the individual sounds of the alphabet as a start at retraining.

2. Speak clearly and in simple sentences; use gestures as necessary.

3. Evaluate which language skills remain intact; speak in very simple sentences, ask the patient to repeat individual sounds, and use gestures or any other means to communicate.
4. Point to the written names of objects and have the patient repeat the name of the object.
5. Have the patient write words and simple sentences

Intellectual Deficits

1. Loss of memory
2. Short attention span
3. Increased distractibility
4. Poor judgment
5. Inability to transfer learning from one situation to another
6. Inability to calculate, reason, or think abstractly

Nursing Interventions

1. Provide information as necessary.
2. Divide activities into short steps.
3. Control any excessive environmental distractions.
4. Protect the patient from injury.
5. Repeat instructions as necessary.

6. Do not create unrealistic expectations in the patient.

Emotional Deficits

(Recognize that pattern is often inconsistent; patient may have good days and bad days or even good hours and bad hours.)

1. Emotional lability (exhibits reactions easily or inappropriately)
2. Loss of self-control and social inhibitions (may speak inappropriately or swear or may expose self or make sexual advances toward nurse)
3. Reduced tolerance for stress

4. Fear, hostility, frustration, anger
5. Confusion and despair
6. Withdrawal, isolation
7. Depression

Nursing Interventions

1. Disregard bursts of emotions; explain to the patient that emotional lability is part of the illness.
2. Protect the patient as necessary so that his or her dignity is preserved; recognize the involuntary bases of this behavior and set limits; anticipate needs.
3. Control the environment and maintain routines as much as possible; remove stimuli that upset the patient.
4. Be accepting of the patient; be supportive.
5. Clarify any misconceptions; allow the patient to verbalize.
6. Provide stimulation and a safe, comfortable environment.
7. Provide a supportive environment; consider pharmacotherapy.

Explain behavior to family as a manifestation of brain injury. Be supportive.

CHART 26–5 • Common Deficits and Emotional Reactions to Stroke and Related General Nursing Interventions (Continued)

Bowel and Bladder Dysfunction	Nursing Interventions
Bladder: Incomplete Upper Motor Neuron Lesion	Do not suggest insertion of an indwelling catheter immediately after the stroke; intermittent catheterization is better than an indwelling catheter.
1. The unilateral lesion from the stroke results in partial sensation and control of the bladder, so that the patient experiences frequency, urgency, and incontinence. (Cognitive deficits affect control.) 2. If the stroke lesion is in the brain stem, there will be bilateral damage, resulting in an upper motor neuron bladder with loss of all control of micturition.	1. Observe the patient to identify characteristics of the voiding pattern (e.g., frequency, amount, forcefulness of stream, constant dribbling). 2. Maintain an accurate intake and output record. *Nursing note:* Incontinence after regaining consciousness is usually attributable to urinary tract infection caused by use of an indwelling urinary catheter.
3. Possibility of establishing normal bladder function is excellent.	3. Try to allow the patient to stay catheter-free: • Offer the bedpan or urinal frequently. • Take the patient to the commode frequently. • Assess the patient's ability to make his or her need for help with voiding known. If a catheter is necessary, remove it as soon as possible and follow a bladder training program (see Chap. 13).
Bowel 1. Altered bowel function in a stroke patient is attributable to: • Deterioration in the level of consciousness • Dehydration • Immobility 2. Constipation is the most common problem, along with potential impaction.	1. Develop a bowel training program: • Give foods known to stimulate defecation (prune juice, roughage). • Initiate a suppository and laxative regimen. 2. Institute a bowel program. Enemas are avoided in the presence of increased intracranial pressure.

plan of care. The case manager is an integral part of the interdisciplinary team who can facilitate access to rehabilitation resources and community-based rehabilitation services. Nursing responsibilities in the rehabilitation process are outlined in Chart 26-6. See Chapter 13 for information about rehabilitation.

The following nursing diagnoses and collaborative problems are often seen in stroke patients and are related to the need for early rehabilitation:

POSSIBLE NURSING DIAGNOSES
• Self-Care Deficits
• Sensory Perceptual Alterations
• Impaired Verbal Communication
• Impaired Physical Mobility
• Altered Urinary Elimination
• Disuse Syndrome
• Altered Thought Processes
• Impaired Adjustment
• Altered Role Performance
• Unilateral Neglect

POSSIBLE COLLABORATIVE PROBLEMS
• Antiplatelet therapy adverse effects

Discharge Planning and Continuity of Care

Discharge planning is taken into account early in the rehabilitative program. The plans for discharge are made with the assistance of the case manager, who assists with continuity and facilitates access to the next level of care, whether rehabilitation or home care. The patient and family should be made aware of community resources. A critical point in discharge planning is to be sure that the patient has an appointment for follow-up so

CHART 26 – 6 • Rehabilitation Strategies Following Stroke

Nursing Responsibilities	Rationale
1. Encourage the patient to do as much of his or her own personal hygiene as possible.	1. Increases independence.
2. Teach activities of daily living (ADLs) with respect to ways to compensate for the patient's disability. (ADLs include dressing, toileting, bathing, eating, gait training.)	2. Provides for alternative methods to overcome disabilities and increases the patient's level of independence.
3. Instruct the patient in bed exercises, such as quadriceps and gluteal setting.	3. Improves muscle tone.
4. Teach the patient transfer techniques (e.g., bed to chair, chair to bed).	4. Increases independence and provides for a greater number of environmental settings for the patient.
5. Provide special skin care, such as lubrication and protection from extremes in temperature, for trophic skin areas.	5. Trophic skin changes are possible with flaccidity.
6. Have the patient dress in his or her own clothes rather than a hospital gown.	6. Improves the patient's self-image and dispels image of the "sick role."
7. Provide for the patient's privacy by screening when he or she is learning new skills (such as relearning to feed self).	7. Preserves the patient's self-esteem and decreases embarrassment if "accidents" happen.
8. Provide emotional support and encouragement.	8. Helps to motivate the patient.
9. Encourage the patient to express feelings.	9. Decreases anxiety and allows for correction of misinformation.
10. Be empathetic with the patient's feelings.	10. Increases the nurse's sensitivity to patient needs.
11. Know what the physiotherapist is doing with the patient.	11. Activities can be reinforced by the nurse.
12. Encourage the family to participate (e.g., demonstrate range-of-motion exercises to the family).	12. Allows family members to feel that they are "doing something to help."

that recovery, new problems, and drug therapy can be monitored (see the earlier section on rehabilitation and the *Post-Stroke Rehabilitation* clinical practice guidelines).

After the patient has been discharged, integration back into community life and roles is important. Rehabilitation continues and is monitored. Depression is common after stroke and is seen in 40% to 50% of patients. Patients and families need to be prepared for this possibility. Pharmacotherapy is quite effective in the treatment of depression. Related nursing diagnoses are listed in the next section.

Patient Education

Patient and family education takes place within a compressed period of time. It is unrealistic to expect that all education can be completed during this short period. Patient education must be viewed along a continuum that extends through the next level of care and in the community by the health care provider. Decide what is critical for the patient to know.

POSSIBLE NURSING DIAGNOSES
• Knowledge Deficit
• Caregiver Role Strain
• Altered Family Processes
• Sexual Dysfunction

POSSIBLE COLLABORATIVE PROBLEMS
• Depression

Medications

The most common drug classifications for patients being discharged with medications are antiplatelets and anticoagulants. Both require special teaching and follow-up. Monitor for obvious and occult bleeding. All patients will need periodic monitoring of coagulation and INR to adjust drug dosage. For patients taking ticlopidine, a complete blood cell count every 2 weeks for 3 months is necessary to monitor for neutropenia. If the patient has not received the drug while in the hospital, he or she needs to be alerted to the possibility of diarrhea or rash. Other medications previously taken before the episode need to be evaluated for continuation. Giving written instructions about drugs, including time and dosage, side effects to expect, adverse reactions, contacting the health provider, and monitoring the schedule, increases adherence to the plan of care.

What to Expect

Both the patient and family need to know what to expect on discharge. The nurse can provide some anticipatory guidance based on the particular needs of the patient. However, the patient and family cannot be prepared for every contingency. It is helpful to plan a time for the nurse to call to assess adjustment to the community and any special problems or concerns. The nurse can triage some problems and manage others completely.

The patient and family need to be aware of community and hospital resources such as stroke support groups, counseling centers, outreach groups, and publications. See "Patient and Family Resources" at the end of the chapter for some helpful booklets and other resources of which patients and families should be made aware.

Recovery

Patients who survive a stroke have some potential for recovery of function. The extent of the stroke and pre-existing disease influence the degree of recovery. Most of natural recovery in motor function and speech occurs in the first 3 to 6 months. However, recovery continues at a slower pace up to a year and beyond with therapy.

REFERENCES

1. National Stroke Association. (1999). *Brain attack statistics*. Englewood, CO: Author.
2. Broderick, J., Brott, T., Kothari, R., et al. (1998). The Greater Cincinnati/Northern Kentucky stroke study: Preliminary first ever and total incidence rates of stroke among blacks. *Stroke, 29,* 415–421.
3. Biller, J., Feinberg, W. M., Castaldo, J. E., Whittemore, A. D., et al. (1998). Guidelines for carotid endarterectomy. *Circulation, 97,* 501–509.
4. Albers, G. W., Hart, R. G., Lutsep, H., Newell, D. W., & Sacco, R. (1999). Supplement to the guidelines for the management of transient ischemic attacks: A statement from the ad hoc committee on guidelines for management of transient ischemic attacks, Stroke Council, American Heart Association. *Stroke, 30,* 2502–2511.
5. Adams, H. P., Brott, T. G., Crowell, R. M., Furlan, A. J., Gomez, C. R., Trotta, J., Helgason, C. M., Marler, J. R., Woolson, R. F., & Zivin, J. A. (1994). Guidelines for the management of patients with acute ischemic stroke. *Circulation, 90*(3), 1588–1601.
6. Adams, H. P., Brott, T. G., Furlan, A. J., et al. (1996). Guidelines for thrombolytic therapy for acute stroke: A supplement to the guidelines for the management of patients with acute ischemic stroke. *Circulation, 94*:1167–1174.
7. Mohr, J. P. (1992). Lacunes. In H. J. M. Barnett, J. P. Mohr, B. M. Stein, & F. M. Yatsu (Eds.). *Stroke: Pathophysiology, diagnosis, and management* (2nd ed., pp. 539–41). New York: Churchill Livingstone.
8. DeGraba, T. J., Fisher, M., & Yatsu, F. M. (1992). Atherogenesis and strokes. In H. J. M. Barnett, J. P. Mohr, B. M. Stein, & F. M. Yatsu (Eds.). *Stroke: Pathophysiology, diagnosis, and management* (2nd ed., pp. 29–48). New York: Churchill Livingstone.
9. Fisher, M. (1991). Atherosclerosis, cellular aspects and potential interventions. *Cerebrovascular Brain Metabolism Review, 3,* 114.
10. Pulsinelli, W. (1992). Pathophysiology of acute ischemic stroke. *Lancet, 339* (8792), 533–536.
11. Back, T. (1998). Pathophysiology of the ischemic penumbra—revision of a concept. *Cellular and Molecular Neurobiology, 18*(6), 621–638.
12. Hossman, K. (1985). Post-ischemic resuscitation of the brain: Selective vulnerability versus global resistance. *Progress in Brain Research, 63,* 3–13.
13. Dutka, A. J., & Hallenbeck, J. M. (1991). Pathophysiology of anoxic-ischemic brain injury. In W. G. Bradley, R. B. Daroff, G. M. Fenichel, & C. D. Marsden (Eds.). *Neurology in clinical practice* (Vol. 2; p. 1354). New York: Butterworth-Heinemann.
14. Hallenbeck, J.M., Dutka, A.J. (1996). Background review and current concepts of reperfusion injury. *Archives of Neurology, 71,* 281–297.
15. Banasik, J. (1995). Cell injury, aging, and death. In L. C. Copstead (Ed.). *Perspectives on pathophysiology* (p. 66). Philadelphia: W. B. Saunders.
16. Pozilli, C., Lenzi, G., & Argentino, C. (1985). Imaging of leukocyte infiltration in human cerebral infarcts. *Stroke, 16,* 251–255.
17. Martin, N. A., & Saver, J. (1999). Intensive care management of subarachnoid hemorrhage, ischemic stroke and hemorrhagic stroke. *Clinical Neurosurgery, 45,* 101–112.
18. Broderick, J. P., Hagen, T., Brott, T., et al. (1995). Hyperglycemia and hemorrhagic transformation of cerebral infarcts. *Stroke, 26,* 484–487.
19. Langhorne, P., & Dennis, M. (1998). *Stroke units: An evidence based approach*. London: BMJ Books.
20. Furlan, A.J. (1992). Transient ischemic attacks: Recognition and management. *Heart Disease and Stroke, 1*(1), 33–38.
21. Yatsu, F. M., Grotta, J. C., & Pettigrew, L. C. (1995). *100 stroke maxims: Stroke* (p. 1). St. Louis: Mosby.
22. Kay, R., Wong, K. S., & Woo, J. (1994). Pilot study of low-molecular weight heparin in the treatment of acute ischemic stroke. *Stroke, 25,* 684–685.
23. Hirsh, J., & Poller, L. (1994). The international normalized ratio. *Archives of Internal Medicine, 154*(3), 282–288.
24. Qureshi, A. I., Luft, A. R., Janardhan, V., et al. (2000). Identification of patients at risk for periprocedural neurological deficits associated with carotid angioplasty and stenting. *Stroke, 31,* 376–382.
25. North American Symptomatic Carotid Endarterectomy Trial Collaborators. (1991). Beneficial effect of carotid endarterectomy in symptomatic patients with high-grade stenosis. *New England Journal of Medicine, 325*(7), 445–453.
26. Barnett, H.J., Taylor, D.W., Eliasziw, M., Fox, A.J., et al. (1998). Benefit of carotid endarterectomy in patients with symptomatic moderate stenosis: North American Symptomatic Carotid Endarterectomy Trial Collaborators. *New England Journal of Medicine, 339,* 1415–1425.
27. Yatsu, F. M., DeGraba, T. J., & Hanson, S. (1992). In H. J. M. Barnett, J. P. Mohr, B. M. Stein, & F. M. Yatsu (Eds.). *Stroke: Pathophysiology, diagnosis, and management* (2nd ed., pp. 1008–1016). New York: Churchill Livingstone.
28. Barnett, H. J. M., Sackett, D., Taylor, D. W., Haynes, B., Peerless, S. J., Meissner, I., Hachinski, V., & Fox, A. (1987). Are the results of the extracranial-intracranial bypass trial generalizable? *New England Journal of Medicine, 316*(13), 800–824.
29. The National Institute of Neurological Disorders and Stroke rt-PA Stroke Study Group. (1995). Tissue plasminogen activator for acute ischemic stroke. *New England Journal of Medicine, 333,* 1581–1587.
30. Bell, T., Kongable, G. L., & Steinberg, G.K. (1998). Mild hypothermia: An alternative to deep hypothermia for achieving neuroprotection. *Journal of Cardiovascular Nursing, 13*(1), 34–44.
31. Maher, J., Hachinski, V. (1992). Hypothermia as a potential treatment for cerebral ischemia. *Cerebrovascular and Brain Metabolism Reviews, 4,* 189–225.
32. Marion, D. W., Penrod, L. E., Kelsey, S. F., et al. (1997). Treatment of traumatic brain injury with moderate hypothermia. *New England Journal of Medicine, 336,* 540–546.
33. Steinberg, G. K., Grant G., & Yoon, E. (1995). Deliberate hypothermia. In R. J. Andrews (Ed.). *Intraoperative neuroprotection* (pp. 65–85). Baltimore: Williams & Wilkins.
34. Kondziolka, D., Weschler, L., Meltzer, C., Thulborn, K., et al. (1999). Phase I safety and effectiveness trial of the cerebral transplantation of LBS neurons in patients with substantial fixed motor deficit following cerebral infarction [abstract]. *Journal of Neurosurgery, 90,* 435A.
35. Gresham, G. E., Duncan, P. W., Stason, W. B., et al. (1995). *Post-stroke rehabilitation* (Clinical Practice Guideline No. 16). (AHCPR Publication No. 95-0662). Rockville, MD: U.S. Depart-

ment of Health and Human Services, Public Health Service, Agency for Health Care Policy and Research.
36. National Stroke Association. (1995). Atherosclerotic intracranial occlusion disease diagnosis, prognosis, and treatment: Part II. *National Stroke Association Stroke Clinical Updates, VI*(4), 13–16.

RESOURCES
Professional
Published Material

BOOKS

Barnett, H. J. M., Mohr, J. P., Stein, B. M., & Yatsu, F. M. (Eds.). (1998). *Stroke: Pathophysiology, diagnosis, and management* (3rd ed.). New York: Churchill Livingstone.

Bogousslavsky, J. (1997). *Acute stroke treatment.* Boston: Blackwell Science.

Bogousslavsky, J., & Caplan, L. (Eds.). (1995). *Stroke syndromes.* New York: Cambridge University Press.

Connors, J.J., & Wojak, J.C. (Eds.). (1999). *Interventional neuroradiology: Strategies and practical techniques.* Philadelphia: W.B. Saunders.

Hachfeld, L. (2000). *Cooking a la heart cookbook: Delicious heart healthy recipes to reduce risk of heart disease and stroke* (3rd ed.). Mankato, MN: Appletree Press.

Sife, W. (1997). *After stroke: Enhancing quality of life.* Binghamton, NY: Haworth Press.

PERIODICALS

Adams, H. P., Brott, T. G., Crowell, R. M., & Furlan, A. J. (1994). Guidelines for the management of patients with acute ischemic stroke. *Circulation, 90*(3), 1588–1601.

Albers, G.W. (1999). Expanding the window for thrombolytic therapy in acute stroke. The potential for acute MRI for patient selection. *Stroke, 30,* 2230–2237.

Albers, G. W., Easton, J. D., Sacco, R. L., et al. (1998). Antithrombotic and thrombolytic therapy for ischemic stroke. *Chest, 114* (Suppl. 2), 683S–698S.

Albers, G. W. (1993). Laboratory monitoring of oral anticoagulant therapy: Are we being misled? *Neurology, 43,* 468–470.

Arvin, B., Neville, F., Barone, F.C., & Feuerstein, G. Z. (1996). The role of inflammation and cytokines in brain injury. *Neuroscience and Behavioral Reviews, 20,* 450–452.

Blank-Reid, C. (1996). How to have a stroke at an early age: The effects of crack, cocaine, and other illicit drugs. *Journal of Neuroscience Nursing, 28*(1), 19–27.

Broderick, J. P., Adams, H. P., Barsan, W., et al. (1999). Guidelines for the management of spontaneous intracerebral hemorrhage. *Stroke, 30,* 905–915.

Bronner, L. L., Kanter, D. S., & Manson, J. E. (1995). Primary prevention of stroke. *New England Journal of Medicine, 333*(21), 1392–1400.

Bussey, H. I., Force, R. W., Bianco T. M., & Leonard, A. D. (1992). Reliance on prothrombin time ratios causes significant errors in anticoagulation therapy. *Archives of Internal Medicine, 152*(Feb), 278–282.

Chimowitz, M. I. (1995). Atherosclerotic intracranial occlusion disease. Diagnosis, prognosis and treatment. Part II. *Stroke: Clinical Updates, 4*(4), 13–16.

Clark, W. M., & Bamwell, S. L. (1995). Interventional neurovascular therapy in cerebrovascular disease. *Stroke: Clinical Updates, 4*(2), 5–8.

Clark, W. M., & Lutsep, H. L. (1999). Medical treatment strategies: Intravenous thrombolysis, neuronal protection, and anti-reperfusion injury agents. *Neuroimaging Clinics of North America, 9*(3), 465–473.

Culebras, A., Kase, C., Masdeu, J.C., et al. (1997). Practice guidelines of the use of imaging in transient ischemic attacks and acute stroke. *Stroke, 28,* 1480–1497.

Dahl, T., Kontny, F., Slagsvold, C.E., et al. (2000). Lipoprotein (a), other lipoproteins and hemostatic profiles in patients with ischemic stroke: The relation to cardiogenic embolism. *Cerebrovascular Diseases, 10*(2), 110–117.

Davis, L. L., & Grant, J. S. (1994). Constructing the reality of recovery: Family home care management strategies. *Advanced Nursing Science, 17*(2), 66–76.

De Graba, T. J., & Pettigrew, L. C. (2000). Why do neuroprotective drugs work in animals but not humans? *Neurology Clinics, 18*(2), 475–493.

Fayad, P, & Awad, I. A. (1998). Surgery for intracerebral hemorrhage. *Neurology, 51*(Suppl. 3), S69–S73.

Fearon, M., & Rusy, K. L. (1994). Transcranial Doppler: Advanced technology for assessing cerebral hemodynamics. *Dimensions of Critical Care Nursing, 13*(5), 241–248.

Feinberg, W. M., Albers, G. W., Barnett, H. J. M., Biller, J., et al. (1994). Guidelines for the management of transient ischemic attacks. *Stroke, 25*(6), 1320–1335.

Furlan, A., Higashida, R., Wechsler, L., et. al. (1999). Intra-arterial prourokinase for acute ischemic stroke. The PROACT II study: a randomized controlled trial. Prolyse in Acute Cerebral Thromboembolism. *Journal of the American Medical Association, 282*(21), 2003–2011.

Ginsberg, M. D., & Pulsinelli, W. A. (1994). The ischemic penumbra, injury thresholds, and the therapeutic window for acute stroke. *Annals of Neurology, 36*(4), 553–554.

Goldstein, L. B. (1995). Common drugs may influence motor recovery after stroke. *Neurology, 45,* 865–871.

Gress, D. R., & Singh, V. (1999). Stroke prevention. *Physical Medicine Rehabilitation Clinics of North America, 10*(4), 827–838.

Hacke, W., Kaste, M., Fieschi, C., Toni, D., Lesaffre, E., & von Kummer, R. (1995). Intravenous thrombolysis with recombinant tissue plasminogen activator for acute hemispheric stroke. *Journal of the American Medical Association, 274*(13), 1017–25.

Hafsteinsdottir, T. B. (1996). Neurodevelopment treatment: Application to nursing and effects on the hemiplegic stroke patient. *Journal of Neuroscience Nursing, 28*(1), 36–47.

Hirsh, J. (1992). Substandard monitoring of warfarin in North America. *Archives of Internal Medicine, 152*(2), 257–258.

Hock, N. H. (1998). Neuroprotective and thrombolytic agents: Advances in stroke treatment. *Journal of Neuroscience Nursing, 30,* 175–184.

Hock, N. H. (1999). Brain attack: The stroke continuum. *Nursing Clinic of North America, 34*(3), 689–723.

Ikeda, Y., & Long, D. M. (1990). The molecular basis of brain injury and brain edema: The role of oxygen free radicals. *Neurosurgery, 27*(1), 1–11.

Kay, R., Wong, K. S., & Woo, J. (1994). Pilot study of low-molecular-weight heparin in the treatment of acute ischemic stroke. *Stroke, 25,* 684–685.

Kay, R., Wong, K. S., Yu Y. L., Chan, Y. W., Tsoi, T. H., & Ahuja, A. T. (1995). Low-molecular-weight heparin for the treatment of acute ischemic stroke. *New England Journal of Medicine, 333*(24), 1588–1593.

Kuether, T. A., Nesbit, G. M., Barnwell, S. L. (1999). Other endovascular treatment strategies for acute ischemic stroke. *Neuroimaging Clinics of North America, 9*(3), 509–525.

Kuster, J. M. (2000). Internet resources for stroke and aphasia. *Topics in Stroke Rehabilitation, 7*(2), 21–31.

Leonard, A. D., & Newburg, S. (1992). Cardioembolic stroke. *Journal of Neuroscience Nursing, 24*(2), 69–78.

Levy, D., Brierly, J., & Plum, F. (1975). Ischemic brain damage in the gerbil in the absence of "no-reflow." *Journal of Neurology, Neurosurgery and Psychiatry, 38,* 1197–1205.

Lugger, K. E. (1994). Dysphagia in the elderly stroke patient. *Journal of Neuroscience Nursing, 26*(2), 78–84.

Mayberg, M. R., Batjer, H. H., Dacey, R., Diringer, M., et al. (1994). Guidelines for the management of aneurysmal subarachnoid hemorrhage. *Circulation, 90*(5), 2592–2605.

National Institute of Neurological Disorders and Stroke, National Institutes of Health, Department of Health and Human Services. (1994). Clinical advisory: Carotid endarterectomy for patients with asymptomatic internal carotid artery stenosis. *Stroke, 25*(12), 2523–2524.

Olsen, T. S. (1989). Improvement of function and motor impairment after stroke. *Journal of Neurological Rehabilitation, 3*(4), 187–192.

Palmer, J. B., & DuChane, A. S. (1991). Rehabilitation of swallowing disorders due to stroke. *Physical Medicine and Rehabilitation Clinics of North America, 3*(3), 529–546.

Perry, I.J. (1999). Homocysteine and risk of stroke. *Journal of Cardiovascular Risk, 6*(4), 235–240.

Pinto, A.M. (1996). AIDS and cerebrovascular disease. *Stroke, 27,* 538–543.

Proot, I. M., Abu-Saad, H. H., de Esch-Janssen, W. P., et al. (2000). Patient autonomy during rehabilitation: The experiences of stroke patients in nursing homes. *International Journal of Nursing Studies, 37*(3), 267–276.

Reeder, G. S., Khandheria, B. K., Seward, J. B., & Tajik, J. (1991). Transesophageal echocardiography and cardiac masses. *Mayo Clinic Proceedings, 66,* 1101–1109.

Sacco, R.L., Kargman, D.E., Gu, Q., et al. (1995). Race-ethnicity and determinants of intracranial atherosclerotic cerebral infarction. The Northern Manhattan Stroke Study. *Stroke, 26,* 14–20.

Sammaritano, L. R., & Gharavi, A. E. (1992). Antiphospholipid antibody syndrome. *Clinics in Laboratory Medicine, 12*(10), 41–59.

Segatore, M. (1996). Understanding central post-stroke pain. *Journal of Neuroscience Nursing, 28*(1), 28–35.

Schievink, W. I. (2001). Spontaneous dissection of the carotid and vertebral arteries. *New England Journal of Medicine, 344*(12), 898–906.

Sherman, D.G., Atkinson, P.R., Chippendale, T., et al. (2000). Intravenous ancrod for treatment of acute ischemic stroke: The STAT study: A randomized, controlled trial. Stroke treatment with ancrod. *Journal of the American Medical Association, 282*(18), 2395–2403.

Shuaib, A. (1994). The role of transcranial Doppler in the study of cerebral vasculature. *Stroke: Clinical Updates, 4*(5), 25–28.

Sisson, R.A. (1998). Life after a stroke: Coping with change. *Rehabilitation Nursing, 23*(4), 198–203.

Taylor, C.L., & Selam, W.R. (2000). Emergency management of ischemic stroke. *Neurosurgery Clinics of North America, 11*(2), 365–375.

Tong, D. C., Bolger, A., & Albers, G. W. (1994). Incidence of transcranial Doppler-detected cerebral microemboli in patients referred for echocardiography. *Stroke, 25*(11), 2138–2141.

Wityk, R,J., & Beauchamp, N.J. (2000). Diagnostic evaluation of stroke. *Neurology Clinics, 18*(2), 1486–1489.

Woods, A. (1999). Patient-teaching aid. "Am I having a stroke"? *Nursing, 29*(12), 32–38.

Websites

See Kuster, J. M. (2000). Internet resources for stroke and aphasia. *Topics in Stroke Rehabilitation, 7*(2), 21—31, for a comprehensive list of websites.

American Stroke Association www.strokeassociation.org

American Heart Association www.americanheart.org/Heart_and_strokeA_Z_guide/stroke.html
7272 Greenville Avenue, Dallas, TX 75231-4596; telephone: (800) 242-8721

National Stroke Association www.stroke.org
9707 E. Easter Lane, Englewood, CO 80112; telephone (800) 787-6537

National Aphasia Association www.aphasia.org
156 Fifth Ave., Suite 707, New York, NY 10010; telephone (800) 922-4622

Family Caregiver Alliance www.caregiver.org
690 Market St., Suite 600, San Francisco, CA 94104; telephone (415) 434-3388

Stroke Information
www.mayo.edu/cerebro/education/stroke.html
Mayo Foundation for Medical Education and Research

Patient and Family

Published Material

American Heart Association. (1994). *Caring for a person with aphasia and stroke.* Dallas, TX: Author.

American Heart Association. (1994). *AHA family guide to stroke treatment, recovery, and prevention.* New York: Times Books.

American Heart Association. (1974). *Stroke: Why do they behave that way?* Dallas, TX: Author.

Gordon, N. F. (1993). *Stroke: Your complete exercise guide.* Dallas, TX: Human Kinetics.

Tanner, D. C. (1997). *The family guide to surviving stroke and communication disorders.* Needham Heights, MA: Allyn & Bacon.

Websites

Stroke Patient Information
www.americanheart.org/Patient_Information/sindex.html.
Stroke and Cerebrovascular Diseases: A Guide for Patients and Their Families.
www.stanford.edu/group/neurology/stroke/strokeinfo.htlm.

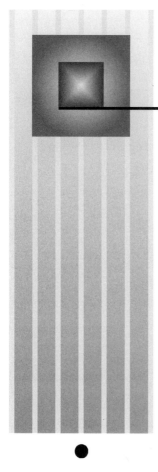

SECTION 8

Nursing Management of Patients With Pain, Seizures, Infections, Degenerative Diseases, and Peripheral Nerve Diseases of the Neurological System

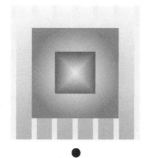

CHAPTER **27**

Management of Chronic Pain: A Neuroscience Perspective

JOANNE V. HICKEY
ROSEMARY P. BROWN

Pain is the most universal of all afflictions. Chronic pain is a complex multidimensional phenomenon that is a significant problem faced by millions of Americans. For many, living with severe pain affects the quality of life of the person and his or her family. The economic impact from traditional and nontraditional treatment, over-the-counter drugs, and loss of productivity in the work environment is estimated at millions of dollars annually. The human misery and suffering caused by chronic pain are immeasurable. The causes of chronic pain are varied, just as the character of chronic pain in an individual is varied. Nurses and other health care professionals involved in neuroscience practice see people who experience chronic pain. Managing people with chronic pain is one of the greatest challenges in health care today. This chapter provides a brief overview of chronic pain management with an emphasis on the role of the nurse as a member of an interdisciplinary team providing medical and surgical management to people with chronic pain.

Pain is an "unpleasant sensory and emotional experience associated with actual or potential tissue damage or described in terms of such damage."[1] Pain is a universal sensation that has plagued mankind since the beginning of time. From medicine men to priests to physicians, relief of pain has been the goal for which generations have searched. The term pain refers to the mechanisms by which noxious stimuli are detected. Pain, however, is more than just detection of noxious stimuli. Noxious stimuli may initiate the pain processes, but the experience of pain depends on many factors, such as experience with the stimuli, the stress or anxiety at the time, and the affective state.

In addition to the general definition of pain, there are distinct definitions for acute and chronic pain. **Acute pain** is defined as "a complex constellation of unpleasant sensory, perceptual, and emotional experiences and certain associated autonomic, psychological, emotional and behavioral responses."[2] Acute pain has the biological function of protecting and alerting the person of potential or real tissue damage. **Chronic pain**, conversely, is described as pain that persists beyond the time when the acute disease course or reasonable time for healing has passed.[2] This time frame is generally considered to be 1 month to 6 weeks. Chronic pain includes pain that is continuous or that recurs at intervals for

months or years. "Chronic pain has no biologic function and causes great social, financial, emotional and physical stress on the patient and family."[3,4] Developing universally accepted terms to describe pain has been difficult, but the International Association for the Study of Pain has attempted to define many of these terms (see Definition of Terms below).

Typically, patients with chronic pain have suffered for years and often present with chronic disability, fear, depression, and pain behavior. **Pain behavior** is a "collection of misdirected activities that are superficially linked to pain but are, often unconsciously, directed at ends other than pain relief."[5] One example of pain behavior is exaggerated complaints of pain to obtain more narcotic medication.

The type of pain treated through neurosurgical procedures is neurogenic pain. **Neurogenic pain** occurs as a result of damage to nerves; it can be peripheral or central in origin. Generally, neurosurgical pain procedures are performed for chronic pain only after all other avenues of pain relief or control have been exhausted.

Neurogenic chronic pain can be caused by a number of conditions and diseases (Chart 27-1). Headache is discussed in Chapter 28, peripheral nerve injuries in Chapter 32, and cranial nerve diseases in Chapter 33.

DEFINITION OF TERMS

The following are definitions of frequently used terms related to pain:

- **Anesthesia dolorosa:** pain in an area or region that is anesthetic
- **Central pain:** pain associated with a lesion of the central nervous system
- **Complex Regional Pain Syndrome (CRPS)-I**, previously called *reflex sympathetic dystrophy:* a variety of syndromes that involve sympathetic hyperactivity associated with persistent pain
- **CRPS-II**, previously called *causalgia:* a syndrome of sustained burning pain and hyperpathia after a traumatic

CHART 27–1 • Common Causes of Chronic Neurogenic Pain

- Spinal cord tumors
- Traumatic spinal injuries
- Intervertebral disc disease
- Spinal stenosis with root compression
- Compression of plexuses
- Thalamic pain syndrome
- Metastatic bone pain (e.g., vertebra)
- Cauda equina disease
- Referred pain
- Peripheral nerve diseases
- Entrapment syndromes
- Mononeuropathy
- Polyneuropathy
- Reflex sympathetic dystrophy
- Causalgia
- Crushing nerve injuries
- Phantom pain

nerve lesion, often combined with vasomotor and psychomotor dysfunction and later trophic changes
- **Deafferentation pain:** pain due to loss of sensory input into the central nervous system, such as occurs with avulsion of the brachial plexus or other types of lesions of peripheral nerves or due to pathology of the central nervous system
- **Dysasthesia:** an unpleasant abnormal sensation, whether spontaneous or evoked
- **Hyperpathia:** excruciating sensitivity to touch
- **Hyperesthesia:** an increased sensitivity to stimulation, excluding special senses
- **Hypoesthesia:** a diminished sensitivity to stimulation, excluding special senses
- **Neuralgia:** pain in distribution of nerve or nerves
- **Neuritis:** inflammation of a nerve or nerves
- **Nociceptor:** a receptor that is preferentially sensitive to a noxious stimulus or to a stimulus that would become noxious if prolonged .
- **Pain threshold:** the least experience of pain that a person can recognize
- **Paresthesia:** an abnormal sensation, whether spontaneous or evoked
- **Trigger point:** a hypersensitive area or site in muscle or connective tissue, usually associated with myofascial pain syndromes

▏▎▍ PAIN THEORIES

Humans have struggled to understand and explain pain since the beginning of time. Some of the earliest pain theories, such as those from ancient Egypt and India, believed that the heart was the center of all sensation and that pain was associated

with demons and gods. This belief lasted almost 2,000 years. It was not until the 17th century that Descartes described some of the beginning concepts of pain pathways from the periphery to the brain. According to Descartes, when the foot comes near a fire, this sensation enters the body and travels up threads to the brain (Fig. 27-1).

The 19th century heralded the study of pain physiology as an experimental science. This research led to the discovery that the dorsal root of the spinal cord was involved with sensory function and the ventral root with motor function. In 1840, Muller wrote that the brain could only receive information about the external environment by way of the sensory nerves. This information, plus discoveries in pain management with morphine, codeine, and regional anesthesia, paved the way for several physiological pain theories. The *specificity theory* noted that there were different afferent sensory neurons for pain and touch. The *intensive theory* supported the idea that any sensory stimulus could become painful if it becomes intense enough.

Debate about these theories and development of several new theories continued into the 20th century. One theory that has become the most widely accepted theory is *the gate control theory* developed by Melzack and Wall in 1965.[18] According to this theory, the central nervous system is surrounded by a barrier that can only be entered by a gate (Fig. 27-2). Pain enters through the gate, and the more pain that is present, the wider the gate opens. The gate can be closed, however, by pulling it shut from the outside (peripheral) or by pushing it shut from the inside (centrally by the brain and

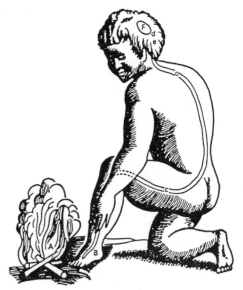

Figure 27–1 • Descartes' (1664) concept of the pain pathway. He writes: "If for example fire (*A*) comes near the foot (*B*), the minute particles of this fire, which as you know move with great velocity, have the power to set in motion this spot of the skin of the foot which they touch, and by this means pulling upon the delicate thread (c.c.) which is attached to the spot of the skin, they open up at the same instant the pore (d.e.) against which the delicate thread ends, just as by pulling at one end of a rope makes to strike at the same instant a bell which hangs at the other end." (From Melzack, R. & Wall, P. D. [1965] Pain mechanisms: A new theory. *Science, 150,* 971–979)

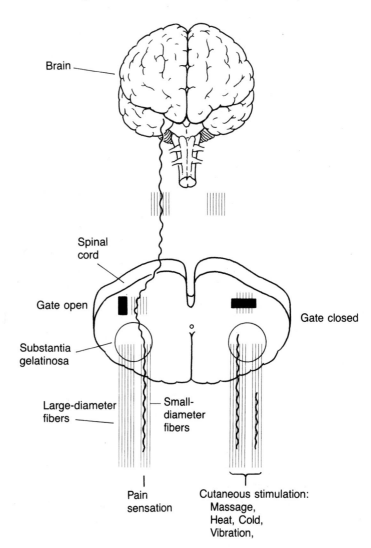

Figure 27–2 • Gate control theory. This shows how thin (tissue damage responding) fibers force open the "gate" into the central nervous system, bringing pain to consciousness. The gate can be pulled shut from the outside, reducing pain, by the activation of large A-beta fibers, rubbing/massage, transcutaneous electrical nerve stimulation, or vibration. The gate can also be pushed shut from inside the central nervous system by various inhibitory systems descending from the brain; some of these inhibitory systems are activated by acupuncture, others by drugs. (From Hudak, C. M. & Gallo, B. M. [1994]. *Critical care nursing: A holistic approach* [6th ed.] [p. 647]. Philadelphia: J. B. Lippincott.)

spinal cord). This theory takes into account the effect of the person's motivational, cognitive, and affective state during the pain experience. According to the gate control theory, the gate can be opened wider by increasing noxious stimulation, anxiety, and depression. The gate can be pushed closed by higher centers of the brain through distraction, relaxation, high levels of endorphins, and enkephalins. The gate can be pulled shut from the periphery through activities such as rubbing and transcutaneous nerve stimulation or vibration.

▌ MECHANISMS OF PAIN

The body has specialized nerve endings involved in the transmission of light, sound, touch, and tissue damage. The nerve endings that recognize tissue damage are called **nociceptors**. Pain can result from stimulation of nociceptors in the skin, viscera, and musculoskeletal structures.

Visceral pain and musculoskeletal pain are not as clearly understood as the physiology behind cutaneous nociception. The cutaneous receptors are affected by thermal, chemical, or mechanical stimulation, which is transmitted through their axons to the spinal cord. These cutaneous receptors have different types of axons: A-beta, A-delta, and C fibers (Fig. 27-3). **A-beta axons** are large, heavily myelinated, and respond to light touch. **A-delta fibers** are smaller, thinly myelinated fibers that conduct "pinprick" or "sharp" pain rapidly. **C fibers** are thin and unmyelinated and transmit burning, aching type pain slowly. For example, a person who burns his or her finger feels immediate pain from stimulation of the A-delta fibers (first pain), followed by a longer-lasting burning sensation from the stimulation of C fibers (second pain).

Tissue damage also causes cell disruption, which leads to release of chemical substances known as *arachidonic acid metabolites*. Prostaglandins and leukotrienes are two of these metabolites. These chemicals result in sensitization of the area and cause previously innocuous stimuli to be perceived as painful. Damaged tissue also releases serotonin, bradykinin, and substance P, which activate nociceptors and further contribute to the pain and inflammation.

Pain impulses enter the spinal cord through the dorsal root synapse in lamina I, II, or V and then cross through the

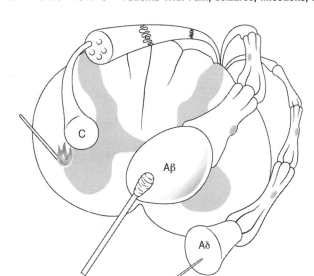

Figure 27–3 • Primary afferent fibers from skin to spinal cord. The largest (Aβ) and most rapidly conducting myelinated fibers are activated by light touch (illustrated by a cotton bud); these are the fibers that are activated by transcutaneous electrical nerve stimulation and vibration. Smaller, more slowly conducting (Aδ) myelinated fibers are activated by pinprick and are involved in acupuncture stimulation. The smallest and slowest fibers (C) are unmyelinated and are excited by tissue damage, here illustrated by a lighted match; they are often called *nociceptors*. (From Carroll, D., & Bowsher, D. [1993]. *Pain management and nursing care* [p. 9]. Boston: Butterworth & Heineman.)

gray matter to the spinothalamic tract. Next, the spinothalamic tract transmits pain to the thalamus. Pain impulses finally proceed to the sensory cortex, frontal lobes, and reticular formation.

▌▌▌▌ MANAGEMENT OF CHRONIC PAIN

The next section examines approaches to chronic pain management and then reviews options in the medical and surgical management of pain.

Multidisciplinary Approach to Chronic Pain Management

A collaborative, interdisciplinary approach to pain control is emphasized in the *Clinical Practice Guidelines* for pain management.[6] Published in 1994, the *Guidelines* are a national standard for chronic pain management. Active participation of the patient and family is required. The goal is to develop an individualized pain control plan that is agreed on by the patient, family, and health care providers. Nonpharmacological and pharmacological therapies to prevent or control pain must be included. After a plan has been developed, the patient's pain must be assessed frequently so that modifications in the plan of care can be made as necessary. Many patients are initially seen and received follow-up care in a pain clinic that offers

a comprehensive, interdisciplinary approach to patient management. Other patients are referred to a pain clinic for an evaluation and recommendations that provide the primary care provider with suggestions for management.

Assessment, Evaluation, and Developing a Plan of Care

Because pain is a subjective phenomenon, it can be challenging to evaluate patients with chronic pain. Instruments such as the McGill Pain Questionnaire (MPQ) may be useful for assessing pain. The MPQ includes 20 categories of descriptive terms addressing the sensory, affective, and evaluative characteristics of pain.[7] In addition to a complete neurological assessment, a pain history must be collected. The following components are included in a pain history:

- **Onset:** Collect a historical sequence of the onset of pain: Were there any precipitating injuries? If so, describe the circumstances and mechanism of injury. Was pain onset gradual or acute?
- **Location:** Draw with your finger where the pain is located. (This can be done as a paper and pencil report on which the patient colors the body areas involved on an anterior and posterior anatomical figure.)
- **Characteristics:** What is the pattern of the pain with time? Is it constant or periodic? What makes it come and go? Does it spread? If so, where? Has it changed with time?
- **Quality:** What does the pain feel like (e.g., stabbing, sharp, dull, "pins and needles," throbbing)?
- **Aggravating circumstances:** What makes the pain worse? What makes it better?
- **Quantity:** How intense is the pain? (Many instruments are available for quantifying the intensity and distress of pain; see Figure 27-4.)
- **Impact:** How does the pain affect your ability to function (activities of daily living [ADLs], job requirements, roles

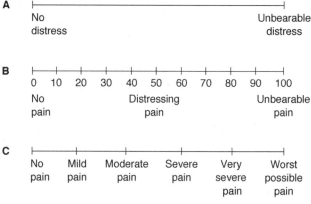

Figure 27–4 • Pain rating scales. Rating scales for measuring pain: (*A*) Visual analog scale; (*B*) numeric pain distress scale; and (*C*) simple descriptive pain intensity scale. (From Acute Pain Management Guideline Panel [1992]. *Acute pain management: Operative or medical procedures and trauma. Clinical practice guideline.* AHCPR Pub. No. 92-0032. Rockville, MD: Agency for Health Care Policy and Research, Public Health Service, U.S. Department of Health and Human Services.)

and responsibilities in the home, family, and community)? How does the pain affect your ability to participate in recreational activities? Are related physiological events associated with the pain (e.g., nausea, vomiting, dizziness, sensory loss)? How do you feel emotionally in response to the pain (e.g., irritable, teary)?

- **Treatment:** How do you treat the pain? Does it work? How much relief do you achieve? What else have you tried in the past? Did it work? If not, why not? If yes, why did you stop using it?

After a complete medical history, pain history, and physical examination have been completed, other discipline-specific data may be added. For example, an evaluation by the pharmacist or physical therapist may be helpful in understanding the pain experience for the individual. After the necessary data have been collected, the interdisciplinary team can confer and develop a pain control plan with the patient and family.

Pain is a collaborative problem requiring a multidisciplinary approach. The nurse as a member of the interdisciplinary collaborative team conducts, collects, and analyzes data to identify nursing diagnoses and develop a nursing treatment plan. The major nursing diagnoses include:

- Acute Pain
- Chronic Pain
- Sensory/Perceptual Alterations

Treatment decisions must be considered in the context of the individual's life and the effect of pain on the quality of life. Many possible combinations of medical and surgical therapies may be helpful for the patient. They are discussed below.

Medical Management of Chronic Pain

Medical management of chronic pain can include nonpharmacological management and pharmacological modalities. In the nonpharmacological approach, there are several traditional and nontraditional methods of managing chronic pain. These are briefly discussed in this section. Often, use of multiple nonpharmacological modalities and pharmacological agents is necessary to optimize patient comfort.

Nonpharmacological Management: Physical and Psychosocial Modalities

The Agency for Health Care Policy and Research has published clinical guidelines for the management of acute pain (1992) and management of cancer pain (1994). The 1994 publication has information related to chronic pain that is helpful.[8,9] Physical modalities include physical therapy, local electrical stimulation, and acupuncture. The major psychosocial modalities include relaxation therapy and imagery, distraction and reframing, biofeedback, patient education, psychotherapy, counseling, and emotional support.

Physical Modalities

Physical Therapy. Physical therapy uses various therapies, such as cutaneous stimulation and exercises designed to decrease discomfort, promote successful engagement in ADLs, and maintain or restore function. Thermotherapy, cryotherapy, massage, and therapeutic exercise are modalities that may be incorporated into the pain management protocol.

Application of dry or moist heat, called **thermotherapy,** can provide analgesic, antispasmodic, and sedative effects.[10] Increasing the temperature of tissue increases blood flow, relaxes motor tone, and increases local cellular metabolism; therefore, this aids in restoring blood flow to tissues and removing waste products. Stretching and active and passive exercise usually follow heat application; these can lengthen and strengthen muscles and tendons and thereby decrease pain. Heat application should be used cautiously in patients with loss of sensation, circulatory compromise, acute inflammation or injury, and malignancy because heat may accelerate cell growth and metastasis.[10]

Cryotherapy, the application of cold, has analgesic, anti-inflammatory and antipyretic effects, and decreased neuromuscular transmission. Initially, cold causes vasoconstriction and decreased nerve conduction, which means fewer noxious stimuli transmissions. This means that the "gate" will not be opened, and pain will not be transmitted to the brain. After the initial response to cold comes the burning sensation that competes with the other pain transmissions to enter the gate. The vasoconstriction caused by the cold also reduces blood flow, which leads to decreased edema, bleeding, and leukocytosis. Cryotherapy should be used cautiously with patients who have circulatory compromise, Raynaud's syndrome, loss of sensation, and cryoglobulinemia.

The primary physiological effect of **massage** is stimulation of peripheral receptors through repetitive and irritative movements of the therapist's hands or massage device. This type of stimulation produces impulses that transmit to the higher brain centers, producing sensations of pleasure or well-being.

Therapeutic exercise is a critical component of all treatment for acute and chronic pain. During the acute phase, exercise is usually limited to range of motion (ROM). However, during the subacute and chronic phases of illness, exercise programs are designed to restore function; increase ROM; decrease muscle spasticity, tension, and contracture; and increase strength and endurance.

Local Electrical Stimulation. The major local electrical stimulation therapy used is called **transcutaneous electrical nerve stimulation (TENS)**. TENS is a method of applying controlled, low-voltage electrical stimulation to large, myelinated peripheral nerve fibers through cutaneous electrodes for the purpose of modulating stimulus transmission and relieving pain.[11]

Acupuncture. **Acupuncture** is an ancient method for the treatment of disease, including pain, that dates back more than 5,000 years in Chinese practice. It is a neurostimulatory technique that involves the insertion of small, solid needles into the skin at varying depths and at specified areas. This drugless, nontoxic, and economical technique has gained acceptance by some as a nontraditional method of managing all types of pain, including chronic. Why it works is unclear.

Psychosocial Modalities

Relaxation Therapy. **Relaxation therapy** is a strategy that can be used to decrease stress and pain and regain self-control. It is believed to decrease pain by causing production of endorphins. Physiologically, relaxation lowers blood pressure, respiratory rate, heart rate, and muscle tension and contraction. There are two categories of mental and physical relaxation. The first category involves muscle relaxation, which then facilitates the response of mental relaxation. Examples of this approach are deep breathing, yoga, and progressive muscle relaxation. Twenty minutes, free from distraction, are necessary for relaxation to occur. A sample of relaxation therapy is as follows:

> We begin by closing our eyes and concentrating on feeling what our body is like when it is at rest. Secondly, we impose tension on it and feel the difference. Then, we relax the body and feel a third quality, that of deep relaxation. Finally, it is possible to discover another state, what we call a "letting go," when the body feels different again.[12]

Relaxation tapes can be purchased in bookstores and health centers for use at home or in health care facilities.

Meditation and Imagery. The second category of relaxation focuses mental relaxation to achieve physical relaxation. **Meditation** requires the ability to concentrate and takes practice. **Imagery** is a cognitive-behavioral strategy of focusing on a personalized pleasant mental image to aid in relaxation. Relaxation techniques are most helpful when combined with personalized imagery.[13]

Distraction and Reframing. **Distraction** is a cognitive strategy of focusing attention on stimuli other than pain or the accompanying negative emotions.[14] Distraction may be internal (e.g., praying) or external (e.g., listening to music, watching television). **Reframing** is a cognitive strategy that teaches the person to monitor and evaluate negative thoughts and images and replace them with more positive ones. For example, if the person is preoccupied with thoughts of being unable to conduct his or her normal business because of pain, substituting self-messages that remind the person that often activities are not negated by pain increases personal control.

Biofeedback. **Biofeedback** is a process in which a person learns to influence two types of physiological responses: those that are not ordinarily under voluntary control and those that are ordinarily regulated, but as a result of disease or trauma, regulation has been interrupted.[15]

Patient Education. Patient education is a cognitive strategy of providing the patient and family with comprehensive and accurate information about pain, pain assessment, and the use of drugs and other methods of pain control with an emphasis on effective management. The goal of patient education is to involve the patient actively in his or her pain management and reaffirm the control of the person to successfully manage self and pain.[16] In addition, providing patients with the names and addresses of community resources can enhance sources of information and support for the patient and family.

Psychotherapy, Counseling, and Emotional Support. Depression, anxiety, and maladaptive coping or behavior are often related to chronic pain. A short or long course of physiotherapy, counseling, structured support, and peer support groups may be helpful to support the person and develop effective coping strategies.

Pharmacological Management: Non-narcotics, Opioid Narcotics, and Adjuvant Analgesics

The pain experience is highly individualized; therefore, drug therapy to decrease the pain experience must also be individualized. Analgesics are the pharmacological mainstay of pain management for acute and chronic pain. Analgesics can be broadly divided into non-narcotics and opioid narcotics. Generally, opioid-narcotic analgesics relieve acute pain or cancer pain, whereas non-narcotics are recommended for chronic pain. Additionally, adjuvant analgesic drugs have analgesic properties or can enhance the effect of the analgesics. The drug classifications included in the adjuvant analgesic drug category are antidepressants, anticonvulsants, and anxiolytics.

Non-narcotic Analgesics

Aspirin and aspirin-like drugs, such as acetaminophen and other nonsteroidal anti-inflammatory drugs (NSAIDs), are the major non-narcotic analgesics. In addition to their analgesic properties, these drugs have antipyretic and anti-inflammatory effects. The one currently used exception is acetaminophen, which has no anti-inflammatory properties. These drugs relieve pain by inhibiting the release of prostaglandins and thromboxane 2, which are associated with pain. Non-narcotic analgesics are most effective for mild-to-moderate levels of pain.

Opioid-Narcotic Analgesics

An **opioid** by definition is any drug, either natural or synthetic, that has similar actions to those of morphine. **Narcotic** can mean an analgesic that has central nervous system depressant effects and can cause physical dependence. Narcotic is also a term that has been associated with a group of illegal drugs, such as marijuana and cocaine. For this reason, opioid is a better term to describe this group of drugs. Opioids act on receptors within and outside the central nervous system. Their effects are analgesia, respiratory depression, sedation, and euphoria. These drugs are effective against moderate-to-severe pain, but there are many side effects, some of which are life threatening; these include respiratory depression, orthostatic hypotension, cough suppression, nausea, vomiting, constipation, and urinary retention. Physical tolerance, dependency, and abuse occur with prolonged use of opioids.

It is generally believed that opioids are best suited for acute pain, but under certain conditions opioids can be beneficial for chronic pain. Some guidelines have been proposed for selection of patients for long-term use of opioid-narcotics:[17]

- Persistent pain is the major impediment to function (pain is disabling).
- Psychological problems are not present or considered pertinent.
- All other analgesic (non-narcotic) medications have failed.
- There is no history of substance abuse.
- A primary care physician will assume responsibility for monitoring the patient and response to the drug.

A frequent drug of choice is methadone (Dolophine) for the following reasons: it has properties similar to those of morphine, a long duration of action, and good oral absorption. Methadone is, therefore, a good opioid choice for long-term chronic pain management.

Adjuvant Analgesics

The adjuvant analgesic drug classes that enhance the effect of analgesics are antidepressants, anticonvulsants, and anxiolytics.

Antidepressants. Depression and chronic pain go hand in hand, with one reinforcing the other. Lack of sufficient norepinephrine and serotonin may be the cause of depression, and these substances play a role in pain transmission. Therefore, depression enhances the pain experience. Amitriptyline (Elavil), doxepin (Sinequan), imipramine (Tofranil), and nortriptyline (Pamelor) are a few of the widely used antidepressants.

Anticonvulsants. Anticonvulsants stabilize the neuronal membrane, reducing neuronal excitability. These drugs are used most frequently for pain that has a sharp, electrical, shooting quality, such as that of trigeminal neuralgia. Carbamazepine (Tegretol) and phenytoin (Dilantin) are two common anticonvulsants used in conjunction with analgesics.

Anxiolytics. Anxiety can increase the perception of pain and can prevent the individual from tolerating pain. The benzodiazepines, such as alprazolam (Xanax), clorazepate (Tranxene), and diazepam (Valium), are common anxiolytic drugs. Ba-

clofen (Lioresal) is a muscle relaxant used to relieve some types of pain associated with spasm and muscle tension.

Surgical Management of Chronic Pain

Surgical procedures for neurogenic pain are directed toward interrupting input of nociceptors. This interruption can occur at different neuronal levels. Pain sensations are transmitted by delta type A and type C fibers from peripheral receptors to the spinal cord. This peripheral tract contains the **first-order neurons**. Pain transmission continues through the dorsal root of the spinal nerve into the dorsal root entry zone gray matter of the spinal cord. The pain transmission pathways in the spinal cord are composed of the **second-order neurons**. The **third-order neurons** transmit the pain sensation from the thalamus to the cortex.

First-Order Neurons

Neurosurgical procedures directed at first-order neurons include neurectomy and rhizotomy. A **neurectomy** is the resection of one or more peripheral branches of cranial or spinal nerves. Neurectomy is a safe, quick procedure requiring only local or regional anesthesia. However, there are several problems with neurectomies. First, peripheral nerves contain motor and sensory input, so motor loss accompanies the loss of pain sensation. Pain relief is often only temporary following neurectomies, and the return of pain can include a new pain syndrome, such as anesthesia dolorosa. Additionally, the specific peripheral nerves are often difficult to isolate.

For these reasons, neurectomies are infrequently performed today. One exception is the peripheral neurectomy for treatment of trigeminal neuralgia (tic douloureux) when gangliolysis has failed or when microvascular decompression is not possible. Table 27-1 outlines post-neurectomy assessment and monitoring.

A **rhizotomy** is the selective destruction of the spinal nerve dorsal root to relieve pain. Indications for a rhizotomy are a limited area of pain and a normal life expectancy. Generally, selective nerve blocks are performed to determine if a rhizotomy *will* be effective. If a patient obtains relief from a selective nerve block, then a rhizotomy should

 Table 27-1 • POSTOPERATIVE OBSERVATIONS AND ASSESSMENT AFTER SPECIFIC NEUROSURGICAL PROCEDURES

PROCEDURE	OBSERVATIONS/ASSESSMENT
Neurectomy	Hematoma, ecchymosis, signs and symptoms of infections, wound drainage, motor and sensory function to the involved area
Rhizotomy	Cerebrospinal fluid (CSF) leakage, wound drainage, signs and symptoms of infection or meningitis, motor and sensory function, respiratory depression (especially in bilateral cervical rhizotomy), and bowel, bladder, and sexual dysfunction (especially in sacral rhizotomy)
Cordotomy	CSF leakage, wound drainage, signs and symptoms of infection or meningitis, hypotension, respiratory depression, urinary dysfunction, ipsilateral motor loss, and Horner's syndrome (complications most frequent with bilateral, open cordotomies)
Dorsal root entry zone (DREZ) therapy/procedure	CSF leakage, wound drainage, signs and symptoms of infection or meningitis, and motor and sensory dysfunction

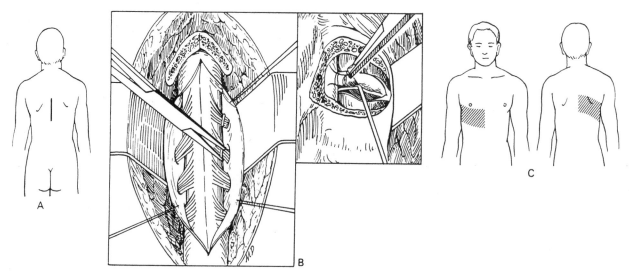

Figure 27–5 • Dorsal rhizotomy. (*A*) Location of midline dorsal incision for T4–T7 dorsal rhizotomy. (*B*) Intradural dorsal rhizotomy with application of metal clip on the rootlets of a root already transected above and being applied to the rootlets of a root below just prior to resectioning them. Inset on the right depicts extradural dorsal rhizotomy showing division of the dorsal root central to the ganglion prior to extirpation of the ganglion by a lesion which will be made just distal to the ganglion. (*C*) Expected area of sensory loss following right T4–T7 dorsal rhizotomy. (From Bonica, J. J. [1990]. *The management of pain* [2nd ed.] [p. 2049]. Philadelphia: Lea & Febiger.)

be effective to relieve pain. Because only the dorsal root is affected, the ventral (motor) fibers are spared. The open rhizotomy procedure requires laminectomies and is performed on the same side as the pain. The dura is opened, and the nerve rootlets are identified. The rootlets are then transected (Fig. 27-5). As a result of a rhizotomy, there is complete sensory loss; therefore, no pain, temperature, or pressure sensations remain intact.

Although these procedures interrupt only sensory input, movements of joints and muscles, a motor function, frequently depend on sensory information. Loss of sensory input can directly result in loss of motor function. For this reason, rhizotomies are generally indicated for thoracic and high cervical pain relief and are not recommended for pain in extremities or low lumbar areas. Rhizotomies have been successful in relieving sacral pain owing to malignancy or postradiation pain. See Table 27-1 for postoperative rhizotomy assessment and monitoring.

Second-Order Neurons

Neurosurgical procedures on second-order neurons involve interruption of the lateral spinothalamic tract within the spinal cord. Cordotomy and dorsal root entry zone lesion surgeries are examples of second-order neuron procedures.

A **cordotomy** is the operative procedure by which the spinothalamic tract is interrupted for the relief of pain. Cordotomies are considered for patients with intractable malignant and nonmalignant pain below the level of the mandible. Cordotomies can be performed as a percutaneous or open procedure. The percutaneous cordotomy can be successfully performed on cancer patients who cannot undergo major surgery (Fig. 27-6). This procedure involves introducing a spinal needle at the level of C1 to C2 with guidance from a myelogram. The anterior border of the spinal cord is visualized and an electrode inserted through the spinal needle; lesions are produced (Fig. 27-7). Access for an open

cordotomy can be through an anterior or a posterior approach (Fig. 27-8). General anesthesia and a laminectomy are necessary. The complication rate is higher for the open cordotomy. The most common complications are hypotension, respiratory depression, urinary tract dysfunction, and ipsilateral motor loss. The result of the percutaneous and open cordotomy is anesthesia *below the level of the lesions.*

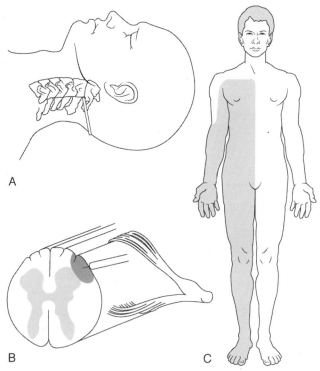

Figure 27–6 • (*A*) Site of percutaneous C1–C2 cordotomy. (*B*) Lesion produced by percutaneous C1–C2 cordotomy. (*C*) Extent of analgesia produced by left C1–C2 percutaneous cordotomy.

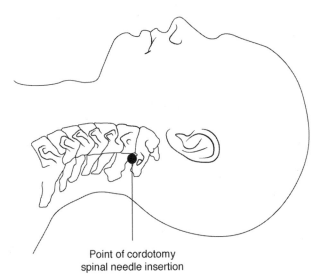

Point of cordotomy
spinal needle insertion

Figure 27–7 • Site of insertion of needle for percutaneous C1–C2 cordotomy.

A **dorsal root entry zone (DREZ)** is an operative procedure that involves making a series of lesions in the DREZ of the spinal cord (Fig. 27-9). These lesions are usually made in the substantia gelatinosa and surrounding fibers. This procedure is indicated for central pain disorders, such as brachial plexus avulsion, postherpetic neuralgia, phantom limb pain, postparaplegia pain, and severe facial pain. This surgery requires laminectomies and general anesthesia. The postoperative period requires 2 to 4 days of bedrest followed by intensive physical therapy. The main complications are wound infection, cerebrospinal fluid leak, and ataxia. Patients who have pain in an extremity with intact motor function may suffer a transient incoordination postoperatively because the spinal cerebellar tract is crossed by the electrode. This usually resolves in weeks to months, but with repeated DREZ procedures, it may become a permanent problem. Table 27-1 shows assessment and monitoring after a DREZ procedure.

Third-Order Neurons

Neurosurgical procedures to relieve pain at the level of third-order neurons are directed at the frontal lobe of the cerebral cortex or thalamus. Cingulotomy and thalamotomy are examples of these procedures. These procedures are done stereotactically or with electrical stimulation.

Cingulotomy. The cingulum is an area in the frontal lobe that is part of the limbic system. Pathophysiology in this area has been associated with the suffering part of pain. Surgical procedures with the creation of lesions in this area are associated with pain relief without measurable deterioration in personality or intellect. The procedure is performed stereotactically through burr holes, in which lesions are created using a radiofrequency technique (Fig. 27-10). The most common indication for a cingulotomy is neoplastic pain associated with depression and suffering. The surgery is contraindicated in patients with bleeding disorders or uncontrolled hypertension. Headache and fever often occur postoperatively, but the greatest danger of the procedure is postoperative intracranial hemorrhage. Other complications include seizures and urinary incontinence.

A **thalamotomy** involves making lesions stereotactically in the thalamus, resulting in interruption of the spinothalamic tract and the absence of pain and temperature opposite to and below the level of the lesions (Fig. 27-11). The most common indication for a thalamotomy is cancer pain. Pain relief is excellent in the early postoperative period, but the relief diminishes with time. Intracranial hemorrhage and infection are rare but dangerous complications of this procedure. Ataxia and mild apathy may occur postoperatively.

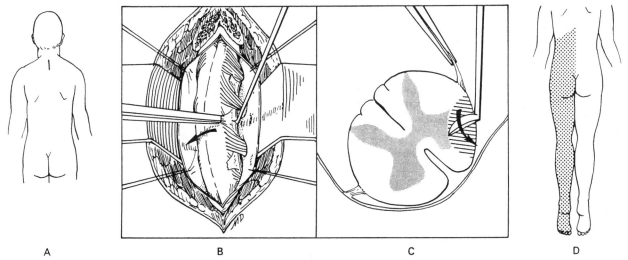

A   B   C   D

Figure 27–8 • (A) Site of open thoracic cordotomy. (B and C). Method of performing open thoracic cordotomy. (B) After T1–T2 laminectomy, the dura is opened and the dentate ligaments sectioned. The linea alba is grasped in a hemostat and the spinal cord is rotated 45°. (C) A special cordotomy knife is used to section the anterolateral quadrant. (D) Extent of analgesia on dorsal surface produced by right T1–T2 open cordotomy. (From Bonica, J. J. [1990]. *The management of pain* [2nd ed.] [p. 2071]. Philadelphia: Lea & Febiger.)

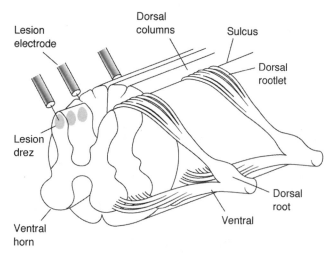

Figure 27–9 • Schematic drawing showing the dorsal root entry zone (DREZ) and the region for DREZ lesions.

General Preoperative Management

Patients hospitalized for a neurosurgical pain procedure must be managed by a multidisciplinary team because chronic pain is a complex phenomenon involving physical, psychological, and emotional components. Typically, neurosurgical pain procedures are not considered the first-line treatment for pain. Therefore, years of a pain syndrome and pain behavior reinforcement may occur before the patient is finally recommended for surgery. People with chronic pain, therefore, often have a history of addiction to pain medications; alteration in functional level; loss of self-esteem and social and financial support; and a history of repeated failed procedures to relieve pain. Comprehensive multidisciplinary pain management is usually found at major health science centers. Therefore, patients may need to travel long distances to centers where these neurosurgical procedures are performed, in which case their support systems may be limited.

A preadmission contact is helpful to provide information about local lodging, the hospital admitting procedure, and a brief description of the hospitalization. This information can be conveyed by telephone, letter, or a patient education brochure. In addition, a clinical pathway can be created for these neurosurgical procedures. This pathway can be shared with the patient and assists greatly in developing realistic expectations and outlining day-by-day activities.

The usual preoperative routines and preparation common for any surgical procedure are followed. In addition, the following baseline data are collected:

- Baseline functional assessment by physical and occupational therapy
- In-depth pain assessment, including pattern, location, associated symptoms, and relieving and aggravating factors (conducted by a professional familiar with detailed pain assessment and patient management)
- Psychological testing (required by some physicians), which can assist with screening for psychiatric diagnosis and as a baseline measure for assessing the treatment protocol

Other specific teaching and points of care include:

- Preoperative teaching is essential; patients need an explanation about the procedure and immediate postoperative management. Realistic expectations about outcomes within a given time frame must be clear to the patient and family.
- Skin preparation depends on the area of the surgery. Typically, skin preparation for stereotactic procedures is done in the operating room. Because the dura is often opened during the procedure, it is common to administer steroids before and often during surgery to decrease swelling and inflammation. High-dose methylprednisolone is commonly used for the DREZ procedure.
- Application of elastic stockings and sequential compression boots is necessary to prevent deep vein thrombosis and pulmonary embolism.
- Patients undergoing lumbar or sacral laminectomies should expect some spasms in the lower back, thigh, or abdominal regions.
- The following should be explained to patients:
  - Log-rolling technique
  - Postoperative pain medication administration
  - Incentive spirometry or deep breathing exercises
  - Postoperative monitoring (vital signs, dressing checks, turning)
  - Importance of maintaining proper body alignment after surgery
  - Pain scale used to quantify the severity of pain
  - Neurological assessment, especially of motor and sensory function

An understanding of what to expect after surgery and the patient's role is important to pain control in the postoperative period because anxiety and fear contribute to pain perception.

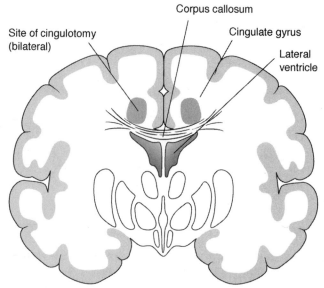

Figure 27–10 • Coronal section of brain indicating sites of lesions for cingulotomy.

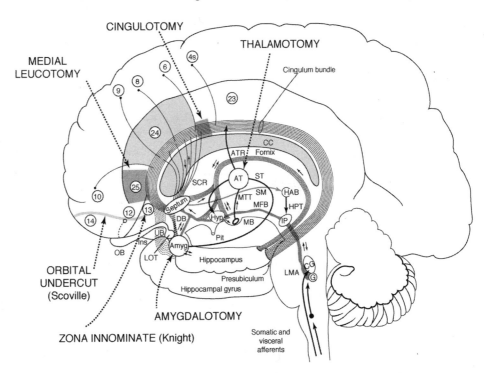

Figure 27–11 • Sites of limbic system surgery. (OB = olfactory bulb; LOT = lateral olfactory striae; INS = insula; UB = uncinate bundle; DB = diagonal band of Broca; AMYG = amygdala; SCR = subcallosal radiations; HYP = hypothalamus; AT = anterior thalamus; MB = mammillary body; MTT = mammillothalamic tract [Vicq d'Azyr's tract]; ATR = anterior thalamic radiations; ST = stria terminalis; HAB = habenula; MFB = medial forebrain bundle; SM = stria medullaris; HPT = habenulointerpeduncular tract [fasciculus retroflexus of Meynert]; IP = interpeduncular nucleus; LMA = limbic midbrain area of Nauta; G = nucleus of Gudden; CG = central gray; CC = corpus callosum.)

General Postoperative Management

After the postanesthesia recovery period, some patients may be transferred to the surgical or neuroscience intensive care unit for 24 hours for respiratory monitoring and pain control. Pain medication is administered during the postoperative period, and pain assessments are made regarding the level of postoperative pain compared with the original pain. Pain control is often best managed by a multidisciplinary pain team, which includes the clinical pharmacist. Some patients experience complete relief immediately after surgery, but for others, pain subsides gradually.

Bed rest may be maintained for 2 to 4 days depending on the type of surgery. For example, after a DREZ procedure, patients typically remain on bed rest for 3 to 4 days. The level of elevation of the head of the bed also depends on the area of the surgery. After a lumbar procedure, elevation of the head of the bed is restricted for 24 to 48 hours to encourage dural healing. All post-laminectomy patients need to be log rolled and wear antiembolic stockings with sequential compression boots. Physical therapy will initially begin on the first postoperative day with gentle ROM and isometric exercises. As the patient is mobilized, physical therapy will increase the level of exercise. Occupational therapy should reevaluate the patient before discharge. Physical and occupational therapists should make recommendations for equipment, home therapy, and a continued exercise program.

Pain control during the postoperative period can be complex because the patient has acute pain from the operative site and remnants of chronic pain. The goal must be to control the postoperative pain. As hospitalization progresses, the question of weaning from previous analgesics for chronic pain must be addressed. Hospitalization time is short, and patients are often discharged with considerable postoperative discomfort. Before discharge, patients should ideally be on oral pain medication and should have

a physician who will assist them through the process of withdrawal from the pain medication. Some patients will require admission to a pain withdrawal center; others will be weaned quickly as their original pain is relieved.

PAIN AND PAIN MANAGEMENT: THE FUTURE

Research into the understanding of the pain phenomenon, its human impact, and treatment options is exciting and is blazing new frontiers of inquiry. The age of molecular biology and neuroimmunology has opened the doors to new understandings about the interplay of the mind on the body and the ability to control pain. These breakthroughs come at a time of a changing health care system and a managed care environment in which treatment options to patients are increasingly controlled by third-party payers. The real challenge is for health care providers to demonstrate the cost effectiveness and improved health that can be achieved for people who suffer from chronic pain.

REFERENCES

1. Mersky, H., & Bogduk, N. (Eds.) (1994). *Classification of chronic pain: Descriptions of chronic pain syndromes and definitions of pain terms* (2nd ed.). Seattle, WA: International Association for the Study of Pain.
2. Bonica, J. J. (1990). *The management of pain* (Vols. I & II, 2nd ed.). Philadelphia: Lea & Febiger.
3. Carroll, D., & Bowsher, D. (1993). *Pain management and nursing care.* Boston: Butterworth-Heinemann.
4. Mersky, H. (1986). Classification of chronic pain: Description of chronic pain syndromes and definitions. *Pain, 3*(Suppl.), SI 225.
5. Hyman, S. E., & Cassem, N. H. (1995). Pain. In D. C. Dale & D. D. Federman (Eds.). *Scientific American medicine* (Vol. III, p. 1). New York: Scientific American.

6. Jacox, A., Carr, D. B., Payne, R., et al. (1994). *Management of cancer pain. Clinical practice guideline.* AHCPR Pub. No. 94-0592. Rockville, MD: Agency for Health Care Policy and Research, Public Health Service, U. S. Department of Health and Human Services.

7. Melzak, R. (1975). The McGill pain questionnaire: Major properties and scoring methods. *Pain, 1,* 277.

8. Acute Pain Management Guideline Panel (1992). *Acute pain management: Operative or medical procedures and trauma. Clinical practice guideline.* AHCPR Pub. No. 92-0032. Rockville, MD: Agency for Health Care Policy and Research, Public Health Service, U. S. Department of Health and Human Services.

9. Jacox, A., Carr, D. B., Payne, R., et al. (1994). *Management of cancer pain. Clinical practice guideline* (p. 2). AHCPR Pub. No. 94-0592. Rockville, MD: Agency for Health Care Policy and Research, Public Health Service, U. S. Department of Health and Human Services.

10. Bonica, J. J. (1990). *The management of pain* (Vols. I & II, 2nd ed., p. 1770.). Philadelphia: Lea & Febiger.

11. Jacox, A., Carr, D. B., Payne, R., et al. (1994). *Management of cancer pain. Clinical practice guideline* (p. 79). AHCPR Pub. No. 94-0592. Rockville, MD: Agency for Health Care Policy and Research, Public Health Service, U. S. Department of Health and Human Services.

12. Carroll, D., & Bowsher, D. (1993). *Pain management and nursing care* (p. 133). Boston: Butterworth-Heinemann.

13. Jacox, A., Carr, D. B., Payne, R., et al. (1994). *Management of cancer pain. Clinical practice guideline* (p. 82). AHCPR Pub. No. 94-0592. Rockville, MD: Agency for Health Care Policy and Research, Public Health Service, U. S. Department of Health and Human Services.

14. McCaffery, M., & Beebe, A. (1989). *Pain: Clinical manual for nursing practice.* St. Louis: C. V. Mosby.

15. Jacox, A., Carr, D. B., Payne, R., et al. (1994). *Management of cancer pain. Clinical practice guideline* (p. 185). AHCPR Pub. No. 94-0592. Rockville, MD: Agency for Health Care Policy and Research, Public Health Service, U. S. Department of Health and Human Services.

16. Jacox, A., Carr, D. B., Payne, R., et al. (1994). *Management of cancer pain. Clinical practice guideline* (p. 83). AHCPR Pub. No. 94-0592. Rockville, MD: Agency for Health Care Policy and Research, Public Health Service, U. S. Department of Health and Human Services.

17. Portenoy, R. K. (1989). Opioid therapy in the management of chronic low back pain. In C. D. Tollidon (Ed.). *Interdisciplinary rehabilitation of low back pain* (pp. 137–157). Baltimore: Williams & Wilkins.

18. Melzack, R., & Wall, P. D. (1965). Pain mechanisms: A new theory. *Science, 150,* 971–979.

RESOURCES

Professional

Books

American Physical Therapy Association. (1985). *Application of TENS in the management of patients with pain.* Alexandria, VA: Author.

Aronoff, G. M. (1999). *Evaluation and treatment of chronic pain* (3rd ed.). Baltimore, MD: Williams & Wilkins.

Blumenkopf, B. (1994). Chronic pain. In S. S. Rengachary & R. H. Wilkins (Eds.). *Principles of neurosurgery* (pp. 48-1–48-9). St. Louis: Wolfe.

Bonica, J. J. (1990). *The management of pain* (Vols. I & II, 2nd ed.). Philadelphia: Lea & Febiger.

Borysenko, J. (1987). *Minding the body, mending the mind.* Reading, MA: Addison-Wesley.

Caillet, R. (1993). *Pain: Mechanisms and management.* Philadelphia: F. A. Davis.

Carroll, D., & Bowsher, D. (1993). *Pain management and nursing care.* Boston: Butterworth-Heinemann.

Nashold, B. S., Jr., & Ovelmen-Levitt, J. (Eds.) (1991). *Deafferentation pain syndromes: Pathophysiology and treatment.* New York: Raven Press.

Philips, H. C., & Rachman, S. (1996). *The psychological management of chronic pain: Treatment manual* (2nd ed.). New York: Springer.

Portency, R. K. & Kanner, R. M. (1996). *Pain management: Theory and practice.* Philadelphia: F. A. Davis.

Periodicals

Gilbert, M., Counsell, C. M., Martin, P., & Snively, C. (1994). Spinal stable pain: Nursing implications. *Journal of Neuroscience Nursing, 26*(6), 347–351.

Iacono, R. P., Guthkelch, A. N., & Boswell, M. V. (1991). Dorsal root entry zone stimulation for deafferentation pain. *Stereotactic Functional Neurosurgery, 59,* 56–61.

Kost, R. G. & Straus, S. E. (1996). Posthepatic neurologic-pathogenesis treatment and prevention. *New England Journal of Medicine, 335*(1), 32–42.

McHugh, J. M., & McHugh, W. B. (2000). Pain: Neuroanatomy, chemical mediators, and clinical implications. *AACN Clinical Issues, 11*(2), 168–178.

Nashold, B. S., Jr., El-Naggar, A. O., Ovelmen-Levitt, J., & Abdul-Hak, M. (1994). A new design of radiofrequency lesion electrodes for use in the caudalis nucleus DREZ operation. *Journal of Neurosurgery, 80,* 1116–1120.

Rawlings, C., III, Rossitch, E., & Nashold, B. S., Jr. (1992). The history of neurosurgical procedures for the relief of pain. *Surgical Neurology, 38,* 454–463.

Richardson, D. R. (1995). Deep brain stimulation for the relief of chronic pain. *Neurosurgery Clinics of North America, 6*(1), 135–144.

Segatore, M. (1994). Understanding chronic pain after spinal cord injury. *Journal of Neuroscience Nursing, 26*(4), 230–236.

Tasker, R. R., DeCarvalho, G. T. C., & Dolan, E. J. (1992). Intractable pain of spinal cord origin: Clinical features and implications for surgery. *Journal of Neurosurgery, 77,* 373–378.

Thomas, D. G. T. (1993). Brachial plexus injury: Deafferentation pain and dorsal root entry zone (DREZ) coagulation. *Clinical Neurology and Neurosurgery, 95*(Suppl.), S48–S49.

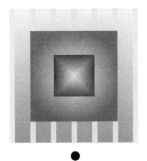

CHAPTER 28

Headaches

JOANNE V. HICKEY

This chapter provides an overview of the most common of human ailments, headaches. Although primary headaches are the focus, a discussion of secondary headaches and how they relate to neurological problems is included.

Headache, defined as diffuse pain in some part of the head or pain located above the orbitomeatal line of the head,[1] is a very common problem experienced by up to three fourths of the population each year. Only 5% seek medical attention, however. Of the 18 million patients who visit health care facilities each year for headache, about half have migraine headaches. The cost of missed workdays and medical expenses associated with headache is about $50 billion annually.[2]

In general, headaches are classified as primary or secondary. A **primary headache** is a headache for which no organic cause can be identified. This category includes migraine, tension-type headache, and cluster headache unassociated with structural lesions or organic causes. About 90% to 98% of headaches are primary. **Secondary headaches** are associated with various underlying primary organic etiologies, such as a tumor or an aneurysm.

In 1988, the International Headache Society (IHS) published the first international headache classification including operational diagnostic criteria for all headache disorders. Translated into many languages, it is accepted throughout the world. Many terms formerly used to classify and describe headaches have been changed in the interest of clarity. The 13 main headache types in the IHS (Table 28-1) provide a framework for this chapter. Identifying the specific type of headache is the key to appropriate treatment and patient education.

The extent of the impact a headache has on a person's life varies greatly. In most instances, a headache is an occasional event accompanied by mild discomfort and relieved by an over-the-counter analgesic. For some people, a headache is a frequent and severe event resulting in disability and a decreased quality of life and often interfering with interpersonal relationships, work productivity, and family life. For others, a headache is a symptom of a serious underlying condition requiring immediate intervention.

HEADACHE: ANATOMICAL CONSIDERATIONS AND PATHOPHYSIOLOGY

Anatomical Considerations

Not all anatomical structures of the head and intracranial space are sensitive to pain. Those structures that do have pain receptors (nociceptors) and are capable of causing pain include the following:

- Extracranial: skin, scalp, muscles, fascia, and parts of the eye and ear
- Meninges: parts of the dura mater at the base of the brain near large vessels
- Cranial nerves: trigeminal, facial, glossopharyngeal, and vagus
- Other nerves: second and third cervical nerves

Those structures that lack nociceptors and are not pain sensitive include the skull, the pia arachnoid, parts of the dura mater, cerebral and cerebellar (parenchyma) tissue, and the ependymal lining and choroid plexuses of the ventricles. The brain itself is not sensitive to pain.

Pathophysiology

Headache is experienced when there is traction, pressure, displacement, inflammation, or dilation of nociceptors in areas sensitive to pain. Pain is transmitted from the periphery by small myelinated fibers and unmyelinated c-fibers. These fibers terminate in the dorsal horn of the spinal cord and the trigeminal nucleus caudalis. Secondary neurons from the dorsal horn reach the thalamus through the spinal thalamic pathways. Neurotransmitters also have a role in pain. Substance P, a neuropeptide, is a pain neurotransmitter for the primary sensory neurons. Interneurons in the dorsal horn use enkephalins and possibly gamma-aminobutyric acid (GABA) as inhibitory neurotransmitters to block pain transmission.[3]

Table 28-1 • INTERNATIONAL HEADACHE SOCIETY CLASSIFICATION OF HEADACHE*

1. Migraine (see Table 28–2)
1.1 Migraine without aura
1.2 Migraine with aura
1.3 Ophthalmoplegic migraine
1.4 Retinal migraine
1.5 Childhood periodic syndromes
1.6 Complications of migraine
1.7 Migrainous disorders not fulfilling above criteria

2. Tension-type headache
2.1 Episodic tension-type headache
2.2 Chronic tension-type headache
2.3 Headache of the tension-type not fulfilling above criteria

3. Cluster headache and chronic paroxysmal hemicrania
3.1 Cluster headache
3.2 Chronic paroxysmal hemicrania
3.3 Cluster headache-like disorder not fulfilling above criteria

4. Miscellaneous headaches unassociated with structural lesion
4.1 Idiopathic stabbing headache
4.2 External compression headache
4.3 Cold stimulus headache
4.4 Benign cough headache
4.5 Benign exertional headache
4.6 Headache associated with sexual activity

5. Headache associated with head trauma
5.1 Acute post-traumatic headache
5.2 Chronic post-traumatic headache

6. Headache associated with vascular disorders
6.1 Acute ischemic cerebrovascular disease
6.2 Intracranial hematoma
6.3 Subarachnoid hemorrhage
6.4 Unruptured vascular malformation
6.5 Arteritis
6.6 Carotid or vertebral dissection
6.7 Venous thrombosis
6.8 Arterial hypertension
6.9 Headache associated with other vascular disorder

7. Headache associated with nonvascular intracranial disorder
7.1 High cerebrospinal fluid pressure
7.2 Low cerebrospinal fluid pressure
7.3 Intracranial infection
7.4 Intracranial sarcoidosis and other noninfectious inflammatory diseases
7.5 Headache related to intrathecal injections
7.6 Intracranial neoplasm
7.7 Headache associated with other intracranial disorders

8. Headache associated with substances or their withdrawal
8.1 Headache induced by acute substance use or exposure
8.2 Headache induced by chronic substance use or exposure
8.3 Headache from substance withdrawal (acute use)
8.4 Headache from substance withdrawal (chronic use)
8.5 Headache associated with substances but with uncertain mechanism

9. Headache associated with noncephalic infection
9.1 Viral infection
9.2 Bacterial infection
9.3 Headache related to other infection

10. Headache associated with metabolic disorder
10.1 Hypoxia
10.2 Hypercapnia
10.3 Mixed hypoxia and hypercapnia
10.4 Hypoglycemia
10.5 Dialysis
10.6 Headache related to other metabolic abnormality

11. Headache or facial pain associated with disorder of cranium, neck, eyes, ears, nose, sinuses, teeth, mouth or other facial or cranial structures
11.1 Cranial bone
11.2 Neck
11.3 Eyes
11.4 Ears
11.5 Nose and sinuses
11.6 Teeth, jaws, and related structures
11.7 Temporomandibular joint disease

12. Cranial neuralgias, nerve trunk pain, and deafferentation pain
12.1 Persistent (in contrast to tic-like) pain of cranial nerve origin
12.2 Trigeminal neuralgia
12.3 Glossopharyngeal neuralgia
12.4 Nervus intermedius neuralgia
12.5 Superior laryngeal neuralgia
12.6 Occipital neuralgia
12.7 Central causes of head and facial pain other than tic douloureux
12.8 Facial pain not fulfilling criteria in groups 11 or 12

13. Headache not classifiable

* Headache Classification Committee of the International Headache Society. (1988). Classification and diagnostic criteria for headache disorders, cranial neuralgias and facial pain. *Cephalalgia, 8*(Suppl. 7), 1–96.

The **ascending pain pathways** from the supratentorial space (the anterior and middle fossa) carry pain sensation by the trigeminal (cranial nerve [CN] V) nerve. Pain sensation from the infratentorial space (posterior fossa) is carried by the glossopharyngeal (CN IX), the vagus (CN X) nerves, and the second and third cervical nerves. The pain pathways ascend through the brain stem to neurons in the midbrain raphe area. From there, they extend to the thalamus, the hypothalamus, and the parietal lobe through the posterior limb of the internal capsule.[4] Serotonin is the primary neurotransmitter in the ascending raphespinal tract. The ascending serotonergic system originates in the midbrain raphe region, innervates the cerebral blood vessels, and is distributed in the thalamus, hypothalamus, and cortex. The major functions of these regions of the brain are cerebral blood flow, sleep, and neuroendocrine control.[3] The **descending pain-modulating pathways** originate in the periaqueductal gray region (PAG) in the midbrain and synapse in the nucleus raphe magnus in the medulla and the dorsal horn. The descending pathways are modulated by norepinephrine, serotonin, and opiates (enkephalins), which produce analgesia by inhibiting pain transmission.

Although there are many theories of chronic headache causation, the precise cause or causes have not been clearly established. The muscle theory is used to explain tension-type headaches as secondary to increased muscle contraction of the scalp and cervical muscles. The vascular theory attempts to provide a basis for understanding migraine and cluster headaches. The neurogenic theory is also used to explain migraine headaches. It suggests that migraine headache is caused by a primary disturbance of brain function.[3] Perhaps one of the most important considerations in understanding headache is the role of serotonin. The amine neurotransmitter serotonin, which is also called 5-hydroxytryptamine and abbreviated 5-HT, is derived from the amino acid tryptophan. Serotonin is widely distributed in the body, with high concentrations found in the gastrointestinal tract (90%), platelets (8%), and brain. Platelets contain all the serotonin normally present in blood.

Migraine Headaches

The relationship between migraine headaches and serotonin is well established. At the onset of a migraine blood serotonin falls, although it is normal between attacks.[3] This is followed by an increase in urinary 5-hydroxyindoleacetic acid, a breakdown product of serotonin that requires platelet aggregation for its release. There are about seven classes of 5-HT receptors in the body, most of which are excitatory.

Controversy continues about the pathophysiology of migraines. Some support the notion that abnormal extracranial and intracranial vascular reactions occur in migraine and other vascular headaches. Narrowing of the blood vessels supplying the brain and the surrounding tissue results in reduced blood flow or **oligemia**. This phase is followed by vasodilation, swelling, and noninfectious inflammation of the blood vessels. Concurrently, platelets clump together during an attack, probably because of exposure to several vasoactive amines, such as serotonin. The role of other vasoactive amines continues to be the subject of research. Further discussion of the basis of headache can be found in the work by Saper and partners[3] and other references cited at the end of the chapter.

▓ CLASSIFICATION OF HEADACHES

Primary headaches include migraine, tension-type, cluster, and miscellaneous headaches unassociated with structural lesions. Additional information on the complete IHS classification and diagnostic criteria is available in other published sources.[1]

Primary Headaches

Migraine Headaches

The term **migraine headache** encompasses various clinical presentations. The diagnostic criteria for migraine both with and without aura are outlined in Table 28-2. By definition, a recurring headache that is moderate or severe and is triggered by migraine-precipitating factors is considered a migraine headache. Seven subtypes come under the broad heading of migraine headaches, including **migraine without aura** (previously called common migraine) and **migraine with aura** (previously called classic migraine). Most patients have migraines without an aura. The characteristics of migraines can vary widely even within the same subtype.

Table 28-2 • INTERNATIONAL HEADACHE SOCIETY DIAGNOSTIC CRITERIA FOR MIGRAINE HEADACHE WITH AND WITHOUT AURA

1. Migraine *without aura*
   A. At least 5 attacks that fulfill criteria B–E
   B. Headache lasting 4–72 hours (untreated or unsuccessfully treated)
   C. Headache has at least two of the following characteristics:
      1. Unilateral location
      2. Pulsating quality
      3. Moderate to severe intensity (inhibits or prohibits daily activities)
      4. Aggravation by walking stairs or similar routine physical activity
   D. During headache at least one of the following:
      1. Nausea and/or vomiting
      2. Photophobia and phonophobia
   E. No evidence of related organic disease
2. Migraine *with aura*
   A. At least 2 attacks that fulfill criteria B and C
   B. At least 3 of the following 4 characteristics:
      1. One or more completely reversible aura symptoms that indicate focal cerebral cortical or brainstem dysfunction or both
      2. At least 1 aura symptom develops gradually over more than 4 minutes or 2 or more symptoms occur in succession
      3. No aura symptom lasts more than 60 minutes
      4. Headache follows aura in less than 1 hour
   C. No evidence of related organic disease

From Headache Classification Committee of the International Headache Society. (1988). Classification and diagnostic criteria for headache disorders, cranial neuralgias and facial pain. *Cephalalgia, 8* (Suppl. 7), 1–96.

Migraines with and without aura are similar except for the obvious absence of the aura in **migraine without aura**. The time frame for migraines is up to 3 days; when they last longer than 3 days, the term **status migrainosus** is used.

Almost half of all patients who have headaches suffer from migraines. Estimates suggest that 23 million Americans currently suffer from migraine headaches, and more than 11 million experience significant headache-related disability.[5] Heredity is a factor in 70% to 80% of sufferers. Migraines affect more than 17% (18 million) of women and 6% (5 million) of men in the United States.[6] Most people with migraine headache experience frequent severe attacks according to the following reported statistics: 25% of women report four or more per month, 35% report three per month, and 40% one or fewer per month.[5] Economic estimates suggest that the cost of migraine in the United States is approximately $17 billion per year.

Migraine Triggers. There are various triggers for migraine headache, including stress, certain foods, weather changes, smoke, hunger, fatigue, and others (Chart 28-1). For women who suffer from migraines, the menstrual cycle is a trigger in about 65%. Migraines occur immediately before, during, or immediately after menstruation. There is complete cessation of headaches during pregnancy in 75% to 80%. Use of oral contraception also affects headaches; 50% of patients have an increase in headaches, 40% report no change, and

CHART 28-1 • Common Triggers That May Precipitate Migraine Headaches

The following factors are common triggers that may precipitate migraine headaches in some people:

FOODS AND BEVERAGES

- Caffeine (coffee, tea, cola)
- Alcoholic beverages, especially red wine and beer (contain tyramine)
- Chocolate
- Foods containing tyramine (strong and aged cheeses, pickled foods, canned figs)
- Nitrites (cured meats)
- Sulfites
- Monosodium glutamate
- Yeast products
- Dairy products

OTHER CONDITIONS

- Stress (a strong precipitator of headache)
- Hormonal changes associated with the menstrual cycle
- Certain drugs such as estrogen and nitroglycerin
- Weather changes
- Decreased sleep or sleep deprivation
- Bright lights
- Fatigue
- Fever

10% report improvement. Stress and depression are powerful causes of migraine headaches. Other triggers include bright lights, sunlight, fluorescent lights, and watching television or movies; sleep deprivation or altered sleep-wakefulness cycles; fatigue; fever; and hunger. Some drugs, such as overuse of ergotamine, and foods, such as red wine and strong cheese, can also trigger a headache. Patients must be educated to avoid circumstances associated with headache.

Migraine Attacks: Phases

One way to consider a migraine attack is through four possible phases: prodrome (premonitory symptoms); aura; the headache; and the postdrome. Patients may have some or all of the phases in their migraine presentation.

Prodrome. **Premonitory symptoms,** experienced by 60% of patients, are symptoms that occur hours to a day or two before a migraine headache. Examples of common premonitory symptoms are depression, irritability, mental slowness, fatigue, sluggishness, yawning, feeling cold, craving special foods, increased thirst, increased urination, anorexia, diarrhea, constipation, and change in one's activity level (hypoactive or hyperactive). A person usually experiences the same prodrome symptoms with each headache.

Aura. Only about 20% of migraine sufferers have an aura. An **aura** is the constellation of focal neurological symptoms that

initiate or accompany an attack. Most auras develop over 5 to 20 minutes and usually last less than 1 hour.[1] Visual disturbances (bright spots, dazzling zigzag lines), often hemianopic, are the most common aura. The most common somatosensory phenomena include unilateral or bilateral numbness or tingling of the lips, face, or hand; slight difficulty in cerebration; paresis of an arm or leg; mild aphasia; slight incoordination of gait; confusion; and drowsiness.

Headache Phase. The headache phase begins with vasodilation, a decline in serotonin levels, and the onset of a throbbing headache. The headache is often unilateral at onset but may be bilateral (40% of patients) either at onset or as the headache intensifies over the next several hours. The headache can begin at any time but most often occurs on rising in the morning. The onset is usually gradual, with the pain peaking and then subsiding. The headache lasts from 4 to 72 hours in adults and 2 to 48 hours in children. Pain is moderate to severe and described as "throbbing" in most people. Simple physical activity or even moving the head can intensify the pain.

In addition to the pain, other symptoms accompany migraine. Nausea occurs in up to 90% of patients, and vomiting occurs in about one third. Many patients experience heightened sensitivity to light, sound, and smell; they seek a dark, quiet room. Other symptoms that may occur are blurry vision, nasal stuffiness, anorexia, hunger, diarrhea, abdominal cramps, polyuria, facial pallor, sensations of heat or cold, and sweating.[7] Local tenderness of the scalp, periarterial edema of the temporal area, and stiffness or tenderness of the neck may occur. Impaired concentration, depression, fatigue, anxiety, and irritability are common. The pain gradually subsides.

Postdrome. After a severe attack, there is often scalp or neck tenderness, anorexia, feeling of exhaustion, irritability, listlessness, impaired concentration, and mood change. In the postdromal period some people feel refreshed or euphoric, whereas others note depression and malaise.[7]

Tension-Type Headaches

Tension-type headaches, previously called tension headache, muscle contraction headache, stress headache, and ordinary headache, represent the second major category of primary headaches. Some physiological evidence suggests that the tension-type headache is a variation of a migraine headache and, as such, it may be reclassified in the future. Table 28-3 gives the diagnostic criteria for episodic tension-type headache.

Tension-type headaches are subdivided into episodic (acute) and chronic headaches. An **episodic tension-type headache** is defined as a recurrent headache that lasts from 30 minutes to 7 days. Pain is bilateral, of mild to moderate intensity, and described as aching, a feeling of tightness, pressure, or constriction, or a viselike feeling around the head. Unlike migraines, it is not accompanied by nausea nor does it intensify with routine physical activity. A tension-type headache may be accompanied by sensitivity to light or sound.

A **chronic tension-type headache** is similar to the episodic tension-type headache except for the time element. A

Table 28-3 • DIAGNOSTIC CRITERIA FOR EPISODIC TENSION-TYPE HEADACHE

A. At least 10 previous episodes fulfilling criteria B–D; numbers of days with such headache is less than 180 days per year.
B. Headache lasts from 30 minutes to 7 days.
C. At least 2 of the following pain characteristics are present:
1. Pressing or tightening (nonpulsating) quality
2. Mild or moderate intensity
3. Bilateral location
4. Not aggravated by walking stairs or similar routine physical activity
D. Meet the following:
1. No nausea or vomiting (anorexia may occur)
2. Photophobia and phonophobia are absent, or one but not the other is present

From Headache Classification Committee of the International Headache Society. (1988). Classification and diagnostic criteria for headache disorders, cranial neuralgias and facial pain. *Cephalalgia, 8* (Suppl. 7), 1–96.

chronic tension-type headache lasts at least 15 days a month during at least 6 months. The bilateral pain is of mild to moderate intensity and is usually pressing or tightening in quality. The pain is neither intensified by routine physical activity nor accompanied by vomiting.

Episodic and chronic tension-type headaches are further classified by whether the headache is accompanied by disorders of muscles around the cranium, such as in the temples and neck. Muscle contraction can be a part of the discomfort experienced in a headache.

In some patients, slight muscle contraction results in pain and headache if, concurrently with muscle contraction, there is also vasoconstriction of the arteries supplying the area. Muscle contraction can be reflexively induced secondary to noxious stimuli from diseases of the eyes, ears, paranasal sinuses, or cervical vertebrae. Anxiety and psychic tension are also common causes of muscle contraction that plague every person living in this complex society to a greater or lesser degree.

Cluster Headaches

The third major category of primary headache is cluster headache (previously called Horton's headache, histaminic cephalalgia, and migrainous neuralgia). These are seen primarily in men between 20 and 40 years of age. A **cluster headache** is an extremely severe, unilateral, burning pain located behind or around the eye. The headache lasts from 15 to 180 minutes, comes in groups, or "clusters," of one to eight daily, lasting up to several weeks or months, and is followed by a period of remission of months to years. Autonomic phenomena associated with the headache include any one or more of the following symptoms: tearing, conjunctival congestion, nasal congestion or runny nose, forehead and facial sweating, miosis, ptosis, and eyelid edema. The headache awakens the person during the night without prodromal signs or aura. Cluster headaches can be triggered by alcoholic beverages or other vasodilating agents such as nitroglycerin.

Miscellaneous Headaches Unassociated With Structural Lesions

This miscellaneous category includes headaches associated with activity such as coughing, exertion, or sexual activity; environmental factors such as cold; and external compression such as experienced when wearing swimming goggles. These types of headaches are not discussed in this chapter.

Secondary Headaches

Other types of headaches are classified as secondary headaches, some of which are included in Table 28-4. Headache can be a *symptom* of an underlying organic problem. There-

Table 28-4 • SELECTED SECONDARY HEADACHES FROM THE INTERNATIONAL HEADACHE SOCIETY*

CLASSIFICATION—HEADACHE ASSOCIATED WITH:	DESCRIPTION OF CAUSES OF HEADACHE
1. Head trauma	Acute and chronic post-traumatic headache with minor or significant head trauma
2. Vascular disorders	Acute ischemic cerebrovascular disease (transient ischemic attacks; thromboembolic stroke), intracranial hematomas, subarachnoid hemorrhage, unruptured vascular malformation (arteriovenous malformation; aneurysm), arteritis, carotid or vertebral artery pain, venous thrombosis, arterial hypertension, and headaches associated with other vascular disorders
3. Nonvascular intracranial disorders	High cerebrospinal fluid (CSF) pressure (benign intracranial hypertension; high pressure hydrocephalus), low CSF pressure, intracranial infections, headache related to intrathecal injections, and intracranial neoplasms
4. Substances or their withdrawal	Acute or chronic substance use (ergotamine induced), acute or chronic substance withdrawal (hangover, caffeine or ergotamine withdrawal, and oral contraceptives and estrogens)
5. Noncephalic infection	Viral, bacterial, and other focal or systemic infections
6. Metabolic disorder	Hypoxia, hypercapnia, hypoglycemia, dialysis, and other metabolic abnormalities
7. Disorder of cranium, neck and other	Disorders of cranial bones, cervical neck, eyes (glaucoma), ears, nose, sinuses, teeth, and temporomandibular joint disease
8. Cranial neuralgias	Compression or distortion of cranial nerves and second or third cervical roots and demyelination, infarction, or inflammation of cranial nerves
9. Headache not classified	All other headaches that do not meet criteria for other classifications are placed in this category.

*Headache Classification Committee of the International Headache Society. (1988). Classification and diagnostic criteria for headache disorders, cranial neuralgias and facial pain. *Cephalalgia, 8*(Suppl. 7), 1–96.

fore, the health care provider must determine whether the headache is part of a primary headache disorder or a sign of another illness. Chronic headaches may be benign or a sign of a serious, life-threatening illness such as a brain tumor, a cerebral hemorrhage, or meningitis. The intensity of headache can be just as great from a benign cause as from a life-threatening illness. Correct diagnosis of the specific headache type is the foundation for selecting appropriate treatment.

APPROACH TO MANAGEMENT OF HEADACHES

In the current managed care environment, patients who seek care for their headaches are usually first seen and evaluated by the primary care provider. If there is an indication that the headache is secondary to some underlying problem, a referral may be made to a neurologist or possibly a neurosurgeon, depending on the underlying problem. For those with primary headaches such as migraines that are intractable to treatment offered by the primary care provider, a referral may be made to a headache clinic. These patients are sometimes seen in the emergency department for relief from severe, intractable pain. The level of care provided for patients with headache depends, of course, on the managed care environment in which they receive health care.

Diagnosis

Accurate diagnosis of headache type is paramount in selecting the appropriate treatment. The primary purpose of the physical examination is to rule out systemic causes for headache. The patient evaluation includes a complete medical history, a family history, a headache history, and a complete physical and neurological examination. The patient's history is the single most important component in diagnosis. From the headache history, the frequency, onset, duration, character, and severity of headache pain guide diagnosis (Chart 28-2). Patients who have difficulty recalling details of their headaches should be encouraged to keep a headache diary (Chart 28-3).

Which diagnostic procedures should be ordered? An exhaustive headache workup is very expensive and most often (99% of cases) identifies no underlying cause for the headache. Clinical judgment and common sense guide the diagnostic workup. The diagnosis of primary headache is usually made on clinical grounds (headache history) and negative findings on both the physical and the neurological examinations. No specific diagnostic tests are available to confirm the diagnosis.

Table 28-5 lists "red flags" noted in the headache workup that suggest the need for further evaluation. Neuroimaging (by computed tomography [CT] or magnetic resonance imaging [MRI]) is the only radiographic procedure recommended through evidence-based practice.[6] An electroencephalogram (EEG) is not indicated in the routine evaluation of headache.[6] Other laboratory studies such as complete blood cell count, erythrocyte sedimentation rate, antiphos-

pholipids, glucose, electrolytes, creatinine, and thyroid panel may be ordered, depending on findings determined by the history and physical examination. Based on the findings and laboratory data, a referral may be made to other specialists or more diagnostic procedures may be scheduled. After the underlying etiology or type of headache is diagnosed, the appropriate treatment can be instituted. The specific treatment options are discussed under the specific type of headache.

Treatment

Overview of Management

Treatment of primary headaches involves a combination of nonpharmacological and pharmacological therapies. **Nonpharmacological therapies** include patient teaching about headaches, control of precipitating factors, stress management, biofeedback, and relaxation techniques. In migraine and tension-type headaches, stress is a frequent cause; thus, causes of stress must be identified and controlled with stress-management interventions. In addition, in tension-type headache, identifying postures assumed throughout the day can often uncover sources of prolonged muscle contraction that can lead to headache. Students, office workers, and those engaged in occupations that require prolonged sitting at a desk or computer are prime targets. Slouching while reading or watching television can also lead to prolonged muscle contraction. Abnormal posture, muscle contraction, and spasms may be the sequelae of previous injury. So-called trigger areas, resulting from previous injury elsewhere in the body, can relay impulses to the central nervous system, producing referred pain to the head. Treatment is directed toward using nonpharmacological interventions such as developing coping mechanisms, engaging in exercise programs, and using ergonomics in workplace design.

Pharmacological therapies include both preventive therapies and abortive therapies to give prompt relief of the headache and related symptoms, such as nausea.

Migraine Headaches

Migraine headaches vary in frequency, duration, and disability among patients. The level and intensity of care depend on the level of disability and the severity of symptoms, such as nausea and vomiting. Preventive therapy should be considered for those patients whose migraine has a significant negative impact on their lives. The goals of long-term migraine treatment include:

- Reduce attack frequency, severity, and disability
- Reduce reliance on poorly tolerated, ineffective, or unwanted acute pharmacotherapies
- Improve quality of life
- Avoid acute headache medication escalation
- Educate patient to manage disease and to enhance self-control
- Reduce headache-related distress and psychological symptoms[6]

CHART 28–2 • Headache History

GENERAL HISTORY

- Were any injuries noted at birth?
- Did you have encephalitis or meningitis, either as a complication of childhood disease or as a separate entity?
- Any history of abnormal nervous system development, such as bed-wetting, sleep disturbances, anxiety reactions (nail biting, untoward fear, and so forth), or fainting?
- Have you had middle ear infections, sinusitis, or surgical procedures involving the ears or sinuses?
- Have you had any injuries to the head, neck, or upper spine?
- Is there evidence now or in the past of cardiovascular disease, such as hypertension, heart disease, or orthostatic hypotension?
- Have you ever had kidney disease, pheochromocytoma, tuberculosis, or tropical infections?
- Have you ever had visual problems, such as astigmatism, dysconjugate gaze, or eye strain? Have you had any eye surgery?
- Have you ever had nervous system disease, such as a seizure disorder, vertigo, visual disturbances (diplopia), or psychiatric or emotional problems?
- Do you see the dentist periodically? Have you had any dental problems?
- Have you ever had arthritis or arthropathies of the neck, shoulder, or upper back?
- Do you have any difficulty with chewing?
- Do you use alcohol, tobacco, or any drugs? What kind? How much?
- Do you have any food, drug, or environmental allergies?
- (With women) Are there any particular symptoms associated with menstruation, pregnancy, childbirth, or menopause that are troublesome?

FAMILIAL HISTORY

- Does anyone in your family suffer from headaches? If so, what is their relationship to you? Describe their headaches.
- Is there a history of seizure disorders, allergies, emotional problems, or depression in your family?

OCCUPATIONAL HISTORY

- What kind of work do you do?
- Describe the physical environment in which you work.
- Are chemicals or fumes present? What kind?
- Do your co-workers complain of headaches?

PERSONAL AND FAMILY RELATIONSHIPS

- What about your life concerns you? (Most often anxiety is associated with loss—death, divorce, separation, independence, and so forth.)
- Describe your overall emotional makeup.
- What do you do to relax? Hobbies? Sports?
- Describe how you react to stress. What body signals tell you that you are in a stressful state?
- How do you get along with family members?
- Are you able to discuss problems with family members?
- What would you most like to change about your life?

SPECIFIC HEADACHE HISTORY

- At what age did the headaches start?
- Where is the headache located (generalized, focal, unilateral, bilateral, frontal, occipital)?
- Describe the type of pain (severe, mild, throbbing, aching, constant or intermittent, and so forth).
- How frequent are the attacks?
- How long do they last?
- What factors are associated with the onset of headache (emotions, intoxication, specific foods, temperature, trigger points, menstruation, stress)?
- What relieves the headache?
- What aggravates the headache?
- What is the usual course of events with the headache?
- What symptoms accompany the headache (nausea, vomiting, visual disturbances, vertigo, watering eyes, flushing, sweating, hemiparesis, numbness, fainting, facial tic)?
- How incapacitating is the headache in terms of your normal activities?
- Are all your headaches the same?
- What do you do to treat the headache? Does it help?

Pharmacological Basis for Migraine Management

Serotonin (5-HT), a potent vasoconstrictor, is an important neurotransmitter in the migraine cascade. At the molecular level, there are at least three distinct types of serotonin receptors: guanine nucleotide G protein-coupled receptors, ligand-gated ion channels, and transporters. There are also other serotonin receptor subtypes.[8] Headaches similar to migraine can be triggered by serotonergic drugs such as reserpine (which releases and depletes serotonin releaser). Two drugs effective in the acute treatment of migraine, dihydroergotamine (DHE, an ergot derivation) and sumatriptan (a serotonin analogue), are agonists at selected receptor sites. It is believed that these drugs block the development of neurogenically induced inflammation by activating prejunctional serotonin heteroreceptors on the trigeminal nerve. This, in turn, blocks the release of neuropeptides, including substance P and calcitonin gene-related peptide, preventing neurogenic inflammation. Nonsteroidal anti-inflammatory drugs (NSAIDs) are also thought to prevent neurogenic inflammation, possibly by inhibiting prostaglandin synthesis.[9] These theories and others suggest that the ergot alkaloids ergotamine and DHE, and possibly sumatriptan, exert their antimigraine effect by

CHART 28 – 3 • Headache Diary

Date	Onset: exact time AM or PM	Ending: exact time AM or PM	Triggers (1)	Prodromal signs (2)	Severity of headache (3)	Location (4)	Quality of headache (5)	Other symptoms	Medication taken, frequency, and route	Pain relief (6)

A series of codes are listed for each numbered heading, such as Triggers. Include all the codes that apply in that category.

(1) Triggers
1. Emotional stress/family related
2. Emotional stress/work related
3. Fatigue
4. Anxiety
5. Menstruation
6. Sleep deprivation
7. Fasting
8. Missing a meal
9. High altitude
10. Physical illness
11. Major life change
12. None

(1) Triggers: Food/Beverage
A. Caffeine (coffee, tea, cola)
B. Chocolate
C. Strong/aged cheese
D. Pickled foods
E. Canned figs
F. Yeast products
G. Dairy products
H. Cured meats
I. Monosodium glutamate
J. Red wine
K. Beer
L. None

(2) Prodromal Signs
1. Depression
2. Irritability
3. Mental slowness
4. Fatigue
5. Sluggishness
6. Yawning
7. Feeling cold
8. Craving special foods
9. Anorexia
10. None

(3) Headache severity scale (rate headache)

1   2   3   4   5   6   7   8   9   10

slight   moderate   very severe

(4) Location of headache (mark location)

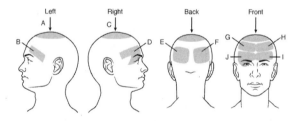

(5) Qualities of headache (include all that apply)
1. Unilateral
2. Bilateral
3. Throbbing
4. Piercing, constant
5. Gradual onset
6. Worse with head movement
7. Worse in lighted room
8. Accompanied by visual changes

(6) Pain relief from drugs scale (rate headache)

1   2   3   4   5   6   7   8   9   10

no relief   moderate   complete relief

---

a receptor-mediated neural pathway in both the central nervous system and the trigeminal nerve, where they block neurogenic inflammation.

Treatment of migraine headache has developed rapidly in the last decade. In addition to new drugs and treatment strategies, new routes of administration including nasal spray, self-administered injections, and rapidly dissolving oral tablets are now available.[10] Drugs and principles of pharmacological therapy for migraine headache are divided into acute (symptomatic) therapy and prophylactic therapy.

Acute Therapy. Acute therapy is directed toward alleviating or significantly limiting a headache that is just beginning or is in progress. Several drugs can be used. Given that patient

Table 28–5 • HEADACHE "SERIOUS SIGNS" THAT SUGGEST THE NEED FOR FURTHER EVALUATION

- "Worst" headache of my life
- Onset of headache after the age of 45 years
- Onset of a different kind of headache
- Headache with findings on the neurological examination
  - Altered level of consciousness
  - Altered cognition
  - Motor weakness, ataxia, or altered coordination
  - Altered sensation associated with headache such as tingling or numbness
  - Cranial nerve deficits such as asymmetrical pupils, extraocular palsies, or decreased hearing
  - Progressive visual deficits
  - Abnormal reflexes
  - Signs of meningeal irritation
  - Abnormal findings on physical examination
    - Fever
    - Hypertension
    - Tenderness or pulsation of temporal arteries

response is highly individualized, the health care provider may need to prescribe various drugs before an effective response is achieved. The most common acute therapy drugs are listed in Table 28-6.

A group of drugs called triptans is currently used to treat moderate to severe migraine. They not only relieve headache symptoms but also alleviate associated symptoms, including nausea, vomiting, photophobia, and phonophobia. This decreases the time needed to resume usual activities. Four drugs within the class of triptans are sumatriptan succinate (Imitrex), zolmitriptan (Zomig), naratriptan hydrochloride (Amerge), and rizatriptan benzoate (Maxalt and Maxalt-MLT). Each of these drugs is available in oral form. Sumatriptan is also available by injectable and intranasal routes. Rizatriptan is available in wafer form, which allows it to be dissolved on the tongue without the need for water.[11] Sumatriptan given by the subcutaneous route offers the most rapid relief to patients who are having a migraine. It works best if taken at the onset of headache and then repeated, if needed, in 1 hour. Some patients do not like to self-inject medication; for them, oral and nasal administration options are available. Rizatriptan taken orally is reported to relieve pain at 1 to 2 hours in a greater percentage of patients. The triptans are effective for about 70% to 78% of patients, which leaves about 22% to 30% nonresponders. Although a patient may not respond well to one drug in the triptan group, other drugs within the group may be effective. Therefore, the triptans should be fully utilized before withdrawing to another approach.

A second group of drugs used for treatment of migraine are called ergots. Ergotamine tartrate, administered orally, sublingually, rectally, subcutaneously, or intramuscularly at the first sign of a migraine headache, may abort the headache. Rectal suppositories are useful if nausea or vomiting occurs. The ergot preparations are therapeutic in two ways:

1. They are alpha-adrenergic agonists and antagonists causing vasoconstriction or vasodilation, depending on the state of the vessel.

2. They block the uptake of serotonin by platelets, thus reducing the precipitous decline of serotonin, a mechanism triggering a migraine attack.

One side effect of ergot preparations is rebound headache, which may occur if the drug is administered for 2 consecutive days or if a certain dosage is exceeded. Ergotism is also a result of drug overdose. After a migraine headache has fully developed, the ergot derivatives are not helpful and analgesics are needed to control the pain.

Migraine Prophylaxis. It is important to consider nonpharmacological treatment before beginning drug therapy or concurrent with drug therapy to manage migraine headaches. According to the evidence-based guidelines, the goals of migraine preventive therapy are to:

1. Reduce attack frequency, severity and duration
2. Improve responsiveness to treatment of acute attacks
3. Improve function and reduce disability

The following considerations guide the decision to embark on a prophylaxis program:

1. Frequency: occurring four or more times per month
2. Disabling: interfering with daily routines despite acute treatment
3. Ineffectiveness of current treatment: drugs for symptomatic treatment are ineffective or contraindicated
4. Untoward events: presence of uncommon migraine conditions such as hemiplegia, migrainous infarction, and the like

The major drug groups used for prophylactic treatment of migraine headaches are beta-adrenergic blockers, serotonin antagonists, antidepressants, and anticonvulsants (Table 28-7). Many of these drugs act by interacting with serotonergic neural systems, either by binding to 5-HT2 or 5-HT2c receptor sites, "down-regulating" the 5-HT2 receptor, or modulating the discharge of serotonergic neurons.[9] Propranolol (Inderal), a beta blocker, is a common first-choice drug for prophylaxis because it is effective and inexpensive. However, it may not be well tolerated because of its bradycardic effect. Other beta blockers can be tried if propranolol is not well tolerated. Another inexpensive and well-tolerated drug is amitriptyline (Elavil).

Tension-Type Headaches

Pharmacological management of episodic and chronic tension-type headaches is directed toward rapid treatment of the attack. The secondary goal is to prevent or reduce the occurrence of headaches. Most tension-type headaches are caused by anxiety, stress, and associated muscle tension. Less often, headache can be attributed to the effects of former injury or poor posture. Stress-reduction, exercise programs, relaxation technique, meditation, topical heat or cold packs, ergonomic principles for work environment, biofeedback, and possibly counseling are important nonpharmacological strategies that should be addressed along with drug therapy.

Table 28-6 • PHARMACOTHERAPY FOR ACUTE (SYMPTOMATIC) TREATMENT OF MIGRAINE HEADACHES

DRUG	DAILY DOSAGE (DIVIDED)	TYPE/ACTION	MOST COMMON SIDE EFFECTS
Non-narcotic analgesics		For mild to moderate headache; take early in the attack; monitor for overuse.	Rebound headache with frequent use
• Aspirin (ASA)	• PO: 650–1,300 mg	• Analgesic and anti-inflammatory effect	• Bleeding disorder; GI distress
• Acetaminophen	• PO: 650–1,300 mg	• Analgesic	• Does not cause GI upset or bleeding; hepatic necrosis
Nonsteroidal anti-inflammatory drugs (NSAIDs)		NSAIDs prevent prostaglandin synthesis by inhibiting cyclooxygenase, a critical element in prostaglandin synthesis; prostaglandin modulates components of inflammation, pain transmission, and platelet aggregation; useful for abortive and preventive therapy	• Limited by GI, liver, and renal side effects
• Ibuprofen	• PO: 400–800 mg		• Better tolerated than ASA
• Naproxen	• PO: 1,000 mg		• Better tolerated than ASA
Narcotic analgesics		For severe headache not controlled by non-narcotics; addictive; use with caution and do not overuse.	• Sedation, confusion, and constipation for both codeine and meperidine
• Codeine/ASA	• PO: 30–60 mg		
• Meperidine	• IM: 75–100 mg		• Sedation, nausea, sweating, vertigo, lethargy, confusion
• Butorphanol	• Transnasal: 1 mg followed by 1 mg 1 hour later	• Narcotic agonist-antagonist analgesic; very addictive; use cautiously	
Antiemetics		Often administered to control associated nausea; taken early in the attack.	Drowsiness, dizziness, confusion, hypotension, insomnia, vertigo
• Promethazine	• PO, PR: 25–150 mg	• Adjunct antiemetic therapy	
• Prochlorperazine	• PO, IM 5–20 mg; PR 25 mg	• Adjunct antiemetic therapy	
		• Parenteral treatment for established headache	
• Metoclopramide	• IM: 25–50 mg	• Adjunct antiemetic therapy; give 15–30 min before DHE or meperidine	
	• PO, IM: 10 mg		
Ergots			Ergots have a cumulative action so must be taken sparingly and as ordered or ergotism (numbness and tingling of fingers and toes, muscle pain, weakness, gangrene, and blindness) will develop. Nausea is a common side effect; need to premedicate with antiemetics.
• Ergotamine tartrate	• PO, SL, PR: 1–4 mg immediately, then 1–2 mg q 30 min (total of 6 mg/attack or 10/mg/wk)	• Abortive treatment for headache unresponsive to nonnarcotic treatment	
		• Take usual effective dose at first sign of attack	
		• Causes cerebral vasoconstriction, which decreases pulsation of cranial arteries	
• Dihydroergotamine (DHE)	• IM, IV: 1 mg; may repeat in 30–45 minutes; may take up to 3 mg/24 hours or 6 mg/wk	• Parenteral treatment for an established headache	*Contraindications:* Diabetes mellitus, sepsis, hepatorenal disease, peripheral vascular disease (PVD), coronary artery disease, hypertension, and pregnancy.
			• Nausea and vomiting; premedicate 10–15 min before with prochlorperazine 5–10 mg PO, IM, or IV; or metoclopramide 10–20 mg PO or 10 mg IM/IV
Other			
• Sumatriptan	• SC: 6 mg, PO: 100 mg; take early in the attack.	• First-line abortive therapy; elective agonist for vascular serotonin receptors; causes vasoconstriction of cranial arteries.	• Both drugs contraindicated in pregnancy, coronary artery disease, PVD, ischemia, and stroke; decreases blood pressure and heart rate
• Isometheptene (Midrin)	• PO: 2 tabs at onset then q 1 h until relief; do not exceed 5/24 hours.	• Sympathomimetic acts as a vasoconstrictor; mild sedative providing tranquilizing effect.	

Table 28-7 • PHARMACOLOGICAL THERAPY FOR PROPHYLAXIS OF MIGRAINE HEADACHES

DRUG	DAILY DOSAGE	TYPE/ACTION	SIDE EFFECTS
Beta blockers • Propranolol • Nadolol • Atenolol • Timolol • Metoprolol	• PO: 80–320 mg • PO: 40–240 mg • PO: 50–200 mg • PO: 10–60 mg • PO: 50–250 mg	• Blocks serotonin receptors; prevents vasodilation; propranolol is first drug of choice for prophylaxis; if it is not tolerated, try others in this class as listed	Bradycardia, fatigue, lethargy, sleep disorders, and depression. Common complaints are gastrointestinal complaints and orthostatic hypotension
Tricyclic antidepressants • Amitriptyline	• PO: 25–150 mg	• Blocks uptake of serotonin and catecholamines centrally and peripherally • Most effective for migraine associated with tension-type headache. • Alternative if beta blockers cannot be taken	May cause dry mouth, urinary retention, and sedation. *Contraindications:* benign prostatic hypertrophy and glaucoma
• Methysergide	• 4–8 mg with meals; must have a drug-free period q 6 mo for 3–4 wk	• Blocks serotonin to prevent early ischemic phase and vasodilation • Stabilizes platelets against release of serotonin • Inhibits release of histamine from mast cells • Potentiates norepinephrine to produce vasoconstriction	• Nausea and vomiting; fibrotic changes in the retroperitoneal and pleuropulmonary tissue, although uncommon, are the most serious complications; monitor creatinine • *Contraindications:* peripheral vascular disease (PVD), coronary artery disease, and pregnancy
Calcium channel antagonist • Verapamil	• 240–640 mg	• Alters calcium flux across smooth muscle • Prevents vasospasm and reactive vasodilation • Drug of choice	*Contraindications:* • Severe left ventricular dysfunction, hypotension, or second- or third-degree heart block • Constipation
Anticonvulsant • Valproic acid (divalproex)	• PO: 250–1,000 mg	• Turns off the firing of serotonin neurons of dorsal raphe which controls pain; particularly useful for chronic headache	• May alter liver function; may cause sedation, hair loss, tremor, and change in cognitive performance

Drug Therapy. Treatment of the mild to moderate pain of episodic headache may include mild analgesics and muscle relaxants. For symptomatic control of headache the following are commonly used: aspirin, acetaminophen, caffeine, a combination of aspirin and caffeine or acetaminophen and caffeine (e.g., Excedrin Migraine, Excedrin E. S., Vanquish, Midol), ibuprofen, naproxen, flurbiprofen, COX-2 inhibitors (e.g., Celebrex, Vioxx), Midrin, and Ultram. Some of these drugs are over-the-counter therapies, whereas others require a prescription. Narcotics should be avoided because of the concern about addiction.

Preventive therapy may also be considered. First-line preventive therapy includes antidepressants known as the selective serotonin reuptake inhibitors (SSRIs). This group includes sertraline (Zoloft), paroxetine (Paxil), and tricyclics such as amitriptyline (Elavil), protriptyline (Vivactil), and nortriptyline (Pamelor). Neurontin (Gabapentin), an anticonvulsant, has also been useful for some patients. Combining drug therapy with counseling may benefit those with frequent headaches. Because pain is interpreted as the presence of a serious problem, headaches may make a person fearful that a life-threatening condition is present. Reassurance helps to relieve such anxiety.

Cluster Headaches

The primary management strategy for cluster headache is to prevent the onset of the headache by eliminating triggers (e.g., alcohol consumption, sleep cycle disturbances, smoking).[3] Because attacks are infrequent and brief, symptomatic treatment is not the main focus of therapy. However, when a patient is experiencing a clustering of headache events, symptomatic treatment is necessary. Symptomatic treatment of cluster headache includes:

- 100% oxygen inhalation using a face mask at 7 L/min for 10 to15 min, preferably at the onset of the attack
- Dihydroergotamine (nasal or parenteral)
- Sumatriptan (subcutaneous or nasal) or other triptans
- Intranasal lidocaine
- Intranasal capsaicin
- Indomethacin (rectal suppository)
- Opioids (rectal/Stadol nasal spray; avoid frequent use)
- Neural blockade (i.e., sphenopalatine ganglion blockade)

For preventive therapy, high-dose calcium channel blockers (verapamil 120-160 mg three or four times a day), lithium carbonate (300 mg three times a day), methysergide, or a short-term course of corticosteroids may be effective. For corticosteroids, prednisone is given for 1 week (40 to 80 mg/d) and is then tapered over the next week.

NURSING MANAGEMENT OF THE PATIENT WITH HEADACHE

Patient management is often a collaborative multidisciplinary endeavor. In this section, the nursing management of patients with headache is briefly discussed, with emphasis on the role of the nurse in patient education. More specific detail is included on migraine and tension-type headaches. Cluster headaches are not discussed further because patient education is very similar to that used in migraine headaches.

Nurses care for patients who have various kinds of headaches. Most patients with primary headaches are managed in the community by a primary care provider or manage the condition themselves. For those with primary headaches that are difficult to control, a neurologist or a multidisciplinary team at a headache center may be necessary. Occasionally, primary headache sufferers go to the emergency department because a severe headache is intractable to the usual acute drug therapy. These people need to be referred for reevaluation. The major role of the nurse working with primary headache patients is patient education for self-management, prevention, and adjustment of lifestyle.

In a hospitalized population, secondary headaches are often symptoms associated with other health problems. Nurses caring for these patients manage headache with analgesics administered on an "as necessary" basis. Patients admitted for other problems may also suffer migraine or cluster headaches. In these circumstances, it may be necessary to consider continuing with headache prophylactic therapy. In addition, the possibility of drug interactions between headache drugs and drugs ordered to treat other health problems should be considered.

Nursing Assessment

A detailed nursing assessment and nursing history are the foundations for planning care. Chart 28-2 provides a sample headache history. The patient is key to providing a detailed history; so take the time to listen and to collect this information. Based on these data, indications for further assessment may be evident. In the hospitalized patient, a headache may be an expected side effect of surgery or an underlying problem. Use of a headache history would not be necessary in those situations.

Nursing Intervention

After the diagnosis of the specific type of headache has been established, the nurse can develop a patient teaching plan to educate the person about how to limit the number of attacks and treat acute attacks with both nonpharmacological and pharmacological methods (Chart 28-4).

CHART 28 – 4 • Teaching Plan for Persons With Migraine Headaches

The following list includes the major points of a teaching plan for persons with migraine headaches:

1. Educate the person about what migraine headaches are and what they are not.
2. Help the person to identify triggers for migraine headache and develop a plan to avoid or ameliorate the triggers (see Chart 28–3).
3. Help the person develop a format for a headache diary.
4. Provide a copy of a tyramine-free diet.
5. Teach stress reduction, stress management, behavioral strategies, and lifestyle changes to minimize the number of headaches.
6. Teach the person about his or her medications including action, how to take the drug, side effects, and how to avoid complications of overuse; include a caution about new drugs included for comorbidity and the possibility of interactions.
7. Teach the person about comfort measures during an attack such as lying down in a dark and quiet room with cold compresses to the head.
8. Suggest resources to help the migraine sufferer learn about migraines, such as:

National Headache Foundation
5252 North Western Avenue
Chicago, IL 60625   (312) 878-7715

Regardless of the type of headache, headaches are most apt to occur when the patient is physically ill, overworked, tired, or under stress. Stress is the major trigger in migraines. Therefore, the nurse should encourage proper diet, adequate rest and exercise, and effective stress management techniques. By helping the patient conduct a self-assessment, the nurse and the patient can identify stressors and particular circumstances that precipitate headaches. This provides a basis for exploring lifestyle changes to minimize these triggers. Appropriate referrals can be very helpful.

Patients should be encouraged to keep a headache diary for reference (see Chart 28-3). The purposes of a headache diary are to:

• Collect data for analysis to demonstrate causal relationships between headache and diet, drugs, physiological activities, emotional responses/states, and lifestyle
• Identify the specific characteristics of the headache
• Document the *individual's* headache pattern and triggers
• Provide a tool to document and alert the patient to the overall circumstances and characteristics of the headache
• Provide the health professional with data for diagnosis and patient education

This diary can be very enlightening to the patient. For example, the chart may reveal that headaches occur mostly on weekends when the entire family is home, or headaches may be noted to occur around the time of menstruation. It is most important to identify any rhythm or pattern in the occurrence of headaches.

For patients who experience fluid retention and weight gain around menstruation, a salt-restricted diet 1 week before menstruation should be encouraged. If this is not helpful, diuretics may be prescribed. Other elimination diets should be encouraged for those patients who have identified relationships between the ingestion of certain foods and beverages and the

occurrence of headaches. The major nursing diagnoses associated with headaches are found in Chart 28-5.

Nursing Management of Patients With Migraine Headaches

Nursing management of the patient with migraine headache is directed toward both symptomatic treatment of the acute attack and possibly prevention strategies. If a migraine

---

CHART 28–5 • Common Nursing Diagnoses Associated With Headache

Nursing Diagnoses (Actual or Potential)	Nursing Interventions	Expected Outcomes
Pain related to (R/T) headache	• Document the characteristics and circumstances of the painful experience • Help the patient identify factors that precipitate headache. • Manipulate the environment to control or prevent headache.	• Pain will be reduced or abolished. • Factors that precipitate headache will be identified and reduced
Ineffective Individual Coping R/T lifestyle stress	• Develop techniques to identify the causes of ineffective coping. • Establish a therapeutic nurse-patient interpersonal relationship. • Assist the patient to gain insight into the cause-effect relationship of ineffective coping. • Assist the patient in developing adaptive coping skills.	• The causes of ineffective coping will be identified. • The patient will gain insight into the effects of ineffective coping. • Effective adaptive coping skills will be developed.
Fluid Volume Excess (Fluid Retention) R/T premenstrual fluid retention	• Help the patient to understand why fluid retention can contribute to the onset of headaches • Identify the signs and symptoms of fluid retention. • Identify any dietary patterns that contribute to fluid retention. • Discuss the purpose of any medications and stress the importance of taking the medications as ordered.	• Fluid retention will be eliminated or controlled.
Sensory/Perceptual Alterations R/T paresthesia and visual alterations	• Document the type and characteristics of sensory/perceptual alterations. • Develop strategies to control or eliminate these signs and symptoms, if possible. • Institute measures to prevent injury. • Collaborate with the physician to provide a therapeutic protocol for treating the problem.	• Sensory-perceptual alterations will be identified and controlled or eliminated. • Precautions for the prevention of injury will be implemented.
Sleep Pattern Disturbance R/T stress and serotonin disorder	• Document the sleep-wakefulness pattern. • Identify factors that prevent adequate sleep. • Develop strategies to overcome obstacles to adequate sleep.	• A satisfactory sleep-wakefulness pattern will be established.
Knowledge Deficit R/T lack of understanding of headache dynamics and treatment protocol	• Identify the specific areas of knowledge deficits or misinformation. • Develop a teaching plan to correct these deficits. • Evaluate the acquisition of new knowledge by the patient.	• The patient will demonstrate a knowledge of headache type, precipitating factors, and treatment.
Anxiety R/T the possibility of headache and the disruption of lifestyle routines.	• Assess the reason for the anxiety. • Help the patient to set realistic goals. • Develop anxiety and stress-reduction strategies.	• Anxiety related to headache or the potential of headache onset will be reduced or eliminated.

headache appears to be developing, abortive drug therapy should be instituted immediately. If the migraine headache becomes fully developed before abortive therapy is instituted, intervention is directed toward acute management, including:

- Providing a darkened, quiet environment
- Elevating the head
- Administering analgesics, antiemetics, and specific migraine drugs

Patient education can be very effective in helping patients to avoid triggers and to adhere to the medication protocol. In addition, because stress is the major trigger for migraine headaches, stress management and relaxation are a necessary part of patient management. The specific stress management plan is based on the patient's personal inventory of stressors and includes strategies designed to reduce or eliminate these stressors. Referrals may be helpful to achieve this goal.

Nursing Management of Patients With Tension-Type Headaches

Most people treat their own tension-type headaches without consulting a nurse or other health care professionals. Over-the-counter drugs such as Excedrin are commonly used. Tension-type headaches are often acknowledged and discussed within the purview of primary care. Fear that the headaches may be "something serious" prompts the discussion. To reassure the patient appropriately, the nurse must be aware of those signs that indicate serious headaches (see Table 28-5). Significantly, a change in the headache pattern can herald a new, possibly serious, condition.

Several of the same principles suggested for migraine headaches are applicable to tension-type headaches. Health promotion through proper diet, rest, exercise, and relaxation should be encouraged. Many people either say that they do not have time for relaxation or do not know how to relax. Understanding that the marvelous machine called the human body has limits of physical and emotional endurance is helpful. Exceeding limits results in danger signals, such as irritability, fatigue, gastrointestinal upset, or headache.

Stress management includes learning new problem-solving skills. This approach requires honest self-evaluation and motivation to alter established behavioral patterns of dealing with stress. Keeping a headache history to note associations of stress and headache is helpful. Even the patient who is certain that no correlations exist may be surprised when confronted with hard data. Encourage the patient to start with one situation that leads to headache and develop alternatives to avoid the usual outcome.

Enrolling in adult education or college courses that focus on self-awareness, self-assertiveness, and stress adaptation is one approach that can help develop support systems for behavioral change. Many self-help books, audiotapes, and videotapes address similar subjects. Biofeedback, relaxation therapy, yoga, and counseling may be necessary for persons who have more than the occasional tension-type headache.

REFERENCES

1. Headache Classification Committee of the International Headache Society. (1988). Classification and diagnostic criteria for headache disorders, cranial neuralgias and facial pain. *Cephalalgia, 8*(Suppl. 7), 1–96.
2. Solomon, G. D., Cady, R. K., Klapper, J. A., & Ryan, R. E. (1997). Standards of care for treating headache in primary care practice. National Headache Foundation. *Cleveland Clinic Journal of Medicine, 64,* 373–383.
3. Saper, J. R., Silberstein, S., Gordon, C. D., Hamel, R. L., & Swidon, S. (1999*). Handbook of headache management: A practical guide to diagnosis and treatment of head, neck, and facial pain* (2nd ed., pp. 32–41). Philadelphia: Lippincott Williams & Wilkins.
4. Aminoff, M. J., Greenberg, D. A., & Simon, R. P. (1996). *Clinical neurology* (3rd ed., pp. 71–93). Stanford, CT: Appleton & Lange.
5. Lipton, R. B. (1997). Prevalence and impact of migraine. *Neurologic Clinics, 15*(1), 1–13.
6. Silberstein, S. D. (2000). Practice parameter: Evidence-based guidelines for migraine headache (an evidence-based review). Report of the Quality Standards Subcommittee of the American Academy of Neurology. *Neurology, 55,* 754–762.
7. Silberstein, S. D., & Lipton, R. B. (1994). Overview of diagnosis and treatment of migraine. *Neurology, 44*(Suppl. 7), S6–S16.
8. Humphrey, P. P. A., Feniuk, W., & Perren, M. J. (1990). Antimigraine drugs in development: Advances in serotonin receptor pharmacology. *Headache, 30*(Suppl. 1), 12.
9. Silberstein, S. D., & Lipton, R. B. (1994). Overview of diagnosis and treatment of migraine. *Neurology, 44*(Suppl. 7), S6–S16.
10. Lin, J. Overview of migraine. *Journal of Neuroscience Nursing, 33*(1), 6–13.
11. Moriarty-Sheehan, M. (2001). Managing migraine: Strategies for successful patient outcomes. *Nurse Practitioner, 26*(Suppl. 4), 1–13.

RESOURCES
Professional

Published Material

BOOKS
Cady, R. K., & Fox, A. W. (Eds.). (1995). *Treating the headache patient.* New York: Marcel Dekker.
Evans, R. W., & Mathew, N. T. (2000). *Handbook of headache.* Philadelphia: Lippincott Williams & Wilkins.
Robbins, L. D. (2000*). Management of headache and headache medications* (2nd ed.). New York: Springer.
Saper, J. R., Siberstein, S., Gordon, C. D., Hamel, R. L., & Swidon, S. (1999). *Handbook of headache management: A practical guide to diagnosis and treatment of head, neck and facial pain* (2nd ed.). Philadelphia: Lippincott Williams & Wilkins.

PERIODICALS
Breslau, N., Merikangas, K., & Bowden, C. (1994). Comorbidity of migraine and major affective disorders. *Neurology, 44*(Suppl. 7), S17–S22.
Clinch, C. R. (2001). Evaluation of acute headache in adults. *American Family Physician, 63*(4), 685–692.
Dalessio, D. (1994). Diagnosing the severe headache. *Neurology, 44*(Suppl. 3), S6–S12.
Gordon, D. L. (1997). Approach to the patient with acute headache. In J. Biller (Ed.). *Practical neurology* (pp. 204–228). Philadelphia: Lippincott-Raven.
Lefkowitz, D. (1997). Approach to the patient with chronic and recurrent headache. In J. Biller (Ed.). *Practical neurology* (pp. 217–228). Philadelphia: Lippincott-Raven.

Lin, J. Overview of migraine. *Journal of Neuroscience Nursing, 33*(1), 6–13.

Lipton, R. B., Ottman, R., Ehrenberg, B. L., & Hauser, A. (1994). Comorbidity of migraine: The connection between migraine and epilepsy. *Neurology, 44*(Suppl. 7), S28–S32.

Lipton, R. B., Stewart, W. F., Diamond, S., Diamond, M. L., & Reed, M. (2001). Prevalence and burden of migraine in the United States: Data from the American Migraine Study II. *Headache, 41*(7), 646–657.

Lipton, R. B., Diamond, S., Reed, M., Diamond, M. L., & Stewart, W. F. (2001). Migraine diagnosis and treatment: Results from the American Migraine Study II. *Headache, 41*(7), 638–645.

Mathew, N. T., Kailasam, F., Gentry, P., et al. (2000). Treatment of nonresponders to oral sumatriptan with zolmitriptan and rizatriptan: A comparative open trial. *Headache, 40*, 464–465.

Markley, H. G. (1994). Chronic headache: Appropriate use of opiate analgesics. *Neurology, 44*(Suppl. 3), S18–S24.

Moriarty-Sheehan, M. (2001). Managing migraine: Strategies for successful patient outcomes. *Nurse Practitioner, 26*(4 Suppl), 1–13.

Peikert, A., Becker, W. J., Ashford, E. A., et al. (1999). Sumatriptan nasal spray: A dose-ranging study in the acute treatment of migraine. *European Journal of Neurology, 6*, 43–49.

Pfaffenrath, V., Cunin, G., Sjonell G., et al. (1998). Efficacy and safety of sumatriptan tablets (25 mg, 50 mg and 1000 mg) in the acute treatment of migraine: Defining the optimum doses of oral sumatriptan. *Headache, 38*, 184–190.

Spencer, C. M., Gunaskara, N. S., & Hills, C. Zolmitriptan: A review of its use in migraine. *Drug, 58*, 347–374.

Weiss, J. (1999). Assessing and managing the patient with headaches. *Nurse Practitioner, 24*(7), 18–35.

Welch, K. M. A. (1994). Relationship of stroke and migraine. *Neurology, 44*(Suppl. 7), S33–S36.

Wilkinson, M., Pfaffenrath, V., Schoenen, J., Diener, H.-C., & Steiner, T. J. (1995). Migraine and cluster headache—their management with sumatriptan: A critical review of the current clinical experience. *Cephalalgia, 15*, 337–357.

Websites

JAMA Migraine Information Center: http://www.ama.assn.org/special/migraine

Migraine Diagnosis: http://www.upstate.edu/haad/hpmidx.htm

AMA Health Insight: Migraine: http://www.ama-assn.org/insight/spec-con/migraine/migraine.htlm

Women's Health Interactive: Health Center/Migraine Headache: http://www.womenshealth.com/health-center/headache/migraine.htm

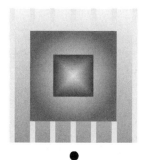

C H A P T E R **29**

Seizures and Epilepsy

JOANNE V. HICKEY

This chapter focuses on the nurse's role in assisting adults to self-manage their epilepsy in the community and on nursing management of the hospitalized adult patient with a seizure disorder. Although seizures and epilepsy are common in children, the special considerations related to children with these conditions are not addressed in this chapter. Other resources, some of which are listed in the Resources section, should be consulted for specific information on childhood epilepsy.

Most people with a seizure disorder are managed in the community by a primary care physician or a neurologist. Some patients who are more difficult to manage may be observed during follow-up at an epilepsy center where a neurologist with a practice focused on seizure management and a multidisciplinary team can provide comprehensive management. In many geographical areas, advanced practice nurses with a focus on seizure management are available to patients and families or as a consultant to other nurses. Almost all nurses who practice in a hospital environment see patients who have a seizure secondary to a primary condition, such as metabolic imbalance. Other nurses may see people with intractable epilepsy who are admitted for surgical intervention. Regardless of the setting in which care is delivered, nurses play an important role in the management and education of patients and their families.

BACKGROUND AND DEFINITIONS

References to epilepsy date back to ancient times, and mystical explanations about seizures continued until the 1870s when Jackson theorized that seizures originated from a localized, discharging focus in the brain. The introduction of the electroencephalogram (EEG) by Berger in 1929 provided the first recordings of epileptic discharges. This landmark event was followed in the 1930s by the work of Gibbs, who correlated the clinical indicators of epilepsy with EEG patterns. The development of classification systems for both epilepsies and seizures has paved the way to better understanding of the variations is clinical presentation. Research focused on the clinical and cellular bases for seizures, new

drugs, and improved management protocols have all contributed to better outcomes for patients subject to seizures.

The following widely accepted definitions of common terms have helped overcome imprecise terminology, which created confusion about seizures and epilepsy in the past.

- **Seizure**: a single (finite) event of abnormal discharge in the brain that results in an abrupt and temporary altered state of cerebral function.
- **Epilepsy**: a chronic disorder of abnormal, *recurrent*, excessive, and self-terminating discharge from neurons. Periods between seizures can vary widely and can be measured in minutes, hours, days, weeks, months, or even years. However, there is repetition of seizure activity at some time in the future, regardless of the interval. Clinically, epilepsy is characterized by *recurring seizures* accompanied by a disturbance in some type of behavior (i.e., motor, sensory, autonomic, consciousness, or mentation).
- **Seizure disorder**: a term adopted by some clinicians when referring to epilepsy. Although this has led to some confusion, the terms *epilepsy* and *seizure disorder* are used interchangeably.
- **Epileptic syndrome**: an epileptic disorder characterized by a cluster of signs and symptoms customarily occurring together.

Epidemiology and Risk Factors

Epilepsy is one of the most common neurological conditions representing a heterogeneous collection of disorders that have in common a recurrence of seizures. About 1.25 to 2 million people in the United States have epilepsy. Approximately 30% of all epilepsies and about 60% of all childhood epilepsies may have a significant genetic susceptibility.[1] The risk of epilepsy is about 1% from birth through 20 years and 3% for the 70-year and older age group. The prevalence and cumulative incidence of epilepsy and partial seizures increase dramatically in the elderly.[2] The prevalence among persons 65 years and older has implications for overall management, especially for education in self-management.

A few basic concepts guide our understanding of seizures in individuals. Anyone can have a seizure, given the right circumstances of central nervous system (CNS) imbalance.

However, there are differences among people in their level of susceptibility or threshold for seizures. Next, there is a high likelihood of a chronic seizure disorder in people with specific conditions such as a penetrating brain injury. Finally, seizures are episodic, suggesting that triggers precipitate seizure activity.[3]

The major risk factors for developing seizures can be classified according to age group. In young adults, trauma, alcohol withdrawal, illicit drug use, brain tumor, and idiopathic causes are the most common. In persons older than 35 years, cerebrovascular disease, brain tumor, alcohol withdrawal, metabolic disorders (e.g., uremia, electrolyte imbalance), Alzheimer's disease and other neurodegenerative diseases, and idiopathic causes rank as the major causes of seizures.[3] The term **idiopathic epilepsy** is used for the 70% of all cases for which no specific causes are identified.

Pathophysiology

Seizures are transient episodes of abrupt and temporary alteration of cerebral function. In recent years, numerous studies have suggested a major role for ligand and voltage gated channels in epileptogenesis. Both sodium and potassium channel subunits and neurotransmitter gated channels (e.g., nicotinic and gamma-aminobutyric acid [GABA] receptors), are implicated in seizures and epilepsy and have been found to be mutated in some familial forms of epilepsy.[1]

Seizures result from an imbalance between excitation and inhibition within the CNS. Excessive excitation or excessive inhibition may occur in focal areas of the cerebral cortex (focal seizures) or over the entire cerebral cortex (generalized seizures). A focal or generalized *increase in neuronal excitability* may result from energy failure of neurons producing transient depolarization or lack of local inhibition. Some seizures may result form *excessive inhibition* of cellular activity producing membrane hyperpolarization and activation of T-type calcium channels. With the opening of T channels, a burst discharge is generated that may be transmitted to the neighboring neurons or, if arising in the thalamus, to the whole cerebral cortex.[4]

Epilepsy can also be viewed as resulting from alterations in membrane potentials that predispose certain hyperactive and hypersensitive neurons to respond abnormally to changes in the cellular environment. The hypersensitive neurons have lowered thresholds for firing and can fire excessively, creating an **epileptogenic focus** from which the seizure emanates. The epileptogenic focus generates large numbers of autonomous paroxysmal discharges that can be enhanced or minimized, depending on the neurotransmitter that is active on the postsynaptic membrane. An epileptogenic focus can induce secondary epileptogenic foci in a synaptically related area and also in opposite cerebral hemispheres through connecting pathways between the same anatomical areas.

On the cellular level, a sequence of events serves to describe how an epileptic episode is initiated. Depolarization associated with ionic imbalances alters the chemical environment of the neurons. As a result, there is an intracellular accumulation of sodium and a depletion of intracellular potassium. At the onset of neuronal stimulation, depolarization is followed by a period of hyperpolarization, which is probably caused by an inhibitory postsynaptic potential. The hyperpolarization is soon replaced by depolarization, which rapidly increases in amplitude. The cell begins to fire repeatedly, thereby producing sustained membrane depolarization and seizure activity. As more is learned about the pathophysiology of seizures, the new knowledge will eventually lead to management that is more effective.[5]

Precipitating Factors: Triggers

In patients with epilepsy, seizures can be precipitated by various stimuli called *triggers*. Sometimes the trigger is very *specific* for a particular person. Common triggers include particular odors, flashing lights, and certain types of music. If a specific stimulus can be identified, then the pattern is called **reflex epilepsy**. Other *general* triggers include fatigue, sleep deprivation, hypoglycemia, emotional stress, electrical shock, febrile illness, alcohol consumption, certain drugs, drinking too much water, constipation, menstruation, and hyperventilation.

Terminology

A few terms describe the general signs and symptoms of seizures:

- **Aura** is a premonitory sensation or warning experienced at the beginning of a seizure, which the patient remembers. An aura may be a gustatory, visual, auditory, or visceral experience, such as a metallic taste or flashing lights. If a patient has an aura, it usually is the same experience each time.
- **Automatisms** are more or less coordinated, involuntary motor activities that occur during a state of impaired consciousness either in the course of or after an epileptic seizure, for which the person is usually amnesic.[6] Several different types have been recognized.[7] Examples of automatisms are lip smacking, chewing, fidgeting, and pacing. Automatisms are often associated with temporal lobe seizures but can also occur with complex partial seizures as well as with other types.
- **Autonomic symptoms** are symptoms that occur as a result of stimulation of the autonomic nervous system (e.g., epigastric sensation, pallor, sweating, flushing, piloerection, pupillary dilation).
- **Clonus** is a term used to describe spasms in which a continuous pattern of rigidity and relaxation is repeated. In the second phase of a generalized seizure, called the *clonic phase*, rhythmic movements are followed by muscle relaxation. In the clonic phase, the process repeats again and again.
- **Ictus** refers to an actual seizure; a seizure may be referred to as an *ictal event*.
- **Postictal** refers to the period immediately after a seizure has occurred.
- **Prodromal** refers to symptoms, such as a headache or feeling of depression, that precede a seizure by hours.
- **Tonus** is the degree of tone or contraction present in muscle when it is not undergoing shortening.

- **Todd's paralysis** is a temporary, focal weakness or paralysis following a partial or generalized seizure that can last for up to 24 hours. The deficit can be correlated with an epileptic focus on the motor strip. Temporary neuronal exhaustion is probably the physiological basis for the deficit.

SEIZURE CLASSIFICATION AND OBSERVATIONS/IDENTIFICATION

Seizures and epilepsy have been classified for clinical and research purposes using several different forms. Most of these are complex and cumbersome to use. In 1981, the International League Against Epilepsy (ILAE) published a modified version of the International Classification of Epileptic Seizures that continues to be a useful classification system (Table 29-1).[8]

The following section briefly discusses partial and generalized seizures. Tonic-clonic seizures, as examples of generalized seizures, are described in greater detail because they are so common. Table 29-2 describes the major subtypes of partial and generalized seizures, and Table 29-3 classifies partial seizures by cerebral lobe involved.

Partial Seizures

Three types of partial seizures are recognized: *simple, complex,* and *evolving into secondary generalized seizures.* Simple and complex seizures are distinguished on the sole basis of consciousness. When consciousness is not impaired, the seizure is classified as a **simple partial seizure**; if consciousness is impaired, the seizure is classified as a **complex partial seizure**.[9] The four subcategories of simple partial seizures are named for the areas of their presenting symptoms: *motor, sensory, autonomic,* and *psychic.* Complex partial seizures include both complex symptomatology and impaired consciousness. Another term for complex symptomatology is *automatisms.* These seizures consist of involuntary, but coordinated, motor activity that is purposeless and repetitive. The final category is a partial seizure evolving into a generalized seizure. These seizures are further categorized based on the type of partial seizure that preceded the generalized seizure (i.e., simple partial seizure only, complex partial seizure only, or simple partial seizure evolving into complex partial seizure).[9] On EEG, partial seizures are noted as focal epileptiform discharges with spikes or sharp waves.

Generalized Seizures

There are six categories of generalized seizures: *absence, myoclonic, clonic, tonic, tonic-clonic,* and *atonic.* Each seizure type has characteristic clinical and EEG findings that are outlined in Table 29-2. The absence seizure is subdivided into typical and atypical absence seizures according to the presence of different EEG patterns and clinical presentation. Clinically, atypical absence seizures have a less abrupt onset and termination and are of a longer duration.[9] The most

 Table 29–1 • CLASSIFICATION OF SEIZURES

I. Partial (focal, local) seizures
  A. Simple partial seizures (consciousness not impaired)
    1. Focal motor (with and without Jacksonian march)
    2. Somatosensory or special sensory symptoms (e.g., Simple hallucinations such as tingling, light flashing, buzzing)
    3. With autonomic symptoms (e.g., as epigastric sensation, pallor, flushing)
    4. With psychic symptoms (disturbances of higher cerebral function)
  B. Complex partial seizures (with impairment of consciousness)
    1. Beginning as simple partial seizures and progressing to impairment of consciousness
    2. With no other features
    3. With features as in simple partial seizures
    4. With automatism
  C. With impairment of consciousness at onset
    1. With no other features
    2. With features as in simple partial seizures
    3. With automatism
  D. Partial seizures evolving to secondarily generalized seizures
    1. Simple partial seizures evolving to generalized seizures
    2. Complex partial seizures evolving into generalized seizures
    3. Simple partial seizures evolving to complex partial seizures to generalized seizures
II. Generalized seizures (generalized bilateral without focal onset)
  A. Absence seizures
  B. Myoclonic seizures
  C. Clonic seizures
  D. Tonic seizures
  E. Tonic-clonic seizures
  F. Atonic seizures
III. Unclassified epileptic seizures (including all seizures that cannot be classified due to inadequate or incomplete data and some that defy classification)

From Commission on Classification and Terminology of the International League Against Epilepsy. (1981). Proposal for revised clinical and electroencephalographic classification of epileptic seizures. *Epilepsia, 22,* 489–501.

common type of generalized seizure is the **tonic-clonic seizure,** formerly called the *grand mal seizure.*

Description of Generalized Tonic-Clonic Seizures

A tonic-clonic seizure progresses through distinct phases including the prodromal, tonic, clonic, and postictal phases. The **prodromal phase** of irritability and tension may precede the seizure by several hours or days. Some individuals experience an aura, whereas in others the seizure begins without warning. Characteristically, the tonic-clonic seizure begins with a sudden loss of consciousness. Neuronal hyperexcitation spreads to the subcortex, thalamus, and upper brain stem, and consciousness is suddenly lost. In the **tonic phase,** there is a major tonic contraction (increased tonus) of the voluntary muscles so that the body stiffens with legs and arms extended. If standing, the person falls to

Table 29 – 2 • MAJOR SUBTYPES OF PARTIAL AND GENERALIZED SEIZURES

TYPE	DESCRIPTION	EEG FINDINGS
Partial Seizures		
Simple partial seizures		
• Motor	• Symptoms depend on the motor region activated • May remain focal or may spread to other areas on the motor strip, a process called "march"; seizures called jacksonian seizures. For example, the seizure may begin in the fingers of one side, and march to the hand, wrist, forearm, and arm on the same side of the body. The particular sequence of involvement is helpful in locating the epileptic foci on the motor strip in the hemisphere opposite the convulsive movement. • Focal motor attack may cause head to turn to side opposite epileptic foci • Todd's paralysis may result; last minutes to hours. • Continuous focal motor seizure is called *epilepsia partialis continua.*	*Applies to all simple partial seizures:* may show abnormal discharges in a very limited region; seizures originating from deep structures may not be noted with scalp electrodes
• Sensory	• Arise from cortical sensory strip. • Usually feels like "pins and needles" or numbness; sometimes, spatial disorientation. • May march to other areas or may become a complex partial or generalized tonic-clonic seizure. • Special sensory symptoms may include visual seizures such as flashing lights or visual hallucinations, auditory seizures with various sounds, gustatory sensations such as metallic taste or primary tastes (salty, sweet, sour, or bitter), or vertigo and floating sensations.	
• Autonomic	• May occur as simple partial seizures.	
• Psychic	• Disturbance in a higher-level function (i.e., distortion of memory), distorted time, feeling of déjà vu, illusions, depersonalization, or hallucinations. • Usually occur with impairment of consciousness and become complex partial seizures.	
Complex Partial Seizures		
One category	• Only symptoms may be impaired consciousness or it may progress to include automatisms; *note automatisms* may occur in partial or generalized seizures. • Simple partial seizure followed by impairment of consciousness resulting in a complex seizure with motor, sensory, autonomic, or psychic symptoms as described above.	*All complex seizures:* generalized 2–4 Hz spike waves
Partial Seizures Evolving to Secondary Generalized Seizures		
One category	Includes seizures that may evolve into generalized seizures: simple partial, complex partial, or simple partial evolving into complex and then to generalized seizures.	
Generalized Seizures		
• Absence seizures *Note:* may be seen along with tonic-clonic seizures	*Typical absence seizures:* common in children; characterized by brief interruption in consciousness without loss of postural control. Typically, there is an interruption of activity with a momentary lapse of consciousness lasting 3 to 30 seconds. If talking, the speech stops or slows; if eating, the hand and mouth stop, and if patient is called, there is no response. • During an attack, the eyes may appear vacant, stare, or roll upward; the eyelids may twitch. • Seizures occur a few times to hundreds of times per day; person may not be aware of them. • People who have several attacks daily most often experience difficulty in learning or employment because of inattention. *Atypical absence seizures*—the lapse of consciousness is usually of longer duration and less abrupt in onset; more obvious motor signs.	*Typical absences:* 3-Hz spike-wave complexes with abrupt starts and stops *Atypical absences:* ≤2.5 Hz; slower spike-and-wave pattern, and more irregular

Table 29–2 • MAJOR SUBTYPES OF PARTIAL AND GENERALIZED SEIZURES (Continued)

TYPE	DESCRIPTION	EEG FINDINGS
• Myoclonic seizures	• Sporadic jerks that are sudden, brief, contractions that are usually symmetrical • When confined to one area, it may be the face and trunk; one or more extremities; an individual muscle; or a muscle group. • Myoclonic jerks are rapidly repetitive or relatively isolated. • Common around time of sleep or awakening; must be differentiated from myoclonic jerks of nonepileptic myoclonus.	Bilateral, generalized epileptiform discharges, typically polyspikes
• Clonic seizures	• Repetitive rhythmic clonic movements that are bilateral and symmetric.	Associated with symmetric spike-wave complexes
• Tonic seizures	• Stiffening of the musculature, mostly of the body, but may also involve the arms.	Low voltage paroxysmal fast activity (10 Hz)
• Atonic seizures	• Abrupt loss of postural muscle tone; last 1–2 sec • Consciousness is briefly impaired, but usually there is not postictal confusion. • Common in children.	Generalized epileptiform discharges (spikes, spike-wave complexes)
• Tonic-clonic seizures	• Most common of the generalized seizures (see p. 621 for detailed description).	Fast high-voltage spikes seen in all leads

Unclassified Epileptic Seizures

One category	This group includes all seizures that cannot be classified because of inadequate or incomplete data. This self-explanatory category is a catch-all for seizures that do not conform to any of the other headings.	

Table 29–3 • SEIZURE ACTIVITY OF PARTIAL SEIZURES (SIMPLE, COMPLEX, AND SECONDARY GENERALIZED) BY LOBE

CEREBRAL HEMISPHERE LOBE	DESCRIPTION
Frontal lobe epilepsy	• Many overlapping syndromes with frequent brief attacks (<30 sec) • Simple complex seizures • Focal motor seizures (from motor strip) • Supplemental area motor seizures • Tonic and postural signs and symptoms with preserved consciousness; frequent falls • Complex partial seizures • Complex motor activity, vocalization, and gestural automatism (may be sexual) • Common to proceed to secondarily generalized tonic-clonic seizures

Mesial temporal lobe epilepsy	• Most common cause is hippocampal sclerosis
	• Mostly complex partial seizures with automatisms and psychic symptoms
	• Often preceded by an aura in 50%–95% of patients; rising epigastric discomfort is the most common aura
	• Seizure may include:
	  Staring
	  Oral or manual automatisms
	  Olfactory and auditory illusions or hallucinations
	  Unilateral dystonic posturing

Parietal lobe epilepsy	• Usually simple complex and secondarily generalized seizures • >75% have somatosensory auras • May have a distorted body image, visual or auditory hallucinations • Usually proceeds to impaired consciousness and contralateral motor activity
Occipital lobe epilepsy	• Most have visual auras • Elemental visual hallucinations (e.g., flashing lights, colored lights) or sometimes blindness, scotoma, or hemianopsia • Eye blinking, nystagmus, head deviation, tonic and clonic eye movement are common • Visual phenomena is usually contralateral to side of the seizure • Often progress to complex partial seizures or secondarily generalized seizure depending on pathways stimulated

the ground. The jaw snaps shut and the tongue may be bitten in the process. A shrill cry may be heard because of the forcible exhalation of air through the closed vocal cords as the thoracic muscles initially contract. The bladder and, less often, the bowel may empty. The pupils dilate and are unresponsive to light. Apnea occurs and lasts for only a few seconds, but the patient may appear pale and dusty. The tonic phase lasts less than 1 minute (average of 15 seconds).

The **clonic phase** begins with a gradual transition from the tonicity of the tonic phase. Inhibitory neurons of the cortex, anterior thalamus, and basal ganglion nuclei become active, intermittently interrupting the tonic seizure discharge with clonic activity. The clonic phase is characterized by violent, rhythmic, muscular contractions accompanied by hyperventilation. The face is contorted, the eyes roll, and there is excessive salivation with frothing from the mouth. Profuse sweating and a tachycardia are common.

In the **postictal phase**, the clonic jerking gradually subsides in frequency and amplitude over a period of about 30 seconds, although it may be longer. The involved cells cease firing. The extremities are limp, breathing is quiet, and the pupils, which may be equal or unequal, begin to respond to the light reflex. With awakening, most patients are confused, disoriented, and amnesic for the event. Headache, generalized muscle aching, and fatigue are common. If undisturbed, the patient often falls into a deep sleep for several hours.

There may also be temporary paresis, aphasia, or hemianopsia. Following a seizure (i.e., generalized or partial), focal weakness, called **Todd's paralysis**, may occur and last up to 24 hours. If it occurs, the focal deficit is important in localization of a focal epileptogenic site.

Because the seizure frequently occurs without warning, it is possible for injury to be sustained from falls or other accidents related to the seizure. Head injury, fracture of the limbs or vertebral column, and burns are examples of serious injuries that may be sustained. Tonic-clonic seizures may occur at any time of the day or night, whether the patient is awake or asleep. The frequency of recurrence can vary from hours to weeks, months, or years.

Status Epilepticus

Although there are many definitions for status epilepticus, one recommendation[10] endorses the following: **status epilepticus** is defined as *either continuous seizures lasting at least 5 minutes or two or more discrete seizures between which there is incomplete recovery of consciousness.*[11,12] The most common cause of status epilepticus is an abrupt discontinuation of antiepileptic drugs (AEDs). Other causes include withdrawal from alcohol, sedatives, or other drugs, or fever.

Clinically, status epilepticus can present with obvious tonic, clonic, or tonic-clonic movements, with subtle twitching of the hand or face, or absence of movement. Absence of observable movement is most commonly seen in hospitalized patients. In this case, the detection of ongoing seizures requires electroencephalography.

With tonic-clonic seizure, the most common type of status epilepticus, the patient is unconscious. Convulsive seizures can be easily observed clinically, but partial seizures are less obvious and more difficult to identify. Subclinical seizures are seizures that do not present with overt clinical signs and symptoms but are apparent on continuous EEG tracing.

Suspicion of subclinical seizure should be considered in patients who seem to be improving generally but have not regained consciousness. Continuous EEG monitoring can assist in the recognition of this serious problem. Therefore, an EEG or continuous EEG monitoring is required for any patient with significant alterations in consciousness or when unconsciousness is sustained.

Status epilepticus constitutes a *medical emergency* associated with significant morbidity and mortality (20%). If not treated aggressively, cardiorespiratory dysfunction, hyperthermia, and metabolic imbalances can develop, leading to cerebral ischemia and neuronal death. Treatment of status epilepticus is discussed later in this chapter.

Epileptic Versus Nonepileptic Seizures

Seizures may also be classified as either epileptic or nonepileptic. Epileptic seizures include partial and generalized seizures discussed earlier. **Nonepileptic seizures** or **nonepileptic events** account for about 20% of referrals to epilepsy centers. Clinically, the signs and symptoms can look like seizures, but there is no epileptogenic origin. Nonepileptic seizures include physiological events, psychogenic events, and malingering.[13]

Cardiac, respiratory, metabolic derangement, and drug toxicity can disturb consciousness as a result of decreased oxygen tension to the brain. Perfusion problems as a result of transient ischemic attacks, stroke, or Stokes-Adams syndrome account for underlying cardiac or cerebrovascular problems. Decreased oxygen tension from poor saturation can result from pneumonia, pulmonary emboli, shunting, or coma. Metabolic causes such as hypoglycemia and electrolyte imbalance can cause nonepileptic events. Toxicity resulting from use of street drugs or prescription drugs, including AEDs, alcohol toxicity, and environmental exposures to toxic substances such as lead can also result in nonepileptic seizures.

Differentiation between nonepileptic psychogenic seizures and epileptic seizures can be made only through analysis of simultaneous EEG tracings and audio-video monitoring during a seizure. The audio-video portion records the behaviors of the peri-ictal events, and the EEG demonstrates the presence or absence of abnormal tracings associated with epileptic seizures. The behavior is triggered by psychogenic internal or external factors. The basis for psychogenic nonepileptic events is secondary gains for the individual such as sympathy or relief from unwanted responsibilities.

Observations/Identification

Physiological causes of nonepileptic seizures must be ruled out with a basic diagnostic workup of a thorough history, physical examination, and laboratory screening.

With nonepileptic psychogenic seizures, the onset is often dramatic, bizarre, gradual, and in the presence of witnesses. By comparison, epileptic seizures are sudden, paroxysmal, and orderly. Emotional upset usually precipitates nonepileptic seizures, and such an episode lasts longer than a true seizure. The dramatic, violent flinging of the extremities, wiry movements, and inconsistent pattern of development are a sharp contrast to the tonic-clonic, orderly, repetitive movements of true seizures. If a scream is heard during a true seizure, it is at the onset of the event. With nonepileptic seizures, screams are usually heard throughout the course of the episode. Observing the features, development, and finale of seizure activity can be most helpful in differentiating between epileptic and nonepileptic seizures.

DIAGNOSIS

The first step in the evaluation of a patient with possible epilepsy is to determine whether the patient did or did not have a seizure. The diagnostic process requires a past medical history and a careful history of the clinical presentation and events related to the alleged seizure. The history is followed by a general physical and neurological examination and diagnostic testing. A prenatal history and achievement of developmental milestones are very important in infants, children, and adolescents. In adults, a history of trauma, drug use, and toxic environmental exposure are critical. Detailed descriptive information about the seizures is collected, including onset and surrounding events such as fever or withdrawal from alcohol, prodromal or aura experiences, precipitating factors, frequency, loss of consciousness, subjective and objective characteristics of the event, postictal behavior, and any injuries associated with seizures. In addition to the usual baseline blood chemistries, a toxicology screen (e.g., drug levels, barbiturates, street drugs, and lead) may be helpful for some, based on history. Other diagnostic tests that may be ordered include:

- Computed tomography (CT) scan
- Magnetic resonance imaging (MRI) (2 to 3 times more sensitive than CT scan in identifying potential epileptogenic lesions)
- EEG
- Video-EEG monitoring with either noninvasive scalp electrodes or deep invasive electrodes
- Possibly a positron emission tomography (PET) scan (limited availability due to high expense)
- Single proton emission computerized tomography (SPECT) scan (helpful for seizure localization and not diagnosis)

Most patients do not require all diagnostic tests listed, whereas others may require additional studies. The objective of the studies is to identify systemic or CNS processes that are manifested, in part, by seizure activity. For many patients, an extensive search for an underlying etiology will yield negative results. The diagnosis of epilepsy is made after ruling out other possible causes (discussed later). The clinical presentation and EEG findings help classify the particular type of epilepsy. Accurate diagnosis of seizure type is important because selection of appropriate drug therapy is seizure-specific in many cases. The EEG is a vital diagnostic procedure because it identifies patterns of abnormal electrical activity that can be correlated with particular types of seizure patterns. An EEG can also aid in lateralization and localization of an epileptogenic trigger focus. However, in

about 50% to 60% of patients with confirmed epilepsy, the interictal EEG can be normal.

Several special techniques are useful in augmenting the data from an EEG. A sleep study, in which there is continuous EEG monitoring, is helpful because sleep activates anterior temporal spike discharges and bitemporal discharges in 80% to 90% of persons with complex partial seizures. The increased interictal epileptiform abnormalities are noted most in non-rapid eye movement (non-REM) sleep. Sleep deprivation also increases the frequency of interictal abnormalities. Extra scalp electrodes, nasopharyngeal electrodes, and sphenoid electrodes help to increase the detection of mesial temporal discharges. The ability to detect and localize abnormal ictal discharges in complex partial seizures is greatly enhanced with the use of invasive procedures such as depth, subdural, and cortical electrodes. Surface electrodes often provide false localization.[14] Simultaneous EEG and audio-video recordings of the patient can distinguish seizure from nonseizure activity and assist in classifying seizure type.

Differential Diagnosis

Given the long list of possible causes of seizure activity, diagnosis can become very difficult. Differentiation between epileptic and nonepileptic seizures (discussed earlier) must be made. Brain tumor, cerebral aneurysm, cerebral arteriovenous malformation, transient ischemic attacks, stroke, migraine headaches, syncope, sleep disorders, myoclonus, cardiac sources, drug and alcohol abuse, drug toxicity, metabolic disorders, breath holding, and psychogenic problems such as anxiety attacks, hysterical responses, and psychosis are some of the possibilities that must be excluded. Nevertheless, accurate classification of seizure type is important to specific treatment choices.

Electroencephalograms and Seizures

The EEG is a diagnostic test during which the amplified electrical potential of the brain is recorded by placing 14 to 21 electrodes on the patient's scalp. Electrodes may also be placed on the cortical surface using an invasive procedure. The tracings reflect the combined electrical activity of several neurons, rather than only one. The basic resting electrical pattern of the brain is altered by opening the eyes, focusing attention on a problem, hyperventilation, photic stimulation, drugs, or sleep. Therefore, recordings are taken at rest, after hyperventilation, during stimulation with a strobe light, and during sleep. The patient must be quiet, relaxed, cooperative, able to follow directions, and seated comfortably in a chair with the eyes closed, although not asleep. The testing room must be shielded from extraneous electrical interference and noise. Often, preparation for the EEG includes keeping the patient awake all night before the recordings. The stress of sleep deprivation is more apt to result in the recording of abnormal EEG tracings.

Even though the EEG is important in diagnosing seizures, these data must be considered in conjunction with other information, including the history, physical examination, and other laboratory studies. Between seizures, normal

EEGs are often recorded in patients with epilepsy. In addition, EEGs that are considered to be "borderline" by one interpreter may be read as normal by another, indicating subjectivity in interpretation.

The tracings for the EEG are made with special ink on electromagnetic paper. The recorded tracings signify the electrical potential difference from the scalp to the ear electrodes and from the scalp to the scalp electrodes. The average EEG consists of 150 to 300 or more pages of recordings, with each page accounting for 10 seconds of tracings. In the normal adult, the most characteristic, normal tracings noted at rest are as follows:

Alpha waves: 8 to 12 Hz (Hz = cycles per minute)
Beta waves: 18 to 30 Hz, a faster wave, seen in the anterior areas of the brain

Both alpha and beta waves are bilaterally symmetrical. Each has its own characteristic shape and amplitude. Changes occur in the normal EEG pattern with various activities. For example, when the eyes are opened, there is an immediate decrease in the amplitude of the brain waves; in the early stages of sleep, the waves slow (lower voltage); and in the later stages of sleep, "sleep spindles," occurring at a rate of 14 to 16 Hz, develop with subsequent higher voltage and slower waves.

Patients with seizure disorders have abnormal recordings on their EEGs. The most common abnormal findings include:

Delta waves: less than 4 Hz with high amplitude; often associated with destruction of brain tissue, such as occurs with infarction, tumor, or abscess (localized over abnormal area)
Theta waves: 4 to 7 Hz (not always abnormal)
Spikes or **sharp waves:** high-voltage, faster waves; asymmetry of frequency and amplitude from one side to the other

On an abnormal EEG, slow and fast waves may be combined in paroxysmal runs, thereby interrupting the normal pattern. These paroxysmal waves are highly suggestive of epilepsy. Recordings taken between seizures in the epileptic patient often include isolated spikes without evidence of a clinical seizure.

TREATMENT

The approach to a patient with a seizure disorder is multidimensional and comprehensive. It includes:[3]

- Treatment of any underlying condition
- Avoidance of precipitating factors
- Suppression of recurrent seizures by prophylactic therapy with AEDs or surgery
- Comprehensive management of physiological and social issues related to having seizures

An individual plan of care must be developed for each patient. If there is an underlying problem responsible for seizures, it must be addressed. For example, if the diagnostic workup revealed a brain tumor as the cause of seizures, the primary problem, the brain tumor, must be treated. Seizures related to the brain tumor can be managed with AEDs. If the diagnosis is epilepsy, identification of the specific type of epilepsy is imperative in developing an effective treatment plan.

After epilepsy has been diagnosed, the patient needs to be made aware of precipitating factors and taught to avoid these situations or conditions. About 75% of patients with epilepsy can be managed satisfactorily with AEDs. Surgery is considered for a small group of patients for whom an epileptogenic focus can be identified or in whom seizures are intractable even with drug therapy. In addition to drug therapy, the management plan must address the behavioral, social, and economic consequences of having epilepsy. For successful adaptation to this chronic problem, it is critical that patients receive education in self-management. Patient counseling and support are also essential components of the management plan.

Medical Management: Drug Therapy

Epilepsy treatment seeks to enable the patient to live as free of the medical and psychosocial complications of seizures as is possible. Pharmacological therapeutics play a large role in helping to achieve this goal. As with any drug therapy, there is concern about side effects, toxicity, ease of administration, efficacy, and effect on different age groups. Management of epilepsy is complicated by the range of age of patients, the number of categories of drugs, and the psychosocial impacts involved.

Effective drug treatment for epilepsy has two goals: to control or reduce the frequency of seizures, and to minimize side effects. AEDs do not cure epilepsy but provide a chemical means of controlling seizures. As with any drug, side effects, such as sedation, may interfere with activities of daily living. Therefore, effective medical management includes the development of an *individualized* drug program that minimizes side effects and supports compliance.

After a diagnosis has been made, the following principles should guide use of drugs:[15]

- Assess the patient (diagnosis of seizure type and classification, patient characteristics such as age and presence of comorbidity, and insurance drug coverage).
- Select the primary drug that is the most effective for the seizure type; monotherapy is preferred, and about 70% of patients with epilepsy can be maintained on one drug.
- Begin with monotherapy and titrate dosage to achieve appropriate blood concentrations and control.
- Consider the pharmacokinetics of AEDs and free AED concentrations.
- Provide patient education.
- Provide follow-up to assess control, tolerance, and side effects.
- Consider the length of time patient has been taking AEDs.

Table 29-4 • ANTIEPILEPTIC DRUGS AND RELATED SEIZURE TYPES*

	PRIMARY GENERALIZED TONIC-CLONIC	PARTIAL (I.E., SIMPLE, COMPLEX, AND SECONDARY GENERALIZED SEIZURES)	ABSENCE	ATYPICAL ABSENCE, MYOCLONIC, AND ATONIC
First-line drugs	• Valproate • Phenytoin • Lamotrigine	• Carbamazepine • Valproate • Phenytoin • Lamotrigine • Phenobarbital	• Ethosuximide • Valproate	• Valproate
Alternative drugs	• Primidone • Carbamazepine • Topiramate • Phenobarbital • Felbamate	• Topiramate • Tiagabine • Primidone • Zonisamide • Gabapentin • Tiagabine	• Methsuximide • Lamotrigine • Clonazepam	• Lamotrigine • Clonazepam • Felbamate

* Data from Holland, K. D. (2001). Epilepsy: Efficacy, pharmacology, and adverse effects of antiepileptic drugs. *Neurologic Clinics, 19*(2), 313–345; Victor, M., & Ropper, A. H. (2001). *Adams and Victor's principles of neurology* (7th ed., p. 357). New York: McGraw-Hill; and Braunwald, E., Fauci, A. S., Kasper, D. L., Hauser, S. L., Longo, D. L., & Jameson, J. L. (2001). *Harrison's principles of internal medicine* (15th ed., p. 2362). New York: McGraw-Hill.

Selecting the Primary Drug Most Effective for the Seizure Type

The classifications of epileptic seizures and epilepsies/epileptic syndromes have made easier the selection of the drug of choice for a given seizure problem. Seizure types and drug of choice plus alternative drug options are outlined in Table 29-4. Table 29-5 lists drugs commonly used to treat seizures and epilepsy. Table 29-6 outlines the management of status epilepticus.

Some AEDs have a narrow spectrum of action and are effective for only a selected seizure type, whereas other drugs are broad spectrum and effective against many different types of seizures. Drugs also have different mechanisms of action. Some types of seizures can be exacerbated by AEDs designed to treat another seizure type. For example, carbamazepine, useful for partial seizures, can exacerbate absence seizures. Phenytoin, phenobarbital, and carbamazepine, which are effective in controlling generalized tonic-clonic seizures and partial seizures, are ineffective for absence seizures and may actually precipitate an increase in their incidence.[15] In addition, with a broad-spectrum drug that can be used for various seizure types, the therapeutic range may differ for different seizure types. For example, blood concentrations for complex partial seizures may need to be higher than the concentration for tonic-clonic generalized seizures.

In addition to a particular seizure type, patient characteristics influence drug selection. The plan of care must be individualized to consider age, co-morbidity, liver and kidney function, previous drug history for allergies, tolerance of side effects, cost, other drug therapy and potential interactions, and child-bearing potential.

Begin With Monotherapy and Titrate the Dosage to Achieve Appropriate Blood Concentrations

The following are important points to keep in mind:[12,13]

• Begin with a single drug, called monotherapy, which is the drug of choice for the particular seizure type.

• Increase the drug gradually over 3 to 4 weeks until seizure control is achieved, intolerable side effects occur, toxicity develops, or the maximum therapeutic range has been reached.

• Recognize that many AEDs are CNS depressants and that drowsiness, lethargy, and tiredness are common in the beginning of therapy; however, these symptoms will usually subside in 7 to 10 days.

• Because of pharmacokinetics (cited later) and variations in requirements for specific seizure types with the same drug, expect to make individual adjustments in dosage.

• Some patients may need more or less than the recommended average therapeutic range for a particular drug.

• Titrate a single drug until maximum benefit is achieved or intolerance or serious side effects occur. If a therapeutic blood concentration has been achieved and seizure control has not been achieved, a second drug may be added. A second drug may be used in combination with the first or replace the first. With replacement, the first drug should be *gradually tapered* after the second drug has been titrated to the desired dosage. This practice is necessary because the sudden withdrawal of a drug can cause status epilepticus, even though a new drug has been introduced in its place.

• If the patient is seizure free, check drug concentration in blood after 5 to 8 half-lives or a period of 3 to 4 weeks. (See Table 29-7 for therapeutic serum concentrations, half-life, and steady state data.)

• The drug's half-life is important because drugs of long duration (phenytoin, phenobarbital) may be taken once daily in some circumstances.

• Have the patient keep a daily *drug diary* routinely, but especially when a new drug is introduced. The diary should include dosage and side effects. The diary is helpful in evaluating the effectiveness of the drug therapy.

Refractory Epilepsy. About one third of patients with epilepsy do not respond well to treatment with monotherapy. It then becomes necessary to try a combination of drugs to control seizures. Although there are no guidelines for combining drugs, in most instances a combination of two first-line

▥▥▥ Table 29–5 • MAJOR ANTIEPILEPTIC DRUGS (AEDs) USED IN ADULTS

GENERIC AND TRADE NAME	ADULT DAILY MAINTENANCE DOSE (mg/d) IN DIVIDED DOSES	MAJOR USES	ADVERSE NEUROLOGICAL EFFECTS	OTHER ADVERSE EFFECTS
Major AEDs Used as Monotherapy				
Phenytoin (Dilantin)	300–400 PO	Generalized tonic-clonic, complex partial, absence, myoclonic	Dizziness, ataxia, nystagmus, incoordination, confusion	Hirsutism, hypertrophy of gingiva, facial coarseness
Valproate (Depakote)	1,000–3,000 PO	Generalized tonic-clonic, complex partial, absence, myoclonic	Ataxia, tremors, sedation	Liver toxicity, GI irritation, weight gain, thrombocytopenia
Carbamazepine (Tegretol, Carbatrol)	800–1,200 PO	Tonic-clonic, complex partial	Dizziness, ataxia, blurred vision, diplopia, ataxia; can interfere with cognitive function in learning situations	Rash, nausea, vomiting, aplastic anemia
Lamotrigine (Lamicatal)	300–500 PO	Focal onset tonic-clonic; atypical absence; myoclonic	Drowsiness, diplopia, dizziness, headache, ataxia	Rash, Stevens-Johnson syndrome
Phenobarbital (Luminal)	90–120 PO; may be given in combination with phenytoin	Tonic-clonic, simple and complex partial	Drowsiness sedation, confusion, difficulty thinking, ataxia	Skin rash
Adjunctive and Special AEDs				
Ethosuximide (Zarontin)	1000–2000 PO	Absence seizures	Ataxia, lethargy headache	Rash; GI irritation, bone marrow suppression
Methsuximide (Celontin)	600–1200 PO	Absence seizures	Ataxia, lethargy headache	GI irritation
Clonazepam (Klonopin)	2–10 PO	Myoclonic seizures, typical and atypical absence	Drowsiness, ataxia, behavior disturbance; seizures	Anorexia
Topiramate (Topimax)	200–400 PO	Focal onset, tonic-clonic	Sedation, fatigue, paresthesias, cognitive effects	Renal stones
Tiagabine	32–56 PO	Focal onset, tonic-clonic	Sedation, confusion, cognitive effects, paresthesias	GI irritation
Gabapentin (Neurontin)	900–3,600 PO	Partial and/or secondary generalized tonic-clonic	Sedation, fatigue, dizziness, ataxia	GI irritation
Primidone (Mysoline)	750–1,500 PO	Tonic-clonic, focal onset	Drowsiness sedation, confusion, difficulty thinking, ataxia	—
Felbamate (Felbatol)	2400–3,600 PO	Complex, partial, tonic-clonic, and atypical absence seizures	Insomnia, dizziness, sedation, headache	Weight gain, decreased appetite, aplastic anemia, liver failure
Levetiracetam (Keppra)	1,000–3,000 PO	Focal onset	Sedation, fatigue, incoordination	Anemia, leukopenia
Zonisamide (Zonegran)	200–800 PO	Focal onset	Sedation, dizziness, confusion, headache	Weight loss
Oxcarbazepine (Trileptal)	900–2,400 PO	Focal onset	Ataxia, fatigue, dizziness, diplopia, headache	Rash, nausea, vomiting, hyponatremia
Antiepileptics Used for Treatment of Status Epilepticus (see discussion of management of status epilepticus for guidelines)				
Lorazepam (Ativan)	0.1 mg/kg IV at 2 mg/min IV	Status epilepticus	Sedation	Respiratory depression, hypertension
Phenytoin (Dilantin)	20 mg/kg at 50 mg/min IV	Status epilepticus	Sedation	Cardiac arrhythmias, hypotension
Fosphenytoin (Cerebyx)	20 mg/kg PE at 150 mg/min IV	Status epilepticus	Sedation	Same as phenytoin
Phenobarbital (Luminal)	20 mg/kg at 50–75 IV	Status epilepticus	Sedation	Respiratory depression, hypotension
Midazolam (Versed)	0.1–0.4 mg/kg/h IV	Status epilepticus	Sedation and neuromuscular blockage	Hypotension, cardiac or respiratory arrest
Propofol (Dipravan)	2–8 mg/kg/h IV	Status epilepticus	Sedation and neuromuscular blockage	Hypotension, cardiac or respiratory arrest

Table 29–6 • MANAGEMENT OF STATUS EPILEPTICUS

TIME LINE IN MIN.	DRUG THERAPY (PROGRESSION ALONG THIS ALGORITHM ASSUMES THAT THE PREVIOUS DRUG ADMINISTERED DID NOT TERMINATE THE SEIZURES)
0–3	**1. Lorazepam (Ativan):** 4–8 mg (0.1 mg/min) IV at 2 mg/min *Note:* additional emergency therapy may not be needed if the seizures terminate *Seizures continue*
4–23	**2. Phenytoin (Dilantin):** 20 mg/kg (about 1 g) in normal saline at a rate of 50 mg/min OR **Fosphenytoin** (20 mg/kg PE (PE = phenytoin equivalent) intravenously at 150 mg/min) *Seizures continue*
22–33	**3. Phenytoin:** (additional) 5–10 mg/kg OR **Fosphenytoin** 5–10 mg/kg PE *Seizures continue* **Proceed immediately to step (6) anesthesia with midazolam or propofol if:** • Patient develops status epilepticus while in the ICU • Has severe systemic problems (e.g., extreme hyperthermia) • Has seizures that have continued for more than 60–90 min
37–58	**4. Phenobarbital:** 20 mg/kg IV at 50–75 mg/min *Seizures continue*
58–68	**5. Phenobarbital:** additional 5–10 mg/kg *Seizures continue* **6. Anesthesia with midazolam or propofol**

Lowenstein, D. H., & Alldredge, B. K. (1998). Status epilepticus. *New England Journal of Medicine, 338*(14), 970–976; and Quality Standards Committee of AAN. (1996). Practice parameter: A guideline for discontinuing antiepileptic drugs in seizure-free patients—summary statement. *Neurology, 47,* 600–602.

drugs (i.e., carbamazepine, phenytoin, valproic acid, lamotrigine) is tried. If this is not effective, adding one of the newer drugs (i.e., gabapentin or topiramate) is suggested. When seizures cannot be controlled by drug therapy, the condition is called refractory epilepsy and surgery becomes a consideration.[3]

Considering Pharmacokinetics and Free AED Concentrations

The pharmacokinetics of AEDs are important to keep in mind. Many AEDs are highly bound to plasma protein. It is the unbound, or "free," concentration that represents the active drug capable of penetrating the blood-brain barrier and interacting with receptor sites. For this reason, patients on high-protein tube feeding will require a higher drug dosage to maintain adequate drug blood levels. Conditions known to alter AEDs' protein-binding capacity are malnutrition, older age, pregnancy, hypoalbuminemia, burns, liver disease, and chronic renal failure. The following are plasma protein binding capacities for selected AEDs:

• Phenytoin and valproic acid (high protein binding)
• Carbamazepine (variable binding)
• Phenobarbital and primidone (minimal binding)
• Ethosuximide (not bound)

Although therapeutic ranges are cited for each drug, patients vary with regard to pharmacokinetics. Therefore, dosage requirements for individual patients vary. For determining dosage, use the gold standard that the patient should become seizure free. The onset of serious side effects or intolerance is a reason to discontinue a drug. Clinical judgment must be used and patient response and blood levels must be monitored to determine the ideal dose and blood concentration for a patient.

Patient Education

Patient education is the cornerstone of drug therapy and promotes a partnership that supports compliance. Patients who understand the purpose of drug therapy and the drugs that they are taking are more compliant. Patient education must be an ongoing process with reinforcement and updates at each appointment. Because many patients are on long-term or life-long therapy, education must also anticipate and prepare patients for developmental changes and changes in normal life routine. If they are to provide comprehensive patient management, health care providers who treat patients with seizures must develop and implement an individualized teaching plan that includes how to initiate and provide ongoing patient education.

Considering Length of Time on Antiepileptic Drug Therapy

Whether AED therapy must be life-long depends on many factors. The American Academy of Neurology has issued these guidelines for exploring discontinuation of AEDs in seizure-free patients:[16] seizure free for at least 2 years; at-

Table 29–7 • THERAPEUTIC SERUM CONCENTRATION LEVELS, HALF-LIFE AND STEADY STATE FOR AEDs FOR MANAGEMENT OF ADULT PATIENTS

DRUG: GENERIC AND TRADE NAMES	THERAPEUTIC RANGE	SERUM HALF LIFE (h)	TIME TO STEADY STATE (d)
Carbamazepine (Tegretol)	4–12 µg/mL	14–25	2–4
Clonazepam (Klonopin)	20–80 µg/mL	24–48	4–5
Ethosuximide (Zarontin)	40–120 µg/mL	60	6–12
Felbamate (Felbatol)	Not established	16–22	3
Gabapentin (Neurontin)	Not established	5–7	1.5
Lamotrigine (Lamictal)	Not established	14	2
Phenobarbital (Luminal)	10–40 µg/mL	90	14–21
Phenytoin (Dilantin)	10–20 µg/mL	10–34	7–28
Primidone (Mysoline)	5–12 µg/mL	4–19	1–4
Topiramate (Topamax)	Not established	20–30	—
Valproate (Depakene, Depakote)	50–150 µg/mL	8–20	1–3

▐▐▐ **Table 29 – 8** • FACTORS TO CONSIDER FOR POSSIBILITY OF AED WITHDRAWAL

	SUGGEST SUCCESSFUL PROBABILITY OF AED WITHDRAWAL	SUGGEST POOR PROBABILITY OF AED WITHDRAWAL
Complete seizure control within 1 year of onset	Yes	No
Combined seizure types	No	Yes
Seizure onset after 2 yr and before 35 yr	Yes	No
Repeated status epilepticus	No	Yes
Normal EEG	Yes	Continued epileptiform activity
Normal MRI	Yes	No
Normal cognitive function	Yes	No

tained complete seizure control within 1 year of onset; the onset of seizure occurred between the age of 2 and up to 35 years; and a normal EEG on AEDs (Table 29-8).[15] Many individual considerations, such as psychological issues and patient comfort, should be included in the decision. However, if the decision is made to discontinue AEDs, a gradual taper must be done.[17] Beyond the need for gradual withdrawal, no agreement exists on the timeframe for drug withdrawal, with timeframes varying from 1 to 6 months in practice.[18,19] The risk of recurrent seizures is approximately 25% for patients *without risk factors* and more than 50% for patients *with risk factors* (Table 29-9). Studies show that 80% of recurrent seizure activity occurs within 4 months after a tapering schedule has been initiated, and 90% occur in the first year.[16,18] Because of the risk of injury to self or others, driving and other potentially dangerous activities should be prohibited for at least the first 4 months after the start of the drug taper.[16,17]

Table 29-5 has been developed to consolidate pertinent data about AEDs. Nursing management associated with a few commonly ordered drugs is discussed below. These drugs include phenytoin, fosphenytoin, carbamazepine, valproic acid, and phenobarbital. In addition, several new drugs approved for use by the U. S. Food and Drug Administration are briefly discussed. More information on drug therapy can be found in Chapter 11.

Phenytoin

Phenytoin (Dilantin), introduced in 1938, is a synthetic drug that is classified as a hydantoin. It is used for the treatment of simple partial, complex partial, and generalized tonic-clonic seizures. It is not effective for absence, myoclonic, or atonic seizures. Phenytoin blocks post-tetanic potentiation (PTP) by influencing synaptic transmission through voltage-sensitive sodium channels.

Pharmacokinetics. Phenytoin is primarily absorbed through the duodenum. There is no first-pass metabolism. Oral absorption is affected by the particle size of the particular brand's formulation so that *there can be variations among brands.* The brand of phenytoin that a patient is receiving should not be switched without careful monitoring.[15] Phenytoin enters the brain quickly and is then redistributed to other body tissues, including breast milk. It crosses the placenta and reaches a state of equilibrium with the mother and fetus. Phenytoin is bound to serum and tissue protein. In the serum, the drug binds primarily to albumin in a predictable, linear fashion provided that the albumin level is normal (see the exceptions in the previous section). Phenytoin is metabolized in the liver and excreted in the urine. At an often unpredictable concentration level, metabolism of phenytoin ceases because of saturation. Any change in dosage at this point will result in significant changes in serum concentrations. In addition, serum concentration does not decline at a predictable linear rate when phenytoin is discontinued. Therefore, serum monitoring is necessary after any dosage change. Because the half-life of phenytoin is 10 to 34 hours (average 22 hours), it may be given once daily.

Administration. Administration of phenytoin may be oral or intravenous (IV). Because the pH of phenytoin is about 12, intramuscular (IM) injection should be avoided to prevent tissue irritation.

Oral phenytoin comes in three dosage forms. The tablets and suspension contain phenytoin acid, whereas the cap-

▐▐▐ **Table 29 – 9** • RISK FACTORS FOR RECURRENT SEIZURES AFTER WITHDRAWAL FROM ANTIEPILEPTIC DRUGS (AEDs)

	LOW RISK FOR RECURRENT SEIZURES	HIGH RISK FOR RECURRENT SEIZURES
Seizure type	Idiopathic seizures	Frequent seizures
EEG on AEDs	Normal	Abnormal
Onset	Childhood	Adolescence
Neurological abnormalities	None	Structural lesion with abnormalities
Control with monotherapy	Well controlled	Difficult to control requiring more than on drug

sules contain phenytoin sodium. Phenytoin sodium is 92% phenytoin. The parenteral form is phenytoin sodium. If they contain equivalent amounts of phenytoin acid, tablets, capsules, and suspension have the same bioavailability. Phenytoin capsules are designated as immediate-release or extended-release. Only the extended-release should be used for once-daily dosing. The suspension form comes in two strengths; either can settle and thus deliver doses of unequal concentration.

To maintain an even blood level, patients on enteral feeding will probably need increased dosage due to the high protein binding of phenytoin. After enteral feeding has been discontinued, the dosage must be decreased. Monitoring phenytoin blood levels provides a guide for adjusting the drug dosage.

If phenytoin is administered IV, it must be administered slowly, at a rate no faster than 50 mg/minute in *a solution of normal saline. Maintaining the proper rate is very important because rapid administration depresses the myocardium and can cause cardiac arrhythmias and cardiac arrest.* If given in solution such as 5% dextrose in water, the drug will precipitate into crystals in the solution. If given by IV push, it must be given slowly (no more than 50 mg/minute); the effect of rapid administration of phenytoin on the myocardium is dangerous arrhythmias. Patients receiving IV phenytoin should also be observed for the development of phlebitis at the IV site.

Drug Interactions. Various drugs in common use can interact with phenytoin:

- Drugs that *potentiate* the action of phenytoin include aspirin, cimetidine, chloramphenicol, felbamate, methsuximide, fluconazole, isoniazid, disulfiram (Antabuse), propoxyphene, sulfonamides, and warfarin.
- Drugs that *decrease* the action of phenytoin include antacids, barbiturates, antihistamines, calcium, calcium gluconate, chronic alcohol, carbamazepine, folic acid, valproic acid, and vigabatrin.
- Phenytoin *decreases* the action of amiodarone, carbamazepine, corticosteroids, cyclosporine, digitalis, dopamine, estrogen, furosemide, haloperidol, oral contraceptives, phenothiazines, quinidine, and sulfonylureas.

Adverse Effects. Lethargy, fatigue, incoordination, visual blurring, higher cortical dysfunction, and drowsiness are related to CNS depressant effects. When serum concentrations exceed 20 μ/mL, patients may experience nystagmus, ataxia, and slurred speech. A morbilliform rash may occur in some patients 7 to 14 days after beginning the drug. The appearance of such a rash indicates that the drug should be discontinued. A lupus-like syndrome has also been reported and is reversible when phenytoin is withdrawn.

Effects seen with long-term, chronic use include gingival hyperplasia (about 50% of patients), decreased cognitive ability, osteomalacia, hirsutism, hypothyroidism, peripheral neuropathy, megaloblastic anemia, blood dyscrasias, and low serum folate concentrations. Periodic complete blood cell counts (CBCs) are important to monitor the development of anemia or dyscrasias. The low folic acid levels respond to folic acid therapy. There is an increased incidence of malformations in children born of women who are taking AEDs.[20]

Fosphenytoin

Fosphenytoin (Cerebyx) is a water-soluble drug that is rapidly and completely converted to phenytoin after IV or IM administration and has a conversion half-life of 8 to 15 minutes. However, protein binding for fosphenytoin is exceedingly high and nonlinear. Therefore, fosphenytoin displaces phenytoin from albumin, thus increasing the unbound phenytoin concentration. This increase in unbound concentration (pharmacologically active form of phenytoin) offsets the delay in phenytoin formation from the prodrug (i.e., phenytoin), making it bioequivalent to phenytoin at 50 mg/minute.[21]

Fosphenytoin is administered IM or IV. Compared with phenytoin, fosphenytoin is rapidly and completely absorbed following IM administration, reaching a peak level in 3 hours. Fosphenytoin is administered in units called phenytoin equivalents (PE, which is the amount of phenytoin to be used) rather than fosphenytoin itself. Fosphenytoin is compatible with standard IV solutions (5% dextrose and water or normal saline [NS]) and can be infused for adults at a rate of 100 to 150 mg PE/kg/minute.[22] The most common side effects are nystagmus, ataxia, and sedation. Although fosphenytoin is more expensive than phenytoin, fosphenytoin is safer and can be administered more quickly. IV fosphenytoin is replacing phenytoin in the treatment of status epilepticus.[22] As with phenytoin, continuous electrocardiograms (EKGs), blood pressure, and respiratory status must be monitored when providing a loading dose of fosphenytoin.

Carbamazepine

Carbamazepine (Tegretol, Tegretol-XR) is a safe drug used as a first-line agent for the treatment of simple partial, complex partial, and generalized tonic-clonic seizures. Carbamazepine can exacerbate absence and myoclonic seizures. The mechanism of action is depression of transmission via the nucleus ventralis anterior thalamus, which acts to decrease the spread of seizure discharge. In addition, it has some depressive effect on post-tetanic potentiation, but to a lesser degree than with phenytoin.

Pharmacokinetics. Carbamazepine has an absorption rate greater than 75%; the dosage peak is reached in 6 to 24 hours. It has a high affinity for lipids that bind to body fat; it also binds to albumin. Carbamazepine is metabolized by the liver.

Administration. Carbamazepine is available only in oral form. It is given in divided doses two to four times daily. Dosage should be adjusted gradually. Because the suspension form of the drug may adhere to the nasogastric tube if not diluted, it is recommended that the suspension form be diluted in an equal amount of diluent before administration with an enteral tube.

Drug Interactions. Some drugs, such as phenytoin and phenobarbital, may interact with carbamazepine by enzyme induction, thus decreasing the concentration of carbamazepine. Other drugs—erythromycin, cimetidine, and isoniazid—interact by enzyme induction; these drugs increase the concentration of carbamazepine. Carbamazepine interacts with other drugs by inducing their metabolism; these drugs include valproic acid, theophylline, warfarin, and ethosuximide.

Adverse Effects. The major dose-dependent side effects are diplopia, nystagmus, ataxia, unsteadiness, dizziness, and headache. Cognitive deficits are minimal, although present. Carbamazepine has been associated with neural tube defects.

Valproic Acid

Valproic acid, which is marketed as both valproic acid (Valproate, Depakene) and divalproex sodium (Depakote), is approved for management of myoclonic, tonic, atonic, absence, and generalized tonic-clonic seizures, and especially for patients with more than one type of generalized seizure. The drug has low toxicity and is well tolerated. Its mechanism of action is unclear.

Pharmacokinetics. Valproic acid is completely absorbed orally when taken on an empty stomach. Its peak concentration is achieved at between 1 and 3 hours. Food delays the time of absorption but does not interfere with the amount absorbed. Valproic acid distributes widely; it is about 90% bound to albumin. The liver is the site of metabolism. At least 10 metabolites of valproic acid have been identified.

Administration. Valproic acid is available in capsule, syrup, and "sprinkle" forms. The tablet form contains divalproex sodium, which must be metabolized in the gut to valproic acid; it is enterically coated to reduce gastrointestinal symptoms.

Drug Interactions. Valproic acid is altered by salicylates, which increase its free concentration. The addition of phenobarbital or phenytoin decreases the concentration of valproic acid.

Adverse Effects. Mild transient drowsiness and minimal cognitive effects are seen with valproate. Hepatic dysfunction, including liver failure, and pancreatitis have been reported. The more common adverse effects include nausea and vomiting, which can be controlled by using enterically coated Depakote or by taking the drug with food. Weight gain, transient hair loss, tremor, and dose-related thrombocytopenia are common. Menstrual disturbances and hyperandrogenism may occur in women. Neural tube defects and congenital abnormalities have been reported in the infants of mothers on the drug.

Phenobarbital

Phenobarbital (Luminal) was introduced in 1912. One of the first drugs available for the control of seizures, it is still widely used as an alternative for generalized seizures, except absence and partial seizures. Other drugs are replacing phenobarbital for treatment of status epilepticus. The drug of choice for seizures in infants, its adverse cognitive and sedative-hypnotic effects make it less than ideal for children and adults. Phenobarbital is a CNS depressant; it elevates the seizure threshold by decreasing postsynaptic excitation, possibly by stimulating postsynaptic gamma-aminobutyric acid (GABA) inhibitor responses.[15]

Pharmacokinetics. Phenobarbital is rapidly and completely absorbed by all routes (oral, IM, rectal). The biphasic distribution includes initial penetration of highly perfused organs, including the brain, followed by even distribution to all body tissues, including fat. By the IV route, peak cerebral concentration is achieved in 3 to 20 minutes. Drugs affecting liver enzymes may alter phenobarbital's metabolism. The elimination pattern of phenobarbital is linear. About 20% to 40% of a dose is excreted through the kidneys unchanged. Urinary pH affects tubular absorption of Phenobarbital, and the amount of excreted drug can be increased by administering diuretics and urinary alkalizing drugs. The binding of phenobarbital to protein is 50%.

Administration. The routes of administration are oral and parenteral. In an emergency, phenobarbital can be given by IV as a loading dose. The half-life of phenobarbital is so long that it can be given as a single daily dose. Because it takes about 3 to 4 weeks to reach steady state, changing doses rapidly is not recommended.

Drug Interactions. Phenobarbital decreases the efficacy of oral contraceptives.

Adverse Effects. The chief adverse effects are sedation, drowsiness, and fatigue. In addition, impairment of higher cortical function and depression of cognitive performance (e.g., learning) are found with the use of phenobarbital.

Newer Drugs

Several new AEDs have been approved by the Food and Drug Administration in the last decade. They include felbamate (1993), gabapentin (1993), lamotrigine (1994), topiramate (1996), tiagabine (1997), levetiracetam (1999), oxcarbazepine (2000), and zonisamide (2000). Their mechanisms of action and uses vary. Felbamate is used as monotherapy in partial-onset seizures and tonic-clonic seizures in adults. Gabapentin is approved for adjunctive therapy for partial seizures in patients 12 year old and older. Lamotrigine is used for treatment of partial seizures in adults and children, whereas topiramate is used to treat partial seizures in adults. Tiagabine is effective as an add-on therapy for partial seizures for adults and children. Levetiracetam and zonisamide are approved for refractory partial seizures. Oxcarbazepine is used as an add-on treatment for partial seizures with or without secondary generalized seizures (see Table 29-5).

Summary of Drug Therapy

Any patient receiving long-term drug therapy should be monitored carefully for the development of side effects or toxicity. Most drugs are metabolized by the liver and excreted by the kidneys. Periodic drug blood levels should be monitored. If anemia or blood dyscrasias are common side effects, a CBC should be done routinely. Folic acid deficiency has also been reported with some AEDs; therefore, folic acid levels should be monitored. Newer drugs have been introduced in the last several years that may be used in controlling seizures that were previously refractory to good control.

Surgical Management

About 20% of patients with epilepsy do not respond well to drug therapy. Those patients who have been given a trial (e.g., 1 year or more) on AEDs and continue to have refractory seizures that impact on their quality of life should be considered for surgical evaluation. Selection criteria are important. Patients who have not responded to medical management of seizure, who have a unilateral focus that will not cause a major neurological deficit if excised, and who have had a significant alteration in their quality of life are good candidates for surgery. Surgery should be preceded by an extensive diagnostic workup that includes electrophysiology, neuropsychology, and imaging studies. All three should suggest an epileptogenic focus. The purpose of surgery is to locate and excise as much of the epileptogenic area as possible without causing neurological deficits.

The presurgical workup is comprehensive and directed at identifying the functional and structural basis of the seizure disorder. The workup includes the following areas:[23]

- In-patient video-EEG monitoring to identify the anatomical location of the seizure site and to correlate behavior patterns with abnormal EEG patterns
- Routine scalp or scalp-sphenoidal recording for localization of lesion
- MRI high resolution with thin slices to localize lesion
- Possible SPECT or PET scans
- Neuropsychological testing
- Possible amobarbital test (Wada's test) to assess language and memory location
- Other tests as necessary

Surgical Procedures

The most common surgical procedure for the treatment of seizures is a cortical excision (lobectomy). A large number of patients with partial complex seizures with a localized focus have that focus in the temporal lobe. With refractory temporal lobe epilepsy, resection of the anteromedial temporal lobe (*mesial temporal lobectomy*) is available. A more limited removal of the underlying hippocampus and amygdala is also available. If scar tissue or other focal epileptogenic area exists, the identified lesion (*lesionectomy*) can be removed. When the cortical region cannot be removed, multiple subpial transection designed to disrupt intracortical connections is sometimes effective in controlling seizures.

A *corpus callosotomy* has been helpful for persons with tonic and atonic seizures. Outcomes vary depending on the type of surgical procedure. For example, outcomes of temporal-lobe resections break down as follows: approximately 68% seizure free, 24% improved, and 8% no improvement at all.[23] Outcomes from surgery are superior to prolonged medical therapy for temporal-lobe epilepsy.[24] Data on corpus callosotomy surgeries indicate that about 8% became seizure free, 61% had worthwhile improvement, and 31% had no improvement.[25] The best results are reported from centers where large numbers of surgeries for epilepsy are performed.

A *hemispherectomy* is reserved for selected catastrophic infant and early childhood epilepsies. Currently, the practice is to perform a modified radical hemispherectomy leaving the frontal and occipital poles in place although disconnected. The response has been good in that about 67% were seizure free, another 21% had a worthwhile response, and 11% had no improvement.[26]

Local anesthesia is used for adolescents and adults unless they have behavioral problems and need to be sedated. In that case, a light general anesthetic is given. Often, the patient *must* be able to follow commands and answer questions during the EEG and cortical stimulation portion of the lengthy surgical procedure. After surgical exposure of the brain surface and depth, electrodes are applied so that an EEG can be taken to identify the epileptogenic focus. Cortical stimulation is used to identify sensory, motor, and speech areas. After the tissue to be excised has been identified, cortical resection is undertaken. Following excision, the electrodes are reattached to determine the presence of any other epileptogenic activity that would require further resection. If the EEG pattern is satisfactory, the patient is anesthetized so that the incision can be closed. Postoperatively, the patient is managed in the same way as any craniotomy patient (see Chap. 15).

Postoperatively and at discharge, the patient continues on an AED, often carbamazepine. EEG recordings are obtained to determine the presence of seizure activity. The decision to discontinue drug therapy after 2 to 4 years is based on an evaluation of the specific patient.

Complications of Surgery

The mortality from a temporal resection is lower than 1%. The complications of surgery include infection; hydrocephalus; cerebral edema, ischemia, or hematoma; hemiparesis or hemiplegia; aphasia; alexia; or visual field deficits. Higher-level functions of cognition, memory, attention, concentration, or language may be affected. In addition, psychosocial impairment such as family interpersonal dynamics, self-esteem, adverse response to treatment failure, and vocational/education disruption are possible.[27]

Vagus Nerve Stimulation

In 1997, vagus nerve stimulation (VNS) was approved for use in the United States as an adjunctive therapy for adults and adolescents over 12 years of age who have partial-onset seizures that are refractory to AEDs. It consists of:[28]

1. A programmable signal generator that is implanted in the patient's left upper chest
2. A bipolar VNS lead that connects the generator to the left vagus nerve in the neck
3. A programming wand that uses radiofrequency signals to communicate noninvasively with the generator

4. Hand-held magnets used by the patient or health care provider to manually turn the stimulator on or off

The mechanism of action is uncertain. The surgical procedure takes approximately 1 hour and can be done under general or regional anesthesia. The procedure is well tolerated except for hoarseness in some cases. Minimal surgical complications have been reported. Several trials report a decrease in frequency of seizures by 25% or more in patients previously resistant to all AEDs. The role of VNS for intractable seizure management is yet to be established.[29]

MANAGEMENT OF SEIZURES AND STATUS EPILEPTICUS IN AN ACUTE CARE SETTING

Most nurses who practice in an acute care setting manage patients who have seizures, regardless of whether they are assigned to a neuroscience unit or to other types of units. Seizures may also occur in community-based settings where such patients are managed. Nurses need to know how to manage seizures and status epilepticus. The following is designed to provide that information.

Managing the Patient During a Seizure in an Acute Care Setting

When a patient has a seizure, the nurse's role is to protect the patient from injury, care for him or her after the seizure, and document the details of the event. In the hospital environment, persons who are at risk for having a seizure are placed on seizure precautions. This means that (1) the side-rails of the bed are up and padded, (2) a suction set-up and plastic oral airway are available at the bedside, and (3) the bed is kept in low position.

Management of the patient during a seizure is directed toward preventing injury and observing for complications. The following points should be observed:

BEFORE AND DURING A SEIZURE
- If the patient is seated when a major seizure occurs, ease him or her to the floor, if possible.
- Provide for privacy by pulling the bed curtains or screen or closing the door.
- If the patient experiences an aura, have him or her lie down to prevent injury that might occur from falling to the floor.
- Remove patient's eyeglasses and loosen any constricting clothing.
- Do not try to force anything into the mouth.
- Guide the movements to prevent injuries; do not try to restrain the patient.
- Stay with the patient throughout the seizure to ensure safety.

AFTER A SEIZURE
- Position the patient on the side to facilitate drainage of secretions.

- Provide for adequate ventilation by maintaining a patent airway; suctioning may be necessary to prevent aspiration.
- Allow the patient to sleep after the seizure.
- On awakening, orient the patient (he or she will probably be amnesic about the event).

Nursing Assessment and Documentation

Collecting data about the seizure requires well-developed observational skills and an understanding of what to look for and how to document observations. It may be helpful to verbalize the observations as events occur. Verbal reinforcement provides for better recall.

The following are several points to consider when organizing information about a seizure:

- Was the seizure witnessed or not witnessed?
- Were there any warning signs or was there an aura?
- Where did the seizure begin and how did it proceed?
- What type of movement was noted and what parts of the body were involved?
- Were there any changes in the size of the pupils or was there conjugate gaze deviation?
- What was the duration of the entire attack and of each phase?
- Was the patient unconscious throughout the seizure?
- Was there urinary or bowel incontinence?
- What was the person's behavior after the seizure?
- Was there any weakness or paralysis of the extremities after the seizure?
- Were there any injuries noted?
- Did the patient sleep after the seizure? How long?

The observations can be recorded in narrative form in the nurse's notes or on a separate seizure activity sheet, which becomes a part of the patient's permanent record. A sample of a seizure activity sheet for generalized tonic-clonic seizures is found in Figure 29-1. Observations are the same for a seizure that was witnessed in a community setting.

Managing a Person During a Seizure in a Community Setting

Seizures may occur in community settings such as ambulatory clinics, work and recreational environments, and the home. The same first aid principles taught to the person and family should be followed by the bystander nurse who comes upon the individual having a seizure. The first aid management of both generalized tonic-clonic seizures and complex partial seizures includes:[13]

First Aid for Generalized Tonic-Clonic Seizures

First aid for generalized tonic-clonic seizures that occur in a community setting is similar to the management of this type of seizure in an acute care setting.

SEIZURE ACTIVITY CHART FOR GENERALIZED TONIC-CLONIC SEIZURES

Patient's Name _____

_____ Age _____

Date	Time	Before		During								After				Nurse's Initials
		Warning Signs	Part of Body Where Seizure Began	General or Localized	Type of Movement	Duration of Each Phase Tonic	Clonic	Level of Conscious-ness	Pupils	Other		Behav-ior	Paral-ysis	Loca-tion of Paral-ysis	Sleep	

Figure 29–1 • A sample of a seizure activity chart.

BEFORE AND DURING A SEIZURE
- The person may fall to the ground, become stiff, and demonstrate clonic movements.
- If the patient is seated, help him or her to lie down.
- Remove eyeglasses and loosen any constricting clothing.
- Do not try to force anything into the mouth.
- Guide the movements to prevent injuries; do not try to restrain the person.
- Stay with the patient throughout the seizure.

AFTER A SEIZURE
- Position the patient on the side to facilitate drainage of secretions.
- Have someone stay with the patient until he or she is fully awake.
- Upon awakening, orient the patient.

First Aid for Complex Partial Seizures

The patient may not seem quite right, engaging in such behaviors as lip-smacking or making chewing motions, walking aimlessly, or not responding to questions (symptoms of automatism).

BEFORE AND DURING A SEIZURE
- Remove harmful objects from the patient's environment or try to coax the patient away from anything that could be harmful.
- Demonstrate a calm manner that does not agitate the patient.
- Do not try to restrain the patient.
- If alone, do not try to approach an angry or agitated patient.

AFTER THE SEIZURE
- Do not leave the patient alone.
- Have someone stay with the patient until consciousness is fully regained; reorient the patient.

When Should You Call for Medical Assistance?

Call for emergency help if

- The individual does not begin breathing after the seizure (cardiopulmonary resuscitation should be activated).

- A generalized tonic-clonic seizure lasts for more than 2 minutes.
- The individual has one seizure right after another.
- The individual is injured.

Managing Status Epilepticus in an Acute Care Setting

Status epilepticus is defined as either continuous seizures lasting at least 5 minutes or two or more discreet seizures between which there is incomplete recovery of consciousness.[10] The most common type of status epilepticus is **tonic-clonic status epilepticus.** In over 50% of cases, status epilepticus is the patient's first seizure.[30] Although there are many types of status epilepticus, the following discussion focuses on the management of convulsive status epilepticus because this form is most common and constitutes a medical emergency.

The initial management of a patient with status epilepticus includes the standard ABCs of life support (supporting respirations, maintaining blood pressure, supporting circulation), administering an AED, finding and treating any underlying cause, and preventing or treating medical complications.

The ABCs of Life Support

Position the patient to avoid aspiration or inadequate oxygenation. A soft, plastic oral airway may be inserted if it is possible to do so without forcing the teeth apart. The airway will need to be suctioned to remain patent. Oxygen is administered at 100% through a nasal cannula. In most instances, patients will breathe on their own as long as the airway is kept patent. Suction the airway to maintain patency. Monitor respiratory function with ongoing pulse oximetry. IV access should be secured, and vital signs and neurological signs should be monitored frequently.

Extreme cerebral hypoxia can result in severe, irreversible neurological deficits. Monitor arterial blood gases because many patients will have a profound metabolic acidosis that corrects itself after seizures are controlled.[10] Support of adequate oxygenation and cerebral perfusion are critical to preventing these serious problems. Monitor glucose by finger stick. Hyperglycemia followed by hypoglycemia is common and needs to be treated. Give 50 mL of 50% glucose for hypoglycemia. Hyperthermia occurs often with status epilepticus. If it occurs, it must be treated aggressively with passive cooling to prevent further ischemia to the brain.

Administering Antiepileptic Drugs

The goal of drug therapy is prompt termination of clinical and electrical seizure activity. The best drug treatment protocol for status epilepticus remains under discussion. Table 29-6 outlines a recommended protocol that proceeds along a timeline and assumes that the previous drug administration did not terminate the seizure.[10,16] If the patient is not already in the intensive care unit, he or she must be moved to that area where intubation, ventilatory support, continuous ECG monitoring, and invasive monitoring can be provided.

Treating the Underlying Cause

The health care provider must try to identify any underlying cause of seizures (e.g., precipitous withdrawal of AEDs, brain tumor) and treat the primary problem. Various possible causative factors are discussed earlier in the chapter.

Preventing or Treating Medical Complications

Adverse physiological consequences of status epilepticus include hypoxia, hypoglycemia, hypotension, and hyperthermia. Severe metabolic acidosis can occur as a result of loss of base reserve. This change may prevent seizure control with anticonvulsants by increasing the amount of potassium in the extracellular space. It may also contribute to cerebral damage. Blood gases should be monitored. Other medical complications that may develop include cardiac arrhythmias, myocardial infarction, and aspiration pneumonia.

Nursing Management of Status Epilepticus

The nurse works as part of a collaborative team in addressing the medical emergency. Goals and responsibilities include:

- Maintaining a patent airway to ensure adequate ventilation
- Suctioning as necessary to prevent obstruction of the airway and possible aspiration
- Providing oxygen by nasal cannula as ordered
- Protecting the IV site to allow for continuous access for medication
- Protecting the patient from injury
- Providing information to the family

ⅢⅢ NURSING MANAGEMENT OF PATIENTS WITH EPILEPSY: COMMUNITY-BASED CARE

In the community, most people with epilepsy are managed by their primary care physicians or by a neurologist. In a managed care environment, more patients with epilepsy, who were previously managed by a neurologist, come under the care of the primary care physician. Those with complicated or intractable epilepsy will probably still be managed by a neurologist or in an epilepsy center.

The role of the nurse in managing patients with epilepsy will continue to be important, and in many settings this role will be expanded. In the community, nursing management is initially directed at assisting with the assessment and diagnostic workup. The components of these activities are discussed in earlier sections. However, the nurse's major role is to provide patient education and patient monitoring. The next section focuses on this aspect of management. The major nursing diagnosis for a newly diagnosed patient with epilepsy is Knowledge Deficit. An individualized teaching plan must be developed (Chart 29-1).

CHART 29 – 1 • Components of a Teaching Plan for Persons With Epilepsy or a Seizure Disorder

DIET/NUTRITION/BEVERAGES

- Eat a well-balanced diet; eat on a routine schedule.
- Avoid excesses of sugar, caffeine, or any other food that may trigger seizures.
- Discuss alcohol consumption with your doctor; if you choose to drink, limit your consumption to whatever your physician recommends. Seizures may be precipitated by alcohol consumption, and even small amounts may trigger a seizure in some people.

GENERAL HEALTH

- Any of the following can trigger seizures in some persons and should be avoided: constipation, excessive fatigue, hyperventilation, and stress.
- Regular exercise is good for general well being and stress reduction. Avoid overfatigue and hyperventilation. Avoid exercise in hot weather; exercise in a climate-controlled environment.
- Regular sleep patterns on a regular schedule are important. Insomnia or awakening tired are indications of insufficient sleep. This may be due to stress, poor sleep hygiene, or a side effect of medication. Determine cause of sleep disturbance and correct it or seek assistance from the health care provider.
- Showers, rather than tub baths, should be taken.
- Good oral hygiene and periodic visits to the dentist are important because gingival hyperplasia can occur from some antiepileptic drugs (AEDs) such as phenytoin.

FEVER AND ILLNESS

- Fever can trigger seizures; the fever and underlying cause must be treated.
- Any prescription or over-the-counter drugs should be reviewed for interaction.
- If antibiotics are ordered, interactions with the AEDs should be evaluated.

ENVIRONMENTAL, OCCUPATIONAL, AND RECREATIONAL RISK FACTORS

- Noisy environments should be avoided; control a noisy environment as much as possible.
- Avoid bright, flashing lights or fluorescent lights, strobe lights, discos, a flickering television, and flashing bulbs on signs or Christmas trees. Tinted glass on the windshield and eyeglasses will help to control glare.
- Use a screen filter on the computer screen to control glare.
- Do not use recreational or street drugs.
- Work or recreational activities that could cause injury if a seizure occurred should be avoided.

- Swim with a "buddy"; help should be available if a seizure occurs.
- Contact sports (e.g., football, boxing) that could lead to unconsciousness should be avoided.

STRESS, ANXIETY, AND DEPRESSION

- Emotional stress is a trigger to seizures; measures need to be taken to uncover the basis for the stress and how this can be decreased. Counseling may be helpful.
- Living with a chronic health problem is stressful and can place a varying degree of limitations on lifestyle. Depression may result. Appropriate psychotherapy through counseling and/or drugs should be provided.

WOMEN'S HEALTH

- There may be an increase in seizures around the time of menses. This should be discussed with your health care provider; some adjustment may be made in your medications.
- If the occurrence of seizures increases around the menses, control other triggers for seizures.
- AEDs decrease the effectiveness of oral contraceptives; intrauterine devices or other contraceptive devices may be preferred.
- The seizure pattern often changes during pregnancy; discuss this with your health care provider.
- Some AEDs can cause birth defects. If pregnancy is planned, it should be discussed with the gynecologist and health care provider following the epilepsy.

LEGISLATION TO PROTECT PERSONS WITH EPILEPSY AND SEIZURE DISORDER

The following laws protect persons with epilepsy or seizure disorders from discrimination:

- Americans With Disabilities Act
- Rehabilitation Act
- Individuals With Disabilities Education Act
- *Legal Rights of Persons with Epilepsy* (1992) is published by the Epilepsy Foundation of America and is a good resource about epilepsy and the law.
- Driver's licenses are controlled by individual states; information on the laws governing driving can be obtained from the Division of Motor Vehicles.

OTHER

- Issues related to marriage, child-bearing, and parenting need to be discussed. Risk factors and questions related to children with epilepsy need a frank discussion.

Patient Teaching: General Points

Patient teaching requires a comprehensive teaching plan to help the patient adjust to the health problem. Family teaching cannot be excluded because the family needs help to adjust to a chronic condition that is, by its very nature, frightening. The family must be instructed in what to do when a seizure occurs, including first aid. The teaching plan is based on a systematic assessment of patient needs. Physical, social, psychological, and vocational dimensions must be considered along with a drug teaching plan.

Each teaching plan is individual, that is, tailored to the needs of the patient and the problems that arise over time. Major points of information that should be presented to the patient are outlined in Chart 29-1. The plan should expand on these points to include the implications that apply to the patient's individual lifestyle.[31] The plan must be revised periodically to update its relevance. Because noncompliance is a common problem, compliance must be evaluated at each encounter with the health care professional. It is important to reinforce information each time the health care provider is seen.

Patients may express concerns about how they will cope with certain aspects of their lives. One common concern of most adults is whether they should reveal their condition when applying for a job. Many report discrimination by employers when they reveal their condition. Those who choose to conceal this information often feel guilty and live in fear that they will experience a seizure on the job or that their seizure disorder will become known to the employer. If a seizure did occur on the job, it could endanger the patient and others, depending on the kind of work that is done. Information that is deliberately concealed is cause for immediate dismissal in most places of employment. It is the patient's decision to determine whether to disclose the epileptic condition.

Patient Teaching Related to Drug Therapy

It is imperative to provide detailed information to the patient and/or a responsible family member about epilepsy and drug therapy. Side effects and signs of toxicity should be discussed. The patient must understand that the drug must be taken as ordered *every day*. The most common cause of seizures in patients who have previously been controlled is failure to take the AEDs. The patient should be asked to maintain a drug chart of time, amount taken, and side effects, along with a record of the frequency and characteristics of any seizures.

Because seizures represent a chronic condition, that is, they are usually not completely arrested, the person must understand the nature of the problem, the precipitating factors, and the adaptations in lifestyle that are required.

The following is an outline of the major points of a drug teaching plan:

- The drug must be taken as ordered to maintain a therapeutic blood level, even if there is no seizure activity.
- AEDs may be necessary for a few years or longer; for some patients, they may be necessary for a lifetime. There are criteria for when and how a trial of drug discontinu-

ation should be managed; discuss this with the health care provider.
- Discontinuation of drugs without the knowledge of the health care provider is the most common cause of seizure activity (e.g., status epilepticus); this should not be done.
- Know the signs of toxicity of the drugs prescribed. Symptoms of toxicity should be reported promptly to the physician.
- Keep drug and seizure charts and bring them with you for your appointment.
- Because there are serious side effects from some drugs, be sure to have blood work done as ordered (e.g., CBC for anemia and blood dyscrasias).
- Because phenytoin is absorbed slowly from the gastrointestinal tract, daily drug schedules can be adjusted for convenience. Missed doses can be "made up" safely.
- Some individuals may be able to take extended-release phenytoin with once-daily dosing; discuss this with your health care provider.
- A Medic Alert bracelet or a card should be carried to indicate a chronic condition. The patient is encouraged to carry a card that indicates that he or she is being treated by a particular physician. If the patient is found unconscious or injured, the physician can be notified.
- Keep follow-up appointments with a health care provider for periodic monitoring and reevaluation.

Special Populations: Women and the Elderly

Two patient populations that have unique needs when discussing epilepsy and seizure disorders are women and the elderly.

Women

Some of the special needs of women are included in the teaching plan in Chart 29-1. Women who have a seizure disorder need anticipatory guidance about contraception and the implications of child-bearing. The effectiveness of oral contraceptives is decreased by AEDs, which induce liver enzymes and increase the rate of metabolism. A sign of ineffectiveness of the oral contraceptive is breakthrough bleeding; an oral contraceptive with a higher estrogen content needs to be taken or other forms of birth control used.

Women taking AEDs who wish to become pregnant should discuss their particular situation with the physician. Myths need to be dispelled and real risks, including risk of teratogenic effects of many AEDs on a fetus, need to be examined. There is evidence that there is a doubling of the rate of malformations in babies born to mothers taking AEDs. Further, the risk may be dose related. A combination of AEDs, especially carbamazepine, phenytoin, and valproate, causes a much higher risk of neural tube defects.[13] The question arises as to what should be done about AEDs if a woman wants to become pregnant. There is no simple answer. The variables include the particular drugs and dosages involved and the severity of the seizure disorder. For some women, discontinuation of the AEDs may be an option. This is a decision that should be made after careful discussion with the physician. After a woman is pregnant, it does no good to discontinue the AEDs.

During pregnancy, many women notice a change in their seizure pattern, which is unpredictable. The increased risk of complications during pregnancy, delivery, and the postpartum period requires that the neurologist or primary care physician and the obstetrician collaborate closely. If breastfeeding is planned, consideration of the effect of the AED in breast milk on the infant needs to be addressed. For details of management, other sources should be consulted.

The Elderly

A high incidence of new onset of epilepsy is found in persons 65 years old and older. The risk factors associated with the increased incidence in this group include stroke, head trauma, dementia, infection, alcoholism, and aging. Of these, stroke associated with paresis and cortical involvement is the leading risk factor for the development of epilepsy in the elderly. Although generalized tonic-clonic seizures are easily recognizable, simple and complex seizures may pose a more difficult problem because of the subtle symptoms and other competing diagnoses. The differential diagnosis includes transient ischemic attacks, syncope, drop attacks, transient global amnesia, psychiatric disorders, and sleep disorders.[32] To make a diagnosis of a seizure disorder, nurses and physicians first need to recognize it as a possibility when evaluating older patients. With seizure disorder in the differential diagnosis, the health care provider is alerted to collect a detailed history from the person and family member and conduct a complete physical and neurological examination. In addition, MRI and an EEG may be useful. It is noteworthy that a normal EEG does not necessarily exclude the diagnosis of epilepsy. An EEG with stresses such as sleep deprivation increases the possibility of observing epileptiform abnormalities. Focal or diffuse slowing on EEG is not necessarily an indicator of epilepsy in older persons. An EEG finding known as **periodic lateralized epileptiform discharges (PLEDs)** is of particular interest; these are abnormal interictal EEG wave patterns characterized by paroxysmal, sharp wave complexes suggestive of an underlying *focal* seizure disorder.[33]

Management consists of treating the underlying problem and choosing the right AED for the seizure type. In choosing an AED for an elderly person, several points should be considered:

- The pharmacokinetics (absorption, distribution, metabolism, and excretion) are altered in the elderly owing to hematological, renal, and hepatic function changes. Before ordering any AEDs, CBC, clotting factors, albumin, liver function studies, and creatinine values should be evaluated to determine whether the AED would have an unusual effect given any abnormal values.
- Many older people are taking several drugs for chronic health problems such as cardiac and respiratory problems. Consider drug interactions when choosing an AED.
- Consider the effect of the drug on cognitive function and balance and how it will affect daily living and patient safety.
- Consider cost. If the drug is too expensive for the patient, compliance will not be maintained.

- Begin with AED monotherapy, starting at a low dose, and titrate slowly to monitor seizure control or toxicity. Monitor the patient for side effects such as folate deficiency with phenytoin. Free AED concentrations should be measured in any patient with renal or hepatic dysfunction who has signs of toxicity when within the therapeutic range.

Long-Term Management of Persons With Epilepsy

Long-term management and periodic reevaluation are necessary with any chronic condition. Because all drugs have side effects and toxicity, patients must be monitored for any signs of toxicity. When adverse reactions occur, medications need to be adjusted or discontinued. Periodic reevaluation provides the opportunity for assessment of emotional, psychological, social, and vocational problems that are apt to develop as the patient adjusts to living with a seizure disorder.

REFERENCES

1. Hirose, S., Okada, O., Kaneko, S., & Mitsudome, A. (2000). Are some idiopathic epilepsies disorders of ion channels? A working hypothesis. *Epilepsy Research, 41*, 191–204.
2. Browne, T. R., & Holmes, G. L. (2000). *Handbook of epilepsy* (2nd ed., pp. 1–18). Philadelphia: Lippincott Williams & Wilkins.
3. Lowenstein, D. H. (2001). Seizures and epilepsy. In E. Braunwald, A. S. Fauci, D. L. Kasper, S. L. Hauser, D. L. Longo, & J. L. Jameson (Eds.). *Harrison's principles of internal medicine* (15th ed., pp. 2354–2369). New York: McGraw-Hill.
4. Benarroch, E. E., Westmoreland, B. F., Daube, J. R., Reagan, T. J., & Sandok, B. A. (1999). *Medical neurosciences: An approach to anatomy, pathology, and physiology by systems and levels* (4th ed., p. 119). Philadelphia: Lippincott Williams & Wilkins.
5. Foreman, P. J. (2001). 14th Annual Houston Epilepsy Symposium: Epilepsy update 2001: Spotlight on new antiepileptic drugs. Houston, Texas, June 2, 2001.
6. Gastaut, J. (1973). Definitions. In *Dictionary of epilepsy, Part I*. Geneva: World Health Organization.
7. Kotagel, P. (1997). Complex partial seizures with automatisms. In F. Wylie (Ed.). *The treatment of epilepsy: Principles and practice* (2nd ed., pp. 385–400). Baltimore: Williams & Wilkins.
8. Commission of Classification and Terminology of the International League Against Epilepsy. (1981). Proposal for revised clinical and electroencephalographic classification of epileptic seizures. *Epilepsia, 22*, 489–501.
9. Benbadis, S. R. (2001). Epilepsy. *Neurologic Clinics, 19*(2), 251–270.
10. Lowenstein, D. H., & Alldredge, B. K. (1998). Status epilepticus. *New England Journal of Medicine, 338*(14), 970–976.
11. Gastaunt, H., & Broughton, R. (1972). *Epileptic seizures: Clinical and electrographic features, diagnosis and treatment* (pp. 25–90). Springfield, IL: Charles C Thomas.
12. Theodore, W. H., Porte, R. J., Albert, P., et al. (1994). The secondarily generalized tonic-clonic seizure: A videotape analysis. *Neurology, 44*, 1403–1407.
13. Gumnit, R. J. (1995). *The epilepsy handbook: The practical management of seizures* (2nd ed., pp. 124–127). New York: Raven.
14. Trescher, W. H., & Lesser, R. P. (2000). The epilepsies. In W. G. Bradley, R. B. Daroff, G. M. Fenichel, & C. D. Marsden (Eds.). *Neurology in clinical practice* (3rd ed., 1745–1779). Boston: Butterworth-Heinemann.

15. Graves, N. M., & Garnett, W. R. (1999). Epilepsy. In J. T. DiPiro, R. L. Talbert, G. C. Yee, G. R. Matzke, B. G. Wells, & L. M. Posey (Eds.). *Pharmacotherapy: A pathophysiologic approach* (4th ed., pp. 952–975). Stamford, CT: Appleton & Lange.
16. Quality Standards Committee of AAN. (1996). Practice parameter: A guideline for discontinuing antiepileptic drugs in seizure-free patients–summary statement. *Neurology, 47*, 600–602.
17. Browne, T. R., & Holmes, G. L. (2001). Epilepsy. *New England Journal of Medicine, 344*(150), 1145–1151.
18. Bana, D. K. (1998). Antiepileptic drug withdrawal–a good idea? *Pharmacotherapy, 18*, 235–241.
19. Spenser, S. S., Spenser, D. D., Williamson, P. D., & Mattson, R. H. (1981). Ictal effects of anticonvulsant medication withdrawal in epileptic patients. *Epilepsia, 22*, 297–307.
20. Holmes, L. B., Harvey, E. A., Coull, B. A., et al. (2001). The teratogenicity of anticonvulsant drugs. *New England Journal of Medicine, 344*(15), 1132–1138.
21. Andrews, C. O., Turnbull, M. D., Paloucek, F. P., et al. (1994). Safety and pharmacokinetics of fosphenytoin following intravenous loading dose administration. *Pharmacotherapy, 14*, 367.
22. Holland, K. D. (2001). Epilepsy. *Neurologic Clinics, 19*(2), 313–345.
23. Engel, J. (1996). Surgery for seizures. *New England Journal of Medicine, 334*(10), 647–652.
24. Wiebe, S., Blume, W. T., Girvin, J. P., & Eliasziw, M. (2001). A randomized controlled trial of surgery for temporal-lobe epilepsy. *New England Journal of Medicine, 345*(5), 311–318.
25. Engel, J. Jr., van Ness, P. C., Rasmussen, T. B., Ojemann, L. M. (1993). Outcome with respect to epileptic seizures. In J. Engel Jr. (Ed.). *Surgical treatment of the epilepsies* (2nd ed., pp. 609–621). New York: Raven Press.
26. Engel, J. Jr. (1996). Surgery for seizures. *New England Journal of Medicine, 334*(10), 647–652.
27. Pilcher, W. H., & Rusyniak, W. G. (1993). Complications of epilepsy surgery. *Neurosurgery Clinics of North America, 4*(2), 312.
28. Schachter, S. C. (2001). Epilepsy. *Neurologic Clinics, 19*(1), 57–78.
29. Wyllie, E. (Ed.). (1997). *The treatment of epilepsy: Principles and practice* (2nd ed.). Baltimore: Williams & Wilkins.
30. Hauser, W. A. (1990). Status epilepticus: Epidemiologic considerations. *Neurology, 40*(Suppl.), 9–13.
31. Shafer, R. O. (1994). Nursing support of epilepsy self-management. *Clinical Nursing Practice in Epilepsy, 2*(1), 5–6.
32. Drury, I., & Beydoun, A. (1993). Seizure disorders of aging: Differential diagnosis and patient management. *Geriatrics, 48*(5), 52–58.
33. Lannon, S. (1993). Epilepsy in the elderly. *Journal of Neuroscience Nursing, 25*(5), 273–282.

RESOURCES
Published Material
Books

Browne, T. R., & Holmes, G. L. (2000). *Handbook of epilepsy* (2nd ed.). Philadelphia: Lippincott Williams & Wilkins.
Wyllie, E. (Ed.). (1997). *The treatment of epilepsy: Principles and practice* (2nd ed.). Baltimore: Williams & Wilkins.

Periodicals

Browne, T. R., & Holmes, G. L. (2001). Epilepsy. *New England Journal of Medicine 344*(15), 1145–1151.
Curry, W. J., & Kulling, D. L. (1998). Newer antiepileptic drugs: Gabapentin, lamotrigine, felbamate, topiramate and fosphenytoin. *American Family Physician, 57*(3), 513–520.
Delanty, N., & French, J. (1998). New options in epilepsy pharmacotherapy. *Formulary, 33*, 1190–1206.
Dichter, M. A., & Brodie, M. J. (1996). New antiepileptic drugs. *New England Journal of Medicine, 334*(24), 1583–1590.
Engel, J., Jr. (1996). Surgery for seizures. *New England Journal of Medicine, 334*(10), 647–652.
Foldvary, N. (2001). Epilepsy: treatment issues for women with epilepsy. *Neurologic Clinics, 19*(2), 491–515.
Lannon, S. L. (1993). Epilepsy in the elderly. *Journal of Neuroscience Nursing, 25*(5), 273–282.
Lowenstein, D. H., & Alldredge, B. K. (1998). Status epilepticus. *New England Journal of Medicine, 338*(14), 970–976.
O'Dell, C., & Shinnar, S. (2001). Epilepsy: Initiation and discontinuation of antiepileptic drugs. *Neurologic Clinics, 19*(2), 289–311.
Schachter, S. C. (2001). Epilepsy. *Neurologic Clinics, 19*(1), 57–78.
Shafer, P. O. (1999). Advances in seizure assessment, treatment, and self-management. *Nursing Clinics of North America, 34*(2), 5–6.
Shafer, P. O. (1994). Nursing support of epilepsy self-management. *Clinical Nursing Practice in Epilepsy. 2*(1), 5–6.
Working Group on Status Epilepticus. (1993). Treatment of convulsive status epilepticus: Recommendations of the Epilepsy Foundation of America's Working Group on Status Epilepticus. *Journal of the American Medical Association, 270*(7), 854–859.

Websites/Contact Information

Epilepsy Foundation of America, Telephone: (800) 332-1000 or (301) 459-3700; http://www.efa.org/ or http://www.epilepsyfoundation.org/gene

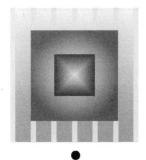

C H A P T E R **30**

Selected Infections of the Nervous System

JOANNE V. HICKEY

Of the many infectious diseases involving the central nervous system (CNS), only the most common are addressed in this chapter. These include bacterial meningitis, viral encephalitis, and the parameningeal infections, as well as brain abscess and extradural abscess. Features of other selected nervous system infections are presented in tabular format. The effects of acquired immunodeficiency syndrome (AIDS) on the nervous system are also discussed.

MENINGITIS

Bacterial Meningitis

Bacterial meningitis is a pyogenic (purulent or suppurative) infection that involves the pia-arachnoid layers of the meninges and the subarachnoid space (SAS), including cerebrospinal fluid (CSF). Infections can occur when bacteria gain access to the meninges through the blood-borne route or through the spread of nearby infections such as sinusitis, mastoiditis, otitis media, osteomyelitis of the skull or vertebrae, or pneumonia. Other sources of CSF contamination are neurosurgical procedures, lumbar puncture, or penetrating head wounds. Infections of the meninges also result from preexisting connections between the CNS and dural defects, congenital sinuses, or occult encephaloceles.[1]

Common Causative Organisms

The common causative organisms for bacterial meningitis tend to differ by age group. In newborns, *beta-hemolytic Streptococci* (Group B) and *Listeria monocytogenes* are the most common etiologies. In older children and adults, *Streptococcus pneumoniae*, *Neisseria meningitidis*, and *Haemophilus influenzae* are the more common causative organisms. *S. pneumoniae* is the most common organism responsible for community-acquired bacterial meningitis. In older adults (50 years of age and older), *S. pneumoniae* is likely to cause meningitis in association with pneumonia or otitis media. In addition, gram-negative bacilli *Enterobacteriaceae* (*Escherichia coli*, *Klebsiella pneumoniae*, *Pseudomonas*, *Enterobacter*, and *Serratia* spp.) are the organisms likely to cause meningitis in

association with chronic lung disease, sinusitis, neurosurgical procedures, or chronic urinary tract infection in older patients (Table 30-1).[2] About 75% of the sporadic cases of meningitis involve infection with *H. influenzae*, *N. meningitidis*, and *S. pneumoniae*. *L. monocytogenes* is now the fourth most common type of nontraumatic or non-postsurgical bacterial meningitis in adults.[3] Except during summer when incidence decreases, the rate of cases of meningitis is constant throughout the year.

Pathophysiology

The *Haemophilus* and *S. pneumoniae* organisms associated with the respiratory tract, and the gram-negative rod organisms, *Enterobacteriaceae*, associated with the enteric tract, often inhabit the nasopharynx and are the major organisms causing bacterial meningitis in children and adults. These bacteria attach themselves to mucous epithelium by secreting a substance known as immunoglobin A (IgA) protease, and enter the bloodstream. In the blood, bacteria are inactivated by complement-mediated bactericidal activity and phagocytosis by neutrophils. However, protection from these mechanisms is afforded by a capsular polysaccharide coating. Bacteria that are able to survive in the circulation enter the CSF through the choroid plexus of the lateral ventricles and other areas of the altered blood-brain barrier. The CSF is an area of impaired host defense because of a lack of sufficient numbers of complement components and immunoglobulins for the opsonization (the rendering of bacteria and other cells subject to phagocytosis) of bacteria.[4]

The pathophysiological events related to meningitis are well described by Roos.[2] Bacteria multiply rapidly in the SAS. Both this multiplication and lysis of bacteria by bactericidal antibiotics cause the release of bacterial cell wall components. These components stimulate the formation of the inflammatory cytokines, interleukin-1 (IL-1) and tumor necrosis factor (TNF) by monocytes, macrophages, brain astrocytes, and microglial cells. Blood-brain barrier permeability is altered; polymorphonuclear leukocytes are recruited. All these events contribute to the formation of purulent exudate in the SAS. Concurrently, IL-1 and TNF induce the formation of molecules that adhere to leukocytes on vascular endothelial cells. This allows neutrophils to traverse the blood-brain barrier. The large numbers of leu-

▌▌▌▌ **T a b l e   3 0 – 1** • CAUSATIVE ORGANISMS OF BACTERIAL MENINGITIS*

DISEASE	ORGANISM	COMMENTS
Pneumococcal meningitis	*Streptococcus pneumoniae* (gram-positive diplococci)	• Found in the young and those >40 yr of age • Most common type of meningitis occurring in adults • Predisposing conditions to pneumococcal meningitis include pneumonia, sinusitis, alcoholism, head trauma, splenectomy, and sickle cell anemia
Haemophilus influenzae meningitis	*H. influenzae* (gram-negative cocci)	• Pediatric problem seen in those 3 mo to 8 yr of age (6–8 mo highest incidence) • Often follows upper respiratory or ear infections
Meningococcal meningitis	*Neisseria meningitidis* (gram-negative diplococci)	• Highest incidence in children and young adults • Petechial rash, purpuric lesions, or ecchymosis develop in 50% of patients • About 10% of affected patients develop a fulminating infection with overwhelming septicemia (meningococcemia); this can create a medical emergency owing to high fever, purpuric lesions, and circulatory collapse from adrenocortical insufficiency secondary to hemorrhage and necrosis of the adrenals (called Waterhouse-Friderichsen syndrome); disseminated intravascular coagulation may also be evident; death can result hours after onset
Other less common diseases	*Staphylococcus aureus* *Streptococcus* group A *Streptococcus* group B *Escherichia coli* *Klebsiella* *Proteus* *Pseudomonas*	• Common in neonates • Often introduced during neurosurgical procedures (especially shunting), lumbar puncture, or spinal anesthesia; seen often in hospitalized neurosurgical patients; head-injured patients, particularly those with cerebrospinal fluid rhinorrhea; or debilitated patients
	Myobacterium tuberculosis	• Secondary infection resulting from bacterial seeding of the meninges from tuberculosis elsewhere in the body • Most common in children • Incidence reflects the rate of tuberculosis in a country (relatively low in the United States)
	Listeria monocytogenes *Salmonella* *Shigella* *Clostridium* *Gonococcus*	• Seen in neonates, the aged, and the immunosuppressed • Rare

* The organisms presented here are responsible for 80% to 90% of the cases of bacterial meningitis worldwide; these organisms are normally found in the nasopharynx of a significant portion of the population. The mechanism by which they cause illness in some people, but not others, is unclear.

kocytes in the SAS add to the purulent exudate and obstruction of flow of CSF. Adhesion of leukocytes to the cerebral capillary endothelial cells increases their permeability and allows plasma proteins to leak through open intercellular junctions. This results in vasogenic brain edema and subsequent increased intracranial pressure (ICP).

In the acute phase of meningitis, the cerebral cortex undergoes little change except for perivascular inflammation with some infiltration into the cortex. In subacute cases, there may be diffuse degenerative changes, with necrosis and glial proliferation within the superficial areas of the brain, spinal cord, or cranial nerves. The optic and acoustic nerves are often affected, although the oculomotor, trochlear, abducens, and facial nerves can also be involved.

The resolution of meningitis depends on the extent of the infection and how quickly effective treatment is initiated. If the process is arrested early, resolution may be complete, without major sequelae. However, the arachnoid layer may undergo fibrotic changes and scar tissue formation. Adhesions and effusions can develop in the SAS, thereby interfering with the normal circulation of CSF. Fibrotic changes in the structures responsible for the production and absorption of CSF may result, contributing to the development of hydrocephalus. Some organisms may produce an abscess. Much of the outcome from bacterial meningitis depends on early and aggressive treatment to prevent the development of complications.

Signs and Symptoms

Although many different organisms are capable of producing meningitis, all produce common signs and symptoms. In infants and very young children, many characteristic signs and symptoms may not occur or may be nonspecific. In such instances, diagnosis can be very difficult. Common symptoms of meningitis in young children include fever, anorexia, vomiting, diarrhea, listlessness, a shrill cry, and bulging fontanels.

In the older child and the adult, the following classic signs and symptoms are noted:

- Headache
- Fever
- Stiff neck/nuchal rigidity and other signs of meningeal irritation
- Altered level of consciousness (LOC) (lethargy, confusion, coma)
- Photophobia

Headache and Fever. The *headache*, which is usually the initial symptom, is described as severe. This symptom is probably attributable to irritation of the pain-sensitive dura and traction on related vascular structures. *Fever* is the rule with bacterial meningitis, and can vary from 38 to 39.5°C (101 to 103°F) or higher. The temperature remains high throughout the course of the illness and can rise to 40.5°C (105°F) and higher in the terminal stages because of decompensation of increased ICP on the brain stem.

Stiff Neck/Nuchal Rigidity, and Other Signs of Meningeal Irritation. A *stiff neck* is an early sign of meningeal irritation. Attempts to flex the neck forward, either actively or passively, prove difficult. This resistance is caused by spasms of the extensor muscles of the neck. Forceful flexion produces severe pain. Two signs of meningeal irritation are Kernig's and Brudzinski's signs. **Kernig's sign** is elicited by flexing the upper leg at the hip to a 90-degree angle and then attempting to extend the knee. In the presence of meningeal irritation, pain and spasm of the hamstrings occur when an attempt is made to extend the knee (Fig. 30-1). The pain is caused by inflammation of the meninges and spinal roots. The spasms are a protective mechanism to deter painful flexion. **Brudzinski's sign** is positive when both the upper leg at the hip and the lower leg at the knee flex in response to passive flexion of the neck and head on the chest (Fig. 30-2). This reflex is caused by irritating exudate around the roots in the lumbar region.

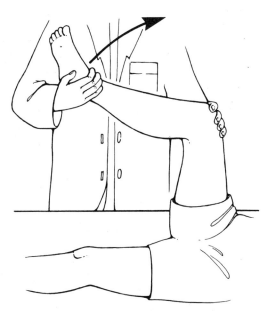

Figure 30-1 • Kernig's sign. With the patient lying on his back, flex one of the patient's legs at the hip and knee. If pain or resistance is elicited as the knee is straightened, this is a positive Kernig's sign, a sign of meningeal irritation.

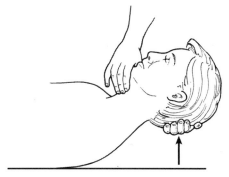

Figure 30-2 • Brudzinski's sign. With the patient lying on his back, place your hand behind the patient's neck and flex the neck toward the sternum. In a patient with meningeal irritation there is neck pain, neck stiffness, and flexion of the hips and knees.

Altered Consciousness. In the very early stages, a shortened attention span and misinterpretation of environmental stimuli are common. The patient becomes disoriented to time, place, and person, is easily bewildered, has poor memory, and appears to have difficulty following commands. Other patients may become restless, agitated, irritable, and disoriented. Adults may progress rapidly from lethargy to stupor and coma. In the older adult, fever, confusion, stupor, or coma is typical.

Other Signs. *Photophobia* is a common sign of meningeal irritation seen in bacterial meningitis, but the pathophysiology for this symptom is not clear. Other signs and symptoms noted include skin hypersensitivity, hyperalgesia, and muscular hypotonia, although motor function is well preserved. Sensory loss does not occur. Seizures occur in 40% to 50% of patients with bacterial meningitis usually within the first week.[1,2] Some patients develop hyponatremia or syndrome of inappropriate secretion of antidiuretic hormone (SIADH) from excessive release of antidiuretic hormone. There are signs and symptoms of water retention, along with oliguria and hypervolemia.

Increased ICP accompanies meningitis because of accumulation of purulent exudate, cerebral edema, and hydrocephalus. Symptoms of brain-stem pressure are reflected in Cushing's response of vital sign changes, such as widening of pulse pressure, decreased pulse, and ataxic respirations. Vomiting is a frequent finding and is related to increased ICP. If the infection is not aggressively treated or response to treatment is poor, cerebral herniation can occur.

Meningococcal Meningitis. Some additional differential signs and symptoms are noteworthy with *N. meningitidis* infection. Petechiae, purpura, or less commonly a morbilliform rash strongly suggest an *N. meningitidis* infection. The petechiae may be seen on the conjunctiva and other parts of the skin and mucous membranes. Disseminated intravascular coagulation (DIC) is most commonly associated with *N. meningitidis*.

Waterhouse-Friderichsen syndrome, a specific combination of signs and symptoms often noted before meningococcal meningitis is evident or diagnosed, is characterized by: chills; fever; headache; malaise; possible joint and muscle pain; petechial hemorrhage, or ecchymosis noted on the skin and mucous membranes; and possible adrenal hemorrhage resulting in adrenal insufficiency followed by hypotension, cyanosis, respiratory distress, and circulatory collapse. If this occurs, immediate administration of adrenal corticosteroids is necessary along with other supportive therapies to treat this life-threatening event.

The need to place a patient on isolation precautions to prevent the spread of disease depends on the type of invading organism and the stage of the illness. For example, in the acute phase of meningococcal meningitis, it is possible to infect others with secretions from the nasopharynx and droplets from the respiratory tract. Meningococci usually disappear within 24 hours of administration of appropriate antimicrobial drugs. Therefore, respiratory isolation of the patient to protect the nursing and health care personnel, visitors, and other patients should be maintained until cultures are negative. The hospital infection control department is the best source of information regarding type and duration of isolation.

Diagnosis

The diagnosis of bacterial meningitis relies on a history, a physical examination, and laboratory data. A history of recent infections, such as those involving the ears, sinuses, or respiratory tract, is of particular interest.

Examination of CSF is the gold standard for the diagnosis of bacterial meningitis. Table 30-2 provides a comparison between the basic CSF criteria for diagnosis of bacterial meningitis and the findings associated with aseptic (viral) meningitis. Procurement of CSF requires a lumbar puncture or sample of CSF from a ventriculostomy. The patient must first be assessed for evidence of elevated ICP, which would be a contraindication for lumbar puncture. If an elevated ICP is suspected, a CT scan may be ordered first. The CT scan is also useful for detection of abscesses and lesions that erode the skull and provide a route for bacterial invasion (e.g., tumors or sinus wall defects). The classic CSF abnormalities noted in bacterial meningitis include:

- Increased opening pressure
- Polymorphonuclear leukocytic pleocytosis
- Decreased glucose concentration
- Increased protein concentration
- Glucose ratio less than 40 mg/dL

- White blood cell (WBCs) count of CSF usually more than 100 cells/mm³ and often more than 1,000 WBCs/mm³
- Protein count higher than 45 mg/dL (most often 100 to 500 mg/dL)

Tests to identify specific causative organisms include gram stain, smear, and culture. Blood cultures may also be of diagnostic value as they are positive in 40% to 60% of patients with *H. influenzae,* meningococcal, and pneumococcal meningitis.[3] For those patients who have received antibiotics, it is more difficult to establish a diagnosis. Newer laboratory techniques are making it possible to detect bacterial antigen in an hour or two. These options include: counter-immunoelectrophoresis (CIE), a sensitive technique that permits the detection of bacterial antigens in the CSF in 30 to 60 minutes; radioimmunoassay (RIA); latex particle agglutination (LPA); enzyme-linked immunosorbent assay (ELISA); and polymerase chain reaction (PCR).[5,6] Finally, measurements of lactate dehydrogenase (LDH) in CSF appear to be of diagnostic and prognostic value in bacterial meningitis. Elevation of total LDH activity is a consistent finding in bacterial meningitis.[3]

Treatment

Because bacterial meningitis is a medical emergency, initial treatment provides general supportive measures, including maintaining blood pressure; maintaining adequate ventilation and a patent airway; treating septic shock; and providing antibacterial drug therapy. Several collaborative problems need to be addressed in the management of these patients:

- Septic shock/sepsis
- Respiratory distress
- Airway patency
- Seizures
- Increased ICP
- Electrolyte imbalance (SIADH, hyponatremia)
- Possibly adrenal insufficiency with meningococcal meningitis
- Hydrocephalus

Drug therapy is based on the identification of the causative organism from CSF analysis, if possible. Alternatively, the

 Table 30–2 • COMPARISON OF THE CLASSIC CEREBROSPINAL FLUID (CSF) FINDINGS IN ACUTE BACTERIAL MENINGITIS AND ACUTE ASEPTIC (VIRAL) MENINGITIS

CSF CHARACTERISTICS	ACUTE BACTERIAL MENINGITIS*	ACUTE ASEPTIC (VIRAL) MENINGITIS
Appearance	Turbid, cloudy	Clear; sometimes turbid
Cells	Increased white blood cells (1,000–2,000 mm³ or more; mostly polymorphonuclear neutrophils)	Increased white blood cells (300 mm³; mostly mononuclear)
Protein level	Increased (100–500 mg/dL)	Normal or slightly increased
Glucose level	Decreased (<40 mg/dL or about 40% of blood glucose level)	Normal
Smear and culture	Bacterial present on gram stain and culture	No bacteria present on gram stain or culture; the virus may be demonstrated by special techniques
Pressure on lumbar puncture	Elevated (>180 mm of water pressure)	Variable

* All patients do not follow this classic profile; about 30% of patients with bacterial meningitis show some of the findings seen in aseptic meningitis.

most likely organism is used for drug selection. The drug should be bactericidal for the suspected causative organism, and treatment should begin while awaiting results of diagnostic tests. The drug prescribed can be changed later based on definitive diagnostic findings. Patient age and known drug resistance patterns in a given area of the country should be considered (Table 30-3 outlines empiric antimicrobial therapy and Table 30-4 has recommendations for drug therapy).

Increased ICP is managed using the usual treatment protocols and elevation of the head of the bed and mannitol (see Chap. 14). Phenytoin is administered prophylactically to prevent seizures. Free water is restricted if hyponatremia is present.

Complications

Complications of bacterial meningitis relate to the type of causative organism and the severity of the illness. Cranial nerve palsies and especially sensorineural hearing loss are common. Meningeal fibrosis around the optic nerve can cause blindness, optic atrophy, or optic neuritis. Hydrocephalus from exudate and meningeal fibrosis can cause dementia, stupor or coma, and paralysis in adults.[3] Other possible complications include personality change, headache, seizure activity, or paresis or paralysis.

Prevention

Bacterial meningitis can often be prevented if the following principles are observed:

- Provide adequate treatment of infections, such as sinusitis, mastoiditis, ear infections, and pneumonias.
- Maintain strict aseptic technique during all intracranial, intraspinal, mastoid, and sinus operations.
- Maintain strict aseptic technique in dressing changes for these procedures.
- Administer prophylactic antibiotics after these procedures.

Table 30-3 • EMPIRIC ANTIMICROBIAL THERAPY FOR BACTERIAL MENINGITIS BY AGE*

AGE GROUP	ANTIMICROBIAL THERAPY
• Adult: 18–50 yr	• Penicillin G or ampicillin or third generation cephalosporin
• Adult: >50 yr	• Third-generation cephalosporin plus ampicillin
• Immunocompromised	• Ceftazidime plus ampicillin or add vancomycin
• Postneurosurgery	• Ceftazidime plus oxacillin or vancomycin plus aminoglycoside
• Basal skull fracture	• Third-generation cephalosporin
• Cerebrospinal fluid shunts	• Vancomycin plus ceftazidime

* Roos, K. L. (1997). Central nervous system infections. In J. Biller (Ed.). *Practical neurology.* (pp. 470–478). Philadelphia: Lippincott-Raven; Adams, R. D., Victor, M., & Ropper, A. H. (1997). *Principles of neurology* (6th ed., pp. 965–741). New York: McGraw-Hill.

Table 30-4 • RECOMMENDED ANTIMICROBIAL THERAPIES FOR BACTERIAL MENINGITIS IN ADULTS BY ORGANISM

ORGANISM	ANTIMICROBIAL DRUG
• Streptococcus pneumoniae	• Penicillin G 20–24 million unit/d IV in divided doses q/4 hr or ampicillin 12 g/d q/4 hr, or ceftriaxone or cefotaxime
• Neisseria meningitidis	• Penicillin G or ampicillin
• Haemophilus influenzae	• Ceftriaxone or cefotaxime
• Pseudomonas aeruginosa	• Ceftazidime 6 g/d q/8 hr
• Listeria monocytogenes	• Ampicillin 12 g/d IV in divided doses q/4 hr
• Staphylococcus aureus (methicillin-sensitive)	• Oxacillin 9–12 g/d IV in divided doses q/8 hr
• S. aureus (methicillin-resistance)	• Vancomycin 1 g IV q/12 hr
• Enterobacteriaceae	• Ceftriaxone or cefotaxime

- Administer prophylactic antibiotics with basal skull fractures, compound skull fractures, dural tears, and injuries causing CSF drainage from the ear or nose.

Viral Meningitis

Viral meningitis, also known as *acute benign lymphocytic meningitis* and *acute aseptic meningitis*, occurs sporadically or as small epidemics. Any number of viruses, such as mumps, enteroviruses (Echo, Coxsackie, poliomyelitis), herpes simplex virus type 2, Epstein-Barr virus, and the arboviruses can be the causative organisms, but no specific organism is identified in most cases. HIV infection can present as aseptic meningitis, especially at the time of seroconversion.[1] All age groups are susceptible, but children are most often affected.

Signs and Symptoms

Signs and symptoms include those of the meningitis syndrome, such as headache, low-grade fever, stiff neck, and symptoms of a systemic or upper respiratory viral illness. Often, a systemic viral infection can be identified.

Diagnosis and Treatment

The CSF is clear with a WBC count typically in the range of 50 to several hundred cell/mm³, predominantly mononuclear cells. The glucose level is normal, and protein is in a range of 50 to 100 mg/dL. A CT scan may be ordered if there is evidence of focal neurological signs.

Treatment of viral meningitis is symptomatic and supportive. Mild cases are managed outside the hospital, but patients with extreme discomfort or excessive vomiting may need hospitalization for symptom management. No drug therapy is effective against the virus. Full recovery is usual within 1 to 2 weeks.

Nursing Management of Patients With Meningitis

Various collaborative problems provide the context of care for patients with meningitis. As a member of the collaborative team, the nurse assesses and monitors the patient throughout the course of the illness, recognizing that the patient is at high risk for complications. Regardless of the etiology of the meningitis, nursing management includes providing supportive care, adhering to specific protocols (e.g., ICP and seizure prophylaxis), preventing complications, and enhancing rehabilitation.

Assessment

In the acute stage of meningitis, the patient is seriously ill.

- Assess vital signs frequently and compare with previous results to detect changes and trends. It is not uncommon for the temperature to reach 40.5°C (105°F). The pulse and respiratory rate are also high in response to the fever. If signs and symptoms of increased ICP are present, the pulse may be depressed and systolic blood pressure elevated.
- Monitor neurological signs frequently. The LOC characteristically deteriorates from confusion to restlessness, lethargy, stupor, and, finally, coma. As the LOC deteriorates, the nurse should assess the patient's ability to protect his or her airway.
- Note signs and symptoms of meningeal irritation as evidenced by nuchal rigidity such as stiff neck, photophobia, pain upon neck flexion, or positive Kernig's or Brudzinski's signs.
- Monitor for evidence of seizure activity and therapeutic levels of anticonvulsant therapy.
- Maintain an accurate intake and output record. A patient with an elevated temperature can easily become dehydrated from profuse perspiration and insensible loss from the skin. Profuse perspiration, oliguria, and dry skin indicate dehydration that requires intravenous (IV) fluid replacement.
- Monitor serum electrolytes for electrolyte imbalances, such as hyponatremia.

Nursing Management

The key points of nursing management of patients with meningitis and the common nursing diagnoses are outlined in Charts 30-1 and 30-2.

Rehabilitation

With meningitis patients, the specific rehabilitative needs depend on the degree of functional disability. Minor functional disabilities may not require any special intervention and improve spontaneously over time with physical activity. Other functional deficits may require an aggressive rehabilitation plan. A comprehensive assessment by the interdisciplinary team is the best means for identifying deficits, determining needed rehabilitation, and setting realistic goals. The nurse works collaboratively with the case manager and other team members to assist in the transition to rehabilitation or home.

ENCEPHALITIS

Encephalitis is an inflammation of the brain caused by viruses (the most common offending organism), bacteria, fungi, or parasites. Some viruses are endemic to particular geographical areas and to particular seasons of the year. There is a lengthy list of specific viruses known to cause viral encephalitis, but only a few appear with appreciable frequency in the United States. Table 30-5 lists and describes the major viruses capable of causing viral encephalitis. Less frequent causes of encephalitis include toxic substances such as lead, arsenic and carbon monoxide; vaccines for measles, mumps, and rabies, which cause postvaccination encephalitis; and viral infections, such as measles, mumps, infectious mononucleosis, and others. The following section addresses encephalitis caused by viruses, the most common cause of encephalitis in the United States.

Signs and Symptoms

The many signs and symptoms of viral encephalitis vary according to the particular invading organisms and the area of the brain involved. The basic syndrome is characterized by fever, headache, seizures, stiff neck, and a change in the LOC, which varies from disorientation, agitation, restlessness, and short attention span to lethargy or drowsiness, and finally to coma. In addition to the wide diversity of levels of consciousness, the patient may exhibit any combination of the following symptoms: aphasia or mutism; motor deficits such as hemiparesis, involuntary (myoclonic) movements, ataxia, nystagmus, ocular paralysis, or facial weakness; or generalized seizures.

Diagnosis is based on the clinical picture, rapid serological assays, and CSF analysis. No specific viral etiology is determined in most cases. CSF findings associated with arboviruses include elevated WBC (mononuclear cells), increase in protein, and normal glucose. There is no definitive treatment or drug therapy for viral encephalitis. Often, the EEG is characterized by widespread slowing. Serological diagnosis depends on a fourfold rise in specific antibody titer, which is often not evident in the acute phase.[1]

The foregoing paints the basic clinical picture of acute viral encephalitis. However, variations in signs and symptoms are noted with specific groupings of viral organisms. The following summarizes cause-specific encephalitis syndromes.

Viral Encephalitis Caused by Arthropod-Borne Viruses

Arthropod-borne viruses causing epidemic encephalitis include Eastern equine, Western equine, Venezuelan, St. Louis, California, and Japanese encephalitis, all spread by mosquitoes. The incidence is more prevalent in late summer and early fall. The severity varies by virus type.

Venezuelan encephalitis is generally mild, Eastern equine and Japanese are severe, and Western equine and St. Louis may be severe. California encephalitis has both mild and severe forms. Western equine and St. Louis encephalitis affect older persons more frequently. The effects of encephalitis on the brain include degenerative changes in the nerve cells, with scattered areas of inflammation and necrosis. There is also some inflammation of the meninges.

Signs and Symptoms

The clinical picture presented by all arthropod-borne viruses in the United States is essentially the same. In older children and adults, the onset is gradual and is characterized by a febrile illness, headache, listlessness, drowsiness, and several days of nausea and vomiting. Seizures, confusion and stupor, stiff neck, muscle pain, ataxia, photophobia, and tremors are then noted. Reflexes are abnormal, and hemipa-

---

CHART 30 – 1 • Summary of the Nursing Management of Patients With Acute Meningitis/Encephalitis

Nursing Responsibilities	Rationale
ASSESSMENT	
• Assess vital signs at frequent intervals.	• Establishes a baseline and provides ongoing data to denote stability, improvement, or deterioration in overall conditions
• Assess neurological signs at frequent intervals.	• Establishes a baseline and provides ongoing data for comparison to determine change
• Assess for signs of meningeal irritation (nuchal rigidity, hyperirritability, hyperalgesia, photophobia).	• Indicates irritation of the covering of the brain and the need for special nursing intervention
• Assess respiratory function (auscultate chest; observe chest movement).	• Alerts the nurse to initiate respiratory support if necessary
BASIC SUPPORTIVE CARE	
• Maintain a patent airway. —Position the patient to facilitate drainage. —Suction as necessary.	• Provides for adequate drainage of oral and nasal secretions
• Maintain adequate oxygenation —Monitor blood gases. —Administer oxygen therapy, as ordered. —Assess the patient for signs and symptoms of dyspnea and cyanosis	• Provides supplemental oxygen to maintain adequate oxygenation
• Administer basic hygienic care.	• Keeps patient dry and comfortable, especially when diaphoretic
• Provide for mouth care every 2 hr.	• Refreshes and moistens the patient's oral cavity, particularly when the temperature is elevated
• Protect the patient from injury by: —Raising side rails. —Keeping the bed low when the patient is left alone —Observing frequently —Protecting the intravenous site or any tubes	• Prevents physical injury to a patient who has a deteriorated level of consciousness and who is often extremely restless
• If the temperature is elevated, measures should be taken to control the temperature, including: —Administering antipyretic drugs, such as acetaminophen (Tylenol), 650 mg orally or rectally —Removing excess bedclothes —Maintaining a cool room temperature (68°F or 20°C) —Giving tepid baths —Using a hypothermia blanket	• An increase in temperature increases the need for oxygen to support increased metabolism. An elevated temperature also increases ICP.
• Control pain of headache, if present, by: —Elevating the head 30 degrees —Applying an ice cap as necessary —Maintaining a quiet, darkened room —Administering analgesics as necessary (e.g., acetaminophen [Tylenol], 650 mg, or codeine, 15–30 mg q 4 h)	• Provides for the patient's comfort and removes major source of restlessness

(continued)

CHART 30–1 • Summary of the Nursing Management of Patients With Acute Meningitis/Encephalitis (Continued)

Nursing Responsibilities	Rationale
PREVENTION OF COMPLICATIONS	
The duration of the acute and chronic phase of meningitis depends on many variables. However, specific nursing protocols are followed to prevent complications.	
• Provide skin care every 2 to 4 hours.	• Prevents skin breakdown; if unable to change position, lubricate, and inspect the skin
—If feverish patient perspires profusely, bed linens may need to be changed to prevent irritation of the skin.	
—Give special attention to bony prominences.	
• If the patient is not able to turn spontaneously, turn him or her every 2 hr.	• Prevents lung congestion, atelectasis, and pneumonia
—If the patient can follow instructions, facilitate deep breathing exercises every 2 hr.	
• Apply elastic hose when maintained on bed rest.	• Improves blood return to the heart and decreases the chances of thrombophlebitis
• Position carefully in good body alignment.	• Prevents development of orthopedic deformities
• Observe for signs of adrenal insufficiency in the patient with meningococcal meningitis (hypotension, respiratory collapse, petichiae).	• Immediate intervention necessary to preserve the patient's life

resis may be present. Residual effects include mental retardation, epilepsy, personality changes with psychosis, dementia, paresis or paralysis, deafness, and blindness.

Mortality rates and the rates of residual effects associated with viral encephalitis from arboviruses vary greatly. Eastern equine encephalitis (50% mortality rate) and Japanese B encephalitis (most common in the world) have higher mortality rates than the Western variety. Although approximately 80% to 90% of patients with Eastern equine encephalitis develop complications, only 5% to 10% of patients with Western equine infections manifest residual effects.

Diagnosis and Treatment

Treatment is supportive and symptomatic. Management of increased ICP is provided. Drugs often administered include steroids to control cerebral edema, anticonvulsants to prevent seizures, analgesics for headache, and antipyretics to control hyperthermia.

Nursing Management

The nursing management for all patients with viral encephalitis is supportive. The basic points of care are outlined in Charts 30-1 and 30-2.

Herpes Simplex Encephalitis

Herpes simplex encephalitis, caused by herpes simplex virus type 1, is the most common sporadic encephalitis affecting all age groups in the United States. There are two types of herpes simplex virus: type 1, which is associated with the common cold sore and is present in most people in the dormant state, and type 2, which is associated with the sexually transmitted genital disease. Herpes simplex virus type 1 is also capable of producing acute encephalitis in the adult. Although the activating principle for the latent virus is not known, some believe it is activated by fever, emotional stress, and infectious diseases. It is also unclear how the virus enters the CNS. Possible avenues include the bloodstream and peripheral nerves.

Herpes simplex encephalitis is a severe, life-threatening illness that causes inflammation of the brain parenchyma. Death occurs in 30% to 70% of patients if treatment is not begun before the onset of coma. The mortality rate is reduced to 28% if treatment with acyclovir (Zovirax) is begun before coma occurs. For those who survive, most are left with serious neurological deficits.

Pathophysiology

The virus attacks the brain and has a particular propensity for the frontal and temporal lobes. The brain or, more specifically, the temporal lobes become edematous, and necrotic areas with or without hemorrhage develop. Once developed, cerebral edema is pronounced with increased ICP and possible temporal lobe herniation.

Signs and Symptoms

Symptoms evolve over a few days and include fever, nausea and vomiting, headache, memory loss, confusion, stupor, coma, and seizures. Some patients also experience symp-

CHART 30–2 • Summary of Major Nursing Diagnoses Associated with Meningitis/Encephalitis

NURSING DIAGNOSES	NURSING INTERVENTIONS	EXPECTED OUTCOMES
Pain (headache, backache, photophobia, and neck pain) related to (R/T) swelling of intracranial contents and irritation of pain receptors	• Assess the location, quality, and severity of pain (cognitively impaired patients may not be able to use the visual analog scale [VAS] to rate severity of pain). • Provide comfort measures, such as positioning, turning, and application of cool, wet cloths to the head. • Control direct light; darken the patient's room. • Assess the need for use of prn analgesics and administer medication as necessary. • Monitor the patient's response to pain and analgesics.	• The patient will report relief or amelioration of pain (documented by the VAS, if possible), or will demonstrate signs of enhanced comfort, such as decreased agitation and ability to sleep.
Altered Tissue Perfusion, Cerebral, R/T cerebral edema and increased intracranial pressure (ICP)	• Elevate the head of the bed to a 30 degree angle. • Keep the neck in a neutral position. • Prevent Valsalva's maneuver. • Monitor neurological signs for evidence of neurological deterioration. • If an intracranial pressure (ICP) monitor is in place, monitor cerebral perfusion pressure (CPP). • Monitor blood gas levels. • Use prn measures to support CPP following parameters set by physician.	• If an ICP monitor is in place, CPP will be maintained at >70 mm Hg pressure. • Neurological signs will reflect stability or improvement.
Hyperthermia R/T infection, inflammation, and pressure on the hypothalamus	• Remove excess bedclothes. • Control room temperature at <70°F. • Apply a cool, wet cloth to the head. • Provide tepid water baths as necessary. • Assess the need for use of prn antipyretic drugs and administer drugs as necessary. • Avoid shivering in the patient.	• Rectal temperature will be maintained at 99°F or lower.
Sleep Pattern Disturbance R/T agitation and/or increased sensitivity to environmental stimuli	• Assess sleep-wakefulness pattern. • Manage the environment to control and decrease environmental stimuli at night. • Make the patient comfortable. • Plan nursing care to provide for uninterrupted quiet and rest.	• At least three sleep periods, lasting 2 hr each, will be experienced during the night.
High Risk for Injury R/T agitation, seizure potential, altered consciousness, and cognitive impairment	• Maintain seizure precautions. • Provide a safe environment (e.g., keep the bed in a low position). • Apply a jacket restraint, as necessary. • Observe the patient frequently. • Assess the need for use of prn orders for sedatives and administer as necessary.	• Physical injury will not be sustained while hospitalized.
Risk for Disuse Syndrome R/T prolonged bedrest	• Develop a turning and repositioning schedule to prevent skin breakdown. • Use supportive devices as necessary. • Apply elastic stockings. • For some patients, alternating compression air boots may be used. • Institute a bowel care program. • Position the patient to facilitate breathing and patency of airway. • Provide a urinary elimination program. • Monitor intake and output, electrolytes, blood gas levels, skin integrity, bowel and bladder elimination pattern, and peripheral tissue perfusion.	• The patient will not develop —Pressure ulcers —Contractures —Deep vein thrombosis —Constipation —Urinary stasis —Atelectasis and pneumonia —Dehydration

Table 30–5 • MAJOR VIRUSES RESPONSIBLE FOR VIRAL ENCEPHALITIS

TYPE OF VIRUS OR DISORDER	SPECIFIC DISORDER OR CAUSATIVE ORGANISM	COMMENTS
Arboviruses (arthropod-borne)		
Altered cycle of infection of mosquito and host	Eastern equine encephalitis* Western equine encephalitis	Early autumn outbreak in Eastern states; year-round incidence throughout country
Mosquito bites infect host, which subsequently becomes infected	St. Louis encephalitis California virus encephalitis	Late summer outbreak throughout the U.S. except on the West coast
Infected mosquito infects host (including humans)	Venezuelan equine encephalitis	Early autumn outbreak in Midwest
	Japanese B encephalitis Murray Valley (Australian X) encephalitis	Year-round incidence in southwestern U.S. South and Central America
Type of virus	von Economo disease, also called encephalitis lethargica and sleeping sickness	Epidemic in U.S. following the influenza epidemic of 1918; has not recurred since 1926
Postviral disease resulting in central nervous system infection	Measles Mumps Chickenpox	
Postvaccination encephalitis	Develops within a week after vaccination for measles, rubella, mumps, or rabies	Appears to be an immune reaction
Other viral infections	Poliomyelitis Rabies Herpes simplex Herpes zoster Infectious mononucleosis	

* Most serious of the arboviruses in the United States; significant mortality rate and serious deficits in many that survive (e.g., retardation, seizures, personality changes, hemiplegia); least frequent arbovirus.

toms of temporal lobe-limbic system deficits, such as olfactory and gustatory hallucinations, anosmia, temporal lobe seizures, periodic bizarre behavioral manifestations, and aphasia.

Cerebral edema and hemorrhage cause an abrupt increase in ICP. Temporal or brain-stem herniation can result. The marked increase in ICP produces coma, causes changes in vital signs, and affects breathing. If the disease is allowed to progress, temporal lobe herniation of one or both lobes occurs, leading to deep coma, respiratory arrest, and death. Death is most apt to occur within the first 72 hours when the cerebral edema is most pronounced.

Diagnosis and Treatment

The diagnosis of herpes simplex encephalitis is difficult to establish in its early stage. By the time a diagnosis is established, it may be too late to benefit the patient; therefore, an aggressive approach to diagnosis is essential. The usual diagnostic workup includes a history and neurological examination; CSF analysis from lumbar puncture; a CT scan or, preferably, a magnetic resonance imaging (MRI) scan; and an EEG. Pressure during lumbar puncture is markedly elevated. Findings on CSF analysis include increased polymorphonuclear cells (early) and lymphocytes, increased protein, normal glucose (usually), and possible xanthochromia if cerebral hemorrhage has occurred. The EEG is often abnormal, with periodic sharp-wave complexes from one or both temporal regions on a background of low amplitude activity.

Recent advances in molecular biology now allow very early detection of deoxyribonucleic acid (DNA) from the

virus in the CSF, and such techniques are routinely used at many centers. Herpes simplex virus itself is difficult to isolate early. Although a fourfold elevation in antibody titer may be seen in the convalescent serum, this is of no help in crucial early diagnosis, and, in fact, may be misleading. For these reasons the detection of viral DNA is an important step in early diagnosis.

Early in the course of the illness, the CT scan may be normal, but the result of the MRI scan is usually abnormal even in the first week of the disease. Hemorrhagic areas in the inferior frontal-temporal region, together with surrounding edema, are usually evident on both studies later in the disease. The EEG may show focal or generalized slowing. Often, there is evidence of seizure activity in the temporal region.

The drug of choice for treatment of herpes simplex encephalitis is acyclovir (Zovirax) 10 mg/kg every 8 hours (30 mg/kg/day) IV for 10 to 14 days. Other drugs that are commonly administered include:

- Dexamethasone (Decadron) in tapering doses to reduce cerebral edema
- Cimetidine (Tagamet) to decrease gastric secretion and prevent development of gastric hemorrhage associated with the use of steroids
- Furosemide (Lasix) or mannitol for diuresis
- Phenytoin (Dilantin) to prevent or control seizures
- Acetaminophen (Tylenol) to control hyperthermia and headache

In addition to drug therapy, treatment is supportive and symptomatic and includes support of respiratory function, an adequate oxygen supply, support of fluid and electrolyte balance, nutrition management, and management of increased ICP.

Nursing Management

Charts 30-1 and 30-2 describe basic principles of management and nursing diagnosis. In some respects management is similar to that of the patient with meningitis. Additional nursing interventions include:

- Monitor neurological signs to detect neurological deterioration; onset of coma indicates a poor prognosis.
- Monitor for evidence of rising ICP; follow treatment protocol to decrease ICP and prevent herniation.
- Isolation is *not necessary*; however, good handwashing technique should be followed.

Prognosis

If the patient survives the acute episode, neurological deficits are common and may include cognitive deficits (e.g., memory, reasoning), personality changes with dementia, seizure disorders, motor deficits, and dysphagia.

OTHER VIRAL ORGANISMS THAT ATTACK THE CENTRAL NERVOUS SYSTEM

A few selected, uncommon diseases caused by viruses are presented in Table 30-6. They include herpes zoster, poliomyelitis, rabies, tetanus, Lyme disease, cysticercosis, and parameningeal infections.

Parameningeal infections are infections that occur in and around the meninges. Three major localized, suppurative lesions in this area are brain abscesses, subdural empyema, and extradural abscesses.

Brain Abscess

A brain abscess is caused by an infection, which extends into the cerebral tissue or by organisms carried from other sites in the body. The major sites of primary infections that extend directly into the brain are infections of the middle ear, mastoid, and sinus. Approximately 40% of all brain abscesses result from middle ear and mastoid infections. Sinus infections (frontal and sphenoid) are responsible for another 10%. A few abscesses occur as a result of intracranial surgery, compound skull fractures, or oral surgery. The remainder of brain abscesses, approximately 50%, are carried by the blood from remote infectious sites. Examples of such sites include generalized lung infection, lung abscess, bronchiectasis, empyema, skin infections, acute bacterial endocarditis, and congenital heart or lung disease with a right-to-left shunt. These abscesses are sometimes called metastatic abscesses.

The location of the brain abscess depends on the source and method of the spread of the infection. Those infections that spread directly from a primary focus create a brain abscess directly adjacent to the primary site. Given that infections around the face spread in retrograde fashion through venous sinuses, an associated brain abscess can be located at some distance from the primary focus.

Pathophysiology

Initially, the infected tissue is soft, edematous, congested, and infiltrated with polymorphonuclear leukocytes. The lesion is poorly delineated and may represent a localized, suppurative encephalitis. Within the next 2 weeks, the necrotic tissue liquefies. The abscess becomes encapsulated by a zone of fibroblasts that surrounds the site and progressively thickens. This wall of granulated tissue is replaced by collagenous connective tissue. The wall is not of uniform thickness and tends to be thinner in its deepest portion. The abscess, which can vary in size and shape, usually lies in the white matter. The deepest thin-walled portion of the abscess lying in the white matter can eventually rupture into the ventricles with catastrophic results. One or more poorly encapsulated daughter abscesses may surround the major abscess, with possible direct communication between them.

Signs and Symptoms

The signs and symptoms of brain abscess can be viewed in two stages: the initial, acute invasion; and the enlarging lesion.

Initial Invasion. The initial invasion corresponds to the initial formation of the abscess. The patient may encounter the following symptoms: headache; chills and fever; malaise; elevated WBCs; and neurological deficits such as confusion and drowsiness, focal or generalized seizures, motor or sensory deficits, and speech disorders. Some patients may be asymptomatic during this period. There may be a history of reactivation of an infectious process in a patient who has had a previous ear, sinus, or lung infection. Symptoms of this earlier recurring infection may be superimposed on the symptoms of brain abscess formation. Symptoms associated with the initial stage may subside temporarily in response to drug therapy.

The Enlarging Lesion. In the second stage, the formalized abscess behaves as a rapidly growing, space-occupying lesion. Within a few weeks, depending on the size of the abscess, the following signs and symptoms may be observed: flulike symptoms; recurrent headache that becomes increasingly severe; confusion, drowsiness, and stupor; focal or generalized seizures; focal deficits; signs of increased ICP; and possible herniation syndromes.

Symptoms According to Abscess Location. Abscesses in particular areas have characteristic signs and symptoms. The following are three common areas of abscess formation with a list of related symptoms:

- **Frontal lobe abscess:** contralateral hemiparesis, expressive aphasia (if the dominant hemisphere is involved), focal or jacksonian seizure, and frontal headache
- **Temporal lobe abscess:** localized headache, upper quadrant visual deficit, contralateral facial weakness, and minimal aphasia

Table 30 – 6 • OTHER SELECTED NERVOUS SYSTEM INFECTIONS

DISEASE/ORGANISM	DESCRIPTION/COURSE	DIAGNOSIS/TREATMENT
Creutzfeldt-Jakob disease; caused by a prion	• Spongiform encephalopathy characterized by progressive dementia, dysarthria, spastic weakness of the limbs, myoclonic jerks, and seizures • 3 years is the average incubation period • Usually occurs in fifth or sixth decade • Vacuolar or spongelike appearance of brain tissue • Death is the final outcome	• *Diagnosis:* confirmed by brain biopsy • *Treatment:* supportive care
Herpes zoster (shingles) (herpes virus-varicella zoster)	• Latent virus from an attack of chickenpox that remains latent in the sensory ganglia • When the host defenses fail, the virus multiplies within the sensory ganglia and is then transported down the sensory nerve and released to the vesicles at the nerve endings • Involves the dorsal root ganglia; follows the sensory distribution of dermatome • An extremely painful affliction in which a rash (vesicles and large irregular bullae on the erythematous base) develops; rash develops from papules → vesicles → pustules → scabs • Some patients may develop postherpetic neuralgia after an attack; otherwise, it is a self-limiting condition • Herpes zoster can attack the ophthalmic branch of the trigeminal nerve and can cause scarring of the eye	• *Diagnosis:* based on clinical findings (vesicles [occurring 2–5 d after pain]); pain along the peripheral nerve) • *Treatment:* acyclovir, 800 mg 5 times a day for 7 to 10 days; isolation not required
Poliomyelitis (caused by one of three polioviruses)—type 1, 2, or 3	• Attacks the motor cells of the anterior horn cells of the spinal cord • Severity varies from mild to paralysis, with death from paralysis of respiratory muscle • Enters through gastrointestinal (GI) tract • Spread through contact with feces and pharyngeal secretions from infected persons	• *Diagnosis:* based on clinical findings and isolation of the virus • *Treatment:* supportive care; may need ventilation support; most patients require extensive rehabilitation; isolation precautions are maintained for a period of time. • *Note:* With the advent of the effective Salk vaccine, incidence of this disease has virtually been eliminated because of mass immunization
Rabies (rhabdovirus) (<10 cases in the U.S./yr)	• An acute encephalomyelitis infection • Transmitted to humans from the saliva of infected animals through bite or contact with saliva • Spread from the wound to the central nervous system by the peripheral nerves • Incubation period varies depending on the distance of the wound from the head • Course of disease —*Early phase:* vague flulike symptoms (headache, malaise, vomiting, fever, drowsiness) —*Second phase:* extreme excitement and salivation, deranged behavior, convulsions, severe and painful spasms of the pharyngeal and laryngeal muscles from slight stimuli or sight of food (lasts 2–7 d) —*Final phase:* onset of coma, followed by cardiac and respiratory arrest	• *Diagnosis:* based on a history of a bite and isolation of the virus • *Treatment:* administration of antitoxin (causes serious side effects); supportive care; isolation required; death may result. Vaccination used even after disease has begun. • *Note:* Vaccination for those traveling to areas of prevalence is encouraged.
Tetanus (*Clostridium tetani*)	• Spread through horse and cattle feces that contaminate soil and objects within the soil • Enters humans from penetrating and crush wounds • Produces three exotoxins that attack the spinal cord and cranial nerves • Causes severe muscle spasms, extreme sensitivity to stimuli, and convulsions • Death may occur from asphyxia	• *Diagnosis:* based on the history and clinical findings • *Treatment:* administration of antitoxin and supportive care • *Note:* Immunization is available (tetanus toxoid and tetanus immunoglobulin)

▊▊▊▊ Table 30-6 • OTHER SELECTED NERVOUS SYSTEM INFECTIONS (Continued)

DISEASE/ORGANISM	DESCRIPTION/COURSE	DIAGNOSIS/TREATMENT
Lyme disease (caused by *Borrelia burgdorferi*)—named for Lyme, Connecticut, where an outbreak first caused attention	• Spirochete transmitted by the bite of an infected tick of the *Ixodes ricinus* complex • Carried on white-tail deer and other wild animals • Course of disease —*Stage 1:* localized erythema migrans, a rash that resembles a bull's-eye; rash fades within 3 to 4 weeks; there may be occurrence of signs of meningitis, radiculitis, and neuritis in an afebrile patient —*Stage 2:* complications may develop—heart block in 10%; Bell's palsy in 10%; other problems may include meningitis, encephalitis, polyradiculitis, or inflammation of the eyes —*Stage 3:* occurs 4 weeks to years after the bite; characterized by arthritis symptoms affecting the large joints and chronic joint pain	• *Diagnosis:* based on a history of bite (which the patient may not recall); elevated titer to Lyme disease after 4 weeks • *Treatment:* —*Stage 1:* azithromycin, amoxicillin, and doxycycline are recommended for treatment of stage 1 to prevent the development of subsequent stages; ceftriaxone is usually given IV in patients with neurological symptoms and helps to resolve symptoms —*Stage 2:* IV administration of 20 million U of penicillin; others recommend tetracycline 500 mg qid —*Stage 3:* controversial; antibiotics are used
Cysticercosis of CNS (caused by *Taenia solium*)	• Most common parasite affecting the CNS • In Central and South America, this is the leading cause of epilepsy and neurological disturbances • Humans who consume raw or undercooked meat from infected animals can become contaminated • When ingested, cyst forms that contains larva; the cyst can lodge in the brain, as well as in other areas • May lodge in ventricles	• *Diagnosis:* Based on multiple, calcified lesions in the brain noted on CT scan or radiological studies • *Treatment:* oral praziquantel, for 3 days; symptomatic treatment of cerebral edema with steroids; surgery may be required to remove intracranial cyst

• **Cerebellar abscess:** postauricular (below the ear) or occipital headache, ipsilateral ataxia and limb paresis, nystagmus and weakness of gaze to the side of the lesion

Diagnosis

The diagnosis of brain abscess is based on the following criteria:

• Identification of a primary infection, such as middle ear, sinus, or lung infection, helps to pinpoint the source of the problem. Chest, skull, and sinus radiographs may be necessary to identify the primary focus of infection.
• On lumbar puncture, the CSF pressure is elevated. Findings on analysis of the CSF include an elevated WBC count from a few to several thousand, with lymphocytes being the predominant cell; elevated protein; and normal glucose. An abrupt onset of coma with a WBC count of 50,000 in the CSF should make one highly suspicious of rupture of an abscess into the ventricles.
• Other laboratory data to localize the lesion include an EEG (area of high voltage over the abscess) and a CT scan.

Treatment. Early diagnosis and prompt antimicrobial treatment are essential. Because anaerobic *Streptococci* and *Bacteroides* are the predominant causative organisms, penicillin G (20 million U) and chloramphenicol (4 to 6 g daily IV in divided doses) are given. In addition, management of the rapidly rising ICP is achieved with IV mannitol, followed by a course of dexamethasone (Decadron, 6 to 12 mg every 6 hours). If this is not effective, surgery will be necessary to remove or aspirate the abscess. If the abscess is well encapsulated, attempts are made to excise surgically both the abscess and membrane totally. If this is not possible, the abscess is aspirated and drained. Injection of the sac with antimicrobial drugs follows. It may be necessary at some future time to drain the sac again because of a build-up of suppurative material.

The use of drugs has greatly reduced the mortality rate from brain abscess. The aggressive treatment of infections that can lead to the formation of brain abscesses has also been a prophylactic aid. The cause of death from brain abscess is the massive increase in ICP and rupture of the abscess into the ventricles. Of the patients who survive, approximately 30% develop neurological deficits, of which focal seizures are most common.

Extradural Abscess

Extradural abscesses may be associated with osteomyelitis of a cranial bone; infection of the sinuses or the ear; or a surgical procedure in which the frontal sinus or mastoid has been opened. A pus pocket accumulates between the bone and dura.

Symptoms include localized pain, fever, tenderness, and purulent discharge. Stiffness of the neck is possible. Localized neurological signs are often absent. If they occur, focal seizures, cranial nerve VI palsy, and decreased sensory perception of the face are the most common symptoms. The only abnormalities noted in the CSF are a few lymphocytes and neutrophils and a slightly elevated protein level.

Treatment consists of antibiotics and surgery for removal of the diseased bone at a future date.

Nursing Management of Patients With Parameningeal Infections

The nursing management of the patient with a brain abscess can be viewed in two stages: the acute initial invasion when the infection organizes into an abscess, and the second stage when the abscess behaves like a space-occupying lesion.

During the initial stage, symptoms correspond to a general systemic infection. If neurological symptoms are present, they can be important in localizing the lesion. Often, symptoms are so general that a diagnosis is unclear. Nursing management during this period includes assessing the patient's condition, managing any presenting symptoms, providing supportive care, and administering drug treatment. If signs of increased ICP are present, follow the basic care outlined in Chapter 14. Seizure precautions are maintained to prevent injury. Noting how a seizure progresses is helpful for diagnosis. Neurological assessment, including assessment for signs and symptoms of meningeal irritation, is important.

Medications ordered are given through IV. As with meningitis, adherence to the administration timetable is imperative for maintaining therapeutic blood levels. Because the drugs used are potent, the patient must be observed for both drug side effects and the development of secondary infections, which can flourish when antimicrobial therapy is used.

In the second stage, the abscess behaves like a space-occupying lesion. Signs and symptoms of neurological deficit must be investigated to make a diagnosis. After the diagnosis is made, appropriate treatment is begun. If surgery is necessary to remove or drain the abscess, nursing management pertinent to the craniotomy patient should be implemented (see Chap. 15).

HUMAN IMMUNODEFICIENCY VIRUS AND ACQUIRED IMMUNODEFICIENCY SYNDROME

Acquired immunodeficiency syndrome (AIDS), a viral infection causing progressive immunosuppression, renders its victims susceptible to various opportunistic infections, malignancies, and neurological disorders. The causative agent is human immunodeficiency virus (HIV). Diagnosis of HIV infection is based on the detection of HIV antibodies in serum using ELISA and Western blot diagnostic techniques.[7] Other tests for HIV infection include the HIV p24 antigen test and plasma PCR assay for HIV RNA.[8,9] Antibodies are usually evident within 4 weeks of inoculation.

The primary target cell for HIV, the CD4-positive lymphocyte, decreases in number over the course of the disease. Because CD4-positive lymphocytes play a major role in initiating and orchestrating other humoral and cell-mediated immune responses, virtually all components of the immune system are affected either directly or indirectly by HIV infection.[10,11] The blood count of CD4-positive lymphocytes (CD4 count) is currently used to stage HIV progression.[12] The revised guidelines from the U. S. Centers for Disease Control and Prevention (CDC) define AIDS as a disorder in any person who has a CD4 count of less than 200 cells/μL or an AIDS-defining illness. This classification provides a standardized way to describe and classify symptoms and diseases (Table 30-7). The rate of progression from one category to another is variable, but 50% of patients progress to active AIDS within 10 years of seroconversion.[13]

Neurological disease at every anatomic level of the nervous system is a common complication of HIV infection, and neurological symptoms may be the initial manifestation of HIV/AIDS.[14] Neurological symptoms occur in at least 75% of AIDS cases, especially when the *CD4 count is low (less than 200 cells/μL)*.[1] AIDS-related neurological lesions may be clas-

Table 30–7 • CENTERS FOR DISEASE CONTROL REVISED CLASSIFICATION FOR HIV-1 INFECTION

CD4 Cell Count	CLINICAL CATEGORIES		
	[A] Asymptomatic	[B] Symptomatic	[C] AIDS-defining
>500/μL	A1	B1	C1[a]
200–499/μL	A2	B2	C2[a]
<200/μL	A3[a]	B3[a]	C3[a]
Category A:	Asymptomatic HIV-1 infection, persistent generalized lymphadenopathy, or acute HIV-1 infection.		
Category B:	Symptomatic conditions other than those in category C, bacterial endocarditis, meningitis, pneumonia, or sepsis, candidiasis (oropharyngeal or vulvovaginal), cervical dysplasia, oral hairy leukoplakia, herpes zoster, idiopathic thrombocytopenic purpura, listeriosis, nocardiosis, pelvic inflammatory disease, peripheral neuropathy.		
Category C:	Recurrent bacterial pneumonia, esophageal or lower respiratory candidiasis, invasive cervical cancer, coccidiomycosis, cryptococcosis, cryptosporidosis, cytomegalovirus including retinitis, HIV-1 encephalopathy, herpes simplex, histoplasmosis, isosporiasis, Kaposi's sarcoma, lymphoma, mycobacterial infection, *Pneumocystis carinii*, progressive multifocal leukoencephalopathy, *Salmonella* septicemia, toxoplasmosis of brain, HIV-1 cachexia.		

[a] AIDS-defining clinical category.

Osenbach, R. K., & Zeidman, S. M. (Eds.) (1999). *Infections in neurological surgery: Diagnosis and management* (p. 228). Philadelphia: Lippincott-Raven.

Table 30–8 • CLASSIFICATION OF THE MOST COMMON AIDS-RELATED NEUROLOGICAL DISORDERS BY ANATOMICAL LOCATION AND PATHOPHYSIOLOGICAL MECHANISM

NEUROLOGICAL DISORDER	PATHOPHYSIOLOGY	ANATOMICAL LOCATION
• Aseptic meningitis	HIV-related	Meninges
• Crytococcal meningitis	Opportunistic infection	Meninges
• Tuberculosis meningitis, encephalitis, or abscess	Opportunistic infection	Meninges or brain
• Cerebral toxoplasmosis	Opportunistic infection	Brain
• Progressive multifocal leukoencephalopathy (PML)	Opportunistic infection	Brain
• Cytomegalovirus	Opportunistic infection	Brain, retina
• Primary central nervous system lymphoma	Neoplasm	Brain
• AIDS-associated dementia	HIV-related	Brain
• Vacuolar myelopathy	HIV-related	Spinal cord
• AIDS polyneuropathy	HIV-related	Peripheral nerves

sified along two complementary schemes: pathogenesis of infection and neuroanatomical location.[15] Table 30-8 outlines the most common AIDS-related neurological disorders using these schemata. These common HIV-related problems, opportunistic infections, tumors, neuropathies, and myopathies, cause altered neurological function and so are frequently seen by neuroscience nurses.

Conditions Directly Attributable to HIV

Some neurological conditions are the direct result of the HIV infection of CNS tissue.[16,17] Peripheral lymphocytes or macrophages infected with HIV enter the CNS through breaks in the epithelial lining of small capillaries and release toxic factors that interfere with cell function.[16] The virus spreads slowly in the brain and eventually causes progressive neurological involvement.[18] The potential sites of nervous system damage are numerous, and the virus has been isolated in CSF, the cerebrum, the cerebellum, the spinal cord, and peripheral nerves.

AIDS dementia, HIV myelopathy, HIV neuropathies, and HIV myopathy are HIV-related problems. These conditions are briefly discussed in this section.

AIDS Dementia

AIDS dementia, also called HIV dementia and AIDS dementia complex, affects about 15% to 20% of AIDS patients. It usually appears after significant immunosuppression has developed, although it may be the initial clinical sign of AIDS.[19] The degree of clinical impairment is disproportionate to the amount of neuropathology noted on autopsy findings. Clinically, cognitive, behavioral, and motor deficits are noted, with memory deficits, inattentiveness, slowness of thought processes, and apathy as common findings. The Price/Brew staging scheme (Table 30-9) is widely used for classification of AIDS dementia.[20] Findings that assist with diagnosis include a CT scan with widened sulci and enlarged ventricles and an MRI with patchy or diffuse white matter changes.[21] Neuropsychological testing is helpful to support the diagnosis and delineate cognitive deficits. Testing can also follow the course of the disease and the response to therapy.[22] With advanced dementia, testing may

not be necessary or possible because of an inability of the patient to participate.

HIV Myelopathy, Peripheral Neuropathy, and Myopathy

A myelopathy, defined as a pathological change in the spinal cord, is often used to denote nonspecific lesions. In AIDS, vascular myelopathy is the most common myelopathy seen and is often seen with AIDS dementia. The clinical signs include a progressive paraparesis, sensory ataxia, and sphincter impairment. On examination, hyperreflexia and spasticity with impairment of joint-position sense are noted.[2]

There are four major HIV-associated neuropathies:[23] HIV distal sensory neuropathy, inflammatory demyelinating polyneuropathy, progressive polyneuropathy, and mononeuritis multiplex. Signs and symptoms vary with the type of neuropathy as follows:

- *HIV distal sensory neuropathy*: stocking-glove sensory loss, symmetrical pain, distal paresthesias (i.e., burning, numbness), and decreased ankle deep tendon reflexes (DTRs)
- *Inflammatory demyelinating polyneuropathy*: progressive

 Table 30–9 • PRICE AND BREW'S STAGING SCHEME FOR AIDS-DEMENTIA COMPLEX

STAGE	DESCRIPTION
0	Normal mental and motor function
0.5–1	(Subclinical) Minimal symptoms without impairment of work function or activities of daily living (ADLs)
1	(Mild) Cognitive or motor deficits that compromise more demanding aspects of work or ADLs
2	(Moderate) Cognitive deficit; patient unable to work or perform more demanding ADLs
3	(Severe) Patient can perform only most rudimentary skills
4	(End stage) Patient has no understanding of surroundings and requires complete care

From Brew, J. B. (1992). Central and peripheral nervous system abnormalities. *Medical Clinics of North America, 76*(1), 63–81.

mild-to-moderate symmetric weakness and paresthesias, mild sensory loss, and areflexia

- *Progressive polyneuropathy*: bilateral lower extremity weakness to flaccid paraparesis, saddle anesthesia, bowel and bladder dysfunction, back pain, urinary incontinence, and decreased ankle and knee DTRs
- *Mononeuritis multiplex*: asymmetrical multifocal cranial and peripheral neuropathy (e.g., facial weakness, wrist drop, foot drop)

Diagnosis is based on clinical presentation, electromyography studies, CSF abnormal findings, and nerve biopsy in the case of mononeuritis multiplex. These neuropathies are painful and include significant disabilities.

HIV myopathy, seen as inflammatory *polymyositis*, can occur at any stage of AIDS. Muscle weaknesses with slowly progressing proximal weakness of the upper and lower extremities are the major clinical signs and symptoms. It presents with subacute, progressive weakness, often manifested by difficulty climbing stairs or rising from a chair. Myalgia, most prominent in the thighs, is common. Physical examination reveals symmetrical, predominantly proximal muscle weakness, usually involving the legs and neck flexors more than the arms. Weakness progresses over months, with waxing and waning. The diagnosis is based on the clinical presentation, electromyography, and elevated levels of creatine phosphokinase.[2]

Opportunistic Infections

Various viral, yeast, and fungal opportunistic infections are seen in AIDS. Those discussed in this section include toxoplasmosis, cryptococcal meningitis, cytomegalovirus, progressive multifocal leukoencephalopathy, and meningeal tuberculosis.

CNS Toxoplasmosis

Toxoplasmosis is the most frequently seen CNS infection in those with AIDS and is associated with a mortality rate of up to 70%.[17] *Toxoplasma gondii* enters the body by ingestion and remains dormant unless immunosuppression permits activation. Diffuse meningoencephalitis develops with cell necrosis progressing to abscess formation.[17] Multifocal, scattered lesions and abscesses appear as masses throughout the cerebral hemispheres. The clinical presentation of toxoplasmosis varies and may include early neurological signs consisting only of myoclonus and asterixis; more often, signs and symptoms developing over days or weeks, including fever, seizures, confusion, and meningeal irritation; and diffuse neurological symptoms followed by focal deficits, including mild hemiparesis, ataxia, limb dysmetria, and cranial nerve palsies.

MRI or CT scan demonstrates characteristic multiple lesions with ring enhancements around lesions. Edema surrounding lesions may produce a mass effect on the brain. Areas affected, in order of frequency, are the basal ganglia; the frontal, parietal, and occipital lobes; and occasionally the cerebellum.[24] Serological studies for IgG antibodies to toxoplasmosis are positive in 85% of cases.[19]

Because of the difficulty of demonstrating the presence of the toxoplasmosis organism and the rapid response to therapy, empiric treatment is begun whenever toxoplasmosis is suspected. Drug therapy includes sulfadiazine 1.5 g PO every 6 hours and pyrimethamine orally with an initial dose of 100 mg followed by 75 mg/day. Anticonvulsants may be ordered to prevent seizures. Clinical improvement and improvement on MRI or CT scan can usually be seen in 1 to 2 weeks. If there is no improvement or if deterioration occurs, stereotactic brain biopsy may be indicated.[25] Pharmacological therapy must be *maintained for life* because of the high probability of relapse of the infection.

Cryptococcal Meningitis

Cryptococcus neoformans, a common fungus found in the soil, enters the body through inhalation and lies dormant. In an immunocompromised host, however, it spreads through the blood and lodges as cysts and small granulomas in the brain parenchyma (e.g., cerebral cortex) or meninges.[17] Cryptococcus invades the brain along penetrating arteries to form clumps of organisms that develop into mass lesions deep within subcortical tissue, especially the basal ganglia.[26]

Most patients with CNS cryptococcosis present with meningitis. Symptoms may be subtle, including fever, headache, and malaise. Meningismus, with altered mental status, occurs in more than half of all patients. Focal neurological deficits including cranial nerve neuropathies and seizures are also seen. The diagnosis is based on MRI, which may or may not demonstrate enhancement of the lesion. Cryptococcal antigen titers are usually positive. If meningitis is present, the organism can be isolated from the CSF. If the lesions are isolated, the CSF may be negative.

Drug therapy includes amphotericin B initially, at 0.6 to 1.0 mg/kg/day, if renal function is normal. For less severe cases, fluconazole 200 mg twice PO for 10 weeks is ordered. The initial therapy must be followed by *lifetime maintenance therapy* with fluconazole 200 mg/day.[19]

Cytomegalovirus

Cytomegalovirus (CMV), which results in a mild mononucleosis-like condition if reactivated, is a member of the herpesvirus family. About 50% of the population have antibodies to CMV. However, in an immunosuppressed host, the organism can lead to encephalitis, meningoencephalitis, retinitis, polyradiculomyelitis, or a multifocal neuropathy.[27] The illness begins with headache, difficulty concentrating, personality changes, delirium, somnolence, and subacute dementia. The onset of dementia occurs earlier in CMV than in AIDS.

The CSF analysis is typically negative. The PCR-based assays are highly sensitive and specific. MRI and CT studies may be normal or may demonstrate periventricular white matter abnormalities, cortical nodules, and hydrocephalus.[28] The encephalitis is often fatal in 4 to 6 weeks. Treatment with foscarnet or ganciclovir by the IV route should be initiated promptly and the dose adjusted based on renal function. After initial treatment, ganciclovir is continued as a maintenance dose.

Progressive Multifocal Leukoencephalopathy

Reactivation of papovavirus (also known as JC virus) in the presence of an immunosuppressed host may lead to progressive multifocal leukoencephalopathy (PML). The reactivated virus affects the astrocytes and oligodendroglia of the hemispheric white matter and results in multifocal demyelinating lesions. PML presents with hemiparesis, aphasia, hemianopsia, ataxia, and other focal deficits.

The MRI demonstrates nonenhanced subcortical lesions, and some patients demonstrate gray matter involvement with ring enhancement.[27] CSF studies are nondiagnostic. Brain biopsy may be useful in atypical cases. Survival after diagnosis is 2 to 4 months. Currently, there is no effective treatment for PML.

Meningeal Tuberculosis

Mycobacterium tuberculosis occurs frequently in people with AIDS. Although generally confined to the lungs, extrapulmonary tuberculosis is seen. CNS involvement by tuberculosis may occur in the form of chronic meningitis, encephalitis, or focal brain abscess. Clinical presentation includes meningeal irritation, headache, and nuchal rigidity. Cranial nerve palsy alone or in combination with hydrocephalus may be seen in relation to basilar adhesive arachnoiditis.

MRI imaging may show meningeal enhancement and intraparenchymal masses with ring or nodular enhancement.[29] CSF analysis may show high protein, low glucose, and lymphocytosis. Acid-fast bacillus (AFB) cultures of the CSF are usually positive.[30] The current treatment for meningeal tuberculosis is isoniazid (INH) 300 mg/day, rifampin 600 mg/day, pyrazinamide (PZA) 20 to 30 mg/kg/day, and ethambutol 15 mg/kg/day for 2 months, followed by rifampin and isoniazid alone for another 4 months.[27] The patient should not be considered contagious unless there is evidence of active pulmonary disease.

Primary CNS Lymphoma

Occurring in 3% of AIDS patients, primary CNS lymphoma is the second most common mass lesion of the brain in these patients after toxoplasmosis. Most such tumors arise from B cells.[27] The clinical presentation includes headache, lethargy, memory loss, and confusion. Cranial nerve deficits and seizures are common. The symptoms may occur acutely or evolve over several weeks.

CT or MRI imaging typically shows single and multiple enhancing lesions that may occur anywhere in the brain parenchyma but have an affinity for the periventricular areas.[31] The CSF findings may be normal or may show elevated protein, mild pleocytosis, and positive cytology. The differential diagnosis includes toxoplasmosis. Because the MRI pattern is not unique for lymphoma, a brain biopsy may be necessary to establish the diagnosis.

The primary treatment for CNS lymphoma includes radiation therapy and dexamethasone. Radiation to the whole brain improves short-term survival up to 6 months. Dexamethasone has a cytotoxic effect against lymphoma and may reduce tumor size and edema. The prognosis is bleak with CNS lymphoma.

Nursing Management of the AIDS Patient With Nervous System Involvement

Although the focus of this discussion is the effects on neurological function, the patient with AIDS must be managed holistically. The nurse is part of a team addressing difficult collaborative problems in a patient at high risk for many complications. Given that most body systems are involved, a comprehensive and individualized management plan is required.

Although AIDS is incurable, many drugs slow viral replication and prolong the period of time before HIV-related symptoms appear. The most commonly prescribed antiviral drugs for AIDS are zidovudine (ZDV), dideoxycytidine, and stavudine. The common side effects of these drugs are listed in Table 30-10. Other drugs to treat specific disease-related problems, such as antiemetics for nausea and vomiting or antibiotics to treat opportunistic infections, are provided as necessary.

Table 30-11 includes many nursing diagnoses related to the neurological complications of AIDS. Patients with AIDS are immunocompromised. Immunosuppressed patients do not demonstrate the cardinal signs and symptoms of infection, such as elevations in temperature and elevated WBC counts. Therefore, the nurse must learn to observe for more subtle signs of infection within the context of immunosuppression.

The following summarizes the nursing focus related to the major categories of neurological problems related to AIDS.

Conditions Directly Attributable to HIV

After AIDS dementia has been established, the nurse must be able to set realistic expectations of performance for the patient and provide a supportive and safe environment. A reasonable amount of stimulation avoids overstimulation that can overwhelm intact coping skills. An assessment of ability to participate in activities of daily living (ADLs) and to maintain safety is necessary. A safe environment must be

Table 30-10 • MEDICATION SIDE EFFECTS

DRUG	SIDE EFFECTS
Zidovudine (ZDV)	Headache, nausea, malaise, myalgias, anemia, neutropenia, myopathy, nail hyperpigmentation
Didanosine (ddI)	Dry mouth, altered taste, nausea, vomiting, diarrhea, peripheral neuropathy, pancreatitis, hepatitis, electrolyte imbalance
Dideoxycytidine (ddC)	Rash, fever, mouth ulcers, peripheral neuropathy, pancreatitis, cardiomyopathy, hyperglycemia
Stavudine (D4T)	Headache, nausea, vomiting, confusion, increased serum transaminase, increased creatine phosphokinase

From Fischl, M. A. (1995). Drug interactions and toxicities in patients with AIDS. In M. A. Sande & P. A. Volberding (Eds.), *Medical management of AIDS* (4th ed.). Philadelphia: W. B. Saunders.

▌▌▌▌ Table 30–11 • NURSING DIAGNOSES RELATED TO NEUROLOGICAL COMPLICATIONS OF AIDS

NURSING DIAGNOSIS	INTERVENTION	OUTCOME
Inadequate Nutrition related to (R/T) decreased intake	Determine reasons for inadequate intake: mouth ulcers, dysphasia, nausea, inability to prepare food.	Meets caloric requirements.
	Determine appropriate nutritional needs (refer to dietitian if necessary).	Weight is stable or increased.
	Provide nutritional supplements, meal preparation assistance.	
	Consider alterations in medication schedules.	
	Assess need for feeding tube or total parenteral nutrition.	
Self Care Deficit R/T cognitive/motor impairment	Assess ability to complete activities of daily living (ADLs).	Patient participates in ADLs at highest possible level of functioning.
	Assist with devices/cues to maintain independence.	
	Provide ADLs which patient cannot do—bathing, dressing, feeding, etc.	
	Be sure patient has adequate supervision/assistance at home.	
Risk for Injury R/T impaired cognitive/motor functioning	Regular assessment of level of functioning.	Self environment is maintained.
	Adequate supervision/assistance with ADLs, meals, medication administration.	Assistance or intervention is provided when appropriate.
	Problem solving and/or direct intervention when unsafe behavior is identified.	
Pain R/T altered sensory perception	Pain assessed regularly using a standard scale.	Pain level is acceptable to patient
	Skin assessed regularly for pressure areas, breakdown.	Medication side effects are tolerable.
	Clothing, shoes do not cause pressure.	
	Pain medications are taken as prescribed and reassessed regularly for most effective management.	
Impaired Social Interaction/ isolation R/T impaired physical mobility and/or cognitive defects	Assess/determine patient's baseline functioning.	Interactions are appropriate for patient's level of disability.
	Determine types of activities appropriate to current level of functioning.	
	Assist patient/family to plan for activities and outings to stimulate interaction.	
	Encourage patient to be as independent as circumstances allow.	
Risk for Infection R/T immunocompromised state	Skin integrity assessed regularly.	Patient does not acquire preventable infections.
	Catheter sites/IV sites are assessed and dressings changed on schedule.	Infections are identified and treatment initiated promptly.
	Appropriate level of medical care is available to patient.	
	New symptoms: fever, chills, local signs and symptoms of infection are promptly evaluated and treated.	
	Good hand washing.	
	Food prepared under sanitary conditions.	
Impaired Physical Mobility R/T motor weakness	Conduct baseline assessment for motor function and reassess regularly.	Patient does not suffer injuries related to weakness or falls.
	Assess for assistive devices such as canes, walkers, bath aids.	Appropriate aids are available.
	Maintain/increase mobility through planned exercise, activity.	Changes in level of function are consistent with overall condition.
	Consultation with physical therapist, occupational therapist as necessary. Assist patient with activities patient cannot do.	
Altered Coping R/T multiple life stressors	Assess current coping of patient and/or family.	Patient is able to identify positive coping skills.
	Assist patient in identifying specific stressors.	Referrals are made to appropriate resources.
	Assist patient in identifying possible resolutions to problems.	
	Refer to appropriate resources: social worker, social services, community based agencies, mental health professional.	
Alteration in Health Maintenance R/T progression of illness	Provide information to patient/family about disease process and treatment options for specific problems.	Patient will contribute to and comply with treatment plan.
	Encourage patient to be actively involved in decisions related to care.	Patient will make informed decisions about medical care.
	Assist patient in identifying resources to meet needs.	Patient will complete advance directives and power of attorney.

Table 30-11 • NURSING DIAGNOSES RELATED TO NEUROLOGICAL COMPLICATIONS OF AIDS (Continued)

NURSING DIAGNOSIS	INTERVENTION	OUTCOME
Alteration in Vision and/or Hearing R/T complications of central nervous system disorders	Assess for degree of vision/hearing loss. Assess environment for hazards and institute measures to ensure safety. Establish alternative means of communication as needed. Use interdisciplinary approach to assist patient with compensatory techniques and devices that promote activities.	Patient remains free of injury. Patient uses compensatory devices to communicate effectively and participate in ADLs.
Decreased Level of Arousal R/T changes in intracranial dynamics	Assess neurological status as condition warrants. Assess cardiovascular and respiratory status regularly. Manipulate environment to deliver appropriate levels of stimulation. Use interdisciplinary approach to prevent complications of immobility. Educate and involve family in care.	Patient will remain free of complications associated with decreased arousal. Patient will progress to highest level of arousal.

provided. Maintaining the patient's dignity in light of cognitive deficits is central to providing care. The family will need help understanding the cognitive deficits present and to learn how to interact with the patient in a satisfactory manner. Anticipatory guidance helps the family plan for future needs.

With HIV myelopathy, HIV neuropathies, and HIV myopathy, sensory abnormalities and pain are common. Pain can be managed with various nonopioid analgesics. Muscle weakness associated with myopathies can result in self-care deficits and impair physical mobility. The physical therapist is helpful in providing assistive devices for mobility. An occupational therapist can assist in recommending both assistive devices and alternative methods of accomplishing ADLs. This information can be incorporated in a plan of care that can be shared with the family caregiver to provide home-based care.

Opportunistic Infections

Patients who have opportunistic infections often receive drug therapy, as already outlined. The nurse assists in providing information about side effects and the need for lifelong therapy in some cases. Because some opportunistic infections result in meningitis, encephalitis, or a space-occupying lesion, all of which lead to increased ICP, monitoring of neurological signs is important to identify deterioration in neurological function related to increased ICP. The usual nursing measures and medical treatment protocol to decrease elevated ICP are employed (see Chap. 14).

Primary CNS Lymphoma

CNS lymphomas result in space-occupying lesions and increased ICP. Nursing management is directed toward management of increased ICP and preventing associated complications, as outlined in Chapter 14.

Summary

The neuroscience nurse may care for a patient who has neurological complications related to being HIV positive or having diagnosed AIDS. However, care must be provided within the context of an incurable disease affecting all body systems, and the nurse must strive for optimal overall outcomes of treatment.

REFERENCES

1. Guberman, A. (1994). *An introduction to clinical neurology* (pp. 419–452). Boston: Little, Brown.
2. Roos, K. L. (1999). In C. G. Goetz & E. J. Pappert (Eds.). *Textbook of clinical neurology* (pp. 842–867). Philadelphia: W. B. Saunders.
3. Victor, M., & Ropper, A. H. (2001). *Principles of neurology* (7th ed., pp. 801–806). New York: McGraw-Hill.
4. Roos, K. L. (1997). Bacterial meningitis. In K. L. Roos (Ed.). *Central nervous system infectious diseases and therapy* (pp. 99–126). New York: Marcel Dekker.
5. Desforges, J. A. (1992). The use of molecular methods in infectious diseases. *New England Journal of Medicine, 327*, 1290.
6. Naber, S. P. (1994). Molecular pathology–diagnosis of infectious disease. *New England Journal of Medicine, 331*, 1212.
7. Saag, M. S. (1997). Quantitation of HIV viral load: A tool for clinical practice? In M. A. Sande & P. A. Volberding (Eds.). *The medical management of AIDS* (pp. 57–74). Philadelphia: W. B. Saunders.
8. Allain, J. P., Laurian, Y., Paul, D. A., et al. (1987). Long-term evaluation of HIV antigen and antibodies to p24 and gp41 in patients with hemophilia. *New England Journal of Medicine, 317*, 1114–1121.
9. Paul, D. A., Falk, L. A., Kessler, H. A., et al. (1987). Correlation of serum HIV antigen and antibody with clinical status in HIV-infected patients. *Journal of Medical Virology, 22*, 257–263.
10. Zunich, K. M., & Lane, H. C. (1991). Immunologic abnormalities in HIV infection. *Hematology/Oncology Clinics of North America, 5*, 215–228.
11. Stein, D. S., Korvich, J. A., & Vermund, S. T. (1992). CD4+ lymphocyte cell enumeration for prediction of clinical course of human immunodeficiency virus disease: A review. *Journal of Infectious Diseases, 165*, 352–363.

12. U. S. Centers for Disease Control and Prevention. (1993). 1993 revised classification system for HIV infection and expanded surveillance case definition for AIDS among adolescents and adults. *MMWR Morbidity and Mortality Weekly Report, 41,* 1–19.

13. Phair, J. P. (1993). Estimating prognosis in HIV-1 infection. *Annuals of Internal Medicine, 118,* 742–744.

14. Levy, R. M., Janssen, R. S., Bush, T. J., & Rosenblum, M. L. (1988). Neuroepidemiology of acquired immunodeficiency syndrome. *Journal of Acquired Immune Deficiency Disease, 1,* 31–41.

15. Price, R. W. (1996). Neurological complications of HIV infection. *Lancet, 348,* 445–452.

16. Elder, G., & Sever, J. (1988). AIDS and neurological disorders: An overview. *Annals of Neurology, 23*(Suppl.), S4–S6.

17. Fisher, E. J. (1995). *Clinician's guide to therapy of adults with HIV/AIDS* (3rd ed.). Richmond, VA: Virginia Commonwealth University HIV/AIDS Center.

18. Levy, J. (1988). The biology of the human immunodeficiency virus and its role in neurological disease. In M. Rosenblum, R. Levy, & D. Bredesen (Eds.). *AIDS and the nervous system.* New York: Raven Press.

19. Cohen, B. (1997). Neurologic complications of AIDS. In J. Biller (Ed.). *Practical neurology* (pp. 479–497). Philadelphia: Lippincott-Raven.

20. Brew, J. B. (1992). Central and peripheral nervous system abnormalities. *Medical Clinics of North America, 76*(1), 63–81.

21. Adams, R. D., Victor, M., & Ropper, A. H. (Eds.). (1997). *Principles of neurology* (6th ed., pp. 742–776). New York: McGraw Hill.

22. Price, R. W., & Worley, J. M. (1995). Management of neurologic complications of HIV-1 infection and AIDS. In M. A. Snade & P. A. Volberding (Eds.). *Medical management of AIDS* (4th ed.). Philadelphia: W. B. Saunders.

23. So, Y. T., Holtzman, D. M., Abrams, D. I., & Olney, R. K. (1985). Peripheral neuropathy associated with acquired immunodeficiency syndrome: Prevalence and clinical features from a population-based surgery. *Archives of Neurology, 45,* 945–948.

24. Houff, S. (1988). Neuroimmunology of human immunodeficiency virus. In M. Rosenblum, R. Levy, & D. Bredesen (Eds.). *AIDS and the nervous system.* New York: Raven Press.

25. Newton, H. B. (1995). Common neurologic complications of HIV-1 infection and AIDS. *American Family Physician, 51*(2), 387–398.

26. McArthur, J. (1992). Neurologic manifestation of human immunodeficiency virus infections. In A. Ashbury, G. McKhanna, & W. McDonald (Eds.). *Diseases of the nervous system: Clinical neurobiology.* Philadelphia: W. B. Saunders.

27. Walter, K. A., Clatterbuck, R. E., & Rigamonti, D. (1999). Acquired immunodeficiency syndrome. In R. K. Osenbach & S. M. Zeidman (Eds.). *Infections in neurological surgery* (pp. 227–239). Philadelphia: Lippincott-Raven.

28. Post, M. J., Hensley, G. T., Moskowitz, L. B., et al. (1986). Cytomegalic inclusion virus encephalitis in patients with AIDS: CT, clinical and pathologic correlation. *American Journal of Roentgenology, 146,* 1229–1234.

29. Kioumeht, F., Dadsetan, M. R., & Rooholamini. (1994). Central nervous system tuberculosis: MRI. *Neuroradiology, 36,* 93–96.

30. Berger, J. R., & Levy, R. M. (1993). The neurologic complications of human immunodeficiency virus infection. *Medical Clinics of North America, 77*(1), 1–21.

31. Taveras, J. M., & Pile-Spellman, J. (1996). *Neuroradiology.* Baltimore: Williams & Wilkins.

RESOURCES

Published Material

Books

Adams, R. D., Victor, M., & Ropper, A. H. (1997). Nonviral infections of the nervous system. In R. D. Adams & M. Victor (Eds.). *Principles of neurology* (6th ed., pp. 695–741). New York: McGraw-Hill.

Bartlett, J. G. (1995). *Johns Hopkins Hospital guide to medical care of patients with HIV infection* (5th ed.). Baltimore: Williams & Wilkins.

McArthur, J. (1992). Neurologic manifestations of human immunodeficiency virus infection. In *Diseases of the central nervous system: Clinical neurobiology* (pp. 1312–1330). Philadelphia: W. B. Saunders.

Osenbach. R. K., & Zeidman, S. M., (Eds.) (1999). *Infections in neurological surgery.* Philadelphia: Lippincott-Raven.

Sande, M. A., & P. A. Volberding, P. A. (Eds.). (1995). *Medical management of AIDS* (4th ed.). Philadelphia: W. B. Saunders.

Periodicals

Barzaga, R. A., Klein, N. C., & Cunha, B. A. (1992). Herpes simplex meningoencephalitis. *Heart and Lung, 21*(4), 405–406.

Cabellos, C., Viladrich, P. F., Veraguer, R., Pallares, R., Linares, J., & Gudiol, F. (1995). A single daily dose of ceftriaxone for bacterial meningitis in adults: Experience with 84 patients and review of the literature. *Clinical Infectious Diseases, 20*(5), 1164–1168.

Loder, P. (1993). HIV infections of the central nervous system: What are the nursing implications? *Nursing Clinics of North America, 28*(4), 839–847.

Minnick, A. (1986). Cysticercosis: Etiology and nursing care. *Journal of Neuroscience Nursing, 18*(3), 135–145.

Morgello, S., DiRocco, A., & Simpson, D. M. (2000). Current views on common neurologic manifestations of HIV. *The PRN Notebook, 5*(3), 19–25.

Myers, F. (2000). Meningitis: The fears, the facts. *RN, 63*(11), 52–57.

Newton, H. (1995). Common neurologic complications of HIV-1 infections and AIDS. *American Family Physician, 51*(2), 387–398.

Peltola, H. (1999). Prophylaxis of bacterial meningitis. *Infectious Disease Clinics of North America, 13*(3), 685–710.

Rosenstein, N. E., Perkis, B. A., Stephens, D. S., Popovic, T., & Hughes, J. M. (2001). Meningococcal disease. *New England Journal of Medicine, 344*(18), 1378–1388.

Simpson, D., & Tagliati, M. (1994). Neurologic manifestations of HIV infection. *Annals of Internal Medicine, 121*(10), 769–785.

Smillova, A., & Walker, E. (2000). Meningococcemia: A critical care emergency. *Critical Care Nurse, 20*(5), 28–38.

Steere, A. C. (2001). Lyme disease. *New England Journal of Medicine, 345*(2), 115–125.

Zackson, R., Calabro, L., & Cunha, B. (1994). Meningitis in adults: Differentiating the sources. *Emergency Medicine, 26*(4), 113–114, 117–118.

Websites

There are an enormous number of websites available for providers, patients, and family members that can be easily accessed.

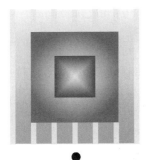

C H A P T E R **31**

Neurodegenerative Diseases

JOANNE V. HICKEY

This chapter covers the five most common neurodegenerative diseases: dementia and Alzheimer's disease, Parkinson's disease, amyotrophic lateral sclerosis, multiple sclerosis, and myasthenia gravis. These diseases are all chronic illnesses with varying patterns of progression over time. Any chronic illness creates strains, stresses, and challenges for the patient and family as well as for the health care system. This chapter begins with a brief discussion of chronic illness and chronic illness management and how these general principles apply to neurodegenerative conditions.

A *chronic illness* is any physical or mental condition that requires long-term (over 6 months) of monitoring and/or management to control symptoms and to shape the course of the disease.[1] It has also been defined as the irreversible presence, accumulation, or latency of disease states or impairments, which involve the total human environment to provide supportive care and self-care, to maintain function, and to prevent further disability.[2] Chronic illness is the epidemic of the 21st century. By 2030, it is expected that 150 million Americans will have one or more chronic conditions. Of that number, 42 million will have activity limitations restricting their ability to work and live independently.[3] Advances in medical science, especially in molecular and genetic research, have greatly increased our understanding of many of the neurodegenerative diseases. Although cures remain elusive, breakthroughs have been made in treatments directed at symptom management.

Several characteristics of chronic illness are important when considering neurodegenerative disorders. A chronic illness tends to include multiple diseases as a result of the impact of the primary disease on other body systems. As chronic illnesses follow uncertain and changing courses, they greatly intrude on the life of the patient and family over a long period (i.e., years). The level of disability waxes and wanes with the course of the illness, which creates a sense of uncertainty. Because of its changing nature, effective management of a chronic illness requires a variety of primary and ancillary services. Chronic illness is expensive to treat and manage, and often third party reimbursement is lacking or very limited. The quality of chronic illness management varies significantly, especially when compared to the high-tech, protocol-driven, hospital-based care that is the hallmark of acute care.

Chronic illness management usually involves home-based care with little use of technology. Day-to-day care is provided by family members in the home setting. Hospitalization, if necessary, is usually short-term and limited to serious relapses or complications related to the disease. Ongoing patient and family education, counseling, and empowerment for self-management are cornerstones of a patient-focused approach. Care focuses on symptom management and interventions to stabilize the disease process and prevent complications. The ultimate goal with chronic disease is adapting to the illness and promoting an acceptable quality of life. This means that care is directed at keeping the patient as independent and functional as possible for as long as possible within the context of his or her lifestyle.

The needs of the patient are best provided for through a collaborative, multidisciplinary, integrated, holistic model with the patient and family as the centerpiece of care. Nurses are an integral part of the health care team and provide comprehensive care and support to both the patient and the family. Unfortunately, much of what nurses do as part of chronic illness care is invisible because outcomes are difficult to measure and attribute to the nurse. Nurses make a major contribution through teaching patients how to integrate their treatment regimens into their lives and how to recognize signs of complications.[1] The nurse's role involves assessing, communicating, teaching, coaching, counseling, role-modeling, comforting, advising, advocating, and coordinating activities and care. Because nurses are attuned to subtle signs that indicate changes in the status of an illness, they can advise the patient when to seek medical assistance. They provide the knowledge and support, both prerequisites to successful adaptation, that assist the patient and family to understand and accept the illness. Assuming a major role for communicating with other team members and community services, the nurse provides for coordination of care through case management and advocacy.

MODELS FOR CHRONIC ILLNESS MANAGEMENT

Several models or frameworks for chronic illness management are available to guide nursing practice. Although acute care is often structured around a medical model based on pathophysiology, diagnosis, and treatment, chronic illness is best structured around a psychosocial adaptation model. The trajectory of illness model provides a framework to guide care for chronic illnesses.[4] A *trajectory* is defined as a course of illness over time, plus the actions taken by patients, families, and health care professionals to manage or shape the course of the illness. To encompass the dynamic and changing character of chronic illness, the concept of *phasing* has been added to trajectory.[1] Nine different trajectory phases, identified by Corbin and Strauss, are briefly described with application to neurodegenerative diseases.[4]

The **pretrajectory phase** includes identification of lifestyle and genetic risk factors that predispose a person to develop a chronic illness (i.e., neurodegenerative disease). It is the ultimate goal of neuroscience research to identify genetic markers and lifestyle characteristics that can be modified before a disease develops. Currently, neuroscience has not developed to this level of knowledge. The next phase is the **trajectory onset**. During this phase, onset of symptoms, seeking medical attention, diagnostic workup, and finally diagnoses occur. The patient begins to learn about the disease and begins to cope with the implications of the illness. In neurological patients, symptoms that cannot be ignored lead to diagnosis, often a frightening term that has no meaning to the patient. The patient begins to learn about what it means to have multiple sclerosis or Parkinson's disease, and what might lie ahead. The **stable phase** is one in which the illness and symptoms are under control and everyday life is being managed within the limitations of the illness. Care is centered in the home. For example, a patient with Alzheimer's disease is functional and has routines and strategies such as a notepad with activities for the day that keep him or her involved in home activities.

The next phase is the **unstable phase**. The symptoms are not under control, and there is an exacerbation of the illness. This is disruptive to carrying out the usual routines at home that have been effective previously. Adjustments are made to return to the normal, stable phase. For example, a previously effective drug schedule for a patient with myasthenia gravis is no longer effective. The patient feels weak and cannot accomplish the home or work activities usually completed. This leads to a search for the cause of this change in status such as an infection, too much anticholinesterase drugs, or emotional stress. The **acute phase** is described as the development of severe and unrelieved symptoms or complications that require bed rest or hospitalization. Normal activity abruptly ceases, and the patient wonders whether he or she will ever recover. For example, a patient with amyotrophic lateral sclerosis develops aspiration pneumonia. A decision regarding a gastrostomy tube placement may need to be made, and the possibility of mechanical ventilatory support may be discussed. A **crisis phase** is a critical or life-threatening situation requiring emergency treatment or care. Everyday life in placed indefinitely on hold. Myasthenic crisis requiring intubation and use of mechanical ventilation is an example with a neurological patient population. The **comeback phase** is a gradual return to an acceptable way of life within the limits imposed by the recovery process and any irreversible losses incurred during the crisis. This phase involves the physical healing, rehabilitation procedures, and psychosocial coming to terms with

the events. It also includes a reentry and adjustment to everyday life and any new limitations.

The **downward phase** is characterized by a gradual or rapid physical deterioration and difficulty with symptom control. It requires alterations in everyday life and loss of some functional abilities. For example, a patient with Alzheimer's disease may now become confined to bed. The final phase is the **dying phase** and includes the final days or weeks before death. The body gradually or rapidly shuts down; the person disengages and comes to closure. In patients with neurodegenerative diseases, often cognitive function has been compromised so that psychological disengagement may have occurred in a previous phase. In other neurodegenerative conditions, the patient is cognitively aware of approaching death and has made decisions for a peaceful death.

The trajectory of illness offers an excellent model to assist the neuroscience nurse in providing care to the patient with neurodegenerative disease. It suggests need for the nurse to provide education, support, and care in each phase of the trajectory. The very nature of a degenerative disease indicates a process of losses. How quickly functional deterioration occurs depends on the particular disease and the individual course. Successful adaptation to chronic illness with an acceptable quality of life is characterized by psychosocial adjustment and an ability to cope with losses while positively reforming intact function. For there to be successful adjustment and adaptation to the illness, each phase of the trajectory requires special work for the patient and family. The nurse can provide the knowledge and skill for this process to occur.

DEMENTIA

Dementia is the generic term that indicates a deterioration of memory and other acquired higher cognitive abilities from a normal premorbid level of intellectual and social functioning.[5] It is a serious and common problem affecting more than 4 million Americans and costing society approximately 80 billion dollars annually for direct and indirect care.[6] The incidence of dementia rises dramatically with age. Its prevalence doubles every 5 years of age so that by age 85, about 30% to 50% are demented.[7]

The *Diagnostic and Statistical Manual of Mental Disorders*, 4th edition (DSM-IV), defines dementia as "the development of multiple cognitive deficits that include memory impairment and at least one of the following: aphasia, apraxia, agnosia, or a disturbance in executive functioning. These deficits must be sufficiently severe to cause impairment in occupational or social functioning, and must represent a decline from a previously higher level of functioning."[8]

The causes of dementia are numerous (Table 31-1) and vary by age group. *Alzheimer's disease* (*AD*), the major cause of dementia accounting for more than half of all dementias, is followed by *vascular dementia* (20% to 25%). In third place is dementia associated with Parkinson's disease (PD) and alcoholism.[9] A newer classification of dementia, *Lewy body disease,* has arisen. Lewy body disease refers to a clinicopathological entity that often occurs in combination with AD, PD, and vascular disease. A Lewy body is an intracytoplas-

▟ Table 31–1 • CAUSES OF DEMENTIA

Major Causes of Dementia in U.S. Population

1. Alzheimer's disease (>50%) of all cases
2. Vascular dementia (20%–25%)
   Multi-infarct
   Diffuse white matter disease
3. Parkinson's disease
4. Alcoholism
5. Drug/medication toxicity*

Other Less Common Causes of Dementia

Degenerative disorders
   Pick's disease, diffuse Lewy body disease; Huntington's disease; cortical basal degeneration; MS; some forms of ALS and PD; and other disorders
Chronic infections
   HIV, Creutzfeldt-Jacob disease, PML, neurosyphilis,* and opportunistic infections (TB, fungal, protozoal);* sarcoidosis*
*Neoplasms**
   Primary and metastatic brain tumors
Toxic
   Heavy metals;* organic toxins
*Vitamin deficiencies**
   Thiamine [B_1]—Wernicke's encephalopathy; Vitamin B_{12} pernicious anemia
*Endocrine and other system diseases**
   Hypothyroidism; parathyroidism; adrenal insufficiency, and renal, liver, or pulmonary failures
Head trauma and diffuse brain damage
   Chronic subdural hematoma;* normal pressure hydrocephalus;* hypoxic brain syndrome; postencephalitis
*Psychiatric disorders**
   Depression; conversion reaction

* Potentially reversible dementia either by category or specific problem.

MS, multiple sclerosis; ALS, amyotrophic lateral sclerosis; PD, Parkinson's disease; PML, progressive multifocal leukoencephalopathy; TB, *Mycobacterium tuberculosis.*

---

mic eosinophilic neuronal body surrounded by a lighter halo seen in some neurodegenerative diseases. Vascular disease and Lewy body disease often occur concurrently with AD.[10] In PD, Lewy bodies are found in neurons of the degenerating substantia nigra. They can also be found in lesser numbers in other central nervous system (CNS) degenerative conditions, and occasionally in the brains of non-parkinsonian elderly persons.[11] Although AD is acknowledged as the most common cause of dementia, many of the remaining cases of dementia are caused by vascular disease and Lewy body disease.

Some dementias are associated with an underlying primary condition and may be reversible with prompt treatment. Common underlying reversal etiologies are drug toxicity, metabolic disorders, and dysfunction in other body systems. In other instances, dementia is a chronic, irreversible condition, resulting in progressive loss of overall cognitive function.

Diagnosis

There is no standard "workup" for dementia, although certain tests should be completed as an initial evaluation of all patients.[12] Early and accurate diagnosis of dementia is im-

portant for several reasons. First, with early diagnostic suspicion, one can avoid overuse of expensive medical resources. Second, the patient can better participate in health care, legal, and financial planning while decision-making capacity is still intact and decisions still reflect his or her wishes.[13] Third, early diagnosis helps to separate dementia from normal aging or "age-related cognitive decline." Older adults commonly have complaints of memory impairment such as difficulty remembering names or appointments or solving complex problems. Memory impairment is also a hallmark of AD. Many people worry needlessly about AD when normal aging is the operative process. Multiple variables, including age, native intelligence, education, normal cognitive demand of work and daily living, nutrition, and psychological well-being, make normal age-related cognitive decline difficult to differentiate from AD. The diagnosis of age-related cognitive decline should not be made without screening the patient for dementia. Table 31-2 lists signs and symptoms that suggest the need to evaluate for dementia. The evaluation should include a careful history, a physical examination including a neurological examination, and diagnostics tailored to the differential diagnoses suggested by the history and physical examination.[12] Figure 31-1 provides a flow chart for the recognition and initial assessment of AD and related dementias.

History and Physical Examination

Some patients seek medical attention for reassurance that they are not suffering from dementia. Other patients, who have dementia, may visit the health care provider reluc-

---

Table 31–2 • CHANGES THAT MAY SUGGEST THE NEED FOR A DEMENTIA WORKUP

Cognitive Changes

Impaired memory (forgets address, phone number); forgetfulness; confusion; difficulty understanding the written or spoken word; word-finding difficulty; lack of knowledge about current activities and events; poor concentration; difficulty recognizing faces and common objects

Change in Daily Function

Self-care and grooming neglect; getting lost in previously familiar surroundings or routes; difficulty managing finances and completing home activities (e.g., cooking, cleaning); difficulty with shopping, using the telephone, or simple problem solving; making mistakes in usual work or volunteer activities

Personality Changes

Social withdrawal; mood swings; loss of appropriate social behavior; loss of self-control; easily frustrated; explosive spells; crying spells

Problematic and Psychiatric Behaviors

Agitation; restlessness; boisterousness; demanding; uncooperative; wandering; sleeplessness; outburst; sexual aggressiveness; verbal/physical abusiveness; safety concerns such as forgetting to turn off stove; losing things such as keys; apathy; depression; suspiciousness; anxiety; fearfulness; paranoia; hallucinations; insomnia

ADLs, activities of daily living; IADLs, instrumental activities of daily living.

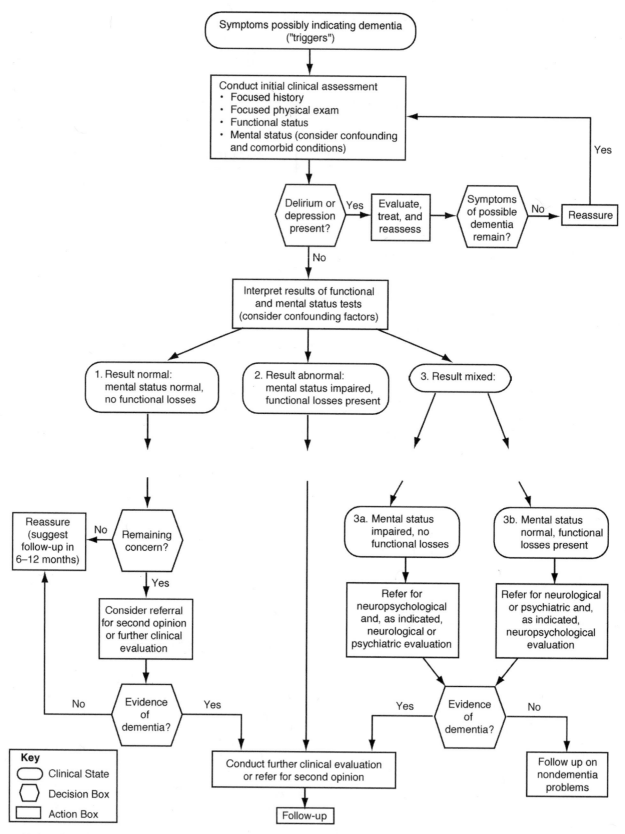

Figure 31–1 • Flow chart for the recognition and initial assessment of Alzheimer's disease and related dementias. (Costa, P. T. Jr., Williams, T. F., Somerfield, M., et al. [1996]. *Early identification of Alzheimer's disease and related dementias. Clinical practice guideline: Quick reference for clinicians, No. 19.* Rockville, MD: U.S. Department of Health and Human Services, Public Health Service, Agency for Health Care Policy and Research. AHCPR Publication No. 97-0703.)

tantly, coming at the insistence of family members. Often a frightening event has triggered the decision to seek medical evaluation. Such an event often involves a threat to safety such as leaving a stove on or becoming lost in familiar surroundings. The patient may try to provide a plausible explanation to downplay the event or show little insight into the concerns expressed by the family.

Screening begins with a complete medical history and detailed description of impairments to function, behavior, and cognition. A careful discussion is conducted with the patient to determine the presence of a progressive decline in memory, personality or behavioral changes, psychiatric problems, or functional deterioration in the ability to conduct activities of daily living (ADLs) and instrumental ADLs, to participate in hobbies and social functions, or to conduct work-related activities. Friends or family members can often provide perspective on troubling events that have occurred as well as on functional and behavioral changes such as forgetfulness. Although the clinical presentation of dementia may vary, depending on the etiology, the diagnostic criteria are consistent.[14] The criteria are well outlined in the DSM-IV. These criteria are found in Chart 31-1. In addition to the interview, various objective rating scales are available to screen dementia in the office setting. A commonly used scale that screens for dementia, the Mini-Mental Status Examination (see Table 7-1), can be completed in 5 minutes in any setting. A score of 24 or higher (range 0 to 30) is generally considered normal, although performance varies depending on age and education.[15]

Although AD is the most common cause of dementia, the differential diagnosis includes many disorders, including neurodegenerative, vascular, neoplastic, traumatic, demyelinating, and genetic disorders.[16] Between 15% to 30% of patients with dementia have a reversible disorder. These include drug effects, metabolic disorders, stroke, vitamin deficiencies, and depression.[17] Therefore, it is important to take a careful medical and drug history to rule out reversible causes of cognitive dysfunction.

The physical examination should include a general systems examination as well as a detailed neurological examination *to detect any focal or generalized neurological signs (e.g., monoplegia, ataxia, myoclonic jerking).* A detailed mental status and cognitive function examination should be conducted. Evaluation of orientation, recent and remote memory, calculation, serial 7s, naming of objects, spelling a word forward and backward, and following simple and complex commands can reveal cognitive deficits. Attention should be given to screening for aphasia (i.e., expressive or receptive deficits), apraxia (e.g., drawing a clock, performing a skilled act on command such as combing the hair) agnosia (e.g., identification of objects), and executive functioning.

Diagnostic Testing

There is no definitive test for dementia or the multiple subcategories of dementia. The use of multiple laboratory tests in the evaluation of dementia is controversial. The health care provider does not want to miss reversible conditions, but sensitivity to cost must be maintained. Each of the multiple tests has a low yield.[9] When the history and physical examination suggest the need for further evalua-

CHART 31 – 1 • Criteria for the Diagnosis of Alzheimer's Type Dementia

A. The development of multiple cognitive deficits as manifested by both
   1. Memory impairment (impaired ability to learn new information or to recall previously learned information)
   2. One or more of the following cognitive disturbances:
     a. Aphasia (language disturbance)
     b. Apraxia (impaired ability to carry out motor activities despite intact motor function)
     c. Agnosia (failure to recognize or identify objects despite intact sensory function)
     d. Disturbance in executive functioning (i.e., planning organizing, sequencing, implementing, abstracting)
B. The cognitive deficits in Criteria A1 and A2 both cause significant impairment in social or occupational functioning and represent a significant decline from a previous level of functioning.
C. The course is characterized by a gradual onset and continuing cognitive decline.
D. The cognitive deficits in Criteria A1 and A2 are not due to any of the following:
   1. Other central nervous system conditions that cause progressive deficits in memory and cognition (e.g., cerebrovascular disease, Parkinson's disease, Huntington's disease, subdural hematoma, normal-pressure hydrocephalus, brain tumor)
   2. Systemic conditions known to cause dementia (e.g., hypothyroidism, vitamin B_{12} or folic acid deficiency, niacin deficiency, hypercalcemia, neurosyphilis, human immunodeficiency virus infection)
   3. Substance-induced conditions
E. The deficits do not occur exclusively during the course of a delirium.
F. The disturbance is not better accounted for by another Axis I disorder (e.g., major depressive disorder, schizophrenia).

tion, laboratory tests, brain imaging, neuropsychological testing and other tests are available.

In addition to the history and physical examination, a routine evaluation includes the following laboratory tests: thyroid function, vitamin B_{12}, complete blood test, electrolytes, Venereal Disease Research Laboratories' (VDRL) testing, and computed tomography and magnetic resonance imaging (CT/MRI). Depending on clues uncovered in the history and physical examination, other optional tests may be ordered, such as liver function, renal function, human immunodeficiency virus (HIV), chest x-ray, lumbar puncture, urine toxin screen, and neuropsychological testing.[9]

The main purpose of neuroimaging (CT or MRI) of the brain is to exclude a focal or generalized structural and potentially reversible cause of dementia. CT or MRI is widely used to exclude brain tumors, hydrocephalus, cerebrovascular disease, or subdural hematoma. Imaging may suggest presence of opportunistic infections in patients at risk for HIV (see Chap. 30). MRI is preferred to detect infarction, small lesions, white matter changes, evidence of normal pressure hydrocephalus, focal atrophy and generalized atrophy, and pathological changes poorly visualized by CT (e.g., base of the temporal lobe and posterior fossa).[16-18]

Neuropsychological testing can make an important contribution to identification of mild dementia and can suggest productive avenues for treatment and management of behavior problems. A battery of tests addressing multiple domains of cognitive function measures the functional level of cognitive abilities and can identify psychiatric manifestations. Neuropsychological testing is helpful to identify dementia among people with high premorbid intellectual functioning.[19] In a patient with dementia, the neuropsychological battery can establish a baseline to monitor disease progression and the effects of treatment. Neuropsychological testing takes several hours to complete and requires the cooperation of the patient.

Treatment and Management

Five major goals guide the treatment and management of dementia. First, treat any underlying causes of dementia. Conditions such as a B_{12} deficiency, low thyroid function, drug toxicity, and brain tumor are treatable, and the treatment may reverse or improve the dementia. Second, problematic behaviors (e.g., agitation, sleep disorder, wandering) that often present safety concerns must be managed. For example, if agitation and wandering behaviors are present, interventions designed to address the underlying cause of these problems must be implemented. Interventions may include cognitive therapy, drug therapy, or a combination of both.

Third, identify and treat depression. Although depression is the most common psychiatric illness in older people, it is often underdiagnosed, especially when concurrent physical illness is present. The diagnosis may be complicated because (1) depression is often mistaken for dementia and vice versa, (2) either dementia or depression may present as the other, and (3) dementia and depression may coexist.[19] There are serious implications for the misdiagnosis of dementia as depression. Inappropriate treatment for nonexistent depression in a person with progressive dementia may exacerbate dementia because antidepressants that have anticholinergic properties may worsen confusion or memory impairment.[19] A change in sleep pattern or appetite, fatigue, behavioral slowing or agitation, complaints of diminished ability to think or concentrate, and apathy are symptoms of major depression and also symptoms of AD. In persons with co-existing depression and AD, failure to diagnose and treat depression may cause unnecessary emotional, physical, and social discomfort for both the patient and family. Additionally, failure to identify and treat depression robs the patient of a higher level of quality of life. Therefore, assessment for depression is an important component of the initial evaluation.

There are a number of standardized scales to detect depression, such as the Geriatric Depression Scale (GDS) and the Center for Epidemiological Studies Depression Scale (CES-D). The GDS uses a 30-item questionnaire with a simple yes/no format. It was developed especially for older people and takes 8 to 10 minutes to administer. The CES-D uses a 20-item questionnaire and takes 5 to 8 minutes to administer. Antidepressant drugs such as selective serotonin reuptake inhibitors (e.g., sertraline [Zoloft]) and tricyclics (e.g. nortriptyline) are examples of drugs commonly ordered. A stable controlled environment helps minimize disorientation, confusion, frustration, agitation, and combative behavior. Too many environmental stimuli, tasks beyond the patient's ability, or unfamiliar surroundings are examples of situations that may precipitate behavioral problems.

Fourth, prepare the patient and family for the future in a supportive, sensitive manner. The type and extent of preparation depends on the diagnosis. Generally, a patient with dementia should make decisions about his or her health care preferences, finances, legal matters, and advanced directives while decision-making capabilities remain intact. The patient and family should receive anticipatory guidance about what to expect in the future and rate of decline that is geared to the underlying cause of the dementia.

Fifth, help the patient maintain the highest quality of life possible for as long as possible. Monitoring should be conducted every 3 to 6 months to reevaluate the patient's and family caregivers' functional levels and to identify new problems that can be addressed to support the patient and family.

The primary health care provider must decide whether he or she will manage the patient alone or whether the patient should be referred to a specialist such as a neurologist. This decision is based on the complexity of the patient, provider comfort, and patient/family wishes. A collaborative interdisciplinary team approach is important to assist both the patient and family over the trajectory of the illness. The role of the nurse is particularly important in providing care for the patient and supporting the family caregiver.

Summary

In summary, the prevalence of dementia, an enormous problem in the United States, is expected to increase as baby boomers age. Dementia is a prominent feature of many diseases. Some of these are discussed in the next section along with treatment and management options.

ALZHEIMER'S DISEASE

Alzheimer's disease is the most common cause of dementia in Western countries. AD was first described by the German psychiatrist Alois Alzheimer in 1907 while treating a 55-year-old woman. The condition was initially thought to represent an uncommon form of presenile dementia, but it has become evident that adults of any age can develop AD, although it most often affects older people.

Signs and Symptoms

Clinically, progressive impairment of short- and long-term memory and cognitive functions is the major feature of AD. Because AD begins with forgetfulness that can be subtle, it can be dismissed easily by the patient and the family. The patient may try to conceal the forgetfulness with excuses, compensating with notes and reminders. Difficulty with new learning, language, and visuospatial function, as well as apraxias and agnosias are features of the deterioration. There is a deterioration in ADLs and instrumental ADLs as noted in work performance and ability to deal with everyday family living and social situations. Some patients have psychiatric manifestations such as paranoia, delusions, agitation, and depression. Appropriate social skills and behaviors may be retained until later stages of the disease. Focal motor or sensory deficits are uncommon. About 8% of patients have seizures. The progressive course continues with the loss of global cognitive function that includes impaired abstract thinking, impaired judgment, and personality change. In the end stage, the patient is bedridden, emaciated, aphasic, and apraxic and lacks control of the body, including sphincters. All cognitive functions and emotional responses are lost. Death is usually caused by an infection, such as aspiration pneumonia.[20]

The DSM-IV outlines the diagnostic criteria for dementia of the Alzheimer type (see Chart 31-1). The average course of AD is 8 to 10 years, although the range is 1 to 25 years.[21] The course of AD is often divided into an early, middle, and end-stages based on the clinical presentation. Chart 31-2 describes the typical behaviors seem in each stage. Various probable and possible risk factors have been identified for AD. They include older age, familial history, genetic factors, perhaps female gender, lower educational level, head trauma with loss of consciousness, myocardial infarction, diabetes mellitus, hypothyroidism, exposure to organic solvents, PD, and Down's syndrome.[20] Protective factors include greater educational achievement, estrogen replacement in women, and use of anti-inflammatory drugs.

Diagnosis

Diagnosis of AD is by exclusion of other causes and is based on a clinical and neuropathological pattern. The definitive diagnosis of AD is made based on meeting the clinical criteria (see Chart 31-1) and histological evidence based on examination of brain tissue obtained from biopsy or autopsy. The histological changes associated with AD include gross, diffuse atrophy of the cerebral cortex with secondary enlargement of the ventricular system. On microscopic examination, there are extracellular neuritic plaques containing $A\beta$ amyloid, silver-staining neurofibrillary tangles in neuronal cytoplasm, and accumulation of $A\beta$ amyloid in arterial walls of cerebral blood vessels.[21] The neurofibrillary tangles and amyloidal plaque deposits are found chiefly in the temporoparietal and anterior frontal regions. The degenerative changes in the basal frontal-temporal region profoundly reduce the content of acetylcholine and the activity of choline acetyltransferase.[22] Other neurotransmitters can be involved, but the loss of acetylcholine occurs early and correlates with the impairment of memory.[22–24] Symptomatic treatment of AD has focused on augmenting cholinergic neurotransmission.[22,24]

CHART 31–2 • Stages of Alzheimer's Disease

The stages of Alzheimer's disease vary from patient to patient, but a few time approximations, as well as characteristic behaviors, can be identified.

STAGE 1: EARLY STAGE—2 TO 4 YR

- Forgetful—may be subtle, may try to cover up by using lists and notes
- Exhibits a declining interest in environment, people, and present affairs
- Demonstrates vague uncertainty and hesitancy in initiating actions
- Performs poorly at work, may be dismissed from job

STAGE 2: MIDDLE STAGE—2 TO 12 YR

- Exhibits progressive memory loss
- Hesitates in response to questions; shows signs of aphasia
- Has difficulty following simple instructions or doing simple calculations
- Has episodic bouts of irritability
- Becomes evasive, anxious, and physically active
- Becomes more active at night owing to sleep-wakefulness cycle disturbance
- Wanders, particularly at night
- Becomes apraxic for many basic activities

- Loses important papers
- Loses way home in familiar surroundings or loses way in own home
- Forgets to pay bills; lets household chores slip and newspapers pile up; does not dispose of garbage; does not take medications
- Loses possessions and then claims that they were stolen
- Neglects personal hygiene (bathing, shaving, dressing)
- Loses social graces; can cause embarrassment to family and friends, which usually results in social isolation of the family and patient

STAGE 3: FINAL STAGE

- Loses much weight because of lack of eating; becomes emaciated
- Is unable to communicate verbally or in writing
- Does not recognize family
- Is incontinent of urine and feces
- Has a predisposition for major seizures
- Grasping, snout, and sucking reflexes are readily elicited
- Finally loses the ability to stand and walk and becomes bedridden
- Death is usually caused by aspiration pneumonia

As previously discussed, the differential diagnosis is problematic in dementias. Some of the difficulty in distinguishing the dementia of AD from dementias associated with other conditions is the lack of clarity of definitions. For example, both delirium and depression can resemble dementia and must therefore be excluded. **Delirium** is a *transient and potentially reversible condition* in which there is fluctuation in levels of awareness (agitation to stupor), hallucinations, and cognitive impairment, particularly memory. The key defining characteristic of delirium is the pattern of *rapid fluctuation of symptoms over a short period of time.* **Depression,** which has many symptoms common to AD (e.g., behavioral slowing or agitation, complaints of diminished ability to think or concentrate, fatigue, changes in sleep pattern or appetite), must be ruled out. It is a common problem seen in older people and is treatable.

CT and MRI are not specific for AD and may produce normal findings in the early course of the disease. As AD progresses, diffuse cortical atrophy is noted and the MRI shows significant atrophy of the hippocampus, an anatomical area associated with memory. Enlarged ventricles are also noted. Imaging is useful to rule out treatable causes of dementia such as a brain tumor or CNS infection. A positron emission tomography (PET) scan, although sometimes ordered, is controversial and not readily available in all facilities. The use of SPECT perfusion imaging has shown promise as a means of earlier diagnosis of AD.[25] Further investigation is needed to determine its use in practice. In the later stages of AD, there is diffuse slowing of the waves on electroencephalogram (EEG). Other laboratory tests are ordered to rule out treatable conditions (see discussion in section on dementia).

Etiology

The cause of AD is unknown. Four susceptibility genes for AD have been identified, which are important to the understanding of the biological basis of AD. Familial AD has an autosomal dominant pattern of inheritance[26] and can be caused by a mutation in the genes for amyloid precursor protein (APP), presenilin-1, or presenilin-2.[27] It is believed that presenilin-1 and presenilin-2 form complexes with at least one other protein, nicastrin, a transmembrane neuronal glycoprotein. These complexes may contribute to the production of Aβ.[28] In both the sporadic and familial forms of AD, the age of onset is modulated by allelic variants of apolipoprotein E (Apo E).[29] Apo E has three alleles: $\varepsilon 2$, $\varepsilon 3$, and $\varepsilon 4$. The $\varepsilon 4$ allele shows a strong association with AD in the general population, including sporadic and late-onset familial cases. In many people with two $\varepsilon 4$ alleles, AD develops at least a decade before it does in those with two copies of $\varepsilon 2$, and $\varepsilon 3$, a condition associated with an onset of disease at an intermediate age.[26,30,31] Intensive research continues on the genetics of AD, with much interest focused on development of an early diagnostic test to identify AD, preventive therapy for those at risk, and cure rather than temporary symptomatic treatment of AD.

Treatment

Unfortunately, there is no cure for AD. Currently, the goal of treatment is to improve or slow the loss of memory and cognition and to maintain independent function for as long

as possible.[22] A multidisciplinary approach meets the changing needs of the patient and the family over the course of the illness. Working collaboratively, the multidisciplinary team (i.e., physician, nurse, social worker, case manager, rehabilitation specialist, neuropsychologist) provides sensitive support and counseling, education, and strategies to control the behavioral manifestations of the disease. Providing support, counseling, and education is an ongoing process to which all team members contribute. Anticipatory guidance to the family helps prepare them for the cognitive and physical decline and for planning ways of managing the patient. There are many patients with AD who do not have family support. They come to the attention of health providers when worried neighbors contact the police to express concern about the patient's safety or behavior. Most patients do not have the opportunity to be treated by a multidisciplinary team in a center dedicated to the comprehensive care of AD. Patients are managed by a primary care provider who monitors the patient (e.g., 3 to 6 months), manages symptoms, and provides support. Management options include drug therapy, and psycho-education and counseling.

Drug Therapy to Slow the Progression of Alzheimer's Disease

A group of drugs classified as cholinesterase inhibitors (anticholinesterases) have shown encouraging results for the symptomatic treatment of impairment in memory and cognitive function for persons with mild to moderate AD. These drugs act to increase cholinergic synaptic transmission by inhibiting acetylcholinesterase in the synaptic cleft, resulting in a decrease in the hydrolysis of acetylcholine released from presynaptic neurons.[22] There are four drugs approved by the Food and Drug Administration (FDA) drugs in this class (Table 31-3).[32] These drugs differ from one another in how they inhibit acetylcholinesterase activity and in side effects.[33] Treatment with cholinesterase inhibitors can begin at any time after diagnosis. Higher doses have the greater benefits and also the more adverse effects. The recommendation is to increase the dose to the maximum tolerable level gradually. Cholinesterase inhibitor therapy is only effective in mild to moderate AD.

The FDA recommends that all clinical trials whose results are to be submitted to the FDA for approval of new AD drugs use the Alzheimer's Disease Assessment Scale, cognitive subscale[34] as the primary outcome measure.[35] In this way, the efficacy of different drugs for their effects on memory and other cognitive function can be validly compared. It is also useful for a health care provider to use this subscale to monitor the effect of a drug on a particular patient. The cognitive subscale includes items that assess memory, orientation, attention, reasoning, language, and motor performance. The range of scores is from 0, indicating no impairment, to 70, indicating severe impairment. In using the scale with AD patients who are not receiving drug therapy, there is an 8% to 10% decline in the score yearly.[36]

Antioxidant drugs have also been used in AD in an attempt to slow progression of the disease. These drugs with their daily total doses include, vitamin E, 2000 U; selegiline, 10 mg; idebenone, 90 to 270 mg; propentofylline, 900 mg; and ginkgo biloba, 120 mg (available in health food stores). In the studies of these drugs, there

Table 31-3 • DRUGS FOR SYMPTOMATIC TREATMENT OF MEMORY AND COGNITIVE FUNCTION FOR MILD-TO-MODERATE ALZHEIMER'S DISEASE

DRUG	ACTION IN ADDITION TO ACETYLCHOLINESTERASE INHIBITION	DOSE/FREQUENCY	COMMON SIDE EFFECTS
Tacrine (Cognex)	Inhibits formation of enzyme-acetylcholine complex	10–40 mg qid	Nausea, vomiting, elevated serum aminotransferase levels
Doneperzil (Aricept)	Inhibits formation of enzyme-acetylcholine complex	5–10 mg qd	Nausea, diarrhea, vomiting
Rivastigmine (Exelon)	Inhibits action of enzyme-acetylcholine complex	1.5–6 mg bid	Nausea, vomiting
Galantamine (Reminyl)	Acts on nicotinic acetylcho-line receptors	4–12 mg bid	Nausea, vomiting, dizziness, diar-rhea, anorexia, weight loss

was no difference in the treatment group compared with the placebo group on the Alzheimer's Disease Assessment Scale, cognitive subscale.[22]

Treatment of Behavioral Manifestations

Treatment of the behavioral manifestations of AD is important in management. Major depression occurs in 5% to 8% of patients with AD, and up to 25% of patients have some depressive symptoms at the time of onset of memory impairment.[37,38] The tricyclic antidepressant (e.g., amitriptyline, imipramine) have not been effective in AD. In addition, some tricyclics like amitriptyline have anticholinergic actions and can cause confusion or orthostatic hypotension.[22] The selective serotonin-reuptake inhibitors (e.g., citalopram, fluoxetine, paroxetine) showed improvement in depression scores on standard depression scales. The side effects noted were insomnia, anorexia, nausea, and diarrhea.

Delusions and psychosis are common and increase with the progression of AD. Use of neuroleptic drugs such as haloperidol and risperidone may be helpful. However, extrapyramidal signs are common side effects. Agitation, another common problem, is treated with benzodiazepines and carbamazepine. Side effects include sedation and ataxia, and both are risk factors for falls. Other nonpharmacological strategies have been developed to assist with problematic behaviors such as wandering and "sundowning."

Psychoeducational Support

When compared with family care for other chronic illnesses of older persons, the progressive dementia of AD is more disruptive to family life, more likely to have negative mental health outcomes for family caregivers, and more of a deterrent to the patient living alone.[39] Research has shown that programs for family education and counseling can decrease the burden of caring and delay nursing home placement of the AD patient.[40]

Nursing Management

Patients with AD are generally managed in the home with the assistance of family, home services, and health care providers. Patient needs vary depending on the stage of disease and individual differences, but the AD trajectory is one of progressive decline to total loss of personality, cognitive function, and independence. Thus, symptoms and management problems vary over the course of the illness. For example, in the middle stage of AD, wandering is a common problem. The person may wander aimlessly within or outside the home or facility, becoming a danger to self. Low-cost, low-tech interventions, such as altering the physical environment so that doors are not readily visible, have had some success in limiting wandering. In addition, use of movement alarms has been helpful in alerting the staff to patients wandering into unsafe or unsupervised areas. Many nursing studies have contributed to better and safer ways of providing sensitive care to patients with AD.

Management of patients with AD is a collaborative multidisciplinary problem directed at providing care for patients with progressive dementia. With the number of patients diagnosed with AD rising, nurses will provide care for AD patients in a variety of facilities and community-based settings. Nurses employed in hospitals have contact with AD patients admitted for other problems such as a fractured hip related to a fall. Nurses based in clinics or community-based care will see patients in nursing homes, day care, and long-term care facilities. Although there is no specific treatment for AD, there are many palliative interventions available directed at maintaining function and independence for as long as possible to provide the highest quality of life possible. Common nursing diagnoses are based on manifestations of the progressing dementia and include:

- High Risk for Injury related to poor memory, judgment, and self-control
- Altered Thought Processes related to cognitive decline
- Self-Care and Self-Management Deficits related to losses of abilities for decision making, assuming responsibility for self, and independence
- Sleep Pattern Disturbance related to agitation and daytime sleeping
- Altered Communications related to cognitive decline
- Social Isolation related to withdrawal and inability to interact with others and the environment
- Caregiver Stress related to ongoing responsibility for the 24-hour care of a family member with progressive dementia
- Knowledge Deficit related to course of AD and management strategies for symptoms

It falls to the nurse to provide support for the patient and family and assist them to deal with the painful decisions that will need attention as the disease progresses. Patients with progressive dementia need to be approached with sensitivity to the ongoing losses incurred with the disease. In mild AD, patients are resourceful and learn to write lists and use other methods for reminders. As the disease progresses, health care providers and family caregivers gradually assume responsibility for structuring the environment and meeting basic and maintenance needs for the patient. Communication skills gradually decline, and the caregiver must learn to anticipate needs and interpret nonverbal cues. Sleep-pattern disturbance is particularly disruptive to other members of the family. Appropriate use of drugs, exercise during the day, and preventing daytime sleeping are helpful strategies in resetting circadian clocks. Agitation and aggressiveness make it difficult to manage the patient and increase the threat to safety for the patient and family members. When this occurs, it can become difficult to manage the patient at home. Again, drug therapy and structured activities are useful interventions to ameliorate these problems.

As the disease progresses, loss of social skills, withdrawal, and impulsive behavior further isolate the patient from interaction with others and the environment. At this stage, the patient will need close supervision, which limits the family's opportunities for social interaction. Finally, keeping the patient safe from injury to self and others is an ongoing concern. Because the patient often lacks insight and good judgment, high-risk situations are not recognized. For example, there will come a point in the illness when a patient should cease to drive. This is often viewed as a major unwelcome loss to independence that is protested by the patient. The health care provider can assist by assuming some responsibility and supporting the family's decision.

The patient and family need support and anticipatory education during the course of this devastating illness. Often, the nurse is called on to provide patient/family education and assist with symptom management issues. The nurse can:

- Encourage the patient to participate in ADLs, hobbies, and community activities for as long as possible to maintain independence
- Encourage the patient to take his or her medications as ordered and monitor for side effects
- Provide the patient and family with specific information about AD in both oral and written forms
- Help the family develop strategies to adequately monitor, supervise, and protect the patient from injury, humiliation, or becoming lost
- Help the family develop strategies to deal with the specific problems of patient management such as insomnia and wandering
- Make the patient and family aware of available community resources and support services, such as the Alzheimer's Disease Association and other support groups
- Encourage the patient and family to make decisions regarding financial matters, advanced directives, end-of-life care, and other matters while the patient still has decision-making abilities intact
- Encourage the patient and family to develop realistic short- and long-term plans

- Help the family understand caregiver stress and options for coping and minimizing stress
- Support the family in decision making regarding the need for institutionalization
- Make referrals to social services and community resources to assist the patient and family in planning for the future

The following are resources for patients and families (there are many resources available on the Internet):

Alzheimer's Association (there are chapters nationwide), 1-800-272-3900, *http://www.alz.org*
Alzheimer's Disease Education and Referral Center, 1-800-438-4380, *http://www.adear@alzheimers.org*

VASCULAR DEMENTIA

The second major form of dementia, vascular dementia, includes two general categories: multi-infarct dementia and diffuse white matter dementia (also called subcortical arteriosclerotic encephalopathy or Binswanger's disease). There is an ongoing disagreement about whether vascular dementia is a distinct disease entity or a complication of cardiovascular or cerebrovascular disease. Because experts also disagree on the basic diagnostic criteria, any discussion of vascular dementia as a disease entity is necessarily uncertain.

When multiple infarcts occur over a period of months or years, a special type of dementia, called *multi-infarct dementia,* may develop together with *focal* cerebral deficits. In some of these cases, the major lesions are found in the white matter, with relative sparing of the cerebral cortex and basal ganglia. This picture of multiple white matter infarcts and lacunae is called Binswanger's disease.[41]

Development of multi-infarct dementia is, in part, related to the amount of damaged cortex incurred over time. Hypertension, coronary artery disease, diabetes mellitus, and previous strokes are common concurrent findings. Clinically, the dementia has a more definite onset and progression pattern than AD. On physical examination, there are focal neurological deficits (i.e., hemiparesis, visual field cuts). An MRI reveals multiple areas of infarction, information that also differentiates multi-infarct dementia from AD. However, AD and multi-infarct dementia may occur concurrently in a patient.

In Binswanger's disease, the subcortical infarctions are found in the frontal lobes and include hypometabolism in the frontal and global cerebral areas.[21] Clinically, there is a slow onset and progression of dementia (unlike other forms of multi-infarct dementia). Symptoms begin with mild confusion, apathy, change in personality, and memory deficit. Later, judgment and self-care deficits are noted; euphoria and aggressive behavior are common.[21] Lateralizing signs are uncommon, but cerebellar signs such as ataxia and gait disorders are common. The patient is at high risk for falls. Urinary incontinence and dysarthria are seen in the advanced state.[42]

Vascular dementia is treated by addressing the underlying causes, such as hypertension, coronary artery disease, and diabetes mellitus. Reversal of lost cognitive function is not probable. Nursing management includes supportive management for a patient with dementia along with supporting adequate hypertension, coronary artery disease, and diabetes mellitus control. The supportive care addresses safety needs, especially risk of falls, meeting basic needs, and providing a structured, supervised environment.

PARKINSON'S DISEASE

Parkinson's disease is the second most common neurodegenerative disease after AD, affecting 2% of people over the age of 65 years.[31] Typically beginning in middle or late life, PD is more common in the 65 and older age group. Approximately 1 million people live with PD in the United States, and with current demographic trends, the number of cases of PD is expected to increase dramatically in the next three decades. Early-onset PD affecting persons as early as their 20s is being recognized with greater frequency. PD is a chronic, slow, progressive disorder caused by loss of dopaminergic neurons in the substantia nigra of the basal ganglia. The major signs and symptoms include tremors, rigidity, akinesia/bradykinesia, and postural deformity (thus the mnemonic *TRAP*). PD shortens life and causes significant disability and decreased quality of life.[43]

Neuroanatomy

Basal ganglia is a collective term for the subcortical motor nuclei of the cerebrum. The structures that compose the basal ganglia include the substantia nigra, striatum, globus pallidus, subthalamic nucleus, and red nucleus. Symptoms of PD are caused by loss of nerve cells in the pigmented substantia nigra pars compacta, including the locus ceruleus in the midbrain. Cell loss also occurs in the globus pallidus and putamen.[44] Depletion of the dopaminergic neurons (pars compacta) of the substantia nigra results in reduction of dopamine, the main biochemical abnormality in PD. Normally, the pars compacta neurons of the substantia nigra provide dopaminergic input to the striatum, a part of the basal ganglia. In PD, loss of pars compacta neurons leads to striatal dopamine depletion and reduced thalamic excitation of the motor cortex.[44]

Pathogenesis

The etiology of PD is unknown. PD is defined by the presence of Lewy bodies and nerve cell loss in the substantia nigra. In the laboratory, parkinsonism has been induced by exposing animals to 1-methyl-4-phenyl-1,2,3,6-tetrahydropyridine (MPTP), a potent neurotoxin that has been sometimes accidentally taken by heroin users. It is this connection that supports a hypothesis that exposures to pesticides and other toxins containing MPTP may be one cause of PD.

Both inherited and sporadic forms of PD have been identified. In both cases, Lewy bodies (eosinophilic intraneural inclusion granules) are widespread within neurons and occur especially in the substantia nigra of the basal ganglia. In PD, Lewy bodies contain α-synuclein. Mutations in the gene for α-synuclein have been found in patients with familial PD.[45] Much about the pathogenesis of PD remains unknown.

Signs and Symptoms

Because symptoms develop insidiously, diagnosis is often delayed, with symptoms often attributed to aging. The disease is progressive, so that eventually the patient's ability to perform ADLs and other independent functions is reduced. Some patients become confined to bed.

The signs and symptoms of PD include the following:

MAJOR MANIFESTATIONS
• **Tremors**
• **Rigidity of muscles**
• **Akinesia/bradykinesia**
• **Postural disturbance and loss of postural reflexes**

SECONDARY MANIFESTATIONS
• Difficulty with fine motor function such as writing and eating
• Soft monotone voice
• Masklike face
• General weakness and muscle fatigue
• Cognitive impairments/dementia
• Autonomic manifestations

Major Manifestations

Tremors. Tremors occur most often in the distal portions of extremities and especially in the hands. A so-called *pillrolling* motion of the fingers is characteristic. Other areas where tremors are seen include the foot, lip, tongue, and jaw. Tremors are present when the hand is motionless and thus are termed *resting tremors* (Fig. 31-2). Tremors are absent during sleep.

Rigidity of Muscles. Muscle rigidity is associated with slowness of voluntary movement (bradykinesia or akinesia). The

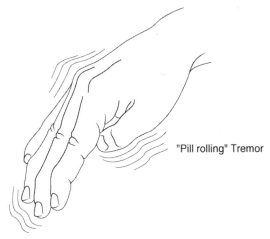

"Pill rolling" Tremor

Figure 31–2 • The tremor in Parkinson's disease is exaggerated by the resting posture, is often relieved by movement, and usually disappears during sleep. The movement of the thumb across the palm gives it a "pill-rolling" character.

muscle feels stiff and requires much effort to move. The patient appears to have difficulty in initiating movement. Because PD patients move minimally when sitting, edema can develop in the feet, legs, hands, and arms. **Cogwheel rigidity** is characterized by ratchet-like, rhythmic contractions, especially in the hand, on passive muscle stretching.

Akinesia/Bradykinesia. The patient has difficulty initiating a movement and then moves very slowly. As a result, difficulty in rising from a chair, getting into a car, and performing ADLs are common. Slow or absent movement renders the patient at high risk for pneumonia, deep vein thrombosis, constipation, and pressure ulcers.

Postural Disturbance, Loss of Postural Reflexes. Patients walk in a stooped-over position with small, shuffling steps and a broad base on turns. The forearms are semiflexed, and the fingers are flexed at the metacarpophalangeal joints. The characteristic appearance and posture of the patient with PD are illustrated in Figure 31-3. After movement is initiated, it frequently accelerates almost to a trot. The patient may fall forward (propulsion) or backward (retropulsion). If pushed, he or she makes no attempt to brace himself or herself or to reach out and stop. As a result, the patient is at high risk for injury. Patients have difficulty in maintaining balance and sitting erect.

Secondary Manifestations

Fine Motor Deficits. Difficulty with fine motor control is seen early in the disease. Handwriting becomes progressively smaller and more difficult to read. Clumsiness and difficulty with ADLs, such as buttoning clothing, is evident.

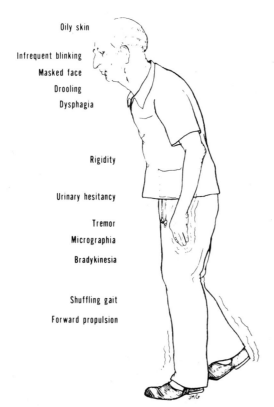

Oily skin
Infrequent blinking
Masked face
Drooling
Dysphagia

Rigidity

Urinary hesitancy

Tremor
Micrographia
Bradykinesia

Shuffling gait
Forward propulsion

Figure 31–3 • The clinical features of Parkinson's disease.

Monotonic Voice. The voice gradually becomes soft to whisper-like, monotonic, and muffled. These changes result in impaired verbal communications.

Masklike Face. The face is expressionless and the eyes stare straight ahead; blinking is less frequent than normal–5 to 10 times per minute rather than the normal 15 to 20 times.

General Weakness and Muscle Fatigue. Initiation of purposeful movement is slow. During movement, the patient may become momentarily frozen. Fatigue is a common complaint, especially when ADLs are attempted. Muscle cramps of the legs, neck, and trunk are common.

Cognitive Changes/Dementia and Psychiatric Symptoms. Cognitive impairments to visuospatial function, executive functions, and memory are common in many patients over the course of the illness. The dementia of PD accounts for 20% to 30% of cases of dementia among persons over the age of 60, and affects 20% to 45% of persons with PD.[46,47] Depression (very common) is seen in over 50% of persons with PD and may even occur before classic symptoms of PD are noted. Hallucinations, delusion, anxiety and apathy are also seen.

Other Common Manifestations. Additional signs and symptoms, many associated with autonomic dysfunction, include the following:

- Drooling: secondary to decreased frequency of swallowing. When the patient awakens, the pillow is wet.
- Seborrhea (oily, greasy skin): probably attributable to hypothalamic dysfunction, which causes release of an increased amount of sebotropic hormone.
- Dysphagia: secondary to the neuromuscular incoordination of the hypopharyngeal musculature. This problem can interfere with normal fluid and dietary intake.
- Excessive perspiration: probably the result of a disorder of the hypothalamic heat regulator mechanism, as well as impairment of perspiration controls. The patient may be diaphoretic even in cold weather and may have a fever in warm weather.
- Constipation: secondary to hypomotility of the gastrointestinal tract and associated with prolonged gastric emptying time. Decreased fluid intake, lack of roughage, and decreased activity contribute to the development of constipation.
- Orthostatic hypotension: probably the result of peripheral autonomic failure noted in parkinsonism. It is also a side effect of levodopa therapy.
- Urinary hesitation and frequency: secondary to autonomic dysfunction. A catheter is rarely necessary.

Scales developed to rate the severity of signs and symptoms of PD objectively are useful clinically and in drug trials for staging the disease and for monitoring deterioration. The categorical, nonlinear scale described by Hoehn and Yahr is frequently used to characterize the severity of illness (Table 31-4).[48] The United Parkinson's Disease Rating Scale (UPDRS) is a sensitive and reliable scale for monitoring response to treatment in drug trials. It has four subscales: cognitive, ADLs, motor examination, and complications of treatment. Items include speech, salivation, swallowing, handwriting, cutting of food and handling utensils, dressing, hygiene, turning in bed, falling, freezing, walking, tremor, and sen-

Table 31-4 • HOEHN AND YAHR SCALE FOR PARKINSON'S DISEASE

STAGE OF DISEASE	DESCRIPTION
Stage I	Unilateral disease
Stage II	Bilateral disease with preservation of postural reflexes
Stage III	Bilateral disease with impaired postural reflexes but preserved ability to ambulate independently
Stage IV	Severe disease requiring considerable assistance
Stage V	End-stage disease, confined to bed or chair

Hoehn, M. M., & Yahr, M. D. (1967). Parkinsonism: Onset, progression, and mortality. *Neurology, 17,* 427–442.

sory symptoms. Each item is scored on a scale from 0 to 4 (0 = normal to 4 = most severe).[49] The scores on the subscales are added to yield a total score (higher scores indicate a higher degree of disability). The scale has good inter-rater reliability. These scales are helpful in clinical practice. In addition, other standardized scales, such as the depression scales previously mentioned, are helpful for assessing and monitoring other symptoms common in PD.

Diagnosis

No diagnostic test is currently available to confirm the diagnosis of PD.[50] MRI imaging is usually normal. SPECT imaging has demonstrated promise in supporting the diagnosis of PD, but it is not commonly used at this time. EEG is not helpful. The diagnosis of PD is made based on history and clinical findings.

Medical Management

Patients with PD require two types of management: symptomatic therapies and preventive or protective therapies. Symptomatic therapies are directed toward ameliorating the symptoms of PD but do not affect the progression of the disease. They include both nonpharmacological and pharmacological interventions. Protective therapies are directed at halting or slowing the course of the PD. Drug therapy plays an important role in both categories of PD management. Several drug groups are present in the symptomatic drug category. It was believed that one drug, selegiline, was the first neuroprotective drug that slowed the course of PD. However, prospective long-term studies (3 years) found no difference between selegiline and placebo.[51,52] Therefore, there is no compelling evidence to support selegiline as a neuroprotective agent.[53,54]

Symptomatic Supportive Approach

Symptomatic, nonpharmacological, supportive therapy is directed toward managing symptoms that are common in PD, such as constipation, perspiration, and urinary dysfunction. Advising on adjustments of lifestyle and preventing complications and injuries are also important. Speech ther-

apy may be recommended for some patients. A comprehensive physiotherapy program that may include gait training, balance maintenance, and exercise can be most helpful in keeping the patient functional. Patient and family education is an integral part of management.

Most patients can be managed at home. Whether home health care or community services are needed depends on the disability associated with the illness and the availability of family assistance. An effective drug program often allows the individual to maintain a near-normal lifestyle. In the advanced stages, management in a nursing home may be necessary if adequate arrangements cannot be made at home. Admission to an acute care facility is necessary only for special problems such as surgery or treatment of complications. Individuals with PD are at high risk for injury because of incoordination, loss of postural reflexes, and rigidity. Injuries, such as a fractured hip, head injury, or spinal fracture, can result from a fall.

Symptomatic Pharmacological Treatment

Although PD cannot be cured or arrested, symptoms can often be controlled with drug therapy. Consideration must be given to timing of drug introduction, selecting the right drug, monitoring and managing side effects, and adjusting the drug schedule for optimal results. The patient and family must be educated about the drugs used, side effects, and precautions to be observed while taking the drugs.

There are five drug classes used in the management of PD: *anticholinergics, antivirals, L-dihydroxyphenylalanine (levodopa), dopamine agonists,* and *monamine oxidase B inhibitors.* These drugs are summarized in Table 31-5. A few additional comments are provided to expand the understanding of drug management.

Once the diagnosis of PD has been made, the severity of symptoms must be assessed and an appropriate management plan developed with the age, lifestyle, and degree of disability kept in mind. The patient and family need to be involved in decision making and educated about the disease and the drugs used. Selegiline is usually begun because it may slow the progress of PD and postpone the need for levodopa. An important decision is when to begin levodopa therapy, especially in younger patients. Although levodopa is the mainstay of drug treatment for PD, it has many side effects and a limited time span for effectiveness. This drug is begun in the moderately symptomatic patient. Although most patients deserve a trial on the drug, those with severe cerebral or cardiovascular disease, psychosis, or severe medical problems need to be carefully evaluated.

Long-term use of levodopa can result in toxicity and unpredictable responses to other drug therapy. The signs and symptoms are listed in Table 31-5. The "on-off" phenomenon, a side effect, is described as a fluctuation in motor function from being ambulatory and active one moment ("on" phase) to being unable to rise from a chair ("off" phase), all within a few minutes.

Patient Teaching for Levodopa. The patient should be made aware of the following limits when taking levodopa:

- Pyridoxine (vitamin B$_6$) is a cofactor of the enzyme dopa decarboxylase. It increases the decarboxylation of levo-

▮▮ Table 31–5 • DRUGS USED IN THE MANAGEMENT OF PARKINSON'S DISEASE (PD)

DRUGS	USUAL DOSE (IN MG) (START WITH LOWER DOSES AND TITRATE TO USUAL DOSE RANGE)	PURPOSE	ACTION	SIDE EFFECTS
Class: Anticholinergics—Helpful in Relieving Tremor in Mild-to-Moderate Disease				
• Benztropine (Cogentin) • Biperiden (Akineton) • Orphenadrine (Disipal) • Procyclidine (Kemadrin) • Trihexyphenidyl (Artane)	• 0.5–2 tid • 1–3 qid • 100 tid • 2.5–10 tid • 2–5 tid	Tremors and rigidity; have little effect on bradykinesia	Muscarinic receptor blockers that penetrate the central nervous system (CNS) and antagonize transmission of acetylcholine by striatal interneurons	Dry mouth, constipation, urinary retention, blurred vision, impaired memory, concentration, hallucinations, and confusion
Class: Antiviral				
Amantadine (Symmetrel)	100 bid or tid	Transient effect on akinesia, rigidity, and tremors	Promotes synthesis and release of dopamine; often taken with carbidopa	Edema of legs; can cause psychiatric problems similar to those related to anticholinergic drugs
Class: Carbidopa/Levodopa—Given in Combination as Sinemet Because Carbidopa is Peripheral Decarboxylase Inhibitor. It Overcomes Peripheral Dopamine Receptor Stimulation and Decreases Nausea, Vomiting, and Orthostatic Hypotension.				
Sinemet, regular and controlled release (CR) Immediate-release • 10-mg carbidopa/ 100 mg L-dopa • 25-mg carbidopa/ 100 mg L-dopa • 25-mg carbidopa/ 250 mg L-dopa CR • 25-mg carbidopa/ 100 mg L-dopa • 50-mg carbidopa/ 200 mg L-dopa	• Usual starting dose is 10/100 tid; increased gradually to 25/250 tid or qid	• Most effective symptomatic therapy for PD but has limitations and produces complications with long-term use • Rigidity and bradykinesia	• Immediate natural precursor of dopamine, which is converted to dopamine by the amino acid decarboxylase; diminished response to drug in advanced stages of PD	Nausea/vomiting, orthostatic hypotension, dry mouth, constipation, dizziness, cough, cardiac arrhythmias, sleep disturbance, and "on-off" phenomenon; hallucinations or confusion
Class: Dopamine Receptor Antagonists—Ameliorate Symptoms by Acting Directly on Dopamine Receptors, Thus Mimicking Endogenous Dopamine. They Can Be Classified As Ergot Derivatives (e.g., Bromocriptine, Pergolide) or Nonergolines (e.g., Pramipexole, Ropinirole).				
• Bromocriptine (Parlodel, analog of dopamine) • Pergolide (Permax) • Pramipexole (Mirapex) • Ropinirole (ReQuip)	• 15–30 mg divided bid or tid • 1.5–3 mg divided bid or tid • 0.5–1.5 mg tid • 3–5 mg tid	• Decreases fluctuation in motor response to L-dopa • Often initial treatment for PD; L-dopa introduced later so that development side effects of L-dopa postponed	• There are three dopamine receptors (D1–D3); various drugs within this group act at different sites • Directly simulates dopamine receptors • Most effective agonists stimulate D2 receptors	Postural hypotension, dizziness, syncope, restlessness, insomnia, hallucinations. Nausea, constipation, urinary frequency
Class: Monoamine-Oxidase B Inhibitor				
• Selegiline (Eldepryl)	5 mg with breakfast and 5 mg with lunch	• Given in early stages to delay need for L-dopa • Increased response to L-dopa	Blocks metabolism of central dopamine; *delays need for L-dopa therapy*	Malaise, dizziness, increased tremors, nausea, restlessness, increased bradykinesia, arrhythmias, orthostatic hypotension

dopa in the liver, thereby decreasing the amount available to be converted to dopamine in the brain. Therefore, patients on levodopa therapy should not take vitamin B_6 or multivitamin preparations that include vitamin B_6.

- Alcohol consumption may antagonize the effects of levodopa and should be avoided.
- High-protein meals block the effect of levodopa when given alone or in combination.[55] Therefore, intake of the following foods should be controlled: milk, meat, fish, poultry, cheese, eggs, peanuts, nuts, sunflower seeds, whole grains, and soybean products.
- Although levodopa is best absorbed on an empty stomach, it may cause nausea; therefore it should be taken with some food to decrease the side effect of nausea.
- Dryness of the mouth can be combated by chewing gum or sucking on hard candy.
- Wearing elastic stockings will help to avoid orthostatic hypotension. Changing positions slowly is also helpful.
- Depression is common and may develop into severe depression with suicidal overtones. The physician should be advised if the patient seems depressed.

Dopa Decarboxylase Inhibitors. One might wonder why dopamine is not given rather than its precursor, levodopa. If dopamine were given orally, it would be metabolized before reaching the brain. Levodopa, however, is able to cross the blood-brain barrier and, once there, become converted into dopamine. For this chemical reaction to take place, the enzyme dopa decarboxylase must be present. In its presence, levodopa converts to dopamine and carbon dioxide, both in peripheral tissue and in the brain.

For the symptoms of PD to be controlled, levodopa must be converted to dopamine within the brain. If the reaction occurs in peripheral tissue, side effects of nausea and other symptoms occur. Inhibitors are given to prevent the conversion of levodopa to dopamine in peripheral tissue. The inhibitors selected to block the dopa decarboxylase enzyme do not cross the blood-brain barrier and thus allow dopamine production in the brain. By using levodopa in combination with dopa decarboxylase inhibitors, the dosage of levodopa can be reduced and side effects can be eliminated or greatly diminished. The inhibitor most often used is carbidopa (Sinemet). When given in combination, the dosage often used is carbidopa, 10 to 25 mg, and levodopa, 100 to 250 mg, three or four times daily.

Anticholinergic Drugs. Anticholinergic drugs are used in conjunction with levodopa or singularly if the patient cannot tolerate levodopa or if symptoms are mild. The drugs most often used are trihexyphenidyl hydrochloride (Artane) (2 to 5 mg three or four times daily) and benztropine mesylate (Cogentin) (0.5 to 6.0 mg daily).

Summary of Drug Therapy. The drugs currently available provide only symptom relief. Protective drugs that alter the underlying progressive disease are still to be developed. In the early stages of PD, when only mild resting tremors are present, anticholinergic drugs are helpful for about 6 to 18 months. As the disease progresses, the patient will need drugs that provide dopaminergic stimulation. Levodopa is the mainstay of drug therapy. The addition of peripheral

dopa decarboxylase inhibitors has helped to control its many side effects (e.g., anorexia, nausea, vomiting). Sinemet combines levodopa and carbidopa in one medication. Treatment of drug toxicity and unresponsiveness to drugs is problematic. Drug therapy may be changed or dosages altered. So-called "drug holidays" of a few days have been suggested, with hospital supervision. The effect of such an approach may improve clinical function, which lasts weeks to months.

Surgery

Surgical treatment of PD has a role for patients with long-standing severe disease who have developed complications to pharmacological therapy (e.g., fluctuations or "on-off" phenomena) and for those who have inadequate symptom control from drug therapy.[56] Ablative procedures and implanted electrical stimulators are options.

Thalamus. A thalamotomy (lesion placed in ventral intermediate nucleus of the thalamus) has been helpful in relieving tremors associated with PD, but it neither relieves other symptoms nor halts disease progression. It is, therefore, not generally used. High-frequency thalamic stimulation using an implanted electrode and pulse generator has gained favor for control of tremors by targeting the ventral intermediate nucleus of the thalamus. A pulse generator is placed in the subcutaneous infraclavicular area and connected to an implanted electrode, which has four contacts that can be programmed in a few ways. An external programming device is used to adjust the stimulus parameters and to turn the stimulator on or off. Complications associated with the technology include paresthesias, ataxia, intracerebral hemorrhage, seizures, and confusion.[56] In addition, infection and technology malfunction are possible. Although helpful for tremors, this option does not provide relief of bradykinesia, an equally disabling problem.

Globus Pallidus. For the patient with severe, intractable tremors, rigidity, or bradykinesia, a *pallidotomy* using stereotactic surgery may be helpful for relief of *all* symptoms for *selected* patients. In this procedure, part of the globus pallidus of the basal ganglia is destroyed using an electrical stimulator. Each side of the brain must be operated on separately. If symptoms are bilateral, an interval of approximately 6 months must elapse before a stereotactic procedure on the other side is considered. At the time of pallidotomy, mapping of the area is also conducted. Mapping consists of identification of optic tracts, sensory and motor tracts, and white matter so that these areas will not be injured during the procedure. Follow-up studies document improved control of the symptoms, although the procedure is not a cure for the underlying disease.

High-frequency stimulations of the globus pallidus internus and the subthalamic nucleus are currently being investigated.[57–59]

Other Potential Treatments. Interest in transplantation of fetal adrenal medulla into the caudate nucleus to decrease the debilitating effects of PD waxes and wanes. The controversy about the ethical implications regarding the use of tissue from aborted fetuses continues. The most recent controversy focuses on use of stem cells. It is unclear how these clashes will be resolved.

Nursing Management

People with PD are usually managed in the community or in long-term facilities. Placement in a long-term care facility may be necessary for end-stage disease when confinement to bed is necessary or dementia makes home management impossible. Nurses provide direct care, support, education, and monitoring of patients over the course of illness, with the goal of helping the patient stay independent for as long as possible. Drug therapy and effective methods of dealing with the symptoms of PD can prolong independence. However, the complications of supportive drug therapy are many and the responses to drugs vary over the course of the illness.

During the long course of the illness, patients need assistance from multidisciplinary professionals to manage symptoms and treatment complications related to PD. Therefore, a collaborative interdisciplinary model of care provides the best outcomes and quality of life for the patient.[60] The nurse is an important member of the team and may be the contact person for the patient and family. Their concerns can often be addressed by the nurse, but there may also be need for referral to other members of the health team.

The following are major nursing diagnoses related to the care of patients with PD:

- Impaired Physical Mobility related to rigidity, bradykinesia, and weakness
- High Risk for Injury from falls related to rigidity, bradykinesia, and weakness
- Impaired Communications related to change in voice (monotone, soft) and difficulty with writing
- Body Image Disturbance related to signs and symptoms of the illness
- Cognitive Deficits related to impaired memory and executive functions secondary to dementia
- Knowledge Deficit related to the disease process and treatment (especially drug therapy)

As the disease progresses, impairment of *physical mobility* is gradual, making it difficult or impossible for the patient to be independent in ADLs and other home and work environment activities. Keeping the patient active and functional for as long as possible is helpful. Physical therapy can recommend an exercise program, and occupational therapy can identify assistive devices that can be used to assist with the accomplishment of tasks. Use of a walker, cane, or other ambulatory assistive device can promote safe ambulation. Integral in working with the patient and family is the concern for injury. As the rigidity, bradykinesia, weakness, and loss of postural reflexes develop, the *risk of falls* in particular is high.[61] A number of nursing interventions can assist in keeping the patient safe. Because most patients live at home, the awareness of the patient and family of risk factors in the home must be heightened.

Both *verbal and written communications* become impaired as the disease progresses. A consultation with a speech therapist can provide strategies to maintain function for as long

as possible. Bradykinesia, a masklike face, drooling, lack of eye blinking, and other symptoms can cause a *body image disturbance*. The patient may withdraw from social interactions and activities that would bring him or her in contact with other people. The change in body image should be explored with the patient. Patients need to be encouraged to interact with others.

Dementia, cognitive deficits, depression, and psychiatric manifestations such as hallucinations are commonly seen with PD. The nurse needs to monitor for evidence of these problems. Depression, for example, can be treated with drug therapy if it is recognized. Discussion with the family may also suggest behavioral or cognitive deficits that can benefit from treatment.

Patient and family education is key to management. The teaching needs of the patient will depend on the stage of the illness and the symptoms at that time. The following are general considerations that should be addressed by the teaching plan:

- Provide a clear explanation of PD and what to expect.
- Give an explanation of the drugs being used, including side effects, toxicity, and precautions (see earlier discussion of patient teaching precautions for levodopa).
- Discuss the high risk for injury (e.g., falls, spilling hot liquids).
- Help the patient and family evaluate the home environment for potential dangers (e.g., scatter rugs, poor lighting, need for hand rails in the bathroom).
- Advise the patient to maintain a weight chart. Weight loss can occur as a result of inadequate nutrition secondary to nausea, vomiting, and dysphagia. Dietary alterations for dysphagia should include soft, ground-up foods and small feedings with limitation of protein.
- Constipation can be managed with the use of stool softeners.
- Urinary problems should be evaluated carefully. Incontinence may be caused by an inability to get to the bathroom fast enough; suggest use of a bedside urinal at night.
- Orthostatic hypotension can be helped by wearing elastic stockings and changing position slowly.
- A bedridden person should change position every 2 hours to prevent skin breakdown, contractures, and pulmonary complications. Deep breathing should be encouraged to avoid lung congestion and pneumonia.
- Range-of-motion exercises prevent stiffness and contractures and are encouraged three to four times daily.
- Speech can be improved by reading aloud, singing, and raising the voice. (Consult with a speech therapist, as necessary.)
- Intolerance to heat is common; temperature control is needed for comfort.
- Using a wide-based (12 to 15 inches) stance improves balance and walking.
- Make the patient and family aware of community resources for PD that can provide educational material, referrals, and community activities such as exercise programs for PD patients. There are often support groups for patients and family members available locally. The following are recognized organizations that are good resources:

- National Parkinson Foundation, Inc., (800) 327-4545, http://www.parkinson.org
- American Parkinson Disease Association, (800) 223-2732, http://www.apdaparkinson.com
- The Parkinson's Disease Foundation, (800) 457-6676, http://www.pdf.org

MULTIPLE SCLEROSIS

Multiple sclerosis (MS) or disseminated sclerosis is characterized by chronic inflammation, demyelination, and scarring (gliosis) of the myelin sheath of the CNS. The manifestations of the disease vary from a benign disease to a rapidly progressive and disabling illness that has a profound effect on physical function and quality of life. The classification of MS is based on its variable clinical courses (Table 31-6). The etiology of MS is unknown, although it is hypothesized that a virus may precipitate an autoimmune response in a genetically susceptible individual. MS has been called the disease of young adults because the highest rate of incidence is between the ages of 20 and 40 years, followed by a gradual decline. The age at onset in men is slightly older than in women.[62]

There are approximately 250,000 to 350,000 cases of MS in the United States,[63] with women being affected about twice as frequently as men. Whites are affected more frequently than any other racial group. Epidemiological studies report that MS is more prevalent in the colder northern latitudes, such as the northern Atlantic states, the Great Lakes region, and the Pacific Northwest, than in southern parts of the United States. In Europe, high-incidence areas include Scandinavia, northern Germany, and Great Britain. Moving to a warmer climate after diagnosis does not arrest the disease.

Pathogenesis and Pathophysiology

The pathological hallmark of chronic MS is the demyelinated lesions or plaques, which are sharply demarcated areas easily distinguishable from surrounding white matter.[64] The composition of a lesion varies depending on its age. In an acute lesion, there is partial or complete damage to the myelin, called *vesicular demyelination*. The damage consists of a breakdown of the myelin sheath that surrounds axon cylinders. As the lesion evolves, there is a proliferation of astrocytes and oligodendrocytes (myelin-producing cells), although many oligodendrocytes are destroyed by the cellular infiltrates of T cells and macrophages. The surviving oligodendrocytes may partially remyelinate affected areas. Long-standing lesions are composed of thick, matted, relatively acellular fibroglia tissue. The axon cylinders of the nerves are relatively spared, preventing wallerian degeneration. Lesions have an affinity for the optic nerves, periventricular white matter, brain stem, cerebellum, and spinal cord white matter. The plaques vary in diameter from 1 to 2 mm to several centimeters.[62,65]

MS affects primarily the white matter of the brain and spinal cord by causing scattered, demyelinated lesions, preventing conduction of normal nerve impulse through the demyelinated zone. Demyelination may have either negative or positive effects on axonal conduction.[62] *Negative conduction abnormalities* are slowed axonal conduction or a complete block in conduction. A conduction block may also occur in response to metabolic derangements or a rise in body temperature. *Positive conduction abnormalities* include generation of ectopic impulses and abnormal "crosstalk" between demyelinated axons. These variations in conduction help to explain the variations in symptoms that occur with MS throughout a day or a week and in relationship to activity (fever and exercise may exacerbate symptoms).[62]

Remission or improvement of symptoms may occur with MS as the result of healing or in response to the conclusion of an acute inflammatory event. Eventually, the axis cylinder of the neuron may become affected, so that disabilities increase and become permanent. At autopsy, multiple sclerotic plaques are scattered throughout the white matter of the brain and cord. The scattering differs from patient to patient, accounting for the variety of presenting symptoms experienced by patients. Some cases of MS are clinically silent, and the presence of the disease process is identified incidentally at autopsy.

Signs and Symptoms

The signs and symptoms of MS vary greatly from patient to patient and can vary over time in the same patient. The most common initial symptoms are: sensory loss (37%), optic

Table 31-6 • FOUR CATEGORIES OF MULTIPLE SCLEROSIS (MS) BASED ON CLINICAL COURSE

TYPE	DESCRIPTION
Relapsing-remitting MS (RRMS) (80% of all cases)	Characterized by recurrent attacks of neurological dysfunction that evolve over days to weeks and may be followed by complete, partial, or no recovery; there is no progression of symptoms between attacks; this pattern is often seen in the early course of the disease and is the most common form seen
Secondary progressive MS	Gradual neurological deterioration with or without acute relapses, minor remissions, and plateaus in a patient who previously had RRMS
Progressive-relapsing MS	From the onset, there is gradual progression of disability; unlike relapsing-remitting MS, there is continuing disease progression without stabilization of the disease
Primary progressive MS	A pattern of gradual neurological deterioration from the onset of symptoms, but with superimposed relapses noted

neuritis (36%), weakness (35%), paresthesias (24%), diplopia (15%), ataxia (11%), and vertigo (6%).[66] There are other sundry symptoms, mentioned below, that occur in 1% to 4% of patients. The multiple signs and symptoms of MS may include the following:

- Sensory symptoms: numbness or sensory loss; paresthesia (burning, prickling, tingling); pain; decreased proprioception and perception of temperature, depth, and vibration
- Motor symptoms: paresis, paralysis, dragging of foot; spasticity; diplopia; bladder and bowel dysfunction (incontinence or retention)
- Cerebellar symptoms: ataxia; loss of balance and coordination; nystagmus; speech disturbances (dysarthria, dystonia, scanning speech, slurred speech); tremors (intentional tremors, described as tremors that increase when a purposeful act is initiated); vertigo
- Other symptoms: fatigue; optic neuritis; impotence or decreased genital sensation and sexual dysfunction; neurobehavioral disorders such as depression or euphoria. Fewer than 4% of patients experience paroxysmal attacks, visual loss, trigeminal neuralgia, facial palsy, and impotence.

Sensory Symptoms

Sensory loss and tingling on the face or involved extremities are common. Loss of proprioception and joint sensation is frequently accompanied by edema of the limb or feelings of constriction. Fifty percent of patients develop objective sensory loss (position, vibration, shape, texture). Pain is uncommon except with flexor spasms of the limbs. **Lhermitte's sign** is described as an electric or shocklike sensation that extends down the arms, back, or lower trunk bilaterally upon flexion of the neck. The sensation probably results from the buckling effect on the dorsal roots of the posterior columns from sclerotic plaques. (Unilateral Lhermitte's sign has been noted in such conditions as cervical spondylosis and narrowing of the cervical spinal canal.)

Motor Symptoms

Motor symptoms often begin with weakness in the lower extremities and complaint of a feeling of heaviness or uselessness of the involved limb. Although complaints initially center on one limb, both limbs are usually involved to varying degrees. Spasticity, with its usual concurrent hyperreflexia, is common. Presence of spasticity often interferes with ambulation and ADLs.

The decline in motor function may last from minutes to hours and is, therefore, not always observed by the physician. Motor function can worsen spontaneously after strenuous exercise, fever, or a hot shower or hot tub bath. This response is called **Uhthoff's sign**.

Incoordination is another frequent symptom. Intentional tremors are noted in the upper extremities. An **intentional tremor** is defined as a tremor occurring when a voluntary act is initiated. The finer the required movement, the greater the tremor will be. In the lower extremities, the incoordination appears as ataxia. Head tremors are not evident until the terminal stages, when the cerebellum is involved. Spastic weakness or ataxia of the

muscles of speech is responsible for the dysarthria common in MS. Speech, in the early stages, is often slurred. Later, it becomes explosive or staccato and unintelligible. **Scanning speech**—slow and measured with pauses between syllables—is seen sometimes with late-stage bulbar involvement if cerebellar ataxia is prominent.

Ocular, Vestibular, and Auditory Symptoms

Optic neuritis, a common early symptom, is evidenced by visual clouding, visual field (often central) deficits, and pain with eye movement; pallor of the optic discs is noted. Diplopia and nystagmus are common. Internuclear ophthalmoplegia of lateral gaze, when noted, strongly suggests MS. The Marcus Gunn phenomenon, related to reduced light perception in the affected eye, is seen with retrobulbar neuritis. Vertigo is a common early symptom usually noted as a mild instability. Vomiting and nystagmus can accompany the vertigo. Deafness is a rare finding.

Paroxysmal Symptoms

Paroxysmal symptoms, which are less common but can occur in MS, include focal or generalized epilepsy, tonic seizures, trigeminal neuralgia, and occasionally, paroxysmal spasms (tetanus-like spasms). The spasms are described as contractions of the hands or feet into a dystonic, sustained, abnormal position and can be very painful.

Neurobehavioral Disorders

Neurobehavioral disorders associated with MS include emotional lability, irritability, apathy, inattentiveness, poor judgment, euphoria, dementia, and cognitive impairment. Depression is very common, occurring in 30% to 50% of patients. Less common are extreme anxiety, bipolar disease, and psychosis.

Other Symptoms

Fatigue is a very common symptom in MS and can range from mild to severely disabling. The basis for fatigue is unknown. Bladder and bowel dysfunction and impotence are common. Bladder retention or reflex emptying is often seen in later stages of MS.

Course of the Illness

The course of MS is varied and unpredictable, as outlined earlier. Symptom clusters have been noted when a particular area of the brain is involved. For example, **Charcot's triad**, which includes nystagmus, intentional tremors, and staccato speech, occurs with brain-stem involvement. Events that may precipitate relapses are menstruation; emotional stress; cold or humid, hot weather; hot baths; overheating; fever; and fatigue. Many relapses last a few days to a few weeks, after which there is complete or incomplete reversal of symptoms. Deficits present after 3 months are usually permanent. Prediction of when the next episode will occur is impossible. Some patients may experience another attack in a few weeks, whereas others may be spared for many years.

Diagnosis

There is no definitive diagnostic test for MS. The neurological history and examination are the cornerstones for diagnosis. There are, however, diagnostic criteria for MS, as well as radiological and laboratory studies to assist in making the diagnosis.

Diagnostic Criteria

The Schumacher Committee on Diagnostic Criteria for MS outlined six clinical characteristics required to diagnose MS, which include:[67]

- Neurological examination that reveals objective abnormalities attributable to the CNS
- Involvement of white matter structures
- Two or more sites of CNS involvement
- Relapsing-remitting or chronic (more than 6 months) progressive course each lasting 24 hours and at least 1 month apart, *or* a gradual or stepwise progression over at least 6 months
- Age at onset of 10 to 50 years
- No better explanation of symptoms

The criteria have been expanded to include data derived from analysis of CSF, evoked potentials, and MRI.

MRI and Evoked Potentials

Wide availability of MRI, a sensitive diagnostic test, has greatly improved the ability to make an accurate diagnosis of MS. Multiple hyperintense lesions, which are best seen on the T2-weighted images, demonstrate multiple foci (Fig. 31-4). A criterion has been established to diagnose MS for people older than 50 years of age and younger than 50 years of age that is based on the size, number, and location of lesions seen on T2-weighted MRI. In MS, evoked potentials demonstrate slow or abnormal

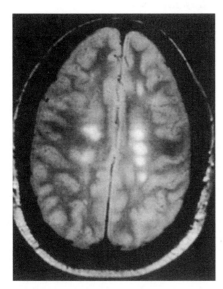

Figure 31–4 • Axial T2-weighted image shows ovoid hyperintense lesions in both hemispheres.

conduction patterns on visual, auditory, somatosensory, or motor pathways.

Laboratory Studies

Laboratory tests may help to establish the diagnosis of MS. Three CSF abnormalities may be noted: mononuclear cell pleocytosis, an elevation in the total Ig, and presence of oligoclonal immunoglobulin. The *mononuclear cell pleocytosis* is usually less than 50 cells/mm³. In rapid progressive MS, the level may reach 100 cells/mm³. The proportion of gamma globulin (mostly immunoglobulin G [IgG]) is increased to values greater than 12% of total protein in about two thirds of patients. The *IgG synthesis rate* represents a calculation of the level of IgG within the intrathecal space. It is increased to more than 3 mg/day in 80% to 90% of MS patients. This rate is a reflection of MRI plaque burden. The *IgG index* indicates the proportion of IgG in the intrathecal space. It is increased to a value greater than 0.7 in 86% to 94% of MS patients.[68]

Oligoclonal bands are discrete electrophoretic bands that are frequently found in the CSF of almost all (90% to 97%) of MS patients. The bands of MS are found only in the CSF when concurrent CSF and serum samples are evaluated simultaneously, and differ from the pattern seen in other inflammatory neuropathies, neoplasms, and systemic immune responses.

Treatment

In the last few years, development in drug therapy options for MS patients has been significant, and research continues on other possible avenues of treatment. The Kurtzke Expanded Disability Status Score, the most widely accepted measure of neurological impairment in MS,[69] is used to compare the clinical effect of current and proposed drugs for treatment of MS. There are two categories of treatment for MS: treatment to arrest the disease process and treatment for symptom management.

Treatment to Arrest the Disease Process

In the United States, three FDA-approved drugs, called the ABCs, are used to modify or arrest the MS disease process for relapsing-remitting MS (RRMS): interferon beta-1a (Avonex), interferon beta-1b (Betaseron), and glatiramer acetate (Copaxone). Ninety percent of MS patients receive one of the interferons as first-line therapy; the other 10% receive glatiramer acetate.[62] Through incompletely understood immune-mediated activities, all three drugs reduce the rate of clinical relapse and the development of new lesions seen on MRI.[64] Table 31-7 summarizes drug therapy options. The cost for any one of these drugs is approximately $10,000/year based on 1999 estimates.[70] Cost is an important consideration in treatment decisions.

Because there are no data on either long-term efficacy and safety or comparative effectiveness, the drugs are considered clinically comparable at this time. Each of these drugs is also used for patients with secondary pro-

▓▓▓▓ **Table 31–7** • DRUG TREATMENT OPTIONS FOR MULTIPLE SCLEROSIS*

DRUG	DOSE	SIDE EFFECTS
For Relapsing-Remitting Multiple Sclerosis (RRMS): Reduces Rate of Clinical Relapse; Reduces the Development of New Lesions on MRI		
Interferon beta-1b (Betaseron) FDA approved in 1993	8 million IU SC qid	Flulike symptoms following injection, which lessen over time for many patients; injection site reactions, of which 5% need treatment; rarer findings: elevated liver enzymes, low white blood count; can cause abortion in pregnant woman
Interferon beta-1a (Avonex) FDA approved in 1996	30 μg IM q/wk	Flulike symptoms of muscle ache, fever, and chills; pain, weakness; rarely, mild anemia, elevated liver enzymes
Glatiramer acetate (Copaxone) FDA approved in 1996	20 μg SC q/d	Injection-site reaction; rarer, an immediate postinjection reaction of anxiety, chest tightness, shortness of breath, and flushing that last 15–30 m
High-dose interferon beta-1a (Rebif) Not FDA approved; available in Canada and Europe	Possible dose-related benefit in patients with more severe disabilities	Injection site reactions and flulike symptoms most common adverse effects; elevated liver enzymes
For Secondary Progressive MS (SPMS): Same as for RRMS but Also Delays Progression of Disability		
Interferon beta-1b (Betaseron)	8 million IU SC qid	As above
Mitoxantrone (sometimes listed as an "off label" treatment option)	Several administration schedules reported in the literature; one example is: 5–12 mg/m² of body surface IV q/3/mo for 2 yr	Amenorrhea, alopecia, nausea/diarrhea, respiratory and urinary infections, anemia, and decreased white blood count
For Primary Progressive MS (PPMS)		
None; offer symptom management therapy		
Therapy for Acute Exacerbations and Relapses: Severity and Duration Reduced With the Use of Glucocorticosteroids		
Methylprednisolone	Various drugs and schedules reported; one example is: 1,000 mg IV qd for 3 d followed by prednisone 60 mg qd for 5 d then taper to 10 mg qd	Fluid retention, loss of potassium, gastric irritation, weight gain, and emotional lability

Data from National Multiple Sclerosis Society. (1999). *Comparing the A, B, and C drugs.* New York: Author; Noseworthy, J. H., Lucchinetti, C., Rodriguez, M., & Weinshenker, B. G. (2000). Multiple sclerosis. *New England Journal of Medicine, 343*(13), 938–952; Van Oosten, B. W., Truyen, L., Barkhof, F., & Polman, C. H. (2000). Choosing drug therapy for multiple sclerosis. In A. Wagstaff (Ed.). *Drug treatment of multiple sclerosis* (pp. 1–16). Auckland, N.Z.: Adis International; Hauser, S. L., & Goodkin, D. E. (2001). Multiple sclerosis and other demyelinating disease. In Braunwald, E., Fauci, A. S., Kasper, D. L., Hauser, S. L., Longo, D. L., & Jameson, J. L. (Eds.). *Harrison's principles of internal medicine* (15th ed., pp. 2452–2461). New York: McGraw-Hill.

gressive MS (SPMS) who have frequent exacerbations. There is no standard time to begin using these drugs. This decision is tempered by the knowledge that formation of neutralizing antibodies may render interferons inactive, leaving the patient without this treatment option in the future.[71] Approximately 35% of patients receiving Betaseron and 24% of patients receiving Avonex develop neutralizing antibodies.[70] A knowledgeable physician is the best person to make these treatment decisions. Careful patient selection and monitoring are critical to patient management.

Several other drugs, called "off-label" treatment options, can be used if there is a poor response or intolerance to the first line interferons. The off-label treatment options include mitoxantrone, azathioprine, methotrexate, cyclophosphamide, intravenous immunoglobulin (IVIg), and methylprednisolone. Use of IVIg dates back about 20 years. The expense of IVIg therapy limits its usefulness.[72] As a group, these drugs modestly reduce the number of exacerbations of the disease. Efficacy, side effects, and cost issues limit their use.

Drug Therapy for Acute Relapses/Exacerbations

A short course of corticosteroids may be given to treat acute relapses and accelerate recovery. The determining factor is the presence of functionally disabling symptoms with objective evidence of neurological impairment. The preferred treatment is a short course of methylprednisolone, 1 g intravenously daily for 3 days, followed by a short prednisone taper. A prednisone taper may begin with 60 mg every day for 3 days followed by decreases in dosage by increments of 10 mg/day. Selection of appropriate drug therapy depends on the severity of the relapse and the resources available to treat the patient with intravenous therapy.

Symptom Management

The management of symptoms associated with MS often requires a collaborative multidisciplinary approach. The major problems requiring management include spasticity, sensory symptoms, urinary problems, tremors, pain, fatigue, and depression. Table 31-8 briefly outlines management.

Table 31–8 • COLLABORATIVE PROBLEMS: SYMPTOM MANAGEMENT IN MULTIPLE SCLEROSIS

PROBLEM	NONPHARMACOLOGICAL THERAPY	DRUGS	SIDE EFFECTS
Spasticity	Physical therapy: exercise program including stretching exercises; splints *Note:* For severe spasticity, *Botulinum* toxin A injections may be used	• Baclofen 5–20 mg bid or tid • Baclofen by intrathecal pump • Tizanidine 4–8 mg tid or qid • Diazepam 2–10 mg bid or qid • Dantrolene 25 mg qd to 100 mg bid or qid	• Exacerbates muscle weakness and ataxia • Less weakness, but more sedation • Use for nocturnal muscle spasm
Sensory symptoms (e.g., burning, itching)	• None	• Amitriptyline 75–150 mg qd in divided doses or 50–150 mg at HS	• Dry mouth, tachycardia, arrhythmias, sedation
Urinary: detrusor hyperreflexia and detrusor-sphincter dyssynergia Urinary urgency, frequency, hesitancy, incomplete emptying	Intermittent self-catheterization	Anticholinergics: • Oxybutynin 2.5–5 mg bid or tid • Prazosin 0.5 mg/d increase to effect	• Dry mouth, tachycardia • Hypotension
Tremors/ataxia	Exercise program and gait retraining	• Clonazepam 0.5 mg/d to 0.5 mg/d tid	• Sedation and muscle weakness
Neuropathic pain (trigeminal neuralgia, and limb pain common)	None	• Neurontin 100 mg tid or qid • Carbamazepine 200–400 mg tid • Amitriptyline 20–30 mg qid	• Titrate slowly to reduce sedation effect • Nausea, vomiting, hypotension, hypertension, fatigue, drowsiness • Use limited because of dry mouth, tachycardia, arrhythmias, sedation
Fatigue	• Rule out other causes (e.g., poor sleep, side effect from other drugs) • Exercise program	• Amantadine 100–200 mg bid • Modafinil 100–200 mg bid	• Depression, irritability, peripheral edema, anorexia • Headache, arrhythmias, nausea
Depression (frequency rate, 25%–55%) • Monitor for signs of depression, including suicide	• Counseling • Psychotherapy	• Citalopram 20 mg qd titrate up to 40 mg qd • Sertraline 50 mg qd; adjust to effect • Fluoxetine 20 mg qd; titrate to effect	• Tremors, somnolence, insomnia • Headache, tremors, insomnia, agitation • Anxiety, insomnia, palpitation, nausea, diarrhea

Drug management begins with an initial dose and is titrated to symptom control and tolerance of side effects. Therefore, close management and follow-up is necessary to achieve optimal results. In addition, patient and family education is very important to manage symptoms and to maintain a reasonable quality of life.

Both nonpharmacological and pharmacological strategies are cornerstones of symptom management. The goal of care is to keep the patient as independent and functional for as long as possible. Although lost motor function usually is not regained, range-of-motion and muscle-strengthening exercises are important to maintain intact function. A physiotherapy program using exercise and ambulatory assistive devices should be designed to maintain function. The physiotherapist can prescribe a brace or support device (e.g., cane, walker), as necessary, to maintain ambulation and independence. If leg spasticity develops, gait retraining designed to develop alternative muscles may be helpful.

Stretching exercises are effective for both spastic arms and legs. With severe spasticity, drugs such as baclofen (Lioresal), diazepam (Valium), and dantrolene sodium (Dantrium) may be beneficial in improving motor function. Baclofen may be given intrathecally using an infusion pump with very good effect. Surgical procedures may be necessary for some patients. To prevent muscle shortening and joint contractures, passive range-of-motion exercises must be a daily part of any patient activity. The patient who is ataxic may be helped by means of gait retraining or by use of a weighted cane or walker to widen the base of support. Weighted bracelets on either extremity are also of value. Occupational therapy provides education and therapy in maintaining ADLs and other instrumental activities of living. Speech therapy is helpful for difficulty in articulation or staccato speech.

Patients with sensory loss must be taught to protect themselves from injury by using their eyes to locate the extremities. The body must also be protected from trauma, heat, cold, and pressure. For patients with paresthesias (abnormal sensations such as burning or prickling), drug therapy may be helpful. Limb pain may be managed with exercise and pharmacological agents. Finally, fatigue and depression are very common. Fatigue is particularly disabling. It contributes to social isolation and depression. Exploration for contributing factors to fatigue helps to identify patterns that may be ameliorated. Risk modification, along with drug therapy, is useful to decrease fatigue. Depression is very common in MS, and the patient, family, and health care providers must be vigilant for signs and symptoms. Approximately 25% to 55% of patients with MS are depressed, and the suicide rate is 7.5 times higher than in the healthy population.[73] The use of standardized depression scales plus monitoring of the patient provides the means for early identification and treatment. Selective serotonin reuptake inhibitors are recommended for treatment.

Nursing Management

Most patients with MS live normal lives between periods of relapses. When relapses occur, most patients are managed in the community by a primary care physician or a neurologist in a clinic. When the physical environment of the home has been adequately adapted, patients with permanent disabilities often live independently with the aid of family members. Some patients with advanced disease are managed in nursing homes. When severe relapses or complications occur, patients are seen in the acute care setting where stays are usually short. Regardless of the setting in which the nurse comes in contact with the patient, it is important for the nurse to assess the patient's understanding of the illness, the factors related to relapse (Chart 31-3), and the need for lifestyle adaptation to live as independently and normally as possible. A teaching plan should be individualized according to the patient's needs.

The significant degree of psychosocial adaptation required of MS patients means that major adjustments must be made over the course of the illness. If permanent disabilities develop, the amount of support necessary from the nurse and other health care professionals increases. Many patients will note a decreased energy level, urinary tract problems, motor deficits, sexual dysfunction, changes in their social and recreational activities, and concerns about roles and employment. Most patients need support in their adjustment process. Some patients need counseling and psychotherapy to deal with behavioral and cognitive deficits.

The nurse, as a member of the multidisciplinary team, plays a key role in patient/family education, symptom management, and support. The major nursing diagnoses include:

• Knowledge Deficits related to lack of knowledge about MS, treatment options, course of illness, and available resources
• Impaired Physical Mobility related to muscle weakness and ataxia
• Self-Care Deficits related to muscle weakness, incoordination, sensory/perceptual deficits, and fatigue
• High Risk for Injury related to weakness, incoordination, sensory/perceptual deficits
• Self-Concept Disturbance related to physical disabilities, altered role performance, and altered self-esteem
• Impaired Home Maintenance related to weakness, incoordination, sensory/perceptual deficits, and fatigue

For the patient with advanced disease, the use of braces and canes and, finally, confinement to a wheelchair may become a reality. These patients need instruction and help in modifying their lifestyles to maintain the greatest level of independence possible. In some instances, the patient will become bedridden. The nurse should modify care depending on the needs of the patient.

Local and national resources are available to assist patients, families, and health care providers through the following:

The National Multiple Sclerosis Society, (800) 344-4867, http://www.nmss.org
The Multiple Sclerosis Association of America, (800) 833-4MSA, http://www.msaa.com

---

CHART 31-3 • Exacerbating Factors in Multiple Sclerosis

The following factors are known to exacerbate symptoms and should be avoided:

• Undue fatigue or excessive exertion
• Overheating or excessive chilling or exposure to cold
• Infections
• Hot baths
• Fever
• Emotional stress
• Pregnancy (should be discussed with the physician to weigh the problems before a decision is made to become pregnant)

AMYOTROPHIC LATERAL SCLEROSIS

Amyotrophic lateral sclerosis (ALS) is a progressive motor neuron disease that involves both the upper and lower motor neurons. It is characterized by wasting of the muscles of the body as a result of destruction of motor neurons in the brain stem and the anterior gray horns of the spinal cord, along with degeneration of the pyramidal tracts. Sensory changes are not a part of the disease. Some muscles become weak and atrophy, whereas spasticity and hyperreflexia are noted in others. Various patterns of involvement can develop, but the classic pattern begins with a combination of weakness with increased tone, atrophy, and fasciculations of the limbs.

The etiology of ALS is unknown, although there is a genetic component in some families. Most cases of ALS are sporadic, although 5% to 10% of cases are inherited as an autosomal dominant trait. In the United States, the incidence of ALS is 3 to 5 per 100,000 people. Men are affected more frequently than women. The most common age group affected is the 40- to

60-year group. ALS is a progressive disease that leads to death from respiratory arrest. The median survival is 3 to 5 years.[74]

Pathophysiology

There are marked degenerative changes in the following structures: anterior horn cells of the spinal cord; motor nuclei of the brain stem (especially nuclei of cranial nerves VII [facial] and XII [hypoglossal]); corticospinal tracts; and Betz's and precentral cells of the frontal cortex. Involvement of the upper motor neurons results in spasticity and reduced muscle strength, whereas lower motor neuron involvement results in flaccidity, paralysis, and muscle atrophy. Functions that are not affected include intellectual ability, sensory function, vision, and hearing. The bowel and bladder are usually spared until very late in the disease.

Signs and Symptoms

The signs and symptoms of ALS can vary from patient to patient. The initial symptoms are usually weakness and wasting of the limbs. A summary of the signs and symptoms follows:

- Muscle weakness, wasting, and atrophy: the muscles most commonly affected are the intrinsic muscles of the hand, as evidenced by clumsiness. The next most commonly affected muscles are the shoulder and upper arm muscles. The lower limbs are affected last; they characteristically feel heavy and are subject to fatigue and easy cramping.
- Muscle spasticity and hyperreflexia
- Fasciculations
- Brain-stem signs evidenced by atrophy of the tongue causing dysarthria. The muscles of speech, chewing, and swallowing are affected so that dysarthria and dysphagia occur.
- Dyspnea that progresses to respiratory paralysis
- Fatigue

Diagnosis

The diagnosis of ALS is made primarily based on the history and a neurological examination that demonstrates upper and lower motor neuron disease.[75] An electromyogram (EMG) is helpful because it will demonstrate fibrillations, which are signs of denervation, muscle wasting, and atrophy. The blood creatine phosphokinase (CPK) level is often elevated. A myelogram may be ordered to rule out other diseases.

Treatment and Management

There is no known treatment to cure this fatal disease. The first drug to slow the deterioration from ALS is riluzole, which was approved by the FDA in late 1995. Riluzole is generally well tolerated. Although the effectiveness of riluzole is not clear, no other treatment is currently available.

Patients must be managed with a multidisciplinary approach that includes the following:

- Physical therapy: range-of-motion exercises to control or improve the weakness or spasticity. Support devices, such as a cervical collar, foot brace, foot drop and finger extension splints, or slings, are useful. A cane, walker, gait training, or wheelchair may be prescribed to assist the patient in ambulation. Although the disease is progressive, therapy optimizes independence for as long as possible.
- Occupational therapy: useful in selecting equipment, such as special eating utensils, and electronic equipment for alternative ways of accomplishing ADLs
- Speech therapy: helpful in giving the patient instruction on projection of the voice; also speech synthesizers and computer technology provide a means to maintain communications
- Gastrostomy tube: if ability to chew and swallow is limited, a gastrostomy tube may be inserted to facilitate nutrition and prevent aspiration.
- Nutrition assessment: to assess caloric needs and modify diet to meet nutrition goals and patient's nutritional needs as they change; educate to prevent aspiration
- Periodic assessment of respiratory function and monitoring of pulmonary function studies including vital capacity; use of respiratory therapy, incentive spirometry, intermittent positive pressure breathing, and suctioning, as necessary
- Respiratory support with a ventilator can be life sustaining; long-term assistive ventilation, when necessary and if desired
- Ongoing counseling, support, and patient/family teaching: the patient and family need support and help in coping with the problems associated with this debilitating, fatal disease.
- Home health referral and assistance with home equipment and community services
- Management of any other health problems or complications precipitated by the disease
- Drug therapy for symptom management includes:
  - Spasticity: diazepam (Valium) or dantrolene sodium (Dantrium)
  - Cramps: quinidine
- Frank discussion for planning and decision-making for the future, including end-of-life care, advance directives, hospice care, and financial, estate, and other issues

Course of Illness

Because the onset of ALS is insidious, the early signs and symptoms may be overlooked. Diverse muscle groups gradually become involved, demonstrating weakness, atrophy, muscle wasting, and fasciculations. As the disease progresses, the arms and legs become severely impaired, and spasticity and hyperreflexia are noted. If the frontal lobe cells are involved, emotional lability may be apparent even though intellectual function is not affected. In the advanced stages, when the brain stem is involved, the muscles of speech and swallowing are affected. Speech is thick and hard to understand, and chewing, swallowing, and managing secretions become very difficult. At the terminal stage, the patient has dyspnea and shortness of breath. Speaking may no longer be possible. Death usually occurs as a result of aspiration, infection, or respiratory failure. ALS is a rapidly progressing disease in which 50% of victims die within 3 years of onset.

Collaborative Problems

No treatment can currently arrest ALS. A collaborative multidisciplinary approach is necessary to meet the needs of the patient and family. The major collaborative problems addressed by the multidisciplinary team include high risk for aspiration pneumonia, loss of ability to speak, muscle spasticity and wasting, malnutrition, respiratory insufficiency, ventilator dependency, depression, and preparation for disease progression and death. The focus of care is palliation and comfort. As a team member, the nurse participates in achieving the following goals:

- Developing and implementing an individualized teaching plan
- Providing information about support groups
- Assisting the patient to be as independent and comfortable as possible for as long as possible through symptom management
- Limiting the development of complications
- Providing ongoing emotional and psychological support for the patient and family
- Making appropriate referrals to other health care professionals and community resources
- Making decisions on desire for a gastrostomy tube and mechanical ventilation, when needed
- Helping the patient to make decisions about end-of life care, advance directives, hospice care, and settling personal affairs
- Preparing the patient for a peaceful death; reassurance of comfort at the time of death

End-of-Life Issues

Key decision points in management must be discussed in advance of a crisis.[76,77] Two key decisions involve insertion of a gastrostomy tube and mechanical ventilation. There comes a time when the patient cannot chew or swallow and protect his or her airway because of disease progression. Because insertion of a temporary feeding tube is inappropriate for long-term management, a surgically placed gastrostomy tube is recommended. Since this is a permanent artificial route for nutrition, the patient must decide whether he or she chooses to accept this approach. Not to accept a gastrostomy will lead to aspiration pneumonia and probable death. The second, more difficult, decision point is related to mechanical ventilation. As the disease progresses, respiratory function is affected. At that point, the decision will be made for tracheostomy and chronic ventilatory support. Unlike other situations in which mechanical ventilator support is temporary, in ALS there will be no reversal of mechanical ventilation. For many patients, permanent mechan-

ical ventilatory support represents an unacceptable quality of life, and they choose not to accept it. Unless these decisions are made proactively, a patient may receive a standard of care that he or she would not have chosen, given an option. Therefore, it is important to address these issues and other end-of-life issues before an emergency arises.

Nursing Management

The nurse's role in managing an ALS patient mirrors the overall needs of the patient and family. Patient problems are numerous in the rapidly developing trajectory of ALS. The major nursing diagnoses relate to the functional losses associated with disease progression and include the following:

- Impaired Physical Mobility related to muscle wasting, weakness, and spasticity
- Impaired Self-Care related to muscle wasting, weakness, and spasticity
- Impaired Communications related to impairment of muscles of speech
- High Risk for Aspiration related to impaired muscles of swallowing
- Ineffective Breathing Pattern related to impairment of respiratory muscles
- Altered Nutrition, Less Than Required, related to inability to swallow

The nurse has special skills and knowledge to assist the patient in finding ways to ameliorate these symptoms in light of a rapidly progressive disease process with continued deterioration of neurological function and increasing disabilities. Psychological and emotional support is very important as the patient adapts to loss of function and approaching death.

Preparation of the Hospitalized Patient for Discharge and Crisis

The patient and family are central to planning for discharge from the hospital. They need to know what lies ahead so that plans can be made to deal with the inevitable. If home discharge is chosen, plans must be made that include the following:

- Patient and family education about treatment protocols and treatment routines
- Home care services and equipment (e.g., suction, oxygen, ventilator, walker)
- Adjustment in household routines and environment
- Arrangement for outpatient services and community resources
- Special therapeutic regimens, such as physical therapy, speech therapy, and occupational therapy
- Spiritual support and counseling
- What to do in an emergency (i.e., aspiration or respiratory insufficiency)
- Continued follow-up and monitoring

- Awareness of the services offered by the National Amyotrophic Lateral Sclerosis Foundation and community support groups
  - Amyotrophic Lateral Sclerosis Association, (800) 782-4747, http://www.alsa.org

Patient and Family Emotional and Psychological Support

The stresses of coping with a diagnosis of ALS and its effects are overwhelming. ALS radically alters roles, relationships, self-concept, self-esteem, body image, finances, and independence. The patient and family need a tremendous amount of support. Depression is commonly seen and needs to be treated. A multidisciplinary collaborative approach is mandatory, and the nurse can contribute to meeting this need as a collaborative group member.

MYASTHENIA GRAVIS

Myasthenia gravis (MG) is a chronic disease of the neuromuscular junction in which an autoimmune process destroys a variable number of acetylcholine (ACh) receptors at the postsynaptic muscle membrane. The hallmarks of the disease are fatigability and fluctuating muscle weakness of selected voluntary muscle distribution, particularly those innervated by motor nuclei of the brain stem (i.e., extraocular, mastication, facial, swallowing and speech).[78] The weakness tends to increase with repeated activity and improves with rest. MG used to have a fatal outcome for many people, but treatment now available is highly effective, although there is no cure. MG is classified as an autoimmune disease, and persons with MG may have other autoimmune conditions. Some patients with MG have a thymoma, which affects the symptoms of the disease.

The prevalence of MG is about 1 per 7,500 people. The National Myasthenia Gravis Foundation estimates that there are approximately 100,000 patients in the United States with the disease. It affects people of all ages, and women are affected more frequently than men by a 3:2 ratio. The highest incidence noted is in women in their twenties and thirties and men in their fifties and sixties.

Pathophysiology

Muscle weakness and fatigability are due to a reduction in the number of acetylcholine receptors (AChRs) sites. This reduction is caused by antibody-mediated autoimmune attacks directed against the sites at the neuromuscular junctions. Which factors trigger and maintain the autoimmune response in MG is still unknown. Studies of muscle biopsy specimens of the neuromuscular junctions of myasthenia patients demonstrate only about one third as many AChRs as in unaffected people. The degree of severity of MG correlates with the number of AChRs. In MG, there is loss of postsynaptic membrane folds and an increase in the gap between the nerve terminal and the postsynaptic membrane.

Muscle contraction is controlled by effective neuromuscular impulse transmission. The effectiveness of transmission depends on the number of interactions between ACh

molecules and AChRs. When ACh binds to the AChR, the receptor's cation channel opens transiently, producing a localized electrical end-plate potential. If the amplitude of this potential is sufficient, it generates an action potential that spreads along the length of the muscle fiber and triggers the release of calcium from internal stores, leading to muscle contraction. At normal neuromuscular junctions, the end-plate potentials are adequate for generation of action potentials consistently. However, at myasthenia junctions, the decreased number of AChRs results in end-plate potentials of decreased amplitude and a failure to trigger action potentials in some fibers. The strength of a muscle contraction decreases given a sufficient number of junctional failures, and muscle weakness is observed. With repeated stimuli, there is a reduction in the amount of ACh and the muscle becomes fatigued. This is compounded by a concurrent decrease in the number of AChRs, resulting in an ACh "run down" phenomenon.[79]

Signs and Symptoms

The onset of MG is usually gradual, although rapid onsets have been reported in association with respiratory infections or emotional upset. The course of the illness is extremely variable. In some patients, the disease is unchanged for months and may or may not progress, whereas in others, there is rapid involvement of other muscle groups. The muscle groups affected have a characteristic pattern. Table 31-9 provides a widely adopted classification for the staging of MG. Early findings in most patients are ptosis and diplopia, which involve the levator palpebrae and extraocular muscles. Ptosis may be unilateral or bilateral and becomes intensified when the patient attempts to look upward. Pupillary response to light and accommodation remain normal. Chart 31-4 provides a clinical classification of MG based on the degree of disability it causes.

Table 31-9 • STAGES OF MYASTHENIA GRAVIS

STAGE	DESCRIPTION OF STAGE	CASES (%)
I	Ocular myasthenia	15–20
II-A	• Mild generalized myasthenia with slow progression • No crises • Responsive to drug treatment	30
II-B	• Moderately severe generalized myasthenia • Severe skeletal and bulbar involvement, but no crisis • Drug response is less than satisfactory	25
III	• Acute fulminating myasthenia • Rapid progression of severe symptoms with respiratory crises and poor drug response • High incidence of thymoma • High mortality rate	15
IV	• Late, severe myasthenia • Symptoms same as stage III, but result from steady progression over 2 yr from Class I to Class II	10

From Osserman, K. E. (1958). *Myasthenia gravis.* New York: Grune & Stratton.

CHART 31-4 • Global Clinical Classification of Myasthenic Severity

Class 0   No complaints, no signs after exertion or at special testing.

Class 1   No disability. Minor complaints, minor signs. The patient knows that he or she (still) has MG, but family members or outsiders do not perceive it. The experienced doctor may find minor signs at appropriate testing, e.g., diminished eye closure, some weakness of the foot extensors or triceps muscles, the arms cannot be held extended for 3 minutes. The patient may have complaints such as heavy eyelids or diplopia only when fatigued, inability to perform heavy work.

Class 2   Slight disability, clear signs after exertion. The patient has some restrictions in daily life, e.g., he or she cannot lift heavy loads, cannot walk for more than half an hour, has intermittent diplopia. Bulbar signs are not pronounced. Family members are aware of the signs but outsiders (inexperienced doctors included) are not. Weakness is obvious at appropriate testing.

Class 3   Moderate disability, clear signs at rest. The patient is restricted in domestic activities, needs some help in dressing, meals have to be adapted. Bulbar signs are more pronounced. Signs of MG can be observed by any outsider.

Class 4   Severe disability. The patient needs constant support in daily activities. Bulbar signs are pronounced. Respiratory function is decreased.

Class 5   Respiratory support is needed.

From Oosterhuis, H. J. G. H. (1984). *Myasthenia gravis.* Edinburgh: Churchill Livingstone.

The next muscles to be affected are the facial, masticator, speech, and neck muscles. When chewing food, the patient becomes tired and must rest. After a few moments of rest, chewing can be resumed, but muscles fatigue quickly again. Because the facial muscle is affected, the mobility and expression of the face are altered. Any attempt to smile looks like a snarl, and there is flattening of the nasolabial fold. The voice is often nasal and weak and fades after talking. There may be problems in managing saliva because of difficulty with swallowing. Food must be eaten very slowly to prevent aspiration.

Generalized weakness develops in approximately 85% of patients.[80] The limb muscles and, often, the proximal muscles, as well as the diaphragm and the neck extensor muscles, are affected. Weakness of the neck extensors causes the head to fall forward. If the shoulder girdle is involved, patients have difficulty keeping their arms above the head when reaching for an object, and with hair grooming. When the intercostal muscles or the diaphragm is involved and breathlessness and dyspnea are present, a condition called *myasthenia crisis* exists. Intubation and mechanical ventilation are necessary. In summary, the muscle groups affected tend to be weaker after use or toward the end of the day when the patient is fatigued. As the disease progresses, muscle fatigue is noted with less exertion and earlier in the day.

Diagnosis

The diagnosis of MG is based on history, physical examination, and confirmatory laboratory testing. The patient usually reports that selected muscles become weak with activity and that a period of rest improves the motor function. However, the muscle becomes fatigued again quickly. On physical examination, there is muscle weakness. MG does not affect reflexes, coordination, or sensory perception. Confirmation of MG is based on results of the following tests: anticholinesterase test; antibody titer for AChRs, repetitive nerve stimulation; and single-fiber EMG

- **Anticholinesterase testing:** The drug commonly used is edrophonium (Tensilon) because it has a rapid onset of 30 seconds and a short duration of about 5 minutes. The test is performed by drawing 10 mg of Tensilon into a syringe and administering 2 mg IV. If no adverse symptoms appear, the remaining 8 mg is injected. If there is improvement in the muscle strength of a previously weak muscle that lasts 5 to 10 minutes, the test result is considered positive.
- **Antibody titer for AChR:** This is conducted by assay of blood. In 80% to 90% of patients with generalized myasthenia, the level of AChR antibody titer is elevated.
- **Repetitive muscle stimulation:** While electrical shocks are delivered to a nerve at the rate of 3 per second, surface electrodes over the muscle record electrical potentials. A rapid reduction of the amplitude of the muscle potential is considered positive.
- **Single fiber electromyography:** This test can detect delay or failure of neuromuscular transmission in pairs of muscle fibers supplied by branches of a single nerve fiber.[20] It is about 99% sensitive in confirming MG.
- **Mediastinal MRI:** An MRI of the mediastinal cavity may be ordered to determine whether the thymus gland is enlarged because many people with MG have a thymoma.

Treatment

Four options are useful for the treatment of MG: anticholinesterase drugs, immunosuppressive therapy, plasmapheresis or IVIg, and thymectomy.[79] After the diagnosis of MG has been established, an *individualized* management plan is developed because no single treatment plan is effective for all patients. The goal of treatment is to achieve a quality of life that is as symptom free as possible.

Anticholinesterase Drugs

Anticholinesterase drugs are the first-line approach for the management of symptoms of MG, although they do not treat the underlying disease. Anticholinesterase drugs enhance the neuromuscular transmission of an impulse by preventing the degradation of ACh by the enzyme cholinesterase (ChE). The ACh inhibitor drug that is the mainstay in managing symptoms of MG is pyridostigmine (Mestinon). Neostigmine (Prostigmin), formerly prescribed, is used much less frequently, and most experts do not include it in their discussions of management. Muscarinic and nicotinic type side effects (discussed later) occur with both drugs. Atropine is the antidote for ChE inhibitor drugs and must be available for any patient receiving anticholinesterase therapy. There is no standard dosage of Mestinon because there are great variations among patients and in the same patient from time to time.

Pyridostigmine (Mestinon). Mestinon, the drug of choice, is available in tablet, syrup, time-release, and IV forms. Its effects begin within 30 to 45 minutes, peak in about 2 hours, and last 3 to 6 hours. The daily dosage and time interval are carefully adjusted, using an affected muscle group to gauge effect. The goal is to produce maximal muscle strength with minimal side effects. For example, if the oropharyngeal muscles are weak, then dosage should be timed to enhance muscle strength optimally at mealtime.[81] The dosage prescribed for most patients falls within the range of 30 to 120 mg every 4 hours orally during daytime hours. Pyridostigmine in 180-mg time-release tablets is sometimes advisable at bedtime for patients who have nocturnal weakness or weakness on arising in the morning.

If ChE inhibitors become ineffective in treating symptoms, then other forms of therapy may be indicated.

The following are common drug-related side effects:

MUSCARINIC-TYPE SIDE EFFECTS
(ON SMOOTH MUSCLE AND GLANDS)
• Gastrointestinal tract: heartburn, belching, epigastric distress, abdominal cramps, increased peristalsis, diarrhea, nausea, and vomiting

• Genitourinary tract: involuntary micturition, increased tone and motility of uterus
• Cardiovascular: bradycardia
• Vision: blurred vision, constricted pupils
• Respiratory tract: bronchoconstriction/bronchospasm, increased bronchial secretions, wheezing cough
• Other: profuse sweating and increased salivation

NICOTINIC-TYPE SIDE EFFECT
(ON SKELETAL MUSCLE)
• Skeletal muscle fasciculations (twitching) and spasms followed by fatigue and weakness

Immunosuppression: Glucocorticosteroid Therapy and Other Agents

For those who do not respond well to anticholinesterase drugs, long-term corticosteroid therapy may be tried (Table 31-10). Prednisone is the drug of choice, producing marked improvement or remission in about 70% to 80% of cases. The choice of drugs depends on an assessment of risks and benefits to the patient and the urgency of treatment.[82] Azathioprine (Imuran) is frequently used with success to treat symptoms of MG. It is the second-line choice after prednisone and a good choice if prednisone is contraindicated. After 1 to 2 years of improvement, the drug can be gradually discontinued. Cyclophosphamide (Cytoxan) is rarely used for treatment of MG because of its high toxicity.

Plasmapheresis and IV Immunoglobulin

Plasmapheresis removes antibodies from the blood. In the case of MG, plasmapheresis removes the anti-AChR antibodies, resulting in short-term clinical improvement. The indications for plasmapheresis are to stabilize a patient in

Table 31–10 • IMMUNOSUPPRESSION IN MYASTHENIA GRAVIS

DRUG	DESCRIPTION	SIDE EFFECTS
Immediate Response		
Intravenous immunoglobulin (IVIg)	• 2 g/kg administered over 5 d	• Headache • Fluid overload • Rarely, renal failure
Intermediate: 1–3 Mo		
Glucocorticoids (prednisone)	• Begin low (15–25 mg/d) and increase stepwise up to maximum improvement or 50 mg/d • Optimal dose is maintained for 1–3 mo • Next an alternate-days schedule is begun • Most patients need some form of chronic therapy	• Peptic ulcer • Hyperglycemia • Fluid retention
Cyclophosphamide (Cytoxan) may be used with glucocorticoids	• Rarely used except if unresponsive to other drugs • 4–5 mg/kg/d in 2 divided doses	• Hypertension • Nephrotoxicity
Response: Long-Term (Months to 1 Yr)		
Azathioprine (Imuran) may be used with glucocorticoids	• Used frequently after prednisone • Range: 2–3 mg/kg total body weight • Monitor white and red blood count • Works in 3–6 mo	• Flulike symptoms (fever, malaise) • Bone marrow depression • Hepatotoxicity • Anorexia, nausea, vomiting
Mycophenolate mofetil	• 1 g bid • Inhibits purine synthesis	• Side effects rare • Diarrhea and leukopenia

myasthenic crisis or to serve as a short-term treatment for a patient undergoing thymectomy. The plasmapheresis is done at the bedside with a blood cell separator machine and albumin as the plasma exchanger. An antecubital shunt provides access. The procedure takes 3 to 5 hours, depending on the weight of the patient. Five exchanges over a 2-week period are the usual regimen. An improvement in muscle strength is usually noted in about 1 to 5 days after the first exchange, but it is temporary.

The indications for the use of **IVIg** are the same as for plasmapheresis: short-term treatment for a serious relapse of MG. IVIg is useful for immunodeficiency and autoimmune conditions and has been used with success in MG. As with plasmapheresis, improvement occurs in a few days.

Thymectomy

Some MG patients have a thymoma, and a thymectomy is indicated. About 85% of patients experience improvement in their MG after surgery, and about 35% have a drug-free remission after the thymectomy. Surgery is planned collaboratively by the surgeon and anesthesiologist because the MG patient is prone to have unpredictable responses to drugs, and the possibility of respiratory failure is always present. Therefore, a thymectomy should only be performed at a designated center with a surgical and anesthesia staff experienced in the perioperative management of the patient.

Cholinergic Crisis Versus Myasthenic Crisis

Two situations can precipitate a crisis that requires respiratory support and intensive care–myasthenic crisis and cholinergic crisis. **Myasthenic crisis** is a sudden relapse of myasthenic symptoms in a patient with moderate to severe myasthenia or generalized myasthenia. A common precipitating event for crisis is infection, although in some instances there is no apparent cause. Even with an increase in medication, the patient can rapidly develop swallowing and respiratory difficulties that may require intubation and ventilation support. Vital capacity and blood gases are often monitored, and many physicians set a predetermined value, such as a vital capacity of less than 1,000, for an elective intubation. By following such a protocol, an emergency intubation is avoided. These patients require intensive medical and nursing management.

There are many drugs that may compromise transmission of impulses across the neuromuscular junction and exacerbate myasthenic muscle weakness. They include neuromuscular blocking drugs such as curare-like drugs; local anesthetics, and antiarrhythmics (quinine, quinidine, procainamide); aminoglycoside antibiotics (gentamicin, kanamycin, neomycin, streptomycin); clindamycin and lincomycin; trimethadione; morphine; chloroquine; beta-blockers; calcium channel blockers; and D-penicillamine. Many other drugs intensify myasthenic weakness. As a rule, MG patients should be observed for deterioration after any new medication is begun. Patient education is critical.

In myasthenic crisis, anticholinesterase drugs are usually ineffective and are therefore discontinued. After the patient is stabilized, drug therapy is reintroduced, and the patient is reevaluated for response. At this time, the best dosage and combination of drugs must again be determined. Concurrently, as motor strength and respiratory function improve, the patient is weaned from the ventilator.

Cholinergic crisis is an event precipitated by toxic effects of ChE-inhibitor drugs and the subsequent muscarinic and nicotinic effects described earlier. It is essentially a problem of overmedication. Muscarinic effects develop slowly. Abdominal cramping and diarrhea are often present for some time before the onset of nicotinic effects, which is rapid. Clinical examination reveals profound, generalized weakness, excessive pulmonary secretions, and impaired respiratory function. Management is similar to that for myasthenic crisis—that is, monitoring of respiratory function for difficulty, possible elective intubation, ventilatory support, and temporary withholding of ChE-inhibitor drugs.

The Tensilon test can be used to differentiate myasthenic crisis from cholinergic crisis. An improvement in muscle strength on injection of the drug suggests myasthenic crisis. If there is no improvement or if there is deterioration in muscle strength, the patient is probably in cholinergic crisis.

Collaborative Problems

The myasthenic patient is usually managed in the community by a neurologist, unless a myasthenic or cholinergic crisis occurs. At that time, admission to an intensive care unit may be necessary, where a multidisciplinary team cares for the patient. In addition, hospitalization is required for a thymectomy. During these times, an endotracheal tube may be necessary and may be used in conjunction with ventilatory support. Management of the myasthenic patient during complications depends on the specific presenting complications. However, assessment and management of muscle weakness, respiratory pattern, airway protection, and drug therapy are major concerns. The nurse provides care for the patient as a member of the multidisciplinary team.[83]

Nursing Management

Careful assessment and monitoring of the *hospitalized patient* is focused on the following areas:

- Assess respiratory function by auscultation and observation and by evaluating respiratory tests for vital capacity and tidal volume.
- Observe for unpredictable responses to drugs used (e.g., excessive sedation, decreased respirations, or agitation).
- Assess the strength of all muscles involved:
  - Respirations: rate, rhythm, quality (labored or smooth), abdominal breathing
  - Voice: quality of voice (whisper, monotone, normal intensity)
  - Hand strength and equality: (ability to hold or pick up objects)
  - Leg movement: ability to move legs freely in bed
  - Extraocular muscles: full range of extraocular movement; presence of eyelid ptosis
  - Head: ability to hold head up

The major nursing diagnoses associated with the management of MG patients include:

- Knowledge Deficit related to the disease process and treatment
- Fatigue related to muscle weakness
- High Risk for Aspiration related to muscle weakness and difficulty managing own secretions
- Activity Intolerance related to muscle weakness and fatigue

Patient Teaching

While the patient is undergoing diagnostic testing or making adjustments in lifestyle or drug schedule, a comprehensive teaching plan should be developed as an important part of nursing management. Encourage living as normal a life as possible. The patient and a responsible family member should be familiar with all drugs being taken, as well as the prescribed dosage and potential side effects. They should also know the signs, symptoms, and differences between cholinergic and myasthenic crises. An Ambu bag and portable suction device should be available at home for patients who are prone to crisis. Provide information about the Myasthenia Gravis Foundation (MGF) and other available resources. The MGF is an excellent resource for educational material and referral information for patients, their families, and health professionals.

- Myasthenia Gravis Foundation of America, Inc., (800) 541-5454, myastheniagravis@msn.com

The following points should be included in the patient teaching plan:

- Wear a Medic Alert bracelet to identify yourself as having MG, and carry a card stating the name of your primary care physician.
- Take medication with bread or a cracker to reduce the risk of nausea and gastric irritation.
- Take the medication long enough before eating to optimize maximal strength of muscles for chewing and swallowing.
- Do not take any over-the-counter medication without your doctor's permission.
- Eat slowly and select a soft diet if you have difficulty in swallowing.
- Relapses of symptoms can be caused by menstruation, infections, extremes in temperature, extensive exposure to sunlight (or ultraviolet light), and emotional stress.
- Provide for adequate rest periods during the day.
- Set priorities and plan ahead so that undue fatigue will not develop. Pace yourself.
- Wear sensible shoes to minimize weakness and loss of balance.

SUMMARY

The most common neurological degenerative diseases and their management have been discussed in this chapter. There are many other disorders too numerous to cover within the limits of this text. However, a common thread for all chronic degenerative conditions is that patient and family education and support are vital to successful adjustment and adaptation. This is true regardless of the course of the chronic illness. Although there may be no cure, the nurse, along with other health care team members, can help the patient maintain the highest level of independence at each stage of the illness. As skills and functions are lost, the nurse can help the patient adapt and compensate for these deficits. Along with the physical adjustment, there is the need for psychological adjustment and mobilization of effective coping skills. The desired outcome of the comprehensive plan of care is to maintain an optimal quality of life for the patient and family.

REFERENCES

1. Corbin, J. M. Introduction and overview: Chronic illness and nursing. (2001). In R. B. Hyman & J. M. Corbin (Eds.). *Chronic illness: Research and theory for nursing practice* (pp. 1–15). New York: Springer.
2. Lubkin, I. (1986). *Chronic illness: Impact and interventions*. Boston: Jones & Bartlett.
3. The Institute for Health & Aging, University of California, San Francisco. (1996). *Chronic care in America: A 21st century challenge*. Princeton, NJ: Robert Wood Johnson Foundation.
4. Corbin, J. M., & Strauss, A. (1988). *Unending work and care: Managing chronic illness at home*. San Francisco: Jossey-Bass.
5. Hamill, R. W., & Pilgrim, D. M. (2000). Geriatric neurology. In W. G. Bradley, R. B. Daroff, G. M. Fenichel, & C. D. Marsden (Eds.). *Neurology in clinical practice* (3rd ed., pp. 2269–2296). Boston: Butterworth-Heinemann.
6. Ernst, R. I., & Hay, J. W. (1994). The US economic and social costs of Alzheimer's disease revisited. *American Journal of Public Health, 84,* 1261–1264.
7. Ritchie, K., & Kildea, D. (1995). Is senile dementia "age-related" or "ageing-related"? Evidence from meta-analysis of dementia prevalence in the oldest old. *Lancet, 346,* 931–934.
8. American Psychiatric Association. (1994). D*iagnostic and statistical manual of mental disorders* (4th ed., pp. 123–163). Washington, DC: Author.
9. Bird. T. D. (2001). Memory loss and dementias. In E. Braunwald, A. S Fauci, D. L. Kasper, S. L. Hauser, D. L. Longo, & J. L. Jameson (Eds.). *Harrison's principles of internal medicine* (15th ed., pp. 148–155). New York: McGraw-Hill.
10. Collerton, D., Davies, C., & Thompson, P. (1996). Lewy body dementia in clinical practice. In R. H. Perry, I. G., McKeith, & E. K. Perry (Eds.). *Dementia with Lewy bodies: Clinical, pathological, and treatment issues* (pp. 171–186). New York: Cambridge University Press.
11. Rodnitzky, R. L. (1995). Clinical correlation : Parkinson's disease. In P. M. Conn (Ed.). *Neuroscience in medicine* (pp. 427–430). Philadelphia: J. B. Lippincott.
12. Devinsky, O., Feldmann, E., & Weinreb, H. I. (2000). *Neurological pearls* (pp. 116–125). Philadelphia: F. A. Davis.
13. Morris, J. C. (1999). Clinical presentation and course of Alzheimer's disease. In R. D. Terry, R. Katzman, K. L. Bick, & S. S. Sisodia (Eds.). *Alzheimer's disease* (2nd ed., pp. 11–24). Philadelphia: Lippincott Williams & Wilkins.
14. Santacruz, K. S., & Swagerty, D. (2001). Early diagnosis of dementia. *American Family Physician, 63*(4), 703–713.
15. Crum, R. M., Anthonym J. C., Bassett, S. S., & Folstein, M. F. (1993). Population-based norms for the Mini-Mental State Examination by age and educational levels. *Journal of the American Medical Association, 18,* 2386–2392.

16. Duara, R. (1992). Dementia. In J. C. Mazziotta, & S. Gilman (Eds.). *Clinical brain imaging: Principles and applications* (pp. 294–349). Philadelphia: F. A. Davis.

17. Gilman, S. (1998). Imaging the brain: Second of two parts. *New England Journal of Medicine, 338*(13), 889–896.

18. Laakso, M. P., Patanen, K., Rickkinen, P., et al. (1996). Hippocampal volumes in Alzheimer's disease, Parkinson's disease with and without dementia, and in vascular dementia: An MRI study. *Neurology, 46,* 678–681.

19. Costa, P. T. Jr., Williams, T. F., Somerfield, M., et al. (1996). *Early identification of Alzheimer's disease and related dementias. Clinical practice guideline: Quick reference for clinicians, No. 19.* AHCPR Publication No. 97-0703. Rockville, MD: U. S. Department of Health and Human Services, Public Health Service, Agency for Health Care Policy and Research.

20. Kukull, W. A., & Ganguli, M. (2000). Epidemiology of dementia. *Neurologic Clinics, 18*(4), 923–950.

21. Bird. T. D. (2001). Alzheimer's disease and other primary dementias. In E. Braunwald, A. S. Fauci, D. L. Kasper, S. L. Hauser, D. L. Longo, & J. L. Jameson (Eds.). *Harrison's principles of internal medicine* (15th ed., pp. 2391–2398). New York: McGraw-Hill.

22. Mayeux, R., & Sano, M. (1999). Treatment of Alzheimer's disease. *New England Journal of Medicine, 341*(22), 1670–1679.

23. Winkler, J., Thal, L. J., Gage, F. H., & Fisher, L. J. (1998). Cholinergic strategies for Alzheimer's disease. *Journal of Molecular Medicine, 76,* 555–567.

24. Francis, P. T., Palmer, A. M., Snape, & Wilcock, G. K. (1999). The cholinergic hypothesis of Alzheimer's disease: A review of progress. *Journal of Neurology, Neurosurgery, & Psychiatry, 66,* 137–147.

25. Jagust, W., Thisted, R., Devous, M. D., Van Heertum, R., Mayberg, H., Jobst, K., Smith, A. D., & N. Borys (2001). SPECT perfusion imaging in the diagnosis of Alzheimer's disease. *Neurology, 56,* 950–956.

26. Prusiner, S. B. (2001). Shattuck lecture—Neurodegenerative diseases and prions. *New England Journal of Medicine, 344*(20), 1516–1526.

27. St. George-Hyslop, P. H. (1999). Molecular genetics of Alzheimer disease. In R. D. Terry, R. Katzman, K. L. Bick, & S. S. Sisodia (Eds.). *Alzheimer disease* (2nd ed., pp. 311–326). Philadelphia: Lippincott Williams & Wilkins.

28. Yu, G., Nishimura, M., Arawaka, S., et al. ((2000). Nicastrin modulates presenilin-mediated notch/glp-1 signal transduction and βAPP processing. *Nature, 407,* 48–54.

29. Saunders, A. M., Strittmatter, W. J., Schmechel, D., et al. (1993). Association of apolipoprotein E allele ε4 with late-onset familial and sporadic Alzheimer's disease. *Neurology 43,* 1467–1472.

30. Farrer, L. A., Cupples, L. A., Haines, J. L., et al. (1997). Effects of age, sex, and ethnicity on the association between apolipoprotein E genotype and Alzheimer disease: A meta-analysis. *Journal of the American Medical Association, 278,* 1349–1356.

31. Martin, J. B. (1999). Molecular basis of the neurodegenerative disorders. *New England Journal of Medicine, 340*(25), 1979–1980.

32. Grundman, M., & Thal, L. J. (2000). Treatment of Alzheimer's disease: Rationale and strategies. *Neurologic Clinics, 18*(4), 807–828.

33. Norberg, A., & Svensson, A. L. (1998). Cholinesterase inhibitors in the treatment of Alzheimer's disease: A comparison of tolerability and pharmacology. *Drug Safety, 19,* 465–480. (Erratum, *Drug Safety, 20,* 146, 1999).

34. Rosen, W. G., Mohs, R. C., & Davis, K. L. (1984). A new rating scale for Alzheimer's disease. *American Journal of Psychiatry, 141,* 1356–1364.

35. Food and Drug Administration. (1991). An interim report from the FDA. *New England Journal of Medicine, 324,* 349–352.

36. Stern, R. G., Mohs, R. C., Davidson, M., et al. (1994). A longitudinal study of Alzheimer's disease: Measurement, rate, and predictors of cognitive deterioration. *American Journal of Psychiatry, 151,* 390–396.

37. Greenwald, B. S., Kramer-Ginsberg, E., Marin, D. B., et al. (1989). Dementia with coexistent major depression. *American Journal of Psychiatry, 146,* 1472–1478.

38. Rovner, B. W., Broadhead, J. H., Spencer, M., Carson, K., & Folstien, M. F. (1989). Depression and Alzheimer's disease. *American Journal of Psychiatry, 146,* 350–352.

39. Gwyther, L. P. Family issues in dementia: Finding a new normal. *Neurologic Clinics 18*(4), 993–1010.

40. Mittleman, M. S., Ferris, S. H., Steinberg, G., et al. (1993). An intervention that delays institutionalization of Alzheimer's disease patients: Treatment of spouse-caregivers. *Gerontologist, 33,* 730–740.

41. Victor, M., & Ropper, A. H. (2001). *Adams and Victor's principles of neurology* (7th ed., pp. 858–859). New York: McGraw-Hill.

42. Chui, H. (2000). Vascular dementia, a new beginning: Shifting focus from clinical phenotype to ischemic brain injury. *Neurologic Clinics, 18*(4), 951–978.

43. Lang, A. E., & Lozano, A. M. (1998). Parkinson's disease: First of two parts. *New England Journal of Medicine, 339*(15), 1044–1053.

44. Aminoff, M. J. (2001). Parkinson's disease and other extrapyramidal disorders. In E. Braunwald, A. S. Fauci, D. L. Kasper, S. L. Hauser, D. L. Longo, & J. L. Jameson (Eds.). *Harrison's principles of internal medicine* (15th ed., pp. 2399–2406). New York: McGraw-Hill.

45. Polymeropoulos, M. H., Lavedan, C., Leroy, E., et al. (1997). Mutation in the α-synuclein gene identified in families with Parkinson's disease. *Science, 276,* 2045–2047.

46. McKeith, I. G., & Burn, D. (2000). Spectrum of Parkinson's disease, Parkinson's dementia, and Lewy body dementia. *Neurologic Clinics, 18*(4), 865–902.

47. Hughes, T. A., Ross, J. F., Musa, S., et al. (2000). A 10-year study of the incidence of and factors predicting dementia in Parkinson's disease. *Neurology, 54,* 1596–1602.

48. Hoehn, M. M., & Yahr, M. D. (1967). Parkinsonism: Onset, progression, and mortality. *Neurology, 17,* 427–442.

49. Robins, A. H. (1976). Depression in patients with parkinsonism. *British Journal of Psychiatry, 38,* 141–145.

50. Colcher, A. (1999). Clinical manifestations of Parkinson's disease. *Medical Clinics of North America, 83*(2) 327–347.

51. Lees, A. J. (1995). Parkinson Disease Research Group of the United Kingdom: Comparison of therapeutic effects of and mortality data of levodopa and levodopa combined with selegiline in patients with early, mild Parkinson's disease. *British Medical Journal, 311,* 1602–1607.

52. Ben-Shloma, Y., Churchyard, A., Head, J., et al. (1998). Investigation by Parkinson's Disease Research Group of United Kingdom into excess mortality seen with combined levodopa and selegiline treatment in patients with early, mild Parkinson's disease: Further results of randomized trial and confidential inquiry. *British Medical Journal 316,* 1119–1196.

53. Munchau, A., & Bhatia, K. P. (2000). Pharmacological treatment of Parkinson's disease. *Postgraduate Medicine Journal, 76,* 602–610.

54. Lang, A., & Lozano, A. M. (1998). Parkinson's dyes: Second of two parts. *New England Journal of Medicine, 339*(15), 1133–1143.

55. Karstaedt, P. J., & Pincus, J. (1991). Protein redistribution diet remains effective in patients with fluctuating parkinsonism. *Archives of Neurology, 49,* 149–151.

56. Aminoff, M. J. (2001). Neurological treatment: Parkinson's disease. *Neurologic Clinics, 19*(1), 119–128.

57. Bejjani, B., Damier, P., Arnulf, I., et al. (1997). Pallidal stimulation for Parkinson's disease. *Neurology, 49,* 1564–1569.

58. Kumar, R., Lozano, A. M., Kin, Y. J., et al. (1998). Double-blind evaluation of subthalamic nucleus deep brain stimulation in advanced Parkinson's disease. *Neurology, 51,* 850–855.

59. Troster, A., Fields, J. A., Wilkinson, S. B., et al. (1997). Unilateral pallidal stimulation for Parkinson's disease. *Neurology, 49,* 1078–1083.

60. Herndon, C. M., Young, K., Herndon, A. D., & Dole, E. J. (2000). Parkinson's disease revisited. *Journal of Neuroscience Nursing, 32*(4), 216–221.

61. Gray, P., & Hildebrand, K. (2000). Fall risk factors in Parkinson's disease. *Journal of Neuroscience Nursing, 32*(4), 222–228.

62. Hauser, S. L., & Goodkin, D. E. (2001). Multiple sclerosis and other demyelinating disease. In E. Braunwald, A. S. Fauci, D. L. Kasper, S. L. Hauser, D. L. Longo, & J. L. Jameson (Eds.). *Harrison's principles of internal medicine* (15th ed., pp. 2452–2461). New York: McGraw-Hill.

63. Anderson, D. W., Ellenberg, J. H., Leventhal, C. M., Reingold, S. C., Rodriguez, M., & Silverberg, D. H. (1998). Revised estimate of the prevalence of multiple sclerosis in the United States. *Annals of Neurology, 31*, 333–336.

64. Noseworthy, J. H., Lucchinetti, C., Rodriquez, M., & Weinshenker, B. G. (2000). Multiple sclerosis. *New England Journal of Medicine, 343*(13), 938–952.

65. Victor, M., & Ropper, A. H. (2001). *Adams and Victor's principles of neurology* (7th ed., pp. 955–975). New York: McGraw-Hill.

66. Compston, A., Ebers, G., Lassmann, H., McDonald, I., Matthews, B., & Wekerle, H. (1998). *McAlpine's multiple sclerosis* (3rd ed.). New York: Churchill Livingstone.

67. Olek, M. J., & Dawson, D. M. (2000). Multiple sclerosis and other inflammatory demyelinating diseases of the central nervous system. In W. G. Bradley, R. B. Daroff, G. M. Fenichel, & C. D. Marsden (Eds.). *Neurology in clinical practice: The neurological disorders* (3rd ed., pp. 1431–1465). Boston: Butterworth-Heinemann.

68. Mitchell, G. W. (1997). Multiple sclerosis. In J. Biller (Ed.). *Practical neurology* (pp. 437–448). Philadelphia: Lippincott-Raven.

69. Kurtzke, J. F. (1983). Rating neurologic impairment in multiple sclerosis: An expanded disability status scale. *Neurology, 33*, 1444–1452.

70. National Multiple Sclerosis Society. (1999). *Comparing the A, B, and C drugs.* New York: Author.

71. Van Oosten, B. W., Truyen, L., Barkhof, F., & Polman, C. H. (2000). Choosing drug therapy for multiple sclerosis. In A. Wagstaff (Ed.). *Drug treatment of multiple sclerosis* (pp. 1–16). Auckland: Adis International.

72. Rolak, L. A. Multiple sclerosis treatment 2001. *Neurologic Clinics, 19*(1), 107–118.

73. Sadovnik, A. D., Eisen, K., Ebers, G. C., et al. (1991). Cause of death in patients attending multiple sclerosis clinics. *Neurology 41*, 1193–1196.

74. Brown, R. J. (2001). Amyotrophic lateral sclerosis and other motor neuron diseases. In E. Braunwald, A. S. Fauci, D. L. Kasper, S. L. Hauser, D. L. Longo, & J. L. Jameson (Eds.). *Harrison's principles of internal medicine* (15th ed., pp. 2412–2416). New York: McGraw-Hill.

75. Belsh, J. M. (1999). Diagnostic challenges in ALS. *Neurology, 53*(Suppl. 5), S26–S30.

76. Rowland, L. P., & Shineider, N. L. (2001). Amyotrophic lateral sclerosis. *New England Journal of Medicine, 344*(22), 1688–1700.

77. Smyth, A., Riedl, M., Kimura, R., Olick, R., & Siegler, M. (1997). End of life decisions in amyotrophic lateral sclerosis: A cross-cultural perspective. *Journal of Neurological Sciences, 152* (Suppl. 1), 593–596.

78. Victor, M., & Ropper, A. H. (2001). *Adams and Victor's principles of neurology* (7th ed, pp. 1536–1547). New York: McGraw-Hill.

79. Drachman, D. B. (1994). Myasthenia gravis. *New England Journal of Medicine, 339*(25), 1797–1810.

80. Grob, D., Arsura, E. L., Brunner, N. G., & Namba, T. (1987). The course of myasthenia gravis and therapies affecting outcomes. *Annals of the New York Academy of Sciences, 505*, 472–499.

81. Sanders, D. B., & Scoppetta, C. (1994). The treatment of patients with myasthenia gravis. *Neurologic Clinics of North America, 12*(2), 343–367.

82. Drachman, D. B. (2001). Myasthenia gravis and other diseases of the neuromuscular junction. In E. Braunwald, A. S. Fauci, D. L. Kasper, S. L. Hauser, D. L. Longo, & J. L. Jameson (Eds.). *Harrison's principles of internal medicine* (15th ed., pp. 2515–2520). New York: McGraw-Hill.

83. Donohoe, K. M. (1994). Nursing care of the patient with myasthenia gravis. *Neurologic Clinics of North America, 12*(2), 370–385.

RESOURCES

Chronic Illness

Corbin, J. M., & Strauss, A. (1988). *Unending work and care: Managing chronic illness at home.* San Francisco: Jossey-Bass.

Hyman, R. B., & Corbin, J. M. (2001). *Chronic illness: Research and theory for nursing practice.* New York: Springer.

Lubkin, I. M. (1990). *Chronic illness: Impact and interventions* (2nd ed., pp. 2–42). Boston: Jones and Bartlett.

Dementia and Alzheimer's Disease

Richter, R. W., & Blass, P. J. (1994). *Alzheimer's disease: A guide to practical management, Part I.* St. Louis: Mosby.

Terry R. D., Katzman, R., Bick, K. L., & Sisodia, S. S. (Eds.). *Alzheimer's disease* (2nd ed.). Philadelphia: Lippincott Williams & Wilkins.

Parkinson's Disease

Dogali, M., Fazzini, E., Kolodny, E., Eidelberg, D., Sterio, D., Devinsky, O., & Beric, A. (1995). Stereotactic ventral pallidotomy for Parkinson's disease. *Neurology, 45*(4), 753–761.

Duvoisin, R. C., & Gage, J. (1995). *Parkinson's disease: A guide for patient and family.* Philadelphia: Lippincott–Raven.

Fitzsimmons, B., & Bunting, L. K. (1993). Parkinson's disease: Quality of life issues. *Nursing Clinics of North America, 28*(4), 807–818.

Laitinen, L. V. (1995). Pallidotomy for Parkinson's disease. *Neurosurgery Clinics of North America, 6*(1), 105–112.

Lang, A. E., & Lozano, A. M. (1998). Parkinson's disease (Part one). *New England Journal of Medicine, 339*(15), 1044–1053.

Lang, A. E., & Lozano, A. M. (1998). Parkinson's disease (Part two). *New England Journal of Medicine, 339*(16), 1130–1143.

Riley, D., & Lang, A. E. (1988). Practical application of a low-protein diet for Parkinson's disease. *Neurology, 38*, 1026–1031.

Taira, F. (1992). Facilitating self-care in clients with Parkinson's disease. *Home Healthcare Nurse, 10*(4), 23–27.

Multiple Sclerosis

Compston, A., Ebers, G., Lassmann, H., McDonald, I., Matthews, B., & Wekerle, H. (1998). *McAlpine's multiple sclerosis* (3rd ed.). New York: Churchill Livingstone.

Francis, G. S., Evans, A. C., & Arnold, D. L. (1995). Neuroimaging in multiple sclerosis. *Neurologic Clinics of North America, 13*(1), 147–172.

Halper J, & Holland, N. J. (Eds.). (1997). *Comprehensive nursing care in multiple sclerosis.* New York: Demos Vermande.

Lublin, F. D., & Whitaker, J. N. (1996). Management of patients receiving interferon beta-1b for multiple sclerosis. *Neurology, 46*(1), 12–18.

Murray, T. J. (1995). The psychosocial aspects of multiple sclerosis. *Neurologic Clinics of North America, 13*(1), 197–223.

Shapiro, R. T. (1994). *Symptom management in multiple sclerosis.* New York: Demos Vermande.

Weiner, H. L., Hohol, M. J., Khoury, S. J., Dawson, D. M., & Hafler, D. A. (1995). Therapy for multiple sclerosis. *Neurologic Clinics, 13*(1), 173–196.

Weinshenker, B. G. (1995). The natural history of multiple sclerosis. *Neurologic Clinics of North America, 13*(1), 119–146.

Amyotrophic Lateral Sclerosis

Kurtzke, J. F. (1991). Risk factors in amyotrophic lateral sclerosis. *Advances in Neurology, 56,* 245–270.

Riluzole for amyotrophic lateral sclerosis. (1995). *The Medical Letter, 37*(963), 113–114.

Tidwell, J. (1993). Pulmonary management of the ALS patient. *Journal of Neuroscience Nursing, 25*(6), 337–342.

Myasthenia Gravis

De Baets, M. H., & Oosterhuis, H. J. G. H. (Eds.). (1993). *Myasthenia gravis.* Boca Raton, FL: CRC Press.

Donohoe, K. M. (1994). Nursing care of the patient with myasthenia gravis. *Nursing Clinics of North America, 12*(2), 370–385.

Drachman, D. B. (1994). Myasthenia gravis. *New England Journal of Medicine, 330*(25), 1797–1810.

Hohlfed, R., & Wekerle, H. (1994). The thymus in myasthenia gravis. *Neurologic Clinics of North America, 12*(2), 331–341.

Hopkins, L. C. (1994). Clinical features of myasthenia gravis. *Neurologic Clinics of North America, 12*(2), 243–261.

Howard, J. F., Sanders, D. B., & Massey, J. M. (1994). The electrodiagnosis of myasthenia gravis and the Lambert-Eaton myasthenic syndrome. *Neurologic Clinics of North America, 12*(2), 305–329.

Maselli, R. A. (1994). Pathophysiology of myasthenia gravis and Lambert-Eaton syndrome. *Neurologic Clinics of North America, 12*(2), 285–303.

Pascuzzi, R. M. (1994). The history of myasthenia gravis. *Neurologic Clinics of North America, 12*(2), 231–242.

Phillips, L. H. (1994). The epidemiology of myasthenia gravis. *Neurologic Clinics of North America, 12*(2), 265–271.

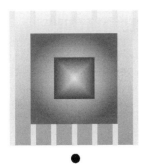

CHAPTER **32**

Peripheral Neuropathies

JOANNE V. HICKEY

This chapter discusses selected peripheral neuropathies commonly seen by nurses in clinical practice. Peripheral neuropathies related to chronic disease such as diabetes mellitus, entrapment syndromes, and Guillain-Barré syndrome (GBS) are included. **Peripheral neuropathy** is defined as a condition in which there is alteration in function and structure of the motor, sensory, or autonomic components of a peripheral nerve. Neuropathies can be classified in various ways.

- By *pathological process:* wallerian degeneration, segmental demyelination, distal axonal degeneration
- By *distribution:* single or multiple peripheral nerves, symmetrical or asymmetrical, proximal or distal involvement
- By *time frame of development:* acute, subacute, chronic
- By *cause:* infections, diabetes mellitus, inflammatory, vascular, among others
- By *clinical presentations:* presenting signs and symptoms including functional losses related to motor, sensory, autonomic, or mixed nerve changes

PATHOLOGICAL PROCESSES

The peripheral nervous system includes cranial nerves, spinal nerves that divide into peripheral nerves, and the autonomic innervation. Peripheral nerves are the major nerves in the extremities and are derived from the associated plexuses (e.g., brachial, lumbosacral). Each peripheral nerve has a well-defined anatomical course within an extremity, supplies a specific area of skin, and provides innervation to specific muscles. The neural vasculature, which nourishes peripheral nerve tissues, is called the *vasa nervorum*. When it is damaged, it ultimately results in nerve ischemia. Most peripheral nerves have both motor and sensory components, although a few are only one or the other. The motor fibers that compose the cranial and peripheral nerves have their origin in the lower motor neurons. A disturbance of function at any point in the peripheral nervous system (i.e., anterior horn cell, nerve root, limb plexus, peripheral nerve, or neuromuscular junction) can disrupt motor function. Disease that primarily affects the muscles can also disrupt function.

In some cases, the proximity of some nerves to bony structures makes them particularly vulnerable to injury.

Although there are several etiologies of peripheral neuropathy, the pathophysiological processes can generally be grouped into three categories: (1) wallerian degeneration, (2) axonal degeneration, and (3) segmental demyelination.[1] An injury that causes interruption between the axon and myelin, as in a transection of a nerve, results in *wallerian degeneration* distal to the injury site. In the distal segment, the myelin and axon degenerate, resulting in a loss of electrical conduction. Regrowth may occur proximal to the transection, but it is slow and often incomplete, and recovery of the nerve is limited. *Axonal degeneration* refers to distal axonal breakdown resembling wallerian degeneration. However, the degeneration is caused by metabolic derangement within neurons (e.g., diabetes mellitus, toxins). The result is denervation of the muscle and muscle atrophy. *Segmental demyelination* (e.g., GBS) results from an injury to the myelin sheath or the myelin-producing Schwann cells. Although the myelin breaks down, there is relative sparing of axons so that no atrophy occurs.

DISTRIBUTION PATTERNS OF PERIPHERAL NEUROPATHIES

Peripheral neuropathies are classified based on the distribution of peripheral nerves involved and the *pattern* of involvement. The classification includes three categories:

- **Mononeuropathy simplex** or **mononeuropathy** involves a single peripheral nerve (e.g., median nerve in carpal tunnel syndrome).
- **Mononeuropathy multiplex** involves several, isolated, unilateral nerves often widely separated by location (multifocal). Mononeuropathy multiplex usually results from disseminated vasculitis, such as seen in association with diabetes mellitus or polyarteritis.
- **Polyneuropathy** describes impairment of multiple peripheral nerves simultaneously, resulting in a symmetrical, bilateral pattern of functional loss, usually occurring distally before proximally. Polyneuropathy is seen with

many systemic processes. The presentation may be mainly sensory (e.g., amyloidosis, leprosy) or mainly motor (e.g., GBS, porphyria).

DEVELOPMENT AND CAUSES

The development of signs and symptoms of neuropathy can be acute, subacute, or chronic. As a general time frame, acute neuropathies have an onset of a few days to a month, subacute develop over weeks, and chronic develop over months to years. GBS is an example of an acute onset polyneuropathy. Subacute onset can be seen in drug-induced (e.g., isoniazid, metronidazole, cisplatin, vincristine, intramuscular injection), environmental toxin—induced (e.g., lead, hexocarbons, organophosphates), and nutritionally induced (e.g., vitamin B deficiency) neuropathies. Malignant diseases (carcinoma, lymphoma), connective tissue diseases (systemic lupus erythematosus, polyarteritis nodosa, scleroderma), and metabolic disorders (diabetes mellitus, uremia, hypothyroidism) are examples of chronic time frame for development. Various causes of peripheral neuropathies are outlined in Table 32-1. Note that an entrapment syndrome refers to a single peripheral nerve. Most of the other categories of peripheral neuropathies present as polyneuropathies.

The categories of etiology for peripheral neuropathy are many and include metabolic/nutritional, drug induced, environmental toxins, idiopathic inflammatory neuropathies, neoplasms, infections, and entrapment syndromes (see Table 32-1).

GENERAL CLINICAL PRESENTATIONS

Disorders of one or more peripheral nerves cause various signs and symptoms that correspond to the anatomical distribution and normal function of the nerve. Some peripheral nerves are purely motor, some are purely sensory, and others are mixed. Diagnostic accuracy depends on a thorough knowledge of specific sensory dermatomes, muscles innervation, reflexes, and autonomic function related to a particular peripheral nerve. The signs and symptoms of a peripheral nerve disorder may include sensory, motor, reflexes, or autonomic/trophic disturbances.[2,3] When *sensory* nerves or components are affected, there is decrease or loss of light touch and pinprick sensation along the involved dermatome. Clinically, tingling, numbness, paresthesias, and dysesthesias are common. *Paresthesias* are unusual sensations such as "pins and needles" whereas *dysesthesias* are unpleasant sensations such as burning. Pain is a feature of some neuropathies, especially if small fibers within the nerves are affected. Examples of polyneuropathies associated with pain include those related to diabetes, alcoholism, porphyria, rheumatoid arthritis, and acquired immune deficiency syndrome (AIDS). Pain is also a common finding with many entrapment neuropathies such as carpal tunnel syndrome.

Involvement of the *motor* fibers of a purely motor nerve or a mixed nerve results in lower motor neuron paresis or paralysis of the muscles innervated by the involved peripheral nerve. Atrophy of the specific muscle groups and related deformities follow. Fasciculations may also be noted. Deep tendon *reflexes* of the involved muscles are decreased or absent. *Autonomic and trophic changes* are noted in the

Table 32-1 • CATEGORIES AND ETIOLOGIES OF PERIPHERAL NEUROPATHIES

Metabolic/nutritional	Common chronic conditions: diabetes mellitus, hypothyroidism, acromegaly, uremia, liver disease, vitamin B_{12} deficiency
Drug induced	*Antineoplastics:* cisplatinum, vincristine
	Antimicrobials: chloroquine, dapsone, isoniazid, metronidazole, nitrofursantoin
	Cardiovascular: amiodarone, hydralazine
	Central nervous system: alcohol, lithium, phenytoin
	Other: cimetidine, colchicine, disulfiram, gold, pyridoxine
Industrial/environmental toxins	*Organic and industrial compounds:* acrylamide, carbon disulfide, dimethylaminoproprionitrile, ethylene oxide, hexacarbons, organophosphates, thallium, trichlorethylene
	Heavy metals: arsenic, lead, mercury, gold, platinum
Connective tissue processes/ vasculitis	Polyarteritis nodosa, rheumatoid arthritis, systemic lupus erythematosus, scleroderma, ischemic neuropathies, critical care polyneuropathy, systemic necrotizing vasculitis, giant cell arteritis, Wegener's granulomatosis
Infections/infectious processes	Leprosy, human immunodeficiency virus; diphtheria, Epstein-Barr virus, rabies, sarcoidosis
Inflammatory processes	Acute idiopathic polyneuropathy (Guillain-Barré syndrome); chronic inflammatory demyelinating polyneuropathy
Neoplasms	Compression and infiltration by tumor, multiple myeloma, nonhereditary amyloidosis
Trauma/compression	Severance, contusion, stretching, compression, crushing, ischemia, electrical, thermal, and radiation injuries and drug injection; stretch injuries from orthopedic traction; compression from prolonged pressure, herniated discs, osteophytes, or fractures
Entrapment syndromes	*Lower extremities:* sciatic and peroneal entrapment syndromes
	Upper extremities: carpal tunnel syndrome, ulnar entrapment syndrome, radial nerve entrapment, thoracic outlet syndrome
Hereditary disorders	Hereditary motor and sensory neuropathies; hereditary sensory and autonomic neuropathies types I–IV, Friedereich's ataxia, porphyria, hereditary amyloidosis

affected area. Skin may become dry, thin, scaly, inelastic, cold, and cease to sweat. The nails may become curved and brittle; nail and hair growth is stunted.

SELECTED PERIPHERAL NERVE CONDITIONS

The following section addresses selected neuropathies related to chronic illnesses, entrapment syndromes, and GBS.

Neuropathies Related to Chronic Disease

Neuropathies related to diabetes mellitus, vasculitis, human immunodeficiency virus (HIV), improper nutrition and alcohol abuse, and metastatic lesions, as commonly encountered in clinical practice, are briefly discussed.

Diabetic Neuropathy

Diabetic neuropathy is a consequence of poor long-term glucose control in patients with diabetes, especially in insulin-dependent diabetes. The pathophysiological processes include either metabolic disturbance with sorbitol and fructose accumulation in the axon or Schwann's cells or occlusion of the small blood vessels.[4] Neuropathies often occur in combination with vascular complications, such as retinopathy and nephropathy. There are several types of neuropathies seen in diabetics, including diabetic polyneuropathy (most common), proximal diabetic neuropathy, autonomic neuropathy, and cranial nerve palsy. They may be seen individually or in any combination.

Diabetic polyneuropathy presents with distal neuropathic pain, paresthesia, stocking sensory loss, and variable weakness that progresses insidiously over the years. In *proximal diabetic neuropathy*, also called diabetic amyotrophy, there is symmetrical or asymmetrical, subacute or slowly progressive pelvifemoral weakness, wasting, and pain. There are two forms of sensory neuropathy based on the type of sensory fibers involved. Large *sensory fiber* involvement results in ataxia whereas *small fiber* involvement results in painful paresthesias or dysesthesia and autonomic instability.[5] A patient may have both forms present concurrently.

Many patients with peripheral neuropathy have some degree of *autonomic neuropathy*. Clinically, pupillary abnormalities, loss of the ability to sweat, orthostatic hypotension, resting tachycardia, gastroparesis, and impotence are seen. For those patients with diabetes and cranial nerve palsy, an oculomotor palsy, usually without pain, may be seen without pupillary involvement. The trochlear and abducens nerves are less commonly affected.

Prevention of neuropathies through tight glucose control is the best approach to patients with diabetes. Daily glucose levels by self-monitoring and periodic glycosylated hemoglobin (A_{1C}) are useful indicators of short- and long-term glucose control. Most of the current treatment of diabetic neuropathy is focused on treatment of pain. No therapeutic modality aside from lowering of glucose levels with insulin or restoring insulin levels with pancreatic transplantation has been shown to reverse the progression of neuropathy after it has begun.[6] The treatment of painful diabetic neuropathies includes amitriptyline (Elavil) 30 to 150 mg at bedtime or nortriptyline (Pamelor) 30 to 150 mg at bedtime. With both drugs, the dosage is gradually increased based on the side effect of morning sedation. Other options include mexiletine (Mexitil) 150 to 300 mg three times daily; phenytoin (Dilantin) 100 to 300 mg at bedtime; or gabapentin (Neurontin) 300 to 900 mg three times daily. Capsaicin (Zostrix) cream applied to the affected area three times daily may provide temporary relief. Special patient education is required with the use of capsaicin that includes washing the hands carefully after use and avoiding the eyes, open areas, and some other parts of the body with the cream. The patient should also be informed that transient burning or stinging occurs with application but will disappear after several days with continued use.[7] Pain is a disabling result of diabetic neuropathy.

Vasculitic Neuropathy

Vasculitis is described as a clinicopathological process characterized by inflammation and necrosis of blood vessels. It may be the predominant feature in some conditions such as polyarteritis nodosa or less obvious in association with other primary conditions, such as systemic lupus erythematosus. Vasculitis is classified from Type I to Type IV as follows:[8]

- Type I: systemic necrotizing vasculitis (e.g., polyarteritis nodosa)
- Type II: hypersensitivity vasculitis (e.g., vasculitis associated with infections, malignancy, connective tissue disease)
- Type III: giant cell arterites (e.g., temporal arteritis and Takayasu's arteritis)
- Type IV: localized vasculitis (e.g., nonsystemic, isolated vasculitis)

Because some forms of vasculitis are treatable if identified early, an understanding of the different types may alert the physician to search for underlying primary conditions that may be controlled or arrested with early identification.[9]

In vasculitis neuropathy, damage to the neural vasculature, vasa nervorum, which normally nourishes peripheral nerve tissue, results in nerve ischemia.[9]

The clinical presentations of vasculitic neuropathies are varied and may include any of the following patterns:

- Overlapping multifocal neuropathies (mononeuropathy multiplex) of varying degrees of asymmetry; differences in sensory and motor deficits between limbs may be subtle
- Multifocal neuropathies occurring simultaneously in different limbs that evolve over days to years
- Distal symmetric, sensorimotor stocking-glove polyneuropathy

A careful medical history is conducted to uncover underlying processes such as malignancy, infection, or connective tissue disease. Because several laboratory studies are useful in ruling out underlying disease processes, the diagnostic net is cast wide. To look for a nonspecific, systemic inflammatory process, erythrocyte sedimentation rate (i.e., "sed rate") and C-reactive protein are ordered. A complete blood count (CBC), blood urea nitrogen (BUN), creatinine, liver enzymes, and urinalysis are ordered. In addition, the antineutrophilic cytoplasmic antibodies (ANCA) test is ordered for polyarteritis nodosa, and the Anti-Hu test for paraneoplastic, small-vessel vasculitis and sensory neuropathy.[10] In addition, nerve conduction studies (NCS), needle electromyography (EMG), and possibly nerve biopsy may be ordered. Treatment depends on the underlying cause, but immunosuppressive drugs such as prednisone and cyclophosphamide may produce remission.[9]

HIV-Associated Neuropathies

Neuropathies are common in HIV-infected patients who may present with neuropathy or develop neuropathy during the course of their illness. The exact pathogenesis of HIV/AIDS neuropathies remains unclear, although factors such as concurrent infection, use of neurotoxic medications, nutritional deficits, and metabolic disorders may contribute to the process. Other possible mechanisms are direct viral infection or cell-mediated immune attack on various components of peripheral nerves.[11]

Distal symmetrical polyneuropathy (DSP) is the most common of the neuropathies seen in patients with HIV/AIDS. The primary symptom of DSP is symmetrical burning pain in the soles of the feet, which is exacerbated by touch or pressure. Stocking and glove sensory loss, distal weakness, and muscle atrophy may occur later in the course. Physical examination of the lower extremities demonstrates a distal to proximal decrease in sensation to pinprick, cold, and vibration, along with hypoactive Achilles tendon reflexes. Nerve conduction studies show mild slowing of maximal conduction velocity with low-amplitude sensory nerve action potentials and minimal denervation on needle EMG. Cerebrospinal fluid (CSF) is usually normal, although a lymphocytic pleocytosis and increased protein may be seen. Treatment is symptomatic with tricyclic antidepressants (amitriptyline, nortriptyline), carbamazepine (Tegretol), phenytoin (Dilantin), and topical capsaicin cream (Zostrex-HP).[12]

Inflammatory demyelinating polyneuropathy (IDP) is an acute monophasic, relapsing, or chronic progressive process that tends to occur early in the course of HIV infection. Symptoms resemble those of GBS. Patients present with progressive weakness, areflexia, and mild sensory changes. The CSF generally shows pleocytosis. Electrophysiological studies generally indicate features of primary demyelination. Nerve biopsy in IDP reveals segmental demyelination and perivascular lymphocytic infiltrates. The pathogenesis has not been proved but may be autoimmune. The clinical course is variable. Patients with acute onset and rapid progression generally do poorly irrespective of therapy and have more residual disability. Chronic IDP is more common in asymptomatic patients with immune systems that are still partially intact. Steroid therapy, plasmapheresis, or both may be effective in restoring motor function. High-dose intravenous immunoglobulin may also be effective.[11] Treatment with zidovudine (ZDV) has been reported to produce improvement in symptoms in some patients, supporting the hypothesis of an infectious cause.

Mononeuropathy multiplex may be noted in the cranial, peripheral, or spinal nerves. Asymmetrical multifocal peripheral and cranial nerve deficits may occur, along with fever, generalized wasting, and CSF pleocytosis. When individual nerve lesions become diffuse or confluent, the course of the disease may resemble that of IDP. Electrophysiological studies may assist in distinguishing the axonal lesions of mononeuropathy multiplex from primary demyelinating pathology. Treatable etiologies of mononeuropathy such as infections related to herpes zoster virus and cytomegalovirus (CMV) must be ruled out. No specific therapy has been identified.[12]

Treatment-associated neuropathies occur in as many as 22% of patients on didanosine (ddI) and 45% of patients on dideoxycytidine (ddC). The specific mechanism by which these two nucleotide analogs cause neuropathy is unclear. This specific toxicity is not associated with the use of ZDV, the other commonly used antiretroviral. Patients complain of painful neuropathy characterized by tingling, burning, or aching, primarily in their feet. Physical examination shows mild sensory loss and diminished ankle reflexes. The degree of neuropathy appears to be dose related and may continue to intensify for 6 to 8 weeks after discontinuing the drug.

Nutritional and Alcohol-Related Neuropathies

The neuropathies associated with malnutrition and alcohol abuse are clinically the same. The most common presentation is sensory or sensorimotor distal polyneuropathy. The insidious course begins in the toes and soles of the feet and progresses in a proximal and symmetrical pattern. The neuropathy may be discovered incidentally while evaluating the patient for another problem such as liver disease, or in response to complaints of neuropathic pain. Sharp or burning pain or aching of the legs and feet may be early complaints progressing to sensory loss.

On examination, the sensory examination is diminished (i.e., light touch, pinprick, temperature, vibration), with greater loss noted in the feet. The legs appear weaker than the arms. Atrophy of distal foot muscles is common. The ankle tendon reflexes are absent. Autonomic disturbances and trophic skin changes are common. Diagnosis is made based on a history of alcohol abuse or malnutrition. In the case of alcohol-related neuropathy, cessation of alcohol consumption is recommended, but this usually requires a comprehensive rehabilitation program. If the neuropathy is due to malnutrition, nutritional support with vitamins is necessary. For example, beriberi is caused by thiamine deficiency and thus requires thiamine. With treatment, slow improvement over weeks and months is possible.

Metastatic Lesions

Sensory and mixed sensorimotor neuropathy may be seen with malignancy, particularly with small cell lung carcinoma. Neuropathy has also been associated with Hodgkin's disease and lymphomas. On laboratory examination, the presence of anti-Hu antibodies is found in the serum. Of interest is that signs and symptoms of neuropathy may precede clinical evidence of a malignancy by months and possibly years.[4] With *sensory neuropathy*, there is progressive sensory loss, paresthesia, "burning" dysesthesia, and sensory ataxia. By comparison, a *sensorimotor neuropathy* includes a distal sensory loss and mild motor weakness of gradual onset. A less common acute severe neuropathy can resemble GBS. Treatment for the neuropathy is primarily with immunosuppressive drugs.

Nursing Management

Neuropathy is common with a number of conditions and, therefore, will be encountered by nurses caring for patients in various settings. The pain associated with neuropathy is a major focus of care provided by the nurse. Pain management is difficult and is compounded by the presence of paresthesias and dysesthesias. In addition, motor deficits interfere with ambulation and other activities of daily living. A careful neurological examination with emphasis on sensory and motor function is essential in determining the degree of discomfort and functional loss present. Education, support, and assistance in modifying any risk factors that contribute to the neuropathy are also important. A focus for ongoing management is helping the patient optimize relief of pain and other sensory discomfort by effective titration of drug therapy. See Chapter 27 for management of pain.

Entrapment Syndromes

In **entrapment syndromes** or **entrapment neuropathies,** a nerve is compressed by the anatomical structure through which it passes. This can occur in areas where peripheral nerves are encased by bone or rigid material, as when cranial and spinal nerves pass through narrow foramina or channels. For example, the median nerve passes between the carpal ligament and tendon sheath of the flexor arm muscles of the forearm and is involved in carpal tunnel syndrome. The narrowness of the foramina and channels, combined with edema from nearby soft-tissue trauma or pressure from a vascular lesion (hematoma or aneurysm), can easily produce a peripheral nerve entrapment syndrome. Ischemia as a cause of peripheral nerve injury is closely associated with compression injuries because compression eventually deprives a nerve of an adequate blood supply. In such circumstances, the etiology of nerve injury is most accurately attributed to the compression-ischemia mechanism. Occlusion of a major artery of a limb can lead to nerve injury because of ischemia. Generally, chronic entrapment syndromes require surgical intervention whereas the neuropathies associated with exposure to toxins, drug therapy, and chronic diseases are managed medically by a neurologist. Carpal tunnel syndrome, ulnar entrapment syndrome (cubital tunnel), and radial nerve entrapment are the entrapment syndromes discussed in this chapter.

Carpal Tunnel Syndrome

In carpal tunnel syndrome, the median nerve is compressed by edema of tissue in and around the carpal tunnel. The median nerve is most frequently entrapped at the wrist

because of its vulnerable anatomical position. It lies between the tendons of the flexor carpi radialis and palmaris longus. The flexor pollicis longus and the flexor digitorum profundus separate the median nerve from the radius. The nerve crosses the wrist level and enters the carpal tunnel, located beneath the transverse carpal ligament. The carpal tunnel is a narrow tunnel through which the median nerve passes. It is bound superiorly by the transverse carpal ligaments and laterally and inferiorly by the carpal bones, including fibrous coverings and interosseous ligaments. If the lumen of this channel is narrowed, the movement of the nerve and muscles is compromised. The result is the development of carpal tunnel symptoms.

Occupation-related activities that require forceful and repetitive movements of the wrists or keeping the wrists in abnormal positions for prolonged periods appear to predispose people to the carpal tunnel syndrome. Such occupational categories include press operators, construction workers who use vibrating equipment, hairdressers, typists, computer keyboarders, and pianists. Women are more commonly affected than men. Several endocrine conditions (e.g., myxedema or acromegaly, pregnancy, and use of oral contraceptives) are also related to this syndrome.

Symptoms of carpal tunnel syndrome include:

- *Sensory loss* in the palmar aspect of the first three and a half fingers and the dorsal aspect of the terminal phalanges of the second, third, and half of the fourth fingers (Fig. 32-1)
- *Pain or paresthesias* in the wrist and hand especially during the night, often awakening the person; although these symptoms are usually confined to the wrist or median-innervated fingers, they may spread upward into the forearm; pain worse on wrist flexion
- *Paresis* of the abductor pollicis brevis and opponens pollicis muscles (difficulty in abducting and opposing the thumb)
- *Wasting* of the thenar hand muscles

As the disease progresses, severe pain and paresthesias accompany the use of the hand during daytime hours. Pain becomes constant, with motor weakness and atrophy. Vasomotor changes are intermittent.

On physical examination, Tinel's and Phalen's signs are positive. **Tinel's sign** is positive if pain and tingling are elicited by tapping over the median nerve at the wrist on the affected side. **Phalen's sign** is positive if tingling and pain occurs in the wrists when they are flexed at right angles for at least 1 minute (Fig. 32-2). There may be evidence of atrophy of the hand muscles. EMG and nerve conduction studies confirm the diagnosis.

Early carpal tunnel syndrome is treated by immobilizing the wrist with wrist splints and using anti-inflammatory drugs to resolve inflammation and edema around the nerve. If nerve injury is advanced, surgery will be necessary to free the median nerve of compression. Most patients do well with surgical decompression.

Ulnar Nerve Entrapment Syndrome

Entrapment of the ulnar nerve in the elbow region is most commonly caused by compression in the *cubital tunnel* that narrows during movement, especially elbow flexion. The roof of the tunnel is formed by the aponeurosis of the flexor

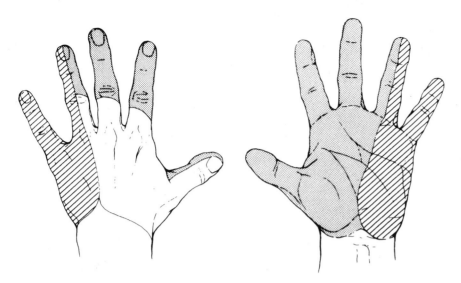

Figure 32–1 • Cutaneous innervation of the hand by the radial (*clear section*), median (*stippled section*), and ulnar (*diagonal lines*) nerves.

carpi ulnaris muscle and the floor formed by the medial ligament of the elbow.[13] The ulna nerve runs through this space and then underneath the flexor carpi ulnaris muscle. Repeated leaning on the elbows, fractures, or bony spurs cause the compression. The signs and symptoms include:[14]

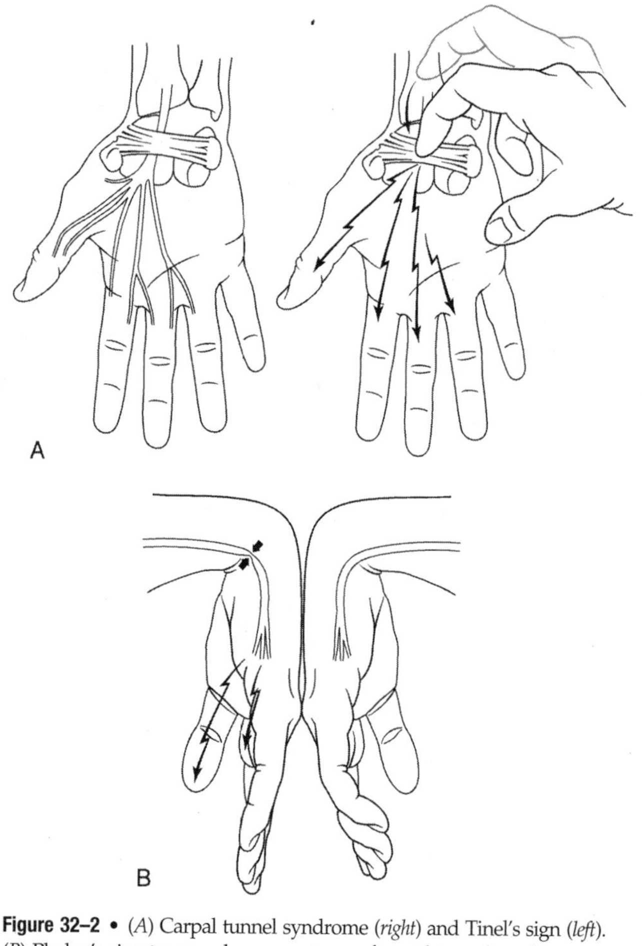

- *Paresthesias and sensory loss* in the fifth finger and medial half of the fourth finger and ulnar part of the hand below the wrist
- *Weakness* of the abductor digiti minimi, adductor pollicis, and sometimes flexor carpi ulnaris
- *Wasting* of the interossei and hypothenar eminence (claw-hand deformity may develop)
- *Pain* in the medial forearm and elbow

The diagnosis is made based on a history and the presenting clinical picture. On physical examination, a taut, palpable, enlarged nerve is noted in the ulnar groove. EMG and nerve conduction studies will localize the lesion to the cubital tunnel.[2] Surgery is indicated to release the nerve.

Radial Nerve Entrapment Syndrome

The radial nerve may be compressed against the humerus by external pressure in the axilla or the spiral groove. Axillar compression can be caused by improper use of crutches. Compression of the spiral groove can occur if a person falls asleep with an arm hanging over a chair. Compression can also occur in a sleeping person under the influence of alcohol who has someone's head against the arm. This prevents the paresthesias from awakening the individual.[13] The radial nerve may also be injured if an arm tourniquet is left on for a prolonged period of time such as during surgery. Signs and symptoms seen with radial nerve injury include:

- *Sensory loss* on the dorsal aspects of the hand, thumb, index, and middle fingers; if the axilla portion is involved, there will be sensory loss on the entire extensor surface of the arm and forearm[2]
- *Paresis* of the triceps with axillary compression only; wrist drop, weakness of finger extensors and brachioradialis for forearm flexion
- *Wasting* of the triceps and posterior surface of the forearm[14]

A

B

Figure 32–2 • (*A*) Carpal tunnel syndrome (*right*) and Tinel's sign (*left*). (*B*) Phalen's sign to reproduce symptoms of carpal tunnel syndrome.

The diagnosis is made based on a history and presenting clinical picture. EMG and nerve conduction studies will localize the lesion to the radial nerve.[2] Surgical exploration may be indicated for pain control and progressive motor weakness.[15]

Nursing Management

Nurses should be familiar with the selected entrapment syndromes discussed in this chapter because they are commonly seen in practice and because nurses have some influence for preventing them. Such is the case with radial compression from improper use of crutches. There are several other entrapment syndromes, including those of the lower extremities, that can be found in medical texts. As with the neuropathies previously mentioned, recognition of the patient who is at high risk for entrapment neuropathies is the first step toward prevention. Pain control and motor weakness are the major problems experienced by the patient. Patient education provides the patient with information on symptom management and corrective interventions to treat the underlying problem.

Guillain-Barré Syndrome

Guillain-Barré syndrome is an acute inflammatory polyneuropathy with an estimated 3,500 cases per year in the United States and Canada.[16] The etiology is unknown but is believed to be an autoimmune response to a viral infection. GBS is a rapidly progressive disorder that primarily affects the motor component of peripheral nerves. (The peripheral nerves include both cranial nerves and spinal nerves.) Most patients give a history of a recent (i.e., within the previous 2 weeks) acute infection, such as an upper respiratory infection, viral pneumonia, or GI infection. In a few instances, the patient has received a vaccination prior to the onset of GBS. As a result of improved respiratory management, most patients survive. Approximately 80% to 90% will have few or no residual disabilities.

Pathophysiology

In GBS, an immune-mediated response triggers destruction of the myelin sheath surrounding the cranial and spinal nerves. The demyelination process is accompanied by edema and inflammation of the peripheral nerves. Collections of lymphocytes and macrophages are allegedly responsible for the actual stripping of myelin from between the nodes of Ranvier. The demyelination of axons results in loss of saltatory conduction. In addition, the inflammatory process may result in varying degrees of axonal injury, which is related to a reduction in amplitude of muscle potential. This signals a poorer recovery. Demyelinization is patchy. The remyelination process occurs slowly.

Syndrome Variants

There are four variants of GBS reflecting the degree of peripheral nerve involvement: ascending GBS, descending GBS, Miller-Fisher's variant GBS, and pure motor GBS.

ASCENDING GBS
- Most common presentation
- Weakness and numbness begin in the legs, then progress upward to the trunk, arms, and cranial nerves
- Motor deficits: paresis to quadriplegia; deficits are symmetrical
- Sensory deficits: mild numbness, which is worse in toes
- Reflexes: diminished or absent
- Respiratory function: respiratory insufficiency occurs in about 50% of patients

DESCENDING GBS
- Motor deficits: initial weakness in the brain stem cranial nerves (facial, glossopharyngeal, vagus, and hypoglossal nerves); then weakness progresses downward
- Sensory deficits: numbness occurs distally, more often in the hands than in the feet
- Reflexes: diminished or absent
- Rapid respiratory involvement

MILLER-FISHER VARIANT OF GBS
- Rare
- Seen as a triad of ophthalmoplegia, areflexia, and pronounced ataxia
- Usually no sensory loss
- Rare respiratory involvement

PURE MOTOR GBS
- Identical to ascending GBS, except sensory signs and symptoms are absent
- May be a mild form of ascending GBS
- Muscle pain is generally not present

In general, GBS is characterized by motor weakness and areflexia. Motor weakness tends to be symmetrical, beginning in the legs and progressing to the trunk and arms. Respiratory failure is attributable to mechanical failure and fatigue of the intercostals and diaphragm. If the cranial nerves are involved, the facial (CN VII) nerve is most often affected. Other cranial nerves that are less often affected are the glossopharyngeal (CN IX), vagus (CN X), spinal accessory (CN XI), and hypoglossal (CN XII). Signs and symptoms of facial nerve dysfunction include an inability to smile, frown, whistle, or drink with a straw. Dysphagia and laryngeal paralysis can develop as a result of paralysis of cranial nerves IX and X. Vagus nerve deficit, if present, is thought to be responsible for the autonomic dysfunction noted in some patients.

When sensory changes are present, paresthesias and pain may be noted. The paresthesia is frequent and temporary and is described as a tingling, "pins and needles" feeling, a heightened sensitivity to touch, or numbness. Sensory changes are often noted in the hands and feet (glove and stocking distribution). About 25% of patients experience pain. Pain is underrated in terms of frequency and intensity. The pain may begin as cramping and progress to frank pain in the arms, legs, back, or buttock. Pain is often worse at night and often interferes with sleep. Analgesics are often necessary to keep the patient comfortable. The pain may be so severe that a morphine drip is necessary.

Autonomic dysfunction is much more common than once thought. The signs and symptoms may include any of the following: cardiac arrhythmias, paroxysmal hypertension, orthostatic hypotension, paralytic ileus, urinary retention, or syndrome of inappropriate secretion of antidiuretic hormone (SIADH). GBS does not affect the level of consciousness, cognitive function, or pupillary signs.

Clinical Course

There are three stages of acute GBS: (1) acute onset, which begins with the first definitive symptom and ends when no additional symptoms or deterioration are noted (lasts from 1 to 3 weeks); (2) the plateau period, which lasts for several days to 2 weeks; and (3) the recovery phase, which is synonymous with the remyelination and axonal regeneration process. In patients who have sustained secondary axonal injury, maximal improvement may take up to 2 years and permanent deficits may result.

Diagnosis

Guillain-Barré syndrome is distinguished from other forms of polyneuritis by its clinical picture. The course and features of the illness are as follows: (1) acute onset, (2) rapid development of weakness and paralysis, (3) involvement of both the proximal and distal limbs, (4) absence of, or slight, muscle atrophy; and (5) absence of other causes.

Diagnosis is based on the clinical presentation just described, a history of a recent viral infection, elevated CSF protein levels with a normal cell count, and EMG studies. Nerve conduction velocities are slowed soon after paralysis develops. If denerved potentials (fibrillations) develop, they will occur later in the illness.

Medical Treatment

Treatment for GBS should be instituted as soon as the diagnosis is made. If treatment is delayed more than 2 weeks after appearance of the first symptom, immunotherapy will not be effective. Either high-dose intravenous immunoglobulin (IVIg) or plasmapheresis is effective in most patients. Steroids are of no benefit. The IVIg is usually given on 5 sequential days for an overall dose of 2 g/kg/of body weight.[16] If the choice of therapy is plasmapheresis, 40 to 50 ml/kg plasma exchange daily for 4 to 5 days is provided. Some patients need a second course of treatments because of relapse. A brief course of treatment with the original therapy is usually effective.[16] Patients with GBS need to be hospitalized and observed carefully for deterioration and respiratory compromise. If this occurs, therapy in an intensive care unit will be necessary.

Respiratory Support

Respiratory mechanical failure secondary to neuromuscular weakness is common in GBS. Vital capacity decreases, the cough weakens, and ineffective airway clearance results. Peripheral alveoli collapse for longer portions of the respiratory cycle, lose their surfactant coating, and remain collapsed. This creates pulmonary tissue that is unventilated but perfused. Pulmonary vascular shunting develops as the vital capacity declines, causing a diminished CO_2 level. The consequences of a lowered vital capacity are atelectasis and probable hypoxemia. Concurrently, the intercostal muscles and diaphragm become fatigued, and tachycardia, dyspnea, and diaphoresis develop rapidly. Some patients will need to be intubated and supported temporarily on a ventilator. To avoid emergency intubation and the increased risk of aspiration, vital capacity is monitored and compared with a predetermined optimal level for the patient (approximately 12 to 15 mL/kg). In a 160-pound person, the target vital capacity is about 1,000 to 1,200 mL. When the patient's vital capacity falls below this level, elective intubation may be indicated. The type of mechanical ventilation usually provided is intermittent positive pressure.[16] Pneumonia related to mechanical respiratory failure is a common complication in these patients.

Some patients require ventilatory support for a short time (less than 2 weeks). However, for those who require extended ventilation, a tracheotomy is necessary. After the patient's illness has stabilized and respiratory function has improved (as evidenced by a vital capacity of 8 to 10 mL/kg), weaning from the ventilator is begun.

The mainstay of treatment is supportive care. Recovery from GBS is usual but takes time. Hospitalization in the intensive care unit usually continues for approximately 2 to 3 months. Supportive care is directed toward preventing complications and maintaining the patient in the best condition possible. In addition to respiratory problems, other complications may include **autonomic dysfunction** (i.e., hypotension, hypertension, cardiac arrhythmias, paralytic ileus, bladder retention, and SIADH), **sleep dysfunction**, possible **pain, nutrition,** and **psychological responses** (i.e., fear, depression).

Management of Complications

Autonomic Dysfunction. Monitoring of autonomic cardiac responses is required so that tachycardia and arrhythmias can be detected early and treatment instituted as necessary. Placing the patient on a cardiac monitor is helpful in identifying cardiac arrhythmias. If paralytic ileus occurs, a nasogastric tube is inserted for gastric decompression. An intermittent catheterization program is instituted to relieve urinary retention. Fluid and electrolytes are monitored for imbalance caused by SIADH. Restriction of free water is common in the event that SIADH develops.

Sleep Dysfunction. A disturbed sleep-wakefulness cycle leads to sleep deprivation. The basis for this problem is unclear, but it contributes to the psychological stress experienced by the patient.

Pain. Pain, the quality of which is described as a "severe charley horse," can be underrated in those 25% of patients who have pain. The pain appears to be worse at night and is not relieved by nonsteroidal anti-inflammatory agents or by non-narcotic agents. Narcotic agents may be indicated for some patients. Administering narcotics with a slow IV drip has yielded good results. Pain can interfere with sleep, although the altered sleep patterns common to GBS patients may also have an autonomic basis.

Nutrition. Patients can rapidly lose weight and muscle mass, leading to weakness, fatigue, and failure to wean from a ventilator. Nutritional support should be aimed toward beginning feeding as soon as is appropriate for the patient.

Immobility. The nursing staff must address problems related to immobility collaboratively. Emphasis should be on such nursing interventions as proper nutrition and maintenance of skin integrity. Minidoses of heparin are administered to prevent deep vein thrombosis (DVT) and pulmonary emboli. The use of compression boots for the prevention of DVTs is controversial, because the boots themselves may apply undue pressure to the sensitive demyelinated peripheral nerves of the leg (e.g., peroneal), leading to palsies. On this basis, heparin is usually chosen rather than compression boots for patients with GBS. Careful positioning and very gradual introduction of limited physical therapy also help to prevent palsies.

Respiratory rehabilitation may take some time and may limit the progress of a rehabilitation program, which includes extensive physical therapy and occupational therapy. Many patients fatigue easily and have a limited tolerance to activity. After respiratory function has been well established, the rehabilitation program can be managed either in a rehabilitation facility or on an outpatient basis.

Nursing Management

Nursing management in the acute phase of GBS includes a comprehensive baseline neurological and respiratory assessment and ongoing monitoring for early recognition of change. Assessment and ongoing monitoring include the following:

RESPIRATORY FOCUS
- Assess respiratory rate and quality frequently.
- Assess vital capacity frequently; know the predetermined value for intubation.
- Monitor the patient for respiratory insufficiency (e.g., air hunger, abdominal breathing, cyanosis, diaphoresis, dyspnea, confusion, and anxiety).
- Monitor perfusion with pulse oximetry.
- Administer oxygen as ordered.
- Be prepared for the possibility of intubation.

NEUROLOGICAL FOCUS
- Assess motor and sensory function frequently.
- Assess cranial nerve function.

OTHER
- Autonomic dysfunction: monitor for cardiac arrhythmias; vital signs indicating hypotension or hypertension; urinary retention.

Initially, neurological assessment is the area of focus in the acute phase. As the signs and symptoms of GBS develop, concern shifts to respiratory insufficiency, and the top priority is providing appropriate support. Many patients will require intubation and ventilatory support. Nursing interventions are directed toward maintaining adequate respirations, maintaining a patent airway, and preventing pulmonary infections.

The patient is maintained on bed rest for an extended period and is, therefore, at high risk for the multiple problems associated with immobility. A major concern is the development of DVTs and pulmonary emboli. As discussed earlier, the physician will probably order minidoses of heparin, rather than compression boots, to prevent DVTs. Special attention to positioning and turning is important to avoid pressure on vulnerable peripheral nerves and to prevent nerve palsies. Other areas of concern include managing paralytic ileus and urinary retention and providing range-of-motion exercises and nutritional support.

The quality and quantity of the pain and fear associated with the acute phase of GBS are unique to this illness. As discussed earlier, those patients who have pain can have such severe pain that only a continuous titration of IV narcotics can give relief. The pain, described as worse at night, interferes with sleep. There may also be some autonomic changes that alter the sleep cycle. The patient experiences sleep deprivation, which also influences the ability to cope with immobility and the powerlessness associated with the illness.

Most patients with GBS are very fearful, often fearing that they are dying. It is often difficult to convince a patient that recovery from GBS is possible. These patients need continued reinforcement that the outcome is optimistic. To be fully conscious and cognitively intact, yet be on ventilatory support, is an overwhelmingly frightening experience. Because some patients are maintained on a ventilator for a few months before weaning is completed, continued support and information is very important throughout the long months of recovery. The book *Bed Number Ten* (see the Resources section) is essential reading for anyone who cares for patients with GBS; it shares the experience and insight of one woman who developed GBS.

As patients move into the plateau and rehabilitation phases of GBS, the nursing focus changes to meet the altered needs of the patient. Many patients will require rehabilitation that extends beyond acute care in the hospital. Multidisciplinary management and planning assist the patient toward an optimal recovery. The major nursing diagnoses related to the nursing management of patients with GBS include the following:

- Risk for Ineffective Breathing Pattern related to neuromuscular weakness of the respiratory muscles (diaphragm and intercostals)
- Ineffective Airway Clearance related to weakness of the cough reflex and the respiratory muscles (diaphragm and intercostals)
- Knowledge Deficit related to acute illness and hospitalization
- Risk for Disuse Syndrome related to immobility secondary to paralysis and confinement of ventilator
- Impaired Verbal Communication related to paralysis of the muscles of speech or intubation
- Pain related to injury to peripheral nerves
- Sleep Pattern Disturbance related to altered autonomic function and pain
- Fear related to illness, hospitalization, treatment protocols, and death

Although patients with GBS who are admitted to the intensive care unit are critically ill, they are conscious and acutely aware of the critical nature of their illnesses. With potential or actual respiratory insufficiency, it is understandable why they are fearful. Maintaining a patent airway and providing respiratory support as needed are the first priorities of care. For those who are intubated, developing a method for communication helps to alleviate fear. The autonomic effects of GBS can be significant. Cardiac arrhythmias and variations in blood pressure are common and continuous EKG and frequent vital sign monitoring is necessary. Patients and families need education and support throughout the illness.

As the patient reaches a plateau and begins to recover, severe pain is common. The pain can be so severe that a continuous morphine drip is necessary to keep the patient comfortable. The morphine also serves to reduce anxiety. An aggressive rehabilitation program is required to help the patient reach optimal recovery. Therefore, a multidisciplinary approach is necessary to provide care throughout the illness trajectory. Patients and families may receive information from the Guillain-Barré Syndrome Foundation:

Guillain-Barré Syndrome Foundation International, P.O. Box 262, Wynnewood, PA 19096, (610) 667-0131

REFERENCES

1. Bradley, W. G., Daroff, R. B., Fenichel, G. M., & Marsden, C. D. (2000). *Neurology in clinical practice* (3rd ed., pp. 2045–2127). New York: Butterworth-Heinemann.
2. Brazis, P. W., Masdeu, J. C., & Biller, J. (1996). *Localization in clinical neurology* (3rd ed., pp. 1–49). Boston: Little, Brown.
3. Simon, R. P., Aminoff, M. J., & Greenberg, D. A. (1999). *Clinical neurology* (4th ed., pp. 159–227). Stamford, CN: Appleton & Lange.
4. Lindsay, K. W., Bone, I., & Callander, R. (1999). *Neurology and neurosurgery illustrated* (3rd ed., pp. 414–447). Edinburgh: Churchill Livingstone.
5. Younger, D. S., Rosoklija, G., & Hays, A. P. (1998). Diabetic peripheral neuropathy. *Seminars in Neurology, 18*(1), 95–104.
6. Gominak, S., & Parry, G. J. (2001). Neuropathies and diabetes. In D. Cros (Ed.). *Peripheral neuropathy: A practical approach to diagnosis and management* (pp. 141–159). Philadelphia: Lippincott Williams & Wilkins.
7. Pearson, L. J. (2000). *Nurse practitioner's drug handbook* (3rd ed., pp. 159–160). Springhouse, PA: Springhouse Corporation.
8. Kissel, J. T., & Mendel, J. R. (1992). Vasculitis neuropathy. *Neurology Clinics, 10*, 761–781.
9. Chad, D. A., Smith, T. W., & Lacomis, D. (2001). Vasculitic neuropathy: Classification, evaluation, and treatment. In D. Cros (Ed.). *Peripheral neuropathy: A practical approach to diagnosis and management* (pp. 160–176). Philadelphia: Lippincott Williams & Wilkins.
10. Younger, D. S., Dalmu, J., Inghirami, G., et al. (1994). Anti-Hu-associated peripheral nerve and muscle microvasculitis. *Neurology, 44*, 181–183.
11. Simpson, D. M., & Wolfe, D. E. (1991). Neuromuscular complications of HIV infection and its treatment. *AIDS, 5*, 917–926.
12. Newton, H. B. (1995). Common neurologic complications of HIV-1 infection and AIDS. *American Family Physician, 51*(2), 387–398.
13. Ross, M. A. (1997). Approach to the patient with upper extremity pain and paresthesias and entrapment neuropathies. In J. Biller (Ed.). *Practical neurology* (pp. 245–258). Philadelphia: Lippincott-Raven.
14. Guberman, A. (1994). *An introduction to clinical neurology* (pp. 237–256). Boston: Little, Brown.
15. Moss, S. H., & Switzer, H. E. (1983). Radial tunnel syndrome: A spectrum of clinical presentations. *Journal of Hand Surgery, 8*, 414–420.
16. Ashbury, A. K., & Hauser, S. L. (2001). Guillain-Barré syndrome and other immune-mediated neuropathies. In E. Braunwald, A. S. Fauci, D. L. Kasper, S. L. Hauser, D. L. Long, & J. L. Jameson (Eds.). *Harrison's principles of internal medicine* (15th ed., pp. 2507–2512). New York: McGraw-Hill.

RESOURCES

Books

Ashbury, A. K., & Hauser, S. L. (2001). Guillain-Barré syndrome and other immune-mediated neuropathies. In E. Braunwald, A. S. Fauci, D. L. Kasper, S. L. Hauser, D. L. Long, & J. L. Jameson (Eds.). *Harrison's principles of internal medicine* (15th ed., pp. 2507–2512). New York: McGraw-Hill.
Baier, S., & Schomaker, M. Z. (1985). *Bed number 10*. Boca Raton, FL: CRC Press.
Bosch, E. P., & Smith, B. E. (2000). Disorders of peripheral nerves. In W. G. Bradley, R. B. Daroff, G. M. Fenichel, & C. D. Marsden. *Neurology in clinical practice* (3rd ed., pp. 2045–2130). Boston: Butterworth Heinemann.
Cros, S. (Ed.). (2001). *Peripheral neuropathy: A practical approach to diagnosis and management*. Philadelphia: Lippincott Williams & Wilkins.
Victor, M., & Ropper, A. H. (2001). *Adams and Victor's principles of neurology* (7th ed., pp. 1347–1445). New York: McGraw-Hill.

Periodicals

Fulgham, J. R., & Wijdicks, E. F. M. (1997). Guillain-Barré syndrome. *Critical Care Clinics, 13*(1), 1–15.
Llewelyn, J. (1995). Diabetic neuropathy. *Current Opinions in Neurology, 8*, 364–366.
Murray, D. P. (1993). Impaired mobility: Guillain-Barré syndrome. *Journal of Neuroscience Nursing, 25*(2), 100–104.
Sternbach, G. (1999). The carpal tunnel syndrome. *Journal of Emergency Medicine, 17*(3), 519–523.
Ziegler, D. (1996). Diagnosis and management of diabetic peripheral neuropathy. *Diabetic Medicine, 13*, S34–S38.

Websites

The Neuropathy Association. http://www.neuropathy.org/explaining/index.html 212-692-0662

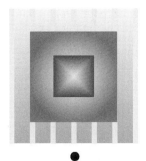

C H A P T E R **33**

Cranial Nerve Diseases

JOANNE V. HICKEY

Certain cranial nerves are especially vulnerable to injury because of their location within the cranial vault. Other cranial nerves, namely, the trigeminal (CN V), the facial (CN VII), the glossopharyngeal (CN IX), and the vagus (CN X), are subject to specific disease processes. Four major cranial nerve diseases are discussed in this chapter: trigeminal neuralgia, Bell's palsy, Ménière's disease, and glossopharyngeal neuralgia.

TRIGEMINAL NEURALGIA

Trigeminal neuralgia, also known as *tic douloureux*, is characterized by intense paroxysmal pain in one or more branches of CN V. The term **tic**, as used in relation to the disease, refers to the paroxysmal contortions of the face in response to the pain. The pain is abrupt in onset, unilateral, and lasts for a few seconds. No motor or sensory deficits are found with trigeminal neuralgia. Terms commonly used to describe the pain are paroxysmal, sharp, piercing, lancing, shooting, burning, and lightning-like jabs. *Status trigeminus*, a rapid succession of ticlike spasms triggered by almost any stimuli, is a rare manifestation of the disease.

Most patients can identify trigger zones, small areas on the cheek, lip, gum, or forehead, which initiate a bout of pain when stimulated. These trigger zones are sensitive to the most minimal of stimuli, such as touch, cold, pressure, or a blast of air. Chewing, talking, smiling, shaving, brushing the teeth, or going out of doors on a breezy day are common activities that may result in acute pain. Trigeminal neuralgia may occur at any age, although it is most common in middle and later life. Women are affected more frequently than men by a ratio of 3:2.

Although the etiology of trigeminal neuralgia is unknown, many contributing factors have been identified. Trauma, infection of the teeth or jaw, and flulike illnesses have been suggested as contributing to the disorder. An elongated, usually atherosclerotic artery adjacent to the trigeminal nerve can cause pressure on the nerve as it exits the brainstem. This pressure seems to be the etiology in most patients. Compression by an aneurysm or neoplasm, arachnoiditis, or multiple sclerosis can also produce the symptoms of trigeminal neuralgia. In making a diagnosis, other etiologies must be ruled out in order to initiate appropriate treatment.

The trigeminal nerve emerges from the pons, passing across the petrous ridge to become the gasserian ganglion, which, in turn, separates into the ophthalmic, maxillary, and mandibular divisions (Fig. 33-1). It is the largest of the cranial nerves, with both motor and sensory components. The sensory fibers relay touch, pain, and temperature sensations, whereas the motor component innervates the temporal and masseter muscles used for chewing, jaw-clenching, and lateral movement. The branch and area supplied include:

- *Ophthalmic:* forehead, eyes (including the cornea), nose, temples, meninges, paranasal sinuses, and part of the nasal mucosa
- *Maxillary:* upper jaw, teeth, lip, cheeks, hard palate, maxillary sinus, and part of the nasal mucosa
- *Mandibular:* lower jaw, teeth, lip, buccal mucosa, tongue, part of the external ear, auditory meatus, and meninges

In trigeminal neuralgia, the second and third branches of the trigeminal nerve are about equally affected. Fortunately, involvement of the first branch is rare, occurring in only about 10% of patients. When the ophthalmic branch is involved, the corneal reflex, a very important protective mechanism, may be lost.

The diagnosis of trigeminal neuralgia is based on the history. The neurological examination is entirely normal except in the patient who has multiple sclerosis or a tumor that compresses the trigeminal nerve.

Course of the Disease

Many individuals with trigeminal neuralgia experience bouts of pain for several weeks or months, followed by a spontaneous remission. The length of remission varies from days to years. With aging, there is a tendency for these remissions to be shorter. The pain causes much suffering and limitation of the activities of daily living (ADLs). Because of the fear of pain, patients may not want to talk, eat, or attend to personal hygiene, such as washing the face, brushing the teeth, or shaving. Some people have become emaciated from not eating in their attempt to keep the face immobilized to prevent triggering pain.

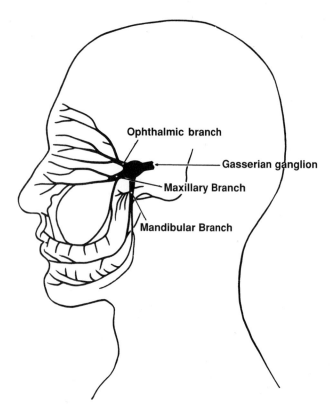

Figure 33–1 • The main divisions of the trigeminal nerve are the ophthalmic, maxillary, and mandibular. Sensory root fibers arise in the gasserian ganglion.

Treatment

The treatment of trigeminal neuralgia includes drug therapy, injection with alcohol or phenol, and surgery. Carbamazepine (Tegretol) is the drug most commonly used to suppress or shorten the bouts of paroxysmal pain. Because carbamazepine can cause myelosuppression and liver damage, patients must be closely monitored with periodic complete blood counts (CBCs), liver enzymes, and liver function tests. If Tegretol is not successful or poorly tolerated, baclofen (Lioresal) and gabapentin (Neurontin) are good choices. Other possible drug choices are phenytoin (Dilantin), capsaicin (Zostrix), clonazepam (Klonopin), and amitriptyline (Elavil).

For temporary pain relief, alcohol or phenol can be injected to block one or more branches of the trigeminal nerve. The injections provide relief of pain that usually lasts from 8 to 16 months. Blocking of the gasserian ganglion provides more permanent control of pain, but the possibility of extraocular palsies, keratitis, blindness, masticator paralysis, and lack of selective cell destruction makes it an unattractive alternative. With both blocking procedures, there is complete anesthesia to a portion of the face. This is most distressing to the patient and explains why the procedure is infrequently used.

The patient with severe pain may be considered for surgery. One possible approach is a percutaneous trigeminal rhizotomy. The most common surgical approach is stereotactic thermocoagulation of the trigeminal roots using radiofrequency energy. Radiofrequency percutaneous electrocoagulation provides lasting relief of pain with limited destruction of the trigeminal nerve. The basic principle is that small, poorly myelinated fibers that carry pain impulses are more sensitive to thermal lesions. With a heat-controlled electrocoagulation instrument, the sensory fibers are sufficiently destroyed to relieve pain without compromising touch or motor function.

A state of sedation and analgesia is achieved by administering small doses of intravenous diazepam (Valium) and fentanyl citrate (Sublimaze) during the procedure. The patient is comfortable but still able to respond verbally to questions. After each lesion is made, the corneal and ciliary reflexes, as well as facial sensation, are checked. Access to the foramen ovale, an opening from which the third branch of the trigeminal emerges, is gained through the cheek. The needle is advanced until cerebrospinal fluid (CSF) is obtained. Radiographic verification of the location within the foramen ovale follows. The electrode is inserted so that the selective electrocoagulation can proceed. The advantages of the procedure are many and include long-term, if not permanent, relief of pain; shorter-term hospitalization (the patient may be discharged the day of the procedure); good toleration by the elderly; no facial paralysis; and intact sensation. Disadvantages include the possibility of puncturing the internal carotid artery and the occurrence of anesthesia dolorosa.

For many patients, microvascular decompression using a posterior fossa craniectomy is becoming the procedure of choice. In this procedure, any blood vessel that appears to be compressing the trigeminal nerve is padded away from the nerve. If no vessel is seen that appears to be compressing the nerve, the trigeminal nerve may be partially cut to provide pain relief. If the nerve is resected at surgery, some sensory loss to the face may be expected postoperatively.

Nursing Management

Trigeminal neuralgia can be very disabling and painful. Fear of triggering spasms may prevent an individual from engaging in ADLs, social and recreational activities, and eating. Nursing management includes identifying trigger points; assessing the frequency of spasms, assessing the effectiveness of drug therapy, providing emotional support, and educating the individual in the ways to avoid triggering spasms. The major nursing diagnoses for patients with trigeminal neuralgia include the following:

- Pain related to spasms
- Knowledge Deficit related to understanding disease and triggers of spasms
- Self-Care Deficit related to fear of triggering pain by touching face
- Altered Nutrition, Less Than Rrequired, related to fear of triggering spasms by chewing or putting food into the mouth
- Social Isolation related to fear of triggering spasm with activity

Specific nursing management after surgery is included in the section on postoperative care.

Drug Therapy

The goal of nursing care is effective pain control. Analgesics, tranquilizers, and antiepileptics are frequently prescribed for this purpose. Drug therapy may be ineffective, and poor pain control may be a disappointing outcome of surgery. In collecting a nursing history, the nurse should carefully question the patient about his or her use of drugs and their effects. The fear that pain that cannot be controlled will be initiated by any activity contributes to the patient's elevated anxiety level.

Postoperative Care

Postoperatively, periodic neurological assessments are conducted. Areas of special focus include the corneal reflex, extraocular movement, and symmetrical facial movement. The sense of taste on the anterior two thirds of the tongue should also be assessed. The motor component of the trigeminal nerve is evaluated by asking the patient to clench the teeth. The contracted masseter and temporal muscles are then palpated to feel the bulk and tightness of the contracted muscles. To test the pterygoid muscles, the patient is directed to open the mouth slightly and press the examiner's finger laterally with the jaw. Weakness of the muscle will result in deviation of the jaw toward the weaker side.

After surgery that has resulted in dissected sensory tracts, the affected side of the face becomes permanently insensitive to pain. The patient is cautioned against rubbing the eye because the protective mechanism of pain, which warns of injury, is absent. The eye is inspected for redness and conjunctival erythema. Because pain sensation is lost on the affected side, routine visits to the dentist should also be scheduled. Artificial tears are instilled into the eyes on the affected side, and the eye is protected from injury. Chewing is prohibited on the operative side until the paresthesia has diminished. A soft diet is ordered.

▌▌ FACIAL PARALYSIS OR BELL'S PALSY

Charles Bell of England first described acute paralysis of CN VII, the facial nerve, in 1821. The facial nerve originates in the pons and emerges from the stylomastoid foramen. It is composed mostly of motor nerves, which supply all those muscles associated with expression on one side of the face. The sensory component innervates the anterior two thirds of the ipsilateral half of the tongue. Because of Bell's interest in this cranial nerve disorder, the disease has been named after him. Bell's palsy may be preceded by symptoms of pain behind the ear or on the face for a few hours or days before onset of paralysis. The disorder is characterized by a drawing sensation on the affected side of the face, followed by paralysis of all ipsilateral facial muscles. The eye does not close and the forehead does not wrinkle (Fig. 33-2). The patient cannot smile, whistle, or grimace. The affected side of the face is masklike and sags, with constant tearing of the eye and possible drooling. The sense of taste for the anterior two thirds of the tongue may also be affected. The diagnosis is based on the history and clinical picture of unilateral CN VII deficits.

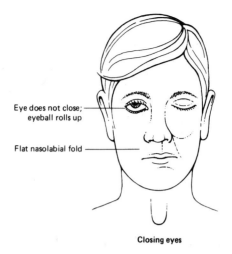

Closing eyes

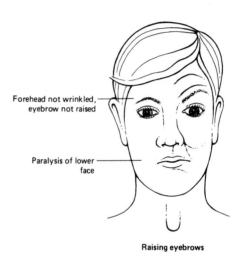

Raising eyebrows

Figure 33–2 • Manifestations of Bell's palsy.

Course and Prognosis

Bell's palsy can occur at any age but is most frequent in the 20- to 60-year-old age group. Both genders are affected about equally. Paralysis may gradually evolve over 24 to 36 hours, or it may be complete upon awakening. Some affected patients do not have complete paralysis but do have weakness. Eighty percent recover completely within a few weeks or a few months. Electromyography studies conducted 10 days after the onset of symptoms can indicate denervation and a prolonged incomplete recovery. Recovery depends on nerve regeneration. Although the etiology of Bell's palsy is unknown, the cause is believed to be an inflammatory reaction. It may also be secondary to other diseases, such as Guillain-Barré syndrome or the mass effect of a tumor.

Treatment

Prednisone, 60 mg daily, is helpful for the first week after the onset of symptoms. In addition, analgesics are given to relieve pain. Gentle massage, moist heat, and electrical stimulation of the nerve are common methods of treatment.

Special facial slings have been developed to support the sagging face. Such a device may be suggested for selected patients. As muscle tone improves, grimacing, wrinkling the brow, forcing the eyes closed, whistling, and blowing air out of the cheeks should be practiced three or four times daily for 5 minutes in front of a mirror.

Nursing Management

Nursing management for patients with Bell's palsy focuses on the major deficits and the need to provide psychological and emotional support. Because the eye does not close, the cornea must be protected from injury and from drying to prevent corneal ulceration and blindness. Instruct the patient to close the eyelid manually. Artificial tears are instilled into the eyes four times daily for lubrication. The eyelids may be taped closed, or an eye patch may be worn for protection. Eyestrain and sunlight are other stressors that may be avoided by wearing sunglasses.

Eating is problematic because the patient is unable to sip through a straw, chew, or control saliva on the affected side. Frequent, small feedings of soft food can be managed. The problems associated with eating are major sources of anxiety and embarrassment. Mealtime, a time of relaxation and socialization for many, becomes a nightmare unless the patient is helped to cope and adapt to the situation.

The simple techniques of moist heat application, massage, and facial exercise can easily be taught to the patient at home. A patient who develops Bell's palsy without other disorders will be treated in the community. If electrostimulation therapy is ordered, it will be provided on an outpatient basis. Patient education for home care outlines eye care and protection, mechanical adjustments of the diet, and a simple physiotherapy and exercise program.

Patients with Bell's palsy need much emotional support to cope with the radical change in self-concept and body image. Fortunately, most patients (80%) recover completely, but this is of little comfort when patients view their distorted reflections in the mirror.

▌▌ MÉNIÈRE'S DISEASE

Ménière's disease is a classic example of a labyrinthine lesion as a cause of true vertigo. The disorder is thought to result from fluid accumulation in the endolymphatic space affecting both the vestibular and cochlear branches of CN VIII. Ménière's disease is characterized by recurrent attacks of vertigo associated with tinnitus and deafness. Tinnitus and deafness may not be evident initially but will gradually increase in severity as the attacks continue.

The vertigo is of the rotational or whirling variety, lasting from minutes to hours and becoming so severe that the patient is unable to stand or walk. Accompanying symptoms include nausea and vomiting, a feeling of fullness in the ears, tinnitus, and rotational or horizontal nystagmus with the slow movement on the ipsilateral side. In most patients, vertigo ceases with complete deafness, although there are exceptions. The attacks vary in frequency and severity, with a possibility of remissions between bouts.

Patients with recurrent attacks are apt to be anxious and in a mild state of disequilibrium.

The hearing loss associated with Ménière's disease may begin early, even before the onset of vertigo. Hearing loss occurs gradually until there is complete unilateral deafness. In 10% of patients, the disorder is bilateral. Both genders are affected with equal frequency. The fifth decade of life is the most frequent time of onset.

Diagnosis

The diagnosis of Ménière's disease is based on the patient's history and the clinical findings of: fluctuating, progressive hearing loss leading to deafness; episodes of vertigo; and significant tinnitus. The disease is usually unilateral and is characterized by periods of remission and exacerbation. Diagnostic testing includes caloric testing and audiometry. The audiometric studies reveal depression of air and bone conduction. Brainstem auditory evoked potentials and magnetic resonance imaging are routinely used to rule out other structural lesions outside the labyrinth that may require specific treatment.

Treatment

During an attack, bed rest is most effective. The patient should be encouraged to try different recumbent positions until one is found that minimizes the vertigo. Antihistamine agents such as meclizine (Antivert), cyclizine (Marezine), or transdermal scopolamine are useful for protracted vertigo. Promethazine (Phenergan) or trimethobenzamide (Tigan) given in 200-mg suppositories is helpful for nausea and vomiting.[1] Mild sedatives and hypnotics are worthwhile in controlling anxiety. If the attacks are frequent and disabling, surgical labyrinth destruction for the patient with unilateral disease and complete deafness is possible. In patients with bilateral disease or incomplete hearing loss, the vestibular portion of CN VIII can be sectioned intracranially or the labyrinth can be destroyed selectively with cryotherapy.

Nursing Management

Most patients with Ménière's disease are treated at home unless admitted for surgery or for other conditions. A major concern is the prevention of accidents from falls because of the vertigo. The nurse should assist the patient in evaluating the efficacy of the prescribed drugs in controlling symptoms. The patient will require much emotional support throughout the illness.

▌▌ GLOSSOPHARYNGEAL NEURALGIA

Glossopharyngeal neuralgia is a much rarer syndrome than trigeminal neuralgia. The two syndromes resemble each other in many respects, however. Similar aspects include attacks of intense, paroxysmal pain; certain activities triggering bouts of pain; no sensory or motor loss of the cranial nerve; and unclear etiology. In glossopharyngeal neuralgia, the paroxysmal pain is located at the base of the tongue and the throat. Pain may also be localized in the ear or may radiate to the ear from the throat. The paroxysmal pain may be initiated by swallowing, talking, chewing, yawning, laughing, sneezing, coughing, or pressure on the tragus of the ear. Many different nerves may be responsible in such cases; it is not necessary to distinguish which nerves are involved because the treatment is the same. The diagnosis of glossopharyngeal neuralgia is based on the patient's history.

Treatment

The same drugs used to treat trigeminal neuralgia are used in glossopharyngeal neuralgia. An intracranial surgical procedure, however, is usually required for long-term relief. The surgery includes division of the glossopharyngeal nerve and upper rootlets of the vagus nerve near the medulla. This posterior fossa procedure carries a small risk of cerebellar and brainstem injury, as well as the risk of injury to the cranial nerves located in the area, but it is usually successful at producing pain relief.

Nursing Management

Nursing management for glossopharyngeal neuralgia is directed toward evaluating the patient's response to drug therapy in terms of pain control and development of side effects. If drug therapy is unsuccessful, the patient will probably require surgery, for it is unlikely that he or she can function very well if swallowing, blowing the nose, and such ordinary activities create pain. These basic activities are necessary to control saliva and maintain nutrition and patency of the upper respiratory tract.

If surgery is performed, nursing management follows the principles outlined for posterior fossa surgery (see Chap. 15).

REFERENCES

1. Victor, M., & Ropper, A. H. (2001). *Adams and Victor's principles of neurology* (7th ed., p. 320). New York: McGraw-Hill.

RESOURCES
Books

Rovit, R. L., Murali, R., & Jannetta, P. J. (1990). *Trigeminal neuralgia*. Baltimore: Williams & Wilkins.
Greenberg, M. S. (2001). *Handbook of neurosurgery* (3rd ed., pp. 373–381). New York: Thieme.
Apfelbaum, R. I. (1999). In R. G. Grossman & C. M. Loftus. *Principles of neurosurgery* (2nd ed., 407–419). Philadelphia: Lippincott-Raven.

Periodicals

Barker, F. G., Jannetta, P. J., Bissonette, D. J., Shields, P. T., Larkins, M. V., & Jho, H. D. (1995). Microvascular decompression for hemifacial spasm. *Journal of Neurosurgery, 82*(2), 201–210.
Broggi, G., Franzini, A., Giorgi, C., Servello, D., & Brock, S. (1993). Trigeminal neuralgia: New surgical strategies. *Acta Neurochirurgica, 58*(Suppl.), 171–173.
Counsell, C. M., Guin, P. R., & Limbaugh, B. (1994). Coordinated care for the neuroscience patient: Future directions. *Journal of Neuroscience Nursing, 26*(4), 245–250.
Levins, T. T. (1994). Bell's palsy versus trigeminal neuralgia questioned. *Journal of Emergency Nursing, 20*(2), 86–70.
Mauskop, A. (1993). Trigeminal neuralgia (tic douloureux). *Journal of Pain and Symptom Management, 8*(3), 148–154.
McConaghy, D. J. (1994). Trigeminal neuralgia: A personal review and nursing implications. *Journal of Neuroscience Nursing, 26*(2), 85–90.
Tien, R. D., & Wilkins, R. H. (1993). MRA delineation of the vertebral-basilar system in patients with hemifacial spasm and trigeminal neuralgia. *American Journal of Neuroradiology, 14*(1), 34–36.
Resnick, D. K., Jannetta, P. J., Bissonnette, D., Jho, H. D., & Lanzino, G. (1995). Microvascular decompression for glossopharyngeal neuralgia. *Neurosurgery, 36*(1), 64–69.
Weir, A. M., Pentland, B., Crosswaite, A., Murray, J., & Mountain, R. (1995). Bell's palsy: The effect on self-image, mood state and social activity. *Clinical Rehabilitation, 9*(2), 121–125.

Index

709